FAMILY HEALTH
MEDICAL ENCYCLOPEDIA

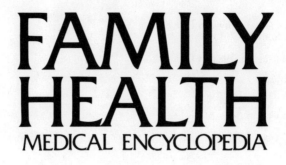

FAMILY HEALTH
MEDICAL ENCYCLOPEDIA

GENERAL EDITOR

Dr. I. A. G. MacQueen
OBE, MA, MD, DPH, FFCM, DSCHE,

PEERAGE BOOKS

First published in Great Britain in 1978 by
William Collins Sons & Co Ltd

This edition published in 1984 by
Peerage Books
59 Grosvenor Street
London W1

© 1978 William Collins Sons & Co Ltd

Reprinted 1985, 1986, 1987

ISBN 0 907 408 84 2

Printed in Czechoslovakia

50 543/4

PREFACE

There are two extreme attitudes to health. One takes good emotional and physical health for granted until illness occurs and then demands speedy and painless cure without much attention to the factors that caused the illness or to the prevention of recurrence. The other attitude is that of the person preoccupied with illness, who places antiseptic on every pin-prick, counts every calorie of diet, and in any illness avidly reads medical textbooks on the chance that the doctor has ignored some diagnostic tool or therapeutic agent.

Between these extremes stand many sensible people – persons who desire to know how their bodies and minds work (but not to the extent of studying textbooks of physiology and psychology), parents who are keen to maintain the mental and physical health of their children (but lack the time to read volumes on child health and child care), people who take reasonable measures to avoid disease or injury (but without making such avoidance the dominating motive of their lives), persons who want to know what to do when confronted with sudden illness (but without embarking on a detailed study of first aid and home nursing), and people who, while hesitating to ask the doctor or health visitor to explain a technical term, would like to ascertain its meaning (but without trying to turn themselves into unqualified health workers). It is for such people that this book has been compiled.

To become a competent doctor, dentist, health visitor, midwife, nurse, or physiotherapist requires long and arduous years of training followed by consolidating experience. So this book is in no sense a substitute for skilled advice on either the prevention or the treatment of disease.

However, a basic knowledge of the structure and functioning of the body and the mind and an understanding of the nature and main causes of disease should be part of the equipment of every educated person. Such knowledge and understanding can prevent the occurence of many diseases and greatly improve the present and future health of individuals and families, and ultimately of the community. It can also be life-saving where serious illness or injury occurs in a remote place with no skilled help immediately available, and can enable the person to seek expert aid when it is required but to do without that aid when it is not needed. Furthermore, when expert help has been sought and obtained some background knowledge can make it much easier to understand and to follow the guidance given.

This encyclopedia attempts to cover the whole field of health and disease, including clinical aspects but with deliberate emphasis on preventive and psycho-social aspects. Care has been taken to make the writing simple and to avoid technical terms wherever possible. While many of the shorter articles inevitably convey the relevant information in a minimum of space, it is hoped that the longer articles are interesting as well as informative.

To facilitate rapid reference the alphabetical method of classification has been employed (except for the appendix on the health services) and cross-references have been restricted as much as possible. In most cases the reader will get the information that he urgently requires by reading a single article.

The book is designed to improve the education for health of the general public and to provide authoritative and up-to-date information for anyone interested in the maintenance of health and fitness, the causes and treatment of disease, the working of the body and the mind, and the functioning of the health services.

Many people played a part in the making of this book. The editor, while unable to thank individually all the persons who offered suggestions or elucidated points, would like to express particular gratitude to three groups: first, to the contributors, listed elsewhere, who not only wrote articles but submitted gracefully to the application of blue pencil and scissors; second, to those who provided or suggested suitable illustrations, especially Dr Margaret Dunn; and third, to Mrs Isobel Reid and other members of the editorial staff of Collins Publishers for a vast amount of help and encouragement.

I.A.G.MacQ.

GENERAL EDITOR

Ian A.G. MacQueen, OBE, MA, MD, DPH, FFCM, DSCHE
Formerly Medical Officer of Health, Aberdeen, and
Chairman, Scottish Council for Health Education.

CONTRIBUTORS

Andrew P. Curran, KSS, BSc, MD, FRCP, FRCP(G), DPH, DIH
Senior Lecturer in Epidemiology & Preventive
Medicine, University of Glasgow

Prof Derek J. Gill, BSc (Soc), PhD,
University of Missouri, Columbia, USA

The late John D. Kershaw, MD, DPH, FFCM
Formerly Medical Officer of Health, Colchester

D. Joan Lamont, SRN, SCM, HV Tutor's Cert, DSCHE
Formerly Head of School of Health Visiting,
Robert Gordon's Institute of Technology, Aberdeen

Robert J. Lumsden, MB, ChB, DPH, MFCM
Formerly Medical Officer of Health, Airdrie

George A. Venters, MB, ChB, PhD, MFCM
Community Medicine Specialist, Lothian Health Board

A

abdomen. The abdomen or belly is the lower part of the trunk bounded above by the diaphragm, below by the pelvic bones, and at the back by the spine and strong muscles, but protected in front only by the muscles of the abdominal wall. It contains the digestive, renal and genital organs, and can be considered as consisting of two parts, the upper abdomen (or abdomen proper) and the pelvis. Broadly speaking, the liver (on the right), the stomach, and the spleen are situated at the top of the abdomen immediately below the diaphragm, which spreads out like a dome and separates the abdomen from the chest. The large intestine lies at each side with a central connecting loop while the small intestine occupies most of the middle. The kidneys and ureters lie at the back, and the rectum, bladder, and internal genital organs (e.g., uterus and ovaries) are mainly in the pelvis.

The muscles of the abdominal wall play an important part in supporting various organs: over-lax muscles may cause organ displacement with repercussions on the efficiency of the particular organ, e.g., lack of support of the intestines leads to constipation. Hence it is necessary to keep these muscles in good tone by suitable exercise and sometimes massage. There are natural weak spots in the abdominal wall through which the intestines can sometimes protrude to form a hernia.

The interior of the abdominal wall is lined with a smooth membrane, the peritoneum, which also passes from the wall to form a suspending and supporting band to cover each contained organ.

Abdominal injuries. The effects of violence to the abdomen depend partly on its nature and degree and partly on whether the muscles are relaxed or contracted. Well developed muscles, if fully contracted, can give considerable protection to the abdominal organs and to the solar plexus. Nevertheless the belly is, with the single exception of the external genital organs, the most unprotected part of the body.

Where violence produces signs of shock these should be treated. Additionally, vomiting, persistent pain, and rigidity of the abdominal wall suggest bruising or rupture of an organ, in which case the victim should be kept warm and moved as little as possible until the arrival of expert help. Where the wall has actually been broken, the patient should be treated for shock, kept warm and at rest with the knees bent over a pillow, and a bandage applied to the wound. In no case should a patient with abdominal injury be given anything by mouth until he has either recovered from signs of shock and from abdominal symptoms, or been seen by a doctor.

Until almost the middle of this century serious abdominal wounds were practically always fatal, but the advent of sulphonamides, antibiotics, and tetanus immunization has now resulted in a high recovery rate.

Abdominal pain. The commonest type of abdominal pain is the griping pain of intestinal colic, generally due to the eating of unsuitable or indigestible food which sets up spasms of the bowel. A laxative produces rapid relief, and meantime the pain can be eased by application of hot-water bottles to the abdomen. Again pain in 'the pit of the stomach' may be due to constipation.

Other causes of pain are more serious. Pain beginning near the navel and then settling in the right lower part of the abdomen may well be appendicitis. Pain under the right ribs may be occasioned by inflammation of the gall bladder. Pain in the lower abdomen may be due to cystitis (bladder inflammation) or in women to inflammation of the ovaries or occasionally simply to menstruation. Pain in the upper abdomen, if associated with eating food, may be due to acidity or an ulcer. Pain, vomiting, and constipation, starting suddenly and causing collapse, suggest peritonitis or intestinal obstruction. Persistent pain, accompanied by wasting and frequent vomiting, may be due to cancer.

In general, unless there is an obvious minor cause for abdominal pain, the symptom should be deemed to need prompt medical attention.

abduct. To move a limb outwards, away from the mid-line of the body.

abiogenesis. Spontaneous generation: the idea that living matter can arise from lifeless material. In the case of multicellular and unicellular organisms down to bacteria this is manifestly impossible: compound organisms (such as man and animals) arise solely from the union of reproductive cells of two parents, (with inheritance determined by the genes contained in the chromosomes of these cells); and unicellular organisms reproduce by simple fission. In the case of certain viruses, however, such as the virus of tobacco mosaic disease, the organism can give every appearance of being a lifeless and inert mere chemical compound and can later, under suitable conditions, become active and multiply.

The modern theory of biogenesis (i.e., that living matter originates only from living matter) owes much to Pasteur.

abortion. Expulsion of a foetus from the womb before it is able to live. It was formerly customary to describe the termination of pregnancy during the first three months as 'abortion' and later termination as 'miscarriage' (if the foetus was not far enough developed to survive) or 'premature delivery' (if the baby was viable, i.e., able to survive). However, the modern tendency is to restrict 'abortion' to artificially induced termination, while all spontaneous terminations before the age of viability are commonly termed MISCARRIAGE.

In countries where artificial termination of pregnancy is illegal, abortion can be very dangerous to the health and even the life of the woman. This applies whether it is conducted surreptitiously by an abortionist, using instruments often under conditions of doubtful cleanliness, or attempted by the woman, using either instruments or drugs. Various countries now deem abortion lawful if the birth would endanger the mother's health, or the health of the unborn child, or the health of other members of the family.

Carried out by a competent obstetrician under good conditions, abortion during the first three weeks of pregnancy is simple and almost without risk, but the danger of complications rises a very little in the fifth and sixth weeks.

Views on the ethics of abortion vary: at one end of the scale are those who hold that even the fertilized ovum is potentially alive and that induced abortion is therefore murder; in the middle are some who regard abortion as justifiable if childbirth would seriously harm the mother's physical or mental health, if the woman is a victim of rape or perhaps if the child is likely to be seriously deformed; and, at the other end, are those who consider an abortion preferable to an illegitimate or unwanted child or to a 'shot-gun' wedding and subsequent divorce.

Even in permissive societies the scales are a little weighted against abortion, because a woman has in a limited space of time to discover that she is pregnant, to decide that she wants an abortion, to find a doctor who will recommend her as suitable and an obstetrician who will carry out the termination. The position may change as a result of the development of prostaglandins which are in effect contraceptives that can be taken after sexual intercourse, but prostaglandins are as yet under experimental trial.

abrasion. The accidental rubbing off, as distinct from cutting, of the surface of the skin or of a mucous membrane. Although slight in itself, the injury can allow the entrance of germs and so lead to an abscess. For a skin abrasion the most effective treatment is to paint it immediately with an astringent and antiseptic fluid and then, if it is large, to cover it with a clean dressing.

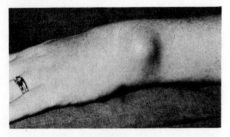

Abscess

abscess. A localized collection of pus, created by germs gaining access to a tissue from an injury or from disease in a neighbouring organ. As pus accumulates it produces reddening,

heat, swelling, throbbing, and pain over the area due to pressure, and general symptoms such as headache and raised temperature. If untreated an abscess will finally burst, but pus formation can be accelerated by poultices or hot fomentations, and once there is evidence of pus the pressure can be relieved by lancing the abscess. Alternatively, an early-stage abscess can often be checked by injections of an appropriate antibiotic, such as penicillin.

abscess, cold. A chronic abscess which develops slowly over weeks or months, produces few symptoms, and is almost always due to tubercular infection. It occurs most frequently in glands, bones, and joints, but is nowadays becoming infrequent.

accidents. Man has always been subject to injuries as a result of inadvertent mishap but the rapid development of machinery and the increase in the complexity of living have converted accidents into the major epidemic of the twentieth century. In the highly mechanized United States, some ten million persons a year (or almost one every three seconds) receive medical treatment following accidents, a third of a million become permanently disabled, and accidental deaths total 100,000. In Britain, rather less mechanized but more congested, the figures are interestingly quite similar when allowance is made for the smaller total population: there are about 28,000 accidental deaths a year in Britain and some two million persons receiving medical treatment in consequence of accidents – about one million following home accidents and one million following all other varieties. The economic cost of accidents, in respect both of loss of productive work and of cost of treatment services, is enormous. Both for that reason and as a common cause of death or disability, accidents constitute a major public health problem in all developed countries and are increasingly regarded as being in considerable measure preventable.

Domestic accidents. These are commoner than all other accidents combined and are the leading cause of death in persons between 1 and 21 years of age and also a frequent cause of death or permanent disability to the elderly. Until the late 1960s they caused more deaths than traffic accidents.

While home accidents are important at all ages and in both sexes, groups of high susceptibility can be identified. Young children are at greatest risk to every type of domestic accident: one-quarter of all home accidents involve children aged 1 to 3 years and another quarter concern children aged 3 to 9 years.

Falls are by far the most common domestic accident, affecting children most of all, while elderly and middle-aged women fall more often than elderly and middle-aged men. In contrast cuts, bruises, crushes, scalds and burns are suffered more frequently by young women than by young men or by middle-aged and elderly people.

Widowed, divorced and separated persons have a disproportionately high number of accidents, and although accidents occur in all socio-economic groups, there is a definite social gradient: the poorer the group, the higher the number of home accidents of all types.

Causes can be classified under three headings. First (and least frequent), housing

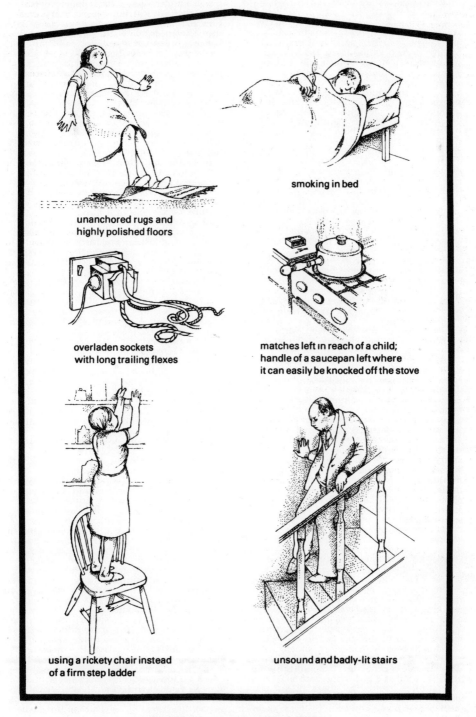

unanchored rugs and
highly polished floors

smoking in bed

overladen sockets
with long trailing flexes

matches left in reach of a child;
handle of a saucepan left where
it can easily be knocked off the stove

using a rickety chair instead
of a firm step ladder

unsound and badly-lit stairs

Common causes of domestic accidents

defects: examples are outside steps without a handrail and dingy entrance halls. Second, defects of furnishing or equipment: instances are highly-polished floors, small unanchored mats, unguarded fires, badly-lit stairs, and long trailing electric wires. Third (and by far the commonest), human defects: in this large group, fatigue is the most frequent cause. Most accidents in adults occur near the end of a period of maximum household activity or shortly after reaching home at the end of strenuous work – with anxiety and emotional upset also appearing as significant factors.

Untidiness and clutter play important subsidiary parts: the adult who is tired or preoccupied will trip over an object left in an unusual position and the toddler will grasp the scissors or pills that have been left in an accessible place. Biological factors are also involved – the helplessness of the baby who can suffocate through inability to turn his head away from a soft pillow, the defective vision of the old person who may walk into the sharp edge of an open door, or the impaired mobility of the cripple increasing his liability to fall over the misplaced article.

On a long-term basis improved house design should reduce accidents, but in the shorter term improved equipment would also do so. Such improvements include adequate lighting especially on stairs, sufficient working surfaces in the kitchen, handrails on outside steps, avoidance of multiple gadgets from a single electric plug and trailing electric wires, fixed guards on fires, and gas taps that cannot be turned on by an exploring small child.

The greatest hope for reduction of accidents, however, lies in education, e.g., teaching the housewife to exercise special care when tired or worried, and teaching her, in anticipation of periods of fatigue or emotional disturbance, to remove potential causes of accidents; persuading her husband to inspect periodically the safety of electrical appliances, windows, and stairs; making persons with elderly relatives aware of common dangers, from the cigarette smoked in bed to the wearing of down-at-heel slippers; and, not least, teaching parents not only to keep medicines, cleansing fluids, sharp articles and matches out of reach of the young child, but also to instruct the child as soon as he is old enough in the safe use of such articles.

The biggest enemy of home safety is complacency – the unexpressed but persistent idea that 'it won't happen to me'. Most workers in the field of home safety have had the experience of ensuring that a householder has a proper step-ladder or pair of steps and then finding the same householder standing on a rickety chair to change a light bulb, or of checking that the medicine cupboard is child-proof and then seeing brightly coloured pills left forgotten on a low table. Nevertheless, reiterated and tactful persuasion can achieve substantial results. There are already towns and counties in which the local health department can claim that, either by the efforts of its own nursing and other staff or by these efforts supplemented by those of voluntary committees, it has succeeded in reducing the incidence of home accidents by more than a third.

Here are a few simple rules for reduction of accidents. Ensure that the stair is well-lit and free from obstacles. Avoid slippery floors and loose rugs without non-slip surfaces. Replace toys and household utensils immediately after use. Keep handles of saucepans turned inwards. Keep hot water, knives, sharp tools, medicines and cleansing fluids out of reach of young children. Keep all medicines in distinctly marked containers. Keep all doors either closed or very fully open. Do not smoke in bed. Ensure that electric wires are in good condition and where practicable keep them short. Ensure that coal fires, gas fires, and electric heaters are adequately protected. Exercise particular care when tired, angry, or distressed.

For treatment of minor injuries received in the home, see FIRST AID.

Industrial accidents. Both in Britain and in the United States industrial accidents are – as compared with home accidents and road accidents – a relatively uncommon cause both of death and of injury. Yet the most curious feature of the hazards of industry is their widely different incidence in countries that correspond broadly in other types of accident. In Britain industrial accidents kill about 700 people each year and injure about 300,000. In the United States (with less than four times the population of Britain) they kill about 15,000 – or twenty times as many as in Britain – and injure fully two million annually. Both countries, as indeed do all states, need to ensure that more extensive measures are applied, although it would seem that in the United States the task will be greater.

Industrial accidents fall broadly into two groups – those involving young workers who do not foresee the particular danger (education at entry to employment would perhaps reduce this group) and those among older workers who appreciate the risk but are unable to take sufficiently swift action to avoid the consequence. The second group might be reduced by adequate safety appliances and, where necessary, by transfer or early retirement of persons no longer agile enough to cope with an inevitable hazard. In both categories accidents to males greatly outnumber those to females.

Traffic accidents. Despite the publicity that attends them, train and aircraft accidents are rarities. Motor accidents in Britain account for more than a dozen times the combined total of all rail and aeroplane deaths and workers in the U.S.A. have calculated that, for every million miles of passenger travel, the passenger death-rate from motor accidents is eight times that from aircraft accidents. Moreover, while these road accidents kill more than 7,000 persons a year in Britain and more than six times that number in the United States, for every person killed in such accidents there are 37 injured.

Except for the numbers killed and injured objective facts about motor accidents are difficult to obtain. Part of the difficulty is that the real cause of a collision involving two drivers and several passengers may be the behaviour of a third driver or of a pedestrian who does not remain available for questioning. More accidents involve collision with other moving vehicles than non-collision, or collision with stationary objects, and a higher proportion occur at night than in daylight. Injured drivers include a disproportionately large number of men under the age of 25 years and considerable, but smaller, numbers of

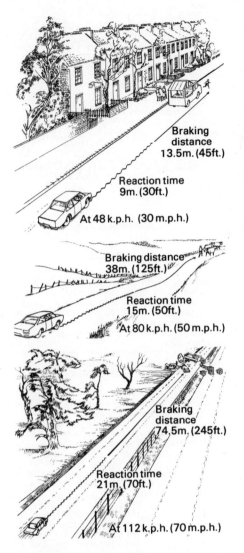

Braking distance 13.5m. (45ft.)

Reaction time 9m. (30ft.)

At 48 k.p.h. (30 m.p.h.)

Braking distance 38m. (125ft.)

Reaction time 15m. (50ft.)

At 80 k.p.h. (50 m.p.h.)

Braking distance 74.5m. (245ft.)

Reaction time 21m. (70ft.)

At 112 k.p.h. (70 m.p.h.)

Emergency stopping times in good road conditions

women in that age group. In relation to total mileage driven the average male driver is involved in almost exactly twice as many accidents as the average woman driver, but this may mean not that men are poorer drivers but simply that they drive more at rush hours and at night. Before the era of breathalyser tests in Britain and elsewhere it was claimed that three-fifths of drivers involved in accidents had been drinking, but no figures were available for the proportion of accident-free drivers that had consumed alcohol. Among injured pedestrians, males greatly outnumber females. There is also a definite social gradient (the poorest most liable to injury) among injured pedestrians, especially children – doubtless because

overcrowded houses, absence of gardens, and mothers at work combine to place more children from poorer districts on the streets.

Essentially there are three ways of reducing motor accidents. The first is by improving roads. Britain has for several decades kept its total of road deaths about level (despite constantly increasing numbers of vehicles) by providing better surfaces and wider roads, by marking danger points, by creating roundabouts to facilitate traffic flow at intersections, by establishing and seeking to enforce speed limits appropriate to particular roads and by separating adequately traffic moving in opposite directions (as on motorways). Some problems of road improvement remain to be tackled, e.g., giving motorists advance warning of sudden fog or ice, and the enforcement during the motorist's nightmare – freezing fog and black ice – of speed limits much lower than those normally applicable to the particular road.

The second method of reduction is improvement of vehicles. Four-wheel brakes, rear-view mirrors, windscreen wipers, and undamaged tyres can prevent many accidents; and most countries are increasingly making it a legal requirement that these should be in a state of efficiency before a car is taken on a public road. Seat belts have proved their value, as have crash helmets for motorcyclists. Other improvements, such as reinforced bumpers and padded and collapsible steering wheels, have been introduced.

The third and probably the most important method is educating the road user and preventing the ineducable road user from driving. In respect of drivers a great deal has already been done. The introduction of driving tests, although standards vary, was an enormous step forward, even though there is something strange in a person today taking a test in which he never exceeds the speed-limit for a built-up area and tomorrow being legally entitled to drive on a motorway. Attempts are being made to identify persons whose impaired health renders them a danger to themselves or others, but moderation seems necessary: for example it would seem an unwarrantable interference with the liberty of the individual to stop from driving a man of 76 who is fully aware of slowed reaction time and decreased vision, who deliberately avoids hazardous situations and has not been the cause of an accident.

In recent years much attention has been paid to alcohol: Sweden attempted – on negligible evidence, for a single whisky may actually improve a driver's efficiency and reaction time – to ban absolutely simultaneous drinking and driving, and in due course had to abandon the experiment; Britain, perhaps more wisely, specified a permissible maximum of 80 mg. per 100 ml. of blood – a reasonable maximum for most people, but a few individuals could drive competently with 100 mg. while a few have impaired concentration and slowed reaction time with only 70 or 75 mg. Unfortunately, fatigue, anger, and distress are as hazardous as alcohol and less easily identifiable. Probably the most hopeful measure for reduction of errors by drivers is the policy – adopted by many insurance companies – of rewarding the accident-free driver by reducing his premium and correspondingly penalizing the driver who has had an accident. Yet, even if this policy were carried to the extent of taking the dangerous driver off the road, there are still no measures to cope with the dangerous pedestrian.

There are courses in schools in the U.S.A. designed to acquaint children with traffic conditions and regulations in the city and such instruction is being introduced into Britain. It could be a useful measure to teach all school children about the stopping distances of cars at various speeds and about the alterations in these distances when a road is wet or icy. Perhaps, too, pedestrians using roads at night should be encouraged – or even required by law – to wear or carry something of light colour. So far we have improved roads, we are improving vehicles, we are in process of improving drivers, but we have ignored pedestrians.

accident-proneness. A liability to road, home, or industrial accidents which is significantly greater than average. Most of us have increased predisposition to accidents at times, in particular when we are tired or emotionally disturbed or when we have consumed too much alcohol; but the term, accident-proneness, is generally reserved for persisting increased liability to accidents.

Scientific investigation of the condition is difficult. Firstly, it involves study of individuals for long periods to differentiate accident repeaters from those who have few or no accidents. Secondly, it requires consideration of degrees of risk, e.g., a taxi-driver has more chance of a traffic accident than has an owner who uses his car about three times a week, and a housewife without outside employment has more risk of a domestic accident than has her husband. Thirdly, it needs detailed investigation of the physical and psychological characteristics of both accident-prone and normal persons.

Defects of special senses clearly play a part: a person with impaired sight, hearing or smell has increased liability to various types of accident. Habitual preoccupation with other matters contributes: the well-known 'absent-minded professor' is a case in point and his equivalent can be found in many occupations. Also there is some evidence that many accident repeaters show more than average aggressiveness, impulsiveness, immaturity, and resentment of restrictions.

In most cases susceptible individuals cannot yet be identified in advance of their first accidents. Counselling of persons who have had one or more home or road accidents might help, and the relating of insurance premiums to previous driving records can discourage accident repeaters from driving.

accommodation. The faculty the human eye possesses of altering its refractive power so that rays of light, whether from far or near, are focused accurately on the retina. The alteration is achieved by means of the elasticity of the lens within the EYE. See also EYESIGHT.

acetabulum. The cup-shaped socket on the PELVIS in which rests the head of the femur or thigh-bone, the two together forming the hip joint.

acetic acid. The active principle of vinegar, prepared commercially by distillation of wood and subsequent separation from tar. The pure form is solid and called glacial acetic acid. In strong solution it is a corrosive poison which is

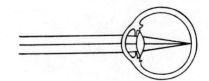

The comparatively slim lens required for distance vision

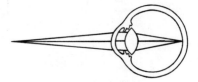

The increased convexity of the lens required for near vision

Accommodation

sometimes used to destroy warts or corns, the adjacent parts being protected with vaseline and the acid applied with a match, generally once daily for several days. In dilute solution, as in vinegar, it may be used as an antidote to poisoning by alkalis, such as ammonia or caustic soda.

acetone. A substance of sweet and sickly smell found in the urine and breath of persons suffering from various wasting diseases, including severe diabetes. It is the product of incomplete oxidation of fats during the digestive process. Commercially produced acetone is commonly used as a solvent for cellulose paints and as a nail varnish remover.

Achilles tendon. The tendon behind the ankle formed from the soleus and gastrocnemius muscles and attached to the heel bone. It may be strained or torn during exercise so that walking and particularly running, become difficult or impossible. Treatment is by rest and possibly physiotherapy.

The tendon gets its name from the Greek hero Achilles whose mother held him by this tendon when he was a baby while she dipped him in the River Styx as a charm to protect him from being wounded. However the heel was thus left vulnerable and eventually he was killed by an arrow piercing the tendon.

achlorhydria. Absence of hydrochloric acid from the gastric juice, with consequent lessening of the digestive capacity. This absence is found in pernicious anaemia and cancer of the stomach, but it is also found in about 5 per cent of healthy young adults and in about 10 per cent of healthy middle-aged people. Where no disease is found, no treatment is usually prescribed.

acholuric jaundice. A hereditary disease in which the red blood cells are abnormally fragile, there is jaundice of the skin and mucous membranes, the spleen is enlarged, and symptoms and signs of anaemia are present, but no bile is present in the urine. Mild cases may need no treatment, but in severe cases removal of the spleen is necessary (because it acts as the destroyer of the fragile red blood corpuscles) and a blood transfusion may be

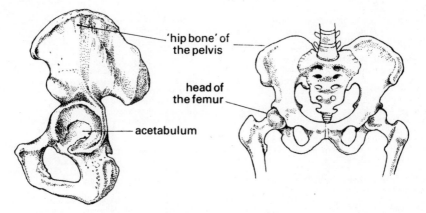

The acetabulum

required to enable the patient to withstand the operation. In general removal of the spleen appears to cure the condition, but if the operation is done in childhood it may increase the liability to infections.

achondroplasia. A hereditary abnormality of bone formation, inherited as a genetic dominant (see GENETICS), which produces the commonest form of dwarfism. The head becomes enlarged with bulging forehead, the trunk may be normal in length, but the arms and legs are grossly stunted. In very severe forms death in infancy is common, but in less severe forms survival into adult life is probable, with height seldom exceeding 120 cm. (4 ft.). There is no treatment. Appropriate contraceptive treatment and GENETIC COUNSELLING could eliminate the condition.

acid. A sour tasting compound which can combine with an alkali to form a salt. While weak acids are sometimes used medicinally, most acids are strong corrosive poisons. Immediate treatment in acid poisoning is to give an alkali (such as milk of magnesia or baking soda in water) and to send for medical aid. An emetic to induce vomiting should not be given. External BURNS caused by acids should immediately have the acid gently washed off and should thereafter be treated like other burns.

acidity. A vague term generally denoting the burning sensation experienced in INDIGESTION and some stomach disorders. Essentially the symptom is due either to excess of hydrochloric acid in the gastric juice or to regurgitation of that juice.

acidosis. A state in which the blood would tend to become less alkaline but for the existence of bodily buffering mechanisms which provide (but use up) an alkali reserve. Acidosis may occur in severe diabetes, certain kidney diseases, and carbohydrate starvation.

In adults it is characterized by drowsiness, sighing respiration and presence of the sweet odour of acetone in the breath; it is prevented by adequate carbohydrate in the diet (a matter of fine judgment in diabetes, where excess carbohydrate is dangerous) and it is treated by giving glucose in solution.

In children it often starts with vomiting and

high temperature (which have, of course, many other causes) and is most often caused by an excessive proportion of fat in the diet.

The immediate treatment consists of rest, ample fluid and glucose; and subsequent attacks can be prevented by adjustment of the diet, bearing in mind both the child's low fat tolerance and his need for sufficiency of the fat-soluble vitamins. In some cases emotional disturbances would appear to precipitate acidosis.

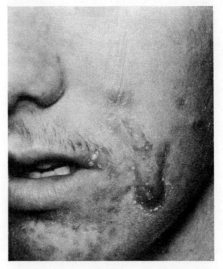

Acne

acne. A skin affection, occurring mostly between 12 and 25 years of age and characterized by pimples and 'blackheads' or comedones which are collections of dried grease in the openings of the sweat glands. They are found especially on the face and neck, caused by overactivity of the sweat glands and believed to be due to a temporary imbalance of the endocrine glands. Acne is difficult to treat, although sometimes helped by frequent washing with mildly antiseptic soap, avoidance of sweet-eating and inclusion of ample fruit and green vegetables in the diet. It usually disappears spontaneously about the age of 25 years.

acne rosacea. A skin condition in which blood vessels, especially of the nose and cheeks, become permanently enlarged, causing a purplish mottling. Possible causes include excess alcohol, chronic indigestion, and prolonged exposure to inclement weather. Provided the patient is willing to co-operate, treatment is possible and includes avoidance of the main cause, moderate use of sedatives, washing the face twice daily with toilet water, and nightly application of an appropriate ointment.

aconite poisoning. Poisoning by an alkaloid contained in the plant known as Wolf's Bane or Monk's Hood, the root of which looks like horseradish. Initial symptoms include tingling in the mouth and throat, followed by numbness. Treatment is by giving an emetic to induce vomiting, keeping warm, and if breathing becomes difficult applying artificial respiration.

acquired characteristics. From the time of Darwin and Galton and by the study of GENETICS it has been fully appreciated that many basic characteristics are inherited (e.g., colour of eyes) but that less basic traits are acquired (e.g., an infant of English ancestry brought up in a Spanish home will speak Spanish as his first language).

Various workers have tried to establish that characteristics acquired by parents and grandparents can be transmitted to children. Concrete proof is difficult because it is necessary first to exclude the influences of environment and personal example; but, despite some interesting recent Russian work, the inheritance of acquired charactistics is regarded by most scientists as not established. For example, if a blacksmith whose father and grandfather were blacksmiths before him closes his forge during the infancy of his son, there is no likelihood that the son will have particularly brawny arms.

acromegaly and gigantism. Related conditions caused by excessive secretion of the growth hormone of the pituitary gland and characterized by abnormal growth of bony and soft parts, especially of the face and limbs.

Gigantism. This condition begins in childhood, before ossification of bones is completed, and produces lengthening of the long bones so that there is an excessive overall height, with very long arms and increased size of feet, hands, and parts of the head.

Normal height varies with at least three sets of conditions: (1) racial inheritance, e.g., most Swedes and Zulus are tall by comparison with Spaniards; (2) personal inheritance, e.g., the child of tall parents is likely to be of greater height than the child of short parents; and (3) nutrition and exercise in childhood, e.g., the undernourished child of tall parents may reach 'normal' stature but in reality be stunted in that he has not reached his genetic potential, and the tall son of apparently 'average' parents may have reached his potential while his parents were really stunted.

Broadly speaking, for persons from Northern Europe, Canada and the U.S.A. a height of over 200 cm. (6 ft. 8in.) in men and 185 cm. (6 ft. 1 in.) in women is considered abnormal. The tallest verified case of gigantism known is an American who, in the fourth decade of this century, reached a height of 271 cm. (8 ft. 11 in.).

Acromegaly. Unlike gigantism, acromegaly starts after ossification is completed and therefore affects bones that can thicken but no longer lengthen. The face becomes enlarged with beetling brow and prominent jaw, and the hands and feet enlarge.

At first there is often increased muscular development in both conditions, and often sexual precosity, followed later by impotence. As the disease progresses headache, stiffness of the spine, and tingling of the extremities becomes common, visual disturbances are fairly frequent and about one-fifth of the cases develop diabetes. If untreated the patient normally dies at between 50 and 60 years from cerebral complications, diabetes, or heart failure. Treatment of the pituitary with x-rays enormously improves the outlook, although it cannot remove skeletal changes that have already taken place. If this irradiation fails, operative treatment is desirable.

acromion. The part of the scapula or shoulder blade that forms the tip of the shoulder.

ACTH. An abbreviation used for the adrenocorticotrophic hormone, nowadays most often shortened to corticotrophin. This is one of the hormones secreted by the anterior lobe of the pituitary gland, and it stimulates the cortex of another pair of endocrine glands, the adrenal glands, to produce other hormones in their turn. These include the corticosteroids, one of which is cortisone, which controls bodily usage of carbohydrate. By a curious 'feed-back' mechanism, deficiency of cortisone in the blood leads to increased production of ACTH, while increase – whether from over-activity of the adrenal cortex or from administration of cortisone – causes a lowering of ACTH.

Where a patient needs steroid therapy and his adrenals are efficient, ACTH can be given by injection – it is useless orally – as an alternative to cortisone, because the injected hormone stimulates the adrenal cortex to produce larger quantities of its own hormones.

Corticotrophin has been used in the treatment of rheumatic fever, rheumatoid arthritis, asthma and some other diseases. Essentially, however, it merely relieves symptoms but does not cure the underlying disease.

actinomycosis. A chronic suppurative disease, occurring mainly in cattle but rarely transmitted to man, and caused by the *Streptothrix actinomyces* or the ray fungus. The commonest site is the jaw, where a hard, tender swelling appears and is sometimes at first wrongly attributed to an infected tooth. Penicillin in high dosage is the drug of choice.

acupuncture. This term is used in two entirely different senses. In Europe and the United States it indicates the insertion of hollow needles into a cavity to permit the draining off of excessive fluid, e.g., in oedema.

In China it has been claimed for at least 2,000 years that absence of pain can be produced by the insertion and vibration of solid needles into carefully chosen points which to Western investigators seem to have no particular relationship to the areas rendered painless. It is

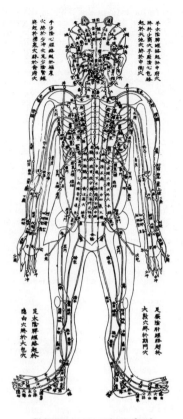

Chinese acupuncture chart

easy for sceptics to dismiss treatment of disease by acupuncture as 'quackery' and to explain any verified cures, as due to spontaneous recovery, good nursing or psychological reaction. It is much less easy to explain away the use of acupuncture to produce analgesia during surgical operation, a method which Chinese doctors claim has the advantage of creating less blood loss than does operation under general anaesthesia.

Cases are on record – watched by reputable British and American physicians – of operation on the right lung being performed on a patient, fully conscious and capable of conducting a conversation during the operation, in whom analgesia was produced by insertion of a two inch needle into a spot over the right biceps and manual rotation of the needle for about ten seconds every half minute; and of operation on the left knee cartilage with the patient rendered insusceptible to pain by insertion of needles in the left ear.

Attempts to repeat analgesia by acupuncture in Europe and the United States have been unsuccessful, and the complexity is increased by the fact that, while Chinese exponents specify points for insertion in great detail, different versions are given by different physicians. Certainly there is no known physiological explanation of why a needle inserted at one point should produce

insensitivity in an area served by entirely different nerves.

It has been suggested that the explanation is entirely psychological, that the patient fully accepts that he will not feel pain and that the site of insertion is irrelevant. Against that view is the detailed specification by the Chinese of points for different areas of the body. Probably complete explanation will have to wait until such time as there is fuller and freer exchange of scientific information between East and West.

acute. A term indicating rapid onset and short duration, in contrast to 'chronic' which implies slower onset and longer duration. In medical usage 'acute' does not carry any implication of severity. A severe case of meningitis and a mild case of the common cold are both termed acute infections.

adder bite. See SNAKE BITE.

addiction. A condition characterized by craving for a particular drug, need for increasing quantities of it, increasing dependence on it and harmful effects. The craving is so strong that a person who cannot otherwise obtain the drug is driven to seek it by criminal means, such as breaking into a clinic or a chemist's shop or stealing to secure money to buy it. The decreasing effect caused by the drug means that the addict requires larger and larger doses. Dependence implies that if the drug is totally withdrawn suddenly the patient has severe withdrawal symptoms and may even die. The harmful effects include deterioration of the personality, inability to work, and ultimately impairment of physical health – largely because the person has neither the inclination to eat adequately nor the money to purchase sufficient food in addition to his drug.

Heroin and morphia are definite drugs of addiction: a couple of doses, many hours apart, as pain-killers, will not produce addiction, but regular dosage for several days almost definitely creates craving and later the other characteristics of addiction. Cocaine and LSD (although the latter is not normally classed as a drug of addiction) lead to craving, increased tolerance and much deterioration of the personality, but rarely to severe withdrawal symptoms.

Alcohol cannot usually be called a drug of addiction since the vast majority of people do not show increasing tolerance but continue to drink the same amounts year after year and do not experience severe withdrawal symptoms if supplies are cut off. In a small minority of drinkers alcohol becomes a true drug of addiction.

The barbiturates are similarly seldom drugs of addiction, although in a few cases they lead to the four classic manifestations.

Tobacco, tea and coffee are not really drugs of addiction: not only do smokers and tea and coffee drinkers tend to consume the same amounts year after year (showing no signs of increased tolerance) but a heavy smoker or a heavy tea or coffee drinker, deprived of supplies, will not commit a crime to obtain them; and withdrawal symptoms are relatively slight.

Addison's disease. A disease caused by decreased or absent secretion of aldosterone by the suprarenal glands, and in most cases due to tuberculosis of these glands. The condition is characterized by slowly increasing general weakness, loss of weight, poor appetite, very low blood pressure and bronzed pigmentation of the exposed areas of skin. It was formerly fatal in one to three years, but cortisone and fluorohydrocortisone have completely altered the outlook. With efficient treatment, usually by mouth every second day, the patient slowly returns to normal weight, regains appetite, gradually loses pigmentation, and can live a reasonably normal life for many years. Since the treatment is replacement of a secretion – not a condition – it must be continued indefinitely.

adduct. To move a limb towards the mid-line of the body.

adenitis. Inflammation of a lymph gland.

adenoids. See TONSILS AND ADENOIDS.

adenoma. Tumour composed of glandular tissue. Adenomata may arise from any gland in the body, and their effect depends on their position and their growth. They do not give rise to secondary growths or involve neighbouring lymph glands, and unless they cause pressure symptoms or disfiguration they are harmless. If completely removed they do not recur.

adenoma sebaceum. A disease, now thought to be of hereditary origin, characterized by the formation of reddish-brown papules on the face and neck, mental deficiency, and frequent epilepsy. No treatment is usually necessary for the skin condition.

adhesions. The uniting together, generally following inflammation or injury, of tissues which should normally be freely movable. They are relatively common after joint injuries, causing stiffness and restriction of movement and, unless prevented by massage and physical treatment while the injury is healing, they may have to be broken down by manipulation of the joint with the patient under an anaesthetic.

Adhesions are also liable to form in the abdomen after operations.

adhesive plaster. A dressing, sticky on the inner side, employed to retain in position the primary dressing of a cut or wound. An adhesive plaster should not be applied directly to injured skin, and before it is applied to healthy skin the skin, if at all hairy, should be shaved. Adhesive plaster commercially prepared with an antiseptic pad is widely used for cuts and other small wounds.

adipose tissue. The technical term for the fat which is distributed under the skin and in the body cavities. It protects against cold, cushions internal organs, and forms a reserve store of food and energy. In starvation and in wasting diseases it rapidly decreases, as it may also do by strict adherence to a diet.

adiposity. Possession of excessive adipose tissue to the extent of OBESITY.

adolescence. The years of transition from childhood to adult life, the period in which the sex glands become active and many physical, emotional and intellectual changes take place. The beginning and end of adolescence vary from person to person, and in general occur earlier in girls than in boys. In recent decades, the very period during which prolongation of education has extended the length of financial dependence on parents, the period of adolescence has become slightly earlier. Although there is some overlapping, adolescence may conveniently be divided into four phases.

1. The pre-puberty phase. This is the period roughly between the ages of 11 and 12 years. A boy grows appreciably, his shoulders broaden, his chest expands and his penis lengthens. A girl has a greater growth spurt, so that her height on average equals that of a boy of the same age and her weight slightly exceeds that of the boy, her hips broaden, her breasts start to develop, pubic hair begins to grow and in some cases menstruation commences. Both sexes become a little resentful of adult control and show more initiative than in earlier years, but are still essentially children.

2. The phase of puberty. At 13 to 15 years a boy's growth continues, pubic hair begins to develop, the voice breaks and he may have nocturnal discharges of seminal fluid ('wet dreams'). At 13 to 14 years a girl's growth spurt continues though slowing down, and menstruation becomes established. Both become interested in members of the opposite sex, very much aware of clothes and teenage fashions, increasingly resentful of the shackles of parental domination and control, although often seeking parental affection and support, and more and more distrustful of their own clumsiness and lack of poise, which are largely due to uneven growth of the arms, legs and neck.

3. Mid-adolescence. Boys of 16 to 18 experience a settling down or stabilization of physiological changes, they begin to need to shave, they start to 'go steady' with a particular girl, they become more independent and claim the right to form their own opinions and use their own judgments, and they have increased social consciousness and idealism with decreased interests in parents and home, although some boys adopt a very protective attitude to their mothers. Girls of 15 to 17 years experience a similar settling down and exhibit the same increased independence and social awareness. They become more self-assured and self-confident, and often have a number of boy-friends. Both sexes display increased curiosity, greater self-consciousness and very strong feelings of right and wrong, with a tendency to deep and distressing mental conflicts.

4. Late adolescence. The boy of 19 to 20 and the girl of 18 to 19 years have reached full physical maturity and have achieved their maximum intellectual capacities and their peaks for analytical thought and for imaginative creativity. While as yet having little experience of life, they are ready for life's responsibilities and are often prepared to 'put the world right'. They tend to be critical of the standards and beliefs of older people and severe in their judgments.

Since these stages overlap considerably, it is perhaps useful to summarize the main characteristics of the turbulent period of adolescence. There is a considerable increase in weight and height, so that an adolescent needs more food than an adult, and there are irregular alternations of energy and fatigue. Day dreaming and fantasy life loom large. There is a growing awareness of the physical self: clumsiness appears as a result of uneven growth and often causes embarrassment, and there tends to be anxiety about social occasions. A marked feature is resentment of parental control, frequently leading to family rows, and yet with the youngster who

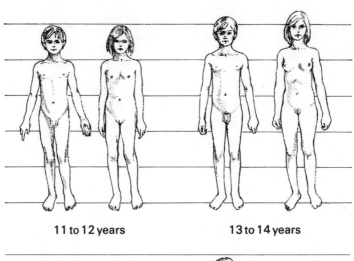

11 to 12 years   13 to 14 years

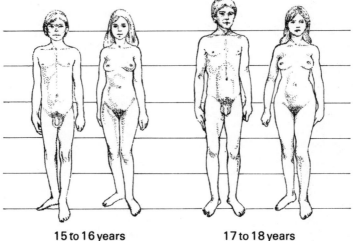

15 to 16 years   17 to 18 years

Stages of adolescence

indignantly rejected parental domination yesterday expecting parental affection and support in the troubles of today. There is at times a desire for solitude. The longing for independence is strong and increases throughout adolescence. The period is characterized by idealism and a tendency to religious and political conversion. There is increasing awareness of the other sex and the phenomenon of falling in love, often with little appreciation of either the imperfections or the interests of the intended partner, and there is a tendency to sexual experimentation. Relationships with parents undergo a change or a series of changes: a capacity to argue develops and is a recognition of the fallibility of adults, sometimes carried to the point where it is assumed that what any adult says will

probably be wrong. Understanding of environmental, social and political matters increases. There is a changed attitude to study – either much greater interest or a complete disinterest.

Yet, despite all these changes, many interests remain unaltered – the book-lover still visits the library and the cricketer still plays. Also the fundamental qualities of the personality do not alter, e.g., the introvert remains introverted.

Adolescence is an era of rapid mood swings, of alternation between dependence and independence and between surging hope and dark despair. Above all, it is an era of loneliness and anxiety. Few adolescents talk freely with adults, least of all with their parents, and many feel misunderstood, anxious, awkward, lonely or impure.

The main developmental tasks of adolescence include: the establishment of relationships with the opposite sex, the achievement of the physical and mental capacity to hold down a job which is recognized by the individual and his associates as worthwhile, the gaining of personal and financial independence and emancipation, and the finding of principles – moral, religious, political, philosophical or pragmatic – by which to live and by which to assess other people.

Success in these tasks and diminution of the turbulence of adolescence depend in considerable measure on three factors – the personality structure (itself conditioned partly by nature and partly by nurture), earlier parental and other relationships, and social and cultural pressures. For example, the development of a self-reliant individual who is no longer dependent on parents and friends is facilitated by security and a loving relationship in childhood, by opportunities to progress gradually and without stress from the safe relationships of the family to association with contemporaries, by friendliness of parents and teachers and by availability of appropriate social contacts. To take a converse example, future attitude to work can be damaged by over-ambitious parents never satisfied with their child's achievements (creating discontent and under-achievement), by parents preoccupied with status and prestige (sometimes producing the drop-out who rejects all traditional values and standards) and by parents who make all decisions, leaving the child with no experience in coping with problems.

Adolescence is a difficult and challenging time both for young people and for their parents, and it is particularly difficult where the period of dependency is prolonged long beyond physiological and intellectual maturation, as happens to some extent with the schoolgirl compelled by law to remain at school, and as emphatically happens with a youngster whose full school education is immediately followed by a university or polytechnic course. The possibilities for conflict, revolt and unhappiness are many. Equally, however, adolescence is a very important period. While it is undoubtedly true that the first four or five years of life are of supreme importance for the foundation both of physique and of personality, and while the next seven years are a vital learning period, it is in adolescence that attitudes are formed or consolidated and emotional forces are guided into right or wrong channels.

Parents, youth leaders, teachers and others dealing with adolescents should remember that adolescents are as a rule easily led (e.g., by appeal to their idealism and sense of justice or by appeal to the reasoning power of which they are so proud) but that no other age-group is harder to drive.

Problems of adolescence. Hormones, intellectual development and emotional changes interact in the production of problems of adolescents, and no classification is really satisfactory. Some of the problems are considered below under four approximate headings – growth, regression, sex and rebellion.

1. Problems related to growth. The prolonged growth spurt means that an adolescent needs to eat more food than an adult and especially requires plenty of meat, fish, milk and green vegetables. So actual malnutrition may arise in an impoverished household or in one in which the parents do not understand the adolescent's needs. Obesity may be created through the satisfaction of hunger by consumption of carbohydrates in large amounts, especially if eating is also employed as a compensation for lack of affection. Under-nutrition may follow obesity as the youngster slims vigorously in an attempt to get rid of podginess and 'puppy-fat'. Uneven growth can create embarrassment over a gawky appearance and clumsy movements. An early or late growth spurt can cause the misery of the tall girl towering above her friends, or of the small boy, with unbroken voice, dwarfed by his classmates.

Most of these problems can be helped by a good diet and reassurance, but all too often parents and other relatives make matters worse by mocking the clumsiness, excessive height or apparent stunting, or by trying to insist that a child embarrassed by appearance nevertheless dons a swimsuit or pair of shorts.

2. Problems related to regression. One of the characteristics of the adolescent is temporary swings back towards the behaviour of childhood. A boy of 14 may at times show less sense of responsibility than displayed three years earlier, a class of 15-year-old girls may giggle in a way that they would not have done at 12, and a youngster of either sex may display a curiously juvenile sense of humour. Such happenings are best regarded as a sort of compensation for physical and intellectual growth by greater expression of childish emotions. If at all possible, the irresponsibility, giggling and juvenile pranks should be quietly tolerated, although this may be difficult in a school where two misbehaving children disturb the progress of an otherwise interested class.

3. Problems related to sex. Most girls nowadays are prepared for mammary development and the onset of menstruation, although the start of bleeding can be terrifying to a girl who has not had the necessary instruction. Boys, however, often receive no preparation for erections, nocturnal emissions and erotic fancies, and are initiated into the mysteries of sex by furtive conversations with other boys or incited to experiment by slightly more mature girls.

Masturbation, a common and usually harmless phenomenon, may give rise to deep guilt feelings.

While the underlying causes of sexual deviation mostly lie in earlier years, sexuality that has previously been repressed may reappear at adolescence in deviant forms, e.g., as MASOCHISM or SADISM. Growth of sexual feelings before a child has ceased to be interested primarily in his own sex may create temporary homosexual relationships, usually only theoretical but occasionally physical.

Love for the opposite sex tends to be romanticized, with no awareness of the other person's imperfections and with exaggerated gloom when these are discovered. A couple may marry at 16 or 17 years without realizing that they have no interests in common, so that teenage marriages have a high rate of breakdown.

The conception of off-spring by unmarried teenagers is in some cases a result of unplanned experimentation, in other cases a symbol of deliberate revolt against the standards of adults, and in yet other cases a consequence of belief in myths that are prevalent (e.g., that a girl cannot become pregnant until she has menstruated several times.)

To a very considerable extent, the sex problems of adolescents can be helped or avoided by adequate sex education in advance, such education including moral and aesthetic aspects as well as anatomy and physiology.

4. Problems related to rebellion. The adolescent is aware of his mental and physical maturity but feels shackled by inexplicable restrictions and regulations, e.g., he can legally marry as soon as he is 16 but he and his wife are legally obliged to attend school until a specified leaving date, and he cannot buy her a glass of beer. He sees some of life's injustices and cruelties, feels that he could put them right, but lacks even a vote. Not least, he is financially dependent.

Inevitably there tends to be conflict with authority, starting usually with small things in the home (such as the time of staying out or the wearing of make-up) but often progressing to a stage in which parents, teachers and policemen are banded together as 'enemies'. Adolescence is above all the period of rebellion and trial of strength, whether evidenced directly by delinquency (which may have its origins much earlier in an unhappy home, lack of love or parental domination) and open clash with authority, or shown indirectly, as when the son of a Conservative MP becomes a Socialist or the daughter of an Anglican clergyman becomes a Roman Catholic or humanist.

Many adolescents, however, achieve the transition from childhood to adult life without clashes with constituted authority and without too many family rows. Sympathetic and understanding parents and early introduction to participation in decision making, together with early training in the use of freedom and the substitution of self-discipline for externally imposed discipline, all play important parts in lessening the problems of adolescence.

adoption. For an illegitimate child whose mother does not wish to keep him (or cannot provide for him), or for a child whose parents have died, a carefully chosen adoption provides a home and a family, with the security and affection that these words imply; and couples who cannot have natural children (whether because of infertility or because of knowledge that one of them is likely to transmit a serious hereditary disease) can satisfy their parental instincts by adopting one or more children.

Careful selection of adopting parents and children is of course necessary. Some adults are unfit to assume a parental role: people who are emotionally immature, over-strict, excessively houseproud or affectionless are examples. Some may be capable of caring for children of their own but unsuitable as adopters: it is often said, for instance, that if the natural child of a couple dies after having become old enough to be recognized as a personality, the parents – if permitted to adopt – tend to contrast the adopted child detrimentally with the one who died. Some children in turn have heredities that make them poor candidates for adoption: serious mental or physical handicaps are an example, although a few prospective adopters actually indicate a desire to adopt a handicapped child. Again a couple may be satisfactory as potential adopters and a child may be suitable for adoption but the particular adults and the particular child may not fit: one would hesitate deliberately to link together adopting parents of academic disposition and sedentary habits and a child whose natural parents were vigorous, athletic and utterly uninterested in books.

In the U.K. adoption arrangements may legally be made only by local authorities and by registered adoption societies (not operating for profit). Attempts are made not only to ensure that the applicants are suitable persons for adoption and that the child is suitable for being adopted but also that they match reasonably. There is a safeguarding period of three months during which the child resides with the applicants, and up to the end of that period the natural parents are free to withdraw their consent to the adoption and the applicants are likewise free to change their minds. After the adoption order is made (at the end of the three months) the child acquires all the rights of a natural child (e.g., in respect of inheriting from the adopting parents) and loses these rights in respect of his natural parents.

The problems of the early years of adoption are sometimes overstated. Certainly the recently adopted child is a 'little stranger', with the new parents knowing little about his high or low intelligence, his quick or placid temper or his resistance or susceptibility to various diseases; but a natural child is also at first very much a stranger who may have inherited qualities from any of his eight different great grandparents; and in a very short time the adopted child is no longer a stranger but a known, accepted and loved member of the family.

Sooner or later the child will learn from some source that he is adopted. To prevent shock it is desirable that the parents should make him aware of the fact at an early age – telling him that he is more fortunate than most children, because most children are just born (with the parents having no choice over sex, colour of hair, and so on) whereas he was deliberately picked out by the parents, with the expressed implication that the parents will therefore love him more than most parents love their children.

adrenal glands. Alternatively known as suprarenal glands, these are important members of the system of ENDOCRINE GLANDS, producing the hormone adrenalin as their principal secretion.

adrenalin. The main hormone produced by the medulla of the suprarenal, or adrenal gland, which is one of the ENDOCRINE GLANDS, and also nowadays manufactured synthetically by chemists. Whether secreted (as in rage and other emotional states) or injected, it raises the blood pressure, mobilizes energy in the form of sugar and dilates bronchial vessels allowing greater use of oxygen. As a natural secretion it is the body's response to fear. As an injected drug it can be life-saving in stimulating the heart muscle in collapse and shock, and is also very useful in acute attacks of asthma.

adulteration. This term is used both for the addition of inferior materials to a food or drug and for the abstraction of any constituent part; examples are the addition of water to milk or the removal of part of the milk fat from milk. In many countries laws exist to prevent or minimize adulteration.

aerobic. Requiring oxygen for existence. Many bacteria are – like human beings – aerobic, and die in the continued absence of oxygen. Some bacteria, however, are anaerobic, not merely not needing oxygen but tending to die in its presence.

aerophagy and gastric flatulence. Aerophagy or air-swallowing consists of air being gulped in and in a few seconds being belched out. It occurs mostly in nervous dyspepsia but is sometimes found in gastric and duodenal ulcer and in angina pectoris. Essentially the patient feels fullness or discomfort, attributes it to 'wind', tries unsuccessfully to belch, swallows air during the attempt and then belches. Treatment consists of explanation and of substituting sweet-sucking or water-sipping for the effort to disperse air. Gastric flatulence includes aerophagy but can also be caused by production of gas by fermentation of food in the stomach.

aetiology. Strictly the study of the causes of any particular disease, but often used loosely as a synonym for 'causes'.

affect. Essentially the effect of any emotion on the mind.

Psychologists often divide personalities into three main types: (1) the cognitive (the thinking, reasoning, logical type whose interests are in theories rather than application, the 'cold' personality whose response to a situation is usually intellectual rather than emotional); (2) the conative (interested in practical results and in active and purposeful activities); (3) the affective (concerned with his emotional reaction to events, and tending either to sympathize with others or to be actively hostile to them). Yet few of us belong solely to one of these types, although one may predominate.

In certain mental disorders the three main types become exaggerated. For instance the schizophrenic has very little affect, shows little affection for others and normally exhibits scant response to emotions: whereas the manic-depressive is dominated by his emotions, and swings rapidly from complete elation to utter dejection.

afterbirth. The name given to the placenta, cord and membranes which attach the unborn child to the mother's womb, and which are expelled shortly after the birth of the child. See CHILDBIRTH.

after-image. A visual impression that outlasts its stimulus. A positive after-image, or weak representation of the original stimulus, can occur after looking at a bright object: e.g., stop reading this, look at an electric light, and you may see an image of the light when your eye returns to the page. A negative after-image is reversed in colour: e.g., stare at a black circle, transfer your gaze to a grey background and you may glimpse a white circle. Similar after-sensations can occur in respect of touch, but not as a rule in respect of hearing.

ageing. The gradual deterioration that occurs in all organized living creatures is occasioned in part by the wearing out of irreplaceable organs and structures. Hence it is inevitable: man is mortal. The deterioration is, however, to some extent a reflection of the life-long battle between the individual and the pressures of his environment, so that it is in part postponed by improvement of the quality of life.

Measured by such standards as 'reaching middle age' or 'becoming elderly' or the ultimate criterion of age at death, persons in a primitive community age more quickly than those in a highly developed society, and (despite the influence of the diseases of affluence, such as those caused by 'rich' diets and stress) the wealthy and the cultured tend to age more slowly than the underprivileged. Yet, within any one single group in any one community, inherited factors (or the influences of early life) are strong: the person whose parents were still physically and mentally active at 70 and whose grandparents were active at 68 is far more likely to be alert at 74 years than his neighbour whose parents were elderly at 60.

The common division into children, adolescents, young adults, the middle-aged, and the elderly (or Shakespeare's division into seven ages) is a loose generalization only. Apart from individual variations and the effects of environment, ageing of body and mind in developed countries is far from uniform: eyesight and hearing are probably at their peak around 14 years, with slight but appreciable deterioration thereafter; intelligence reaches its maximum around 16 years but its decrease over the next fifty years is very slight; lung capacity and cardiac output fall rapidly after the age of 30 while reaction time shows trivial reduction until after the age of 75. In general it is true to say that in most cases any physical or mental diminution is balanced in whole or in part by increased experience and skill. We might consider, for example, that a rifle-shooting marksman was 'getting beyond his best' at 26, that a boxer was nearing retirement at 34, that a statesman or an academic could reasonably be given a new post at 60, and that an otherwise healthy car-driver could safely have his licence renewed at 74.

The physical changes of ageing are, nevertheless, obvious – slight decrease in elasticity of skin and arteries beginning in the thirties, slower movements from the forties, in women the menopause in the late forties, and the muscle-shrinkage and bent backbone of old age. Mentally there are parallel, but rather later changes: a gradual decrease in tolerance, a slow narrowing of interests, and as ageing progresses some failure of recent memory and some exaggeration of the attitudes or prejudices held in earlier life. Simultaneously there comes an increased amount of susceptibility to illness and an increased number of medical consultations and hospital admissions.

Yet ageing is by no means all loss. The referee of 45 is neither less happy nor less useful than the sportsman of 30; the professor of 60 balances by greater knowledge and wider experience the slightly higher intelligence of his colleague of 40; and, just as the young adult is released from the turmoils and stresses of adolescence, the person of 'retirement age' comes to terms with life, has no more problems of ambition and promotion and, by the very narrowing of his interests, sometimes produces his best work.

Senility is a term employed for extreme old age accompanied by decay of mental and physical powers. There is no clear borderline between senility and normal old age, but the former is essentially a caricature or exaggeration of the latter. For instance, wrinkling of the skin, difficulty in standing upright, impaired vision, poor hearing and frequent passing of urine are all features of normal old age but are found to greater extent in senility; and mental deterioration, tedious repetition, loss of recent memory and lack of ability to concentrate, while all features of senility are to some extent found also in normal old age.

The truly senile person may collect rubbish, hide away money and food, wander outdoors in his night clothes, and become incontinent. Often, however, apparent senility is in some measure a result of poor nutrition, loneliness or lack of interests; and timely attention to these matters may prevent or postpone senility or may transform apparent senility into normal old age. Of particular importance in the apparently senile is attention to eyesight and hearing. Proper glasses and an efficient hearing aid may transform an apparently senile person into a reasonably normal senior citizen.

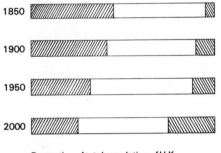

Proportion of total population of U.K.

under 20　　　　　over 65

ageing population. In industrialized countries until this century and in less developed countries until very recently, death rates in infancy, childhood and middle age were high, so that survival into old age was something of a rarity. In 1850, for example, only 5 per cent of the population of Britain and 3 per cent of the population of the United States were above the age of 65 years. Improved living conditions and preventive and curative services (notably immunization procedures, and the discovery of vitamins and antibiotics) have completely altered the pattern of survival. By the 1960s several countries had more than one-tenth of their inhabitants aged over 65 and young deaths are steadily becoming fewer. Given a continuation of existing trends a reasonable forecast of the population structure of a developed country around A.D. 2000 would be that 25 per cent would be dependent young (under 20 years), 50 per cent of working age (20 to 60), and 25 per cent of retirement age.

The changing age structure is already beginning to dominate medical and social planning. More and more attention has to be paid to disabling and chronic diseases. The housing shortage of many countries is occasioned essentially by the new phenomenon of the simultaneous existence of two and even three generations of adults. There is ever increasing need for geriatric hospital beds, for old people's homes, and for the development of 'sheltered housing' where old people can live within call of immediate help, but nevertheless continue to care for themselves for considerably longer than they could in the isolation of their own home.

In general, increased survival has been followed by reduced birth rate and decrease in family size, but only after a considerable time lag. Hence, various countries are faced in the 1970s with the problem of providing sufficient adults to undertake the care of a large population of children (e.g., teachers) and sufficient adults to look after a growing number of old people (e.g., nurses) at a time when there is a fall in the total number of adults of working age available to assume these tasks in addition to undertaking the productive work of the country.

agglutination. The clumping together of bacteria by substances in the blood of persons who have – or have had – the relevant bacterial disease. The Widal test for typhoid is one of the many agglutination tests employed in modern medicine.

Apart from agglutination thus produced, similar clumping can occur when blood of different groups is mixed.

agoraphobia. A form of NEUROSIS characterized by morbid and irrational fear of open spaces. The name is derived from the Greek words *agora,* the market place, and *phobia,* fear.

agranulocytosis. A condition characterized by diminution of the granular white blood corpuscles, with high temperature, development of ulcers and a high death-rate. The main cause is an abnormally sensitive reaction to certain drugs, e.g., chlorpromazine, amidopyrine, antihistamines and sulphonamides. Manifestations include rigors, pains in the limbs and throat, prostration, high temperature and the formation of ulcers.

Prevention is achieved essentially by warning each patient receiving drugs associated with agranulocytosis to report immediately if any of the symptoms develop. Treatment consists of rapid withdrawal of the offending drug and injections of hydrocortisone or ACTH. About three-quarters of untreated cases die, but early treatment reduces the death rate to about one-quarter. The risk of agranulocytosis is one of the reasons why certain non-addictive drugs remain available only on medical prescription.

ague. An old-fashioned term to denote fevers characterized by alternating paroxysms of cold and of heat and sweating. While the differentiation of fevers without characteristic rashes was very difficult until about 1900, the fever generally indicated by the word 'ague' was malaria.

air. The normal atmosphere consists of about 21 per cent oxygen, 78 per cent nitrogen, with argon, carbon dioxide, and rarer gases making up the remaining 1 per cent.

All animals, including people, require oxygen for the functioning of their RESPIRATION. Exhaled air contains only about 16 per cent of oxygen and some 5 per cent of carbon dioxide, and is heavily saturated with water vapour. Plants, under the influence of sunshine, on the other hand, absorb carbon dioxide and liberate oxygen. The nitrogen in the atmosphere simply dilutes the oxygen.

Unduly moist air retards evaporation from the skin, hampers respiration and impairs the oxygenation of the blood, thus reducing the capacity for both physical and mental activity. Hence one can play cricket or baseball in a hot, dry atmosphere, but cannot undertake any prolonged strenuous activity in a warm, humid atmosphere.

Increased water vapour and decreased oxygen, as in badly ventilated rooms, lowers working capacity and produces headache and breathing difficulty, going on in very extreme cases to air-hunger and even to coma, and ultimately to death. Bad VENTILATION is also associated with high incidence of sore throats and infections of the upper respiratory tract. Increased carbon dioxide, while a useful measure of air pollution, is not itself harmful. Many of the harmful effects formerly attributed to excess of carbon dioxide are now known to result from stagnation and lack of movement of air.

air hunger. Difficulty in breathing, shown by gasping for breath, due to lack of oxygen in the blood and consequently in the tissues, known as ANOXIA. It occurs in various heart and kidney diseases and also in acidosis. Treatment with oxygen and carbon dioxide relieves the attack but recurrence is likely unless the underlying condition can be cured.

air swallowing. See AEROPHAGY.

alastrim. A mild form of SMALLPOX alternatively called variola minor, caused by a virus which breeds true (i.e., never produces ordinary smallpox). Although it is appreciably less infectious than ordinary smallpox, produces a less profuse rash, causes less pitting, and has a much lower mortality, it is nevertheless a serious and highly infectious disease. The viruses of smallpox (*Variola major*) and alastrim are closely related, and vaccination against one also protects against the other.

albinism. A hereditary condition caused by absence of the enzyme required to form the pigment that is normally found in the skin, hair, and eyes. In albinos the hair is white, the skin very white and sensitive to sunlight, and the eyes pink owing to light shining through the colourless iris to the blood-vessels behind. Albinos often have to wear tinted spectacles and to avoid strong sunshine. The condition is inherited as a recessive character; see GENETICS.

albumin. The main protein contained in the blood. It helps to maintain the osmotic pressure of blood (see OSMOSIS). Where albumin is diminished – as in starvation, certain diseases of the liver (which normally manufactures albumin) and severe albuminuria – there is retention of fluid in the tissues and therefore oedema.

albuminuria. Presence of albumin in the urine. It occurs in most fevers and in various diseases of the heart and kidneys. Testing regularly for albuminuria is important in pregnancy because its presence may indicate disordered kidney function requiring skilled treatment.

alcohol. Any of a large group of organic hydroxides. The simplest chemically is methyl alcohol (wood spirit), a colourless, highly poisonous liquid distilled from wood. When drunk it produces unconsciousness without any preceding feeling of elation, it can create temporary or permanent blindness, and it may cause death. Methyl alcohol is not further considered in the paragraphs below.

Usually by 'alcohol' is meant the second simplest of the group, ethyl alcohol, a colourless liquid produced by fermentation of substances containing starch (e.g., barley, wheat, rye, potatoes) and used since history has been recorded to remove shyness or inhibitions and to induce a festive atmosphere. Simple fermentation produces a solution containing not more than about 12 per cent alcohol (e.g., beers and unfortified wines) because above that level the ferments become inactive. More concentrated solutions are prepared by distillation (e.g., whisky, brandy, gin, and vodka).

Since alcohol is very rapidly absorbed from an empty stomach it has value, taken in small quantities, as an immediate source of energy in some situations (although it should never be given to persons suffering from exposure on the hills), and since it promotes the flow of gastric juice it is commonly taken as an appetizer before or with meals. Normally, however, it is taken for its social and emotional effects. It induces a feeling of relaxation, lowers nervous tension and irritability, and reduces self-criticism. Other effects include a slight quickening of the heart beat and a dilating of blood vessels.

In appreciable quantity it impairs concentration, judgement, and self-control. The individual, while still apparently sober, may become – according to temperament – excitable, garrulous, quarrelsome or depressed; his reaction time is slowed and his manual skills and co-ordination of movements become less good. Larger amounts produce signs of drunkenness, including slurred speech and staggering gait, and often depression, while in still larger quantity, alcohol produces stupor and unconsciousness.

In general, absorption of alcohol is slowed by the presence of food in the stomach, especially milk or oil, hence the custom of eating oily hors d'oeuvres at the beginning of a meal. Absorbed alcohol is broken down at a fairly constant rate of 15 to 20 mg. per 100 ml. per hour (so that a man who had reached a level of 150 mg. would become legally fit to drive in about four or five hours). The effects of a given quantity of alcohol vary greatly with the individual (some people have 'no head for spirits' while others remain sober after large quantities) and with the person's previous familiarity or unfamiliarity with alcohol in general and with the particular variety of spirit consumed. Effervescence, as in whisky and soda, accelerates the effects, as does mixing of products of grain (e.g., whisky, vodka) and grape (e.g., brandy); so does cold air, so that the habit of 'one for the road' is to be deprecated.

While drinking is in general a controversial subject, its most controversial aspect is the relationship of alcohol to traffic accidents. Considering the speed at which cars are able to travel, anything that reduces a driver's reaction time or impairs his judgement is clearly liable to increase the danger of accidents. There is general agreement that the drunken driver is a menace and should be put off the road. Unfortunately there is no agreement as to what quantity of alcohol significantly impairs judgement or slows reaction time. Some workers claim that at around 25 mg. alcohol per 100 ml. blood (or very roughly the level produced in a man of average size by an ordinary single whisky) reaction time is actually improved, and that significant slowing does not appear until the level is about 100 mg.

The problem is extremely complicated because the blood level produced by a constant dose of alcohol varies with such factors as body size of the drinker, duration of period since drinking and stomach contents at time of drinking. Also, even if allowance is made for all known factors, there appears to be very considerable individual variation. For the safety of the public the permitted level of alcohol must clearly be low enough to allow for the reasonably worst combination of these various factors, but to set the level below that at which there was any possibility of reaction time being slowed would be merely repressive legislation. Nevertheless, some countries have tried making illegal the consumption of any alcohol at all for some hours before driving, but Sweden – the pioneer in this legislation – found its 'no alcohol for drivers' law unhelpful and rescinded it. Some European countries have established a legal limit of 50 mg. but when other factors (e.g., density of traffic) are taken into account evidence is lacking that the 50 mg. limit is safer than the present U.K. limit of 80 mg.

Continued heavy drinking for years can produce inflammation of the stomach (gastritis) and scarring of the liver (cirrhosis), together with brain deterioration. Additionally, since alcohol consumes or inactivates vitamin B_1, prolonged high consumption of alcohol may cause symptoms of deficiency of that vitamin.

While drunkenness is disgusting and alcoholism is a serious disease, the desirability or otherwise of moderate drinking is highly controversial. A few drinks can enliven a social occasion, and there is no indication that emotionally stable persons harm themselves by moderate indulgence. On the other hand, persons of unstable or inadequate personality may become utterly dependent on alcohol.

Alcohol and disease. Alcohol is useful in various conditions – to reduce fever by dilating the skin blood vessels and permitting easier access of air, to stimulate failing heart or respiration, to promote sleep at night, and to produce immediate warmth or relaxation of tension. It is definitely undesirable in cases of head injury and abdominal injury, is inadvisable in gastritis and gastric ulcer, and is considered by some experts to be detrimental in serious disease of the heart, cardiovascular system, or kidneys.

Since alcohol enlarges the small blood vessels in and near the skin and therefore increases heat loss from the body it should not be given to a person suffering from exposure to cold while he or she is still exposed.

In sudden excess it can cause intoxication, in the early stages of which the person may become aggressive and try to pick quarrels, or maudlin and tell his secrets to strangers, or over-generous and give away his possessions, or depressed and even attempt suicide, while in a later stage his speech is indistinct and his gait reeling. Unrepeated intoxication is not a disease. It is an episode, indicating that a youth has not discovered his limits, that an older person has over-used alcohol under abnormal stress, or that an individual has inadvertently mixed his drinks. Repeated intoxication is an indication that an individual cannot drink safely at all and is one form of ALCOHOLISM.

Even though not becoming an alcoholic, the habitual drinker, while deriving certain real or imagined benefits from his habit (such as personal pleasure, relief from worry and easing of social intercourse), runs certain risks. The first risk, often forgotten, is similar to that of the habitual eater of sweets or cakes – that of obesity, with consequent strain on heart and kidneys. Alcohol is a food, providing calories and energy; so that if alcohol does the work normally done by carbohydrates, the carbohydrates eaten are largely unused and deposited in the tissues as fat. Exact calorie values for any fixed quantity vary, being highest for spirits, less for fortified wines, and lowest for light white wines and some varieties of beer. Roughly, 30 ml. (1 fluid oz.) of whisky contains 60 Calories, or about the same as three times that quantity of milk.

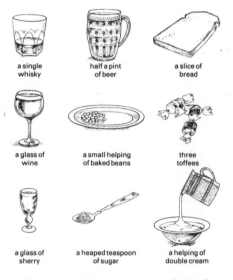

a single whisky

half a pint of beer

a slice of bread

a glass of wine

a small helping of baked beans

three toffees

a glass of sherry

a heaped teaspoon of sugar

a helping of double cream

These items all have approximately equal Calorie content

Alcohol, especially undiluted spirits, can cause inflammation of the lining of the stomach. Continued heavy drinking over a long period can produce cirrhosis of the liver, peripheral neuritis, and brain damage. A series of bouts of heavy drinking can lead to tremors of the hands, loss of appetite, and finally the hallucinations known scientifically as delirium tremens and colloquially as the blue devils.

Some workers have suggested that a healthy man of average size can normally consume a daily ration of 45 to 50 ml. of whisky or a bottle of unfortified wine without damage to physical or mental health; but individual variation is considerable, and no dependable norm is possible.

alcoholism. Dependence upon alcohol to such extent as to interfere frequently or persistently with bodily or mental health, with interpersonal relations, or with working capacity. There are several types of which two will be mentioned here.

1. Episodic bouts of heavy drinking: the individual becomes completely drunk at intervals (e.g., about once a month), 'sleeps it off', perhaps wakes with a hangover but is sober in the considerable periods between bouts. Treatment of the episode involves letting the individual rest, sometimes giving a sedative to counteract restlessness, keeping him warm and offering adequate liquid, preferably with vitamins B_1 and C. Treatment of the condition is as indicated below, but – while far from easy – is less difficult than is that of the 'alcoholic who is never drunk'.

2. Persisting and increasing inability to abstain: the individual is perhaps never intoxicated, especially in the early years of his disease, but meets every fresh situation (from the emergence of a problem to the arrival of a visitor) with a drink, consumes gradually larger and larger quantities, and passes from heavy social drinking to secret drinking, e.g., having an extra glass before his guest arrives or after the guest leaves. Excessive expenditure on alcohol and a developing lack of interest in spouse and family often lead to marital unhappiness, causing in turn more drinking. Work begins to suffer, leading to lack of promotion and sometimes to unemployment, with further drinking as a compensatory mechanism. If untreated the individual steadily deteriorates over a number of years. It is important to note that, while he displays a poor memory, a lowered working capacity, and often garrulousness or irritability, he may never be intoxicated and may not be recognized by neighbours and workmates as an alcoholic.

The wife (or occasionally the husband) of an alcoholic suffers enormous distress and is as much in need of help as the alcoholic. If, as often occurs in the second type mentioned above, the drink problem is unrecognized by relatives and neighbours the woman may be at her wit's end to know where to turn for aid. On the one hand she, more than anyone else, may be the person able to persuade her husband that he needs treatment and should seek either medical aid or the help of an organization such as Alcoholics Anonymous (branches of which now exist in about a hundred countries) and during treatment her help and support will be invaluable. On the other hand she may utterly fail to motivate her spouse, the situation may become increasingly intolerable, and for her own and her children's sake she may ultimately have to consider separation. Before taking such an extreme step and abandoning the husband as beyond redemption she should certainly discuss the situation with her doctor or with her health visitor or with an appropriate social worker: the mere airing of the situation will bring her a measure of relief, and an emotionally detached person with professional knowledge may be able to suggest to her a useful reorientation of her tactics to persuade her husband that he needs treatment.

Social patterns such as the spirit drinking of Scotland and Ireland play a part in the creation of alcoholics. So do ready availability – there is a high incidence in bar tenders – and loneliness, as illustrated in the alcoholism among men whose occupations necessitate frequent appreciable absence from their homes.

Principally, however, alcoholism is a reflection of personality defect: the individual is unable to cope with life's problems and resorts to heavier and heavier drinking as an escape mechanism. The main hope for the long-term prevention of alcoholism probably lies in the fostering of good personality development in children – providing an atmosphere of security and demonstrated affection in which the child can develop but encouraging him in large measure to make his own decisions and experiments, with the result that he gradually acquires self-confidence and self-discipline.

Treatment of an alcoholic involves recognition – by the doctor, by other health and social workers, by the employer and especially by the spouse and family – that he is ill, not wicked, and needs help, not moralizing. Cure is impossible unless the patient actually desires to be cured. Where he has such a desire, he has to be 'sobered up' in a hospital or elsewhere and weaned completely from his drinking: an ex-alcoholic cannot as a rule ever become an ordinary social drinker but either must abstain or relapse into alcoholism. Drugs like antabuse, which create unpleasant sensations if alcohol is subsequently consumed, may aid the weaning process but, if treatment is to succeed, the patient will require a great deal of help with his emotional and social problems. Short of providing that help over a long period, treatment of the alcoholism alone is merely seeking to remove his escape mechanism, and as such is likely to be doomed to failure, as alcoholics are notoriously cunning in outwitting their watchers. The patient, as in other personality problems, must be brought to recognize the underlying reason for his condition and encouraged either to overcome it by other means or to accept it.

aldersterone. A hormone, produced by the cortex of the adrenal gland (an ENDOCRINE GLAND) responsible for regulating the excretion of sodium and potassium by the kidneys. Diminished secretion is found in Addison's disease.

alimentary canal. The DIGESTIVE SYSTEM: the musculo-membraneous tube through which food enters the body, in which the food is digested, and from which the remains are excreted as faeces. The canal comprises mouth, pharynx, oesophagus (gullet), stomach, duodenum, small intestine, large intestine, rectum, and anus.

alimentary system. A term used to describe not only the alimentary canal but also the other organs concerned with digestion, e.g., salivary glands, pancreas and liver.

alkalaemia. Increase in the alkali reserve of the blood. It can occur through over-breathing in cases of hysteria or through ingestion of large quantities of alkali, as in cases of peptic ulcer. Symptoms include headache, nausea, vomiting, loss of appetite, and slow, shallow respiration. Immediate treatment is by acid sodium lactate, followed by treatment of the causal condition.

alkali. A substance that neutralizes acids, the general principle being that an acid and an alkali combine to form a salt and water. Strong alkalis, such as caustic soda, can produce severe burns. Milder alkalis, such as sodium bicarbonate, can effectively neutralize acids if given early enough.

The blood and digestive fluids are all slightly

alkaline, with the exception of the acid gastric juice, and in the treatment of indigestion alkalis such as sodium bicarbonate (baking soda) are often used to neutralize the gastric hydrochloric acid.

alkaline poisoning. Strong alkalis such as caustic soda or potash are corrosive poisons, which can cause death but generally cause thirst, repeated vomiting, and symptoms of shock. Emetics should not be used because they bring the poison up to the throat. Treatment involves inducing the patient to swallow a weak solution of vinegar or lemon juice and counteracting shock by warmth.

alkaloids. Naturally occurring substances, derived from plants, containing nitrogen and having certain properties of alkalis. Many of them are highly poisonous in appreciable doses but have medical uses in appropriately small quantities.

The ones in most frequent use are the main pain-killing drugs, morphine, heroin and codein (all obtained from opium poppies). Others of medical significance include digitalin (from foxgloves), atropine (from deadly nightshade), quinine (from cinchona bark) and strychnine (from the seeds of an eastern tree). Gradually, however, as science advances, many of the alkaloids are being replaced in medical practice by newer synthesized drugs which have a similar effect but with a greater margin of safety.

allergen. A substance which can give rise to an allergic reaction.

allergy. The term was first used in 1905 to indicate an exaggerated susceptibility to certain foreign proteins. The individual, having become sensitized to a protein in a particular food or in a particular variety of pollen or in a particular dust, produces antibodies against it; and the combined presence of the protein and the antibodies causes release of histamine from the tissues – resulting, according to the tissues involved, in asthma, hay fever, nettlerash, migraine, or angioneurotic oedema. The symptoms – from the weal of nettlerash to the tightening of bronchioles in asthma – are essentially due to production of histamine.

Recent investigations show that not all the offending substances (allergens) are proteins. Some are simpler substances which combine with proteins in the body to form 'new' foreign proteins.

The causes of allergy are complex. In many cases a hereditary or familial factor is present but not necessarily related to any one allergic disease: e.g., the father suffers from hay fever and the son from asthma. Physical factors, in particular the presence of the allergen, åre clearly important. Emotional factors, such as home tensions disturbing young people, may predispose the individual to an allergy, and in a high proportion of cases emotional factors also play a considerable part in precipitating attacks, sometimes even in the absence of the allergen; a person allergic to cats may develop an attack on seeing a picture of a cat. The typical victim of allergic diseases is described as intelligent, over-anxious, and highly strung. To add to the complexity, hypersensitivity may develop in the course of an infection: for instance, rheumatic fever, while initially due to streptococcal infection, is probably in part an allergic condition.

Where the allergen can be identified two courses of action are possible. First, where practicable the allergen and the patient can be separated: the man sensitive to eggs or feathers can stop eating eggs or exclude feather cushions from his house; and the person allergic to pollen can move from the country to a town. Secondly, the patient can be gradually desensitized by graded doses of the allergen.

Antihistamines are very effective in some allergic diseases (e.g., hay fever) but useless in others (e.g., asthma). Where the allergen cannot be identified and antihistamines are unsuccessful one can only provide symptomatic treatment (e.g., adrenalin or ephedrine for asthma) and attend to the emotional factors. The latter may require anything from simple reassurance and explanation to full-scale psychotherapy.

alopecia. Loss of hair, BALDNESS.

altitude sickness. An unpleasant condition, sometimes serious and very occasionally fatal, occurring as a result of insufficient oxygen in the tissues as a consequence of the low atmospheric pressure of high altitudes.

As a result of the lowered concentration of oxygen in the mountain air, the red blood corpuscles cannot absorb enough oxygen in the lung-capillary exchange. Because of this deficiency, the breathing is quickened (to try to obtain more oxygen) and the amount of carbon dioxide in the blood is reduced. While there is much individual variation, common symptoms include breathlessness, lethargy, irritability, impaired judgement and muscular weakness.

Since modern aeroplanes are pressurized, the condition does not normally occur during flight, but quite often arises in people who have newly arrived at a high altitude, e.g., over 1500 metres (5000 ft.). Persons arriving at a place very considerably higher than that in which they previously resided are wise to refrain from all strenuous activity for the first forty-eight hours to give their bodies time to adjust to the new circumstances – and people with any disease of the heart should not travel to a high altitude without first seeking medical advice.

alveolus. A small cavity. The term is used both for the socket of a tooth and for the many tiny air-pockets in the lungs from which oxygen diffuses into the blood capillaries and carbon dioxide passes from the blood to the respiratory channels for excretion in the breath.

amaurosis fugax. Temporary blurring of vision associated with stooping or exercise. It is a symptom, rather than a disease, and implies that there exists swelling of the head of the optic nerve as a result of raised intracranial pressure. The symptom calls for prompt medical attention because unless the pressure is relieved, there is a likelihood that blindness will follow.

This blurring of vision on stooping is quite unrelated to occasional DIZZINESS on suddenly standing, which is caused by sudden changes in intracranial pressure.

amaurotic family idiocy. A hereditary disease of infancy characterized by progressive diminution in sight (amaurosis), progressive bodily paralysis, and progressive mental impairment. The condition usually leads to death within three years. A similar condition, also hereditary but occurring later in life and less rapid and less often fatal in its course, is known as Tay-Sachs' disease.

ambivalence. Conflicting emotions, usually resulting in an alternation of affection and resentment.

To some extent this is a normal happening. At times most of us are angry and impatient with our closest relatives and best friends, with love temporarily replaced by irritation, and at these times we tend to be harsher towards them than we would be towards mere acquaintances who did exactly the same things to annoy us. This minor ambivalence is very common between children who are the best of friends today, not on speaking terms tomorrow and again close friends next week. Between adults with deep affection for each other it is generally tolerated, the person who is faced with unexpected anger either waiting patiently for the storm to pass or else 'clearing the air' with an open row followed by reconciliation. Where minor ambivalence between adults has serious results, such as the breakdown of a marriage, the consequence is not so much the result of temporary resentment as of human stubbornness, with neither party willing to say, 'The fault was mainly mine.'

Where minor ambivalence can be harmful is in the relationship between adults and their children. If a child is mildly rebuked for his behaviour on Monday, tries the same behaviour experimentally on Thursday and finds it tolerated, and is then severely punished for the identical behaviour on Saturday, simply because the parent is irritated and resentful, his sense of justice becomes confused, he may become suspicious of his parents and his personality development may be harmed. Yet probably not one parent in a hundred can honestly claim that he is always consistent and never lets resentment temporarily replace affection.

More serious ambivalence, such as frequent alternation of affection and concern for the well-being of a friend and jealousy of (and even hatred for) that friend, is not only detrimental to human relations but is also a common cause of neurosis, since it is an expression of unresolved conflict. Here psychiatric treatment often helps, but it may sometimes be necessary for the persons to sever their connections, giving up the companionship and solace of affection in order to be rid of the damaging effects of jealousy and hatred.

amblyopia. Loss of sight, partial or complete, without apparent disease of the eyes. It can occur after a stroke, or after poisoning by alcohol (especially methyl alcohol), lead, arsenic, or occasionally tobacco. It may also occur as a result of a squint when the sight of one eye is suppressed in order to prevent double vision. Depending on the cause, it may be temporary or permanent.

amenorrhoea. Absence of menstrual periods between puberty and the menopause. Primary amenorrhoea, where menstruation has never occurred, may be due to maldevelopment of the uterus or ovaries, or to anaemia, or – more rarely – to inflammation of the vulva or disturbance of the endocrine glands. Secondary amenorrhoea, in which menstruation ceases, is usually due to pregnancy but is sometimes caused by anaemia, shock following severe emotional upset, or premature menopause. Treatment depends on the cause.

amentia. Failure of cerebral development in the womb or in early childhood, arising from disease, injury, or hereditary defect. See MENTAL DEFICIENCY.

amino-acid. A weak organic acid containing nitrogen and forming, with other amino-acids, the essential structure of PROTEINS. Human proteins contain some twenty-two different amino-acids, eight of which cannot be synthesized in the body and must therefore be provided in the diet. These are the essential amino-acids. No single protein contains all the essential amino-acids, although egg albumin with seven comes fairly near; but most good mixed diets contain enough of all eight.

A diet composed largely of maize is short of tryptophane, and lack of tryptophane along with lack of the vitamin nicotinamide causes the disease pellagra. Phenylketonuria is an inherited inability to deal with the amino-acid phenylalanine, and can be successfully treated only by supplying a diet lacking that amino-acid.

ammonia. A colourless, pungent smelling gas, generally used in watery solution for household purposes. If drunk accidentally it is a corrosive poison, best treated by giving a dilute solution of vinegar, lemon juice or orange juice, and by keeping the patient warm.

amnesia. Complete loss of memory in respect of a period of time. It may be current, i.e., an inability to retain new impressions, or retrograde, as in loss of memory for events leading up to a head injury. 'Middle-aged amnesia' is the term used colloquially for the gradual deterioration of memory that occurs as one ages. There is, as yet, no known treatment, although some drugs are under trial.

amniocentesis. See PRENATAL DIAGNOSIS.

amnion. The membraneous bag which forms within the uterus to enclose the developing unborn child. The bag is filled with a clear fluid which protects the foetus and maintains it at an even temperature. See CHILDBIRTH.

amphetamines. A series of drugs which, in contrast to the barbiturates, stimulate the central nervous system, temporarily reduce fatigue, lessen appetite, and produce a sensation of well-being. Various amphetamines have been employed to create additional energy (e.g., in battle situations), as aids to slimming, and as treatment for depression and epilepsy. For all these purposes they have now been virtually abandoned as they are mildly but definitely habit-forming and, because of this risk of addiction, they are obtainable on prescription only. Almost the only remaining medical uses of amphetamines are for the treatment of barbiturate poisoning and in some mental diseases. Illegally, however, they still circulate and are known by such names as 'purple hearts', 'black bombers' and 'speed'.

Excess of amphetamine leads to excitement, tremor, euphoria, and dilated pupils, passing with larger doses to anxiety, hallucinations, and uncontrolled movements. In most cases the only immediate treatment required is rest and sometimes a mild sedative, but if the addiction is well established its cure may be difficult.

ampicillin. A synthetic derivative of penicillin which, unlike penicillin itself, is not inactivated by gastric juice and is therefore effective by mouth. It is effective against a wide range of organisms and is particularly useful in urinary infections and in typhoid and paratyphoid.

amputation. The surgical removal of a part of the body, such as a limb. Amputation becomes

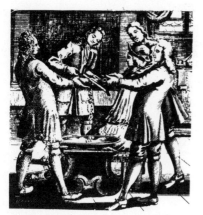

An eighteenth century amputation

necessary when there is irremediable damage from a road, industrial or other accident, or from such conditions as gangrene, frost-bite, cancer or advanced arteriosclerosis.

Before deciding whether to amputate, the surgeon has to consider the chance of recovery without the operation, the danger to life or to other parts of the body in the absence of operation, the patient's occupation and leisure interests, the availability of an artificial replacement and the ability of the patient to withstand a serious operation. It is also important that before amputation the patient is fully informed about the necessity for the operation, the availability of an artificial replacement and the extent to which the replacement will fulfil the functions of the amputated part.

amyl nitrite. A yellowish liquid, which will evaporate very rapidly, normally supplied in small capsules and inhaled after crushing in a handkerchief. By dilating the coronary arteries amyl nitrite relieves the pain of angina pectoris within seconds. Because it raises the tension in the eyes it should be avoided for patients with glaucoma. With that exception it is useful for all sufferers from angina, but it causes headache in some individuals.

anaemia. Bloodlessness, and in particular shortage in the blood of haemoglobin, the oxygen-carrying pigment contained in the red blood corpuscles. The mass of disease known collectively as anaemia is most easily classified by cause.

1. Excessive loss of blood corpuscles. This occurs in severe haemorrhage, excessive menstruation and 'hidden' bleeding (e.g., into the stomach following consumption of too much aspirin). Here the blood cells and haemoglobin are at first reduced equally, but, as the bone marrow vigorously produces replacement red blood corpuscles, these recover first – so that blood examination reveals an adequate number of corpuscles but with abnormally little pigment.

2. Excessive destruction of red blood corpuscles. In sickle-cell anaemia, an hereditary abnormality of the haemoglobin with an increased fragility of the cells (found in about 1 per cent of all inhabitants of the U.S.A.

and in fully 8 per cent of American negroes) the red blood corpuscles are shaped rather like sickles. Normally red blood corpuscles are destroyed and replaced about every four months, but in cases of excessive destruction they have a life of only one month and the bone marrow cannot manufacture new corpuscles speedily enough to keep pace with the destruction. Children suffering from the disease have signs and symptoms of anaemia, usually enlarged spleens, and bouts of fever and of pain in muscles and joints. The disease is progressive and usually leads to death before the age of 30 years. There is as yet no satisfactory treatment.

3. Iron deficiency. There is in this case insufficient iron in the diet for proper production of cells, so that the red blood corpuscles are small and the amount of haemoglobin in them is low. This anaemia of poverty and poor diet is by far the commonest anaemia in western countries. For instance, it affects fully 20 per cent of British women aged 20 to 50 years (i.e., roughly of menstruating age) and is also not uncommon in men and in children. It is, of course, preventable by proper diet.

4. Lack of vitamin B_{12} in the diet or of folic acid. This variety, known as pernicious anaemia, was deemed inevitably fatal until 1926, when it was found to be treatable with large doses of raw liver, and has been relatively easy to treat since the isolation of vitamin B_{12} in 1948.

5. Suppression of red blood cell formation by the bone marrow. This aplastic anaemia is rare but inevitably fatal unless the marrow recovers its ability to manufacture corpuscles; however, in order to afford a chance of such recovery the patient can be temporarily kept alive with blood transfusions.

6. Other types. These are such conditions as the anaemia that follows prolonged low-grade poisoning by lead, arsenic, or mercury, or the anaemia associated with various chronic diseases.

In general, irrespective of type, anaemia is characterized by signs and symptoms of oxygen lack. There is pallor of the skin, especially noticeable on the lips and eyelids, where the skin is thin; the patient feels tired and listless; the pulse is full and soft; both pulse rate and respiration rate increase unduly on very slight exertion, and ankles tend to swell. Some minor signs help to differentiate the types, e.g., the varieties caused by excessive destruction of blood corpuscles often show a yellowish, jaundiced appearance; for accurate differentiation, blood counts and haemoglobin estimations are essential.

Treatment varies according to the type. In the commonest of all varieties – the iron deficiency anaemia of poverty or poor diet – it is necessary to treat the patient for months with a digestible iron salt (such as ferrous sulphate tablets, 200 mg. thrice daily after meals) and simultaneously – and afterwards – to ensure that he eats a good, mixed diet, including a sufficiency of meat and green vegetables.

anaesthesia. Generalized or localized insensibility to pain, induced by drugs. The anaesthetic properties of nepenthe were mentioned by Homer, early physicians in several countries rendered patients insensible through inhalation of the vapours of a type of hemp, and mandrake preparations were much used in medieval times. Yet to all intents general anaesthesia, and the more delicate surgery that it rendered possible, started only about 130 years ago.

As early as 1800 Sir Humphrey Davy, experimenting on nitrous oxide, discovered its pain-killing properties and suggested that it might be used in surgery; but the advance of medical science requires not only discoveries in the laboratory but courageous use of such discoveries, and more than forty years elapsed before any such use was made. In 1846 W. T. Morton publicly demonstrated the use of ether anaesthesia before physicians and surgeons in Massachusetts and at about the same time in Connecticut H. Wells began to employ nitrous oxide. Sir James Y. Simpson, having previously used ether anaesthesia in midwifery practice, announced his discovery in Edinburgh in 1847 of the anaesthetic properties of chloroform which had first been manufactured by Liebig in 1831. Some churchmen and others opposed the employment of anaesthetics in childbirth but their use may be regarded as having become established when Queen Victoria accepted chloroform for the birth of Prince Leopold in 1853.

The main early anaesthetics were: nitrous oxide (laughing gas), a very light anaesthetic still sometimes used in dentistry and midwifery but unsuitable for lengthy surgical operations; ether (technically di-ethyl ether), a colourless volatile liquid the vapour of which was administered by inhalation, the liquid being dropped on gauze held over the nose and mouth; and chloroform, a colourless volatile liquid the fumes of which when inhaled produced deep unconsciousness and muscular relaxation. All had disadvantages, for example chloroform had a fairly narrow margin of safety and was liable to produce nausea and vomiting after consciousness was regained.

In recent decades anaesthesia has made vast progress and most modern general anaesthetics are given not by inhalation but by injection. The patient usually loses consciousness even before the syringe has been withdrawn from his arm, has no nausea or vomiting after the operation and is not unknown to enquire on wakening, 'When are you going to start the operation?' Sodium pentothal, cyclopropane and trichloroethylene are examples of modern general anaesthetics.

Local anaesthesia has also made enormous advances. It consists essentially of injecting – and temporarily deadening – the nerve which transmits sensation from the operation area to the brain, or temporarily abolishing sensation in the lower limbs by injection into the spine, or for very brief anaesthesia 'freezing' the surface of the skin. It is possible, for instance, to perform under local anaesthesia a cataract operation with the patient not only fully conscious but actually · unaware of the operation taking place. Of many local anaesthetics administered by injection probably the best known is procaine hydrochloride (novocaine), and the spray most commonly used to 'freeze' the skin is ethyl chloride.

One consequence of the progress of anaesthesia from the simple dropping of chloroform or ether on to a mask has been the .

rise in status of anaesthetists from assistants to the surgeons to their equals as members of a full medical speciality.

anal canal. The narrow muscular passage leading from the rectum to the exterior at the contracted orifice called the anus. It is about 3.5 cm. (1.5 in.) long, is lined with mucous membrane, and has a rich blood supply. Where a vein in the area becomes varicose it is termed a haemorrhoid or PILE.

anal fissure. An ulcer or abrasion at the lower end of the anal canal, causing sharp pain during and after defecation. In mild cases regulation of the bowels by laxatives and application of vaseline may effect a cure. In more severe cases a small surgical operation is required.

analgesia. Reducing or relieving pain by drugs. In the past, when complete suppression of pain was virtually impossible, the term was often used as synonymous with both general ANAESTHESIA (rendering the patient stuporous or unconscious) and local anaesthesia ('freezing' skin or temporarily paralysing appropriate nerves). Nowadays it is usually restricted to the use of pain-deadening drugs which neither cause sleep and stupor (as the narcotics do) nor the complete unconsciousness of general anaesthesia. The border between analgesics and narcotics is vague, however, because large doses of some analgesics create sleepiness and narcotics may relieve pain without actually causing sleep.

There is a vast number of pain-reducing drugs ranging from aspirin to heroin and some, such as opium, have been known and used for centuries. The analgesics in common use are derivatives of salicilic acid (e.g., aspirin), phenazone (e.g., amidopyrine), and phenacetin (e.g., paracetamol). These drugs provide temporary relief from pain and are extremely useful, but they do not themselves cure diseases.

In a terminal illness there seems no reason why the patient should be allowed to suffer, but in illnesses from which recovery is expected the stronger pain-killers have to be used with discretion. To let a patient endure prolonged agony is not only inhumane but very damaging to the sufferer, but to use strong drugs too frequently may produce addiction, and an overdose can cause death. For these reasons household supplies of such drugs should always be kept in a safe cupboard out of reach of children.

anal pruritis. Itching of the anus. In many cases the itching starts from a transitory cause and continues because of the patient's scratching. Other causes include threadworms, piles, and fistula, or fissure, dermatitis and more rarely disturbance of the intestinal bacteria following the use of an antibiotic. Cleanliness and careful but gentle drying sometimes effect a cure; and application of steroids is often helpful.

anal spasm. Painful contraction of the muscle controlling the orifice of the anal canal may arise from anal fissure, or fistula, or pruritus. Apart from attention to the cause, treatment usually involves keeping the motions soft by laxatives.

anal fistula. An unnatural channel from the anal canal to the exterior. It is generally caused by an abscess which, through pressure of pus, makes its way to the surface and is thereafter prevented from healing by constant reinfection

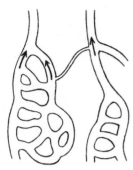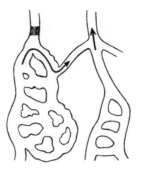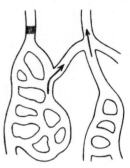

Anastomosis

of the raw surfaces by the passage of faeces. Treatment is surgical.

anaphylaxis. Abnormal sensitivity to a particular protein, an extreme form of allergy. This rare condition occurs mainly in relation to SERUM treatment. A person with this abnormal sensitivity who is given antitoxic serum may react very sharply to the protein contained in it, with bronchi going into complete spasm, and may even die unless given an immediate injection of adrenalin.

anastomosis. Linking of the branches of one blood vessel to another. In anatomy the term is employed for natural connection which, if one vessel is obstructed, enable another vessel to supply blood to the part. In surgery the term is usually applied to an artificially created connection between two tubular structures: for instance, in disease of the liver excessive blood in that organ may be reduced by connecting the portal vein (the vein of the liver) to the vena cava (the main vein of the body).

anatomy. The science concerned with the structure, form, arrangements and relationships of all parts of the body. Accurate anatomical information is clearly essential for the surgeon, but knowledge of anatomy and of physiology (the science of how the parts of the body work) is also vital to the physician.

Until the sixteenth century doctors usually relied not on what they saw but on what had been dogmatically stated by Galen in the second century or by Avicenna's eleventh century translation of Galen. Galen not only based his description of human anatomy simply on the dissection of animals but at times ·distorted the facts to fit his theories. For a science based solely on observation, anatomy developed very slowly; it had its true beginnings in the sixteenth century with actual dissection of human bodies and drawings and descriptions (by Leonardo da Vinci among others). Anatomy became a real science when Vesalius in 1543 published his *De Humani Corporis Fabrica,* which incidentally corrected some 200 of Galen's errors. But for half a century thereafter authoritarian statements, backed by ecclesiastical and secular power, continued to hold sway.

Histology, or microscopic anatomy, the study of the cellular structure of tissues and organs, developed largely in the eighteenth century, and comparative anatomy, the study

of the structure of various animals, is essentially a product of the nineteenth century.

Perhaps the main error of medical education in the first two-thirds of this century was an over-emphasis on anatomy. Only in very recent years has it been appreciated that knowledge of psychology and sociology is no less essential for medical and nursing students than is knowledge of anatomy.

See individual entries for anatomical description of the various structures in the body.

androgen. A male sex hormone. Androgens include testerone, produced in the testicles, and several hormones produced by the cortex of each of the adrenals, two ENDOCRINE GLANDS. Androgens are also produced in small amounts in the ovaries of women.

Insufficient secretion of androgens in a boy prevents the development of such male characteristics as deepening of the voice, facial hair and enlargement of the sex organs. The condition can sometimes be helped by injection of androgens. Excessive secretion in boys, as occurs in certain tumours of the adrenals or the testes, causes precocious puberty.

Excessive secretion in females results in virilization, i.e., increased muscular development, growth of facial hair and enlargement of the clitoris, part of the female genital tract. Treatment varies with the cause.

anencephaly. Failure of the brain to develop while the unborn child is still in the uterus. The condition, while rare, is usually fatal.

aneurine. A name for vitamin B_1. See THIAMIN and VITAMINS.

aneurysm. A bulge in the wall of an artery. Aneurysms are often classified according to shape: fusiform, tapering towards the ends; saccular, forming a pouch; and dissecting, where the cavity develops between the coats of an artery. All types result from the combination of a weakening of the arterial wall and a rise of the blood pressure to a greater extent than the wall can resist.

Congenital aneurysms usually affect the arteries at the base of the brain. Traumatic aneurysms can result from any penetrating wound, such as a shotgun injury, and most often occur in the limbs. Syphilitic aneurysm, mostly of the aorta, was formerly quite common but has become extremely rare. So-called degenerative aneurysms develop mostly

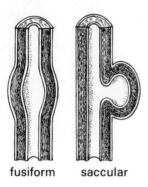

fusiform   saccular

Two kinds of aneurysm

in early middle age in men who follow strenuous occupations such as dock labourers.

Where the bulge is in an accessible position the diagnosis is obvious: there is, in the line of an artery, a swelling which pulsates with each beat of the heart. Less accessible aneurysms can be shown by injecting a radio-opaque substance into the blood vessels in order to make them visible on x-ray in the process known as angiography.

Symptoms are generally due to pressure, e.g., an aortic aneurysm may press on the gullet, wind-pipe and laryngeal nerve, causing difficulty in swallowing, breathlessness and a barking cough. In untreated cases there is about a 50 per cent chance of rupture, when profuse haemorrhage may cause death.

Surgical treatment is sometimes practicable – tying off the aneurysm, or even tying the artery above and below it and then connecting the two parts of the artery by a tube. Sometimes, too, an attempt may be made to produce a clot which gradually increases until it fills the sac and prevents further growth. It has to be remembered, however, that an aneurysm in one artery often indicates that the arteries in general are in poor condition.

angina pectoris. Severe paroxysms of pain over the breast-bone, sometimes spreading down the left arm or occasionally both arms. The pain comes on during or immediately after exercise, bringing all activity to a sudden stop and tending to produce expectation of death. It usually passes off after a few minutes.

As a rule, angina is a condition of men rather than women, of middle age rather than of youth and of 'white-collar' workers rather than labourers. The agony, the consequent ashen-grey face and restrained breathing and the rapid relief after rest make the condition easily recognizable, although·obviously other causes of chest pain should be considered when a diagnosis is being made.

Angina is a symptom, not a disease. It implies that the heart muscle is receiving insufficient oxygen (usually because of arteriosclerosis of the coronary arteries) and that the nerve-endings are being stimulated by the incomplete products of combustion of foods.

Treatment of individual attacks is by rest as soon as the first suggestion of pain appears, and by administration of drugs that rapidly dilate the coronary arteries. A 0.5 mg. tablet of glyceryl trinitrate chewed or sucked under the tongue will stop an attack within two minutes: and amyl nitrite capsules, broken into a handkerchief and inhaled, can be even quicker although in some people they produce other symptoms. A person subject to angina should always carry appropriate tablets or .capsules, as prescribed by the doctor.

General management has to be adapted to the frequency and severity of the attacks, the patient's occupation and socio-economic status and even his temperament. Broadly, he should be encouraged to find a compromise and to limit his physical and mental activities to what he can do without producing an attack, but not to limit them more than is necessary. He should seek to avoid hurry, excitement and emotional tension and should, so far as is practicable, cultivate a philosophical attitude to life. Frequent small meals are usually better than occasional large ones, and while alcohol in moderation is not harmful, tobacco is inadvisable. Sedatives at night may be useful.

Prevention of angina is essentially prevention (ten or twenty years earlier) of the underlying coronary disease. Possible measures include taking of reasonable and moderate exercise; avoidance of obesity; limitation of sugar intake; and limitation or avoidance of tobacco. Avoidance wherever possible of abnormal emotional, mental and physical stress also contributes greatly to the prevention of angina.

angiography. A method of showing defects such as aneurysms by x-rays. An iodine compound is injected into the suspected vessel before it is x-rayed and renders the vessel temporarily opaque to the rays, so that it shows up clearly.

angioma. An overgrowth of capillary blood-vessels, commonly known as a naevus or BIRTH-MARK.

angioneurotic oedema. A condition, probably hereditary, in which swellings appear on the skin and mucous membranes. The swellings – raised patches, usually hot and red but occasionally cold – occur chiefly on the face and hands and appear suddenly, most commonly after emotional disturbances. The swellings appear to be the result of dilation of capillaries and release from them of histamine or a histamine-like substance. The condition is related to allergy.

Where the underlying cause is physical a search for the allergen can be useful, with the idea of removing it from the individual or the individual from it. In psychosomatic cases sedatives (e.g., barbiturates or bromides) may be helpful. Irrespective of the cause, antihistamine drugs (e.g., anthisan) are valuable in attacks; an injection of the hormone adrenalin can also produce a dramatic improvement as it constricts the capillaries which have become dilated.

ankle. The joint formed by the lower ends of the tibia and fibula and the upper surface of the astragalus. The joint is of the hinge variety, permitting only two movements – flexion (bringing the foot nearer to the front of the leg) and extension or plantar flexion (straightening the ankle with the toes pointed downwards). The capsule of the joint is strengthened by several important ligaments.

The common injuries of the ankle are sprain and fracture.

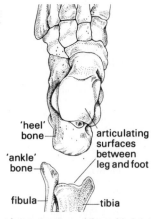

'heel' bone

'ankle' bone

articulating surfaces between leg and foot

fibula — tibia

The bone structure of the ankle joint

Abrupt twisting of the ankle (as in a fall) tears the tendons and ligaments, causing a sprain, characterized by swelling and tenderness. A sprain is best treated by cold compresses followed by strapping for several days. Elastoplast perhaps gives more support to the injured ankle than does a crepe bandage.

Less common is the fracture-dislocation of the ankle known as Pott's fracture, in which the foot is twisted outwards, the fibula on the outer side of the leg is broken, and the tibia on the inner side may or may not be broken. The injury may occur from direct violence, as when a wheel passes over the leg, but is more often the result of indirect violence, e.g., stepping off a pavement without noticing. Symptoms include pain, partial loss of power in the leg, tenderness and swelling.

Differentiation between a fracture and a sprain is not easy, but in a sprain the foot is usually twisted inwards; any apparent sprain with pain and tenderness persisting for twenty-four hours should be x-rayed.

Splinting and bandaging of the leg are essential in cases of fracture, and in most cases the leg will need to be placed in plaster for some weeks, during which the patient will have to use crutches for walking.

It is said of Percival Pott (1714-88), surgeon at St. Bartholomew's Hospital, London, who studied ankle fracture after having personal experience of it, that he sustained the fracture when crossing London Bridge, purchased the nearest available front door, had himself placed on it, and asked to be carried to Guy's Hospital, saying that the only good surgeon at St. Bartholomew's had just broken his leg.

ankylosis. Loss of movement of a joint through the joint surfaces becoming united by fibrous tissue, cartilage or bone. Fibrous ankylosis, occurring for example after prolonged immobilization of a joint in treatment of a fracture, can be treated by massage and movement. If these measures fail the fibrous adhesions can be broken down under general anaesthesia. Cartilaginous ankylosis, e.g., from fusion of two neighbouring cartilages in arthritis, and bony ankylosis, occurring where disease or

operation has denuded a joint of cartilage, both produce complete immobility of the joint. They must either be left and the immobility accepted, or treated by surgical operation. Since a functionless joint is often preferable to a painful joint, ankylosis is sometimes deliberately produced by surgery to relieve persistent pain.

ankylostomiasis. see HOOKWORM DISEASE.

anodyne. An old name for any drug that relieves pain. See ANALGESIA.

anopheles. The generic name for a type of mosquito. One variety of the genus, *Anopheles maculipennis,* can transmit the parasite of MALARIA.

anorexia. The technical term for loss of APPETITE. It occurs temporarily in several acute fevers and toxaemic conditions, may be a result of certain anxiety states, or may also be the first sign of cancer of the stomach.

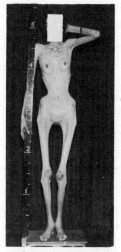

Anorexia nervosa

Anorexia nervosa. A dangerous condition of psychological origin, this chiefly occurs in women aged 15 to 25 years. It is a form of neurosis, characterized by extreme indifference to eating, restless energy, and increasing loss of weight. The condition is essentially a psychological refusal to accept adult life, with rejection of food serving as a symbolic rejection of adult sexuality. Treatment usually involves separating the woman from her relatives and providing skilled psychotherapy and appropriate drugs. Most cases recover after some months, but a considerable minority continue to have eating difficulties and about 10 per cent die, usually from infections due to lowered resistance.

anosmia. Loss of the sense of SMELL. Temporary forms are usually due to disease of the mucous membrane of the nose, e.g., partial anosmia occurs during a severe cold in the head. Anosmia of longer duration is generally a result of damage to the olfactory nerve (which carries sensations of smell from the nose to the brain) by, for instance, head injury or brain tumour. Our appreciation of different tastes is very dependent on the sense of smell so that the loss of that sensation also reduces our enjoyment of food. Heavy smoking is said to dull the sense of smell but not to the extent of causing anosmia.

anoxia. Insufficiency of oxygen in the blood. See ASPHYXIA.

antabuse. Antabuse or disulfiram is a drug used in the treatment of alcoholism. When it is present in the system consumption of alcohol produces nausea or actual vomiting. In extreme cases its use can be dangerous to life and it is, therefore, applied less often than in the past.

antacid. Any drug that neutralizes the acid of the gastric juice. See INDIGESTION.

antenatal care. See PREGNANCY, health in.

anthelmintics. Drugs employed to kill intestinal worms. The essential requirements for an anthelmintic are that it is poisonous to the particular type of worm, that (in the dosage used) it is not poisonous to man, and that it is only slowly absorbed from the intestine, because otherwise it will not have time to act on the parasite. Examples are male fern for tapeworm, oil of chenopodium for hookworm and santonin for roundworms.

anthracosis. A disease of the lungs and bronchi, caused by inhalation of coal dust and fairly common in miners. Repeated inhalation of coal dust causes excess fibrous tissue in the lungs, persistent bronchitis and ultimately emphysema. Treatment is very difficult and unsatisfactory. Prevention depends on suppression of dust, e.g., by water-drilling in mines and by hydro-blasting instead of shot-blasting.

anthrax. An infectious disease of farm animals sometimes called wool-sorter's disease, caused by a germ – the bacillus *anthracosis*. It is very occasionally transmitted to man from the hair, wool, hide or flesh of infected animals and from manufactured products produced from infected raw material. In man the incubation period varies from one to seven days and this rare disease appears in one of two main forms: (1) the malignant pustule – a severe, localized and often painless inflammation generally at the site of a cut or abrasion through which the germ entered; this is the commoner form and is dangerous unless treated. (2) A fulminating pneumonia, when the germs have been inhaled or swallowed, which is generally fatal unless treated.

For treatment Schlavo's antiserum, in use for many years, is now superseded by a combination of penicillin and streptomycin. The patient, being highly infectious, is nursed in isolation, with the attendants wearing gloves and masks.

Preventive measures include identification, slaughter and either incineration or burial in lime of infected animals; immunization of animals deemed exposed to infection; thorough disinfection of effluents and trade wastes from premises in which contaminated hides or hair have lain; disinfection of hair and bristles from sources suspected of contamination; rapid identification and treatment of the disease in man; and isolation of the infected person until he has recovered.

The bacillus was the first bacterium to be identified (1849). Under adverse conditions it forms a spore which can be killed only by burning or by special measures such as steam under pressure as it is remarkably resistant to heat and disinfectants. Of all living organisms the anthrax spore is probably the one that clings most tenaciously to life.

anthrycide. A relatively new drug which cures several diseases caused by trypanosomes affecting cattle and horses and, sometimes, man. In addition to the curative effect, a single injection of the drug appears to confer an immunity lasting for several months.

Apart from its life-saving importance to humans for preventing or curing sleeping sickness, the drug seems likely to improve substantially the prospects of meat production in some of the African countries – a point which is important in that world population is making increasing demands on the world supply of meat.

antibiotics. Drugs produced from living organisms which prevent the growth and reproduction of other organisms. Thus the mould *Penicillium* prevents the growth of many bacteria, and penicillin is the drug manufactured from the mould. The inhibiting effect of the mould was noted by Alexander Fleming in 1928, and in 1941 H. W. Florey and E. B. Chain produced penicillin and used it on patients. Several different penicillins have since been prepared, some taken by mouth and others only by injection.

Other antibiotics include streptomycin (effective against the tubercle bacillus and in particular altering tuberculous meningitis from an invariably fatal to a curable disease), chloramphenicol (useful in typhoid) and terramycin (effective against the rickettsia of typhus).

While antibiotics are unquestionably life-saving drugs and while they have had an effect on mortality second only to vaccines and vitamins, three points should be noted. Firstly, many of them can have serious side-effects, e.g., streptomycin can cause permanent deafness and chloramphenicol can cause fatal aplastic ANAEMIA. So antibiotics should not be needlessly used for minor infections that will yield to other treatment. Secondly, inadequate use of an antibiotic may create a resistant germ that has, in effect, developed an immunity. For instance, penicillin was at first completely effective against staphylococci (the commonest cause of septicaemia) and gonococci (the cause of the commonest of the venereal diseases), but sheer under-treatment of patients has produced many strains of staphylococci and gonococci resistant to penicillin. Thirdly, while appropriate antibiotics can cope with most bacteria, spirochaetes and rickettsia, most of them appear to have no effect on viruses.

Strict control of their use is therefore of great importance and for that reason they are obtainable only on a doctor's prescription.

antibody. A protein formed in the body to counteract an invading foreign protein which has acted as an antigen. The antigen may be a bacterium, an allergen or an organ transplanted from another person.

For example, in diphtheria the toxin produced by the invading germs acts as the antigen, and the untreated person will die unless antibodies and antitoxin are produced in time to destroy the germs and toxin. In the serum treatment of diphtheria the defence mechanisms of the body are assisted by the injection of serum very rich in antitoxin: blood is drawn from the vein of a horse that has previously been immunized against diphtheria, and the serum is separated and concentrated. In immunization against diphtheria the body is 'tricked' into forming appropriate antibodies and antitoxin by injection of inactivated toxin. Thereafter the body, having learned the art of producing these, retains its capacity to produce them, so that if actual diphtheria germs later invade and start to produce toxin they are very promptly counteracted.

anticoagulant drugs. Drugs which reduce the natural tendency of the blood to clot, e.g., when the circulation, is slow or the blood vessels narrowed. In coronary thrombosis, for instance, these drugs are often used to prevent further clotting in the blood vessels supplying the heart and the lungs. Heparin is perhaps the quickest acting of the anticoagulant drugs but has to be given by injection and is very costly, so that where practicable a slower acting substitute taken by mouth replaces heparin after the first few four-hourly injections.

Anticoagulant drugs are not advisable if the patient suffers from diseases of the liver or kidneys.

antidote. A substance which neutralizes or counteracts the effect of a poison. Apart, however, from acids and alkalis, few poisons have specific antidotes.

antigen. A substance, usually a protein foreign to the body, which stimulates the production of ANTIBODIES. Thus a bacterium in addition to creating illness will stimulate the growth of antibodies and if these are produced quickly enough they may kill the invaders and end the disease, even without any treatment. Similarly the injection of killed bacteria, which are harmless but contain the same protein, causes production of antibodies which can destroy invading bacteria of the same type: this is essentially the mechanism used in immunization.

In allergic diseases pollens, fungi and dust particles may act as antigens and the antibodies produced cause physical reactions.

antihistamine. A substance acting against HISTAMINE, which is found in nettles and insect stings, and released when tissues are damaged, e.g., by burns. The released histamine causes narrowing of the bronchioles (and hence asthma), widening of small blood vessels with leakage into the tissues (and hence urticaria and inflammation) and various allergic manifestations. Antihistamine drugs combating these effects are very useful in nettlerash and hay fever, and also sometimes relieve travel sickness. They are less effective in asthma.

Antihistamines often cause drowsiness and therefore should not be taken shortly before driving a car. In excess they may produce excitement, tremors and convulsions, with some danger of choking, and very rarely they cause agranulocytosis.

antimony. A poisonous semi-metal resembling arsenic. Salts of antimony, especially tartar emetic, are used in the treatment of several tropical diseases, including kala-azar, oriental sore, sleeping sickness (trypanosomiasis) and fluke worm infection. Antimony and its salts cause vomiting, diarrhoea and collapse if the medicinal dose is exceeded. In suspected antimony poisoning the patient should be kept warm and given milk if he can drink. Medical aid should be summoned speedily.

antipyretic. The term applied to drugs which lower the temperature of the body in fevers. Aspirin, phenacetin and phenazone are examples. While these drugs have other functions, they are now seldom used simply as antipyretics. In general, moderate fever in an infection is a protective response by the body, and high fever responds better to cold or tepid sponging than to antipyretic drugs.

antiscorbutic. Foods or chemical preparations containing vitamin C (ascorbic acid), the essential factor to prevent or cure SCURVY (also known as scorbutus). Among the richest natural antiscorbutics are lemons, oranges and blackcurrants. See VITAMINS.

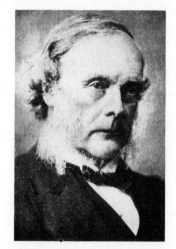

Joseph Lister, founder of antiseptic surgery

antisepsis. Procedures designed to destroy bacteria or to prevent their growth. The term was used by Sir John Pringle in 1750, but the real pioneer of antisepsis was Joseph Lister who in the 1860s introduced the cleaning of surgical instruments with disinfectants, the spraying of operating theatres and wards, and the covering of wounds with carbolic dressings. These measures enormously reduced mortality from 'hospital gangrene', from puerperal fever (childbirth fever) and from wounds on the battlefield. Surgery had become painless following the introduction of anaesthetics about 1846; following the introduction of antisepsis it became relatively safe.

Yet under controlled conditions, such as those of an operating theatre, antisepsis was only a second best. In particular application to the tissues of too strong an antiseptic could damage them, while too weak an antiseptic might fail to kill some of the bacteria. Hence asepsis, i.e., complete avoidance of all possible exposure to germs, gradually replaced antisepsis in surgery.

In uncontrolled conditions, as in the home, antisepsis still has a very important role. The ordinary procedure for treating an open wound is to remove dirt by gently washing with soap and water, and then to apply a mild antiseptic such as tincture of iodine or hydrogen peroxide. Babies' feeding bottles and other domestic implements are sterilized by well-recognized commercial antiseptics or, where appropriate, by boiling, and disinfectants are in common use in sick-rooms and lavatories, while minimal doses of specified antiseptics are used to preserve various foods.

Chemical antiseptics are essential for many purposes, but although heat is seldom effective unless the infected material can be boiled, the value of sunshine as an antiseptic should never be forgotten. Articles which would be damaged by boiling or by the use of strong chemical disinfectants can often be adequately sterilized by exposure to sunlight for a few hours.

antispasmodic drugs. Drugs which relieve spasm of a muscular organ. For instance, adrenalin and ephedrine relieve the spasm of the small bronchioles in asthma, and derivatives of opium reduce spasm of the intestine, kidney and ureter.

antitoxin. A substance formed in the blood, as a result of germ infection, for the purpose of neutralizing the toxin produced by the particular germ. An antitoxin is produced in the event of disease but may not be formed quickly enough to affect the outcome.

If a person or animal is given small, graduated doses of a known toxin, antitoxin is produced without the development of the disease. Not only is the person or animal rendered immune to the disease, but the blood serum of the immune individual can be used to provide a starting dose of antitoxin for somebody infected by the particular germ. This is the basis of the serum treatment of diphtheria, botulism and tetanus. A horse is usually selected, simply because it is a large animal which can supply a goodly quantity of blood; the horse is immunized with graded doses of toxin; when immunity has developed, blood is withdrawn, essentially as in the case of a person giving blood for a transfusion; the serum is separated off and concentrated; and the antitoxin is then ready for injection into a person suffering from the disease. Serum treatment has saved innumerable lives, although for many infections it has been replaced by treatment with appropriate antibiotics.

Part of the basis of active immunization against bacterial infections is injection into a healthy person of killed germs or inactivated toxin. The body is 'deceived' into manufacturing the appropriate antibody or antitoxin, so that the person becomes protected against the particular disease.

antrum. A cavity or air-cell in a bone. The term is especially used for the mastoid antrum, an air-cell in the bony process behind the ear. The cavity is connected with the middle ear by a small passage. Hence inflammation of the middle ear can develop into mastoid disease.

anus. The orifice at the lower end of the digestive system through which semi-solid waste matter (faeces) is discharged.

anxiety states. Intense and persisting fear or worry in the absence of obvious reason for anxiety. We all have momentary irrational fears and most of us at times fears of longer duration but demonstrable cause; but the worry in an anxiety state not only lacks obvious cause (or persists with slight change of direction if the apparent cause is removed) but also dominates the person's whole existence. The sufferer has great difficulty in facing the ordinary stresses of life, lacks powers of concentration and effort, may be emotionally uncontrolled and may suffer from palpitations, breathlessness, loss of appetite, heart pains, sleeplessness and in some cases irregular beating of the heart. In other words, the anxiety state – which may apparently be related to work, to sexual relations, to physical health or simply to a deep, undefined dread – affects not only the mind but also the cardiovascular, digestive and nervous systems.

Anxiety states quite often occur in association with heart disease, asthma and peptic ulcer, and in women are sometimes associated with the menopause, but are also common in persons with no recognizable organic disease. The origin often lies, decades back, in insecurity or lack of affection in childhood. In other cases anxiety states arise from STRESS caused by overwhelming current financial problems or problems of personal relationships.

Simple reassurance is seldom effective. Tranquillizers and sedatives may be of some use in mild cases, and practical advice and help can be greatly beneficial in anxiety due to current problems. Where the main causes lie in childhood, however, it is necessary for a psychotherapist to unearth the basic fear or root conflict (which may well be hidden in the unconscious and quite unrealized by the patient) and to bring this to consciousness so that it can be discussed rationally. With adequate psychotherapy fairly rapid recovery is likely.

Anxiety states are not uncommon in children, where they may be accompanied by bed-wetting, nightmares, vomiting and diarrhoea. Investigation and treatment at a child guidance clinic are required.

Despite the enormously successful work of Freud and his successors, anxiety states are among the most under-treated of serious diseases. Too often the physician, having found no underlying organic disease, merely exhorts the patient to 'Pull yourself together', whereas in reality the patient is incapable of doing so until the root cause has been unearthed.

aorta. The main artery of the body, conducting oxygen-rich blood from the left side of the heart to all parts of the body. The aorta leaves the left ventricle where its opening is guarded by a semilunar valve; it then gives off two small branches, the coronary arteries, which supply blood to the heart muscle; after arching over the base of the heart, it gives off three branches from the arch, namely the innominate (which divides into the right common carotid and the right subclavian), the left common carotid and the left subclavian; it then runs downwards through the thorax and abdomen, giving off various branches to supply the viscera; and finally in front of the fourth lumbar vertebra, it divides into the right and left common iliac arteries (each of which divides into an internal and an external branch).

Diseases of the aorta include arteriosclerosis (by far the commonest), aneurysm, and a congenital narrowing termed coarctation. Diseases of the semilunar valve are (1) aortic incompetence: deformity of the valve cusp with enlargement of the opening; and (2) aortic stenosis: narrowing of the valve cusp.

aperient. See LAXATIVE.

aphasia. Loss or impairment of the ability to speak. The commonest causes are cerebral haemorrhage, embolism, thrombosis and tumours, all of which can interfere with the areas in the left cerebral hemisphere of the BRAIN associated with speech. In motor aphasia, where the outgoing tract is damaged (i.e., the nerve transmitting the impulses which control the physical action of speech), the patient cannot speak but may understand and can sometimes write. In sensory aphasia, where the damage is to the the incoming tract (i.e., the nerve transmitting the sensation of the sound of speech), the patient cannot understand speech but may retain the power of uttering words and even of reading aloud, but with no understanding of what he is reading.

Management must vary with the cause, but often there is some spontaneous recovery as the original condition subsides.

aphonia. Loss of voice, usually due to some disorder in the vocal cords. An acute form is found in laryngitis, and a more persisting but less complete variety is found in persons who habitually over-use their voices. Aphonia is also a common symptom in hysteria. For inflammatory aphonia rest of the voice is essential and steam inhalations of friar's balsam may help.

aphrodisiac. The term, derived from Aphrodite, the Greek goddess of love, is used for any food, drink or drug believed to stimulate sexual desire or sexual activity. Over the centuries there have been extraordinary numbers of alleged aphrodisiacs, such as caviar, wheat-germ oil and celery, but none of these are of proved value, while cantharides simply acts by irritating the whole urinary system, and alcohol increases sexual desire but reduces sexual performance. In short, there is really no evidence that aphrodisiacs exist except to the extent that, where impotence or sub-fertility is due to deficiency of a hormone (e.g., testosterone, the testicular hormone), appropriate dosage of the hormone may restore normal sexual feeling and power.

As a rule, impotence and lack of orgasm respond to psychiatric treatment, not to drugs.

apomorphine. An alkaloid derived from morphia. When injected under the skin it rapidly induces vomiting so that it is useful in cases of non-corrosive poisoning.

apoplexy. A condition, colloquially called 'stroke' in England and 'shock' in Scotland, caused by interruption of the normal circulation in the brain. The three usual causes are: (1) cerebral haemorrhage, the bursting of a small blood vessel in the brain; (2) cerebral embolism, the blocking of a blood vessel by an obstruction, e.g., a fragment of a diseased heart valve; and (3) cerebral thrombosis, the blocking of a vessel by the formation of a clot.

The immediate treatment is to loosen constrictive clothing (e.g., the collar) to turn the head to the side, reducing the danger of the patient choking, and to summon the doctor. See STROKE.

apothecary. An old-fashioned term for a pharmacist. Until less than 200 years ago most doctors left surgery to barbers and the preparation and supply of drugs to apothecaries, the physicians concerning themselves mainly with abstract theories and – according to widespread opinion – fees. In general, the wealthy man who was sick consulted a physician and the poor man visited an apothecary.

apothecaries' weights and measures. A system of weights and measures used for drugs and medicines in the English-speaking countries. Until a few years ago a complicated double system existed in Britain and the U.S.A., whereby most long-established medicines were prescribed and dispensed in apothecaries' weights and measures, while new drugs were usually reckoned in the metric system. The older measures are, however, in process of disappearing and will soon merely be of historical interest.

Weights
20 grains = 1 scruple (1.29 grammes)
3 scruples = 1 drachm (3.88 grammes)
8 drachms = 1 ounce (31.1 grammes)
Measures
60 minims = 1 fluid drachm (3.55 millilitres)
8 fluid drachms = 1 fluid ounce (28.4 millilitres)
20 fluid ounces = 1 pint (568 millilitres) Britain
16 fluid ounces = 1 pint (455 millilitres) U.S.A.
Approximate equivalents
1 grain = 0.06 grammes or 60 milligrammes
15 grains = 1 gramme
1 minim = 0.06 millilitres
16 minims = 1 millilitre
1 pint (British) = 0.6 litres
Rough domestic equivalents
Tumbler = 10 fluid ounces (280 millilitres)
Tea cup = 5 fluid ounces (140 millilitres)
Tablespoon = ½ fluid ounce (14 millilitres)
Dessert spoon = 2 fluid drachms (7 millilitres)
Teaspoon = 1 fluid drachm (3.5 millilitres)
Drop (of water) = 1 minim (0.06 millilitres)

Since domestic utensils vary considerably in size, these equivalents are only approximate.

appendicectomy or **appendectomy.** Surgical removal of the appendix as in acute or chronic appendicitis. Although both terms are to be found on both sides of the Atlantic, appendicectomy is commoner in Britain and appendectomy in the U.S.A.

appendicitis. Inflammation or abscess of the appendix, the commonest emergency of abdominal surgery. The condition, rare in primitive societies, seems to be associated with refined, low-residue diets. If bacteria and faeces enter the appendix, it – along with the adjacent peritoneum – become inflamed, and if the condition is untreated general peritonitis may follow with serious danger to life.

The main symptom of appendicitis is severe abdominal pain, usually at first generalized but settling in a position low on the right. There is marked local tenderness which is important in diagnosis, and nausea and vomiting may occur. Treatment is essentially by immediate surgical removal. This was considered a dangerous operation sixty years ago but is nowadays regarded as simple, straightforward and practically devoid of risk to life; persons unfit for operation sometimes respond to antibiotics.

Chronic appendicitis is a condition in which the diseased appendix causes vague and usually intermittent abdominal pain and tenderness. Diagnosis of a 'grumbling appendix' is not easy, but when it is made the obvious remedy is surgical removal.

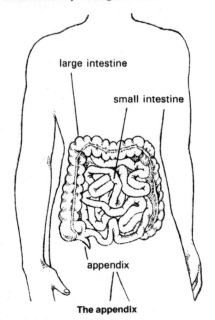

large intestine

small intestine

appendix

The appendix

appendix. A small blind tube, 7 to 10 cm. (3 to 4 in.) long, leading from the caecum at the junction of the small and large intestine. It has no known function and is probably a vestigial structure, i.e., a now needless organ left over in the course of evolution. It only becomes important when germs and faecal matter enter from the caecum and produce APPENDICITIS.

appetite. Desire for food and drink. Appetite should be differentiated from hunger. The latter, physical need for food, occurs when the stomach is empty and is accompanied by hunger pangs produced by contractions of the muscles of the stomach. By contrast, appetite can be present when the stomach is full and absent when it is empty although, fortunately, appetite and hunger normally coincide.

Appetite is in part created by sight: an interesting, well-cooked meal, pleasantly displayed and served in clean and cheerful surroundings, is more likely to stimulate appetite than is distasteful-looking food, badly served. In part it is created by the smell and taste of food: attractive food stimulates the secretion of salivary and gastric juices which are necessary for digestion. In part it is dependent on mental states: few of us have much desire for food when very angry or deeply grieved, although some people who feel unloved or bereaved develop a habit of eating in compensation for lack of affection, and voracious appetite immediately before death – 'grave greed' – is not unknown. Appetite is the spark which sets the digestive machinery in motion: when Macbeth told his guests, 'Let good digestion wait on appetite' he stated a physiological fact.

Loss of appetite is most commonly a result of worry, apprehension or emotional upset, so disturbing and emotional topics should be avoided at meal-times and, where practicable, there should be a period of relaxation before a meal. Mental fatigue, physical exhaustion and impairment of the senses of smell and taste (as in the common cold) are other causes of poor appetite. Excessive smoking may also reduce appetite, as may eating between meals, too much alcohol, constipation, septic conditions of the gums and teeth, and various diseases of the stomach, liver and kidneys. Loss of appetite persisting for more than a few days requires medical attention. See also ANOREXIA.

Increased appetite may be found in cases of dilated stomach and in pregnancy, and, as already mentioned, it occurs in some people who are unhappy. It is also sometimes found in diabetes and hyperthyroidism, which results from goitre.

Perverted appetite, a desire to eat rare or strange things, is one of the symptoms of several mental diseases and also occasionally occurs in pregnancy.

arcus senilis. A white crescent appearing just below the upper margin (and later just above the lower margin) of the cornea of the eye. It is caused by fatty deposits in the corneal tissue. It does not increase and does not interfere with vision but is one of the recognized signs of advancing years.

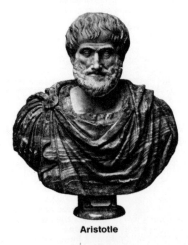

Aristotle

Aristotle. The son of a Macedonian physician in the fourth century B.C. and tutor to Alexander the Great, Aristotle was the most notable collector and systematizer of knowledge in the ancient world, and in many ways the founder of the scientific method. His classification of animals and his account of embryology, based on the development of the chick, came very near to suggesting the theory of evolution over two thousand years before Darwin. In large measure he was the creator of formal logic, stressing that all scientific theories must spring from the evidence of observation. Yet the very definiteness of his views and the logical method of their expression perhaps harmed the development of the sciences for the next eighteen hundred years, making them essentially deduction from accepted (and sometimes faulty) premises, instead of induction following new experimentation.

arm. In ordinary speech the arm is the whole upper limb, but in descriptive anatomy the term is restricted to the part extending from the shoulder to the elbow (i.e., excluding the forearm). Its bone is the humerus, which joins with the scapula above, forming a swivel joint that can move in any direction, and with the radius and ulna below, forming a hinge joint. Its muscles are the deltoid over the shoulder, the biceps in front and the triceps behind; and its main blood supply is from the brachial artery.

armpit. The deep space, otherwise known as the axilla, between the upper chest wall and the upper part of the arm. It is enclosed by the pectoral muscles in front and the latissimus dorsi muscle behind. It contains the nerves and blood vessels for the upper limb and also a group of lymph glands; these can become inflamed from infection spreading upwards from the hand and may also be infected from the breast.

Crutch palsy is a condition of temporary paralysis of the arm from pressure of a crutch on the nerves in the axilla. Careful padding of the crutch will prevent the condition.

The axilla is well equipped with sweat glands and therefore needs frequent washing to remove perspiration and reduce odour.

arrhythmia. Any variation from the ordinary rhythm of the heart, which is normally regular in time and force. Arrhythmia is produced by any condition which interferes with the normal beating of the heart. Examples are: sinus arrhythmia (the normal variation caused by breathing, more rapid during inspiration and slower during expiration), extrasystoles (where there is an occasional premature beat followed by the missing of a normal beat), auricular fibrillation, auricular flutter, heart block and paroxysmal tachycardia.

arsenic. A crystalline metal, used from early times as a medicine and as a poison. In very small doses it has an alleged tonic effect, and an arsenical preparation, neoarsphenamine, was the standard treatment for syphilis until the era of antibiotics.

Arsenical poisoning causes vomiting and diarrhoea, numbness of the feet, muscular cramps and collapse. Until recently treatment consisted mainly of giving an emetic (to get rid of arsenic not yet absorbed) and keeping the patient warm, but a relatively new drug, BAL (British Anti-Lewisite or dimercaprol) has proved useful in poisoning by organic arsenical compounds.

Arsenic is used in insecticides and in the manufacture of glass and various pharmaceuticals, and accidental poisoning is largely from inhalation of dust. Preventive measures include (1) substitution, where practicable, of non-toxic substances, (2) exhaust ventilation, (3) use of protective clothing, including masks where appropriate, and (4) periodic medical examination tk detect skin pigmentation and other early signs of chronic arsenical poisoning.

arteriosclerosis. Hardening and thickening of the coats of arteries, with consequent loss of the elasticity of the coats. This makes the arteries (1) narrower, so that increased pressure by the heart is needed to push the blood through, (2) brittle, and therefore liable to rupture, and (3) rough, with danger of blood clotting on the roughened surface.

Causes. The condition, the commonest vascular disease in developed countries, is primarily due to the deposit of minerals and fatty particles in the arterial walls, it both causes high blood pressure and is exacerbated by high blood pressure. The disease is frequent in persons whose diet is rich in foods containing large quantities of animal fats (e.g., fat meat, butter and cream) and it is thought that the saturated fatty acids in these foods raise the level of blood cholesterol and facilitate the depositing of fatty particles. Hence the partial substitution of foods containing unsaturated fatty acids (e.g., vegetable oils) should decrease arteriosclerosis. However, although the disease seldom produces symptoms until middle age, the substitution should be made much earlier, to prevent the early deposits which precede symptoms by many years.

Not all experts fully accept the cholesterol theory. Some maintain that excessive carbohydrates and resulting obesity are as potent factors, that heavy muscular work raises the blood pressure and throws strain on the vessel walls, that mental stress plays a considerable part probably by raising the blood pressure, and that heavy smoking is a factor. Others suggest that arteriosclerosis is simply a degenerative condition towards which some people inherit a tendency; but while the condition undoubtedly runs in families, the explanation may lie in family dietetic habits.

There are some associations between arteriosclerosis, coronary thrombosis, high blood pressure and chronic nephritis; almost certainly all four have several factors causing them, the main single one probably being high blood cholesterol.

Symptoms. Common early symptoms include loss of physical and mental vigour, giddiness, headache and attacks of breathlessness. Often, however, there are no specific symptoms until the arterial and blood pressure changes cause a major catastrophe, such as coronary thrombosis or cerebral thrombosis (STROKE).

Treatment. While a single, badly affected artery can be surgically repaired or replaced, there is no cure for generalized arterial thickening, but much can be done to check its advance and to prolong useful life. In particular, no extra strain - as from violent excitement or violent exercise - should be thrown on the heart and blood vessels, diet should be moderate, and alcohol and tobacco should be limited. Anticoagulant drugs may reduce the risk of clotting; and, although the body requires a fairly high blood pressure because of the narrowness of the vessels, drugs that reduce the pressure may be used in moderation.

Prevention. In the present state of knowledge the best preventive measures would appear to be: (1) avoidance of excessive animal fat from childhood or adolescence onwards, but bearing in mind the need for sufficient quantities of the fat soluble vitamins; (2) avoidance of excessive carbohydrates; (3) reasonable and regular exercise but avoidance of extreme muscular strain; (4) avoidance or limitation of smoking; and (5) avoidance of mental stress and emotional disturbance. Inevitably some people would consider that complete acceptance of these preventive measures would make life too dull and that a workable compromise is necessary to limit the risk of arteriosclerosis without damaging the quality of life.

artery. Any vessel carrying blood away from the heart. The pulmonary arteries convey blood to the lungs to receive oxygen. All other arteries carry oxygenated blood from the heart to the tissues.

The arterial system can be considered as resembling a tree with the aorta as its trunk; the carotids (to the head), subclavians (to the arms) and common iliacs (to the legs) as its main branches; thereafter it divides into smaller and smaller branches which end in numerous 'twigs' called arterioles. These in turn lead to a mesh of capillaries from which the oxygen and carbon dioxide exchange with the tissues takes place.

Each artery has an outer coat of connective tissue, a middle coat of elastic and muscular tissue, and an inner coat of fine cells which do not allow the blood to clot.

When cut across, arteries do not collapse, so that injury to an artery causes dangerous bleeding. Arterial bleeding is characterized by being bright red and spurting in jets coinciding with the heart-beat. Bleeding from a small artery can be stopped by applying pressure directly on the artery over the cut end nearer the heart. To stop bleeding from a large artery it is necessary to apply considerable pressure at a point where the artery lies close to a bone. In some instances where there is a good alternative blood supply by ANASTOMOSES (e.g., in the scalp) there is blood loss from both the severed ends.

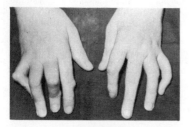

Arthritic hands

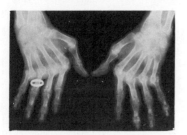

X-ray of arthritic hands

arthritis. Inflammation of a joint. It may be acute or chronic and due to many different causes, ranging from infection of joints and their related structures by identifiable

organisms to the destruction of joints which occurs in certain diseases of the nervous system. Examples of infective forms are tubercular arthritis, gonococcal arthritis (arising from gonorrhoea), and streptococcal arthritis (resulting from infection from a wound) but antibiotic treatment has greatly reduced the risk of such diseases affecting the joints.

The term is most often used in reference to three common crippling diseases: rheumatoid arthritis, osteo-arthritis, and gout.

articulation. See JOINT.

artificial insemination. The introduction of male seminal fluid into the genital tract of the female by artificial means for the purpose of producing conception and pregnacy.

The procedure was first developed in Denmark and is mainly used in veterinary practice for stock-breeding purposes, so that the characteristics of a champion animal can be transmitted to the progeny of many more females than he could sire naturally. There are also considerations related to economics and convenience.

Artificial insemination (which is carried out at the time of ovulation) has only a limited place in human reproduction. The semen of the husband can be used (artificial insemination-husband: AIH) when a husband is fertile but impotent, or semen of a donor (AID) when the husband is infertile. However, AID is fraught with medico-legal difficulties, for any offspring is technically illegitimate.

artificial pneumothorax. Artificial pneumothorax is the condition which results when air is deliberately introduced into the chest (pleural cavity) to produce collapse of one lung. The procedure is intended to put a diseased lung at rest in order to encourage healing, to promote the collapse and obliteration of infected cavities, and to minimize any tendency to bleeding from damaged areas.

It was formerly much used in the treatment of pulmonary tuberculosis particularly if the disease was present in one lung only but early diagnosis and the use of effective antibiotic drugs has now resulted in its virtual abandonment for most cases. It may also be employed in the treatment of bronchiectasis.

artificial respiration. In cases of asphyxia from various causes such as drowning, suffocation, exposure to poisonous gases, narcotic poisoning, and electrocution, a patient's natural respiration may have stopped but his heart and circulation and the vital processes of his central nervous system may not yet be incapable of recovery. If some form of 'breathing' can be contrived so that his blood receives a continuing supply of oxygen there is a chance that his life may be saved.

The various methods of doing this are known as 'artificial respiration' by which inspiration (breathing in) and expiration (breathing out) are artificially induced.

Although there are resuscitation appliances available for the maintenance of respiration, the nature of the emergency is such that it brooks of no delay. Treatment should be commenced forthwith and *must not be delayed* in anticipation of the arrival of skilled help and special equipment.

No matter which procedure is employed it is essential to make sure that there is a clear air-

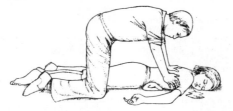

Artificial respiration: Schafer's method

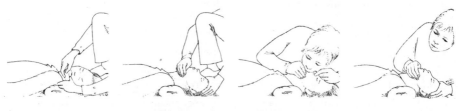

Mouth-to-mouth resuscitation

way and that the upper part of the respiratory passages is not obstructed by a sagging jaw, by the tongue, or by dentures or any other item which should always be looked for and removed. In cases of drowning it is essential as a first step to eliminate water from the air passages by tilting the patient's head downwards and compressing the chest.

The patient should also be treated in reasonably open surroundings where there is adequate fresh air, and it is advisable to take steps to conserve body heat by the use of blankets or some improvised additional covering.

Manual methods. These all make use of the principle that some exchange of gases in the blood supply within the lungs can be achieved by alternate compression and relaxation of the chest wall. They differ only in how this is done.

1. Hall's method. The patient is placed on his face and then rolled on to one side and a little beyond (inspiration) and then back on to the face (expiration).

2. Silvester's method. The patient is placed on his back with a pillow under his shoulders. His arms are raised above his head (inspiration) and then lowered on to the chest with a compressing movement (expiration).

3. Howard's method. The patient is placed on his back with a pillow under his waist. The operator kneels astride and with both hands and spread fingers alternately compresses the lower part of the chest (expiration) and allows it to spring back (inspiration).

4. Schafer's method. The patient is laid face downward with the head turned to one side. The operator kneels astride and with both hands and spread fingers placed on the back leans forward with his arms straight and compresses the chest by his weight (expiration). He then removes the pressure he is exerting and allows the chest to expand (inspiration).

In all these methods the movements should be repeated between ten and fifteen times per minute. If natural respiration shows signs of re-

starting, the movements should be synchronized with the patient's efforts.

The best procedure is probably Schafer's, which is effective and least fatiguing for the operator.

Eve's rocking stretcher. This is a very effective method which operates on a slightly different principle. It requires some equipment which may readily be improvised.

The patient is secured face-down by legs and arms to a stretcher or plank, which is then balanced at its mid-point on a trestle. When tilted head down to 45 degrees the abdominal contents push on the diaphragm and compress the lungs (expiration). The stretcher is then tilted feet down to the same extent, the abdominal contents move downwards, drawing the diaphragm down also and air is drawn into the chest (inspiration).

Mouth-to-mouth resuscitation. This is the method popularly known as the 'kiss of life', and is really not so much mouth-to-mouth as mouth-to-nose. It is efficient and its use is indicated if there is any suspicion of fractures or other injuries.

After making sure that there is a clear airway and that the head is tilted back the operator holds the patient's mouth closed. He then applies his lips to the patient's nose and blows. The patient's chest rises with the insufflated air (inspiration), and is then allowed to relax again (expiration). As in the other methods this is repeated between ten and fifteen times a minute. The procedure may be made rather more aesthetic by the use of a simple plastic tube known as a Brook Airway which should form part of any First Aid kit.

Mechanical methods. A variety of special devices is available ranging from an airway with bellows to more elaborate mechanical equipment (e.g., iron lung) which may also be capable of supplying additional oxygen or oxygen and carbon dioxide mixtures. Most ambulances now carry such appliances as standard equipment but their safe and successful use requires some training and experience.

If natural respiration is not speedily restored the question then arises as to how long attempts at artificial respiration should be prolonged. In the absence of any professional advice it would be reasonable to assume that death had occurred if no response was obtained after one hour. In cases of poisoning from drugs, however, there may be severe depression of the respiratory centre and it would be wise to persist until the patient comes under hospital treatment.

artificial sweeteners. Synthetic compounds of no food value used to sweeten foods and drinks. Diabetics, who have to restrict their intake of sugar, either have to consume their food and drink unsweetened or to use artificial sweeteners. Persons who are overweight often employ these sweeteners as a convenient method of slightly reducing their calorie intake: for a person who drinks six cups of tea or coffee daily, with one teaspoonful of sugar in each cup, the substitution of a sweetener represents a reduction of about 150 Calories each day.

The most commonly used sweeteners are saccharin and the commercial preparations made from it. Another group of sweeteners, cyclamates, are now restricted in many countries because large amounts have been shown to have harmful effects on animals, although these effects have not been fully proved in man.

Ascheim-Zondek test. A test described in 1927 by two German gynaecologists for the early diagnosis of PREGNANCY.

ascites. The accumulation of free fluid within the abdominal cavity.

Causes. These may be simply classified as follows: (1) infections of the peritoneum (the membrane lining the abdominal cavity) such as tuberculosis or malignant diseases; (2) obstructions of the venous blood flow through the liver (the portal circulation) as in cirrhosis; (3) congestive cardiac failure; (4) chronic kidney disease, and (5) some types of severe anaemia.

Treatment. This is directed to the underlying disease, but the amount of accumulated fluid and the resultant abdominal distension may be very great and may produce symptoms such as difficulty in breathing with impairment of circulation and digestion in a purely mechanical way, because of the weight and pressure. When this occurs relief can be given by 'paracentesis', a simple operation for withdrawal of fluid through a hollow needle.

A salt-free diet and the administration of diuretics to increase the flow of urine from the kidneys may help to slow down the rate at which fluid re-accumulates.

ascorbic acid. Diets inadequate in fresh fruit and vegetables ultimately result in scurvy. This was recognized at least 150 years ago, and sailors were given a daily issue of lemon or lime juice to compensate for the lack of some unknown but obviously essential substance not provided by their sea-going rations. This substance was given the name vitamin C (see VITAMINS) and in 1937 research showed that it was ascorbic acid, a precise and relatively simple chemical compound.

Oranges, lemons, tomatoes, cabbages and other green vegetables are among the best natural sources of this vitamin but it is readily destroyed by overcooking, especially in the presence of air and of alkalis such as sodium bicarbonate.

In man the daily requirements of ascorbic acid are 1mg. per kg. body weight and about twice that amount for babies and pregnant women.

Vitamin C is not stored in the body and a higher intake is desirable during infective illness when the rate of utilization tends to increase. There is also a claim that doses of 1g. or more per day prevent or cure the common cold.

asepsis. The system of surgical practice which aims at the total exclusion of micro-organisms from the tissues during any surgical procedure.

Louis Pasteur (1822-95) a French chemist and bacteriologist, showed that wound infection was due to the action of bacteria, and Joseph Lister (1827-1912) exploited this discovery by introducing the use of antiseptics in surgery. These were various chemical substances, initially carbolic acid, which inhibited the growth of micro-organisms and thus prevented them from causing suppuration by multiplying in wounds to which they gained access.

This was antisepsis and it suffered from the disadvantages that it was neither completely effective nor free from the risk that the chemical agents themselves might also damage the tissues.

It was therefore the logical next step to try to destroy potential causes of infection before they reached a wound, and to do this by a method which did not also carry a risk of tissue damage. This procedure became known as asepsis.

Bacteria are to be found everywhere and during surgical operation there is a risk that they may gain access to a wound from the environment, from the person and clothing of the attendants, and from the surgical instruments and dressings. In an aseptic technique it is necessary that all these possible sources of bacterial infection should receive attention, and so operations are now carried out in specially designed operating theatres, which can be thoroughly cleaned and disinfected. The most modern also have arrangements for filtering or sterilizing the air. The surgeons and nurses change their outdoor clothing and after prolonged washing and scrubbing of their hands and arms array themselves in gowns, overboots, caps, masks, and rubber gloves, all of which have been previously sterilized and rendered germ free by autoclaving – a process of disinfection using steam at raised temperature and pressure.

Surgical instruments and dressings are usually similarly sterilized, although alternative methods may be used for instruments which could be damaged by heat. Increasing use is also being made of disposable small instruments, such as syringes and needles, which can be discarded after a single use. These are supplied commercially in sealed outer covers, having been sterilized after enclosure by the application of gamma radiation.

aspergillosis. A type of long-lasting chest infection due to invasion of the lung by fungi of the genus *Aspergillus*. The fungi grow in mouldy grain, and the disease is acquired either by chewing such grain or by inhaling its dust.

The disease mainly occurs amongst workers in grain stores, flour factories, malting floors and so on, and pigeon fanciers are traditionally liable because of the practice of feeding young birds by transferring grain from their own mouths.

Both from symptoms and x-ray the disease is liable to be confused with pulmonary tuberculosis but laboratory examination of the sputum should ensure a correct diagnosis. For treatment various antibiotics have been claimed to be helpful, steroids are sometimes used and an aspergillus vaccine is occasionally tried.

asphyxia. The condition which results when any interference with any stage of respiration denies the body tissues an adequate and continuous supply of oxygen.

In normal respiration air of an acceptable quality is taken into the lungs by the muscular efforts of the chest and diaphragm. It enters the body by the mouth or nose, and passes by the larynx, trachea, bronchi, and bronchioles to the terminal air passages and air sacs (alveoli) of the lungs. In the alveoli an exchange of gases takes place between the blood and the inspired air. Reduced haemoglobin in the pulmonary circulation absorbs oxygen, and carbon dioxide is given up from the plasma for exhalation. All this depends on nervous control by the respiratory centre in the brain and on the ability of the heart to maintain an adequate circulation of blood.

Causes. With this summary in mind the causes of asphyxia can readily be appreciated:

1. Obstruction to air-flow: smothering; obstruction by foreign body; throttling, strangulation, hanging; inhalation of vomit; fluid in the air passages as in drowning; injury and swelling of tissues from disease, burns, scalds, and corrosive poisons.

2. Quality of inspired air: irrespirable gases; rarefaction of the atmosphere as in mountaineering or high-altitude flying.

3. Failure of inspiratory effort: fixation of chest and abdomen by pressure as in burial by debris, crowd accidents, and overlaying of infants; penetrating wounds of chest causing pneumothorax; paralysis of voluntary muscles, as in poliomyelitis and injuries to the spinal cord.

4. Failure of respiratory exchange: disease of lung such as pneumonia; inadequate circulation as in heart failure; interference with oxygen-carrying capacity of haemoglobin as in carbon monoxide poisoning.

5. Impairment of respiratory centre: narcotic poisons; head injuries; intracranial disease.

In acute asphyxia the patient struggles for breath, respiratory movements become violent, the face becomes livid and neck veins appear engorged. This first stage may last for about three minutes until unconsciousness occurs; respiration now ceases but the heart will continue to beat for a variable period and recovery may still be possible if the cause of the asphyxia can be removed and ARTIFICIAL RESPIRATION begun.

Some types of asphyxia require tracheotomy intubation and mechanical assistance with respiration.

In asphyxia of gradual onset due to disease the treatment is that of the underlying disease and the administration of oxygen may help.

Everyone really dies of asphyxia in the end as terminal cardiac failure occurs.

Asphyxia of the new-born. Before birth the infant receives its oxygen supply from the maternal circulation. The oxygen is exchanged for carbon dioxide across the placenta, supplied on one side by maternal blood, and on the other by the infant's blood stream which reaches it and returns by the umbilical cord. At birth there is an abrupt change because this method of gaseous exchange ceases, the accumulation of carbon dioxide in the infant's blood then stimulates his respiratory centre, and he tries to breathe air in the normal manner.

If at any stage before delivery this process is initiated prematurely, the infant is born with a deficiency of oxygen and an accumulation of carbon dioxide in the blood stream and is thus in a state of asphyxia.

The chief causes of interference with the placental circulation before birth are prolonged labour, premature separation of the placenta, and pressure on the umbilical cord or its twisting or expulsion before the birth of the baby. The administration of drugs to the mother may impair the respiratory centre of the infant. However, even in the absence of any of these causes the premature infant may be born in an asphyxiated state because of the inherent feebleness of its circulation.

Asphyxia may also result from the inhalation of mucus or amniotic fluid during the infant's initial attempts to breathe, from brain damage during delivery, or from a failure of the lungs to expand properly.

It is usual to distinguish two types of asphyxia, namely, (1) asphyxia livida, in which the infant's circulation is adequate and the symptoms are due mainly to the lack of oxygen, and (2) asphyxia pallida, in which the oxygen lack is part of a general state of collapse brought about by the stresses of the delivery.

aspiration. The act of sucking out fluids or gases from a vessel or cavity.

aspirin. Originally a proprietary name, 'Aspirin' is a synonym for acetylsalicylic acid, much used as a household remedy. It acts by allaying pain and diminishing fever and it is particularly helpful in rheumatic conditions.

A gastric irritant, it may cause indigestion or gastric haemorrhage, and in some sensitive persons it produces skin-rashes or asthma. It should not be given to infants and only with caution to small children. Household supplies of the drug should be kept out of reach of children owing to the substantial risk of accidental poisoning.

Symptoms of aspirin overdosage in a child include drowsiness, pallor and heavy breathing. In an older child or an adult these symptoms are often accompanied by dizziness and a sensation of alarm. Very rarely a rash appears on the skin. The immediate treatment of overdosage is to wash out the stomach with a 0.5 per cent solution of sodium bicarbonate (baking soda).

asthma. A respiratory disease characterized by recurrent paroxysmal attacks of difficulty in breathing, usually accompanied by wheezing, cough, and a sense of constriction of the chest. It may be associated with bronchitis but true bronchial asthma can occur quite independently.

It is due to spasm of the muscular fibres in

the walls of the smaller air passages in the lungs (bronchioles). This reduces the size of the airway and impedes the respiratory air flow, particularly when breathing in. Activity of these muscle fibres is controlled by nervous impulses reaching them from the autonomic, or involuntary, part of the nervous system, particularly the vagus nerve.

Causes. The asthmatic attack is therefore brought about by factors which influence this nervous control. Amongst these are: (1) direct irritation of the bronchial mucous membrane; (2) reflex irritation from disease elsewhere, especially infection in the nose and throat; gastric irritation; intestinal infection; and (3) sensitivity or allergy: individual patients may be sensitive to a great variety of substances such as pollens, animal dandruff, hair and feathers, certain foods, moulds, house dust, and so on; house dust has frequently been shown to contain products of the house mite. Finally, (4) psychological factors such as sudden severe emotion, fear, anxiety, anger, and more deep-seated personality disorders undoubtedly play a part in precipitating some attacks.

Asthma may occur at any age but it is common in children, when it is often associated with eczematous dermatitis. It is more common in males. A hereditary tendency is well-recognized and often the patient's personality is of a definite type – highly strung and of general nervous instability.

Treatment. The acute attack usually responds quite dramatically to the administration of adrenalin, ephedrine, antihistamines, or the use of inhalations based on measured doses of newer drugs such as iso-prenaline or cromoglycate; but the long-term treatment of the condition is difficult and unrewarding.

Skin tests should be used to detect any specific allergen and positive results followed up by desensitization. Any source of infection should be searched for and eradicated. Breathing exercises are sometimes helpful. Otherwise the indications are to attend to general health and hygiene and to provide drugs such as inhalant sprays for either routine use or relief of symptoms.

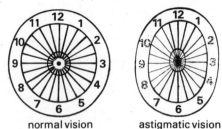

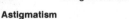
normal vision   astigmatic vision

Astigmatism

astigmatism. A defect of EYESIGHT in which the front of the eye is not curved uniformly so that the whole of an image cannot be brought into focus

astringent. Substance which, when applied to skin or mucous membranes, contracts blood-vessels and secretory ducts (so limiting haemorrhage or discharge) and which shrinks swollen membranes.

Those used to arrest superficial bleeding are given the special name of 'styptics' – e.g., alum and ferric salts.

Some astringents and where they act are: (1) on blood vessels – cold compresses; adrenalin; stypticin. (2) On skin ulceration – preparations of lead sub-acetate; silver nitrate; zinc sulphate (lotio rubra); calamine lotion. (3) On mucous membranes – alum; tannic acid. (4) On nose and throat – sprays of ephedrine. (5) On conjuctiva – zinc sulphate eye drops.

ataxia. Incoordination of voluntary movement characterized by an unsteady gait, lack of precision in hand and arm movements and inability to stand steady with the eyes closed (Romberg's sign).

There are three principal causes: (1) organic disease of the central nervous system affecting the cerebellum or the sensory pathways in the spinal cord (locomotor ataxia in the third stage of syphilis is the classic example of a disease affecting the spinal cord in this way), (2) disturbance of the balancing mechanism of the internal ear occurring in Ménière's disease and other types of vertigo, and (3) functional disorder of the nervous system due to the effect of alcohol or other drugs.

atelectasis. Incomplete expansion of one or both lungs. This is a relatively common cause of perinatal death, the infant failing to breathe properly and so to expand the lungs. It can often be successfully treated by artificial expansion of the lungs through a tube passed down the trachea. In adults and older children atelectasis can occur through blockage of an air-passage, e.g., by pressure of a tumour or by inhalation of a foreign body. In such cases treatment varies with the cause.

atheroma. Thickening and degeneration of the inner coat – and less often of the middle coat – of arteries, occasioned largely by wear and tear, and encountered mainly in old people and in persons with high blood pressure. Since the condition interferes with the passage of blood along the arteries it to some extent also creates high blood pressure and is one of the factors in causing ARTERIOSCLEROSIS.

atherosclerosis. See ARTERIOSCLEROSIS.

athlete's foot. A disease of the feet (and occasionally of the hands) characterized by white, sodden-looking skin on the inner surface of the foot with groups of blisters especially between the toes. The condition is an infection, due to a fungus closely allied to that of RINGWORM, and can spread wherever people mix in bare feet, e.g., at swimming baths. Excessive perspiration appears to render feet more susceptible.

Prevention includes adequate cleansing and disinfection of the surfaces liable to carry the infection. Daily applications of magenta paint are commonly recommended for treatment. The washing of sweaty feet both night and morning and the changing of socks daily assist both prevention and treatment.

atlas. The first cervical vertebra, i.e., the top-most of the bones forming the spinal column. It consists of a complete ring of bone, supports the head, and permits backward and forward movements of the head. Sideways movement of the head is really permitted by the second vertebra, the AXIS.

atomic bomb, effects of. A nuclear explosion differs in several important respects from that of a conventional high explosive bomb. The nuclear devices used in attacking Japan in 1945 had an explosive force equal to twenty thousand tons of TNT. Much more powerful weapons have since been developed with energy-yields in the range of one to fifty megatons of TNT - a megaton being one million tons. Nuclear bombs are thus many thousand times more powerful than the largest practicable high explosive bombs and in addition the temperature at the centre of the explosion is some millions of degrees Centigrade, compared with a maximum of 5,000°C. in a conventional explosion.

A large proportion of the energy of a nuclear explosion is therefore emitted as heat and light and is referred to as 'thermal radiation'.

Blast and thermal radiation differ from an ordinary bomb only in scale; but atomic bombs also emit invisible penetrating and harmful gamma rays (akin to x-rays) and atomic particles called neutrons. These constitute the 'initial nuclear radiation' but the area of explosion is subsequently contaminated by 'fission products' which are also widely dispersed as 'fallout' and continue to emit similar harmful radiation for about two years. This effect is known as 'residual radiation'.

The effects of an atomic explosion may therefore be summarized in relation to blast, heat, and radiation.

The blast wave. Blast travels outwards at the speed of sound and causes the initial damage to buildings. With a megaton bomb there will probably be total obliteration within a one-mile radius from the explosion centre; irreparable damage between one and two miles; severe damage between two and five miles; light damage between five and ten miles. Blast alone can cause personal injury by compression and damage to internal organs, by shearing of soft tissues, and by rupture of ear-drums, but individuals near enough to suffer these effects are more likely to be fatally burned by thermal radiation.

Thermal effects. The thermal radiation from an ordinary bomb is insignificant except quite close to the explosion but with an atomic bomb very large amounts of energy are emitted and propagated with the speed of light to distances of ten miles or more. Anything combustible will burst into flames, and so numerous fires develop.

People in the open receive third degree burns (charring) up to eight miles away; second degree burns (blistering) at eight or nine miles; and first degree burns (reddening) up to fifteen miles. These are 'flash burns' and can be avoided by any light shielding, even clothing, but as the clothing ignites 'flame burns' ensue.

Radiation effects. Atomic radiation damages living matter by 'ionization' and the immediate result is 'radiation sickness' whose severity depends on intensity of exposure.

These are four forms the effect of radiation can take: (1) cerebral form - very large amounts of radiation cause convulsions, coma, and death in a few days, (2) enteric form - nausea, vomiting, diarrhoea, and usually rapid deterioration to death within fifteen days, (3) bone-marrow form - nausea and vomiting for some days; a latent period of three weeks followed by anaemia, and (4) non-apparent form - no clinical symptoms but temporary reduction in white cells of blood.

In the longer term, cases of ultimately fatal leukaemia may begin to occur after two years and may continue to be discovered for many years after the initial exposure.

atrium. One of the muscular chambers of the HEART, often called an auricle.

atrophy. The shrinkage or wasting of any cell, tissue, limb, or organ.

Atrophy may be local or generalized and the latter in particular is part of the normal process of ageing. Some examples will illustrate the principles of other more specific causes.

1. Disuse atrophy: limbs which are splinted for long periods or immobilized by disease rapidly show muscular wasting.

2. Interference with nerve supply: damage within the brain (as in cerebral vascular disease such as cerebral haemorrhage) or in the spinal chord (as in poliomyelitis) cause paralysis and muscular atrophy. In other nervous and muscular diseases degeneration of spinal nerve cells produces a similar result.

3. Interference with blood supply: vascular disease can reduce blood flow to any part and impair its nutrition; this is especially important in the coronary vessels of the heart. Local pressure (as with a cervical rib) can act similarly.

4. Absorption of bone: old persons develop bone wasting leading to fractures from trivial causes and atrophy of jaw bones leads to loss of teeth.

5. Toxins: atrophy of optic nerve transmitting impulses of sight from the eye; acute yellow atrophy of the liver; inflammation of various nerves as in lead poisoning.

6. Infections: peripheral nerve lesions as in leprosy; degeneration of muscle in typhoid fever.

atropine. An alkaloid which is the active constituent of belladonna, a medicinal agent originally derived from the deadly nightshade plant although other sources are now used commercially.

Atropine is an important drug and its therapeutic effect is due to its selective action on the vagus nerve, which is inhibited. It is therefore employed to cause relaxation of involuntary muscle, i.e., the muscles of the body (mainly in the digestion system) which cannot be controlled at will. Atropine is particularly useful in such conditions as renal or intestinal colic, gastric ulcer and bronchial spasm associated with asthma. It is also prescribed before operation to reduce bronchial secretion and before certain eye examinations to dilate the pupil.

Undesirable side effects include increased pulse rate, dryness of the mouth, and inability to focus near objects.

It is a powerful and poisonous drug, effective in very small doses (0.3 to 0.6 mg.). Symptoms of over-dose are alarming, with mental confusion, hallucinations, high temperature, blurred vision, a hot dry skin (due to inhibition of sweating) and sometimes a rash resembling scarlet fever. Treatment includes giving an emetic to induce vomiting, keeping the patient warm and providing ample hot fluids such as strong coffee.

aura. Any peculiar sensation or phenomenon preceding an attack of an illness such as epilepsy or migraine.

In the case. of an epileptic fit, general symptoms such as headache, irritability, elation, or lethargy may be experienced some days before an attack, but usually the premonition is more immediate and takes the form of hallucinations of sensations such as visual images, strange noises and smells.

The aura which precedes attacks of migraine is very often visual, with flashes of dazzling light and dark and bright spots.

auricle. One of the muscular chambers of the HEART more correctly known as an atrium.

auricular fibrillation. A type of disordered heart action. The normal heart beat is a regular rhythmic contraction of the auricles followed by similar contraction of the ventricles. Impulses causing this originate in the 'pacemaker' of the HEART and pass in sequence to auricles and ventricles along a band of specialized muscle fibre. The rate and intensity of the impulses are determined by nervous and chemical stimuli influencing the pacemaker.

If this conducting band of specialized muscle is damaged by cardiac disease the regular co-ordinated contractions of the auricles become irregular, uncoordinated, and excessively fast. This is auricular fibrillation. The rate, rhythm, and force of ventricular contraction are also disordered by the imperfect impulses, causing the pulse to be weakened and irregular.

autism. A condition in which a child appears aloof and cut off from the world, with no apparent emotion (except occasional outbursts of rage), no indication of affection or response to affection, stereotyped mannerisms, an interest in toys rather than people and an avoidance of eye contact. Because the child does not listen to speech his speech is usually retarded and he is sometimes, wrongly, thought to be deaf; and in the past many autistic children have been falsely diagnosed as mentally defective, although, apart from speech problems, they show no indications of low intelligence.

There has been relatively little research into this fairly rare but serious condition. Some workers regard it as due to deprivation of affection, with the child given intellectual stimulation but little more. Others deem it a form of infantile SCHIZOPHRENIA and probably a result of hereditary factors. As yet no adequate preventive measures exist, but with skilled management the outlook – formerly very bleak – can be greatly improved and an autistic child can often grow into an adult capable of earning his living and maintaining a reasonable existence.

Further progress in the prevention or treatment of autism would seem to require the combined skills of geneticists, paediatricians, nurses, teachers and social workers, with psychologists perhaps playing an important part.

auto-intoxication. A state of poisoning produced by some uneliminated toxin generated within the body.

Intestinal auto-intoxication formerly had something of a vogue as a supposed cause of vague ill-health rather like 'biliousness'. It was claimed that symptoms such as headache, lassitude, and loss of appetite were due to the contents of the lower bowel being retained longer than normal and undergoing abnormal decomposition whereby harmful poisons

entered the blood; but there is no real evidence that this occurs.

The term has largely fallen into disuse and should not be used for specific examples of toxaemia such as uraemia.

automation. The manufacture of articles by electrical, mechanical, hydraulic or electronic processes, and ultimately the substitution of machines for work that previously involved unskilled human labour. In the highly developed countries automation is already beginning to have appreciable socio-economic effects. For example, a factory that formerly required twenty skilled workers and a thousand unskilled workers may now need thirty skilled workers and only forty unskilled persons, so that already there is a shortage of skilled staff and considerable unemployment among the unskilled.

The answers to the complicated problems of increasing automation would appear to be (1) relatively slow transition from manual to automatic work, (2) better general education so that some who would have lacked opportunity in the past can become professional workers or skilled technicians, (3) reduction of working hours with employment of relatively more people, and (4) education of the public for increased leisure and use of leisure.

In countries like the U.K. we are already seeing some results of automation, such as persistent shortages of nurses, doctors, etc. through diversion of a higher percentage of intelligent youngsters into industry and commerce, and, coupled with that shortage, large pools of unskilled unemployed persons through one machine doing the work of many men.

automatism. A state of impaired consciousness in which a person acts in an apparently conscious manner but with no recollection afterwards of having done so. It occurs particularly after seizures of EPILEPSY and is of medico-legal importance when used as a defence against allegations of crime or indecency.

Somnambulism or 'sleep-walking' is another example of automatism; and likewise the true alcoholic after even a mild debauch may recover days later unaware of what he has done in the interval.

autonomic nervous system. See NERVOUS SYSTEM.

auto-suggestion. A form of self-hypnotism. Certain psychosomatic diseases may be due to, or influenced by, psychic or emotional factors affecting the subconscious so that the patient experiences bodily symptoms which his conscious mind regards as 'real'. Auto-suggestion attempts to reverse this process by enforcing a conscious effort to appreciate the psychic or 'unreal' nature of the symptoms in the expectation that if the patient is really convinced at the level of conscious thought, the subconscious mind will accept that its apprehensions are unfounded. Conditions which may fall into this category include certain cases of gastric ulcer, asthma, migraine, and many skin diseases.

The most notable exponent of the technique of auto-suggestion was Professor Emil Coué (1857-1926), a French psychotherapist who claimed to have cured his own asthma by frequently repeating to himself the words 'Every day in every way, I am getting better and better!' The use of this formula became widely known as 'Coué-ism', and was a popular therapy of the 1920s.

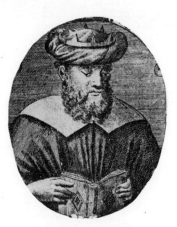

Avicenna

Avicenna. Known by his countrymen as Ibn Sina (980-1037), the greatest of Persian physicians and the dominating figure in medicine for at least six centuries.

Even if some of his romantic adventures and his fondness for the wine-jug and dancing-girls have been magnified by the mists of time, Avicenna stands out as an extraordinary, multi-faceted genius. He was several times grand visier, or, as we would say, prime minister. He made significant contributions to mathematics, astronomy, physics, philosophy, poetry and music. Medically he cured monarchs and treated the poor free in order to extend his knowledge of disease. He wrote the *Canon,* which remained for many hundreds of years the standard text-book in the medical schools of Asia and Europe.

The *Canon* is not merely a comprehensive outline in about a million words of all that was best in Greek, Roman and Persian medicine: at least some things in it are thought to be original. In hygiene he extended and advanced the best practices of the Romans, and he was probably the first person to recognize the existence of water-borne infections. His study of symptoms was brilliant. His sections on child care could still usefully be read. His treatments were a curious mixture of rational and often highly effective measures and of procedures that we now deem absurd.

He lived at a time when all European learning was centred on theology, with scientific study totally rejected, so that his is the greatest name in medical history between Galen, in the second century, and the re-awakening of scientific enquiry in the Europe of of the Renaissance. His influence on Asian medicine is still strong and as one medical historian puts it – 'Avicenna has been sleeping since the year 1037, but he still treats all the invalids of Persia'.

axilla. See ARMPIT.

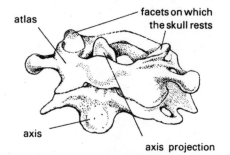

atlas — facets on which the skull rests

axis

axis projection

The atlas and axis vertebrae

axis. The second cervical vertebra, i.e., the second bone from the top in the spinal column. It has a small projection on its upper edge which lies in a hollow of the atlas (the first cervical vertebra). The skull and atlas can move around this, enabling the head to be turned to right and left.

B

baby. The human infant from birth until it begins to walk and becomes a 'toddler'.

A still-born baby is a child born dead after a pregnancy lasting long enough for viability – about twenty-eight weeks. Premature and post-mature babies respectively are those resulting from pregnancies shorter or longer than the normal period of about 280 days. A dysmature baby is one whose development at birth is less advanced than expected from its gestational age – the 'small-for-dates' baby.

See also articles on INFANCY, INFANT, POST-MATURITY and PREMATURITY.

bacilluria. The presence of bacilli in the urine. The term is properly applied to a urine which contains bacilli but no pus cells, indicating that the kidney is passing bacilli derived through the blood stream from an infective condition elsewhere and not originating in the urinary tract. The organism most commonly present is *Escherichia coli.* The presence of typhoid bacillus in the urine is also sometimes a problem in 'typhoid carriers' as a possible means of transmitting infection.

bacillus. A term commonly used for any rod-shaped micro-organism or bacterium but scientifically a member of the genus

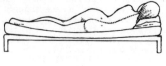

wrong

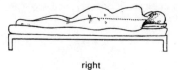

right

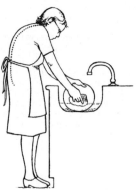

wrong

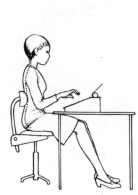

right

wrong

right

The right and wrong way of doing things

Bacillaceae of which *B. anthracis* is an example. See BACTERIA.

backache. Backache is a symptom and not a disease in itself. The term is used in a general way to describe pain and disability related to the spine and particularly the so-called 'low back pain' of the lumbar region and sacral part of the pelvis.

It is common in middle-aged and overweight women and is a major cause of industrial disability in manual workers. (In the latter, because of the subjective nature of the complaint, it often causes difficulty in the certification of incapacity if there are inadequate physical signs.) However, every effort must be made to reach an accurate diagnosis as an essential prerequisite for the proper management of what can be a very disabling condition.

Anatomy. Any rational discussion of the cause must be founded on the anatomical features and relationship of the parts involved. These will be taken as including the pelvis, the lumbar vertebrae, their ligaments and muscles, and the abdomino-pelvic organs which can cause 'referred pain' in the back.

The SPINAL COLUMN of this region is composed of the five lumbar vertebrae, the sacrum (which

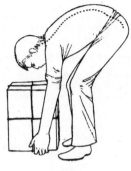

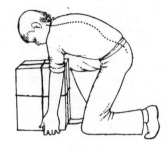

wrong   right

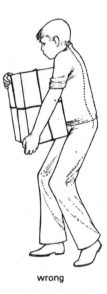

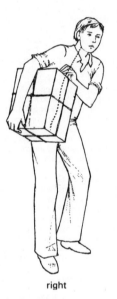

wrong   right

The right and wrong way of doing things (contd.)

forms the rear wall of the pelvis and is attached to it by the sacro-iliac joint on each side) and the tail-piece or coccyx. Between the lumbar vertebrae lie the cartilagenous discs. The bony vertebral arch below the level of the first lumbar vertebra protects the nerve fibres coming from the spinal cord, and these emerge, pair by pair, between the vertebrae and from openings on the sacrum.

These bones are supported and laced together by fibrous ligaments and attached to this composite structure are the muscles which provide the power for voluntary movement – bending forwards (flexion), backwards (extension), and sideways (lateral bending) and also some rotation.

Accurate diagnosis by physical examination depends on an assessment of the effect of these movements supplemented by neurological tests and x-ray investigation. Movements are tested by voluntary action – the patient performing the action unaided – and by passive movement – the doctor moving the limb without the aid of the patient. There must also be a careful external inspection with the patient suitably undressed to detect any other feature such as skeletal asymmetry or muscle-wasting.

Causes. With these anatomical considerations in mind the following can be enumerated:

1. Lumbago. Fibrositis or 'muscular rheumatism' affecting the lumbar muscles.

2. Lumbar back-strain. A localized rupture of some of the lumbar muscle fibres. There is usually a localized point of tenderness and resistance to only some directions of passive movement, contrasting with the generalized pain and spasm of lumbago.

3. Lumbo-sacral strain. Damage to the ligaments supporting the lumbo-sacral joint with localized tenderness over the joint and general restriction of movement. It is usually due to

lifting stresses, especially with a bent back, and it is the commonest cause of chronic disability in the overweight person.

4. Sacro-iliac strain. Similar causes affecting the joints between the sacrum and pelvis. Usually on one side only, the point of maximum tenderness is off-centre to the affected side; bending forward and to the affected side are painful and restricted. The condition is sometimes seen in people who have to work standing with their weight mainly on one leg, e.g., dentists, or in cases where the legs are of unequal length.

In the foregoing it is often possible to make a diagnosis on clinical grounds alone, but x-ray examination may show up the following:

5. Osteo-arthritis of the spine. The movements of the lumbar spine are limited, and x-ray will show osteoporosis and bony outgrowths.

6. Prolapsed intervertebral disc. (Commonly known as 'slipped disc'.) Excessive strain may rupture the fibro-cartilaginous pad between vertebrae, and portions of it may protrude to cause pressure on the related spinal nerves emerging between the vertebrae. This is also a common cause of pain radiating down the leg in the regions served by the sciatic nerve (sciatica).

7. Spondylolisthesis. In this condition there is developmental defect of a vertebra, usually the fifth lumbar, so that it does not retain its proper position in relation to the sacrum.

8. Other bone disease. The spine is a common site of osseous tuberculosis, and in malignant disease secondary tumour deposits may be seen on x-ray examination.

9. Other causes. Any investigation must include search for causes in the abdominal and pelvic organs. The commonest abdominal causes are diseases, such as infection or abscess of the kidney and related tissues together with malignant disease of any organ.

In the female there may be pain, usually felt in the sacro-iliac joints, resulting from the laxity of ligaments which occurs during and after childbirth. Pain may also be felt in the back from pelvic infection, a displaced uterus, or tumours of the uterus and ovaries.

Treatment. This depends entirely on professional determination of the underlying cause and only some general principles can be stated. Lumbago generally responds rapidly to rest, analgesics, and local heat, although it is prone to recur. Lumbar back strain is dealt with similarly but lumbo-sacral and sacro-iliac strain will probably require some form of supportive corset.

Prolapsed disc can often be relieved by traction and subsequent support but some cases come to operation for removal of the damaged disc and surgical ankylosis.

Osteo-arthritis is an established chronic condition for which not a great deal can be done except to provide support to limit painful movement. Spondylolisthesis is treated by surgical ankylosis. Tuberculosis of the spine requires prolonged immobilization and anti-tubercular drugs.

Pelvic and abdominal conditions call for local treatment where this is possible.

Prevention. Since causes are numerous, prevention is highly complex. To take some examples, sacro-iliac strain can in large measure be avoided by teaching people who

have to lift heavy weights how best to do so; the backache caused by a displaced uterus can be avoided by post-natal examination of the woman and attention being given to the displaced organ. Tuberculosis of the spine can be prevented by general measures for the prevention of tuberculosis, and osteo-arthritis can be made less common by attention to weight and posture.

backwardness in children. At birth the human infant displays only reflex activity of a primitive protective nature such as the 'grasping reflex' (the well-known strong grip with which a tiny baby will clutch an offered finger) and Moro's 'startle reflex' (an outward movement of arms and legs in response to, say, a knock on the side of the cot). From birth to adolescence the child continues to grow and develop, and its normality or otherwise can be assessed by its physical, intellectual, and social progress.

A child who fails to reach developmental status appropriate to chronological age is regarded as 'backward' or retarded. The term is conventionally restricted to delayed development of physical and intellectual skills. Retarded growth in itself is 'dwarfism' and delayed emotional progress is better referred to as 'IMMATURITY'.

In a child of school age 'backwardness' implies a limitation of intellectual ability or a retardation of educational progress likely to preclude education in a normal class. In general, 'backwardness' implies a retardation less marked than that indicated by 'MENTAL DEFICIENCY'.

Causes. Some cases are genetic in origin and the commonest of these is mongolism (or Down's syndrome). Others such as phenylketonuria, galactosaemia and hypothyroidism (cretinism) are due to faulty METABOLISM and relatively uncommon but it is important that they should be recognized early so that suitable treatment can be given before irreparable brain damage occurs. Most of these, if untreated or untreatable, really fall into the more extreme category of mental deficiency.

However, many more cases of mental retardation are due to adverse influences such as toxaemia infection and anoxia, either recorded or presumed, which may affect the child before, during, or immediately after birth. The frequent association of physical defects such as congenital heart disease and brain or nerve damage confirm some such specific causation.

There is, however, a normal range of intelligence in the individuals of any community, from the dullards to the very clever, and some children regarded as backward are really within the normal intellectual range. They have potential within the lower levels of the normal range of intelligence but their progress may have been impaired by social deprivation or emotional difficulties. With appropriate and understanding care and education they have good prospects of improvement.

Another important group comprises children who have no intellectual defect whatever but have been held back by some physical handicap affecting their sensory or motor functions, such as deafness, defective vision, or paralysis. They respond to appropriate treatment – once recognized. (In the past this has too often failed to happen.)

Developmental assessment. A suspicion of backwardness is aroused when either the mother or (in Britain) the health visitor notices that a child is failing to reach the 'milestones' of its development during infancy and pre-school years at the expected age for any particular achievement. Points to note are when the child starts to smile, sit, stand, walk, speak, feed himself, and become toilet trained. Other guidelines are his response to visual and auditory stimuli, his attention to sounds, the ability to follow with his eyes, his use of meaningful phrases and sentences, and his readiness to play with building bricks. Feeding difficulties, sleeping difficulties, irritability, or undue placidity also require consideration in forming an assessment of mental deficiency.

Although observations of this kind have a reasonable predictive value, a more formal plan of developmental assessment is desirable for all children, and well-organized child welfare schemes are providing this to an increasing extent. In recent years there has been a greater use of intelligence tests designed for all ages.

The practice of paediatrics is developing the sub-specialities of neo-natal and developmental paediatrics. The neo-natal paediatrician is in a favourable position to identify the 'at risk' child, whose future development may have been prejudiced by adverse occurrences before or during birth. The developmental paediatrician is responsible for organized 'developmental screening' (which ideally should provide for assessment at 6 weeks, 6 months, 10 months, 18 months, 2 years, 3 years and 4½ years of age) and has the skill and experience to detect promptly any deviation from normal and the opportunity to initiate any treatment which may help to ensure that the child will achieve the maximum performance of which he is potentially capable.

bacteria. Minute living organisms of vegetable nature, bacteria are visible only microscopically. Properly, they are only one sub-division of the 'fission-fungi' but the term is generally used as synonymous with 'microbes' or 'germs' and it is in this sense that they are described here. From bacterium is also derived bacteriology or the general study of all forms of micro-organisms.

Bacteria are found in air, water, soil, on the skin and hair of animals including man, and particularly in the intestinal tract, and they are found too wherever there is death or decomposition, and often in disease. They are responsible for the spoilage of food, and effects such as the souring of milk and the putrefaction of cheese and meat are everyday examples of their action. Some are associated with specific diseases and are called 'pathogenic bacteria'. Many of the bacteria found in man are harmless – or even beneficial – but others cause disease.

Bacteria are exceedingly small, single-celled plants without chlorophyll and of various shapes. Round ones are called 'cocci', straight or curved rods are respectively 'bacilli' and 'vibrios'. Spiral or undulatory forms are 'spirilli'. The latter are mobile but some of the rod-shaped forms have whip-like extrusions of their protoplasm, called flagellae, which also serve for propulsion.

Under favourable conditions of food supply, moisture, and temperature, bacteria multiply rapidly and their 'colonies' become visible to the naked eye. Most species require oxygen for their development (the aerobes) but some cannot tolerate oxygen and are classified as anaerobes. They reproduce by swelling and then simply dividing into two at intervals of about every two hours, so that one bacterium on Monday morning may have given rise to four thousand by Tuesday morning and to several millions by Wednesday morning. However, some also reproduce by spores, which are rounded bodies appearing at the end or in the middle of a bacterium. Spore-formation is a response to an insufficient food supply or other adverse influences and enables life to be maintained until conditions become more favourable.

Bacteria in nature. Bacteria obtain their food-supply by breaking down organic matter, particularly the dead tissues and waste products of animals and plants, and by doing this the constituent elements are liberated to re-enter the cycle of growth and decay. The most vital of these is nitrogen. By bacterial action ammonia is released from dead protein and further oxidation forms the nitrates necessary for soil-fertility and plant growth.

Some bacteria can also extract nitrogen from the atmosphere. They grow in root nodules on certain plants, particularly the legumes and clovers. These plants can be grown on poor soils and ploughed in to improve fertility for better pastures and heavier food crops. All these soil bacteria are essential to cultivation and indeed (as a link in the 'nitrogen cycle') to life itself.

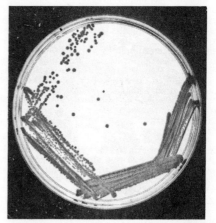

Bacteria: a culture growth of *Candida albicans*

Bacteria in industry. Many traditional crafts and industrial processes depend on bacteria. Examples are the making of cheese and wine, brewing, the maturation of silage, the decomposition of pectin in plant tissues as in flax-retting, the manufacture of alcohol, glycerin, acetic acid, citric acid and lactic acid, the production of enzymes and antibiotics, and many others. The biological treatment of sewage is another of their indispensable uses.

Bacteria and disease. Until the nineteenth century infectious diseases were a mystery, with theories of their cause based on superstition and misconception. Only better microscopy reinforcing the inspiration and work of pioneers like Pasteur and Koch led to the correct appreciation of the part played by the presence of micro-organisms in the animal body as the agents causing disease.

These 'pathogenic' micro-organisms vary considerably. There are protozoa, fungi, and viruses in addition to bacteria which can invade the body and multiply within it to cause illness, and often death, by tissue destruction and the effects of their toxic products.

The list of bacterial diseases in man is a long one and the following merely indicates the variety of well-known conditions which have a bacterial origin:

1. Wound infections: local sepsis due to staphylococci or streptococci; septicaemia from the same organisms; tetanus; anthrax.

2. Cardiac infections: bacterial endocarditis.

3. Respiratory tract infections: scarlet fever; diphtheria; pneumonia; tuberculosis; whooping cough.

4. Intestinal infections: typhoid and paratyphoid fevers; cholera; bacillary dysentery.

5. Urinary tract infections: gonorrhoea; intestinal organisms.

6. Central nervous system: cerebro-spinal fever; other forms of septic meningitis.

7. Generalized infections: plague; glanders; undulant fever.

Infection. When bacterial invasion of the body tissues takes place the result is disease. The process is spoken of as 'infection' and the organism responsible is deemed 'pathogenic' or capable of producing disease.

But 'pathogenic' is not a rigid term as applied to a particular micro-organism. It is often only pathogenic to a particular animal species, and its capacity to cause disease, even in that animal, is determined by various factors such as its present virulence, the numbers of bacteria present in the infective matter, the path of infection, the local tissue resistance of the victim, and his state of immunity.

If an individual is in a healthy or resistant state even large quantities of virulent bacteria can be destroyed by the body defences before damage occurs.

If, however, the bacteria gain a foothold they exercise their harmful effects by means of their toxins which are of two kinds – exotoxins and endotoxins – and the difference is fundamental for treatment. Exotoxins, as in diphtheria or tetanus, can be neutralized by a suitable antitoxin, but organisms producing harmful effects by endotoxins must themselves be attacked and the prospect of doing this successfully has been greatly improved for most common bacterial diseases by the development of ANTIBIOTIC drugs.

The manner in which the body overcomes infection by its own efforts or is protected from it artificially is dealt with in the article on IMMUNITY.

bacteriology. Literally, bacteriology is the study of BACTERIA and their effects but it is a relatively young and growing science which embraces much more than is implied by even the popular and imprecise meaning of bacteria. Microbiology is a newer and better term for a subject which can include the natural history and behaviour of all minute plants and animals.

Since bacteria are so tiny, the development of bacteriology has been greatly dependent on the parallel development of the microscope from the primitive one first constructed by the Dutch naturalist van Leeuwenhoek in 1683, magnifying only some 100 times, to the instruments of today with their much greater power and much better definition.

A magnification of 1000 is the practical maximum for a microscope dependent on visible light because of the limitations imposed by the wave-length of the light itself, and this is insufficient for the study of viruses and of the finer detail of larger organisms. For these purposes there is now the electron microscope using not light but an electron beam focused by magnetic fields. This has provided a further tenfold increase in magnifying power.

The practice of bacteriology is, essentially, dual-purpose. Firstly it is engaged in the purely academic task of discovering, isolating, identifying, and classifying the immense range of living creatures which are the subject of its study. Secondly it is concerned with how its systematic knowledge of bacteria, their properties and effects, can be employed in the useful arts and in the elucidation of the causes of disease in order to develop methods of prevention, diagnosis and treatment.

The better microscopes of the late nineteenth century enabled bacteriologists to see bacteria and to describe their shapes and general appearance, but it soon became evident that this was not sufficient. To study them effectively there was a need to be able to identify them positively, to isolate separate species, and to determine their individual characteristics and behaviour, both in the test-tube and in relation to other living organisms.

A simple but fundamental advance was the introduction of the plate culture by Koch (1881). In nature, and in liquid media, the problems of separating and differentiating various kinds of bacteria were insuperable. By spreading material containing bacteria in a thin layer on a sheet of solid nutrient material composed basically of gelatin and peptone, and then incubating it, the individual bacteria grew into separate visible colonies from which samples could be taken for sub-culture and further study.

Almost as important was the discovery by Weigert (1871) that bacteria took up aniline dyes or stains in different ways and this not only made them easier to see microscopically but helped in their primary classification.

Once bacteria could be obtained in pure culture further methods for their identification became possible. These were largely based on the characteristics of their metabolism such as their ability to ferment various sugars, their selective growth on special media, and on their reaction with other living organisms. During their growth bacteria produce complex protein substances called 'antigens'. Injected into an animal these stimulate production of antibody in the blood serum which is specific for a particular antigen. Serum containing antibody will react with antigen to form a precipitate, and with a suspension of the original organism will produce clumping (or agglutination) of the suspended organisms. Procedures of this kind proved to be a particularly sensitive means of determining identity. Another important discovery was that bacteria themselves are parasitized by virus particles known as 'bacteriophages' and the presence of these even enables different strains of the same bacterium to be traced.

Practical applications. Many traditional crafts and industrial processes depend on bacteria – wine making, cheese-making, and the manufacture of vinegar and glycerin to mention only a few. Bacteriology has demonstrated how these operate and now provides the means for scientific control and improvement.

In medicine the examination of discharges from a patient enables an infective illness to be accurately diagnosed. In some diseases such as diphtheria, tetanus, and anthrax the administration of antiserum prepared by bacteriological methods provides a means of treatment. A wide range of diseases can now be prevented by the giving of inoculations whose efficiency and safety again depends on bacteriological control. On a community scale bacteriology plays a part in the control of epidemics.

Scope. Because of the ubiquity of bacteria and other micro-organisms, such as protozoa, fungi and viruses, and their widespread influence on human interests it is clear that bacteriology or microbiology has now become a subject too large to be encompassed as a single speciality. Many workers now concentrate their attention on separate aspects related to medicine, veterinary medicine, industrial processes, soils, dairy practice and IMMUNIZATION. Obviously this is a trend which will continue to grow.

balance. The sense of balance is maintained mainly by the three semi-circular canals at right angles to each other in the inner EAR. Movement of the head in any direction causes movement of the fluid in one or more canals, from which nervous impulses are passed to the brain which then directs appropriate muscles to adjust the position of the body. Balance is also assisted by vision and by pressure of the soles on the ground, but in general any disturbance of the sense of balance is due to factors affecting the inner ear.

balanitis. An acute inflammatory condition affecting the mucous membrane of the head of the penis and accompanied by pain, swelling, and purulent discharge. It is usually associated with gonorrhoea, but poor hygiene and a redundant or unretractable foreskin may predispose to an infection caused by other pus-forming organisms.

baldness. The lack or loss of hair, known medically as alopecia. It occurs almost exclusively in males (although it appears in some women after the menopause) and may commence quite early in adult life with atrophy of the hair-follicles (see HAIR). No specific cause is known and a tendency to early loss of hair is merely an inborn characteristic of the individual. Sometimes, but by no means always, it is associated with seborrhoea in which inflammation around the follicle may hasten the process.

Baldness usually follows a familiar pattern, with thinning of the hair on the temples and top of the head gradually extending until the crown is quite hairless or covered only by downy growth while the sides and back remain comparatively normal. No known treatment has any real success.

Apart from classical baldness, a temporary or permanent hair-loss may occur from toxic influences e.g., acute infections such as typhoid fever and poisoning from arsenic or thallium. X-rays produce a similar result.

A special variety of baldness is alopecia areata where the hair falls out in patches. The cause of this is equally obscure but the condition tends to occur in neurotic subjects and may be related to the influence of nerves on the nutrition and maintenance of normal conditions in the scalp tissue. However, re-growth usually takes place spontaneously, and treatment by stimulating applications, which increase blood flow in the scalp, may help to hasten a cure.

bandages and bandaging. Bandages are strips of material used for binding up any part of the body, and bandaging is the procedure of applying them in the proper manner.

Purposes of bandaging. (1) To maintain in position a dressing, splint, or other application; (2) to maintain a limb or other part of the body in a desired position; (3) to supply support or pressure, as in varicose veins; (4) to limit the collecting of tissue fluids after injury; and (5) to prevent or control haemorrhage.

Types of bandage. Bandages are of many types, materials, and sizes, adapted to the purpose for which they are required, and may be either inextensible or elastic. Those commonly employed in modern practice are (1) cotton bandages of varying densities of weave – gauze, muslin, and calico; (2) flannel or domette (cotton warp; woollen weft) bandages; (3) crepe bandages with natural elasticity from the nature of their weave; (4) elastic adhesive bandages; (5) rubber bandages – used for arrest of haemorrhage; (6) plaster-of-paris bandages used for supporting fractures; and (7) tubular gauze bandages which require a special applicator.

Bandages are now manufactured in metric sizes and the commercial range for ordinary cotton is 2.5 cm., 5.0 cm., 7.5 cm., and 10 cm. in width by 5.0 m. in length. They are supplied rolled ready for use and usually known as roller bandages.

Special bandages. (1) triangular bandage – an isosceles triangle of calico with base of 127 cm. and sides of 90 cm. It is versatile and is extensively used for first aid work. (2) Many tailed bandage, for chest and abdomen. (3) Four-tailed bandage, for jaw. (4) T-bandage, for perineum. (5) Capelline bandage, a double-headed roller bandage used for the scalp.

Principles of bandaging. The availability of loosely-woven and extensible materials which readily conform to the shape of the body has greatly reduced the degree of skill which bandaging formerly required, but the correct application of an ordinary roller bandage is still something of an art which needs practice and some study of the technique employed. More detailed instructions can be found in any good First Aid manual.

There are, however, four standard bandaging procedures which can be readily adapted to various situations.

1. The spiral bandage. Stand facing the part to be bandaged with a bandage of suitable width in the hand nearest the outer side of the limb and with the unrolled part of the bandage uppermost so that it will unroll readily. Start from below and bandage from within outwards

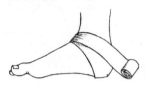
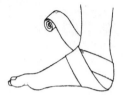
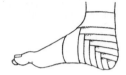

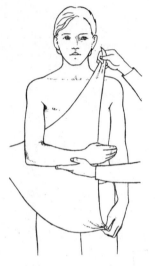
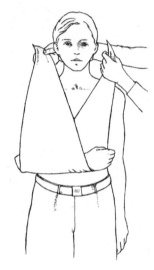
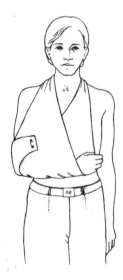

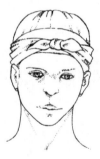

Bandaging

over the front of the limb. After fixing the tail of the bandage by two superimposed turns proceed up the limb covering two-thirds of the preceding turn. This procedure can be continued on a part of uniform girth but when the limb widens the bandage will not lie flat and it is then necessary to introduce 'reverses'. To do this the last turn is fixed by the thumb of the disengaged hand and the bandage is allowed to turn over so that it forms a fold with the edge against the thumb; the inner surface of the bandage thus becomes the outer. Another turn is taken and the process repeated, care being taken to keep the reverses in line. Finally the bandage is tied off by splitting the end and knotting or secured with a safety-pin.

2. The figure-of-eight bandage. This is used for ankle, knee and elbow joints. Starting with two turns round the joint the bandage is applied in widening loops alternately above and below the joint. The centre point of the '8' is kept in front of the elbow and ankle and behind the knee.

3. The spica bandage. A modified figure-of-eight bandage used for shoulder and hip and also for the thumb. For the shoulder start with spiral turns round the upper arm till the armpit is reached. Then carry the bandage over the shoulder, across the back, under the opposite armpit, across the chest, over the injured shoulder, under the armpit of the same side, and so back to the starting point. This procedure is repeated until the shoulder is covered. In other situations the figure-of-eight is made round thigh and pelvis or thumb and wrist.

Cautions. Never bandage a limb below the lower level of a splint and always on completion of a bandage inspect the extremities of a limb to see that the circulation is not impaired. By pressing on the nails and then releasing the pressure it can be judged if blood flow is satisfactory.

barber's rash. An infective condition of the skin of the face affecting the 'beard region' where there are hair follicles. There are three main types according to the infecting organism. Streptococcal infection causes superficial crusting, as in impetigo, and ringworm of the beard (*Tinea barbae*) may be either scaly or suppurative. Sycosis barbae is usually due to infection with staphylococci often from the patient's own nostrils, and caused by minor injury during shaving. Papules and pustules appear in the beard area, often with reddening of the surrounding skin.

Treatment is by application of an appropriate antibiotic twice daily for about a fortnight with avoidance of shaving or the use of an electric razor. Hygienic precautions should include the use of personal towels and their disinfection before laundering. Most cases clear up readily. In the very occasional case that does not respond to treatment the patient may have to be advised to discontinue shaving and grow a beard.

barbiturates. A large and varied group of drugs which reduce the activity of the central nervous system. They are organic compounds derived from barbituric acid, which is a condensation product of urea.

The earliest drug of the group to be used in medicine was barbitone (or diethyl barbituric acid) which originally appeared under the trade-name Veronal.

Types. Barbiturates may be classified according to their pharmacological action:

1. General anaesthetic agents. Preparations given intravenously to produce short term general anaesthesia. They are extensively used in dentistry and in minor surgical procedures. Examples are thiopentone sodium, hexobarbitone sodium, and thialbarbitone sodium marketed under various trade names.

2. Hypnotics and sedatives. The distinction between a hypnotic and a sedative is largely a matter of dosage. Hypnotic doses directly induce sleep but the same drug in lesser dosage may be prescribed simply to induce mental relaxation, lessen emotional tension, and decrease anxiety.

Barbiturates of this group also differ in their duration of action and this can be a factor in deciding which particular preparation should be given. (1) Long-acting: phenobarbitone and derivatives; also used as anti-convulsants; (2) medium-acting: allobarbitone, butobarbitone and amylobarbitone; (3) short-acting: cyclobarbitone, quinalbarbitone, etc.

3. Tranquillizers. These are used when it is desired to calm anxiety without noticeable sedation or impairment of mental function but there are better drugs for this than the barbiturates.

Some compound preparations are available in which an attempt has been made to counteract the sedative effect of a barbiturate by adding a cerebral stimulant so that there is a period of sedation and reduction of anxiety, followed – as the second drug takes effect – by rapid restoration of full mental activity. In general, however, these preparations are not very useful.

Use. Barbiturates undoubtedly have a legitimate place in medical practice but their use needs careful consideration and control.

In some individuals they produce undesirable side-effects such as nausea, diarrhoea, lassitude, vertigo, and skin eruptions. In the elderly they often cause mental confusion. Their effect is enhanced by simultaneous consumption of alcohol, and this is not always appreciated by persons driving motor-vehicles.

Tolerance to their use is easily acquired and there is a temptation to employ increasing doses. They are also cumulative and carry a serious risk of accidental or suicidal overdosage. Poisoning by barbiturates leads to breathing becoming slower and also shallower and may lead to coma. These conditions require intensive and skilled treatment, but despite this many fatalities still occur.

In relation to drug dependence barbiturates now cause considerable concern. Psychic dependence is a continuing demand for the administration of a drug either for pleasure or for the avoidance of discomfort, and the very widespread use of barbiturates is in many instances an example of this.

The size of the problem can be seen from the fact that in Britain 6 per cent of the total number of prescriptions written is for drugs in the barbiturate group. It is also estimated that there are at least 600,000 regular users of barbiturates of whom 100,000 are dependent.

barium. In its pure state barium is a pale yellow metallic element classified with the other alkaline earth metals magnesium, calcium, and strontium. In nature it occurs as 'heavy-spar' or barytes, which is barium sulphate, and as the mineral witherite, mainly barium carbonate.

Its soluble salts are poisonous and are not now employed pharmacologically, with the possible exception of barium sulphide, which may be used in depilatory creams.

Barium sulphate has however an important medical use in diagnostic x-ray work as it provides the radio-opaque constituent of 'barium meals' and enemata. The gastro-intestinal tract is not itself opaque to x-ray, but the barium sulphate in the tract makes it visible on the x-ray plate.

barley water. A bland drink made by the infusion of 30 g. of pearl or prepared barley in

0.5 l. of boiling water (1 oz. to 1 pint). It may be used in the treatment of gastro-intestinal disorder in infants or invalids and is a convenient mild diuretic in kidney disease or inflammatory conditions of the urinary tract. It may be sweetened or flavoured by the addition of lemon juice. Commercial preparations of barley water are readily available.

Barlow's disease. A deficiency disease of infancy characterized by a tendency to haemorrhage into the skin and from mucosal surfaces, and by disorders of bone development. Also known as infantile SCURVY, it is due to a deficiency of vitamin C in the diet. Although breast milk generally contains adequate amounts of this vitamin, the artificially-fed infant requires supplementary vitamin C in the form of orange juice or equivalent proprietary preparations.

basal metabolism. See METABOLISM.

battered baby. A child who has been subjected to violence from a parent. The frequency of such cases has been slow to gain recognition because of a natural reluctance to believe that any parents could maltreat their children, but it has been suggested that up to 10 per cent of cases of serious childhood injury reaching hospital may be due to this cause. The battered baby syndrome, however, includes lesser injury, and the child who shows frequent bruising, and who apparently fails to thrive at home may equally be a victim of parental abuse and neglect.

The parents of such children fall into three overlapping groups: some 4 to 5 per cent have been shown to have psychopathic personalities, a large number are emotionally inadequate or emotionally immature (often as a result of deprivation in their own childhood) and many, while apparently normal and well-adjusted, are harrassed to the point of frenzy by abnormal local or domestic circumstances.

For recognizing children 'at risk' the British health visitor is in a key position: her nursing training is supplemented by her further training in psychology and social science; in addition she has unique knowledge of the families she is visiting and unrivalled access to their homes without being sent for. Unfortunately, however, many mothers who have struck or felt strongly tempted to strike their babies are overwhelmed by guilt feelings, considering their conduct (or contemplated conduct) monstrous and unnatural. So, instead of confiding their impulses to the health visitor in order to get support and help, they try to conceal their aggressive feelings and to hide minor violence, without realising that the same circumstances that created the impulse to violence may recur, and on that later occasion they may seriously hurt the child.

Where a child is identified as being 'at risk', whether by the mother wisely confiding or by the health visitor observing signs of aggression or potential aggression, prevention is still far from easy. The harrassed parent of reasonable maturity can at least be given help and support during times of crisis and can sometimes be afforded considerable relief by the older children being admitted to a day nursery or nursery school; the less mature or inadequate parent can also be helped by these measures, by counselling by the health visitor, and sometimes by being given an address or phone number to contact in moments of despair; but it is difficult to aid a psychopath (or two psychopaths, since like tends to marry like) and removal of a child deemed to be 'at risk' is generally impracticable until there is clear evidence that child abuse has actually taken place.

Collaboration between health visitors, social workers and general medical practitioners is obviously desirable and can appreciably reduce baby battering, but two types are probably unpreventable: (1) where the parent has shown no previous signs of abnormal aggression and the child has no unexplained bruises, but sudden circumstances reduce the parent to such a state of harrassment that serious violence occurs; and (2) where a child is suspected to be 'at risk' but parents decline help, and evidence to justify removal is lacking.

BCG vaccination. The initials stand for Bacillus of Calmette (1863-1933) and Guérin (1816-95), French bacteriologist and surgeon respectively. The bacillus itself is derived from a culture of the bovine variety of the tubercle bacillus rendered harmless by prolonged breeding under laboratory conditions. The BCG vaccination is preventive; inoculation against TUBERCULOSIS uses a living suspension of this harmless organism.

To explain the procedure it is necessary to say something about the natural history of tuberculous infection. Under ordinary living conditions every individual is likely sooner or later to acquire an infection caused by the tubercle bacillus. The risk of this is diminishing but until tuberculosis is completely eradicated it will continue to exist. The first exposure to infection, although it produces a definite tissue reaction is not necessarily followed by disease and in most cases the 'primary complex', usually in the lung and associated lymph glands, heals without incident. Recovery is accompanied by a degree of immunity to re-infection and by development of allergy to 'tuberculin', a product of the tubercle bacillus.

The immunity although substantial is not absolute and if an individual is subsequently re-exposed to massive infection or if his resistance is lowered by other factors, re-infection may still occur. The disease process is then of a different pattern, determined by the pre-existing allergy and may cause local destruction of tissue without any spread along the lymphatic vessels.

Thus BCG vaccination is an attempt to produce this relative immunity in a controlled fashion and at the most advantageous time, having regard to the risks of infection and the susceptibility of the subject.

Mention has been made of allergy or sensitivity to tuberculin, and the detection of this by means of the tuberculin test is an essential part of BCG vaccination, because it is both undesirable and unnecessary to vaccinate persons who have already been infected. The test also provides a means of checking that vaccination has been successful in inducing the altered reactivity associated with immunity.

There are several varieties of the tuberculin test based on pricking the skin (von Pirquet); application onto the skin (Moro, Hamburyer, 'patch' tests); or injection into the skin (Mantoux, Heaf, 'Tine-test,' and modifications). The most reliable is the Mantoux test, in which a measured quantity of a standard concentration of tuberculin is injected into the skin of the front of the forearm and the result examined in seventy-two hours. An area of redness and thickening constitutes a positive result.

The detailed procedure for BCG vaccination is therefore as follows: (1) Mantoux test, (2) read result, (3) if positive – no further action, (4) if negative – give standard dose of vaccine, (5) six to eight weeks later repeat Mantoux test to determine whether the previously negative result has converted to positive, indicating acquirement of immunity.

There remains the still mildly-controversial question of whom to vaccinate. Clearly tuberculin negative contacts should be done and also other persons at special risk, such as nurses and medical students. In addition most experts now recommend and offer general routine vaccination of the pre-adolescent about the age of 14 in order to ensure good protection during the years of greatest susceptibility. On the other hand some advocate vaccination of the infant at birth but the arguments against this are substantial and the reasons in favour have lessened as the level of community infection has declined.

Although BCG vaccination was introduced by Calmette in 1921 its general acceptance took a long time because of doubts about its safety and efficacy. Some of the opposition and prejudice stemmed unfairly from what was known as 'Lübeck disaster.' In Lübeck in 1933, 251 infants were given by mouth what purported to be a BCG vaccine. Because of a manufacturing error the vaccine contained virulent tubercle and 77 infants died. This unfortunate accident engendered unfounded fears which persisted for many years.

In modern practice the procedure is now regarded as effective, safe, and practically trouble free.

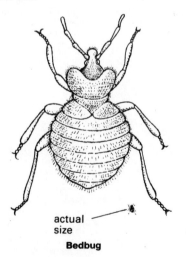

actual size

Bedbug

bedbugs. Nocturnal insect parasites infesting unclean houses. The bedbug (*Cimex lectularius*) is 4 to 5 mm. long, reddish-brown in colour, broad and flat and has a prominent beak-like proboscis, which it uses to suck blood from its human hosts in bed at night. It lives in mattresses, in crevices of bedsteads, behind

loose wall-paper and in cracked plaster; it prefers fairly warm conditions in the region of 10° to 21° C. (50° to 70° F.), and it has a characteristic musty smell.

The female lays some 200 eggs at the rate of four or five a day. These hatch in six days and the nymphs subsequently develop into adult insects.

Bedbugs can be eradicated by cleanliness and good standards of housekeeping combined with the use of a reliable insecticidal spray and powder based on pyrethrin/DDT.

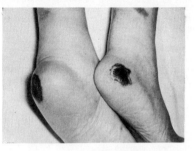

Bed sores

bed sores. Sores or ulcers occurring in persons confined to bed for long periods and caused by continued pressure interfering with circulation of blood to the compressed tissues. Common sites are the back, buttocks, heels and elbows. Bed sores are in the main preventable by good nursing, including seeing that sheets are not crumpled, regular and frequent changes of the patient's position and careful washing and very gentle drying of the compressed areas. Further preventive measures are: gentle massage of these areas to stimulate blood circulation; application of methylated spirit and zinc and boracic ointment; and, if reddening appears, cushioning of the part, e.g., by use of an air-ring or by air-beds or water-beds for long-term patients. Where bed sores have occurred, treatment is difficult; if there is no infection, spraying with a 5 per cent solution of tannic acid may help; and if infection is present, a penicillin cream may be useful.

bedwetting. Most children are dry at night by about the age of 2½ years. Substantial continuation of bedwetting, known medically as nocturnal enuresis, after that age, or reversion by a child previously dry, may indicate disease of the kidney or bladder, but is far more commonly of psychological origin. In such cases, the child is subconsciously seeking to return to the more protected life of babyhood, because he feels unprotected, insecure, or unloved often through no fault of the parents but because of such factors as the birth of a younger child or the mother's return to work.

Scolding and punishment merely aggravate the situation, and fluid restriction in the evening seldom helps. After the situation has been ignored for six months or so in the hope of spontaneous recovery, and after medical examination has excluded physical causes, the child may need expert psychological examination (e.g., at a child guidance clinic) so that his insecurities and frustrations can be identified and removed gradually.

bee sting. See BITES AND STINGS.

behaviour. The ways in which people (or animals) conduct themselves in relation to others or to their physical or social environment, and also the ways in which they react to stresses and to abnormal situations.

Sources of behaviour. It is only in recent decades that psychologists have begun to appreciate the enormous complexity of sources of behaviour.

The simplest theory of human behaviour is that it is normally rational: we do things initially as a matter of trial and error, and then persist in the actions that lead to satisfactory results. Obviously reasoning plays a substantial part in shaping our behaviour. We decline to trust a particular man because he has cheated us in the past and we infer that he might do so again, and we put on a raincoat because our experience suggests to us the likelihood of rain. Yet we do not necessarily take adequate exercise or cut down cigarette smoking despite knowing that the one is good or the other bad for us. Much of our behaviour is not based on reason.

The behaviourist school, led by Pavlov and later Watson, has shown that much behaviour can be traced to past training and experience; and indeed, if this were not so, our entire educational system would be valueless. Our religious and political philosophies, for example, are in most cases based either on views and attitudes acquired in childhood or, perhaps less frequently, on sharp revolt against those of childhood. Yet to attribute behaviour simply to an extension of conditioned reflexes is to ignore thought, feeling, emotion and virtually every creative impulse.

Freud and the psychoanalysts demonstrated that a considerable part of our behaviour is based on ideas and experiences that have been repressed into the unconscious. The existence of unconscious mental activity is revealed by the common practice of 'sleeping on a problem', and many of our likes, hates and fears are explicable only on the ground of influences below the level of consciousness.

Sociologists and social psychologists have stressed the large part played by cultures and sub-cultures. Even the person who prides himself on his independence is greatly influenced by the values and judgments of those with whom he is – or has been – associated.

Not least, our behaviour is influenced by the hormones produced by the endocrine glands. A woman of nervous type is more nervous during and immediately before menstruation and some women are capricious in the early months of pregnancy.

Also, just as mind influences body, body affects mind. When very tired we are irritable and may behave unreasonably. When recovering from influenza we tend to see the gloomy side of any situation.

A doctor who seeks to cure a patient of a painful condition has a relatively easy task, because the patient is strongly motivated to follow the advice given. By contrast any health worker who aims to alter the attitudes and behaviour of a person who is not yet ill has to be aware of the complexity of the sources of behaviour.

Behaviour disorders. These are conditions in which behaviour is considered objectionable by a person's associates or by society at large. Examples are outbursts of destructiveness, stealing in a law-abiding community and sexual conduct regarded as intolerable by the current standards of the district. The relationship to standards should be noted: for example, wife-beating is abnormal behaviour in most social groups today but not in all, and the whipping of erring servants was regarded as normal conduct in the eighteenth century.

As indicated above, a number of factors influence an individual's behaviour; these include standards learned in childhood, experiences of later life which have a psychological influence, and variations in psychological make-up – which, in turn, are governed by factors as widely differing as the daily alcohol intake and the functioning of the ENDOCRINE SYSTEM. In recent years it has been increasingly recognized that behaviour disorders may also be the outcome of social interactions.

In the past the tendency has been to account for behaviour disorders as being either the result of unusual chemico-physiological disturbances (such as are caused by alcohol or drugs) or of psychological problems such as repression or conflict, or of brain damage. To a great extent most cases of behaviour disorder probably spring from these causes (see FREUD, NEUROSIS and PERVERSION). However, nowadays a small additional group is recognized: in Russia people who hold unorthodox and inconvenient views are, by very definition, deemed mentally sick; and in the Western World it is far from unknown for families to reject an 'unacceptable' member by negotiating with the medical profession until an acceptable label of some form of mental illness is adopted.

The work of child guidance clinics has to some extent clarified abnormal behaviour in children, but – despite our increasing knowledge of hormones and the central nervous system on the one hand and of psychological and social interaction on the other – the appearance of extraordinary behaviour in a previously 'normal' adult is in many cases still something of a mystery.

belching. The sudden expulsion of wind from the stomach otherwise known as eructation. The gas may arise from fermentation within the stomach or from the swallowing of air.

belladonna. An extract from the deadly nightshade plant, containing ATROPINE. It was so named from its one-time use in the Middle East to enhance the brilliance of ladies' eyes, since it causes the pupil to dilate.

Bell's palsy. See FACIAL PARALYSIS.

bends. See DECOMPRESSION DISEASE.

benign. Essentially harmless. A benign tumour neither invades adjacent organs nor gives rise to new tumours (secondaries) in other parts of the body. Any symptoms that it produces, e.g., from pressure, are purely the result of its size and position, and if it is removed the tumour is permanently cured.

benzedrine. A drug, amphetamine sulphate, occasionally used in the treatment of mild depressions and of behaviour disorders in children. It is also sometimes employed, in combination with menthol, for treatment of the common cold and of sinus inflammations. Because it has a mild tendency to cause

ADDICTION it is tending to fall into medical disuse.

bereavement. The loss, through death, of a key figure in a person's life.

Personal aspects. When one is bereaved, grief and mourning are inevitable although varying with the closeness of the emotional relationship. There is often a withdrawal of interest from the ordinary affairs of life, a preoccupation with memories of the deceased person, a great feeling of loneliness and frequently weeping, sleeplessness and loss of appetite.

The feelings of unhappiness and even of desolation are natural, and no attempt should be made to hide grief. The grief has to be 'worked through'. In most cases the bereaved person will begin to take an interest in ordinary matters and return to a state of mental equilibrium in about a month, but it does no good to tell such a grief-stricken person that he will get over it. Quiet sympathy and kindness are helpful and, for those who are religious, visits by their clergyman are often useful. Where a husband or wife has died and the surviving spouse may have to move from their home, no immediate decision should be taken: the bereaved person is often in no condition to take decisions, and the sorrowing is sometimes less painful amid the memories – both pleasant and sad – stimulated by the previously shared home.

The visits of friends and relatives, important during the weeks of acute mourning, are no less important later, because the widowed person often finds a marked reduction in the number of friends – not only because some couples have been more interested in the partner who died but also because an unattached person can make an inconvenient number at a dinner table.

It is important to realise that, where the departed person has been much loved, grieving is psychologically necessary. The mourner has to do what has been called his 'grief-work' to enable him in due course to adapt to the loss and to fill the emotional gap.

The two types of mourner likely to need medical – or psychiatric – help (apart from the possible prescription of sedatives during the period of sleeplessness) are the person who shows no return towards normality after six or seven weeks, and the person who apparently utterly suppresses his grief, to all appearance simply coping with the problems of living without any remembrance of the departed loved one.

Social aspects. During the last hundred years there has been a considerable increase in longevity in sophisticated western industrialized social systems. More and more resources have to be devoted to the care of old people and these have to be provided by a proportionately declining work force with pensions and medical care for the elderly imposing an ever increasing burden on a country's gross national product. While the average age at death has increased the comparative advantage of women over men has not changed appreciably. Generally speaking, women tend to experience the consequences of bereavement for a longer period of time than is the case for men who lose their wives.

Used to living with one person for the majority of their adult life, in bereavement people are suddenly faced with the need to adjust to the circumstances and status of a single person. Western societies are erected upon the institution of marriage where occupational roles and social activities are built around the husband and wife as a complementary unit. When the husband dies income from his employment ceases and often a pension stops or falls sharply, and when the wife dies, the widower may have to employ domestic help at considerable cost. On top of this sudden crisis of income is the additional trauma of having to adjust to a single as opposed to a paired condition. However the widowed try to manage their situation, the circle of friendships and acquaintances is likely to diminish almost in spite of any attempt made to preserve them; many social activities and relationships are based on the assumption that two people will be involved, and a widow or widower becomes an awkward encumbrance in social arrangements. In addition to personal grief, financial insecurity, a loss of independence and a degree of social isolation are the frequent consequences of the loss of one's life partner.

The institution which is the major mechanism for handling the consequences of bereavement is still the family. While some relatively affluent couples may retire to 'pensioners' towns', such as Eastbourne, wives on the loss of their husbands frequently return to the families of their offspring. In working class communities the relationship between 'mum' and her married daughters is frequently very close and never severed by the marriage bond. In these circumstances the relationship continues throughout the life of the parents and that of the family or families of the younger generation which are formed as the children grow up and marry. Most widows and widowers are therefore cared for by their relatives, usually daughters and sons-in-law during the final stages of the life cycle.

Support services to families caring for old people are woefully inadequate and when the demands, in terms of time and effort, of providing for the elderly become too great they are removed to nursing homes or to hospital geriatric wards. It is time western societies recognized this progression and increased the facilities available to care for the elderly in non-institutional settings, while recognizing that the last stage of the life cycle is likely to be spent in a hospital for the chronic sick; the facilities therein should make as pleasant as possible the transition from life to death.

beriberi. A disease of malnutrition due to deficiency of vitamin B_1. The disease is characterized by inflammation of the nerves, disturbed sensation, weakness of muscles, heart weakness, and shortness of breath. There is a 'dry' form with increasing weakness and pains, especially of the calf muscles, followed by muscle wasting. The 'wet' form shows oedema of the legs, breathlessness, rapid pulse rate and sometimes palpitations. There is also a 'mixed' form, combining these features, and an infantile form, characterized by generalized oedema, deficient amount of urine, vomiting and lack of appetite.

It occurs mostly in countries in which the staple diet is polished rice, i.e., rice from which the husks (which contain vitamin B_1) have been removed. Prevention is by substituting unpolished for polished rice and by adding to the diet other foods rich in B₁. Treatment is similar, with additional B₁ for some days or weeks (according to severity) at first by injections and subsequently by mouth. A condition rather similar to beriberi is found in some alcoholics, both because they deprive themselves of adequate food and because alcohol to some extent destroys the vitamin.

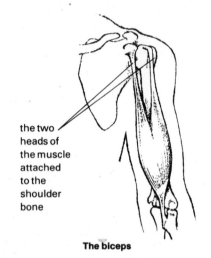

the two heads of the muscle attached to the shoulder bone

The biceps

biceps. Two headed. The term is commonly used as the name for the large muscle that lies superficially on the front of the upper arm, with two tendons to the scapula (or shoulder bone) and a single tendon at the other end attached to the radius. The muscle semi-rotates the forearm, bends the elbow, and helps to flex the shoulder joint.

Another biceps muscle is the biceps femoris, running from the buttock and the back of the thigh down to the fibula in the lower leg; it is concerned with bending the knee.

bifocals. Spectacles in which each lens consists of a part for distant vision and a part for near vision. They are normally unnecessary where glasses are required for only one function, such as motoring or reading, but they can be extremely useful where rapid alternation of close and distant vision is needed, as for example in the case of a lecturer who requires both to see his notes and to see his students. A person wearing bifocals for the first time is liable to make occasional mistakes for a few days, inadvertently trying to use the distance lens for near vision or the close lens for distant vision. Some care is therefore desirable at first when descending stairs or crossing streets, but in almost all cases the difficulties disappear within a week.

bile. A yellowish-brown substance of bitter taste, secreted by the liver and collected and concentrated in the gall-bladder. It is utilized in the digestion of fats and the absorption of fat-soluble vitamins and also in the extraction of waste product from the liver. In certain conditions bile pigment is deposited in the skin, giving rise to the yellowish appearance known as jaundice.

bilharziasis. A disease, otherwise known as schistomiasis, caused by invasion of the body by parasites called fluke worms. The FLUKES have a complicated life cycle and, if swallowed by man, the adults settle in the bladder or intestine, and their spiked eggs irritate the organ before leaving the body in urine or faeces. The disease – common in Africa, the Far and Middle East, and South America – causes bleeding into the urine or symptoms of dysentery.

Eradication is possible by sanitation and health education, or by removing the snails which carry the flukes by chemical treatment of the water. Treatment of the disease is by antimony salts or lucanthone.

biliary colic. The intense pain which arises if a gall-stone is forced through the narrow bile duct towards the intestine. The pain persists until the stone either reaches the intestine or is surgically removed. The blocking of the duct may produce jaundice.

bilious attack. A vague term generally applied to the headache, discomfort, and vomiting that occur in inflammation of the stomach following dietetic indiscretions. The explanation of biliousness is that the liver normally transforms toxic products of digestion into substances that can be excreted by the kidneys, but if these toxic products are in greater quantity than the liver can control they remain in the circulation and cause headache and depression. Simultaneously, the liver produces excess bile in an effort to deal with the toxic products, and the excess bile in turn leads to nausea and vomiting. Prevention is by avoidance of over-indulgence in fatty or greasy foods and moderation in consumption of alcohol.

biopsy. Removal of a tiny piece of tissue from the living body for laboratory examination to determine, for example, the presence or absence of a particular disease or to decide whether a tumour is malignant or benign. In suspected tumours of the skin or of the mucous membrane of the mouth it is very easy to scrape off a minute portion. For less accessible situations special instruments may be required. For instance, a bronchoscope can be used not only for a visual inspection of the bronchi but for the taking of a tiny portion from a bronchus.

birds and disease. Birds eaten as food are neither safer nor more dangerous than other animals. Both can acquire the organisms that cause various diseases, and in both cases inadequate cooking can leave the germs alive. Because of their feeding habits ducks are alleged to be particularly common sources of intestinal infections. It is essential to thaw out frozen poultry for twenty-four hours before cooking, otherwise the cold will protect the germs in the meat. About 4 per cent of British wood pigeons suffer from an avian (or bird) form of tuberculosis: until recent years it was thought that humans were immune to this variety of tuberculosis, but it is now known not only that the avian form can occasionally infect man but also that the avian germ is particularly resistant to antibiotics.

The droppings and cage-dust of infected parrots can transmit psittacosis, a dangerous disease with symptoms like a mixture of typhoid and pneumonia, and various cage-birds can produce ornithosis, a severe form of pneumonia usually contracted by inhalation, e.g., of dust from a budgerigar's cage.

birth control. Deliberate prevention of the union of the sperm and the ovum within the body of a woman after sexual intercourse.

History. Contraceptive methods are probably as old as the earliest population explosions that produced an excess of people over food and resources. The ancient Chinese used withholding of ejaculation (coitus reservatus) and drugs designed to terminate pregnancy. Early Indian writings contain recipes for rendering 'those with gazelle eyes' unfruitful. In the third century B.C. Jewish women wore sponges and did physical exercises to expel semen and had the approval of the law. The Greeks and Romans relied more on abortion and infanticide, though Soranus about A.D. 120 gave in his *Gynaecology* a long description of contraceptive measures, better than anything produced in the next 1700 years. The Arab-Persian civilization was familiar with withdrawal (coitus interruptus) among other methods. Neither Mohammed nor Christ mentioned contraception, and the disapproval of some Christians stems from St. Augustine (who actually directed his attacks mainly on the use of the 'safe period') and St. Thomas Aquinas.

At first fairly uncertain, birth control became substantially more scientific in seventeenth century France. In the U.K. Place's advocacy of the sponge and withdrawal (1823), and in the U.S.A. Owen's plea for the condom and the sponge (1831) led to violent accusations of destroying morality, and attempts to open birth control clinics led to arrests, the latest being in Connecticut in 1961. The legal battle was won in Britain when Charles Bradlaugh and Annie Besant were acquitted in 1878 of publishing an 'obscene' book and yet as late as 1886 a doctor was struck off the Medical Register for publishing a handbook on contraception. Marie Stopes opened a clinic in London in 1921; the Church of England gave limited approval in 1930 and unqualified approval in 1958. The introduction of oral contraceptives in 1956 enormously simplified birth control.

Desirability. In respect of need or desirability birth control falls essentially into four groups: (1) family avoidance, e.g. in carriers of serious hereditary defects; (2) family postponement, e.g., in a young couple seeking to acquire some savings before having a child, or in unmarried people who seek to have intercourse without its consequences; (3) family spacing, e.g., to avoid the mother becoming exhausted or some members of a large family of young children becoming neglected; (4) family limitation, e.g., when a couple have had the number of children they desire, or when a still-birth or the birth of a deformed child has made them aware of a hereditary risk (though this does not imply that all still-births or all handicapped children are the result of genetic defects).

From a national or international point of view birth control should be encouraged because (1) world population is fast outstripping natural resources; (2) children with serious genetic defects (e.g., cases of spina bifida, schizophrenia, mongolism and phenylketonuria) survive in increasing numbers as antenatal care and obstetrics improve; they create enormous physical and emotional problems for the parents who have to care for them and constitute a growing burden on the community; and (3) the rearing of unwanted and neglected children again constitutes a heavy burden on society, while a child brought up in a nursery, orphanage or foster home is often psychologically disadvantaged. Most people appear to accept the general case for birth control, but some would restrict it to married couples (leaving the one-parent child to pay for the sins of his father and mother) and some (despite St. Augustine's attacks on the use of the 'safe period') would restrict the methods to those provided by nature.

In relation to family spacing and limitation it is important to get rid of the idea that a woman cannot become pregnant while breast-feeding a baby. Fertility is lessened in these circumstances but conception is perfectly possible. Perhaps the need for the mother to avoid pregnancy during breast-feeding and thereafter to have some months rest is the most obvious example of the desirability of birth control in cases with neither hereditary defect nor excessive existing family.

'Natural' methods. Those methods that require no artificial or mechanical intervention to avoid conception.

1. Continence (complete absence of intercourse) is obvious but is psychologically frustrating to a young and highly-sexed couple living together and can even cause nervous breakdown. It is practicable for unmarried persons 'going steady', but inhibitions are sometimes temporarily removed (e.g., by a combination of alcohol, opportunity and deep affection).

2. The 'safe period' or 'RHYTHM METHOD' is based on the idea that the female ovum is ripe for reception of a sperm between the tenth and the eighteenth day after the beginning of menstruation, so that the avoidance of intercourse during these nine days should prevent pregnancy. Unfortunately, not all menstrual cycles are at regular twenty-eight day intervals, and in some women the 'dangerous period' extends from the sixth to the twentieth day after the start of menstruation (or roughly half the month). There are even recorded cases of conception before the sixth and after the twentieth day. Broadly use of the 'safe period', if carefully calculated in a regular woman, removes about three-quarters of the risk of pregnancy.

3. The 'temperature method' is an attempt to pin-point the time of ovulation (i.e., the beginning of the 'danger period') by noting a slight rise in temperature; but the rise is only about 1° C., and many other factors can cause or prevent such a small rise. This method, despite its scientific appearance, is no better than the use of the 'safe period'.

4. Withdrawal (coitus interruptus) of the penis before climax is reached is somewhat uncertain because some seminal fluid may be discharged before withdrawal. Also withdrawal may place considerable psychological strain on both partners.

Mechanical methods. Those methods that require artificial intervention to prevent conception.

1. The condom or male SHEATH of appropriate size, rolled or slipped over the erect penis, is much more reliable than any

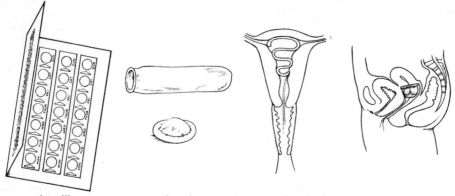

| the pill | sheath | intra-uterine device | cap |

Methods of birth control

'natural' method. Provided the sheath is not torn, and provided spermicidal douches or creams are used if there is any suspicion of a leak, the method is 95 per cent effective. Curiously the condom is known in Britain as 'the French letter' and in France as 'la capote anglaise'.

2. The 'cap' pessary of rubber and the 'Dutch' or steel spring pessary, both inserted while the woman is in a squatting position, aim to shut off the vagina from the cervix of the uterus, thus preventing the sperm and the ovum from coming together. Pessaries are highly reliable, especially if used smeared with a spermicidal jelly or cream, and followed by douching, perhaps twelve hours after intercourse and before removal of the pessary. In some cases, however, they irritate the soft tissues.

3. Although invented as early as 1909 the INTRA-UTERINE DEVICE was for some reason little used until the second half of this century. It is generally inserted by a doctor (requiring considerable skill for insertion), can be left in for long periods, and is more reliable.

Oral contraceptives. In the last twenty years oral contraceptives, containing minute quantities of the female hormones oestrogen and progesterone, have come to dominate the field of birth control. They have a success rate of over 99 per cent, and in fact conception while using 'the pill' is almost always due to human error, e.g., forgetting to take a daily pill, although some modern varieties provide sufficient 'carry-over' to minimize the risk of a one-day omission. There are many varieties, so that side effects can be eliminated by giving each woman an oral contraceptive that suits her.

Oral contraceptives with relatively high oestrogen content were virtually abandoned before 1970, in which year a very large scale investigation showed that they had a danger to health approximating to one-tenth of the danger created by a pregnancy; by contrast the same investigation and other studies have not shown any dangers in respect of the oral contraceptives in common use, although there

are a few disease conditions which render these contraceptives undesirable for persons with these particular diseases. In highly developed countries (e.g., Western Europe and North America) millions of women have used oral contraceptives during the last dozen years, so that their effects are at least as well known as those of any other modern medicines.

Permanent methods. While oral contraceptives are ideal for family postponement or family spacing, it seems unfortunate that a woman who has completed her family by the age of 28 or so should have to take oral contraceptives for another eighteen years. So increasing attention is now being paid to the cutting or tying of the male or female tubes.

In the male, sterilization is carried out by the very minor and painless operation of vasectomy. Using a local anaesthetic the surgeon makes a small cut in the scrotum, either removes a tiny portion of the vas deferens or ties it with a ligature, and repeats the process on the other side. The whole operation, including the time waiting for the local anaesthetic to take effect, is over in fifteen to twenty minutes, the man normally leaves the clinic or hospital within an hour of entering it and is usually fit for work on the next day or sometimes even the same day. It takes two to three months for the spermatozoa already in circulation to die off, but thereafter the man is completely sterile. He can still feel sexual desire, have erections and ejaculate semen, but the semen contains no spermatozoa.

Vasectomy has the limitation that it is permanent (if a portion of the vas is removed) or difficult to reverse (if the vas is tied) but it is the simplest form of sterilization, much easier and more rapid than ligation of a woman's uterine tubes.

The operation is becoming increasingly popular with men who have fathered the number of children that they desire.

Despite the ancient, mediaeval and even early modern fondness for more drastic procedures, such as castration, vasectomy was unknown until less than a hundred years ago.

Indeed it is a sad commentary on medical knowledge that as late as 1686 a textbook – *De Morbis Foemineis* - suggested making men sterile by cutting the veins behind the ear, in the belief that semen was produced in the brain and descended through these veins.

In the female, sterilization is carried out by cutting and tying – or in some other way closing off – the Fallopian tubes. The cutting and tying method requires abdominal operation but less complicated procedures now involve operating through a small stab-wound with the use of a laparoscope (a sort of periscope) to seal off the tubes either by diathermy or the application of special clips under direct vision. Both methods leave the woman with unaltered sexual feelings and menstrual periods but with the ova no longer able to travel to the womb. Other possible procedures are still on trial.

While some doctors themselves provide birth control advice and treatment, increasing numbers of individuals seek the expertise available at family planning clinics. These clinics of course provide both privacy and confidentiality. In the British cities with the most highly developed contraceptive services, and with parallel health education about these services, the birth rate has fallen by as much as 20 per cent, creating in these cities a stationary population as opposed to a constantly expanding one.

birth marks. Congenital blemishes of the skin, falling into two types. The vascular naevus is a small cluster of tiny blood vessels. Of these the red 'strawberry mark' often fades after some years, while the purple 'port wine stain' usually remains. The pigmented naevus or mole is essentially a cluster of pigment cells.

Many, but not all, birthmarks decrease in size as the child grows older, but if they remain disfiguring plastic surgery or cautery treatment can be effective, although in many cases a cosmetic preparation can hide them. There is no foundation for the superstition that birth marks are caused by events which took place during pregnancy.

bites and stings. An insect which stings is acting malevolently in self-defence but one which bites is merely being a parasite and feeding on the blood or juices of a host which it is against its own interests to injure.

Insect bites. These can cause trouble in various ways. After puncturing the skin the insect injects a salivary secretion into the victim in order to assist the sucking process and this causes irritation and local swelling, even when there are no complications. However, the bites may become septic because of infection introduced from the mouth parts of the insect or by scratching. Bites should not be scratched; calamine lotion or antihistamine creams will allay irritation.

In tropical countries many insects harbour in their secretion organisms of serious disease which are thus inoculated into the host. Mosquitos, biting flies, fleas, lice and ticks are known carriers of a great variety of tropical diseases and so in tropical and sub-tropical areas the potential risks of insect bites should be appreciated and appropriate measures adopted to avoid being bitten. In addition, as a precautionary measure, drugs should be taken which will act against infection with malaria should this occur.

Animal bites. Unless there is a reason to suspect that the animal suffers from rabies, an animal bite should simply be thoroughly washed with a mild disinfectant solution, or – failing that – with soap and water, and thereafter treated like any other wound.

Diseases transmitted by the bites or stings of certain infected insects and animals are considered elsewhere. See MALARIA, YELLOW FEVER, TYPHUS, and RABIES.

Stings. The word 'sting' refers either to the specialized organ of attack or else to its effect on the victim. Bees, wasps, and hornets are the only important examples in temperate regions. These stings usually cause only sharp pain and local swelling or sepsis but can be dangerous in the mouth or at the top of the throat where swelling may cause difficulty in breathing. In such cases a doctor should be summoned urgently, since an injection of adrenalin or an intramuscular antihistamine or (in cases of extreme respiratory difficulty) a tracheotomy operation, may be life-saving. Occasionally signs of shock and collapse appear, in which case whisky or sal volatile should be given. It should however be emphasized that these are extreme rarities: nineteen stings out of twenty cause only minor irritation.

In most cases a bee-sting is best treated by gently removing the sting (if it can be seen) and applying a mild alkali such as baking soda. Antihistamine drugs may also help to relieve the symptoms.

Like most insect stings wasp stings cause a release of histamine but, unlike most other insects, wasps inject an alkaline venom and therefore a mild acid, such as vinegar, should be applied.

Where a person is allergic to a sting venom and cannot change his residence to an area in which a sting is unlikely, a desensitization course may be required. See ALLERGY.

In sub-tropical and tropical countries the scorpion is feared. It holds on with its feet and stings with its pointed tail. It frequently kills children from resultant respiratory paralysis and even adults can be very ill. Local treatment employs ammonia with novocaine and adrenalin to relieve pain. A specific antivenene is available.

Other hazards are the giant centipede, and some tropical fish such as the sting-rays which have poisoned barbs in their dorsal fins. Jellyfish can give particularly painful stings; these are probably best relieved by mild acids such as vinegar, skin irritation due to the stinging nettle is caused by formic acid and can be relieved by alkaline applications. See also SNAKE BITES.

Black Death. A particularly infectious and virulent form of PLAGUE that destroyed about a third of the world's population in 1346-51.

When Pope Clement VI asked for the number of the dead, the statistics that he received accounted for 42,836,486 corpses, including more than 25 million in Europe; but modern investigators assess the total at around 60 million for Europe and Asia or roughly half the entire populations of these continents.

Terrible stories are told of the Black Death – of villages with a single survivor, of ships that drifted through the seas with lifeless crews, of entire Jewish communities burned to death in the belief that they had caused the plague, of the collapse of law because there were no officers to enforce it, of unbridled debauchery and every variety of sexual perversion, and of doctors and priests fleeing wildly from the pestilence. It is significant of the medical knowledge of the time that Europe's foremost surgeon, Guy de Chauliac – who, although in terror, did not flee – attributed the Black Death to 'The grand conjunction of the three superior planets, Saturn, Jupiter and Mars, in the sign of Aquarius'. More than five centuries were to pass before it was realized that it was due to the grand conjunction of virulent organisms, rats and fleas.

black eye. Darkening of the eyelids and surrounding skin and reddening of the conjunctive of the eye following an injury. Essentially the mechanism is the same as in a bruise elsewhere, but there is much loose skin in the eyelids in which blood can easily accumulate. A cold, wet cloth applied to the eye is the best immediate treatment, in spite of the quite false reputation of raw steak.

blackhead. Glands producing oil (sebum) to lubricate the skin release it through pores which sometimes become plugged by dried skin and other debris. When this happens the area around the gland becomes inflamed and the typical red spot with a black centre is produced. Sometimes infection occurs with pus being formed as is seen in ACNE.

black vomit. Black or dark-brown vomit, often described as 'coffee-grounds'; the indication is that blood has entered the stomach and been partially digested before being brought up. Possible causes include gastric and duodenal ulcer, acute gastritis, and – more rarely – cancer of the stomach. Medical consultation is advisable.

blackwater fever. A rather infrequent but often fatal complication of MALARIA of the falciparum type. It is characterized by blackening of the urine through blood pigment which has passed through the kidney filters. It is thought that the condition is associated with frequent but insufficient treatment of bouts of malaria by quinine. Blood transfusion helps, and kidney failure should be treated in the usual way.

bladder. A flexible muscular bag that serves as a reservoir for the urine secreted by the kidneys. The bladder is connected to the kidneys by two tubes, the ureters, and to the exterior by a passage, the urethra, with the outlet from bladder to urethra guarded by a circular muscle, the sphincter. When empty, the bladder lies wholly in the pelvis, but as it becomes distended its upper end rises several inches into the abdomen. The adult bladder can hold almost half a litre (1 pint) of urine.

After the bladder has become appreciably distended from the continuous trickle of urine from the kidneys, the muscular walls begin to resist, producing the desire to pass urine. In a baby the subsequent relaxation of the sphincter is purely a reflex action, and the voiding of urine follows; but as a child ages this relaxation of the sphincter comes increasingly under control of the will. If the sphincter is deliberately not relaxed, the signal from the bladder muscles ceases but, as distension increases, is later renewed. If the signal of muscle resistance is repeatedly ignored, reflex emptying ultimately supersedes voluntary control.

Incontinence is loss of control over the sphincter muscle and it occurs when the bladder is irritated (e.g., by inflammation or stone or enlarged prostate) or when the sphincter is paralysed (e.g., in certain diseases of the spinal cord). Incontinence in children usually takes the form of bedwetting but the elderly may also experience an occasional involuntary voiding of urine.

Diseases. Common diseases of the bladder include the following. (1) Cystitis or inflammation – infection of the bladder, commoner in women than in men because the female urethra is shorter and so gives less protection against entrance of bacteria. The main symptoms are frequency of urination and some pain. (2) Stone from the kidneys or ureters; usually indicated by considerable pain, bleeding into the urine, and frequency. (3) Tumours also occur, the most common being the benign papilloma, characterized by painless bleeding into the urine; cancer of the bladder, much less frequent, is initially hard to differentiate from papilloma. (4) Rupture of the bladder also occurs, generally as a result of violence.

bleeding. Any form of external or internal passage of blood from the arteries, veins, or capillaries. For immediate treatment see FIRST AID. See also HAEMORRHAGE.

The term also means a medically-prescribed release of blood by application of leeches or by cutting a vein. In the seventeenth and eighteenth centuries this was a standard treatment for many diseases, but far from helping, it usually simply increased the weakness of patients. The treatment has almost died out, except that venesection is occasionally used in a few conditions in which the veins are over-filled with blood.

bleeding disease. See HAEMOPHILIA.

blepharitis. Inflammation of the eyelids, characterized by swelling, redness, and in chronic cases thickening of the lining mucous membrane. It may be caused by infection, allergy or malnutrition and is often associated with dandruff. Treatment will vary with the cause.

blindness. Lack of sight in both eyes or in one. Perhaps the greatest triumph of health services has been the effective transfer of blindness from a condition of youth to one of old age. Some of the very numerous causes, listed here, fall into four principal categories.

Loss of vision from infancy. By far the commonest cause of blindness in children in developed countries until the last forty years was ophthalmia neonatorum, i.e., transmission of gonococcal infection from the mother to the baby during the birth process. Another cause of blindness in babies that has almost disappeared in the last fifteen years is retrolental fibroplasia, created by giving excess oxygen to premature babies. Such few cases of blindness as are now found in young children in developed countries are mostly hereditary, such as hereditary cataract and amaurosis. These can be reduced by genetic guidance and family planning.

Gradual loss of vision in one or both eyes. In several less-developed countries the commonest cause of blindness is still trachoma, which affects all age groups but in developed countries impaired or absent vision is now primarily a condition of old age. Glaucoma is essentially a disease of the over-sixties, although its early stages are said to be present in about 5 per cent of persons aged 45 to 50 years: while it is not yet preventable, it can be controlled and usually blindness avoided. Cataract responds to surgical treatment, and amblyopia of the tobacco or the toxic variety responds to discontinuing the intake of the causing factor. Atrophy of the optic nerve and tumour of the pituitary gland also cause gradual loss of sight.

Sudden blindness of one eye. This may be caused by thrombosis of the vein draining the retina (the light-sensitive inner layer of the eye), embolism of the retinal artery or by detachment or degeneration of the retina.

Sudden blindness in both eyes. Sun-blinding is the result of looking directly at the sun – the intense brilliance of the light burns the area of the retina it shines on and the tissues can never recover. It is, therefore, extremely important always to shield the eyes with smoked glass if, for instance, watching an eclipse. Other causes of sudden blindness are uraemia, diabetes and of course, injury. In a very few cases of blindness, where the defect is caused by cornea (the transparent front covering of the eye) becoming opaque, sight may be restored by a corneal graft, replacing the damaged cornea with a clearly transparent cornea from a donor eye.

Social aspects. In the past partially-sighted or totally blind people were to be found in every age group but in the developed countries today the highest incidence of blindness tends to occur among the elderly. Blindness, therefore, like other degenerative diseases, has to be discussed mainly in relation to the process of ageing and the various circumstances in which the elderly find themselves.

Expert medical advice and treatment can prevent blindness in many cases or limit it to partial loss of sight. Where the condition is unprevented or unpreventable it is important that the person, while still partially sighted, should learn to make full use of his other senses and also to be systematic, e.g., counting the steps as he walks down stairs, and placing his pipe and matches in a fixed and safe position where he can find them without using his eyes.

When blindness has developed he should promptly seek to become registered as a blind person, so as to gain such advantages as the chance of being trained for appropriate work and then helped to find a job, visits by experienced home workers for the blind whose advice can be very valuable, and in some countries free radio licences and reduced postage rates for embossed literature. If he is still relatively young and active, his mobility will be greatly improved by the acquisition of a guide dog, specially trained in the U.K. by the Guide Dogs for the Blind Association. Even if fairly old but mentally alert he should certainly be prepared to learn braille in which many books are published.

The situation of people who lose their sight in old age is very different. Some degree of isolation, both physical and social, is often associated with growing old (see BEREAVEMENT). The loss of any of the senses is likely to increase the problem of social isolation, and the partial or total loss of vision may cause old people to withdraw even further into themselves. This may be particularly distressing since medical and social services are not particularly well equipped to help the elderly blind person, and a person who is becoming sightless has usually no advance knowledge of blindness that he can use in trying to adapt.

The organizations, mostly voluntary, which exist to help blind people tend to place the elderly at the bottom of their lists of priorities. These organizations, while sometimes subsidized by public funds, are dependent largely upon voluntary contributions to continue their work. It is easier to persuade people to give money to a good cause if it is suggested that the afflicted can be helped and trained to fend for themselves and to make a positive contribution to the economic sector. Consequently organizations for the blind have tended to focus their efforts on the young person who can be trained in some economically productive role.

The elderly blind have greater needs which are more difficult to deal with without there being much possibility for helping such people to lead a socially 'useful' life. Their mobility may already be impaired so that the usefulness of guide dogs is limited, even assuming an old person is fully capable of caring for a dog. Like most elderly people the blind or partially sighted wish to remain in their own homes for as long as possible, which means that assistance has to be brought to them rather than their travelling to (or living in) a centrally based institution.

Gradually more resources are being devoted to the care of the elderly. In Britain retired people are regularly contacted by health visitors although the case loads of these health and social workers are far too high for them to be able to provide a complete service. A vast expansion of resources devoted to the care of the elderly is desperately needed and an increasingly important element in their work will be the care of the blind or partially sighted. Clearly the major priority is to reorganize the medical and social services in such a way that the service is taken to the patient rather than the latter being expected to come to a general practitioner's surgery, a hospital, or a social work agency.

blister. A small area of the skin in which the surface layer is raised and contains fluid; it is caused by heat or friction. In general a blister is best left unbroken and treated by application of calamine lotion. Where it has broken it should be covered with lint spread with zinc or boracic ointment.

blood. The fluid, contained in arteries, capillaries and veins, which transmits oxygen and nutritive substances to the various tissues and conveys waste materials from the tissues to the lungs (in the case of carbon dioxide) and the excretory organs. Blood makes up approximately one-fourteenth of the weight of the body, or about 5 litres (8 pints) in the case of an average adult male.

Blood consists of a large number of red cells, and smaller numbers of white cells and of tiny bodies called platelets, all floating in a pale, yellowish, clear liquid, the plasma.

1. Plasma is the sticky, amber-coloured fluid which carries not only the blood corpuscles but also various raw materials and waste products. Plasma contains proteins – albumin, globulin and fibrinogen – which are formed mainly in the liver. These protein molecules are too large

normally to pass through the walls of the capillaries. The presence of albumin is important to the function of OSMOSIS and deficiency leads to an accumulation of fluid in the tissues known as oedema. This occurs in certain diseases of the liver (where not enough is formed) and of the kidney (where albumin passes to the urine). Globulin is associated with immunity to certain infectious diseases. Fibrinogen is altered by a ferment released by the platelets when blood is shed. It forms threads of fibrin, and these, entangling corpuscles in the network of threads, form a clot. (Serum is plasma which has no fibrinogen, i.e., it is the fluid which separates from a clot.)

2. Red blood corpuscles (erythrocytes) are circular, concave discs, normally about five million to each cubic millimetre of blood. They are manufactured in the bone marrow, and each corpuscle when worn out – after some three to four months – is destroyed by the spleen. Red blood corpuscles are essentially envelopes containing an iron compound, HAEMOGLOBIN, which combines with oxygen in the capillaries of the lungs and in due course gives up oxygen to the tissues. Haemoglobin cannot be formed without an adequate supply of iron, and red blood corpuscles cannot mature without vitamin B_{12}. Red corpuscles are about a thousand times as numerous as white ones.

3. White blood corpuscles (leucocytes) are slightly larger and much less numerous than red cells, roughly about eight thousand to the cubic millimetre. They, like red corpuscles, are formed in the bone marrow and they constitute the main defence mechanism of the body. They gather rapidly at the site of infection by bacteria or invasion by a foreign body, and they have the power of surrounding bacteria and ultimately destroying them. Leucocytes are of two main types: granulocytes (which on being stained show small scattered granules in the cell) chiefly concerned with protection against bacteria; and lymphocytes (where on being stained the cell is seen to be largely occupied by a nucleus) which play a considerable role in resistance to virus diseases and also in chronic infections. Moderate increase in leucocytes is a healthy response to infection, and identification of such increase – by spreading a drop of suitably diluted blood thinly on a glass slide, staining appropriately and counting the cells – gives a useful clue to the presence of infection. Ungoverned over-production of white corpuscles is characteristic of a cancer-like disease, leukaemia.

4. Platelets (thrombocytes) are very much smaller than red or white corpuscles and are involved in the clotting of shed blood. They release a hormone which helps to convert fibrinogen to fibrin. A disease with abnormally slow blood clotting time is known as haemophilia.

Blood tests. These fall into three main groups – haematological (or study of the state of the blood itself), chemical (or investigation of its contents) and bacteriological (or study for organisms or antibodies). Many tests require merely a single drop of blood, obtained by pricking the finger lightly with a needle. Others need several millilitres of blood, obtained by inserting the needle of a syringe into a vein. Some of the tests most commonly undertaken are: (1) measuring the amount of haemoglobin by an instrument called a haemoglobinometer; (2) counting under a microscope the numbers and types of red and white cells in a suitably diluted and stained drop of blood spread on a glass slide; (3) studying the normality or abnormality of the cells so seen; (4) calculating the rate at which red blood corpuscles settle in blood diluted with sodium citrate; (5) estimation of clotting time; (6) determination of amount of blood sugar; (7) estimation of blood urea; (8) examination of blood for parasites (e.g., in suspected malaria); (9) blood culture (for organisms); (10) Widal test (for present or past typhoid or paratyphoid fever); (11) Wassermann test (for syphilis); and (12) determination of blood group.

Blood diseases. The various forms of insufficiency of red blood corpuscles are discussed under ANAEMIA. Polycythaemia, excess of red blood corpuscles – one of the few conditions for which bleeding is still used – is thought to be due to excessive activity of bone marrow, and is hereditary in some cases. Excess of white corpuscles is considered under LEUKAEMIA, and hereditary tendency to uncontrollable bleeding is discussed under HAEMOPHILIA. For poisoning of the blood by germs or their toxins see SEPTICAEMIA and TOXAEMIA respectively.

See also CIRCULATION OF BLOOD and BLOOD GROUPS.

blood groups. Until 1900 all red blood corpuscles were deemed identical, and blood transfusion (life saving in persons who had lost a great deal of blood) had occasional unexplained fatalities, in which the blood of the patient appeared to agglutinate (or clump) the transfused cells.

In that year Karl Landsteiner (1868-1943), a New York pathologist, and other workers elsewhere, showed that individual blood samples could contain two factors (agglutinogens), A and B, and that these factors could cause red blood corpuscles from a different sample of blood to clump together. These factors occurred singly or together or were absent, and so four groups were possible A, B, AB or O. Similarly it was shown that serum from blood could be grouped in terms of agglutinins named anti-A and anti-B.

Group A, found in about 42 per cent of Western Europeans, will mix with blood containing A but will cause clotting if mixed with blood of group B; Group B, found in about 9 per cent, will similarly mix with B but will cause clotting if mixed with A. Group AB, the 'universal recipients', will accept without clotting blood from any group, and constitute about 3 per cent of the population, and Group O, the 'universal donors', blood from any group; can safely provide blood to any group and make up roughly 46 per cent of the population. Diagnosis of these groups made blood transfusion vastly safer. Forty years later Landsteiner and Weiner discovered that irrespective of these four main blood groups there is another variation: the RHESUS FACTOR. They showed that 83 per cent of the population are Rhesus positive (Rh+ve) and 17 per cent are Rhesus negative (Rh-ve).

A Rhesus negative person who has a transfusion of Rhesus positive blood, or more commonly a Rhesus negative woman who bears a Rhesus positive child (inheriting the factor from his father), is likely to form an antibody which reacts with a further contact with Rhesus positive blood, e.g., in a transfusion or a subsequent pregnancy.

Apart from implications both for blood transfusions and in obstetrics, the discovery of the four main types and the Rhesus sub-types is of considerable value in paternity cases, since a child inherits its blood grouping from either father or mother. To give two examples: if mother and child are both of group A, Rhesus +ve we have no evidence, because the child has inherited from the mother; but if the mother is of group A, Rhesus +ve and the child of group AB, Rhesus -ve, we have quite a bit of information about the father.

blood heat. The normal temperature of the blood is about 37. 7° C. (100° F.) but the body temperature in health is about 36 to 37.2° C. (98 to 99° F.) and is conventionally taken as 36.7° C. (98.4° F.). The circulating blood maintains the body at very constant TEMPERATURE.

blood pressure. The pressure at which the heart pumps blood into the main arteries. The extent of this pressure depends principally on two factors – the force of the muscular pump of the heart, and the calibre, elasticity and resistance of the arteries. The blood pressure is normally measured at two points of time, namely that of maximum heart contraction (systolic pressure) and that of maximum relaxation (diastolic pressure).

Measurement. This is carried out on a SPHYGMOMANOMETER, invented in 1896 by Riva-Rocci (accounting for the symbolic R-R used in some countries as the unit of blood-pressure measurement). An inflatable cuff is wrapped around the patient's arm and air pumped into it until it constricts the arm sufficiently for the pulse-beat to be stopped. This air pressure is meantime also raising a column of mercury against a scale and the blood pressure is recorded according to the height of the column of mercury. Thus in a healthy young adult at rest the average systolic pressure is equivalent to a column of 120 mm. of mercury, and the average diastolic pressure is equivalent to 80 mm. of mercury. There is, however, considerable individual variation, especially in respect of the systolic pressure. To an experienced examiner the PULSE can give an accurate assessment of the blood pressure.

High blood pressure. The pressure rises temporarily during exertion and in emotional disturbance. A sustained rise in blood pressure is perhaps the commonest pathological condition found in highly developed countries and is associated with excess worry and mental activity, over-eating and perhaps lack of physical exercise.

Causes of raised blood pressure include hardening of the arteries (arteriosclerosis) so that the heart has to work harder to pump in the same amount of blood, certain diseases of the kidneys with poorer blood flow through them, and occasionally increased stickiness of the blood (as in polycythaemia). Symptoms sometimes include headaches, giddiness and heart pains, but often a rising blood pressure is symptomless. A mild rise of pressure in middle-age is probably best ignored as merely a 'normal' feature of modern life: in millimeters of mercury the average systolic pressure is sometimes described as '100 plus number of years lived'.

Serious and increasing rise of pressure – and especially of diastolic pressure – indicates risk

of a cerebrovascular incident, such as a stroke. Such continuing rise therefore demands a revision of life's routine to diminish both mental and physical strain, in the hope of stopping or slowing the increase. Certain drugs that act on the sympathetic nervous system (e.g., guanethidine and methyldopa) can also be used in moderation to lower the pressure, but it has to be remembered that in general the pressure has risen because it is needed to force the blood into hardened arteries, and that too vigorous reduction of the pressure can do more harm than good.

Low blood pressure. A temporary fall in blood pressure can occur on suddenly standing up (because the reflexes have not yet adjusted to the changed posture and too much blood at first drains towards the feet) and is also found in shock. Permanently low blood pressure is characteristic of Addison's disease and also occurs in some prolonged debility states.

Blood pressure in pregnancy. During a normal pregnancy the blood pressure does not rise, and indeed a rise in blood pressure is an indication that a pregnancy is not proceeding normally and that skilled help is needed. During the actual labour the pressure rises but rapidly falls again after the birth.

blood spitting. See HAEMOPTYSIS.

blood tests. See BLOOD.

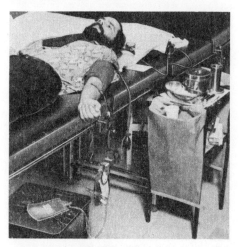

A blood donor

blood transfusion. The procedure by which blood from a donor is transfused to the circulatory system of a patient in order to restore loss of blood-volume resulting from haemorrhage and shock or to improve states of severe anaemia. In 'exchange-transfusions' all the blood of a patient is replaced by donated blood and this expedient is employed in new-born infants suffering from the effects of RHESUS incompatibility and also in certain cases of poisoning and liver disease.

Although now a commonplace of surgical and medical practice blood-transfusion had a stormy history. It really begins with Harvey's discovery of the circulation of the blood in 1628 and subsequent experiments by members of the Royal Society of England as described by

Pepys in his Diary for 14th November, 1666. Many other attempts were made both in England and France and the first account of successful human transfusion appears in *The Lancet* for 1829. Thereafter some general use ensued, principally by obstetricians, but it remained a hazardous and uncertain procedure until two fundamental discoveries were made.

In 1901 Landsteiner showed that blood contained agglutinins which 'clumped' the cells of unmatched blood and this was followed by elucidation of the blood groups A, B, AB, and O worked out by Jansky (1907) and Moss of Baltimore (1910). The second discovery was that blood could be prevented from clotting by the addition of sodium citrate. Citrated blood was first used by Professor Agote of Buenos Aires in 1914 with complete success, and this advance, allied to accurate grouping and cross-matching, finally assured the simplicity, certainty, safety, and efficiency of a life-saving measure now essential to modern practice.

When blood is to be collected from a healthy donor an arm vein is usually made to stand out by the application of a tourniquet; a needle is inserted and blood allowed to run through the needle and a tube into a suitable receptacle where clotting is prevented by the addition of a small amount of sodium citrate. The citrated blood can be stored for several weeks at 3 to 4°C. (i.e., the temperature of an ordinary domestic refrigerator), and then when required can be run slowly into the vein of a person of similar BLOOD GROUP.

The discoveries first of the inherited blood group systems and then of the Rhesus factor have together removed the former dangers of blood transfusion. Freed from these dangers it is extremely useful – indeed life-saving – after accidents and injuries involving heavy loss of blood. Virtually all general hospitals now have 'blood banks', with stored blood of various groups available for immediate use when required

Very rarely (only, in fact, in the combination of a serious condition and an unusual blood group) is blood transferred directly from donor to recipient. The blood bank system is more suitable for the donor who can give his blood at a time convenient both for him and for the hospital staff; it is better for the staff, since when a transfusion is urgently needed they do not need to await the arrival of an appropriate donor; and if there is any doubt about the donor's health it allows time for investigation.

blood vessels. A collective name for the arteries (which carry blood from the heart), the veins (which return blood to the heart) and the capillaries (through which occurs interchange with the tissues of oxygen, nutrients and waste products). See CIRCULATION OF BLOOD.

blue baby. A new-born child with a bluish complexion, indicating unsatisfactory oxygenation of the blood in consequence of a congenital heart defect, e.g., a communication remaining between the right and left sides of the heart so that the oxygenated blood to be pumped around the body is contaminated by the deoxygenated blood which has returned from the body to the heart en route for the lungs. Until the 1950s this condition was usually fatal, but modern surgical techniques can nowadays successfully cope with the abnormality.

blushing. Reddening of the skin, especially of the face and neck. In persons of nervous or excitable temperament any emotional disturbance – painful or pleasurable – may cause a dilation of the capillaries of the skin, resulting in production of a rosy colour. Of the many causes of flushing perhaps the commonest are: (1) temporary hormonal imbalance in adolescence; (2) similar imbalance at the menopause, and (3) anxiety states. In the first two cases the condition passes in time, and in the third the treatment is that of the underlying condition.

While not a serious condition and seldom unattractive, flushing places its victim in the position that the existence of strong emotion is revealed to the observer.

boils. Small abscesses commencing in a hair root and usually caused by a staphylococcus. A single boil is painful while the damaged tissues, leucocytes and bacteria are forming pus that is at first under tension. In due course the stretched skin breaks or the boil may be opened surgically to let the pus escape. The pus drains out and the lesion heals. Poultices may expedite the pus formation. Apart from lancing the boil when pus is definitely present, interference is undesirable. In particular, squeezing a boil not only damages the tissues but may send infectious material inwards.

A series of successive or simultaneous boils implies lowered vitality of the skin and suggests (1) chronic serious disease (e.g., of the kidneys), (2) extreme physical or mental exhaustion, or (3) faulty feeding. Apart from seeking for an underlying cause, building up the general health and attention to skin hygiene, the individual may benefit from injections of a suitable antibiotic.

bone. Bone is composed of two layers of tissue: externally, a dense, ivory-like shell of compact bone, traversed only by very narrow channels (the Haversian canals) in which run the nourishing blood vessels and lymphatics; and internally a spongy or porous network, the cancellous bone, rich in blood vessels and supporting the red bone marrow. A bone is surrounded by a tough, fibrous membrane called the periosteum. Sensation apparently from the bone really comes from the nerves in the periosteum.

Bones are classified into long, short, flat and irregular. A long bone (e.g., femur or thigh-bone) consists of a shaft and two expanded ends. Short bones (e.g., those of the wrist) consist of cancellous bone thinly encased by compact bone. Flat bones (e.g., those of the skull) are composed of outer and inner tables of compact bone with layers of cancellous bone sandwiched between. Irregular bones (e.g., the vertebrae) are simply those that do not conform to any classification.

Bones form the skeletal framework about which the body is moulded. They give protection to the vital organs, and they permit the body and limbs to be moved in various directions by the action of the muscles.

Formation. Bone tissue develops from cartilage and this begins early during pregnancy, but as late as the time of birth some bones are still entirely cartilaginous. Growth of the bone, which requires the availability of sufficient calcium (and also vitamin D to permit absorption of calcium) depends on the activity

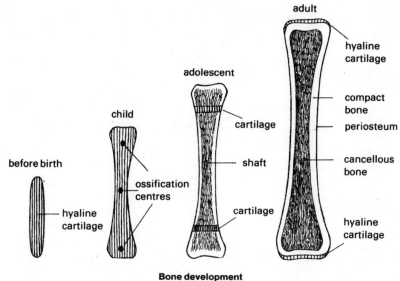

Bone development

of cells called osteoblasts. These extract calcium phosphate from the blood.

In young children bones consist largely of cartilagenous tissue, and under strain they bend rather than break. With advancing years bones come to contain more and more calcium phosphate and become more brittle.

Disorders. Bone is subject to the same type of disorder as most other tissues, but is more rigid, so that if it yields at all it breaks, so that the edges of an abscess cannot close, and so that in inflammation there is no space for expansion. Also bone lacks nerve endings, so that (unless the periosteum is affected) bone diseases are painless.

Some of the commoner bone disorders are: fracture; periostitis (inflammation of the periosteum); osteomyelitis (inflammation of the bony substance itself); tuberculosis (now becoming rare); of the malignant tumours carcinoma is usually secondary to primary cancer elsewhere, but sarcoma sometimes starts in bone. See also RICKETS, ACROMEGALY and OSTEOMALACIA. Abnormal fragility of bones is fairly common in old people (see OSTEOPOROSIS) and is occasionally found as a hereditary condition in children (see OSTEOSCLEROSIS FRAGILIS).

borborygmus. A rumbling noise arising in the bowel from intestinal indigestion.

Bornholm disease. A disease caused by a virus and characterized by high temperature, headache, severe pain in the muscles of the chest and abdomen, inflammation of the throat and sometimes pleurisy and mild meningitis. The condition generally clears up in two or three days but recurrence a few days later is quite common. Analgesics are needed to relieve the pain but there is no known specific treatment and no known method of prevention.

bottle feeding. Where the mother has an illness that renders breast-feeding undesirable, e.g., heart disease or pulmonary tuberculosis, or produces inadequate milk, or has working commitments that prevent complete BREAST-FEEDING, partial or total bottle feeding may be needed.

Modification of liquid cow's milk may be attempted at home – seeking to reduce the high protein and mineral content of cow's milk to about the levels of human milk (by addition of sterile water), to raise the low carbohydrate content (by addition of lactose) and to make the curd more digestible (by addition of sodium citrate); but proprietary dried milks (and in the U.K. National Dried Milk) make the required modifications more accurately and under conditions of guaranteed sterility. If the directions on the tin are strictly followed, and not varied except on the advice of a doctor or health visitor about the particular needs of an individual child, an infant can be very satisfactorily fed by bottle.

It is important that the baby be held in the arms while feeding, both for emotional stimulation and because it is dangerous to leave a baby sucking from a bottle attached to a pillow. The teat must of course be of the right size for the infant's mouth and the hole should be large enough for the milk to drop out when the bottle is inverted but not large enough for it to flow out. Bottles and teats should be carefully washed and scalded after each feed or else washed in a suitable disinfectant – all the various commercial preparations widely advertised for this purpose are satisfactory – and then rinsed in boiled water to remove traces of the disinfectant.

Vitamin supplements are needed, but to avoid risk of over-dosage of vitamin D the amount of that vitamin in any proprietary milk used should be known and taken into account.

The gradual introduction of other foods should be similar to that for breast-fed babies.

In the U.K. advice on bottle feeding (and breast-feeding) and weaning is readily available from health visitors. See also INFANT FEEDING.

botulism. Food-poisoning caused by the micro-organism *Clostridium botulinus* and its toxin. It is often fatal but cases are extremely rare. The name derives from *botulus* (Latin – a sausage) and out-breaks of 'sausage-poisoning' have been recorded from Germany and Central Europe since the sixteenth century.

Nowadays, botulism is mainly associated with vegetables and fruits which have been inefficiently canned or bottled. The organism will survive to multiply and produce toxin if the temperature attained in the pack is not high enough to kill it. Because of this, home-canned produce is a special risk and should always be re-cooked before consumption. Home-canning is commoner in U.S.A. than in Britain and a significant number of cases occur there.

Unlike other food-poisoning, gastro-intestinal symptoms are usually slight. Instead, botulinus toxin damages the nervous system. Onset occurs with dizziness, double vision, laryngeal paralysis, and loss of voice. The vital centres of the brain controlling the heart and respiration may be affected.

An antitoxin is available but unless the disease is promptly recognised opportunity for effective administration is easily lost. Treatment otherwise mainly consists in maintaining respiration and combating collapse.

The sinister reputation of botulism is largely due to an isolated dramatic incident which occurred at Loch Maree in Ross-shire in 1922. Anglers were given luncheon sandwiches made with wild duck paste. This was infected with *Cl. botulinus* and all eight members of the party were dead within a week.

bowel. The part of the digestive system which extends as a musculo-membranous tube from the lower opening of the stomach to the anus. It occupies most of the abdominal cavity and comprises the small and large intestines.

The small intestine comprises convolutions of some 1 m. (20 ft.) named successively duodenum, jejunum, and ileum. It digests fats and absorbs nutriments including those derived from earlier digestion in the stomach.

The large intestine is about 1.5 m. (5 ft.) in length and named successively as ascending, transverse, and descending colon and finally rectum. The junction between small and large intestines is the ileo-caecal valve.

The colon absorbs water from the fluid material reaching it from above and forms waste-matter into a semi-solid state suitable for evacuation as faeces.

Obstruction. Any hindrance to the normal onward progression of the foodstuffs passing through the intestine. This may be acute or chronic, and can occur at any point in the small or large bowel; the chronic type is always liable to become acute.

Causes are varied, including strangulated hernia; intussusception (part of the bowel becomes telescoped within a lower part); volvulus (the bowel becomes twisted); peritoneal bands and adhesions; impaction of foreign bodies; stricture (due to bowel disease); tumour (particularly carcinoma of the lower bowel), and, occasionally, congenital abnormalities.

Symptoms such as colicky pain, vomiting, shock, abdominal distension, tenderness and rigidity are suffered. The muscular efforts of the intestine, attempting to overcome the obstruction, may be seen on the abdominal surface as 'visible peristalsis'. Treatment is

always surgical and acute obstruction calls for emergency relief.

bow legs. Lateral curvature of the legs so that the knees are widely separated when the ankles are in contact. The condition is due to rickets and is preventable by proper diet and adequate vitamin D.

In young children, cases generally improve under skilled supervision, combined with temporarily keeping the weight off the legs, and correction of dietary deficiencies. Adult cases in which permanent deformity has resulted from subsequent ossification may require surgical correction.

BP and BPC. These abbreviations signify respectively the British Pharmacopeia and the British Pharmaceutical Codex.

The Pharmacopeia, published every five years by the General Medical Council, is a descriptive list of 'official' drugs and products used in medicine. It details tests for the determination of identity and purity, specifies standards of strength and activity, and gives instructions regarding the preparation and dosage of formulations suitable for clinical use.

The Codex is published by the Pharmaceutical Society of Great Britain and gives similar information about many other useful medicaments not listed officially in the Pharmacopeia.

brachial neuritis. The nerve trunks of the arm originate from the brachial plexus at the root of the neck and extend downwards as the brachial, median and ulnar nerves.

The plexus and individual nerves are sheathed in fibrous tissue which extends also between the nerve fibres. Acute or chronic inflammation of this connective tissue produces brachial neuritis.

Neuro-fibrositis, a more general name, is usually due to obscure infective or toxaemic conditions, loosely described as rheumatism, and may also be caused by injury or strain. There is pain and tenderness of the affected nerve, and sometimes muscular twitching, cramp, and tingling. Treatment is by rest, application of heat, and analgesics.

bradycardia. Slowness of the heart beat. The usual pulse-rate is 72 beats per minute but a rate of 50 may be found in perfectly healthy athletic subjects, and old people often have slow pulse-rates.

Bradycardia may however indicate disease, especially 'heart-block', where heart-muscle damage causes irregularity of the impulses stimulating contraction of the ventricles. It occurs also in toxic conditions such as uraemia and jaundice; as an indication of heart complications in severe fevers, notably diphtheria and typhoid fever; in hypothyroidism; in poisoning by morphine and other depressant drugs; after excessive dosage of digitalis; and in increased intracranial tension.

brain. The brain is the complex mass of nervous tissue at the upper end of the spinal cord of vertebrates.

As animals evolved the simple reflex control provided by the spinal cord alone became inadequate for the needs of increasingly complicated organisms as they adapted themselves to live more freely, more safely and more successfully within their environment.

In the nervous system this adaptation took place by the expansion of the upper end of the

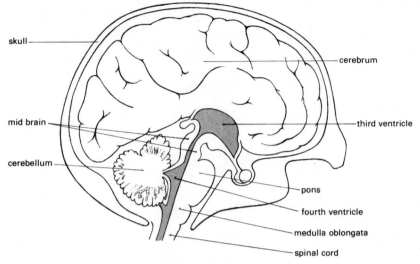

skull

cerebrum

mid brain

third ventricle

cerebellum

pons

fourth ventricle

medulla oblongata

spinal cord

Brain: anatomy

spinal cord in order to provide the additional nervous equipment needed to develop and maintain an independent and purposeful existence.

This upper expanded portion of the central nervous system is known as the encephalon or brain, and in man and all the vertebrates it is contained within the skull or cranial cavity. Its relative size in various animals is an indication of their status on the evolutionary scale and the human brain is by far the largest relative to body-size.

Inside the cranial cavity the brain is encased by three separate layers of membranes or meninges named, from the outside inwards, the dura mater, the arachnoid mater and the pia mater. The dura is tough and fibrous and represents the periosteum of the inner surface of the skull. It also provides four partitions (or septa) which extend into the cavity and form smaller spaces to accommodate and support the sub-divisions of the brain. The arachnoid is a more delicate membrane and between it and the pia (a layer containing blood vessels closely attached to the brain surface), is the sub-arachnoid space containing cerebro-spinal fluid. This fluid layer helps to cushion the brain against impact and sudden movement.

The substance of the brain is composed of grey matter and white matter with blood vessels and a small amount of connective tissue.

Grey matter is composed of nerve cells which originate and receive nerve impulses; white matter is made up of nerve fibres whose function is to transmit nerve impulses from point to point. The proportions and relationships of grey and white matter vary in different parts of the brain.

Parts of the brain. In a simplified description of the brain, the parts from below upwards are:

1. Medulla oblongata. Although continuous with the spinal cord below and only 3 cm. long its minute anatomy is very complex. Within it, nerve fibres from the right side of the fore-brain cross over to pass to the left side of the spinal cord and vice-versa. This is known as the pyramidal decussation and explains why damage to the fore-brain causes paralysis on the opposite side of the body. The medulla also contains the nuclei of the last eight cranial nerves.

2. Pons and cerebellum (or hind-brain). In front of the medulla is the pons, a broad, rounded mass of nerve fibres running transversely and connected below the medulla, above to the fore-brain and behind to the cerebellum which is an egg-shaped mass behind the medulla, and arranged in layers of both grey and white matter.

3. Mid-brain. This is a further short constricted section of the main axis. It is continuous below with the medulla but at its upper end it divides to form two large branches, the cerebral peduncles, which carry fibres to each of the cerebral hemispheres.

4. Cerebrum (the cerebral hemispheres or fore-brain). This is much the largest part of the brain and occupies most of the cranial cavity. It is divided from front to back into two hemispherical masses of nervous tissue known as the right and left cerebral hemispheres and at the bottom of this central fissure is a broad band of communicating fibres, the corpus callosum.

Each hemisphere is in turn divided by grooves called sulci into four main lobes – frontal, temporal (at the side), parietal (on the top), and occipital (at the back).

The surface of the hemispheres or cerebral cortex is made up of grey matter and is arranged in a complicated pattern of ridges and furrows called respectively convolutions and gyri.

The cerebral hemispheres each contain a cavity, the lateral ventricle, occupied by the vascular choroid plexus which produces the clear CEREBRO-SPINAL FLUID. The lateral ventricles unite below as the third ventricle and the fluid passes down through a channel

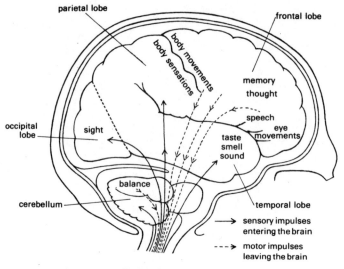

parietal lobe

frontal lobe

body movements

body sensations

memory
thought

speech

occipital lobe

sight

taste
smell
sound

eye movements

balance

cerebellum

temporal lobe

→ sensory impulses entering the brain

---→ motor impulses leaving the brain

Brain: physiology

(Sylvian aqueduct) to the fourth ventricle behind the medulla and from there by an opening to the general sub-arachnoid space.

The PINEAL GLAND and the pituitary gland are both ENDOCRINE GLANDS which form part of the structure of the brain.

Functions of the brain. The individual areas of the brain all have very specific functions.

1. Cerebrum. Removal of the cerebral lobes in an animal deprives it of volition and intelligence. Flourens (1794-1867), the French physiologist, held that the cerebrum was a unitary organ like the liver and that all of it was involved in any mental process so that mental capacity was reduced proportionately to the tissue removed. An opposing school of thought dominated by Sir David Ferrier (1843-1928), born in Aberdeen and professor of neurology at Kings College London, held that different functions of the brain were located in precise areas.

In 1881 the Third International Medical Congress was held in London and at a dramatic session contributed to by F. L. Goltz (1834-1902) of Strasbourg in support of Flourens' theory and by Ferrier, the overwhelming experimental evidence advanced by the latter carried the day for cerebral localization.

We now know that all the higher functions of the brain can be referred to specific cortical areas and in very general terms that the frontal lobes are concerned with memory and thought, the parietal with motor function and sensation, the temporal with taste, smell and hearing and the occipital with sight.

2. Mid-brain. In the region of the third ventricle are other important nerve centres, the thalamus, hypothalamus and basal ganglia. These are concerned with functions carried on automatically below the level of consciousness. The thalamus is the chief relay station of the sensory systems and receives impressions from cord, cerebellum, and cranial nerves; the hypothalamus regulates metabolism, stabilizes temperature and integrates the functions of the organs in the body, and the basal ganglia regulate muscle tone and co-ordinate voluntary movement.

3. Cerebellum. The cerebellum receives linking fibres from cerebrum, cord, and the vestibular part of the acoustic nerve and is concerned with reflex maintenance of balance and posture.

4. Medulla oblongata. Apart from its function as the main connection between the cord and the upper brain and as the site of the crossing of both motor and sensory fibres, the medulla is of supreme importance because it contains all the 'vital centres' and the nuclei of all but the first four pairs of cranial nerves. These vital centres are concerned with respiration, blood pressure, and heart action.

Cranial nerves. Arising from the medulla and from the base of the brain are twelve pairs of cranial nerves all concerned with vital functions and sense-organs. Some are motor (i.e., stimulating muscles to act), others are sensory (i.e., transmitting sensations to the brain) and some contain both motor and sensory fibres. Within the brain their origins, terminations and connections with each other are complex, so that active co-ordination can occur. The nerves pass through openings in the skull.

By enumerating them from below upwards it can be seen that there is a pattern of increasingly specialized function paralleling the upward evolutionary expansion of the central nervous system:

Twelfth: hypoglossal – motor nerve of tongue

Eleventh: spinal accessory – movements of soft palate and head

Tenth: vagus – influences action of organs

Ninth: glosso-pharyngeal – sensory to tongue and assists swallowing

Eighth: acoustic – hearing and balance

Seventh: facial – motor nerve to muscles of face and mouth

Sixth: abducent – eye movements

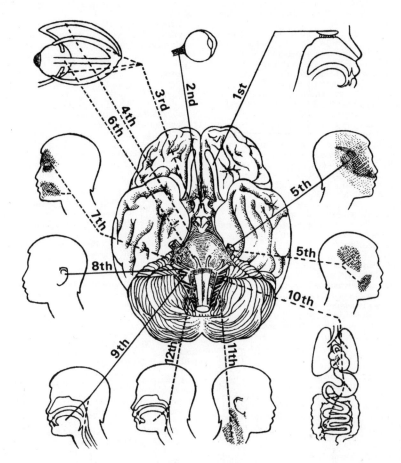

Brain: cranial nerves

Fifth: trigeminal – sensory to face and motor to muscle of mastication
Fourth: trochlear – eye movements
Third: oculomotor – eye movements
Second: optic – sight
First: olfactory – smell

Disease. Because of its complexity the brain is subject to many diseases and only some of the commonest are here mentioned.

1. Infections. Inflammation of the brain substance, encephalitis, may occur in various virus diseases, e.g., poliomyelitis, rabies and encephalitis lethargica (sleepy sickness). Inflammation of the surrounding membranes, meningitis, may be due to invasion by bacteria or viruses or, in the tropics, trypanosomes. All are serious but can be cured by modern treatment, mostly with antibiotics.

2. Arterial disease. There are three forms of stroke: cerebral haemorrhage, where a small artery (weakened by arteriosclerosis and overstressed by high blood pressure) ruptures causing bleeding into the brain substance; cerebral thrombosis where blood clots in a small vessel, depriving a part of the brain of nourishment; and cerebral embolism, where a particle (e.g., an air bubble) causes similar blockage. Again, rupture of a weak part of a blood vessel may cause bleeding between the layers of surrounding membrane (sub-arachnoid haemorrhage).

3. Tumours. Primary tumours, gliomas and mengingiomas, are not uncommon, and secondary tumours may occur from spread from elsewhere in the body. Whether actually destroying brain tissue or merely acting by pressure they cause many variable symptoms, e.g., headache, personality changes, fit paralysis and blindness.

4. Degeneration and atrophy. Many poison (e.g., lead) produce brain degeneration and a general atrophy of the brain occurs in senile dementia, chronic alcoholism, and advanced untreated syphilis.

5. Congenital abnormalities. Hydrocephalus is an example of a developmental anomaly.

6. Injuries. These are not uncommon, particularly in traffic accidents.

brain fever. An old-fashioned term signifying the delirium associated with infections of the brain and its enclosing membranes (meninges), or with toxaemia from acute fevers. See MENINGITIS.

breast. The breasts or mammae are glands accessory to the female reproductive system, producing milk for the nourishment of the infant. In the male they are rudimentary.

The weight and size of the breasts differ in individuals and at different periods of life. Developing as reproductive capacity is established, they enlarge during pregnancy and lactation, and atrophy in old age.

They consist of a glandular mass supported by fibrous tissue and rounded by fat. The gland tissue has many small lobes and from each arises a secretory duct known as a lactiferous tubule. There are between fifteen and twenty such ducts which open on the surface at the nipple, but within the nipple each has a small dilated section or ampulla, which serves as a milk-reservoir. The nipple is encircled by a coloured area of skin known as the areola.

When stimulated the nipple undergoes some erection so that it may be more readily grasped by a suckling's lips.

Diseases. Inflammatory conditions of the breast are mostly associated with lactation. Infection enters through a grazed nipple to cause either inflammation (acute mastitis) or mammary abscesses at various levels – sub-areolar, intra-mammary, or sub-mammary.

Chronic mastitis is related to the changes which occur in the breast after lactation and towards the end of reproductive life. Overgrowth of connective tissue constricts the glandular tissue and ducts and may give rise to cysts.

Tumours are frequent; if non-malignant they are mainly composed of glandular and connective tissue. The commonest malignant tumour is CANCER; it usually produces contraction and indrawing of the breast rather than enlargement. Paget's disease of the nipple is a cancer arising within the lactiferous ducts of the nipple.

breast feeding. There are strong arguments for continuing to advocate breast feeding, but despite professional support it has nevertheless become increasingly unfashionable. The composition of human milk provides for the optimum nutrition of the human infant, and it is also sterile, conveniently available at the correct temperature as required, and free of cost. Also, the act of breast feeding forges a psychic bond between mother and infant which is beneficial to emotional development. In addition to this, although many children thrive completely satisfactorily on artificial feeding, there is a greater risk of malnutrition and infection through carelessness while preparing the bottles and filling them.

Lactation. Under hormonal influence, the breasts, soon after conception, prepare for subsequent lactation, but actual secretion of milk is inhibited until after the birth. The stimulus of suckling also encourages output. Immediately after childbirth the breast secretes only colostrum, a fluid especially rich in protein and not requiring digestion. This provides the infant's needs for the first two or three days until its digestive system is operative. It also provides temporary immunity to some infections as it contains substances from the mother's blood plasma. By the third day

swelling of the breasts occurs and normal milk secretion begins.

Adequate lactation is conditioned by both physical and psychic factors. Good health, contentment, lack of fatigue, a liberal well-balanced diet with ample protein and a sufficient fluid intake are obvious requirements, but pleasure in nursing, determination and optimism are thought to influence by reflex the production by the pituitary gland of milk-forming hormone, while grief and worry inhibit this.

Methods of regime. Mothercraft lectures during pregnancy should encourage a determination to breast-feed and should include instruction in the technique of nursing and the care of breast and nipples.

After washing the breasts and nipples the mother should sit comfortably in a low chair with her infant in the crook of the arm on the side being used. The breast is supported with the other hand and the skin above the nipple retracted by thumb to avoid obstruction of the infant's nostrils.

Hospitals and professional advisers favour their individual regimes but the following is typical:

Starting six to twelve hours after birth, three feeds of a few minutes at each breast are given each day during the first and second days, or until full lactation commences. During this period the infant obtains only small amounts of colostrum and its fluid requirements should be made up by sterile water from a spoon. When lactation is established the breasts provide about 425 g. (15 oz.) of milk per day, rising to 550 to 700 g. (20 to 25 oz.) at one month, 700 to 850 g. (25 to 30 oz.) at three months and 850 g. to 1 kg. (30 to 35 oz.) at six months. Thereafter the quantity declines.

There is difference of opinion about regular and 'on-demand' feeding, but regularity may be better both for emotional development and for the digestive tract. For the first two months three-hourly feeding is usual, (6 a.m., 9 a.m., 12 noon, 3 p.m., 6 p.m., 10 p.m.) changing to four-hourly at six to twelve weeks. One breast may be used alternately at each feed of about twenty minutes, or ten minutes given at each breast. The use of one breast is said to be preferable because the end-milk is richer in fat. The infant ingests air during suckling and should be 'posseted' – set upright and allowed to 'break wind'.

If there is any anxiety of UNDERFEEDING, suggested perhaps by the infant failing to thrive, it is important to ascertain how much milk a breast-fed infant is actually getting. This is done by a 'test-feed' i.e., weighing the baby on an accurate scale before and after a feed. If insufficient, a 'complementary feed' can be given by bottle after each breast feed, or a 'supplementary feed' replacing one or more breast feeds.

Breast feeding is inadvisable if the mother is suffering from malnutrition, general illness, tuberculosis, chronic nephritis, severe heart disease or puerperal psychosis. It is equally inadvisable if the infant suffers from prematurity, brain damage or other mental abnormality, hare-lip or cleft palate.

If the mother does not wish to breast-feed, lactation may be checked by giving several doses of oestrogen. Without such help there may be swelling and pain in the breasts for a few days but, lacking in stimulus of suckling, the breasts gradually return to normal over several weeks.

breathlessness. Distressed respiration or dyspnoea, although temporary breathlessness after considerable exertion is a normal phenomenon and is therefore not dyspnoea. The basic cause of dyspnoea is over-stimulation of the respiratory centre in the brain by excess of carbonic acid in the blood. This implies that oxygen is not easily leaving the lungs (as in asthma), or is not being carried by the blood at sufficient rate (as in defective circulation), or is not being conveyed in adequate amounts by the blood (as in anaemia), or is limited in quantity (as occurs in high altitudes).

Respiratory distress may affect breathing in (inspiration) and breathing out (expiration) unequally. Obstructive causes tend to produce inspiration dysponea; lung damage mostly affects expiration. In other conditions there is no marked difference.

A complaint of breathlessness requires investigation, and appropriate treatment can only be decided after a precise diagnosis of its cause.

breath, offensive. A more formal term for offensive breath is halitosis. Common causes are septic conditions of the mouth, nose, or naso-pharynx – e.g., bad teeth, unhealthy gums with pyorrhoea, mouth ulceration, diseased tonsils, and certain chronic nasal conditions. Mild offensiveness is sometimes due to gastric disorder or constipation.

Excessively putrid breath occurs in such lung conditions as bronchiectasis or lung abscess. Some general diseases, such as uraemia or diabetes, may produce characteristic odours, as may certain drugs.

bronchi. The bronchi are part of the main air-passages and arise in mid-chest by sub-division of the trachea or windpipe.

The right bronchus divides into three branches which enter the root of the right lung and pass to the upper, middle, and lower lobes. The left bronchus divides into two main branches to enter the upper and lower lobes of the left lung. Within each lung, these main branches divide and sub-divide throughout the whole organ to form the intrapulmonary bronchi or 'bronchial-tree', conveying air to all parts of the lungs, the fine terminal branches being known as bronchioles.

In detailed structure the bronchi consist of three layers: an outer layer of fibrous tissue, containing rings of cartilage which keep the airway from collapsing; a layer of smooth muscle-fibre which controls the calibre of the airway; and an internal of muscous membrane, lined by special cells which keep the airway moist and help to expel secretion.

Bronchitis, or inflammation of the bronchi, is one of the commonest maladies, readily caused by a wide variety of physical agencies or infective processes.

bronchial cyst and fistula. See GILLS.

bronchiectasis. A lung condition in which the bronchi or larger air-passages become dilated, either in their length (cylindrical bronchiectasis), or irregularly to form cavities (sacculated bronchiectasis). It is due to two factors: weakening of the bronchial wall by chronic bronchitis; and forced inspiration after coughing, especially if peripheral parts of the

lung are damaged by disease and cannot expand freely.

Purulent secretion accumulates in the dilated parts and this erodes and further weakens the bronchus, establishing a vicious circle. There is often offensive sputum and offensive breath due to decomposition of pus which has not been coughed out.

The treatment is that of chronic bronchitis. Postural coughing may help the evacuation of sputum, and pneumothorax or other surgical procedures are occasionally used in selected cases.

bronchitis. Inflammation of the bronchi. Acute bronchitis is very common, especially where winter conditions are inclement, and is sometimes called the 'English disease' and chronic bronchitis follows repeated attacks of the acute form. Acute bronchitis is due to infection by some bacterial or viral agent. The windpipe is generally affected as well and if infection extends downwards to the smaller air-passages the disease becomes indistinguishable from broncho-pneumonia. An attack usually begins suddenly with malaise, fever, chest pain, breathlessness, and a dry ineffective cough. Sputum later becomes copious – moist and frothy at first but becoming pus-like. A typical attack without complications lasts about seven to ten days. Acute bronchitis may also be caused by inhalation of dust or of irritants such as smoke or chemical vapours.

Treatment is by bed rest and the administration of antibiotics. Poultices, cough-mixtures, and medicated inhalations, although rather old-fashioned, still give some relief from symptoms.

In chronic bronchitis, the bronchial walls become thickened and fibrotic, and the mucous glands and the cells lining the bronchi degenerate. Long-standing chronic bronchitis may lead to emphysema, pulmonary fibrosis, and bronchiectasis, which in turn affects the circulation to the lungs, so that a degree of right-sided heart failure (corpulmonale) may eventually develop.

The patient with chronic bronchitis complains of his 'chest' – persistent cough, expectoration, and breathlessness on exertion. The cough varies in severity, usually recurring each winter. Smoking is undoubtedly a contributory cause.

Treatment of established chronic bronchitis can only be precautionary and soothing. A mild winter climate, avoidance of chill and exposure, cessation of smoking, attention to diet and general regime, antibiotics or vaccines, may all help to prevent worsening of the condition. Attacks, when they occur require treatment as acute bronchitis.

broncho-pneumonia. An inflammatory lung condition in which infection spreads from the terminal air-passages (bronchioles) to the air-sacs (alveoli) and thence to the surrounding tissue, producing a patchy type of consolidation (lobular pneumonia), in contrast to the massive consolidation of a whole lung lobe which occurs in ordinary lobar pneumonia. It can begin as a primary broncho-pneumonia, especially in children, but many cases are secondary to other disease such as whooping cough or measles.

Broncho-pneumonia is a common sequel to many debilitating diseases and often hastens death in the aged. Treatment nowadays is usually by antibiotics.

brucellosis. Undulant or Malta fever. An infection, caused by *Brucella abortus,* mainly from the milk of infected cattle, sheep and goats and characterized by continued or intermittent fever, headache, profuse sweating and joint pains, all of which may last for days, months or occasionally years. The disease is transmitted to man from the milk of infected animals, from contact with the tissues or discharges of such animals (e.g., in the case of veterinary surgeons) and very infrequently by airborne spread. There is no evidence of the infection passing from man to man.

Diagnosis is difficult clinically because the symptoms are vague and intermittent so it usually depends either on blood tests which show a rise in antibodies or on laboratory isolation of the infectious agent.

Prevention depends finally on either (1) ascertainment of all infected animals by blood tests and elimination of these animals by segregation or by slaughter, or (2) immunization of all calves, etc., in any area in which the disease is present. Pending such measures imperative steps are pasteurization of milk and other dairy products from cows, sheep and goats, or boiling of milk if pasteurization is impracticable; great care should be taken by veterinary surgeons and meat inspectors to avoid infection.

Treatment prospects have improved in recent years: tetracycline, or another suitable antibiotic, usually cures the disease in about three months, but relapse occurs in quite a proportion of cases.

bruises. A bruise or contusion is a superficial injury caused by impact or other external violence without actually breaking the skin. This results in damage to tissue and blood-vessels immediately beneath the skin and blood infiltrates the area. If an actual rupture of the underlying tissues occurs, blood may accumulate in the resultant space to produce a haematoma.

The signs of a bruise are obvious, with discoloration and swelling, but the possibility of associated damage to underlying organs and other structures must always be considered.

The amount of subcutaneous bleeding and of swelling varies a great deal not only with the degree of violence, but also with the part of the body injured. Where the tissues are lax the amount of bleeding is correspondingly greater, and it may track along beneath the skin by the influence of gravity and according to the surrounding anatomical structures, so that the discoloration (or ecchymosis) may appear elsewhere than at the actual site of injury.

Bruises undergo changes in colour as the blood within them disintegrates and becomes re-absorbed. At first they are of a dark purplish-blue colour which gradually alters over a week or so to various shades of brown and green and then to a pale yellow before disappearing completely.

In the initial stages, bruises are best treated by cold compresses and firm bandaging in order to limit bleeding. Later on, when the bruising is no longer painful, the absorption of effused blood can be hastened by massage. A localized haematoma, which may remain tense and painful for some time, can be relieved, and recovery hastened, by aseptic draining.

bubo. An inflammatory swelling of the lymphatic glands in the groin (inguinal lymphadenitis). The term is sometimes also applied to a similar condition in the armpit but not correctly because 'bubo' is derived from *boubon,* the Greek word for groin.

Inguinal bubo is due to some infective condition in the related lymphatic drainage area. In the classical bubo of bubonic PLAGUE it is caused by the entry of the bacillus through bites from infected fleas. The common causes are more mundane, ranging from septic sores on feet and legs, to various forms of venereal disease. Certain tropical diseases such as filariasis and sleeping sickness produce similar swellings.

The treatment is that of the underlying condition but the bubo may form pus and require surgical drainage of the resultant abscess.

bubonic plague. An epidemic disease due to infection with *Pasteurella pestis,* the PLAGUE bacillus.

Bubonic plague is of great historical significance, and many classical outbreaks are recorded: it occurred amongst the Philistines after they defeated the Israelites at Ebenezer (I. Samuel ch. 5); it stopped the seventh Crusade at Tunis in 1270; it was the cause of the Black Death which raged in Europe from 1346 to 1351 (invading England in 1348) and which eventually killed 25 million people – a quarter of the population of Europe.

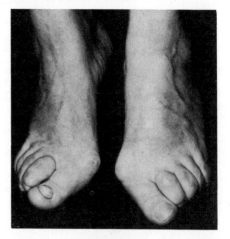

Bunions

bunion. A condition, usually found over the joint at the base of the big toe, in which there is thickening both of the skin and of the head of the metatarsal bone. The main cause is the wearing of shoes which are too short or too narrow at the toes, so that the big toe is forced out of position towards the other toes. Prevention is essentially by wearing wide enough shoes. Where the condition has developed, treatment may include wearing socks like gloves with a compartment for each toe, or inserting every morning a piece of lint between the great toe and the next toe. In very severe cases operative treatment may be required.

burns and scalds. Exposure of any part of the body to excessive heat causes injury to the tissues. With flame or dry heat the result is a burn; hot liquids and hot moist vapours, such as steam, produce a scald. Burns may also be caused by acids, alkalis, electricity, friction, and exposure to sources of radiant energy, such as excessive sunlight, ultra-violet light, gamma-rays and x-rays.

Heat injury is described according to the severity of tissue reaction and damage. The classification of burns, ranging from 'first degree' to 'sixth degree' was originally proposed by Baron Dupuytren (1778-1835), a celebrated French surgeon, and is still in current use, although to some extent the area of a burn is more important than its degree.

First degree: reddening and congestion of the skin; no tissue destruction.

Second degree: blistering of skin.

Third degree: cuticle and outer layer of the true skin is destroyed but the deeper papillae with nerve-endings survive. Since these are then left exposed, this grade of burn is very painful and causes considerable shock.

In these three degrees of burn, sufficient skin-cells survive to ensure healing by natural multiplication of cells without recourse to skin-grafting.

Fourth degree: the whole thickness of skin and subcutaneous tissue are destroyed.

Fifth degree: muscles are destroyed.

Sixth degree: a whole limb is charred or disorganized.

Clinical features. Apart from the tissue destruction described above, the immediate danger of a severe burn is the amount of constitutional upset. Shock and collapse are related more to the area of a burn than to its depth, and require immediate treatment. Later on there will be absorption of toxins from the burned areas, manifested by raised temperature and pulse-rate, and often delirium. Further complications may ensue, such as broncho-pneumonia and suppression of urinary excretion.

In cases which survive, inflammation (usually accompanied by infection) gradually leads to separation of dead tissue as sloughs, leaving an ulcerated surface which eventually heals. If not skin-grafted, the resultant scarring may produce contractures and deformity.

Treatment. Local treatment depends on the severity of the burn and on its extent. The objects are to allay pain and to prevent secondary infection of the burned area.

Immediate treatment: separate the casualty from the danger, bathe the damaged part freely in cold water to reduce the pain and heat, and then apply a non-sterile dressing and cover this with available soft materials, such as cotton-wool and a bandage.

For minor burns of small extent, initial cleaning with a mild antiseptic or normal saline (i.e., 1 teaspoon of salt to 0.5 l. (1 pt.) of water) followed by the application of medicated tulle, is simple and effective. The tulle is an open-weave gauze impregnated with soft paraffin and an antibiotic. If saline or antiseptic is not immediately available, the burned part may be held under cold running water for a few minutes. Any blister which may develop should not normally be drained.

In more severe burns, and in superficial burns involving large areas of skin, the immediate need is to initiate adequate treatment against SHOCK and possible complications. Such patients should be sent to hospital, and the first aid treatment is therefore just to cover the burned areas with a sterile, or at least clean, dressing. The dressing may be either dry or moistened with normal saline or a weak solution of sodium bicarbonate – say 2 teaspoonfuls to 0.5 l. (1 pt.) of water. Measures to combat shock should also be initiated by keeping the patient warm and giving hot sweet drinks.

In hospital it will probably be necessary to give intravenous infusions of saline or plasma. For local treatment, various centres have their own favourite regimes.

At a later stage, whole-skin destruction will necessitate skin-grafting.

Acid burns. Corrosive acids cause tissue damage with much the same effect as a burn by heat, but continue to act harmfully until removed or neutralized. Such injuries should therefore first be sluiced freely with clean or sterile water, saline, or a weak alkaline solution of sodium bicarbonate (2 teaspoonfuls to 0.5 l. (1 pt.) water). Thereafter a moist dressing can be applied using the same alkaline solution.

Alkali burns. Corrosive alkalis, such as caustic soda, also cause tissue damage with much the same effect as a burn by heat, and they too continue to act harmfully until removed or neutralized. Such injuries should therefore first be sluiced freely with clean or sterile water, saline, or a weak acid solution of vinegar (2 tablespoonfuls to 0.5 l. (1 pt.) water). Thereafter a moist dressing can be applied using saline or the vinegar solution.

Eye burns. Burns of the eye are always potentially serious since even small superficial injuries involving the cornea will impair subsequent vision. The eyelids automatically protect the eyes, which themselves often escape even in extensive facial burns, but a hot 'spark' may enter and cause injury. More common are the effects of splashes of caustic materials – acids, alkalis, quicklime, etc.

It is essential to wash out the harmful substance *immediately:* lay the patient down, hold the eyelids open, and pour plenty of plain water over the eye, or put the face in a basin of water and open and shut the eyelids while submerged. For acid injuries, a solution of 1 teaspoon of sodium bicarbonate to 0.5 l. (1 pt.) of water can be used for washing out, and for alkalis (including quicklime), a weak acid solution of 1 tablespoonful of vinegar to 0.5 l. (1 pt.) of water.

Speed is vital, and the value of immediate washing out with plain water outweighs delay in obtaining more precise antidotes. In all cases the subsequent first-aid treatment is to instil a drop of castor or olive oil, apply an occlusive pad and bandage, and send the patient to hospital.

bursa. A pouch, or sac-like cavity in the tissues, lined by synovial membrane (as in joint-capsules), and containing synovial fluid as a lubricant. Its purpose is to minimize friction of the tissues at points subject to pressure or movement. Bursae are found in many parts of the body as normal anatomical structures, between muscles and tendons, and between bony prominences and the skin.

Familiar examples are the bursae over the knee (pre-patellar bursa), the elbow (olecranon bursa), and over the bony points carrying one's weight when seated (ischial bursa). These frequently become inflamed in BURSITIS.

Repeated pressure and friction may also lead to the development of bursae not normally present, and therefore called 'adventitious bursae'. Examples are those which appear in the scalp and over the shoulder blades and upper spine in porters who carry burdens on their heads and backs; over the ankle bones in tailors and others who sit cross-legged; and over the outer side of the great toe as bunions.

bursitis. Inflammation of a bursa. The sac of a bursa subjected to repeated small injuries may become inflamed and distended by an excessive development of the fluid within the bursa, usually mixed with blood. Deposits of fibrin from the blood produce a thickening of the bursal wall with a diminished capacity to re-absorb the excess fluid.

Swellings thus develop in familiar sites, as 'housemaid's knee', 'miner's elbow' and bunions.

Initially these may respond to rest and draining of their contents but resistant cases will require removal of the sac. Bursae may become infected and develop pus, when they will also need surgical treatment.

Bursitis can also occur in general diseases such as gonorrhoea and syphilis, and in tuberculosis in proximity to infected joints.

byssinosis. A condition of diminished chest expansion and emphysema, characterized by paroxysmal cough and respiratory difficulty resembling that of asthma. It occurs among persons who have for long periods breathed the dust from cotton and cotton fabrics, and is ascribed to moulds present in these materials. Byssinosis is in part preventable by measures for the reduction of the dust, and regular medical examination of cotton workers can usually identify the disease in the early stages, when treatment is still relatively easy. The first essential of treatment is to separate the patient from the cause, and to deal with any associated condition (e.g., bronchitis); but in advanced stages the condition is usually permanent.

C

cachexia. A severe state of ill-health accompanied by constitutional disorder and serious malnutrition. It develops in chronic wasting diseases such as pulmonary tuberculosis, malignant conditions, prolonged sepsis and fevers, hyperthyroidism and other endocrine disorders, toxaemia from various causes, and some kinds of chronic poisoning.

caecum. A musculo-membraneous pouch situated down on the lower right of the abdomen and forming a cul-de-sac at the beginning of the large intestine. It receives the contents of the small intestine through the ileo-caecal valve before their onward passage through the colon.

At its lower extremity it terminates as a tube of much reduced calibre which is the appendix, often affected by appendicitis.

caesarean section. Delivery of a child by an incision through the abdominal and uterine walls instead of by the natural passage.

The name is traditionally due to the Roman historian Pliny who relates that Julius Caesar was delivered in this manner. Certainly, such sections did occur in ancient times, usually to save the child when a mother died in an advanced stage of pregnancy. Persons so delivered were known as Caesones and regarded with some superstitious awe. In his play *Macbeth,* Shakespeare exploits this idea. In the dramatic climax, Macbeth, who had been told by the witches that 'none of woman born' could harm him, is slain by Macduff, who had been 'from his mother's womb untimely ripp'd'.

Nowadays, caesarean section is a routine and safe surgical procedure employed in obstetric situations where normal delivery might carry risk to mother or baby. It may be carried out if one or more of the following conditions apply: contracted pelvis; disproportionately large babies; obstructive position of the placenta (placenta praevia); ante-partum haemorrhage; toxaemia or other disease of the mother; rupture of the uterus; and more rarely, tumours or congenital abnormalities of the uterus interfering with the normal mechanism of labour.

caffeine. A white crystalline alkaloid substance contained in tea and coffee. A cerebral stimulant and mild diuretic, it is a common constituent of analgesic powders because of its reputed effect in relieving the migranous type of headache.

Aspirin compound tablets (BPC) contain aspirin, phenacetin, and 30 mg. of caffeine. The official dose of caffeine is 60 to 300 mg.

There are two other official preparations: caffeine citrate (120 to 600 mg.) and effervescing caffeine citrate (4 to 8 g.) which mixed in water, makes a pleasant effervescent drink with some reputation as a 'pick-me-up'.

caisson disease. Known also as 'diver's paralysis' or 'the bends', this condition affects workers under compressed air who return too rapidly to normal atmospheric pressure. See DECOMPRESSION DISEASE.

calcification. The deposition of lime salts in body-tissues. Calcification is a normal process in the growth and development of bones and teeth when calcium salts, mainly phosphate and carbonate, are laid down in an orderly fashion. Calcium metabolism is controlled by activity of the parathyroid glands and by the availability of dietary vitamin D.

Calcification also occurs pathologically, and in general, dead or degenerating tissue tends to become impregnated by lime salts; this type differs from ossification since the lime salts are without definite structure and may produce harmful mechanical effects both to the tissue which they occupy and to its surroundings.

calcium. A hard, yellowish, metallic element, always found combined with another element. It occurs as deposits of calcium carbonate (limestone, chalk, marble) or calcium sulphate (gypsum, alabaster); it is widely distributed in the soil and is a mineral constituent of all plants and animals.

The body requires calcium particularly for the formation of bones and teeth. Milk and vegetables are good sources but it is abundant in any ordinary diet. However, its proper utilization requires an adequate intake of vitamin D, otherwise children suffer from rickets and older persons develop osteomalacia. Calcium metabolism is also influenced by the parathyroid glands, over-activity of which decalcifies bone. Under-activity lowers serum calcium to produce the condition known as parathyroid tetany.

calculus. A concretion occurring abnormally in hollow organs or in ducts as the result of the deposition of mineral salts or organic material. See STONE.

caliper or **calliper.** A caliper or walking-caliper splint consists of a padded ring which encircles the upper thigh and rests against the bony prominence in the lower buttock which is the ischial tuberosity of the pelvis. To this ring are attached two metal bars (usually adjustable in length), one on each side of the limb. Angled lower-ends fit into the heel of the patient's boot and thus his weight is transmitted through the caliper and not through the limb. Such a splint is used after fractures and joint disease so that walking is possible without crutches or risk of injury to diseased or healing parts. The same principles of caliper splintage or traction are used elsewhere. Digital fractures are an example.

The term 'calipers' is also used as a name for various measuring devices, basically resembling a pair of mathematical dividers, but of suitable size and design to facilitate the measurement of dimensions with clinical importance such as pelvic diameters, depth of chest, and skin-fold thickness.

callosity. A circumscribed thickening of the outer layer of the skin, occurring as a protective reaction to friction, pressure, or other chronic irritation. Callosities are commonly seen on the feet, on the hands of manual workers, on the shoulders of porters, and so on.

Callosities are generally painless, and require no treatment, but sometimes a sac, containing synovial fluid, develops beneath them to form an adventitious BURSA, which may become inflamed and infected and require to be dealt with surgically. A CORN is another type of painful callosity. It has a central, inverted core of overgrowth which presses on the sensitive deeper layers of the skin, causing pain and discomfort.

Calorie. For measuring quantities of heat the scientific unit is the gram-calorie; this is the amount of heat required to raise the temperature of one gram of water by one degree centigrade.

Food is the fuel which the body requires for its energy; since foods vary in the amount of energy which they liberate when 'burned' or metabolized, it is usual to express their food-value in this respect in units of heat. For this purpose the gram-calorie is an inconveniently small unit, so the heat-equivalent of foods are stated in Calories (capital C); these are kilogram-calories, equal to 1000 gram-calories. In the future a new unit of measurement, the KILOJOULE will be used more frequently to measure food values.

Dietary needs in terms of Calories and the Calorie values of individual foodstuffs are explained in the articles on DIET and NUTRITION.

cancer. Any malignant tumour or unregulated growth of tissue is commonly called 'cancer' but scientifically there are three types according to the cells of the tissue involved. The cells which cover the outer surface of the body and line internal passages and closed cavities are called epithelial cells: malignancy in these cells is known as carcinoma. In other body cells it is sarcoma. Malignant proliferation of certain blood cells is seen in leukaemia.

Cancer is essentially the unregulated and unrestricted growth of new cells to form tissue which lacks the useful function of its parent tissue and serves no purpose; which disorganizes the structure and function of the part of the body where it arises; which invades adjacent tissues; and which tends to spread to other organs by blood-borne metastases.

Cancer occurs in man and all vertebrate animals. An incidence of about one in twenty of the population is increasing slowly, but the increase is probably more apparent than real, due to better diagnosis and because more persons now survive to reach the older cancer-prone age-groups.

Causes. Although world-wide and massive cancer research has so far failed to demonstrate exactly why cells should behave in this way, nevertheless much is known about predisposing factors. A theory put forward by Conheim (1839-84) that cancers arose from inclusions of embryonic tissue has now been discarded as a general solution. Cancer of the stomach has been shown to occur more frequently in persons of certain blood groups, but cancer is not hereditary in the true sense and any hereditary influence is apparently due to some genetically determined variation in resistance to environmental factors, whose importance is undoubted. Scrotal carcinoma in chimney-sweeps has long been recognized as due to irritation by soot, and there are many other organic chemicals which tend to induce carcinoma, for example: the polycyclic hydrocarbons derived from tar; benzyprene in cigarette smoke (which has been incriminated as a cause of lung cancer); and naphthylamine solvents used in the rubber industry (which cause carcinoma of the bladder).

Mechanical and physical factors may also induce cancer: a jagged tooth or ill-fitting denture may produce a chronic mouth ulcer which refuses to heal and undergoes malignant change; and skin cancer can be due to prolonged x-ray exposure. Since 1911 it has been known that virus material can induce malignant changes in animals (Rous' chicken-sarcoma).

More recent work by Burkitt on a type of lymphoid tumour found in parts of Africa also suggests the influence of a transmissible viral agent.

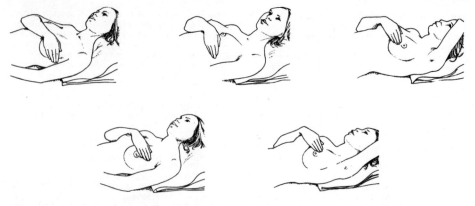

Self examination for breast cancer. Lie down with a cushion under one shoulder. Using the flat of the fingers rather than the tips, first check into the armpits for any 'lump' and then work carefully round the breast, always stroking from the edge towards the nipple. Change the cushion to the other side and repeat the test.

The final explanation of cancer development requires further study.

Signs and symptoms. Because pain is a late feature, cancer is often neglected until the prospects of successful treatment are imperilled. In view of the importance of early treatment, attention may here be called to some warning signs, although it must be understood that there are other possible explanations of each sign listed below, so that, while indicating the desirability of skilled investigation, these signs do not necessarily indicate the existence of cancer.

On external surfaces any thickening of the tissues or any persisting sores and ulcers should arouse suspicion. Internal cancers are insidious but weight loss and anaemia in an older person need investigation, especially if accompanied by any of the following:

1. Breast: tumour; skin-puckering; retraction of, or bleeding from, the nipple.
2. Gastro-intestinal tract: persistent digestive symptoms; abdominal pain; constipation; 'tarry' stools indicating internal bleeding; fresh blood; alternation for an appreciable time between constipation and diarrhoea.
3. Respiratory system: cough; pain; breathlessness; blood-stained sputum; persistent hoarseness or difficulty in swallowing.
4. Bladder: blood in the urine.
5. Female genital tract: irregular bleeding or its persistence after the menopause.

Prevention. Known hazards, such as those noted above, should be avoided, but in general the prospect of successful treatment depends on early detection.

Cancer detection clinics were pioneered by the American Cancer Society in 1920. The essentials are a careful clinical history and examination; x-ray of chest; blood examination of faeces for occult blood (i.e., blood that is not obvious on inspection). For the female, CERVICAL CYTOLOGY (the 'cyto-test'), when a smear is taken from the uterine cervix for microscopic examination, is now widely available, and simple self-examination for breast cancer is carried out easily at home.

Treatment. The basic treatment for early accessible cancer is surgical removal with dissection of related lymph-glands. Deep x-ray therapy and radium application are used as alternative or auxiliary procedures.

Chemical methods are being developed. Such drugs may be antimetabolites (which inhibit nucleic acid synthesis), cytotoxins (which act on formed nucleic acid), radio-isotopes (for special tumours), steroids (which influence antibody response), antibiotics (e.g., actinomycin C in Hodgkin's disease) or other drugs such as methylhydrazine derivatives or vincristine sulphate.

cancrum oris. A very severe infective STOMATITIS with ulceration and gangrene of the lips and cheeks.

canine teeth. The single-cusped or pointed teeth (the Latin *caninus* means 'dog-like') of which there are two in each jaw situated on each side between the last incisor tooth and the first pre-molar tooth. In children they erupt at about the eighteenth month and their permanent replacements appear at the age of 11 years.

They occupy an important position in the dental arch between the front and back teeth: premature loss of deciduous (or 'baby') canines is particularly detrimental to satisfactory alignment of the permanent teeth, because the incisors and pre-molars tend to encroach on the space needed for the permanent canines. These subsequently grow in faulty positions, necessitating orthodontic treatment.

cannabis. A drug obtained from the Indian hemp plant (*Cannabis sativa*). The dried flowering tops contain a resin, cannabinol, and are used to make cigarettes (reefers). Cannabis is also called marihuana and another preparation using resin from the whole plant is known as hashish. The drug is taken to produce the pleasurable effects of a mild intoxication in which the user feels elated.

The possession and use of cannabis are now illegal in most countries and the United Nations Commission on Narcotic Drugs considers cannabis abuse a form of addiction likely to be a forerunner of dependence on more dangerous drugs. This view has been challenged on the grounds that cannabis is a less antisocial drug than alcohol. Nevertheless, it has powerful effects on the central nervous system and psychotic illness has been caused by its excessive use.

Legalization of cannabis, leading to widespread use of the drug as a substitute for alcohol, would certainly bring its own problems, and should perhaps continue to be resisted by society.

cantharides. The 'Spanish fly' is really a beetle, *Cantharis vesicatoria*, one of numerous species of small, brightly-coloured blister beetles common in southern Europe. Their bodies contain a substance, cantharadin, a powerful irritant, which causes inflammation of the skin and blistering.

The beetles are found in early summer, feeding on the leaves of trees and shrubs. As a commercial undertaking, they are collected and dried and various official pharmacopeial preparations – plasters, tinctures, and ointments, whose active ingredient is cantharadin – are made from the dried beetles for use in medicine.

Blistering is now an out-moded procedure, but these medicaments were once much used as counter-irritants. Acetum cantharadini is still employed to encourage hair-growth in baldness but its efficacy is doubtful, while its reputation as an aphrodisiac simply depends on irritation of the entire urinary system. When absorbed, cantharadin is an irritant poison with severe effects on the gastro-intestinal and urinary tracts. The use of its various preparations requires care.

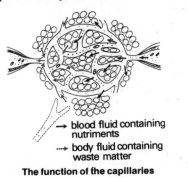

→ blood fluid containing nutriments
⇢ body fluid containing waste matter

The function of the capillaries

capillaries. The minute blood-vessels which connect the terminal branches of the arteries (arterioles) to the small radicles of the venous system (venules) and which form a network in most parts of the body. The blood can thus circulate through the tissues to provide food and oxygen, arriving from the heart by the arterial system and returning through the veins.

Similar small vessels are found in the lymphatic system and are known as lymphatic capillaries.

capsule. Anatomically, a capsule is any fibrous or membraneous sac enclosing an organ or part of the body. Examples are the kidney and spleen, most joints, and the lens of the eye.

Capsules are also used in pharmacy to enclose various drugs. Amylnitrate is dispensed in thin-walled capsules (0.2 ml.) enclosed in absorbent fabric. They are crushed between finger and thumb and the vapour

inhaled to relieve anginal pain. Officially these are called 'vitrellae' to distinguish them from gelatine capsules in which many medicines for oral use are now supplied, especially if they have a nauseating taste or are unsuitable for moulding into tablets. Somewhat similar are cachets made of two watch-glass shaped halves of soluble wafer-paper between which the drug is enclosed. These are used when a bulky dose is required (1 to 2 gm.).

Both gelatine capsules and cachets are intended to be held momentarily in the mouth till moistened and softened and then swallowed whole.

carbohydrate. An essential component of our food, carbohydrates are organic compounds containing carbon, hydrogen, and oxygen.

In terms of the diet, carbohydrates are the starches and sugars, almost entirely of vegetable origin, and they provide the greater part of the energy requirements of the body. In the process of digestion both the starches and the more complex sugars are broken down to glucose which is absorbed and stored in the liver and muscles until required as fuel by the tissues.

carbohydrate intolerance. Inability to digest and absorb carbohydrate. Signs and symptoms include flatulence and distension of the abdomen (both due to formation of gas from the undigested carbohydrate), watery diarrhoea (from partly broken down carbohydrate), and in due course weakness (from insufficient supplies of energy), enlarged liver (from disturbed storage of carbohydrate) and acidosis (from fermentation). The cause of the intolerance is either faulty secretion of the digestive juices which normally break down sugars and starches to simpler sugars (monosaccharides) for absorption, or inability of the digestive tract to absorb monosaccharides.

Treatment depends on the cause but may consist of supplying drugs to replace or stimulate the faulty digestive juices, of giving drugs which slow the movement of food in the digestive tract and so provide more time for absorption, or of removing ordinary starches and sugars from the diet and substituting the simplest of sugars, glucose.

carbolic acid. An organic compound distilled from coal-tar. Also known as phenol, it is a powerful antiseptic, disinfectant, and germicide. In its pure state it forms colourless crystals which always absorb moisture; they then form an oily liquid with a characteristic odour.

Carbolic acid is mainly of interest because it was the antiseptic used by Joseph Lister (1827-1912) in developing his system of antiseptic surgery. However, it has disadvantages in relation to toxicity and tissue damage and has largely been superseded by safer compounds.

The disinfecting value of a substance is expressed as its Rideal-Walker coefficient which uses carbolic acid as a standard of comparison.

carbon monoxide. A colourless gas, odourless, poisonous and lighter than air, produced by the combustion of carbon in a limited supply of oxygen. It is poisonous because it combines with the haemoglobin of the blood to form the stable, bright-red compound carboxy-haemoglobin which can no longer carry oxygen to the body tissues, and so death results from a form of asphyxia. A concentration of 10 per cent in the atmosphere is highly inflammable and a concentration of 1 per cent is definitely dangerous to breathe.

Carbon monoxide is used in industry as a fuel and as a reducing agent (e.g., in iron-smelting). It is also a constituent of motor vehicle exhaust gas; defective exhaust systems or running engines in closed garages are therefore potential hazards.

Although in many places coal-gas is now being replaced by natural gas, which is mainly methane and relatively harmless except in high concentrations, domestic coal-gas contains carbon monoxide and it is therefore frequently a cause of accidental deaths resulting from carelessness or misuse, and is often used in suicide attempts.

In chronic, low-grade poisoning (as from a persisting small gas leak) the main signs are pallor, headaches and signs of anaemia. Acute poisoning is characterized by headache, nausea, vomiting, staggering gait, muscular weakness and mental confusion (a general picture resembling drunkenness), often continuing to coma and death.

In rescue work the wearing of a respirator, or failing that a wet cloth round the mouth and nose, is important: the intending rescuer may otherwise become a second victim.

On entering a room filled with coal-gas the rescuer should open the windows widely before doing anything else, and he should in no circumstances use a naked light. Having opened the windows and dealt with any immediate source of gas (such as a tap left on) he should get the victim into the open air, loosen clothing, especially round the neck, apply artifical respiration and send an available person for a doctor because administration of oxygen is likely to be necessary.

Whether gas poisoning is fatal or not, the question of accident, suicide or murder inevitably arises. Accidental poisoning is common from a leaking pipe or from gas turned off at a meter or main, or may be due to occupants of a room failing to turn off the tap when the flame goes out. Suicide may be indicated by the position of the victim, e.g., lying with the head in a gas oven. Murder is fortunately rare but its appearances usually counterfeit those of accident or suicide.

Producer gas is a mixture of carbon monoxide and nitrogen made by passing air over red hot coke. Water gas is a mixture of carbon monoxide and hydrogen made by passing steam over red hot coke.

Strict safety precautions are essential in industries using carbon monoxide and in the domestic use of coal gas.

carbuncle. An area of localized infective gangrene resulting from invasion of the subcutaneous tissues by bacteria, most commonly *Staphylococcus aureus*.

This can appear anywhere but is most often seen on the back and over the back of the neck as an extension of a BOIL. A hard painful discoloured swelling develops, followed by the appearance of pus, sinus formation and sloughing of tissue. Constitutional symptoms may be severe and carbuncles of the face carry a special risk of venous thrombosis which may spread to blood-sinuses in the brain or cause generalized pyaemia. Debilitated and diabetic patients are particularly susceptible.

Treatment requires draining away the pus, removal of dead tissue and antiseptic packing with prompt administration of appropriate antibiotics. General health also needs consideration.

carcinogen. A substance liable to cause cancer.

carcinoma. The scientific term for CANCER, i.e. malignant disease arising from epithelial cells which form such tissues as skin, mucous membranes and secretory glands. Carcinomata may be further qualified to indicate the type of cell or organ involved, as for instance squamous (flattened cells) carcinoma, or bronchial carcinoma. Malignant change in supportive tissues is known generally as sarcoma.

cardiac. Concerning the heart.

cardio-vascular disease. Disease affecting the heart and blood vessels. The term is generally used in a more restricted sense to describe degenerative changes occurring in the arterial system and thus affecting the heart by increasing its work and diminishing its blood supply.

The arterial changes are mainly of two kinds. In sclerosis, high blood pressure leads to hardening, inelasticity, and narrowing of arteries. In atheroma, degeneration of the artery lining is followed by the appearance of deposits and accumulation of cholesterol, fatty substances and lime-salts, which narrow the vessel and may ultimately block it. The conditions may coexist and are of special importance in relation to coronary heart disease, which in the U.K. causes about one-quarter of all male deaths and a smaller but increasing proportion of female deaths.

It has been shown that a diet high in animal fat is associated with a high blood-cholesterol level and that the latter is in turn associated with increased numbers of deaths from coronary thrombosis. Many other contributory factors such as stress, obesity, cigarette-smoking, excessive sugar consumption and soft drinking water have also been incriminated to a greater or lesser degree.

However, it does appear to be worthwhile to advocate a diet relatively free from animal fats ('saturated fats') and low in cholesterol. Some of the unsaturated fatty acids, as found in margarine, and particularly linoleic acid, are 'essential fatty acids' (EFA). These are precursors of a newly-discovered class of hormones known as the prostaglandins. As these have some remarkable physiological effects, including reducing blood pressure and lessening the 'stickiness' of blood platelets, it may well be that the substantial replacement of animal fat by unsaturated fats of vegetable origin will in the long term reduce the incidence of cardio-vascular disease. Reduction of cigarette-smoking and obesity may also help.

caries. Usually this term refers to dental caries, which is the gradual dissolving and decay of the enamel and dentine of the TEETH by acid substances in the mouth, a process prevented or reduced by DENTAL HYGIENE.

Caries of bone is the decay and gradual disintegration of bone structure in the presence of chronic infection such as osteomyelitis or tuberculosis of bone.

carminatives. Drugs reputed to relieve flatulence by assisting the expulsion of gas from the stomach and intestines. They act by stimulating the muscle of the gastric and intestinal walls. Most of the usual carminatives contain volatile or 'essential' oils obtained from a variety of aromatic plants such as aniseed, peppermint and ginger.

'Carminative' is derived from the Latin word for 'charm', which may explain the diminishing importance of these medicaments in modern medicine. If they are employed at all their use is traditional and their value as flavouring agents is probably greater than their therapeutic activity.

carotid arteries. The principal arteries supplying blood to the head and neck. They arise as the right and left common carotid arteries but both divide at mid-neck level into the external and internal carotid arteries. The external branch supplies the exterior of the head, face and neck, while the internal branch supplies the brain and other structures inside the skull.

Both the internal and external carotid arteries are easily divided by a stab-wound behind the angle of the jaw, producing instant unconsciousness and usually fatal haemorrhage. This method of silently killing sentries is taught to troops raiding enemy territory.

carriers of disease. During an attack of infectious disease the organism responsible is present in the body of the sick person and can usually be detected by test during the illness. However, in some infections the germ can exist, or continue to exist, within the body of the host without producing obvious symptoms of disease. A person harbouring an organism in this way is a 'carrier', defined as being the apparently healthy host of a germ normally capable of causing disease.

The carrier state may develop after an actual attack of disease, and such carriers are called consequential carriers and classified as convalescent, chronic, or permanent carriers according to the duration of their infectivity. Contact carriers are persons harbouring an organism and who are known to have had contact with a case of disease. In independent carriers there is no knowledge of contact with any case.

Carriers are a risk to the community because the organisms they carry, although harmless to the carrier, may cause disease in other persons. The carrier state is particularly liable to occur in relation to diphtheria, typhoid fever, food-poisoning 'salmonellosis', bacillary dysentery, cholera, cerebro-spinal fever and streptococcal infections of the respiratory tract.

The control of any epidemic of these diseases should include a rigorous search for carriers amongst the contacts of known cases, and they too should be prevented from spreading the infection more widely. In a serious outbreak of diphtheria in Manchester during 1971 intensive examination of contacts identified a considerable number of carriers. Their isolation played an important part in limiting the epidemic.

Chronic carriers frequently present health authorities with a difficult problem, particularly in relation to typhoid fever and other salmonella infections. Such persons must be excluded from occupations involving food handling and must be instructed about their need for scrupulous personal hygiene.

In typhoid fever, the carrier state may persist for months or years, the organism continuing to be excreted from the bowel or in the urine. The source of the infection in the excretion from the bowel is often from a diseased gall-bladder and surgical treatment may be required before non-infectivity is achieved. The excreted material from such carriers should be sterilized by disinfectants before disposal into the drainage system.

Legal powers exist in many countries for the control of carriers likely to be a danger to the community.

cartilage. More familiarly known as gristle, cartilage is a firm, tough, elastic, translucent tissue devoid of blood vessels and nerves. In the body it is found in joints, in the discs between vertebrae, in the rib cartilages, in the larynx and trachea, and in the ears and tip of the nose. In general it increases flexibility.

There are several varieties of cartilage. Hyaline cartilage is mainly found in joints where the requirements are smoothness and resilience. White fibro-cartilage and yellow fibro-cartilage contain fibrous tissue in order to ensure additional toughness and elasticity.

The 'torn cartilage' which troubles footballers is one of the crescent-shaped structures of white fibro-cartilage which are present in the knee-joint. The 'slipped disc' of back injuries represents some form of damage to the pads of white fibro-cartilage, which lie between the vertebrae of the spine.

case-history. An account of previous illnesses and other major happenings in the life of the patient as an aid to the diagnosis and treatment of a current illness. In many physical diseases a detailed case-history (or anamnesis) is just as important as a full clinical examination, and in mental, psychosomatic and stress diseases the physical examination may reveal much less than the case-history. A study in 1976 of general practice in Britain and the U.S.A. suggested that, while doctors in both countries consider case-history important, those in the U.S.A. devoted more time to case-history and less time to physical examination than their colleagues in Britain.

castration. The procedure by which animals are deprived of their sex-glands (testes or ovaries) and so rendered sterile.

It is widely used in animal husbandry, particularly for male animals, to render them more manageable and more easily domesticated, and to improve and quicken their development as food animals for slaughter. Castrated horses, bulls, rams, boars and cocks are known respectively as geldings, bullocks, wethers, hogs and capons. The operation in the male is simple and the various methods employed are still fairly primitive and traditional. Female castration or 'spaying' is more difficult because of the position of the ovaries in the abdomen, but it is common in pigs, the castrated sow being known as a gilt.

Human castration used to be extensively practised in Africa, Asia and under the Roman and Byzantine empires to provide eunuchs to look after harems. It was also employed in Italy until at least the eighteenth century to prevent breaking of the voice in boy singers since the range and timbre of a boy's voice allied to adult lung-power was particularly effective. Some Italian castrated singers were internationally famous, notably Carlo Farinelli (1705-82). The practice was continued until late in the eighteenth century and the castrato Pergetti was heard in London in 1844.

catabolism. Every living organism depends for its survival on continuous internal chemical activity which provides its requirements for energy, growth, repair and the break-down and replacement of worn-out tissues. The sum of these chemical processes is known generally as METABOLISM, but they can be divided into those which involve the building up of complex compounds from simpler materials and those which involve the reverse process. Reactions involving building up are called synthesis or anabolism, and decompostions are called catabolism. The most familiar example of the latter is the break-down of food by the process of digestion.

catalepsy. A nervous disorder producing a trance-like state in which the patient is unable to move or feel. Pulse and respiration are slowed and the body surface is cold and pale. The voluntary muscles are not paralysed: it is the will to move them that is lost. As a result limbs can be placed in unusual positions which will be rigidly maintained, as if the patient were a wax figure. Repeat attacks usually occur and the catatonic state may last from a few minutes to several days.

Catalepsy may occur as a manifestation either of hysteria or of schizophrenia. The differentiation of these two causes is often very difficult especially in the early stages of schizophrenia, and experienced psychiatric assessment is essential.

Catalepsy should not be confused with the very similar-sounding term cataplexy.

catalyst. A substance which, without itself being altered in the process, causes or assists a reaction between two or more other substances.

cataplexy. A condition in which there is a sudden loss of posture often as a result of some strong emotion. The muscles which control posture suddenly relax and the patient sinks limply to the ground fully conscious but unable to speak. Complete recovery ensues within a few minutes.

Cataplexy is usually classified with the minor epilepsies, but it is not generally agreed that it is a true epileptic phenomenon. It represents a sudden inhibition of brain function, whereas epilepsy results from a sudden and uncontrolled discharge of nervous energy.

Cataplexy should not be confused with the very similar-sounding term catalepsy.

cataract. An opacity of the crystalline lens of the eye, or of its capsule, causing blurring of vision and, if untreated, blindness.

In senile cataract opacity develops very slowly as a degenerative process in later life.

Infants may be born with congenital cataract which perhaps results from adverse antenatal influences. Traumatic cataract can follow bruising or penetrating injury; diabetic cataract may be a complication of severe untreated diabetes; glass-blower cataract is an industrial hazard of long exposure to excessive light and radiant heat, and occurs in such trades as glass manufacture and iron smelting.

The treatment is to remove the opaque lens surgically and compensate for the loss of focusing power by prescribing spectacles with a suitable convex lens to restore clear EYESIGHT.

A primitive operation known as 'couching' was formerly used in India and other tropical

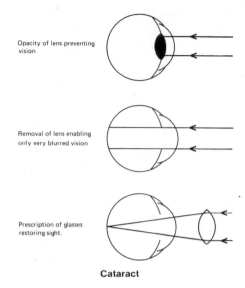

Opacity of lens preventing vision

Removal of lens enabling only very blurred vision

Prescription of glasses restoring sight.

Cataract

countries where cataract is common. The lens was merely displaced to the bottom of the eye by puncture and dislocation. In the classical operation the 'ripe' cataract is extracted through an incision at the edge of the cornea leaving the lens capsule behind. In the intra-capsular operation lens and capsule are extracted together. This makes possible earlier operation but not without some additional risk of failure through loss of vitreous humour and a partial collapse of the eye.

catarrh. Inflammation of a mucous membrane usually accompanied by excess secretion of mucus.

The term is most often used to mean inflammation of the upper respiratory tract which, as the 'common cold', runs its course in two stages. The mucous membrane is at first congested, swollen, hot and dry, and then subsequently produces a free mucoid or watery discharge, which may become purulent before drying up as the inflammation abates.

Repeated attacks may lead to a condition of chronic nasal catarrh often associated with some residual infection of the sinuses or with nasal polyps.

Other types of catarrh are hay fever, bronchial catarrh, gastric and intestinal catarrh and vesical catarrh – inflammation of the bladder.

Efficient nose-blowing, compressing each nostril in turn and vigorously expelling air through the other nostril, can sometimes prevent the development of nasal catarrh; and douching with a solution of bicarbonate of soda, common salt and borax is worth trying in early cases.

catgut. A cord-like material manufactured from sheep intestine and used in many operations as SUTURES and ligatures for stitching wounds and tying-off blood vessels. Its advantage over other materials such as nylon thread is that it is gradually absorbed by the tissues and therefore does not require removal.

Catgut is available in different thicknesses

and with different rates of tissue absorption to suit the particular needs of any operative procedure. Plain catgut is absorbed in five to seven days. Chromic catgut, tanned by chromium trioxide, is obtainable with absorption periods of ten to forty days.

cathartic. See LAXATIVE.

catheter. A tubular instrument designed to be passed into the urethra or external urinary passage in order to release urine from the bladder in cases of retention.

A female catheter is a short, straight, or slightly curved tube of glass or metal, but male catheters differ very much in design and material according to the needs of the particular case.

The term catheter has been extended to include tubes used for other surgical and medical purposes. Ureteric catheters are passed into the ureters in order to examine the function of each kidney separately. Endo-tracheal catheters may be used in anaesthesia. Cardiac catheters are passed along veins to enter the heart for the investigation of cardiac abnormalities. Eustachian catheters are used to blow air into the middle ear via the Eustachian tube. Uterine catheters are used to inject medicaments into the uterus.

cat-scratch fever. A viral disease most commonly occurring as a complication of scratches from cats although other animals and insect-bites may also occasionally be responsible.

A minor inflammatory reaction around the scratch with swelling, erythema, ulceration, or papule formation appears at the site of the wound. The related lymph-glands become swollen and tender and may suppurate and there may be moderate fever of an undulating character. The condition usually subsides spontaneously in two or three weeks and it is not much influenced by treatment although it may be possible to alleviate constitutional symptoms.

It is an uncommon disease but on principle scratches should be properly cleaned and disinfected as a precaution. A skin test may be used to pin-point the diagnosis since cat injuries may also become infected, resulting in ulceration.

caul. Within the womb the unborn child is enclosed in the amniotic sac and surrounded by amniotic fluid. During labour the amniotic sac is forced downwards and helps to open the neck of the womb. After that the sac walls (membranes) rupture, the amniotic fluid escapes, the child is born, and the membranes and placenta follow during the third stage of labour. If the membranes fail to rupture, as occasionally happens, the child may be born still enclosed in membrane. This is being 'born with a caul', which is harmless.

In the past superstition attached to this occurrence, and the dried caul or membrane was prized as a charm capable of conferring eloquence or preserving seamen from drowning.

cauliflower ear. A popular descriptive term for the final results of a neglected haematoma of the external ear ('auricle'). Blows on the ear may result in bruising which causes small veins to break so that blood escapes between the cartilaginous substructure of the ear and the over-lying skin. This blood is only slowly absorbed, and with softening of cartilage and subsequent fibrosis the ear becomes shrunken and twisted.

Immediate injury should be treated by cold compresses and a firm bandage to limit the bleeding, but any residual fluid swelling of effused blood should be drawn off to secure its removal before degeneration and contracture damage the shape of the ear.

In normal persons, haematoma auris or 'prizefighter's ear' usually only occurs after blows of considerable force, but it is sometimes seen to arise spontaneously in the elderly insane.

causes of disease. Disease – lack of health of body or mind – is hard to define. It is fundamentally a condition in which the functioning of the body or of some of its parts or organs is disturbed or deranged. The causes of the derangement are very numerous, sometimes overlapping, sometimes poorly defined, and therefore difficult to classify.

Disease has afflicted man, and indeed all living organisms, from the earliest times. Appreciation of its causes has gradually expanded with increase of scientific knowledge. Diseased persons are no longer regarded as being afflicted by magic or evil spirits nor would we now be satisfied to coin names like 'influenza' or 'malaria' which only concealed ignorance of real causes behind a suggestion that the conditions were due to some malign influence or to the miasmas – *mal'aria* (bad air) – of the Roman marshes.

Classification of disease. There are many possible approaches to the classification of disease. The anatomist is interested in the part of the body affected, the pathologist in the disease process, the clinician in both. Even the jurist has a different outlook. These points were made by William Farr (1807-83) in his report as Registrar General of England and Wales in 1856.

Diseases are now classified in accordance with the *International Statistical Classification of Diseases, Injuries and Causes of Death,* but although this is essential for statistical purposes it is both too detailed and too obscure to illustrate the factors which cause disease.

In considering disease as a whole, it is possible to identify three main types of causes of physical disease in addition to the separate entities of social and mental disease.

Some diseases are essentially due to inheritance. Others that become manifest in later life are due to the biological processes of ageing and degeneration. Between these two extremes is a wide variety of other conditions which are caused by harmful agencies derived from 'the total environment', where this term is used in the widest possible way to include anything at all which adversely affects the normal functioning of the body. It would be an attractive theory to maintain that there was a unity covering all three groups, and it is not without supporting evidence.

We know that gene changes can be brought about by outside influences, and so genetically-determined diseases may represent the inherited adverse effects of a distant past. Similarily it is well known that ageing tissues become increasingly vulnerable to environmental influences, including stress and injury, and that they gradually lose their powers of recuperation, repair, and restoration. It is not beyond possibility that means may yet be found of identifying, and then delaying or neutralizing, the factors leading to the changes in ageing tissues.

Genetically-determined diseases. Genetic diseases and congenital abnormalities are becoming steadily more important. This is partly because of the successful control of many other diseases caused by external factors but also because, with improved recognition and treatment, many more cases of inherited disease survive to adult life. This has important implications for future generations, because these diseases are passed on in accordance with Mendel's principles of GENETICS. Briefly these are that defective genes may be dominant, recessive or sex-linked, affecting the influence they have on the developing embryo.

The list of diseases related to genes is now a large and growing one but some of the more common conditions include achondroplasia, Huntington's chorea and some types of muscular dystrophy (which are generally dominant), cystic fibrosis, familial mental defect associated with blindness, phenylketonuria and glycogen-storage disease (which are genetically recessive), and haemophilia, which is sex-linked.

Partial or complex inherited factors can cause pyloric stenosis, spina bifida, hare-lip, cleft palate, congenital hip disease, some other congenital malformations, diabetes, schizophrenia and manic-depressive psychosis.

Chromosome abnormalities take the form of abnormalities of structure or number. The best known is the condition of mental deficiency known as mongolism, where there is an extra no. 21 chromosome (trisomy 21).

Exogenous diseases (*external causes*). These are the diseases brought about by harmful influences derived from 'the total environment'.

The group therefore includes the effects of parasites and infection by protozoa, fungi, bacteria, and viruses. It covers also conditions caused by dietary deficiency, unsuitability or excess, injurious atmospheric or climatic conditions, harmful living and working conditions, the action of poisonous substances, and the effects of injury.

The so-called psychosomatic or stress diseases are also primarily external in origin. The body normally reacts to stress in a physiological way. If it over-reacts, or reacts abnormally, or is forced to react excessively or for too long a period, its capacity for normal functioning is disturbed and the effects are shown in susceptible organs. The best known psychosomatic diseases are probably duodenal ulcer and migraine.

Degenerative diseases. Functioning is impaired as tissues age and change in character. So older persons become the victims of such chronic conditions as cardio-vascular degeneration, osteo-arthritis, malignant disease, and senile dementia.

It will be obvious that the sections of this classification are not mutually exclusive. To take an example, asthma is largely caused by allergy to a particular external substance but also has important psychosomatic elements and often runs in families. Cancer is perhaps another case in point. There is so far no evidence of it being hereditary but predisposition may have some genetic basis: we already know that certain types of cancer are common in persons of particular blood groups; environmental influences are certainly the main causes in such instances as the lung carcinoma of cigarette smokers and the bladder tumours of rubber-workers; and it is a matter of common knowledge and experience that malignant conditions occur predominantly in older persons.

Social diseases. So far, consideration has been restricted to conditions of disease in which there are demonstrable changes of some sort. Nevertheless society is becoming increasingly concerned with other departures from the normal.

The World Health Organization has defined health as 'a state of complete physical, mental and social well-being and not merely the absence of disease or infirmity'.

If absence of social well-being is thus being regarded as akin to disease any consideration of the causes of disease must also include some reference to our present basis of society. It would seem to be an inescapable conclusion that the manner in which it operates is responsible for the increasing proportion of its numbers who, as isolates, delinquents, neurotics and hypochondriacs, can certainly be regarded as socially sick although not physically ill.

cautery. Any instrument or device used to apply heat to the tissues in such intensity as to burn them.

Cauteries are sometimes employed to stimulate the healing of inactive ulcers but their main use is in the arrest of haemorrhage. Multiple small bleeding points which are difficult to reach or control can often be effectively dealt with by searing and so closing the vessels.

cell. The basic structural and functional unit of the living matter (protoplasm) which forms the tissues of animals and plants.

Like knowledge of bacteria, knowledge about cells and their characteristics has been largely dependent on advances in microscopy because most cells are of microscopic size. However, the yolks of birds' eggs are in fact single cells, and cell size actually ranges from less than one-thousandth of 1 mm. to the yolk of the ostrich egg.

Typical structure. Living cells, with only a few exceptions, have a standard fundamental structure. The main body of the cell consists of protoplasm, a sticky colloidal fluid known in this context as cytoplasm and contained within an outer wall, the cell membrane. Protoplasm consists of water, protein, fatty substances, starches and sugars, with various inorganic and organic salts.

Within the cell, and concerned with the regulation of cell activity, is a denser globular structure called the nucleus. This is made of chromatin, which holds the genetic information necessary to determine the specialized characters and function of the cell.

Chromatin is the name given to the nuclear material generally, in recognition of the fact that it stains readily with basic dyes when prepared for microscopic examination (the term derives from the Greek *chroma*, meaning 'colour'); but this rather unimaginative name does less than justice to its complexity. With the help of the electron microscope the complexity is gradually being unravelled in the separate science of molecular biology.

Chromatin is mainly made up of protein,

deoxyribonuclecic acid (DNA) and ribonucleic acid (RNA): DNA is a highly complex molecule and its structural arrangement is responsible for providing the 'code' which determines the hereditary characteristics and individuality of a cell and ensures that its regulated growth and function conform to an appropriate pattern.

Cell repoduction. In the animal body all tissues and organs originate from the female germ-cell (ovum) after it has been fertilized by a germ-cell from the male (spermatozoon). Thereafter the fertilized ovum multiplies by simple divisions into an enormous number of daughter cells which become modified in size, shape and other characteristics according to the sites and functions for which they are destined.

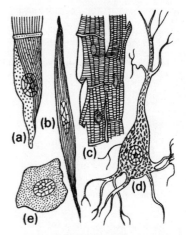

Types of body cell: (a) ciliated epithelial from trachea; (b) involuntary muscle; (c) heart muscle; (d) nerve; (e) epithelial from mouth.

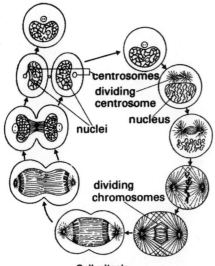

Cell mitosis

Before cell division the nucleus undergoes a complicated process known as mitosis in order to ensure that each daughter cell has an identical share of the chromatin material and especially of DNA by which its own invariability will be assured. In mitosis the nuclear material becomes divided into small pieces called chromosomes. These each divide into pairs which draw apart, and the nucleus and its surrounding protoplasm then divide into two. So each daughter cell is provided with the same number of chromosomes as the original cell.

A modification of this process is required before fertilization. It will be obvious that when two cells unite the resultant cell would have twice the proper number of chromosomes. The germ cells therefore undergo meiosis in which the number of chromosomes which each contributes is reduced to one half so that a new sexually-reproduced cell has the proper number of chromosomes for the species; how this influences inheritance is the study of GENETICS.

Tissue formation. Cells are single units but they combine in multicellular organisms and become specialized for particular purposes.

A typical animal body contains a large variety of cells with particular characteristics all of which have arisen by repeated division from the original fertilized ovum.

They include epithelial and endothelial cells covering the outside and lining the inside surfaces of the body, cells for skeletal tissues such as bone and muscles, cells for the nervous system, and cells for all the diverse organs such as heart, lungs, blood, liver, kidney, glands and so on.

cellulitis. A spreading inflammation of the cellular tissues deep in the skin resulting from invasion by micro-organisms. It may proceed to suppuration, sloughing or gangrene.

It is particularly likely to occur with penetrating wounds, in lacerations where there is damaged tissue, and in patients whose general resistance is low as a result of other disease. The affected part is red, hot, tender and swollen and there is usually considerable constitutional upset.

The treatment is incision to secure adequate drainage of infected matter, the removal of damaged tissue, and the giving of appropriate antibiotics to combat the infection.

central nervous system. The brain and spinal cord. See NERVOUS SYSTEM.

cerebellum. The part of the brain lying within the lower rear part of the skull. It consists of a central and two lateral lobes, and is concerned with balance and the maintenance of posture.

cerebral embolism, haemorrage and thrombosis. See STROKE.

cerebrospinal fever. A serious disease due to infection of the membranes of the brain which is alternatively known as meningococcal MENINGITIS. It usually appears as sporadic cases, probably infected from symptomless carriers of the organism, but epidemics occur under conditions of over-crowding, especially of sleeping quarters.

The incubation period is short (one to three days) and the onset is usually abrupt with high temperature, intense headache, and mental confusion. Severe cases may show a rash of tiny red spots. These are the basis for the synonym 'spotted fever'. Characteristic diagnostic signs are that the neck and legs become rigid and the whole body tends to be arched backwards.

In the past about half the victims died but the antibiotic treatment now available has greatly improved the outlook even in severe cases. There is as yet no effective vaccine and the most important control measure is prevention of overcrowding in living quarters and working places. Patients should be isolated until twenty-four hours after the start of antibiotic treatment.

cerebrospinal fluid. The fluid which surrounds the brain and spinal cord forming a water bed for their protection. Its function is to cushion the brain and cord against sudden movement and to equalize changes in pressure.

In various diseases such as meningitis, poliomyelitis, and syphilis, changes occur in the chemical nature of the fluid, white blood cells appear, and fluid pressure increases. These alterations are of diagnostic importance and can be demonstrated in a specimen of fluid obtained by lumbar puncture.

Obstruction of the flow of cerebrospinal fluid may cause hydrocephalus. See also BRAIN, diseases of.

cerebrovascular. Concerning the blood vessels which supply the brain.

cerebrum. The upper and largest part of the BRAIN occupying most of the cranial cavity, and larger and more complex in man than in other mammals.

cervical. Concerning the neck, or concerning a neck-like structure, e.g., the neck of the uterus.

cervical cytology. A rapid and easy method of detecting the very beginning of cancer of the cervix of the uterus long before the condition is dangerous.

Essentially where cancer of the cervix is developing the cells become abnormal in appearance and only later become cancerous.

In cervical cytology the doctor or nurse takes, absolutely painlessly, a tiny scraping – called a cervical smear – from the mucous membrane of the cervix. The specimen so obtained is stained and then examined under a microscope. In the overwhelming majority of cases the cells so examined are normal, but in a tiny proportion of cases they show abnormality and therefore render operation desirable before the cells actually become cancerous.

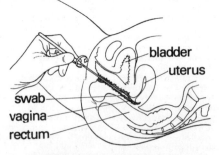

Taking a cervical smear

In the Canadian province of British Columbia persuasion of women to have cervical cytology as a routine measure every few years has virtually eliminated cancer of the cervix, and some towns and counties in Britain that were pioneers in this field also reported a drastic reduction in the disease. In most countries the examination is now advised for women every three years.

Cervical cancer is commonest in mothers of several children and especially in women of the lowest socio-economic groups; but unfortunately these are the very people least likely to respond to invitations to visit clinics or doctors' consulting rooms for cervical smears. So in large measure the reduction of cervical cancer depends on person-to-person persuasion by health workers.

cervical rib. An abnormal extra rib arising in relation to the seventh cervical vertebra.

It is usually bilateral and is more common in women. It is often not discovered until the age of puberty but at that age the ribs, which are cartilage in childhood, become hard and bony, and the bones of the shoulder may be pulled down by breast development so that symptoms ensue from pressure on the artery and nerve supplying the arm.

The pulse is weakened and the arm may become cold, blue, and swollen with fluid from interference with its circulation. Effects on the nerves include neuralgic pain, tingling and numbness, with weakness and wasting of the muscles of the hand.

The only effective treatment is surgical removal of the rib.

cervix. The lower segment of the uterus or womb.

It is about 2.5 cm. (1 in.) long with a central canal, and it projects downwards into the vagina as a narrow cylinder with a rounded end.

The cervix is frequently the site of disease.

Chronic cervicitis may result from the infection of a tear occurring during childbirth and may persist to cause shallow ulcerated areas (known as cervical erosions) producing discharge and discomfort.

The lining cells of the lower part of the cervix are very susceptible to malignant change, so carcinoma of the cervix is also not uncommon. Regular examination of the characteristics of these cells by means of CERVICAL CYTOLOGY (the 'cyto test') provides a means of detecting any potentially dangerous developments in time to ensure successful treatment.

chafing. Abrasion and superficial inflammation of the skin produced by friction. This can occur in various ways and the chafing produced by rough wet clothing at points of movement such as the neck or wrists is a matter of common experience.

Less obvious however are the effects of rubbing between opposed skin surfaces as sometimes seen in obese persons where rolls of flesh overlap, beneath heavy and pendulous breasts, and in the groins of babies. In such circumstances the skin secretions are prevented from drying so that the superficial cells become softened; this increases the friction and aggravates its effect.

Chafing also occurs over 'pressure points' especially the heels and sacrum, of persons confined to bed, and may be the first stage of an ultimate bed sore.

Treatment is really a matter of proper hygiene. The areas affected should first be carefully washed and dried to get rid of debris which would otherwise form a lodging for micro-organisms. Subsequent application of a skin lotion to dry and harden the skin can be followed by the use of a dusting powder to minimize friction.

For the patient in bed suitable pads should be used to provide protection from the effects of pressure and friction.

chancre. The primary sore resulting from infection with the organism which causes SYPHILIS. In acquired syphilis the initial site of infection in both men and women is usually in the genital area, but chancres are occasionally also seen on the lips, breasts, fingers and indeed any part of the body. The risk of infection by contact is considerable.

chancroid. A venereal disease, sometime called soft sore, which is much less common than gonorrhoea and less well known than syphilis. Infection is almost always through sexual intercourse and, after an incubation period of one to five days, a red papule appears in the genital area; this breaks down to form a painful ulcer and the lymph glands of the groin become swollen. The discharge of pus may infect the surrounding skin to produce further chancroids. There is often general disturbance and a raised temperature.

The disease responds well to sulphonamides and to streptomycin. After treatment there should be blood tests at intervals for three months because syphilis may also have been contracted at the same time, but its presence masked by the chancroid.

change of life. A colloquial expression for the MENOPAUSE.

chapped skin. A superficial disorder of the skin characterized by the occurrence of cracks and fissures of its outer horny layer. It affects exposed areas, especially the fingers, hands, forearms and face.

External irritants such as friction, cold, dust and injurious chemicals cause thickening of the horny layer. Because of its inelastic nature this readily cracks to produce fissures which are painful because the sensitive lower layers of the skin are exposed.

When the condition is extensive it may be due to ichthyosis or to a form of dermatitis (eczema), but many persons have 'chaps' in cold weather without these being regarded as due to specific skin disease.

Treatment should comprise the protection of the skin from any irritant including cold and the application of a glycerin-based lotion of which many examples are available commercially. Greasy applications are less suitable.

chemotherapy. The treatment of a disease by using chemicals to kill the germs which are causing it.

The German scientist Paul Ehrlich (1884-1915) conceived the idea of developing drugs which destroy specific disease-producing germs. His search for these 'magic bullets' was rewarded in 1907 by the discovery of arsphenamine ('Salvarsan 606') which proved effective against syphilis. Unfortunately this initial success was a solitary triumph until 1935 when Domagk published the results of his experiments with a dye, sulphamido-chrysoidin ('Prontosil') which had overcome streptococcal infections in mice. In the following year it was shown that part of the Prontosil molecule was as effective as the parent substance and from this discovery came

the sulphonamide drugs. Meantime Sir Alexander Fleming in 1928 had noticed the antibacterial effect of a mould, *Penicillium notatum,* although his observation was not followed up by the actual manufacture of penicillin until 1942.

These discoveries were the foundation of chemotherapy and over the past thirty years a great range of similar substances has become available based either on substances derived from sulphanilamide (the sulphonamides) or on substances produced by living organisms (the antibiotics). The treatment of disease caused by germs is now dominated by these two groups of drugs.

Antibiotics act by competing with germs for some organic substance which both require for their metabolism. This however is not without potential effects on the patient as well. Successful treatment depends on administering such doses as will not deprive a patient's system of some essential substance. For instance para-amino-benzoic acid, an essential vitamin to both man and microbe, may be destroyed by sulphonamides; and two antibiotics, aureomycin and chloromycetin, have been shown to damage foetal cells as well as bacteria. Fortunately these effects are generally far outweighed by therapeutic value and on this margin rests the clinical safety of these drugs.

Their remarkable success against the majority of harmful germs has however tended to obscure some of their limitations. Their action is purely antibacterial, they do not counteract toxins previously produced by the germs, and they have no beneficial effect on the patient's general resistance, or on his ability to develop immunity. In a disease such as typhoid fever where a toxin is released when the germ dies, effective chemotherapy may temporarily worsen a patient's condition, so initial dosage needs care. In any infection final cure also depends on destruction of organisms by white blood corpuscles and a favourable outcome requires that the body's own defences are not grossly impaired by other causes such as chronic disease or malnutrition, otherwise stalemate may occur with the infection not becoming worse but not being removed. Moreover other diseased conditions predispose to infection and relapse. Unless such underlying disease conditions can be corrected a risk of relapse will persist despite apparent success at the earlier stage. So chemotherapy is only one factor in an ordered plan of treatment.

Individual antibiotics differ in potency, toxicity, and range of activity, and in their ability to create drug-resistance in the invading germs. All these factors require consideration. Toxicity may be a particular problem. It may be specific, as in the effect of streptomycin on the auditory nerve, or general, due to unwanted impurities as with polymixin. With penicillin, acquired sensitivity may produce drug-rashes. Even the sulphonamides may cause agranulocytosis (impaired white cell function) or deposit crystals in the urinary tract. Another simultaneous disease such as renal insufficiency may aggravate these effects.

Drug resistance is a complex subject. The emergence of resistant strains is probably due to successive generations of bacteria gradually developing immunity to the particular antibiotic. The logical answer to this is to endeavour to destroy all the germs at an early stage and this requires dosage or combinations of drugs.

Chemotherapy is not a complete form of treatment. The patient's own resistance must be sustained by rest, diet and fluids, by the neutralization of toxins and the correction of metabolic deficiencies, and sometimes by surgical removal of damaged tissue. Lack of attention to these points courts failure, as do faulty dosage schedules, inaccessibility of the seat of infection, and ending the treatment too early.

Chemotherapy despite its potency requires to be used with discrimination. Many mild infections are probably best treated only by reducing the symptoms, and not by immediately deploying the full panoply of the chemotherapeutic armoury.

chest. A familiar name for the thorax, the bony cage of the upper part of the body containing the heart and lungs. It is formed behind by the twelve thoracic vertebrae of the spine from which twelve pairs of ribs sweep round to join the sternum or breast-bone in front. Its narrow upper opening is occupied by the structures of the neck and it is closed below by the diaphragm which forms its floor.

Its shape may be altered in disease · and various deformities are characteristic of rickets; in emphysema the chest is enlarged, a condition known as 'barrel-chest'.

The chest is an essential part of the mechanism of the RESPIRATORY SYSTEM.

Cheyne-Stokes respiration. A pattern of breathing in which there is a regular cycle of variation in volume. In each cycle, the breathing increases in depth until it becomes noisy and distressed. Respiration then gradually diminishes until for thirty seconds or more there is a pause, followed again by gradual increase. Various modifications of this pattern are also loosely referred to by the same term.

Cheyne-Stokes breathing occurs in cases of coma, head-injury, 'stroke', increased intra-cranial tension, hyperpyrexia, and in many heart, lung and kidney diseases as death approaches. It is due to disturbance of the part of the brain which controls respiration, and it is always of grave significance.

John Cheyne (1777-1836) and William Stokes (1804-1878) were Scottish and Irish physicians respectively.

chickenpox. The common name for varicella, a mild but highly infectious disease mainly affecting children and caused by the varicella virus. The same virus is found in shingles (herpes zoster) and in some cases of encephalitis.

Chickenpox is world-wide in distribution and endemic in all large populations. Epidemic outbreaks occur at irregular intervals with greatest prevalence in the autumn. Infants are rarely affected, because of temporary inherited maternal immunity, and most cases occur in children under 10 years. Adult cases are uncommon but tend to be more severe.

Infectivity. In its early stages chickenpox is very infectious, spread occurring from case to case by inhalation of 'droplet' respiratory spray. Dried crusts of skin are also regarded as infective. Patients are infectious from about one day before the appearance of the first vesicles to a week later. Outbreaks in children's hospitals are common usually as the result of the admission of an unsuspected case in the pre-eruptive stage.

The incubation period of the disease is normally a fortnight with extremes of eleven and twenty-three days, and isolation should be maintained until all the crusts from the pustules have separated.

Clinical features. Older children may initially have some malaise and rise of temperature with a pinkish general rash for twenty-four hours, but usually the disease is simply heralded by appearance of the typical skin eruption. This appears as 'crops' of clear vesicles (blebs) which become pustular and then dry up to form scabs. The crops appear on successive days for about three days, usually on the back, chest and abdomen, face, scalp and limbs in that order.

In most cases there is little or no general disturbance and children make an uneventful recovery but complications, although rare, are not unknown especially if the patient was already not well.

In varicella haemorrhagica there is haemorrhage not only into the vesicles but also into the skin and mucous membranes, and this type is often fatal. The same is true of varicella gangrenosa where secondary infection of the vesicles causes ulceration and intense toxaemia. Encephalitis is also rare and the outlook for recovery is generally favourable.

Treatment. The ordinary routine case requires very little active treatment. The application of an antiseptic paint may help to prevent secondary infection of the vesicles. If there is any suspicion that this is occurring antibiotics are given.

Differentiation from . smallpox. This can sometimes be a pressing administrative problem. Diagnosis turns on the early symptoms, the vaccination state, and a careful study of the rash, especially its character, distribution and progress. Laboratory tests to identify the virus are also available.

chilblains. An inflammatory condition of the skin generally occurring on exposed parts of the hands and feet as a reaction to cold.

It is a disturbance akin to Raynaud's disease in which the arterioles are constricted while blood stagnates in the dilated capillaries to the detriment of skin nutrition. The affected parts are swollen, reddened, shiny, itchy or painful, and superficial ulceration may ultimately occur.

Effective management is essentially preventive: susceptible areas should be adequately clothed in cold weather. There is no specific internal treatment but calcium lactate or gluconate with additional vitamin D or vitamin K is commonly prescribed. Treatment of the affected area which is designed to improve blood flow is sometimes helpful. Friction, infra-red radiation, paraffin-wax baths, diathermy, counter-irritation with tincture of iodine, and exposure to ultra-violet light all have their advocates. The distressing irritation from chilblains may be relieved by painting them with compound tincture of benzoin to which menthol has been added.

Patients with chilblains are often anaemic as well and this possibility should be investigated and corrected if necessary.

childbirth. The process of parturition, i.e., the act of giving birth to a living child. Delivery of a dead child whose intra-uterine development

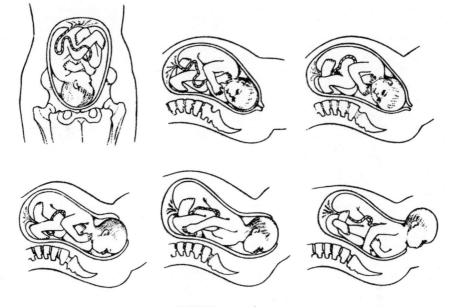

Childbirth: normal

has continued long enough for viability (6½ months) is known as a still birth; expulsion of a less mature foetus is an abortion or miscarriage.

Childbirth occurs as the climax of PREGNANCY. The whole products of conception and pregnancy – foetus, amniotic fluid, placenta, and membranes – are normally expelled and separated from the uterus by the physiological processes of labour affecting the mother. The course of events from the onset of labour until the mother is able to resume her normal activities is generally referred to as her CONFINEMENT.

Onset of labour. Labour occurs spontaneously after a gestation period of about 280 days. The exact causes of onset are still imperfectly understood. Older theories postulated the influence of reflex irritability of uterine muscle, uterine distension at term, and degenerative changes in the placenta which stimulates uterine muscle. While these factors may be relevant, it is now considered that the onset of labour is largely due to hormones.

Course of labour. It is usual to divide labour into three stages: (1) dilatation – from the onset of true labour pains to full dilatation of the cervix (twelve to eighteen hours); (2) expulsion – from full dilatation to expulsion of the child (two or three hours with a first child; often much shorter in later pregnancies); (3) delivery – from birth of child to expulsion of placenta or 'afterbirth' (half to one hour).

First stage: The mother experiences periodic pains due to contractions of the uterus. The contractions bring about dilation of the neck of the womb as the amniotic fluid within its membranous sac is forced down to act as a fluid wedge. Dilation is usually accompanied by a slight discharge of blood-stained mucus known as the 'show'. When full dilation is achieved the amniotic sac ruptures leading to a gush of amniotic fluid – the escape of the 'forewaters'. Premature rupture of the membranes may occur if the position of the baby is abnormal (e.g., in breach presentation).

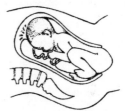

Childbirth: breech presentation

Second stage: After rupture of the membranes labour pains often cease temporarily but then begin again with greater force and frequency and develop a 'down-bearing character'. The abdominal muscles begin to play a part.

In a normal delivery the child is born as a 'head down' or vertex presentation and with its face directed backwards in relation to the mother. In this position its head passes most easily along the birth canal formed by the pelvis and the associated soft tissues.

The final obstacle to the child's delivery is the perineum or area of tissue between the anus and vaginal opening. The perineum gradually thins out and stretches. It may tear or require to be divided surgically, the operation of episiotomy.

As soon as the head is born, the shoulders, trunk and limbs follow without great difficulty and the actual birth is concluded by tying and cutting the umbilical cord.

Third stage: After the birth of the child there is a short cessation of pains but the uterus soon begins to contract again and can be felt through the abdominal wall as a hard and solid mass. Its contractions ultimately expel the placenta and the remains of the ruptured amniotic sac (otherwise known as the 'membranes').

Management of childbirth. The conduct of labour is a matter for the professional expertise of the attendants. In most advanced countries the great majority of mothers are now being confined in hospital where the necessary skill and facilities are assured.

The two essentials for safe childbirth are the recognition of abnormalities in time to deal with them in the most appropriate manner and the maintenance of a strict technique to avoid the risk of infection reaching the birth canal or uterus.

Much can be done to minimize the actual pains of labour. Anaesthesia in childbirth was pioneered by Sir James Y. Simpson, the discoverer of chloroform, but this substance because of its inherent risks is now seldom or never employed. Scopolamine-morphine narcosis or 'twilight sleep' enjoyed a vogue for some time but the favoured methods of obstetric analgesia now rely on inhalation procedures employing automatic devices suitable for unskilled use. The first of these inhalers supplied nitrous oxide gas as the anaesthetic agent but a more compact apparatus which has largely superseded it relies on the vaporization of tri-chloro-ethylene (Trilene).

The use of inhalation analgesia in this way under patient-control and with supervision by the midwife has greatly served to minimize the immemorial pangs of childbirth. See also CAESARIAN SECTION.

Diseases. These include the factors complicating labour and certain other conditions arising between the start of labour and the end of the puerperium.

The first group is usually sub-divided into faults in 'the powers', in 'the passages' and in 'the passenger'.

Successful labour depends essentially on the expulsive force exerted by the uterus with assistance from the abdominal muscles. This may be inadequate (primary uterine inertia) in nervous women because of the inhibitory effects of fear, in cases of malpresentation where the normal stimulus of the descending head is lacking, or in over-distension of the uterus as in hydramnios (when there is excessive amniotic fluid), or in cases of twin pregnancy. Secondary amniotic fluid, or twin pregnancy. Secondary uterine inertia occurs in a uterus exhausted by prolonged effort to overcome some obstructive difficulty.

Faults in the birth canal are numerous and varied. The most common is some form of contracted pelvis but malposition of the uterus, rigidity of the cervix and other soft parts, and tumours of the uterus may all cause difficulty in childbirth.

In the present context the 'passenger' is the child and its surrounding amniotic sac filled with amniotic fluid. The amniotic sac or 'membranes' may be unduly adherent to the uterus, sometimes as a result of previous inflammation of the lining of that organ, or of earlier haemorrhage; or the sac may rupture prematurely. Both conditions may delay labour but disproportionate size or faulty positioning of the child are more usual causes. Other complications related to the child are congenital abnormalities and prolapse of the umbilical cord.

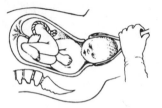

Childbirth: forceps delivery

Apart from faults in the powers, the passages or the passenger, the most serious complication of labour is haemorrhage occurring either during labour or immediately after. Haemorrhage during the birth usually occurs because the placenta is so situated that it is ruptured during the delivery. Haemorrhage after the birth occurs at the end of labour from an exhausted uterus or as a result of damage to the soft tissues.

After delivery the most serious risk is infection of the raw surface of the genital tract to cause puerperal pyrexia or puerperal fever.

Eclampsia is more properly a disease of pregnancy but may first show itself during the puerperium. Another condition, fortunately rare, is puerperal insanity which though usually short-lived can be very distressing. Sudden deaths are occasionally recorded from pulmonary embolism where air or amniotic fluid has entered the venous blood stream from the open uterus sinuses.

No attempt has been made here to deal with the treatment of any of the conditions described. With adequate pre-natal care and skilled professional attendance at the delivery the aim should be to avoid or at least anticipate the difficulties.

child guidance. Many children suffer from disorders of personality and conduct which influence their attitude to everyday life and prevent them from making a satisfactory and acceptable adjustment to the demands of the society in which they live. There is a great variety of indications of such personal maladjustment.

The young child may develop undesirable habits such as thumb-sucking, nail-biting, bedwetting, masturbation, eccentricities of movement, or whims about food, and may show abnormal personal characteristics in the form of excessive shyness or aggression, oversensitiveness or obstinacy, seclusiveness or quarrelsomeness, laziness or restlessness, timidity and exaggerated fears – to name only a few.

The school age child may similarily come to notice because of 'school phobia', truancy, lying, stealing, destructiveness, bullying, temper-tantrums, rebellious outbursts or sexual misbehaviour.

Child guidance is a service, still in a developing and evolutionary phase, which recognizes that many of the difficulties of the maladjusted adult have their roots in infancy and childhood. It therefore seeks to identify those children with abnormalities of attitude and behaviour, who – at home, at school, or in the community – are in some sort of conflict with their environment. It also owes a great deal to the concepts of psychology elaborated by Sigmund Freud (1856-1939).

In some instances problem children may in fact be suffering from mental illness or mental defect, but these are the province of the psychiatrist or mental deficiency specialist. Child guidance is primarily concerned with children who are capable of more or less normal development.

History. Organized child guidance began in America; Europe and Great Britain were relatively late in recognizing its importance but the difficulties disclosed by the evacuation arrangements of the Second World War gave it considerable impetus and facilities now exist in most education authority areas.

In America its origins stem from the work of Dr William Healey and his associates who in 1909 started a juvenile psychopathic clinic and institute in connection with the Chicago Juvenile Court. This was followed by the Judge Baker Foundation in Boston (1915) and later by an expanding series of clinics elsewhere.

In Britain the work was pioneered first at the Tavistock Clinic of Dr Crichton-Miller, a clinic which was already caring for functional nervous disorders in adults. It received an impetus (1921) from the Commonwealth Fund which inaugurated a five-year plan for grants to demonstration clinics, notably the London Child Guidance Clinic with its home in Canonbury. Other clinics rapidly developed in the provinces, and in Scotland the Glasgow Notre Dame Clinic became particularly well-known.

Child guidance clinics. Most of the work of these clinics is with children of school-age. For the behaviour problems of the infant and pre-school child useful advice is in most places readily available from an ordinary child health clinic where there will be a doctor experienced in paediatrics and health visitors with the opportunity and insight to appreciate the family background, and with the ability and knowledge to explain to mothers the needs of their offspring for love, talk, play, company, consistency, and the avoidance of over-protection, over-dependency, over-strictness, or over-indulgence.

It is generally older children with behaviour difficulties related more to the outside world who eventually reach the child guidance clinic, brought by parents or referred by teachers, probation officers, church and social agencies, or sent more formally from the courts or children's panels.

Team work. In child guidance every child who comes to notice has to be considered not in isolation but in relation to the setting or situation in which he lives. It is unhelpful to label a child as a thief, truant or coward without undertaking a thorough study of the social and psychological factors which have made him what he appears to be.

Child guidance therefore requires to be a team effort in which the paediatrician, the child-psychiatrist, the psychologist and especially the social case-worker all play their respective parts, with the health visitor and the general practitioner also involved.

Diagnosis. A physical examination is an essential part of the investigation because mood and behaviour are influenced by health. The fatigue of chronic illness is different in quality from that of an anxiety state; the restlessness of chorea can be confused with the overactivity of mental stress; apathy and dejection may be created by hormone imbalance as well as by psychological factors; allergies may indicate psychosomatic instability; bodily conformation has been shown to be correlated with mental make-up.

A full history of the child should include an account of his medical, developmental, psychological and educational progress from his earliest years.

These medical aspects of the case require to be supplemented by the investigations of the social case-worker, by school reports, and by the views of the psychologist who has at his disposal a wide range of scientific techniques for the investigation of intellectual capacity and personality.

Treatment. A linking together of all the investigations, either by consideration of reports by a case conference, or more usually by informal disussions between members of the team, will enable a diagnosis to be made and a plan of treatment decided. The diagnosis will normally fall into three categories: (1) that the problem is purely intellectual and that the remedy lies in remedial educational measures with the assistance of the psychologist and his facilities for continuous constructive help; (2) that some environmental adjustment and parental enlightment can be undertaken by the social worker or health visitor, or (3) that an established neurosis exists which will require psychotherapy from the psychiatrist.

In this context psychotherapy can range from play therapy, either alone or in groups, through simple talks, suggestion, re-education and reinforcement of the personality, to the more advanced forms of analysis which seek to explore the unconscious mechanisms of conduct and behaviour.

Community aspects. The pressures of modern society have their effects on children as well as upon adults, and child guidance has come to be regarded as an essential community service concerned not only with the disturbed child but with the general application of the principles of mental hygiene. It has effected the general principles of social work and it is the basis for new legislation.

The problems of personality are receiving more attention; parent-teacher associations play a role in this and enlightened industrialists have come to see the value of similar contracts for adults between management and workers.

The principles and technique of mental hygiene are equally applicable in the world at large. Personality studies would avoid much of present-day stress at work and lessen the resultant need for treatment and rehabilitation.

The growing emphasis on educational and preventive work is designed not only to help the school-age child but to provide vocational guidance for his future based on the ideal of giving to everyone a stable adjustment to life by equating its demands to individual interest and capacity.

child health services. Services provided with the aim of safeguarding and improving the physical and mental health of children, monitoring their development, guiding parents as to requirements for good development and identifying and rectifying diseases and disabilities.

There is no real difference in meaning between child health services and paediatrics, though the first term is generally used for the health monitoring and improvement of the child who is not ill (i.e., preventive paediatrics) while the second is sometimes restricted to curative aspects (i.e., clinical paediatrics). The development of the services and their enormous achievements are disussed under PAEDIATRICS. The present article deals with the services as applying to the individual child.

In many countries the services are centred on the home in the early years of childhood and on the school in later years. In the pre-school period there are two key figures: (1) a qualified nurse with subsequent training in psychology, human development, sociology and health teaching, known in the U.K., South Africa and Nigeria as a HEALTH VISITOR and elsewhere identifiable under other names, and doing much of her work in the child's home; and (2) a qualified doctor, often specialized in preventive paediatrics (e.g., the child health medical officer of the U.K.), occasionally a paediatrician dealing with both healthy children and sick children, and sometimes an unspecialized general practitioner, and in all these cases usually seeing the child in health centre, clinic or consulting room. In the school period the key figures are the school doctor and school nurse who may be the same people as in the pre-school stage or they may specialize entirely in children of school age.

In some areas the health visitor sees the parents in the prenatal period, sharing with the midwife guidance on the hygiene of pregnancy, advising the prospective parents about the child's future physical and emotional needs, persuading them to attend an appropriate health class or discussion group, discussing the preparation of any older child for the baby's arrival, and tactfully inducing the mother to think (when she has more time than after the birth) about such relevant matters as the avoidance of home accidents, the value of immunization and the question of spacing of children. In other areas these important educational opportunities are lost, and the health visitor pays her first call after mother and child have left the maternity hospital.

At the first visit and to some extent at later visits she examines the baby carefully for abnormalities and, gearing her teaching to the apparent needs and capacities of the mother, begins systematic guidance as well as answering questions raised by the mother. In general she tries to use anticipatory guidance, e.g., to deduce that the Smiths will tend to be over-strict disciplinarians and to help them to realize before any problems of discipline arise that a child needs some freedom to investigate and to learn by trial and error, and similarly to deduce that the Greens will tend towards over-indulgence and therefore to make them aware of the need for a few rules and a kindly guiding authority. She also encourages the parents to attend the appropriate health centre or clinic for medical examination and for immunizations, to take advantage of any relevant health discussion group provided in the neighbourhood and, if she has found any signs of disease or abnormality, to seek treatment promptly.

The doctor undertakes comprehensive developmental assessment of the child at periodical intervals, gives or arranges for appropriate immunizations and tries to ensure that any physical or mental abnormality or any sensory defect (e.g., impaired hearing) receives remedial or supportive treatment. If he is specialized in healthy children he does not himself undertake treatment but refers the child to the appropriate general practitioner or (usually via the GP in the U.K.) to a paediatric physician, paediatric surgeon, child psychiatrist or child psychologist.

In advanced countries dental services are often available for all children and other specialized services (e.g., those of orthoptists, who train inefficient eye muscles) may be provided.

After the child enters school there is usually a routine medical overhaul to detect abnormalities missed earlier or recently developed, and one or more routine medical examinations later, together with specially arranged examination on request by parent, teacher or school nurse. Additionally there are periodical dental inspections by a dental officer or dental hygienist and general health surveys from time to time by the school nurse or school health visitor. There are frequent discussions between doctor and nurse on the one hand and teacher on the other to ensure that the educational provisions are matched to the health and capacity of the child: to give a simple example, to ensure that a short-sighted child is encouraged to wear his glasses and is not seated at the back of the classroom. Both the nurse, especially if she is a qualified health visitor, and to a smaller extent the doctor are likely to be involved in health education in the school, and they have obvious roles in relation to school hygiene and the control of infectious diseases. Vocational guidance is still in its infancy but at least specific disabilities of school leavers are identified, so that, for example, a colour blind child does not seek to become a taxi driver. See also SCHOOL HEALTH SERVICES.

This general picture applies with minor modifications to several countries in the Commonwealth and broadly similar comprehensive schemes are to be found in the Scandinavian countries and in the Communist Bloc countries of Eastern Europe. In the U.S.A. provision of child health services is very uneven – of the highest standard in some areas but virtually absent in many city slums. Many countries of the Third World still face the problems with which Europe and America had to grapple a century ago, namely poverty, malnutrition, ignorance, exploitation of children in a period of early industrialization, and almost total absence of skilled preventive and curative workers.

Even in advanced countries problems largely associated with poverty are far from solved, e.g., prevention and early detection of disability, reduction of home and road accidents and reduction of serious hereditary diseases. The increase in affluence has created problems of overnutrition and dental caries, while behaviour disorders have hardly been tackled. There has been an enormous reduction in child deaths (e.g., in babies from one in six to one in sixty, and even lower in Sweden) and great improvement in the physical health of children, and much credit is due to health visitors, child health medical officers, obstetricians, midwives, paediatricians and general practitioners; but vast potentialities for future improvement remain. Among the basic difficulties are the following.

1. A minority of affluent and educated parents regard health visitor calls and clinic attendances as appropriate only for 'the poor'; but it is often the children of such parents who become overnourished or who develop behaviour disorders through over-forcing, over-emphasis on tidiness or lack of opportunity for self-expression and development of initiative.

2. While parents of low socio-economic status mostly accept health visitor visits and derive benefit from advice given, many of them are reluctant to attend health centres or consulting rooms, even for immunizations, so that in some districts only a minority of children receive routine developmental assessment and half of them remain exposed to risk of preventable infections.

3. Guidance on the spacing of families tends to come too late, when there are too many young children in the family, so that the mother is exhausted and older children are partially neglected because of the greater needs of younger brothers and sisters.

4. Genetic counselling tends to be sought and given after a seriously diseased child has been born, instead of before the first child is conceived by parents of doubtful family history.

5. A vociferous minority oppose health advances, e.g., vaccination and immunization, fluoridation of water and provision of oral contraceptives.

6. In many areas opportunity is not taken to advise expectant mothers, before they become preoccupied by the needs and demands of the young baby.

7. Health visitors are in short supply but there is an ambivalent attitude to their provision. For instance, in the U.K. in 1976 the government committed itself to a substantial annual rise in the number of health visitors, but some health boards (financed from government funds) met financial stringency by actually leaving health visitor vacancies unfilled so that quite a number of newly qualified health visitors could not obtain posts.

8. Argument continues about whether preventive paediatrics should be undertaken by doctors specializing in normal children, by paediatricians who deal mostly with sick children, or by general practitioners who deal mostly with sick people of all ages; and some doctors resent the increased status and competence of the public health nurses.

These difficulties, however, should not blind us to the enormous successes of the child health services.

childhood, psychology of. Psychologists and psychiatrists agree that the personality, character and mental health of a child, and of the adult which he becomes, are influenced profoundly by parental attitudes during the formative years from birth onwards and also by the relationships which he makes with brothers, sisters and playmates. The mother, or failing her some permanent mother substitute, has the greatest opportunity of moulding and influencing his psychical development. She is best situated from the very beginning to provide the comfort and security required. Some of the psychological factors affecting infant development are dealt with in the article INFANCY, PSYCHOLOGY OF but between the ages of 1 and 5 years the child begins to emerge as an individual, and character formation can be significantly affected for good or ill by the pattern of his upbringing. Faulty physical development from malnutrition or neglect is now relatively rare but it is just as important that parental care should help children to develop with healthy minds and balanced personalities. The adult who has grown up with undesirable social attitudes – such as hostility, agressiveness, self-assertion or timidity, inability to work reliably and conscientiously or to accept responsibility, lack of initiative or unwillingness to face new experiences with resolution, resource and adaptability – is as a rule showing the end-results of misunder-standing or mis-management in childhood.

Behaviour problems. Many mothers are troubled by what they regard as wilfully deviant behaviour by their children. Destructiveness, temper-tantrums, persistent disobedience, lying, bullying or stealing are symptoms of basic unhappiness. Punishment is usually of little avail. Compliance may be enforced by pain or fear but only at the cost of inducing an attitude of mind which may show as withdrawal, an increasing sense of inferiority, a reluctance to think and act independently, a fear of criticism or ridicule, or a readiness to deny before accusal. It is necessary therefore to seek for the real causes of misbehaviour. A child may be resentful over displacement in favour of a new baby or over-excessive parental discipline or from being bullied and teased by elder brothers and sisters. He may not have adequate outlets for his growing curiosity and sense of exploration or he may not have the scope for play and the play-material appropriate to his age. On the other hand he may be so over-protected and over-indulged that he feels his lack of independence. Physically he may be getting too little rest or be subjected to too much excitement.

Jealousy. The toddler sees a new baby as a threat to his security and may seek to regain attention by unconsciously trying to become a baby himself again. He will refuse to play, cling to mother, develop food-fads or refuse to eat, suck his thumb or become incontinent. Punishment does not help; it only reinforces his conviction that he is unloved. Verbal reassurance is equally unsuccessful; active demonstrations are required. He should be involved in the new family situation and encouraged to help with the new baby as for instance in bathing and feeding. Jealousy also promotes quarrels between children and one child should never be held up as a model to the others. This only increases antagonisms and conversely makes the model vain and self-righteous.

Fear. Children should be helped to face life with courage. Basically they are rather fearless and the mother who over-protects is undermining this attribute and will induce either resentment of domination or inability to face life without help. It is right to safeguard them unobtrusively from real dangers but constant admonishments to take care and the encouragement of fear-reactions to objective situations such as lightning, dogs, policemen or doctors only causes harm. The consistently timid child has subjective fears. He lacks self-confidence because in some way his sense of security has been destroyed often by parental treatment where impatience, anger, criticism and constant correction have engendered a feeling that whatever he does cannot gain for him the approval or love which he craves.

Negativism. This may be defined as contrariness or behaviour in which requests or commands are bluntly refused.

Around the age of 2½ years negativism is not naughtiness but a normal stage of development. The previously docile and dependent child has begun to realize that he has a choice. Where previously he obeyed instructions without thought, he now delights in saying 'I won't'.

Punishment is undesirable and struggles of will between parent and child are harmful to both. The wise parent, recognizing the beginnings of the stage, will make life more tolerable for himself by minimal interference with the child's activities, and, where a request must be made, by framing it such a way that there is a choice: e.g., instead of 'Put your toys away now', asking 'Which one do you want to put away first?' Where the parent receives an actual refusal, the best plan is to ignore it and to divert the child to another topic.

When an older child reverts to a negativistic stage, parents and teachers, before seeking psychological help, should ask themselves, 'Am I creating this by inadvertently ordering almost every detail of the child's life?'

Play. Play is not just a childish method of passing the time. It is fundamental to a child's exploration of his environment, and playthings matched to his growing capacities help him to do this. Up to 9 months or so a baby enjoys rattles or bright dangling objects and soon after he will achieve satisfaction by hammering with a spoon, banging blocks together, or playing with soft toys. By 15 to 18 months he is ready for peg-boards, a posting-box, or insert cutouts. The toddler needs pushing and pulling toys, blocks to build, a sand-box and tins or floating toys and water-play. There is a need for vigorous movements and large toys, and modern housing often makes this difficult. Confinement to a play-pen frustrates the need for adventure and exploration. Throwing out toys expresses resentment of restriction or conversely the reaction may be one of sulkiness, withdrawal and lack of interest.

Constructional toys and painting books are needed by the 4 year old child, and he should be allowed to carry out his own plans in order to encourage independence. Help should be given only if asked for and must not become interference. Too much passive amusement submerges the creative urge which expresses itself in childhood as imaginative play, and life becomes boring and meaningless.

General. The understanding mother will find many other ways of influencing her child's development: by involving him in household activities such as shopping, by teaching table-manners and skills, by conversation and stories, and by encouraging questions and providing patient and accurate answers. Pets are another good idea. They satisfy two very strong natural tendencies – the desire for

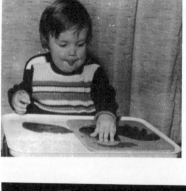
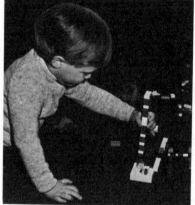

Childhood psychology: Jamie (aged 2 years 4 months) and Paul (aged 3 years 10 months) each playing with a toy well chosen for his age.

possession and the desire to protect – and they also inculcate a sense of responsibility.

Preparation for the change from home (where the child is very central) to school (where he is one of a group) is also important.

Apart from formal education a school should strive to encourage a sense of duty and responsibility and should foster feelings of accomplishment. Particular care is necessary with several types of child, e.g., the unintellectual and unathletic child who may feel a failure, the very bright child who may become bored, and the child with a minor disability, such as obesity, who may be mocked by his mates.

Parents should be on their guard about over-forcing a child and about making him feel a failure by expressions of dissatisfaction with his progress. The child who feels a failure may react with hostility to both school and parents, and may develop antisocial tendencies in an attempt to gain recognition. See also INFANCY, PSYCHOLOGY OF and PARENT AGE AND CHILD CARE.

children, behaviour disorders. A diverse group of socially unacceptable behaviour patterns in children. Causes may be of a social and/or psychological nature, while other, co-existing, physical or mental handicaps may contribute and complicate the situation. See BEHAVIOUR DISORDERS.

children, diseases of. Disorders usually only encountered in infancy or childhood. They include all classes of illness, from infections to tumours. Many of the infectious diseases which used often to be fatal are now preventable by routine immunization in infancy, and have thus been virtually eliminated from developed countries; these include whooping cough, diphtheria, and poliomyelitis. Less serious complaints, however, such as chickenpox, still cause widespread illness, while some less common diseases, such as leukaemia, still generally lead to death.

It is also recognized that many 'adult' diseases often run a quite different course in children and should properly be regarded as children's diseases, needing treatment employing paediatric skills.

chill. A sensation of cold accompanied by involuntary shivering or shaking, and skin pallor. When associated with an elevation of temperature in the interior of the body, it may indicate the invasion of the blood by toxins, signifying the early stages of an infectious disease. Chill in this sense is especially characteristic of malaria and pneumonococcal pneumonia.

Preventive measures include the wearing of protective clothing against the elements and the suppression of malaria with drugs. Specific treatment depends on the identification of the cause, and might therefore include the use of anti-malarial or antibiotic drugs, as well as general measures of rest, appropriate fluid intake, and diet.

In popular usage a chill also implies a respiratory (or sometimes a gastric or urinary tract) disorder, held to be caused by exposure to cold and damp. Hence the term includes a host of complaints.

Chinese medicine. A system of traditional and irrational medicine has prevailed in China from earliest times. According to legend it was originated by Fu Hsi (c. 2953 B.C.). It was developed by the Emperor Shen Nung under inspiration from the great Taoist god P'an Ku and later by Huang Ti (2698-2598 B.C.). The latter was the Yellow Emperor and traditionally author of the medical work *Nei Ching* but it is not really certain that this is earlier than the third century B.C. Subsequent Chinese medical literature relies greatly on the precepts of the *Nei Ching* but two other original works were the *Mo Ching* (the *Pulse Classic* of A.D. 300) and the *Golden Mirror*, a compilation of medical traditions of the Han dynasty produced about A.D. 1700.

Over the centuries any change has simply elaborated ancient theories. Although some infiltration of Western ideas began in the nineteenth century they gained little acceptance and traditional methods are still widely practised. However there has long been real concern for those who were ill, and in ancient China institutions for the sick grew up in association with monasteries as 'Houses of Benevolence'.

Medical thinking was based on Taoist philosophy which held that orderly existence depended on a balance between two fundamental opposing principles – Yang and Yin. Yang was associated with masculinity, light, sun, dryness and the south, while Yin

represented femininity, darkness, earth, moisture and the north. Health, character, and success of all kinds were determined by the relative preponderance of Yang or Yin and Chinese medicine aimed at their control.

Religious teaching forbade dissection and the Chinese conception of anatomy held that the body enclosed five elements – wood, fire, earth, metal and water – and twelve channels. The elements were influenced by five planets, five atmospheric conditions and similar groups of colours, tones, and smells. Any inconvenient anatomical knowledge was adapted to fit this cosmic system. There were for instance five organs which stored but did not eliminate; five which eliminated but did not store; 365 bones and 365 joints; and three 'burning spaces'.

Traditional physiology held that the blood-vessels contained blood and air in proportions determined by Yang and Yin which circulated in the twelve channels, controlled the pulse, and in combination with blood passed continuously round the body. This assertion by the *Nei Chang* has been advanced as a claim for precedence over William Harvey who described the circulation of the blood in 1628.

Chinese diagnosis lays stress on history-taking with minute enquiry about dreams, tastes, smells and other sensory impressions and on observation of voice, complexion, and tongue. Great attention is also paid to the pulse which is taken at the wrist with three fingers and three degrees of pressure and at ten other sites. The findings can thus be combined in great variety both for diagnosis and for the assessment of treatment, and this may take hours.

Treatment is based on a complex range of medicines embodying a great variety of remedies from vegetable, animal, human, and mineral sources. It also employs MOXIBUSTION and ACUPUNCTURE. Famous herbals of the past were collated by Li Shih-chen in the *Great Herbal* of the sixteenth century. Its fifty-two volumes have been frequently revised and reprinted and are still in use. Drugs are intended to restore the harmony of Yang and Yin and since their effects are also related to the five planets and the whole five-grouped theory of anatomy, prescribing is incredibly complicated.

Some Chinese drugs have, however, been adopted by Western medicine. Examples are rhubarb, iron, castor-oil, kaolin, camphor, cannabis, chaulmoogra oil (for leprosy) and the plant Ma Huang (*Ephedra vulgaris*), source of the valuable drug ephedrine.

A particularly prized and expensive Chinese remedy however is ginseng root (Sang) obtained from two species of *Panax* (from the Latin *panacea*, meaning 'cure-all'). These are *P. quinquefolius* and *P. ginseng*. Some ginseng is now grown in America and exported to the East and this cultivation has a chequered history of exploitation and speculation but the reputed value of the drug as a diuretic and aphrodisiac is exaggerated.

Hydrotherapy is also used; cold baths for fevers are recorded from 180 B.C.

Moxibustion utilizes small cones made from the powdered leaves of mugwort or wormwood (*Artemisia moxa*) which are applied to the skin and ignited, the ashes then being rubbed into the resulting blister. Other substances are also used and many applications at selected sites may be made simultaneously.

In acupuncture needles are inserted into various parts of the body to affect the distribution of Yang and Yin in the channels and spaces. The procedure dates from at least 2500 B.C. and there are many treatises on its use giving instructional diagrams based on a bronze figurine of A.D. 860. It is a form of treatment still widely used, and even in the West there are some exponents of 'fringe' medicine prepared to accord it a degree of acceptance.

More rational ideas are now eroding traditional Chinese practice, especially in the larger centres. Perhaps the most surprising fact is that the older methods have persisted so stubbornly in a nation which has not taken three thousand years to follow the West in other directions and which has already acquired the technological competence to master the secrets of nuclear science and engineering.

chiropodist. A person specialized in the care and treatment of minor foot disorders. In most of the developed countries schools of chiropody are subject to formal approval (just as are medical, nursing and dental schools) and the person who duly qualifies from such a school, usually after a course lasting for three years, then becomes a registered chiropodist. Chiropody, however, is still a young profession, and in most countries there are still some chiropodists who are permitted to continue in practice but whose professional training would today be deemed inadequate either in length or in quality.

Chiropody services are now an established part of general health services and recognized as an essential part of over-all medical care; but in countries like the U.K. and the U.S.A. there is taking place both an extension in the training and legitimate expertise of chiropodists and an enlargement of the scope of their work. Twenty years ago chiropody was largely a 'comfort' service for pensioners with painful feet, in at least some cases suffering from defects that could have been prevented by health education and advice about suitable footwear earlier in life. Today, while the average chiropodist probably spends more than half of his time with the elderly, he is increasingly concerned with the foot health of younger people.

Besides dealing with conditions that affect the soft tissues of the feet (e.g., corns) and the nails (e.g., ingrowing toe-nails), matters of little medical significance, a chiropodist is now involved in the treatment of (1) foot disabilities directly associated with general medical and surgical states; (2) structural and functional disturbances of more importance, such as club foot, abnormalities of the arch of the foot and deformities of the toes; and (3) infections resulting from sepsis, foot warts and ringworm.

A chiropodist also prepares and provides chiropodial appliances, and is increasingly being assisted by chiropody attendants with more limited routine skills and by chiropodial appliance technicians. Not least, chiropodists should be involved in preventive chiropody – such as inspecting children's feet for incipient disorders and taking part in education on foot health, but of course this involves the training of some chiropodists in the methods and skills of health education.

In several developed countries there has been a tendency to remunerate doctors and dentists well, nurses rather badly and chiropodists very badly, with the result that there are insufficient chiropodists for a growing service that is greatly needed both for the foot health and comfort of the people and to conserve the time of dermatologists, orthopaedic surgeons and general practitioners.

choking. Partial or complete suffocation. It may be caused by (1) mechanical obstruction, through inhalation of a foreign body or from external pressure on the larynx or trachea; (2) spasm of the larynx caused by an irritating gas or liquid; or (3) excessive secretions from the inner surface of the lungs, which accompanies acute left heart failure.

Relief of choking is directed at removal or treatment of the specific cause. In cases of immediate obstruction a hard slap between the shoulders may dislodge the obstruction. In severe cases emergency measures such as tracheotomy or artificial respiration are sometimes required

cholecystitis. Inflammation of the gall-bladder. There are two main types: (1) acute: usually caused by impaction of a gallstone in the duct of the gall-bladder or, occasionally, by infection, and (2) chronic: usually caused by long-standing presence of gallstones within the gall-bladder.

Acute cholecystitis is usually treated by general medical measures involving bed rest, adequate fluid intake, and analgesics, while chronic cholecystitis generally necessitates surgical removal of the gall-bladder.

cholera. An acute infectious disease of man, caused by cholera bacteria, and occurring in epidemics chiefly in Asia. It is characterized by a profuse watery diarrhoea and a state of collapse, and is rapidly fatal if untreated. Spread occurs by faecal contamination. The great nineteenth century epidemics in Europe followed in the train of Mecca pilgrimages, and were only controlled when specific sanitary precautions amongst pilgrims were enforced. Recent spread to Europe and Africa has accompanied the arrival of mass air travel, an example being the 1973 outbreak in Italy with about 130 cases and 27 deaths.

Preventive measures include the control of people's movement to and from infected areas, measures of personal hygiene, and the use of anti-cholera vaccines, though the latter are not yet especially effective. Prompt treatment with bed rest and adequate fluid replacement usually leads to complete recovery.

In archaic use the term cholera indicated a variety of gastro-intestinal disturbances.

cholesterol. A naturally occurring substance found in all animal fats and oils including the blood and most bodily tissues. It plays an important part in metabolism, being related to the bile acids, the sex hormones, and vitamin D.

Its level in the blood plasma is fairly constant for each individual, but shows wide variation between individuals. There are characteristic changes of level in certain diseases: it is low, for example, in hyperthyroidism, and high in hypothyroidism and untreated diabetes mellitus. The association of raised plasma cholesterol levels with an increased incidence of heart diseases and arteriosclerosis has lead to their treatment with specific cholesterol-lowering drugs, as well as to the increasing adoption of low cholesterol diets (particularly in the U.S.A.). These include the use of unsaturated fats (as in margarine and corn oil) rather than animal fats. Evaluation of such measures in the prevention of these diseases is complicated, and may take many years to complete.

chorea. A disorder characterized by irregular, involuntary, twitching movements of the limbs or facial muscles.

Sydenham's chorea, also called St. Vitus' dance, is an acute, toxic or infective disorder of the nervous system, usually associated with acute rheumatic fever. The characteristic movements of the face and fingers often spread to the limbs and trunk, and there is weakness and incoordination of voluntary movements, and emotional instability. The disease chiefly affects children aged 5 to 15, and girls twice as frequently as boys. It disappears in sleep and responds to treatment of the underlying cause, including rest in bed, skilled nursing and, usually, tranquillizers.

A completely different disease, HUNTINGTON'S CHOREA, is an inherited chronic disorder.

choroid. The middle coat of the EYE, lying between the sclera and the retina, and composed of arteries, veins and capillaries.

choroiditis. Inflammation of part or all of the choroid, usually affecting the underlying retina. The effects depend on the area involved, and may sometimes involve partial or complete loss of vision. Choroiditis may be associated with an infective or non-infective general disorder, or with other eye disease or injury.

Treatment consists of eradicating the underlying cause, if known, and employing drugs to restrict inflammation, relieve pain, and control any infection. Prolonged rest is occasionally required.

chromosome. One of a number of small, rod-shaped bodies present in each cell of the body and carrying certain genes which determine a person's inherited characteristics. In human beings every cell except the ovum and sperm contains twenty-three pairs of chromosomes: a woman's cells contain twenty-two pairs of ordinary chromosomes (autosomes) and one pair of sizeable sex-chromosomes commonly called X-chromosomes; and a man's cells contain twenty-two pairs of autosomes, a single X-chromosome and a much smaller chromosome called the Y-chromosome.

In preparation for reproduction the pairs of chromosomes divide. The ovum contains twenty-two autosomes and one X-chromosome. The sperm contains twenty-two autosomes and either an X- or a Y-chromosome. When the ovum is fertilized by a sperm, if the sperm happens to contain an X-chromosome, the result will be a girl (twenty-two pairs of autosomes, one of each pair from each parent, and two X-chromosomes, one from each parent). If on the other hand the sperm contains a Y-chromosome, the result will be a boy (twenty-two pairs of autosomes, one X-chromosome from the mother and one Y-chromosome from the father).

From the genes, situated along the chromosomes, derive the inheritance of all predetermined characteristics, e.g., colour of hair and blood group.

Dominant inheritance occurs where a stronger gene (e.g., for achondroplasia, Huntington's chorea or diabetes insipidus) is inherited from one parent and a weaker gene (e.g., for normality in respect of the particular condition) is inherited from the other. The child will show the effects of the stronger gene, i.e., suffer from the disease. If the affected child reaches adult life, clearly half his sperms will contain the dominant (stronger, abnormal) gene and half will contain the recessive (weaker, normal) gene. So, if he marries a normal person, on average half his children will be affected (inheriting the dominant gene from him and a normal gene from the other parent) and the other half will be unaffected (inheriting normal genes from both parents).

In the case of recessive inheritance a weaker gene (e.g., for cystic fibrosis, phenylketonuria or deaf mutism) is inherited from one parent and a stronger gene (e.g., for normality) is inherited from the other. The child will appear normal, but if he reaches adult life half his sperms will contain the weaker (recessive, abnormal) gene and half will contain the normal (dominant) gene. So, if he marries a normal person, on average half the children will be normal (with normal gene from each parent) and the other half will appear normal but be capable of transmitting the condition (having normal gene from one parent and recessive gene from the other). If the apparently normal person (with normal and recessive gene) marries a similar person, it is likely on average that a quarter of their children will be normal (inheriting normal gene from each parent), half will appear normal but be capable of transmitting the condition (inheriting a dominant normal gene from one parent and a recessive abnormal gene from the other) and a quarter will suffer from the disease (inheriting the abnormal gene from both parents). Dominant and recessive inheritance are rather more fully considered in GENETICS.

X-chromosome. As indicated above, a girl inherits one X-chromosome from each parent, and a boy inherits an X-chromosome from his mother and a Y-chromosome from his father. Where one of the mother's two X-chromosomes is recessive for a disease (e.g., haemophilia) the girl inherits a normal (dominant) X-chromosome from her father (and therefore will not show the disease) but has a 50 per cent chance of inheriting a normal or recessive X-chromosome from her mother. In adult life the ovum of the girl who had normal inheritance from both parents will clearly contain either a normal X from the father or a normal X from the mother, but the ovum of the girl who inherited the recessive X-chromosome from her mother has equal chances of passing to her ovum a normal X-chromosome (from her father) or the dangerous X-chromosome (from her mother). In other words the daughter of a mother who is a carrier of haemophilia has a one in four chance of being a carrier in turn; but, since a female has two X-chromosomes of which the normal one is dominant, neither she nor her daughters will themselves show the disease.

On the other hand, if the mother is a carrier (with one normal and dominant X-chromosome and one recessive abnormal X-chromosome), on average half the sons will inherit Y-chromosome from the father and the normal X-chromosome from the mother (and therefore be normal) and the other half will inherit Y-chromosome from the father and the abnormal X-chromosome from the mother (and therefore suffer from the disease). This situation in which a quarter of the daughters are carriers and half of the sons are sufferers is what is termed sex-linked inheritance. Where the father is a sufferer from haemophilia, his sons will be normal (inheriting Y-chromosomes from the father) but his daughters will be carriers (inheriting the abnormal X-chromosome from the father and a dominant normal X-chromosome from the mother).

Y-chromosome. As mentioned above, the male sperm is of two types, one containing twenty-two autosomes and a sizeable X-chromosome (leading on fertilization of the ovum to a female child) and the other containing twenty-two autosomes and a small Y-chromosome (leading on fertilization to a male child). So sex is determined at the moment of conception and depends solely on which of the father's sperms reaches the ovum.

Unlike the larger X-chromosome, the Y-chromosome is not notably associated with transmission of hereditary disease.

Spermatozoa containing the Y-chromosome of maleness are a shade lighter and more motile than those containing the X-chromosome. So on average something like 110 to 120 boys are conceived for every 100 girls. Males, however, are the weaker sex even before birth. Male babies are slightly more subject to miscarriages and stillbirths than are female babies. At birth the ratio is about 104 boys per 100 girls. In the long era of high baby and child mortality more boys died than girls, the sexes became about equal in numbers by 15 or 16 years and from about 20 years there were more women than men. In the improved preventive and curative services of today there are still more deaths of boys than of girls but there are far fewer deaths, so that males are more numerous than females up to the age of 35 years, and it is likely that in another decade males will be more numerous up to the age of 40.

This change in the sex-ratio has important implications. For instance, 'surplus' females are no longer available to staff such professions as nursing and teaching or to provide maid-servants for the wealthy; a child today is more likely to have a bachelor uncle than a maiden aunt; there are increasingly fewer unmarried daughters to care for elderly parents; and, just as male deaths in 1914-18 resulted in increased numbers of women entering formerly male occupations (e.g., as doctors, lawyers and secretaries), so the relative fall in the numbers of young women is causing the appearance of men in previously female occupations (e.g., as nurses, primary school teachers, etc.).

Some sociologists even associate the altered sex-ratio with changes of behaviour: when there were over 100 female adolescents for every 100 male adolescents virtually every man who desired to marry could secure a mate; but when there are only 98 females for every 100 males, and very attractive career prospects open to some of the 98 without need for matrimony, males have to compete for mates – a fact which may explain many changes of behaviour, from the wearing of brighter clothing to the increase in aggressive actions.

chronic. A longstanding condition. The term relates to duration only and does not imply that the condition is permanent or incurable.

chyle. A form of LYMPH, found in the lymph vessels of the small intestine after the absorption of fat from foodstuffs. Milky-white in appearance owing to the presence of emulsified fat, chyle passes into the veins by the way of the thoracic duct.

chyme. Food, partly digested in the stomach, liquid in form, and brown or grey in appearance, passing into the intestines for the completion of digestion.

cigarettes. See SMOKING.

circulation of the blood. Until three and a half centuries ago Galen's curious idea persisted, namely that there existed between the right and left sides of the heart a permeable septum (i.e., partition) through which blood oozed. There were vague questionings of this unproved (and baseless) theory from one or two physicians of the Persian-Arab civilization, and in the sixteenth century a definite indication of the circulation was made by Michael Servetus, who was subsequently burned at the stake. But the real discoverer of the circulation of the blood was WILLIAM HARVEY (1578-1637) who published his description in 1628. It is indicative of the state of learning at that time that the teaching of Harvey's 'doctrine' was forbidden by the Paris Medical Faculty and that in Britain, where Harvey had reached his conclusions by careful dissection and research, he was 'disproved' within two years by a doctor who undertook no personal investigation but merely assembled a mass of quotations from various ancient authorities. However, the spirit of the age favoured scientific investigation and Harvey's proofs became accepted.

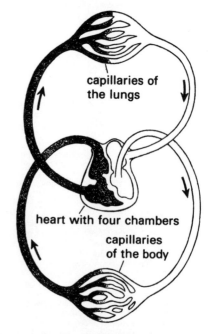

labels: capilaries of the lungs · heart with four chambers · capillaries of the body

Diagramatic scheme showing continuous blood flow round the circulatory system.

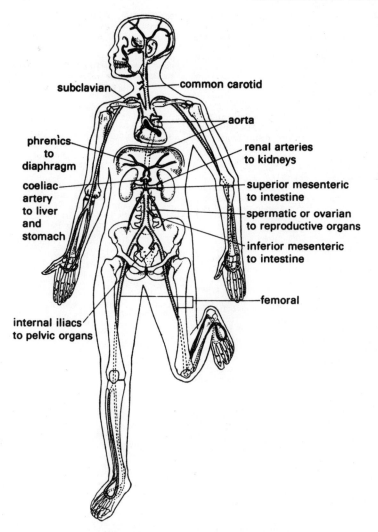

subclavian — common carotid

aorta

phrenics
to
diaphragm

renal arteries
to kidneys

coeliac
artery
to liver
and
stomach

superior mesenteric
to intestine

spermatic or ovarian
to reproductive organs

inferior mesenteric
to intestine

femoral

internal iliacs
to pelvic organs

The circulatory system, showing the main arteries

From the heart the blood makes a double circuit. Venous blood, containing carbon dioxide and other waste products and coloured dark because of the interaction of carbon dioxide and haemoglobin is brought to the right auricle from the superior vena cava (which drains venous blood from the head and arms) and the inferior vena cava (which drains from the rest of the body). It passes to the right ventricle and then travels by the pulmonary artery and its branches (the only arteries containing venous blood) to the lungs. In the capillaries of the lungs there is an interchange of gases: carbon dioxide passes out to the alveoli of the lungs and is subsequently breathed out, and oxygen passes in, interacting with the haemoglobin and giving the oxygenated blood (arterial blood) its bright red colour.

The oxygenated blood is carried by the pulmonary veins (the only veins containing arterial blood) to the left auricle, passes to the left ventricle and is from there pumped into the AORTA, the main artery of the body. From branches and sub-branches of the aorta the arterial blood passes to capillaries in the various muscles and tissues of the body. From the capillaries the oxygen is removed to supply the needs of tissues and organs, and carbon dioxide and other waste products enter the capillaries, so that the blood becomes venous blood. The capillaries carrying venous blood unite into small veins and these into larger veins which in due course empty into the superior and inferior vena cava.

So for the transport of oxygen and carbon dioxide there are really two circulations: venous blood travelling from the right side of the heart to the lungs, gaining oxygen and returning as arterial blood to the left side of the heart; and arterial blood pumped from the left side of the heart to the tissues, losing oxygen and travelling as venous blood to the right side of the heart.

There is also a third circulation. Blood from the stomach, pancreas, spleen and intestines travels by veins to the liver. In the capillaries of the liver glycogen is extracted from the blood for storage or returned to the blood for use in the tissues, and the blood with its glycogen adjusted to balance needs is returned by the hepatic veins to the inferior vena cava. This third circulation is termed the PORTAL CIRCULATION.

circumcision. The operation of cutting away part or all of the foreskin (prepuce) of the penis. The origin of this practice is probably very ancient, circumcision having been practised as a ritual in diverse cultures, performed before or at puberty. Its practitioners attach profound religious significance to the ritual. The Ethiopians, the Jews, and a few other peoples practise it at birth; when performed at puberty it represents the beginning of initation into manhood.

It has been widely practised in some countries (e.g., the U.S.A.) as a hygienic measure, the circumcised seldom suffering from inflammation of the glans penis or from carcinoma of the penis. The other possible benefit (protection against carcinoma of the cervix of the uterus among women who consort only with circumcized men) is unproven and the subject of considerable current research.

cirrhosis. A progressive liver disease in which normal liver tissue is partially destroyed and replaced by non-functional tissue. It leads to impaired liver function, frequently resulting in jaundice and other complications. Its most frequent cause is alcoholism (in all except alcohol-free cultures), though it is uncertain whether alcoholism leads to cirrhosis through a direct effect on liver tissue or because of an associated nutritional deficiency. It is also caused by obstruction of the bile ducts and is an occasional late effect of infective hepatitis.

Prevention depends mainly upon control of alcohol intake. Alcohol avoidance and vitamin supplementation form the basis of treatment.

cisternal puncture. The passage of a hollow needle through the junction of the skull and spinal column into the subarachnoid space surrounding the cerebellum and medulla of the brain, in order to draw off cerebro-spinal fluid or inject (for diagnostic purposes) material opaque to x-rays. Less commonly it is used to inject antibiotics to treat meningitis.

claudication, intermittent. Attacks of lameness and pain, especially in the calf muscles, brought on by walking. The symptoms increase as walking proceeds until further progress is impossible, but after a short rest, during which the symptoms cease, walking becomes possible again. Intermittent claudication is caused by limitation of blood supply to the leg muscles due to narrowing, by ARTERIOSCLEROSIS, of the arteries of the legs. It is the commonest symptom of a process involving the whole arterial system, and is therefore commonly found in people suffering from heart disease and cerebrovascular disease. No specific treatment exists, though

weight control may be helpful, and cigarette smoking is particularly discouraged.

claustrophobia. An irrational dread of being within walls, or of being shut in a room or confined space. Like other obsessional neuroses it generally starts in early adult life. In Britain, treatment is usually by psychotherapy and tranquillizers, though treatment by psychoanalysis, by hypnosis, and by behaviour therapy is also practised. About 70 per cent of patients recover or become much better within a year or two, whatever treatment is given; the outcome does seem to depend much more on the duration of the illness and the previous personality and circumstances of the patient than on the form of treatment employed.

clavicle. See COLLAR-BONE.

clawfoot. An exaggeration of the normal arch of the foot to give a hollow foot so that the weight of the body is taken on the point of the heel and the balls of the toes. This rare defect, encountered at birth, is treated by manipulation and the application of plaster casts.

cleft palate. See HARE-LIP AND CLEFT PALATE.

clergyman's throat. Prolonged hoarseness and tickling cough, usually due to excessive voice strain, as is liable to occur in public speakers, clergymen, teachers and others who frequently have to address large groups, but also occasionally caused by excessive use of tobacco or over-indulgence in alcohol. See PHARYNX, DISEASES OF.

climacteric. As far as women are concerned, this is a synonym for the MENOPAUSE or 'change of life', the cessation of the child-bearing phase in a woman's life, occurring normally between 40 and 50 years but very occasionally earlier or later. The 'change of life' should certainly not be regarded as the beginning of old age – the average menopausal woman has a third of a century ahead of her – but as the start of a new phase in which there is no longer monthly physiological preparation for child creation and subsequent childbirth.

There is a similar crisis which affects most men in middle life, generally between 45 and 60 years of age, resulting from their increasing realization of their own mortality in association with a waning of their physical powers. The often sudden appreciation that he can never hope to achieve all that he had once dreamt of doing, together with the prospect of an apparently steady and relentless decline of his faculties, precipitates depression or unexpected uncharacteristic behaviour in a few seemingly well-adjusted individuals. For some men the crisis provides the incentive for a sensible re-planning of their lives: most just muddle through.

Reproductive ability is not lost at the male climacteric as it is in women; in common with women, men suffer no dimunition of sexual drive at this time unless psychological disorders supervene. The preparation of men and their families to anticipate and prevent the problems of the male climacteric is virtually non-existent in Britain.

climate and health. The influence of climate on health is far less marked nowadays than when Hippocrates wrote his *Airs, Waters, Places* about 2400 years ago. Double glazing and central heating can make life perfectly tolerable within the Arctic Circle, while air coolers and humidity extractor fans can do the same thing in the tropics. Drainage of swamps and use of insecticides can reduce – or even abolish – the danger of such diseases as malaria and yellow fever in warm climates, while suitable clothing (even including clothing with an incorporated electric battery) can lessen the risk of frostbite in cold countries.

Nevertheless it is still in large measure true that tropical heat is associated with increased incidence of food-borne and insect-borne infections as well as with such perils as snake bites and scorpion stings, that a warm humid atmosphere tends to render very difficult the taking of physical exercise and so tends to stunt the growth of children, that cold and damp climates are associated with high incidence of bronchitis and rheumatic diseases, that mountainous regions with reduced atmospheric oxygen are deemed unsuitable for persons suffering from various diseases of the heart, and that dry sunny climates are often advised for asthmatics if they can afford to change their home and place of work.

In general life in a temperate climate has health advantages over life in a tropical or arctic climate, but the powers of adjustment of robust young adults to climate changes are remarkable. In the Second World War troops from Britain and other temperate countries remained in good health in the biting cold of Iceland and in the tropical heat of Burma. By contrast elderly people are much less adaptable: British persons who have emigrated to Australia or Southern Canada and seek to retire to their native country often find the climate too cold, and the writer knows two couples who sought to retire from Shetland to their native Aberdeen and found Britain's most northerly and most bracing large city 'impossibly relaxing and warm'.

The remarkable adaptability of man – as opposed to most animals – in his younger years is largely due to the sweat glands which enable him to get rid of varying amounts of moisture and heat as circumstances demand. In humid tropical heat a thoroughly acclimatized man can get rid of at least a litre of sweat each hour, and of course requires compensatory additional intake both of water and of salt.

It is probably fair to say that man can now occupy with reasonable health and comfort the whole of the earth's surface except the extreme polar regions, mountainous territory more than 3,600 m. (12,000 ft.) above sea-level and the centres of large deserts.

clothes, women's. Men's garments may occasionally be dictated by convention (e.g., full evening dress in hot weather or in an internal temperature of 27 °C., which is 80 °F.) but are in general selected for comfort and protection and vary little from decade to decade, recent changes being in the direction of brighter colours rather than differences of texture or construction. By contrast women's garments are to some extent at the mercy of the mysterious dictates of fashion, varying (as Byron wrote over 150 years ago) 'From Eve's fig leaf down to the petticoat hardly less scanty of days less remote'.

Fortunately the tyranny of the steel or whale-boned corset which constricted the abdominal muscles appears to be a thing of the past, as is the tight garter which was a former common precipitating cause of varicose veins. In general women's clothes in the 1970s are satisfactory from the aspect of health: often of cellular fabrics, giving warmth in cold weather and coolness in hot weather; light, thin and loose indoors and for outdoor use in warm weather, allowing adequate ventilation of bodies and aeration of skin, and in sunny weather allowing contact of the sun's rays with arms and neck; and with heavy coats, trousers, etc. available for outdoor use in cold weather. On average women's clothes nowadays tend – with the possible exception of footwear – to be more sensibly adapted to climatic variations than those of men; but one still meets women, especially of the older generation, who 'stifle' in a warm room because of heavy underwear and then wonder why they develop respiratory infections and rheumatic pains after going outside – with perhaps a 22 °C. (40 °F.) temperature drop – with only a thin coat as additional protection.

clothing and health. In place of the fur and feathers of animals and birds man needs clothing for protection against both heat and cold. He also uses clothing for decoration and satisfaction of social conventions, and sometimes fashion dictates the type and nature of clothing with little regard to its protective functions.

In a climate in which the temperature remains high even at night it is sometimes alleged that clothing has no health function – that, where used, it is employed simply to indicate status or rank, or for ornamentation, or to conform with the conventions or moral standards of a particular society. Yet clothing affords considerable protection against both sunshine and heat. Dark clothes in particular help to obstruct undesired rays both of light and of ultraviolet, clothes that leave a layer of still air next to the body protect from heat as well as from cold, and clothes that absorb sweat facilitate heat loss. The African of the Congo, with heavily pigmented skin and to some extent protected by dense foliage from the direct rays of the sun, can perhaps afford to wear the minimum clothing (e.g., a loin cloth) that convention demands; but the Arab of the Sahara, with much less protecting pigment and much less sun-obscuring foliage, requires his layers of protective clothing.

Where the temperature is usually high during the day but low at night further problems arise. The person whose thin external garment gave some protection from sun and heat and whose single layer of underclothing facilitated absorption of sweat needs additional protection from the sharp winds of morning or evening.

Man's conquest of the temperate zone and subsequently of cold zones has depended primarily on the wearing of clothing which would retain body heat. The provision of adequate shelter and heating is also important but people migrating northwards had to live in a colder climate while building their houses.

The five main substances used in clothing are wool (from which are made flannel, worsted and alpaca), silk (which can be taken to include satin, velvet and crepe), linen, cotton (including fustian and muslin) and man-made fibres (including artificial silk, rayon and nylon). For provision of warmth in cold climates these have been mentioned in roughly descending order: wool (followed by silk) is a poor conductor of heat and therefore tends to retain bodily heat, while linen, cotton and cellulose allow heat to escape. A layer of intervening still air is, however, an even worse conductor of heat than wool, so 'cellular' underclothing preserves heat still better.

Ideally for cold weather underclothing should be of loosely woven wool, with retained layers of still air, and it is preferable to wear two layers of underclothing rather than one to improve retention of air (e.g., vest and shirt); the outer garment should be wind-proof to prevent too rapid changes of air, and water-repellent to prevent soaking; however, completely waterproof material will prevent loss of water vapour, so it should not be worn for any long period of time.

For coolness in warm climates absorption of moisture from the sweat is important. Wool absorbs moisture better than cotton, linen or silk, so that – contrary to popular belief – loose-fitting woollen underclothing is probably best for persons exercising freely in a warm atmosphere. On the other hand, warmth at night is maintained by bedclothes and, since the sleeper should not perspire, linen or cotton nightwear is clearly preferable.

Britain in the 1970s is tending to follow America in respect of warmer houses, restaurants, offices, trains, etc. than in the past. This change implies that British people require for their health to be aware of the increasing difference between the temperature indoors and that outside, especially during the colder months of the year. For internal conditions they require less and lighter underclothing than in the past (many British people are considerably overclothed in their warm homes and offices), and for transfer to the colder outside temperatures they require substantial additional clothing – pullovers, heavy overcoats and scarves. A British person in 1955 perhaps passed, in winter, from a home or office temperature of 16.5 °C. (62 °F.) to an outside temperature just on freezing point, and he could afford merely to don an overcoat. A similar person today perhaps passes from a home or office temperature of 22 °C. (72 °F.) to the same external temperature at freezing point: he should consider whether he is not often overclothed in the home or office and so relatively underclothed when he passes to the outside.

club foot. Technically called talipes equinovarus. A deformity of the foot long known to be due to faulty development before birth and nowadays recognized as being hereditary in origin. The deformity, which occurs rather more frequently in boys than in girls, consists in the sole of the foot being turned inwards and the heel drawn up, so that the person walks on the outer border of the foot on which corns tend to develop.

If the condition is identified early it can sometimes be cured by manipulation, splinting and massage. If it is not identified for a couple of years or so, surgical reconstruction of the joints of the foot may be required, and even after the operation special footwear may be needed. If untreated it causes life-long deformity, as in the case of the poet Byron.

coal gas poisoning. See CARBON MONOXIDE.

coal miner's lung. A disease of the lungs and bronchi arising from prolonged inhalation of fine particles of coal dust, creating breathlessness and chronic bronchitis.

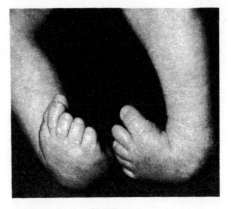

Club foot

Preventive measures include ventilation of mines and wet-drilling. Where the condition is identified in an early stage a change of occupation is desirable.

cocaine An alkaloid, derived originally from the leaves of the coca plant in Bolivia and Peru, sometimes used in ophthalmology, dentistry and nose and throat surgery to produce local anaesthesia, but seldom employed internally because of the great danger of addiction. Habitual use of cocaine causes temporary feelings of elation, severe craving, and ultimately complete deterioration of the personality.

coccus. A micro-organism whose shape is spherical, or nearly so. Cocci are microscopically small (often about one-thousandth of a millimetre in diameter) and they have characteristic patterns of growth, appearing as pairs (diplococci), clumps (staphylococci), or long chains (streptococci).

Various species are responsible for numerous important diseases. Certain diplococci cause pneumonia, gonorrhoea, and cerebrospinal fever. Superficial infections of the skin and subcutaneous tissues, and localized deep infections of bones, joints, and internal organs, are usually due to staphylococci. Streptococci are associated with scarlet fever, tonsillitis, respiratory tract infections, endocarditis, wound infections, post natal infections, and spreading septicaemic conditions generally.

coccydinia. See COCCYX.

coccyx. The lower end of the spinal column. It is a triangular bone beyond the sacrum and consists developmentally of four tiny vertebrae that are fused together. It is all that remains in man of the tail of animals.

Coccydinia, which is pain in the area of the coccyx, is sometimes the result of injury, e.g., a fall, but is more often a neuralgia of the nerves in that neighbourhood. In some cases it is a neurotic symptom. Treatment varies with the cause and no single treatment is of guaranteed efficiency. Surgical removal of the coccyx is a last resort which should not be used until less dramatic remedies have proved unsuccessful.

cochlea. The true organ of hearing (organ of Corti). It consists of a spiral tube resembling a snail-shell and forms part of the inner EAR.

cockroaches. The inch-long black beetle (*Blatta orientalis*) and the smaller and lighter German roach (*Blatella germanica*) are among the most widespread of household pests. They are potentially dangerous because of their opportunities for crawling over food and because they can carry germs on their feet and in their intestines. Cockroaches feed on fermented garbage as well as on clean food and they frequent such unsavoury places as cesspits and drain manholes.

Eggs are laid in batches of fifteen to thirty, and incubation takes about ten weeks. Young cockroaches pass through a series of moults but become mature in six months, and the adults live for several years.

Infested sites, e.g., behind stoves and other fixtures or behind skirting boards, should be treated weekly with a suitable insecticide powder, and the treatment should continue for fully six months. Sodium fluoride in 50 per cent strength is perhaps the most useful powder, but several effective commercial preparations contain benzene hexachloride.

codeine. A white crystalline compound, derived from morphia but not possessing its addictive qualities, much used in tablet form to relieve mild pain and in cough mixtures to reduce unproductive coughing. However it also slows the movements of the muscles of the intestine and so may cause constipation, and it often tends to cause slight drowsiness.

cod-liver oil. A pale yellow liquid of fishy odour and unpleasant taste obtained from the fresh liver of cod fish. It is a very rich source of vitamins A and D, and was formerly much employed for the prevention of rickets and – perhaps less effectively – for the treatment of children suffering from bronchitis, tuberculosis and various other diseases. Because of its unpalatable taste it was often given combined with malt or orange juice, or as an emulsion. In general cod-liver oil has now been replaced by purer, more concentrated preparations of fat-soluble vitamins.

Cod-liver oil also has some value as an external application for the treatment of slowly healing wounds or ulcers.

coeliac disease. A wasting disease of childhood in which the lining of the intestine is damaged by gluten (a protein found in wheat, barley and some other cereals) so that it fails to absorb fats and calcium properly. The condition appears between the ages of 6 and 24 months; the child loses appetite and ceases to thrive, and diarrhoea develops with large, pale, offensive stools containing much unabsorbed fat. If the disease is untreated signs of vitamin deficiency and anaemia appear; there is considerable emaciation and the abdomen becomes very distended. A minority of cases die but the majority ultimately recover although they may be permanently stunted in consequence of having had a year or so of malnutrition during what should have been an important growth period. Such stunting is also common if treatment is started late.

Early treatment with a gluten-free diet, which means eating cereals only when the gluten portion has been removed, and some attention to vitamin supplements together with initial restriction in the amount of fat eaten, usually result in complete recovery with ultimate ability to assimilate ordinary food. The required duration of treatment varies from under six months to over two years and is best estimated by trying the child every few weeks with a little ordinary flour and watching the state of the stools.

coitus. Sexual intercourse, or the act of sexual union. Intercourse is preceded by arousal, a stage of sexual excitation, during which the penis of the male, by engorgement with blood, becomes enlarged, erect, and capable of penetrating into the vagina. In the female similar engorgement causes the thick folds of skin at the entrance to the vagina to swell and turn outwards, so that the opening is exposed; there is also an increased secretion of mucus which lubricates the parts and facilitates penetration. Since female arousal is generally less immediate, preliminary 'love-play' will ensure mutual readiness.

After penetration, rhythmic movements by the man, to which the woman responds, increase excitation until the culmination of orgasm is reached. In the man this is accompanied by reflex ejaculation of semen, and in the woman by pleasurable muscular spasms, primarily in the genital area but sometimes spreading more widely.

Ideal coitus should aim at achievement of simultaneous orgasm and this calls for forbearance and an understanding approach by the man, since female orgasm is generally attained less rapidly. Prolongation of arousal, with variations in position and technique, will help to ensure the mutual release from tension, and the pleasurable feelings of relaxation and refreshment which should follow.

coitus interruptus. An unreliable non-medical method of CONTRACEPTION. At intercourse the penis is withdrawn as ejaculation is about to occur, so that semen is discharged well outside the vagina. It requires considerable self-control on the part of the man 'being careful', and tends to diminish sexual satisfaction in both partners.

There is a substantial failure-rate, variously quoted as 5 to 20 per cent, because motile sperms may be present in the man's mucus even before climax; or because ejaculation may have been gradual and not appreciated as a well-defined climax; or finally because sperm deposited at the vaginal entrance may still succeed in ascending to the cervix by their own motility.

Coitus interruptus may also be psychologically harmful by increasing feelings of emotional insecurity and contributing to frigidity and failure of female orgasm.

cold, the common. Technically termed coryza. A catarrhal inflammation of the nose and upper respiratory passages, characterized by a feeling of chilliness, watering nose, sneezing, watering eyes and general discomfort. A cold usually lasts three to five days, although the French have a saying that a cold lasts two weeks when treated and fourteen days when not treated.

Most cases of coryza are due to a virus and therefore infectious, so that the sufferer should remain at home in the interests of others as well as for his own comfort. It appears, however, that some colds are allergic in nature and not infectious.

Frequent colds may arise as a result of debility, lowered general resistance, adenoids or minor deformities of the nose or throat. Certain families have more than their average share of colds, whether from poorer nutrition or from similarities in their nasal passages. By contrast some people appear to have a high natural immunity.

Colds are no more common in the Arctic than elsewhere and quite infrequent in open-air sanatoria, although in any one climate they are more frequent in winter than in summer, perhaps because of more accumulation of people indoors, less ventilation and easier transmission of infection.

Aspirin tablets and warm drinks promote perspiration and make the patient feel a little better, and cough medicines may be required when the catarrh reaches the larynx and bronchi. Anti-coryzal vaccines are under trial but the outlook is not very hopeful since coryza itself does not confer any lengthy immunity and since infectious colds may well be due not to one virus but to a series of broadly similar viruses. Decongestant nasal sprays may also give relief but proprietary medicines to be taken by mouth often contain drugs which interact with alcohol – a popular remedy – so that alcohol should be avoided if these are taken.

cold, effects of. A cold environment causes the blood vessels near the surface of the skin to contract thus decreasing the loss of body heat; it also reduces the conducting capacity of nerves so that the cold portion of the body becomes numb. This is made use of in some forms of local anaesthetic when the skin is temporarily 'frozen' for small surgical procedures. If the cold is extreme the fingers, toes and ears may become damaged by FROSTBITE. Raynaud's disease (pallor and purpling of the fingers and toes) and chilblains (patches of itching, bluish-red, cold skin) are precipitated in susceptible persons by cold.

A cold environment also causes increased secretion of the thyroid hormone and of adrenaline, which in turn increases heat production by combustion of carbohydrate and fat – as if the body were attempting to compensate by deliberately raising its heat. Shivering is essentially a result of this increased heat production. Body hair becomes erect with the appearance of 'goose-pimples' in an attempt to trap still air in the spaces thus formed next to the skin and, as air is a poor conductor of heat, this prevents heat-loss from the body.

If severe cold continues, the body's balancing attempts ultimately cease, the whole body begins to cool (hypothermia), the person usually falls asleep, and he is likely to die when his temperature falls below 20 °C. (68 °F.).

Inability to withstand cold, and thus the risk of HYPOTHERMIA, is particularly marked – and particularly dangerous – in babies and old people. Heat is produced by the body in proportion to its weight, but lost in proportion to its surface area: a man who weighs 68 kg. (11 stones) is roughly eight times as heavy as a baby weighing 9 kg. (20 lb.) but only has approximately four times as much body surface area. The baby is thus much more susceptible to cold than the man. In old age ability to generate body heat is reduced so that the elderly are less able to withstand cold. Sensible use of CLOTHING and DIET are important.

cold feet. A source of considerable discomfort, cold feet are also a frequent cause of chilblains. The essential underlying cause is poor circulation either of blood or of lymph. This poor circulation is less often due to cardiovascular disease than to the impeding of the circulation by tight belts at the waist, tight garters on the legs or constricting shoes. Treatment consists principally in removing the cause, but additionally vigorous exercise and a diet containing adequacy of calcium and vitamin D are thought to help.

cold sores. See HERPES.

colic. Irregular, painful and spasmodic contractions of the muscular tissue in hollow organs, most commonly in the intestine. Intestinal colic is usually due either to inflammation from an irritant or to pressure from indigestible material in the bowel, but is occasionally caused by poisoning of the nerves (as in lead poisoning) and is sometimes a symptom of other conditions such as appendicitis and intussusception. The degree of pain varies from slight spasms of little more than discomfort to almost intolerable paroxysms.

Treatment varies with the cause. In cases due to an irritant a fairly mild laxative may suffice to remove it, and meantime hot fomentations may help to reduce the pain. Repeated attacks of colic call for medical advice.

Colic may also arise in the gall bladder, the stomach and the kidneys.

colitis. Inflammation of the colon, characterized by uneasy feelings in the lower abdomen accompanied by occasional sharp pains. Colitis may be acute – a result of bacterial or other food poisoning – in which case acute diarrhoea is a symptom; or it may be chronic, associated with chronic constipation or over-use of laxatives.

Prevention of acute colitis is mainly a matter of good hygiene on the part of all persons handling food.. The treatment is obvious – temporary cessation of solid food, supply of ample fluids to prevent dehydration, a laxative to remove the irritant and in severe cases of bacterial origin an appropriate antibiotic which is not easily absorbed from the intestine.

Since the chronic variety of colitis often occurs in nervous, over-anxious, obsessional persons, psychological treatment is necessary in many cases. Additional possibilities in treatment include antispasmodic drugs such as hyoscyamus and bromides, colonic lavage with alkaline fluids, and mild laxatives.

colitis, ulcerative. A severe persistent inflammation of the intestine, occurring mostly in women aged 25 to 40 years, and thought to be due primarily to bacterial infection although the bacteria appear to invade mucous membranes already damaged by some unknown process. There may be an allergic factor involved, and many experts believe that an emotional factor plays a part in the cause, although it is equally true that the symptoms can cause emotional upset.

Symptoms – lasting over many months – include irregular bouts of high temperature, and long continued diarrhoea and painful motions, with blood, pus and mucus in the stools. If the condition is untreated the diarrhoea leads to dehydration and emaciation and the continued small loss of blood leads to anaemia.

Treatment is difficult but includes a period of rest in bed with warmth, an easily digested diet with little indigestible residue, colonic lavage, antibiotics to combat infection and in some cases corticosteroids. Occasionally surgical treatment is needed.

collagen diseases. Collagen is a protein and is the main constituent of the connective tissue found in ligaments, tendons and capsules of joints. The molecules of the protein are structurally like three-stranded ropes.

Disorganization of the collagen fibres is in some cases a hereditary condition, in others a sequel to inflammation and in yet others perhaps simply a result of ageing; and the diseases caused by the disorganization are numerous and vary with the age of the patient and with the parts of the body affected. Marfan's syndrome, characterized by excessive growth of the length of fingers and toes and to a lesser extent of the length of arms and legs, is an example of a collagen disease inherited as a Mendelian dominant (see GENETICS), and so is gargoylism, in which the patient has an abnormally large head and a saddle-shaped nose. Lupus erythematous, manifested by raised temperature, skin eruptions and joint changes resembling those of arthritis, is a collagen disease of inflammatory origin. Some forms of rheumatism are thought to be associated with degeneration of the collagen fibres.

In general CORTICOSTEROIDS suppress symptoms in the collagen diseases but do not cure the underlying conditions.

collapse. This term and the term SHOCK are both applied to a state of exhaustion and prostration which results from acute circulatory failure with great reduction in the amount of circulating blood. After sudden injury or extensive burns or scalds the condition is called shock; when it appears in the course of an exhausting illness it is called collapse.

collar-bone. A long, doubly curved bone otherwise known as the clavicle that forms part of the shoulder girdle. It is affected by two particular types of injury resulting from a fall on the shoulder – dislocation at its joint with the sternum in adults, and fracture in children or adolescents. Fracture may also be caused by a fall on the outstretched hand. Treatment of dislocation is rarely required but treatment of fracture requires the application of a figure-of-eight bandage for about a month.

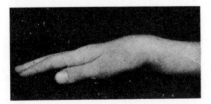

Colles' fracture

Colles' fracture. As originally described by Abraham Colles in 1814 a Colles' fracture was of the lower end of the radius bone about 1½ inches above the wrist. The term is now usually applied to the very much commoner fracture – generally due to a fall on the outstretched hand – of the radius about half an inch above the wrist joint. The fracture is usually transverse, and the small fragment of the radius that is

broken off is displaced backwards, rotated and tilted.

If no doctor is at hand padded splints should be applied to the inside and outside of the wrist and an arm-sling used to support the forearm. Early manipulation is, however, important to place the broken fragments in a position in which they can heal without deformity. Thereafter the wrist is normally placed in plaster for a few weeks.

colloid. A substance of an even gluey consistency and made up of very large molecules.

colon. The large bowel – that part of the DIGESTIVE SYSTEM into which the small bowel opens and in which the waste products of the bowel become transformed from a fluid into a solid or semi-solid stool by the absorption of water. It is a large tube which starts in the lower right hand side of the abdomen, passes up under the rib cage on the right (the ascending colon), crosses from right to left in the upper part of the abdomen (the transverse colon), travels down on the left hand side of the abdomen (the descending colon) into the pelvis where it becomes the pelvic colon and ends by becoming continuous with the rectum.

colostomy. The operation of making an artificial opening into the intestine to permit evacuation of faeces. This operation is usually performed when an obstruction in the large bowel prevents the normal passage of waste products through the anus. It may be a temporary measure in an acute obstruction but in some patients has to be permanent. In the latter event there is a wide range of appliances – belts, bags etc. – which minimize the inconvenience of what is essentially an abdominal anus.

Persons with a colostomy can lead a normal life but require moral support while learning to cope with what is, for them, an entirely new method of waste disposal. Such support can be obtained from others who have had and adapted to the operation and also from voluntary organizations.

colostrom. The first milk produced by the mother after the birth of her child. It differs from all subsequent milk in that it has a higher protein content and less sugar. In some animals, probably including humans, it appears to be of major importance in that the mother transfers antibodies to her offspring in this 'milk', in effect providing temporary immunization to diseases to which the mother has acquired a resistance.

colour blindness. A visual defect in which the sufferer cannot distinguish between different colours or perceives them differently from the normal person. About 8 per cent of the male population and 0.4 per cent of women have some defect of colour vision. The rarest type is the person totally unable to distinguish colour, but most colour blind persons can differentiate some shades.

Red-green colour blindness is the commonest type. In this condition sufferers have very little colour discrimination at the red end of the spectrum and thus are unable to distinguish between red, green and brown. More rare is the 'blue blind' person who cannot distinguish blue from green but has normal discrimination at the end of the spectrum. In contrast with the other forms, blue blindness is as common in women as in men, but other forms may be recessive sex-linked characteristics (see GENETICS) carried on the x chromosome and consequently are more likely to be found in men; a woman only suffers if she had a carrier mother and an affected father.

colour vision. There are many theories of colour vision which can shed light on the nature of colour blindness. Specific cells in the retina of the EYE (the cones) appear to contain pigments sensitive to colour. There are three types of these, those sensitive to red, those to green, and those to blue. Red-green colour blindness is due to lack of the red or green sensitive pigments while lack of the blue gives rise to blue-green blindness. Persons who perceive colours differently from normal individuals are thought to have abnormal amounts of pigment in the colour sensitive cones.

coma. A state of deep unconsciousness in which the individual is unresponsive to any form of stimulus. It can arise as a result of illness, severe intoxication by drugs or drink, or serious head injury. It frequently occurs just prior to death in patients who have been ill for a long time.

comedo. A BLACKHEAD.

communication. The transfer of meaningful information. It should be noted that communication is not necessarily verbal: without the patient having uttered a word the doctor sees from the facial expression that the patient disagrees with a particular suggestion; the health visitor interprets the client's look as indicating a lack of comprehension; and the lecturer while still speaking realizes that he has roused the enthusiasm of most of his class but has merely bored two members.

Communication is nearly always two-way: the commonest error made by beginners in the personal health services is to assume that they can spend most of their time informing the client or patient, whereas with experienced workers the patient or client may well do considerably more than half of the talking. In the case of teacher and student the latter may already be enthusiastic, and prepared to listen to an orderly succession of dogmatic statements because he wants to pass his examinations, but in most of the situations involving health workers or social workers the client needs ample opportunity to express his doubts, hesitations, disagreement or misunderstanding: the most lasting effect is usually achieved not when the expert tells the client what to do but when expert and client, by discussing together, enable the client himself to evolve an appropriate course of action.

Three common causes of failure of communication are as follows.

1. Use of technical terms or terms with a more precise meaning in the health professions than in ordinary speech. The patient may fear that to ask the meaning of a word that he feels he ought to know would display excessive ignorance on his part, or he may simply guess the meaning and perhaps guess it wrongly, or he may not realize until later that the meaning escaped him. Also while concentrating on an unfamiliar term he may lose the thread of what is being said next.

2. Continuation by the expert without pauses for query, argument or request for elaboration. The professional worker who speaks continuously for twenty minutes, otherwise

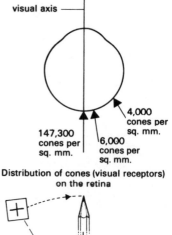

Distribution of cones (visual receptors) on the retina

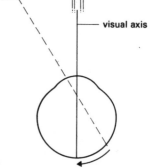

An in eresting experiment: on several pieces of white paper the size of postage stamps, draw a cross, each in a different colour; while looking fixedly at a pencil about 30 cm. (1 ft.) from the face, move the papers in turn towards the pencil from the side. It will be noted that the colour of the cross cannot be distinguished until the paper is close to the pencil, i.e., until the point on the retina which is stimulated has a high density of cones.

Colour vision

than to a group of persons who are already highly motivated, is not really communicating but merely displaying his erudition.

3. Attempting to convey too many separate ideas. Most of us, when we are confronted with a subject of which we have no appreciable previous knowledge, find it difficult to grasp many new ideas in rapid succession.

In the U.K. HEALTH EDUCATION of individuals and families has achieved very considerable success (e.g., in reducing infectious diseases both by guidance on personal hygiene and by persuasion about immunization, and in improving the management of young children) largely because of successful communication between health visitor and client.

Until recent years, however, the health education of sizeable groups was relatively unsuccessful, largely because of past failure to appreciate that skill in communication – including the extracting no less than the imparting of information – is just as important for the educator as is special knowledge of the particular subject. Similarly the criticism has been levelled at British hospitals that, while they provide efficient treatment during the patient's period of residence, they often discharge him with scanty and inaccurate insight into the nature and extent of his disease and little idea of how best to rearrange his life to lessen the likelihood of it recurring or being aggravated.

communications in health services. the transmission of information related to health from one individual or organization to others within the context of organized health services.

Because of the organizational complexity and the comprehensively providing nature of any national health service, communication within it never stops. There are many headings under which aspects could be considered. Convenient groupings for the purposes of this article are: communication between the patient and the service, communication concerned with the continuous provision of the services, and communication aiming at the changing of behaviour.

1. Communication between the patient and the service. The network of communication processes surrounding the act of patient care is learned informally both by the student doctor and nurse (and by those workers after qualification) and by the patient seeking their aid. Whom to ask to perform various services, what and how to fill in forms to have various treatments and investigations carried out, how to question and answer the patient, doctor, or nurse are all learned 'on the job' rather than by formal teaching of students.

While it is easy to identify what form to send to the x-ray department to have a particular film taken, the process of communication between doctor and patient, of ensuring that the patient understands what is being said to him and, equally important, that the doctor understands what the patient is saying to him, is only learned by observation. Most doctors start with the disadvantage that they belong to different social groups from their patient: 80 per cent of doctors in Britain for example come from fairly affluent and educated families, but these families constitute only about 20 per cent of the population. Consequently the social language of doctors (and in part of nurses) is different from that of many patients, and in addition many medical terms are incomprehensible to the average layman. Therefore, with the best will in the world, the doctor is a disadvantaged communicator with his patient.

A further problem arises in that professions tend to be secretive about their own private body of knowledge, but wilful denial of information to the patient is much less likely to occur than mutual misunderstanding, except in situations in which the information is likely to be unpleasant for the doctor or the recipient.

It is to be hoped that the inclusion of sociology into the medical and nursing curricula will enlighten members of the health professions to the fact that communication is a real and difficult problem and that the increasing of their contact with people in less artificial environments than the hospital will help comprehension. Already it is notable that professionals in contact with patients or clients in their own homes (e.g., health visitors in the U.K.) communicate more easily and more successfully than do their hospital colleagues.

2. Communication concerned with the continuous provision of services. Much of the communication related to patient care occurs on an informal and predominantly verbal level.

Some events demand immediate action and usually there are well established channels and end points of communication that allow an adequate professional and community response. Certainly most regions have well defined contingency plans for a major disaster, specifying who should be notified and when, so that appropriate persons and resources will be available when required. Less dramatic emergencies are constantly occurring which require a co-ordinated response from persons in various professions, e.g., the notification of infectious disease or the occurrence of a serious road accident. Local exigencies usually dictate the patterns of communication in such emergencies but they are always clearly defined and usually one individual (such as, in Britain, the medical officer of health of yesterday or the community medicine specialist of today) organizes the informing of all parties likely to be immediately involved.

However, the bulk of communicating between different branches of the health and allied services is done on paper, either from the outset or as a back up to a conversation. Such communications have the advantage of acting as a record as well as providing information for immediate use. Records are the tools by which the health of the community is monitored and the efficacy of health care is measured.

Channels of communication exist so that the administrators (medical, nursing or lay) with responsibility for the health of the community can determine what is happening and also enlighten the community they serve. Various returns are made to these officers from diverse sources, such as notifications of births and deaths from hospitals and general practitioners, of infectious disease from laboratory services and doctors, of children seen at schools, of babies and mothers at clinics, and of immunizations given; from such communications they build up a composite picture of the health of the community. In the light of this picture they inform the public when urgent action is needed, and submit special and annual reports to the employing authority.

Central government in many countries also demands information on the running of services at a local level and various returns are statutorily required from all portions of the health service. Such returns can relate specifically to a patient or an episode, e.g., the school record for each child or summaries of the activity of a hospital over a period of months.

3. Communications directed towards the changing of behaviour. This is a ponderous way of saying health education, and health education is a two-way process. It is a responsibility of any health service to try to persuade the community to live as healthy a life as is possible while the community also has the responsibility of ensuring that the professionals in the health service are

constantly informed as to the priorities and views of the community or its representatives.

There are many ways in which ideas for improving health can be communicated to the public. Depending upon the message to be conveyed the technique will differ. Information should normally be conveyed in a non-threatening environment, on a personal basis, when the individual is at ease and receptive, e.g., information on child feeding and management is best provided in the patient's home both before and after the child is born, and this health educational function is a well recognized part of the work of the British health visitor. She has always to bear in mind that to give factual information is the smaller part of her task; her difficult job is to alter behaviour and established habits and attitudes.

For topics such as sex education or contraceptive advice small groups may be more effective in that various attitudes and ideas emerge and possible problems and solutions can be discussed by the participants. Although small groups afford the best means of communicating ideas, because misapprehensions are readily perceived and clarified and the content of the message adapted to the level of understanding of the recipient, the mass media provide a useful reinforcing stimulus to ideas implanted by personal contact. However, they are inefficient means of primary communication of more than the most basic information because they afford the recipient no means of asking questions and are pitched at the average rather than the individual. On the other hand they are allegedly more economical of staff than individual or small group teaching in that the message, however ineffectively, is transmitted to a large number of people.

The converse process to professionals educating the community is communication of ideas and expectations by the community to doctors and nurses. We have already considered the inbuilt difficulties that put barriers to communication between doctor and patient. There is also no explicit definition of what the community wants of the doctor other than by the statements of novelists such as Alexander Solzenhitsyn in his book *Cancer Ward*, and the occasional pronouncements of investigating sociologists. Social definitions of expectation occur by default in that procedures are set up to investigate complaints and the sorts of medical behaviour that society will not tolerate are thus defined. Hippocrates and history have provided the health profession with a code of ethics, but on the whole it is still doctors who decide what the public expect of doctors, and the same gap in communication exists at an organizational level as can occur at an inter-personal level. An encouraging though comparatively modern phenomenon is the development of organized bodies of patients in societies such as the Multiple Sclerosis Society and the British Diabetic Association in the U.K. This trend allied with the increasing awareness of the rights of the consumer may eventually lead to better communication at an organizational level between society and the health professions. See also HEALTH EDUCATION and HEALTH VISITOR.

community health services. Since 'community' may imply anything from a tiny hamlet to a vast city and since 'health' is sometimes used in the sense of maintaining or promoting good health and is at other times employed as an omnibus term to cover both health and disease, the superficially simple term 'community health services' has several different meanings, three of which are indicated below. Moreover, whether the term is used for local services that safeguard health, for local preventive and curative services outside hospital, or for all the health and disease services in a particular district, exact demarcation from education services, social services and general environmental services is very difficult.

It is, for instance, arguable whether the portion of health education involving school children is (like other portions of health education) primarily a health service or primarily an education service, or whether child guidance clinics should be administered by health authorities or by education authorities. Home help services, day and residential nurseries, hostels for old people and centres for the mentally or physically handicapped can all be regarded as serving purposes connected with health and disease or connected mainly with social welfare. Some aspects of housing pertain largely to health, and the eradication of bovine tuberculosis and brucellosis is of profound importance for human health, but not every facet of housing or every aspect of animal well-being can be deemed a health service.

In different countries the exact borderlines of health, education, social and general environmental services vary, and the boundaries tend to be determined rather by tradition and administrative convenience than by any logical decision. To take one example at random, in the U.K. fully nine-tenths of applications for the aid of home helps emanate from health visitors, home nurses and general medical practitioners (i.e., from health workers) and increase or decrease in the amount of help needed depends largely on changes in health, but the home help service is administered by social work departments.

1. Where 'health' is interpreted in its positive sense, i.e., as good health in contrast with both absence of health and actual disease, community health services are the services provided within and by a community for the purpose of safeguarding and promoting health. These often include health education (of individuals and groups and also by use of mass media), antenatal care (though decisions about financial allowances and welfare foods are generally taken at national or state level), maternity services (in the home or in hospital), health visiting of mothers and children (and sometimes of other groups), infant and pre-school health services (such as child health clinics), immunization and vaccination, school health services, family planning services, 'well women clinics' and cervical cytology, control of infectious diseases, port health services, environmental health services and in some countries services to maintain the health of the elderly (e.g., pre-retirement courses, advice by dieticians, counselling by health visitors and other health workers, chiropody services, etc). Apart from the need for arbitrary boundaries dividing community health services from education, social and environmental services, demarcation problems arise in the case of

services that are designed partially for prevention and partially for treatment, e.g., the work of orthoptists and physiotherapists.

2. Quite often 'community health' is understood as including both the promoting and safeguarding of good health, and the treating and supporting in their own homes of people in bad health. In such circumstances the term 'community health services' comes to include, in addition to the preventive services mentioned above, such items as home nursing services, ambulance services and in some countries the services of non-hospital medical and dental practitioners. Apart from the need for differentiation from educational, social and environmental services, this interpretation of community health services looks simple, covering all medical, nursing and allied services (preventive or curative) outside hospital. There are difficulties however. For instance, in some eastern European countries doctors and nurses working in the community tend to be replaced by hospital-based or clinic-based doctors and nurses who come into the community for part of their time; in some states of the U.S.A. the general medical practitioner has almost disappeared, and in the U.K. many general practitioners are primarily oriented to cure and care, lacking both skill and interest in health education and preventive techniques, and in some cases spend part of their time working in hospital. Again, because maternity hospitals, hospitals for infectious diseases and tuberculosis sanatoria have obvious community functions, they are sometimes split off from other hospital services and deemed part of the (non-hospital) community health services.

3. In some countries an attempt has been made to integrate all the hospital and non-hospital health and disease services, so that the term 'community health services' means all the services falling under the jurisdiction of the health authority for a particular district, often with a sizeable general hospital as its focal point. Here, apart from the needs for lines of demarcation from educational, social and environmental services, the meaning is clear but in practice the term is often meaningless. A community health service employing for a single community several thousands of persons from many different health professions (and complicated by persons from any one profession having different and non-interchangeable skills) has to be divided into sections for efficient administration. The differences between the persuasive skills and sociological knowledge of preventive workers and the clinical skills and therapeutic knowledge of doctors and nurses working in the field of cure or care make the functional division obvious. So we tend to find, for example, within the integrated service for a community a principal nursing officer (community) and a principal nursing officer (hospital). Moreover, this administrative reversal of integration is probably necessary: on a long-term basis prevention is generally cheaper as well as pleasanter than cure, and to employ one extra preventive worker (whether health education officer, health visitor or preventive-minded doctor) today may well save the need for a dozen extra treatment workers in ten years time. But hospital services employ vastly more medical, nursing and other staff than do non-hospital services, consume far more money, and have a glamour and an immediate urgency. So, in the absence of this administrative reversal of integration, the preventive and health-promoting parts of the service could easily be eclipsed and swamped by the larger component.

Irrespective of which definition of community health services is used and irrespective of exact dividing lines from other services, the services should clearly cover the individual from before conception (e.g., family planning services and genetic counselling) to the grave (e.g., enabling a person at the close of life to die with dignity and without undue pain). Their comprehensiveness varies greatly according to the degree of enlightenment of the local or national community in which the person lives, the extent of funds available, the amount of emphasis placed on health and disease services in comparison with other demands on the public purse (e.g., defence, education and housing), the relative amounts of stress laid on health-promotion, prevention, cure and care, and not least the numbers – in relation to population – of the various workers involved in promotion of health, prevention of disease, treatment, and support.

complex. A system of repressed and usually unconscious feelings and ideas, often derived from experiences in early childhood, giving rise to patterns of behaviour at variance with those that would be expected from the person's cultural background and social circumstances. A very simple example may be given first: an intelligent and inquisitive 3-year old enters a dark cellar, the door swings shut behind him, he cannot open it and for a time his cries are unheard; thirty years later he has completely forgotten that half hour of terror but he has a persisting and apparently irrational fear of the dark. Other examples are the man who habitually shrinks from responsibilities for which his education and experience would seem to fit him, the woman who becomes panic-stricken in a thunderstorm, the person who has an irrational hatred of members of a particular race and the person who obtains sexual pleasure in an abnormal way.

Essentially complexes are an antisocial or pathological equivalent of sentiments and dispositions. When the mind of the child is still being shaped he acquires various dispositions and sentiments (e.g., a disposition to be fair-minded and a sentiment of loyalty to his family) and is later unaware that he has acquired these through a mixture of example, precept and personal experience. Simultaneously he may acquire abnormal or pathological dispositions – complexes – which create tendencies to anxieties, phobias and other types of unacceptable behaviour.

Clearly we can to some extent prevent the development of complexes by seeking to avoid in children the type of happening that gives rise to them, by being careful to minimize (rather than accentuate) any infirmity or deficiency of a child, and by trying in the presence of children to avoid showing exaggerated reactions of anger, fear or depression; but probably very few adults have had such perfect childhoods that they have adsolutely no complexes. Indeed, some complexes probably arise simply as a result of physical defects or infirmities, e.g., very small people are often unduly aggressive.

In many cases a complex creates abnormal behaviour only during periods in which it is precipitated by unusual circumstances. In these cases we can try to avoid or minimize the particular circumstances. The person terrified of trains can avoid travelling by rail and the person afraid of responsibility can take a routine job.

Where a complex creates seriously abnormal behaviour or deep personal unhappiness elaborate psychological treatment is required. Changing the physical or social environment will not alter a sexual deviation or a persisting depression or an irrational hatred of a particular religion. To change these attitudes we have to search for the long-forgotten causes of the complex and then to attempt the difficult task of eradicating these causes.

complexion. The colour, texture and appearance of the skin, especially òf the face.

While the texture varies considerably in different persons and reacts differently to exposure to fresh air and to cleansing processes, in general fresh air, some sunlight and thorough cleanliness are necessary for the health and beauty of skin. Some people with very fair skin react to strong sunshine by rapid soreness and burning and need very gradually increased exposure so that protective pigment can be slowly formed. A few people have skins easily irritated by cold winds and have to learn to wrap up well and to avoid needless exposure to wind. A small number have skins that are irritated by soaps containing free alkali and may need special cleansing creams followed by washing with superfatted toilet soaps. Persons with abnormally dry skins – i.e., skins deficient in natural oily secretion – may also require the application of creams or other artificial lubricants. It should be emphasized, however, that these abnormalities are rare and that for the vast majority of people the care of the skin simply implies regular washing with soap (preferably a toilet soap) and hot water (preferably soft water such as rainwater) and a reasonable amount of exposure to fresh air.

Since the skin is part of the living body its appearance and texture depend not only on skin care but also on general health. Sallowness and pustular spots are often indicative of excessive intake of sweet foods and fatty foods, of insufficiency of fruit and green vegetables, and of constipation. A reddened, blotchy face with purplish nose is typical of alcoholics, though there are other conditions which cause this appearance. Pallor suggests lack of fresh air, or anaemia, or, if extreme, advanced cancer. High-coloured cheeks and mottling of the skin over the cheek bones suggests heart disease. A yellow tinge suggests jaundice but a sallow and almost yellow hue is sometimes seen in persons whose skin is returning to normal after a holiday in an area of bright sunshine. There are also a number of other conditions in which the complexion gives a clue to underlying disease.

Broadly these points apply whether the person's natural skin colour is white, brown, yellow or black, but it is clearly difficult for a person accustomed only to one natural colour to assess health from the skin of a person of different natural colour. In such a case he has to rely more on smoothness and texture than on colour.

compression of the brain. Pressure on the brain as a result of a fall, blow or other head injury, so that a depressed piece of bone or a clot of blood from a torn blood-vessel presses on the delicate brain tissue. There are sometimes no symptoms for several hours while the pressure is building up, but in due course the patient becomes deeply unconscious, with heavy breathing, full and slow pulse, and unequal pupils. In such cases operation is urgently necessary to relieve the pressure and to stop any bleeding inside the skull.

The condition has to be differentiated from CONCUSSION. In concussion there is a commotion of the brain cells, leading to a dazed state or unconciousness, but often responding to the patient being simply put to bed in a darkened room with ice-bags, if available, applied to his head. In compression the pressure on the brain goes on building up and in the absence of urgent surgical relief the patient is likely to die.

From these points it follows that a person who has sustained any severe injury to the head should, even if he is conscious and lucid immediately after the injury, be kept under observation for several hours, preferably in a hospital with facilities for brain surgery.

conception. The union of the sperm and the ovum within the body of a woman, whereby she becomes pregnant.

Although if intercourse has taken place only once in the relevant weeks the date of conception is generally presumed to be that of the intercourse, there can actually be a period of several days between the two events. After intercourse the spermatozoon propels itself upwards at a speed of 2 to 3mm. per minute. If the ovum is already in the uterus the sperm may push its way into the ovum within an hour or two of the sexual act. On the other hand, if the ovum has not yet reached the uterus – and the process of ovulation occurs only once a month starting thirteen to fifteen days after the end of menstruation – the sperm can remain alive for several days and can still fertilize the ovum.

The ovum during its journey to the uterus has divided, losing half of its chromosomes. So at the moment of conception the sperm has twenty-three somatic chromosomes and either a single male or a single female sex chromosome, and the ovum has twenty-three somatic chromosomes and one female sex chromosome. So there is no possibility of continuing life of the ovum or sperm alone.

The sperm is about one-twentieth of a millimetre long and the ovum is a sphere of about one-fifth of a millimetre in diameter. It is a matter of philosophical rather than medical argument whether life can be considered to begin when the head of the sperm enters the ovum, producing a single cell with the forty-eight chromosomes of the human species; or two months later when the embryo is about 25 mm. long, the head is assuming a human shape and the tail of the embryo is beginning to disappear; or after five months when the foetus is abòut 200 mm. long and might possibly survive if separated from the mother.

The duration of PREGNANCY, normally given as 273 days, is subject to some variation: at the one extreme a fully developed child has been born as early as the 240th day and at the other extreme a child apparently not post-mature has been born as late as the 313th day. However, although a day or two of that variation is explicable by differences in the time of conception, the bulk of the variation probably depends on individual factors. For instance there is some evidence that in a fatty uterus development of the foetus tends to be a little slower than in a normal uterus.

concussion. A shaking of the brain cells, e.g., as a result of a blow or a fall. In slight concussion there may be a dazed feeling or a short period of unconsciousness, the victim may have no recollection of the injury and he may act automatically for some hours afterwards. In severe concussion there may be deep and prolonged unconsciousness.

Rest, quiet and, if available, application of icebags to the head may be all that is needed; but the person should be kept under observation for several hours because of the possibility that he is also suffering from COMPRESSION OF THE BRAIN, a condition which requires urgent surgical treatment.

condom. See SHEATH.

condylomata. Rounded, fleshy-like swellings of mucous membrane, occurring in the secondary stage of SYPHILIS, and most often found round the anus, between the buttocks and in other warm and moist parts of the body. The surface of a condyloma often breaks down so that serum leaks out, and the condyloma then becomes the most infectious of all syphilitic lesions.

As the syphilis is treated the condylomata usually slowly disappear, but in a few cases they require removal by application of caustics or by cutting.

confinement. The period during which a woman is in bed through giving birth to a child. The term is often used as synonymous with labour but strictly should include not only the period of the actual labour but also the days of restoration of strength after the birth of the child.

Calculation of the probable date of the start of confinement is best done by reckoning from the first day of the last menstrual period, a date which the patient may remember. Allowing 5 days for menstruation, a further 2 days as an average time before coitus occurs and 273 days for the normal development of the unborn child, we can estimate that labour will probably start about 280 days after the beginning of the last menstrual period; but this is only an approximate date and is liable to considerable alteration. Labour may occur several days earlier than expected, or up to three weeks later, the explanation of the second feature being that conception occurred not soon after the last period but shortly before the first period missed. As pregnancy progresses rough checks may be attempted by measuring the height of the top of the uterus or by trying to count from the date of quickening, but in general these do not give more accurate results than simply calculating from the last period.

Health education, improved antenatal care, anaesthesia and improved obstetrics have during the present century enormously reduced the dangers and the discomforts of confinement. It is fair to say that in a developed country, provided various factors apply, confinement can be anticipated as a normal and not particularly unpleasant happening. These factors are (1) that genetic counselling, if required, has reduced the likelihood of inherited abnormalities, (2) that guidance about family planning has made pregnancy in women over 40 years a rarity and (3) has eliminated the formerly common finding of a woman exhausted by a series of pregnancies only about a year apart, (4) that antenatal care has been adequate and has devoted due attention to both emotional and physical health, (5) that medical and obstetrical supervision have been satisfactory during the pregnancy, and (6) that arrangements are available for coping immediately with any complication arising during or just after labour. Where these factors all apply the mother's chance of speedy restoration to normal health and fitness is considerably better than 999 out of 1,000, and the chance of a living and healthy baby is more than 99 out of 100. By contrast we can recall the statement of Medea in Euripides' play 2,400 years ago – a statement that would still have been valid in the U.K. and U.S.A. a century ago: 'I would rather stand in the battle line thrice than once bear a child'.

Perhaps indeed, when all credit is given to immunization against various infections and to education thereon, to the reduction of various nutritional diseases in the developed countries and to the virtual eradication of many so-called 'dirt' diseases, the greatest achievement of the health-educative and disease-preventive services has been to change confinement from a traumatic experience with considerable risk to the mother and high risk to the child to a normal and unhazardous event of life.

conflict. In normal speech the term means any fight, struggle or clash of opposed principles. In psychology and medicine it refers specifically to the distressing internal situation where a person's strong desires are in opposition either to the codes of the society in which he lives or to deep-rooted parts of his own personality.

The first of these is easily understood. For instance, in time of war a man who has either an intense disbelief in the violent taking of life or a strong instinct of self-preservation finds himself in conflict with the general wave of patriotic and military enthusiasm, and usually resolves the conflict in one of three ways – by resisting the opinions of his associates (and becoming a conscientious objector), by submitting to them (and reluctantly joining the army) or by escaping (retaining his pacifist views without publicly expressing them and contriving to find a job which will exempt him from military service). Another example might be where a woman whose religion forbids divorce strongly wishes to marry a divorced man; she usually either resists the dictates of her religion or sadly abandons the idea of the marriage. These external conflicts occasionally remain unresolved and can lead to illness, but in the vast majority of cases one or other of the opposing forces gains the victory, so that the conflict ends, the person becoming either a conformist or a rebel.

Rather less easy to understand is the purely internal conflict. To take an example, when Shakespeare's Lady Macbeth plots to murder Duncan she is unconcerned with the views of her associates (so long as they remain ignorant of her action) but, when she tells Macbeth that she would have slain the sleeping Duncan but for the fact that he looked like her own father, she is exhibiting an internal conflict, the conflict that ultimately drives her mad. Part of her personality – ambition, power-drive – wants to kill Duncan and part revolts against the deed.

Few if any people go through life without conflicts. Many a highly sexed man of high moral principles has at some point in time felt a strong desire to make love to a woman other than his wife; many a normally honest but impecunious person has been under deep temptation after finding a note-filled wallet in the street. However, in most cases the conflict ends fairly quickly with the submission of one side or the other. The person either bows to the codes of his associates or the laws of the community or the sentiments and moral views that he has developed from childhood, conforming perhaps with some regret, or else he resists these and follows the dictates of the strong emotion, rebelling perhaps with some remorse. In submission he may ease his frustration by a transfer mechanism: for example, the man whose strong power-drive has urged him to seize an opportunity to damage his immediate superior may, after resisting that impulse as contrary to his whole ethical code, ease his frustrated power-drive by bullying his subordinates or his children.

Where neither side submits he may use an escape mechanism. He may succeed in repressing from his conscious mind the forbidden desire, though it may sometimes emerge in distorted forms in dreams. Alternatively he may seek to escape the conflict – by physically removing himself from the circumstances (as with the person who suddenly throws away a good job and leaves the district), by hysteria or psychosomatic illness, by day-dreaming and fantasy, by over-indulgence in alcohol, or more usefully by transfer of his energies to an absorbing hobby. Clearly the use of an escape mechanism can be either helpful or harmful, and in relation to the conflict itself it can be successful or unsuccessful.

The most dangerous situation, however, is where there is neither submission of one side or the other nor any successful escape mechanism but continuation of the unresolved conflict, for instance the women with aged and dependent parents and a fiancé who has accepted a promotion post a hundred miles away, who neither accepts nor rejects marriage and change of residence but remains undecided, worried and miserable; or the teacher who decides that he has become dull, uninspiring and disliked by his pupils but who neither makes up his mind to try to change his job or his methods nor faces the fact that not all teachers are brilliant and that he must be content to be a rather poor member of his profession; instead he just broods constantly, with increasing feelings of guilt and unworthiness. Such continuation of conflict is the commonest cause of anxiety neurosis and indeed of other forms of psychoneurosis.

Where a stable personality has been formed in childhood – by influences such as physical and emotional security, demonstrated affection, consistency, adequate opportunity to explore and investigate, opportunities to take decisions, kindly and not excessive discipline, suitable playthings and playmates, and plenty of praise and encouragement – the conflicts that arise later are likely to be satisfactorily resolved, whether by submission of one side or by successful use of an escape mechanism.

If a conflict remains unresolved, discussion either with a trusted friend or with a professional worker of known integrity (e.g., a health visitor or a social worker) sometimes helps, both by bringing the issues clearly into the victim's consciousness and because the dispassionate listener may be able to indicate additional aspects sufficient to tilt the victim's mind towards resolution of the conflict in one direction. Unfortunately, however, in many cases of unresolved conflict the roots lie deep, so that extensive psychological or psychiatric treatment is needed.

confusional psychosis. Clouding of consciousness with disorder of memory and of sense of time and place, difficulty in recognizing people and places and (frequently) hallucinations, all in consequence of poisoned or exhausted brain cells. The term is sometimes reserved for the milder forms of DELIRIUM but essentially the conditions are the same.

congenital. A term applied to disease and deformities existing from birth. In general the word covers three kinds of disorder of differing origin: (1) the enormous number of hereditary (i.e., inherited) conditions, e.g., spina bifida, phenylketonuria and deaf mutism; (2) conditions acquired during the mother's pregnancy, e.g., the various defects that are associated with the mother suffering from German measles (rubella) during the early months of pregnancy; and (3) conditions acquired during the actual passage of the child through the birth canal, e.g., ophthalmia neonatorum acquired from a mother suffering from gonorrhoea.

Deformities acquired as a result of faulty obstetrical procedures or faulty care immediately after birth, e.g., blindness as a result of excessive administration of oxygen or head injuries through badly applied forceps, are not usually classed as congenital.

conjunctivitis. Inflammation of the conjunctiva, i.e., the membrane which covers the front of the eye. The conjunctiva, although exposed to many sources of irritation and inflammation, is well protected, first by the mobile action of the eyelids which close very rapidly in hostile environments such as a cloud of dust, and second by the secretion of tears, by which foreign matter is quickly removed from the front of the eye to the tear duct. Nevertheless, conjunctivitis is not infrequent, especially in the young and especially during the dry sunny months.

The causes are numerous, perhaps the commonest being measles, in which conjunctivitis is really part of the disease. There are also several varieties of the condition.

In the most usual form of conjunctivitis, sometimes called the catarrhal type, the symptoms include smarting of the eye, a sensation of sand or grit beneath the eyelid, reddening of the eyeball and excessive watering or flow of tears. Where the pain is appreciable or where the condition does not clear up without treatment in a couple of days medical advice should be sought.

constipation. Failure to pass solid waste matter known as stools or faeces. There are many causes but basically they can be grouped into causes resulting from dietary deficiencies, from mechanical obstruction to the passage of food along the bowel, or from faulty bowel habits.

The waste is the indigestible part of food and if the diet is high in foodstuffs which can be absorbed and low in vegetable fibre (such as is found in fruits, bran and vegetables), which cannot, there may be insufficient bulk of waste in the bowel to form more than the occcasional stool. Starvation also causes constipation for obvious reasons.

Mechanical obstruction can occur because of narrowing of the bowel tube, by inflammation, tumour or external compression from fibrous bands. It can also occur from the accumulation of hard lumps of waste (faecoliths) in the bowel itself. Apart from the last cause, such mechanical obstruction usually requires an operation to remedy it.

Faulty bowel habits are the main cause of constipation in Western society. A mythology has persisted about the desirability of evacuation of excrement with monotonous, preferably daily, regularity. However, metabolisms and diets differ and one man's constipation may be another's regularity. Preoccupation with a daily performance causes some people to resort to laxatives, an artificial means of producing a stool. The most harmless of these increase the bulk of the stool, for instance, bran or mineral salts are not absorbed by the bowel and ensure a copious stool because they require water to dissolve them. Others, such as senna and cascara, increase the physical movement of the bowel causing it to hurry along the reluctant faeces. This 'flogging' of a bowel that is functioning normally can give rise to a vicious circle because a bowel that has been stimulated unnecessarily relaxes after the stimulus disappears and, as the faeces due 'tomorrow' were passed 'yesterday', there is, naturally, a pause in bowel activity. But this produces the anxiety that led to the use of the laxative in the first place and a repeat dose may be taken until the bowel responds not to natural needs but to the periodic dose of purgative. If this dose is taken regularly the patient should be regular, perhaps unnatural, but regular.

Children. There are rare anatomical causes in new-born children but the commonest cause in infancy is insufficient food. It can occur in both breast-fed and bottle-fed infants receiving an adequate diet for different reasons. In breast-fed children, because human milk is a minimum roughage diet, it is perfectly reasonable for a child to go for a week without passing a stool. Cow's milk, the basic source of nutrition for bottle-fed children, contains more protein and calcium than human milk. These consituents are less well coped with by the infant bowel and can lead to hard stools that the child cannot pass.

In older children constipation can occur because they are too preoccupied to go to the toilet: if the stimulus of a full rectum is ignored, such neglect can become increasingly easy because the muscle of a loaded rectum becomes sluggish. If the child finds it painful to defecate (as can occur with a tear in the skin of the anus), postponement leads to chronic constipation. Such tears commonly result from the passage of hard stools. Therefore, to prevent habitual constipation, children should be encouraged to respond promptly when nature calls.

constituents of food. See FOOD.

consumption. See TUBERCULOSIS.

contact lenses. Transparent structures that are applied close to the eye to correct defective vision. Because of their close contact with the surface of the eye they can be uncomfortable to wear, but 80 per cent of users can wear them for twelve to eighteen hours without discomfort.

They can be rigid and made of a plastic called methacrylate, fitting over the entire globe of the eye or only over the transparent part (the cornea). About 90 per cent of contact lenses are of this corneal type and 1 per cent of the larger type. The rest are 'soft' contact lenses which are made of a type of plastic which can absorb a certain amount of moisture and is softer and easier to tolerate than the harder type of lens. However, they are slightly larger, more fragile, less easy to sterilize and twice as expensive as the more conventional ones.

Contact lenses have the advantage that they are almost invisible and they can be used in occupations and sports in which spectacles would be cumbersome; in addition there are certain uncommon defects of vision which cannot be corrected adequately by spectacles for which contact lenses improve the sight.

contagious diseases. A category of infectious illnesses transmitted mainly by direct physical contact with an infected person; consequently they are usually diseases of the skin (with the exception of venereal diseases). The types of infectious organism that can be spread by touch include viruses (e.g., warts), bacteria (e.g., impetigo, erysipelas), funguses (e.g., ringworm, or athletes foot) and free living animals (such as the mites that give rise to scabies and the lice producing infestations of the hair on the head and body).

Contagious disease is much less common than it used to be, because of greatly improved living standards, better personal hygiene, and more effective specific treatments. However there is a depressing recent increase in the amount of infestation by head lice because of the fashion of long hair and the emergence of a species of lice which is resistant to insecticide. Such parasites are nearly always with us and local epidemics can occur because the apparent absence of such organisms results in the lowering of the guard of the health professions and the 'rarity' of such infections may lead to misdiagnosis.

contraception. The deliberate prevention of fertilization of the egg cell. There is a variety of methods depriving the male cell (spermatozoon) of access to an ovum and they are discussed in the article BIRTH CONTROL.

contusion. See BRUISE.

convalescence. The period after an illness or operation during which the patient recovers strength. With the increasing tendency towards active rehabilitation after illness, rather than waiting passively for recovery, and the increasing recognition of the dangers of prolonged bed rest there has been a steady fall in the period of time allotted by doctors for convalescence for nearly all illnesses. Also the increased availability of effective therapies, e.g., penicillin for pneumonia, and better pre-operative and post-operative treatments, means that patients are less debilitated and so will require less time to recover.

convulsion. Violent uncontrolled movement of a muscle or group of muscles or even all the muscles in the body; it may be accompanied by loss of consciousness as in the case of major epilepsy.

Children, and particularly infants, are much more liable to convulse than adults. If they are feverish they may have a convulsion, and the onset of an acute infection may be heralded by a convulsion, but these feverish convulsions become less frequent as the child grows older and generally do not recur in adulthood. Less frequently convulsions can occur because the blood calcium is low (as in rickets) or as the result of breath-holding attacks.

When alterations in the level of consciousness occurs, the convulsions are usually caused by brain damage of some sort, either (1) physical such as after injury or (2) biochemical, as can occur when the body accumulates large amounts of toxic products of metabolism because of failure of the kidney or liver to function properly. Convulsions can also occur without loss of consciousness because of increased muscular activity, such as shivering, or increased nervous excitability, as can be seen in tetanus.

Care. The important points in looking after someone who is unconscious and convulsing are to make sure that he does not strike any sharp object or edge, does not choke, and does not bite through his tongue. The patient is best lain on side or face and a gag put between his teeth. Fingers are unsuitable for gags and a spoon covered with a handkerchief is an adequate emergency substitute.

coprophilia. An abnormal interest in and liking for filth, particularly excrement. While most children are naturally interested in their own waste products and 'school boy' humour is notoriously pre-occupied with faeces, an abnormal interest may persist into adulthood and may take the form of sexually deviant practices.

corn. A localized, thickened area of skin caused by the pressure of tight or ill-fitting shoes. It can be hard or soft but the hard ones are much commoner.

Hard corns are usually formed over the outer parts of the little or big toe on the upper surfaces of the other toes. Pressure causes hardening of the skin till eventually a horny cone is formed with its flat base on the outside and its apex pointing inwards. This apex will cause pain whenever any pressure is put upon it and if infection of the corn occurs such pain can be excruciating.

It is possible to remove corns by paring them with a knife after softening by immersion of the foot in warm water for a period. Pain can also be relieved by placing a ring of felt around the base of the corn so as to prevent pressure from being applied to its centre.

Soft corns occur between the toes and probably do not result from increased pressure. The overgrowing skin is white and sodden because of the presence of sweat and their removal is best undertaken by a chiropodist.

Corns are better avoided than treated, and the best means of prevention is to wear appropriately fitting shoes that do not rub against the toes. Unfortunately fashion does not always follow the dictates of common sense.

cornea. The curved transparent structure, through which we see, covering the iris and pupil of the EYE.

Influence of cholesterol level, cigarette smoking and high blood pressure.

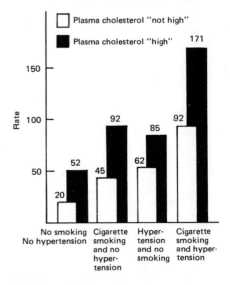

coronary thrombosis. The blocking of the arteries supplying the heart muscles (or myocardium) so that insufficient blood reaches the muscles of the heart. The condition is related to heart attack. It may occur gradually in one vessel in which case dilatation of others can maintain a satisfactory blood flow, but it usually causes ischaemic heart disease, i.e., the disability arising from reduction or arrest of blood supply to the myocardium. Coronary thrombosis is now the largest single cause of death in men in Western society. Over one-third of all male deaths between the ages of 35 and 65 years are from ischaemic heart disease, and, while it is more common in men than women under the age of 45 years, after the menopause the rate of disease in women begins to equate with that of men. It is a dangerous disease, being fatal in 10 per cent of heart attacks occurring in persons under the age of 40 years, in 30 per cent of attacks between 40 and 70 years, and in 50 per cent of attacks in persons over 70 years of age.

How it occurs. The basic degenerative process affecting the blood vessels is atherosclerosis, a hardening and internal narrowing of the arteries because of the accumulation of cholesterol (a compound derived from fat) under the internal lining of the arteries and the deposition of successive layers of other blood constituents on top of this to form a plaque. Eventually such raised plaques are to be found under the lining of all the larger blood vessels. This process of atherosclerosis is a gradual one and there is evidence that it occurs to some extent in all men and most women over the age of 20 in Western society.

Unfortunately the coronary arteries are peculiarly liable to plaque formation because they are subjected to much physical movement on account of the regular contraction of the heart. Slight physical injury to the lining may be one of the stimuli to cholesterol, and disturbances of flow through increased turbulence help the process of plaque formation. The blood flow in the coronary arteries is uniquely turbulent because it is very much reduced during the contraction of the heart muscle.

Ultimately deposition of further layers of the assortment of cellular and fatty substances results in increasing 'silting up' of the artery and reduction of its internal diameter so that insufficient blood can get through to provide adequate nutrition for the heart muscle. If this narrowing is a gradual process the sufferer will notice pain only when he taxes his heart by physical effort. Typically, on exertion such a person will feel a dull tightness over the front of his chest, perhaps spreading up into the neck and chin or down into the arms, and this pain will disappear soon after the exertion stops. This pain is called angina. Such 'early warning' pain is useful in that it allows the sufferer to know what amount of effort his heart muscle can tolerate. Drugs that dilate the coronary blood vessels will also give relief from this pain, and the most commonly used of such drugs are nitroglycerine derivatives.

Sudden narrowing can occur without warning and usually results in severe pain and distress in the sufferer, although it is not uncommon for 'silent' heart attacks to occur in which the patient feels no discomfort. With the cutting off of blood flow to a part of the heart muscle the deprived muscle dies (becomes infarcted) although a certain amount of blood supply may persist because of links (collateral anastomoses) between the smaller blood vessels supplied by different branches of the main arteries. The dead muscle tissue is replaced with fibrous tissue which cannot contract and extend; consequently the remaining heart muscle must work harder to maintain an adequate cardiac output. There is some reserve in the myocardium and, provided the amount of infarcted tissue is not too great, it is possible for the individual to recover to such an extent that his physical capabilities are as good as, or occasionally even better than, they were before the attack. However a very severe first attack may cause so much damage as to leave a heart that cannot cope without the use of drugs (such as digitalis) and leave the sufferer severely incapacitated, a cardiac cripple.

The acute attack. This can be a terrifying experience in which the sufferer feels agonizing pain or tightness across the chest and sometimes in the arms and neck. He is pale, sweating, and short of breath with a weak rapid pulse. He should be made to sit down (not lie down), be reassured as much as possible and kept warm. Spirits may be given in moderation and a doctor should be sent for immediately. Because the myocardium is damaged it may be very irritable and contract irregularly or stop altogether. If the person becomes suddenly unconscious, stops breathing and is pulseless (the weak pulse is best felt in the neck) he should immediately be laid on his back on a hard surface, with care during this process not to bang or jerk the head. The head should be turned to one side, and a sharp hard blow struck on the bottom part of the breast bone just above the hollow between the lower edges of the rib cage. If no pulse is felt after this, then cardiac massage must be started. If there is only one person present, he should try both cardiac massage and mouth-to-mouth resuscitation at about the ratio of ten beats to one breath.

Cardiac massage is accomplished by the masseur kneeling by the side of the patient with both arms fully extended placing the heel of one hand on top of the other on the lower left hand side of the breast bone and then putting his full weight on his extended arms at a rate of 70 to 100 beats per minute. This pushes down the breast bone and compresses the heart, forcing blood from it into the general circulation. If two people are present one can feel for a pulse in the root of the neck and, if this is felt, the massage is effective. If not, the hands should be moved to a position in which pressure produces a pulse. The other person should also be inflating the lungs of the patient by mouth to mouth breathing. See ARTIFICIAL RESPIRATION.

Such measures should be persisted with until the patient's pulse is felt and he begins to breathe. Should he become pulseless again, the same procedures must be resumed. If the patient fails to respond after fifteen to twenty-five minutes there is little likelihood that he will revive.

Prevention. One of the basic steps in the production of atherosclerosis is the deposition of cholesterol. Measures to diminish the level of cholesterol in the blood of the population (e.g., by reduction of animal fat eaten) may be tried, but are not easy because they demand substantial changes in dietary habits and because some people with different metabolisms can keep blood cholesterol low in spite of a high fat intake. Nevertheless, raised blood levels of cholesterol and other fatty compounds indicate a predisposition to heart disease, and these levels can be lowered by diet and certain drugs.

Diets that diminish blood cholesterol and fat levels are those which are low in animal fats and high in unsaturated vegetable oils. Their value in the prevention of heart disease in populations is still arguable though studies in institutions indicate that the frequency of ischaemic heart disease is diminished in groups on such diets. It is of course essential to ensure that a person on such a diet receives sufficient quantities of the fat-soluble vitamins.

Smoking, particularly in the younger age groups, is associated with an increased likelihood of heart disease although the causal link is unclear. Consequently abstaining from smoking should diminish the chance of a heart attack.

There is some evidence that the incidence of heart disease is higher in districts with a soft water supply than those with harder water but the nature of the link between hardness of water and freedom from thrombosis is not yet established.

High blood pressure and obesity are associated with many increased health risks. As obesity may be an indicator of indolence and consumption of atheroma-causing foodstuffs it would seem logical to recommend that weight loss be suggested to the overweight, while the control of high blood pressure certainly reduces the likelihood of strokes (which arise from diseased blood vessels in the brain) and may have a similar influence on the coronary vessels.

It seems likely that lack of exercise predisposes to coronary thrombosis, and the taking of exercise by the customarily sedentary is to be encouraged. Brief periods of taxing exercise are probably to be preferred to the sustained gentle sort such as is provided by jogging, etc., but should not be undertaken until the flabby subject has been restored to some degree of fitness.

One school of thought holds that excessive mental stress plays a big part in causing the disease; that it occurs largely in persons working overhard in an effort to secure promotion, or under constant tension through holding jobs beyond their capacities, or suffering from domestic or marital difficulties; and that features like over-smoking and over-eating are merely compensatory mechanisms. If this is the case, preventive measures should include the fostering of good emotional health and personality development in childhood (so that the person becomes able to withstand life's normal stresses) and emphasis on the importance both of healthy exercise and of leisure interests. It should also be remembered that the early years are the best time to start prevention of obesity (since fat children become fat adults) and discouragement of cigarette smoking.

To summarize, prevention can be considered under two heads. Long-term prevention, or keeping a healthy heart healthy, involves attention to the whole pattern of living. It includes, for example, measures to foster development of a personality that can cope with normal stresses, to encourage development of eating habits that neither create obesity nor raise the blood cholesterol and to dissuade the taking up of cigarette smoking (see HEALTH EDUCATION). More commonly prevention is applied to the person who already has a raised blood pressure or anginal pain on effort. Here it induces attempts to modify stress factors, cultivation of a philosophical attitude to life, reduction of obesity, limitation of animal fat in the diet, curtailing or cessation of smoking, and the giving of appropriate drugs to reduce blood pressure and to decrease the risk of clotting.

corpuscles. The term is used for the small round cells of the BLOOD (and also for the specialized nerve endings which are sensitive to pressure).

corrosive. A chemical which destroys the substance of the tissues. Medically, the term is usually applied to a group of poisons which act by burning into the tissue; they may be splashed or spilt upon the body and occasionally they are swallowed – more often by accident than intent because their effects cause intense pain. Strong acids, such as nitric, hydrochloric and sulphuric acid, alkalis, such as caustic soda or potash, and salts, such as mercury chloride or sodium hypochlorite (bleach), are the commonest corrosive substances. Caustic soda is particularly dangerous if it is splashed into the eye. It

should immediately be washed out with clean water and medical aid sought. If such substances are swallowed the person should be given liberal amounts of water immediately and egg white in milk if available. He should not be made to vomit and medical attention should be sought at once.

The late result of swallowing corrosives may be severe scarring of the throat and gullet, so much so that it can become completely obstructed. In view of the damage done to tissues both immediately and in the long term by such substances, prevention is important and eminently possible by the wearing of appropriate goggles or clothing when working with corrosive substances, by storing them only in distinctively marked containers, and above all by making sure that they are inaccessible (particularly to children) when not in use.

cortex. The outer layer or part of an organ. The term is commonly applied to the brain, the kidney and the adrenal gland. In the brain it is applied to the convoluted folds that form the outer part of the brain as distinct from the more central larger concentrations of grey matter. In the kidney the term is applied to the paler outer part of the kidney and similarly in the adrenal gland.

corticosteroids. A group of chemical substances (hormones) produced by the outer part (the cortex) of the adrenal gland. They are liberated on occasions of stress and controlled by ACTH from another of the ENDOCRINE GLANDS, the pituitary. In general, they suppress inflammatory response and reduce allergy: they also increase resistance to stress and affect the state of the mind.

Some corticosteroids such as aldosterone have an affect on the excretion of salt by the kidney and can be produced in excess in such conditions as tumours of the adrenal gland. Yet others affect the sexual characteristics and if they become unbalanced they can lead to virilization of women with the appearance of beards and deepening of the voice, while others can cause the reverse process in men with the appearance of breasts and loss of facial and body hair.

Besides being necessary as replacement therapy in Addison's disease, they are used in the treatment of some inflammatory diseases such as rheumatoid arthritis and the collagen diseases; in acute allergic states such as asthma, drug reactions and serum sensitivity; in some skin disease, leukaemia and other blood disorders, Hodgkin's disease, ulcerative colitis, and acute gout. Their effect is also of value in organ-transplantation, in that they suppress the response of the body to foreign tissue.

Cortisone. This corticosteroid was originally extracted from animal adrenal glands but was first manufactured in 1937, and since then it has been made on an increasing scale; production was simplified by the discovery that the tortoise plant (*Testudinaria sylvatica*) which grows abundantly in South Africa, contains in its bulky rhizome (elephant's foot) a substance which can be used as an advanced starting-point.

Cortisone and its derivatives are powerful drugs and prescribing them involves risks which must be taken into account when deciding on their use. Their many unwelcome side-effects include decreased resistance to infection which may reactivate old disease (e.g., tuberculosis); osteoporosis; other tissue changes which may aggravate peptic ulceration; retention of water and sodium with weight-gain and hypertension; changes in fat deposits in the body with development of 'moon-face' and 'buffalo-hump'; mental changes; and sex-hormone effects such as the appearance of facial hair in women, acne, loss of sexual desire and cessation of menstruation. They also weaken natural adrenal gland activity so that treatment once established can only safely be withdrawn very gradually.

In carefully-selected conditions, corticosteroids are undoubtedly of great benefit in a variety of distressing and disabling states but prolonged treatment requires that the balance of advantage and disadvantage should be well-considered and that patients should be made aware of potential risks. They should also carry Steroid Warning Cards to guard against the risks of sudden withdrawal of treatment in any accidental circumstances.

corticotrophin. See ACTH.

cortisone. See CORTICOSTEROIDS.

coryza. The common COLD.

cosmetics. Substances prepared to improve the appearance of the user by their effects on the health and beauty of the complexion, eyes and hair. Although they were probably used in prehistoric times in China, the earliest recorded use of such substances was in Egypt about 3000 B.C. where crude (and toxic) paints were employed to enhance the beauty of the eyes and give the skin of the face a smooth texture and colour. Scented oils and ointments were also used to improve the appearance and texture of the skin. While attractiveness is a matter of century and culture, spotty, dry, rough skins have never been in favour and the present cosmetic industry follows the same aims as the Ancient Egyptians by producing materials to obtain, or give the illusion of, soft smooth skin of whatever shade is in fashion, eyes that are lustrous and sparkling, and glossy well-groomed hair.

The skin can be cleaned and preserved so that it either retains the healthy suppleness of youth, or is disguised; and various creams, emulsions and lotions will achieve these desirable ends.

Soap is an effective cleanser but tends to remove the natural oils and so dry the skin. Consequently special toilet soaps are produced that contain oils to replace those removed by the detergent in soap. Alternatively there are cleansing creams that remove grime without drying the skin and help to keep it soft. They are mostly based upon a mixture of soft paraffin (vaseline), mineral oils and perfumed slightly astringent solutions such as rose water. Other creams clean and leave a residual film of a protective oily compound (vanishing creams) that will minimize the drying of the skin. 'Nutrient' creams contain lanolin in addition and serve to lubricate the skin, giving the appearance of smoothness. They do not feed the skin; they only oil it.

Foundation creams can camouflage obvious defects in the skin and also provide a smooth surface on which powders may be applied to ensure the appearance of an attractive complexion. Powders also produce a matt surface which may be desirable and can be obtained in a variety of shades according to the dictates of fashion and the preference of the user.

Pigment-containing creams or soft waxes are also applied, more or less as paints, especially on the lips and round the eyes. They have little protective or lubricant function.

The cost of cosmetics varies greatly and their efficacy, other than by disguise, is a matter of debate. However they are probably cheaper than pregnancy which, while improving the texture of the skin, may not enhance the silhouette!

costs of health services. Whether paid by individual consumers (and by charity in the case of the impoverished) or largely by taxation, health services cost a sizeable slice of the gross national product – over 7 per cent in the U.S.A. and 6 per cent in Britain. In this article the British costs are given as illustrative.

The health services of the United Kingdom are an enormous industry employing the whole-time equivalent of almost a million people. Taking figures for slightly before the 1974 integration of services, the equivalent of 790,000 whole time staff were employed in hospitals (including 350,000 nurses, 274,000 ancillary and domestic workers, 57,000 administrative and clerical staff, 44,000 technicians and 29,000 doctors); 53,000 were employed by Executive Councils (including 25,000 general medical practitioners and 12,000 general dentists); 29,000 were employed by Local Health Authorities (with health visitors, midwives and home nurses constituting the largest groups) and 90,000 were in Social Work Departments (including home helps and the staffs of old people's homes and nurseries).

Published figures are inevitably in areas but those for 1971-72 show that in that year the health and personal social services cost £2,698 millions, or about 5.7 per cent of the gross national product (GNP), or very nearly £50 per head of population. Out of this massive total figure over 58 per cent (£1,549 millions) was expended on hospitals, 24 per cent on Executive Council services (with pharmaceutical, general medical and general dental the largest components in descending order), 11 per cent (£276 millions) on personal social services and only 5.4 per cent (£146 millions) on Local Health Authority services. Of this last sum approximately one half was spent on ambulance services (in England and Wales) and home nursing, leaving exactly 2.7 per cent available for all other Local Health Authority services, including antenatal and child health clinics, immunization and vaccination, family planning services, health visitors, midwives, dieticians, health education services of all varieties, and so on.

Slightly less than 5 per cent (£131 millions) of the total expenditure was recovered in direct charges to recipients of services, the biggest elements being charges for personal social services (e.g., home helps) and for dental and ophthalmic services. National Health Service contributions by individuals accounted for roughly 9 per cent, about 16 per cent came from local authority rates and consolidation grants to local authorities, and just over 70 per cent was a direct charge on the Government.

The services have been subject to criticism on three main grounds – that they are too dear, that they are too cheap and that their allocation is faulty.

Too expensive? Total costs, and in particular costs of the hospital component, soared in the early years of the National Health Service, with the rising expenditure justified by the claim that before 1948 many people simply did not receive adequate health care, but with counter claims that in the first few years some members of the public abused the 'free' service. However, a specially appointed committee (the Guillebaud Committee) in the middle 1950s could find no evidence of extravagance or abuse in any branch of the service.

Since then there have been further large increases in costs. For instance, using staff numbers because monetary figures are distorted by inflation, the number of hospital doctors in whole time equivalents rose by a third between 1965 and 1972 (from 22,123 to 29,360), and in the same period the number of hospital nurses again in whole time equivalents rose by almost a third (from 264,683 to 350,333). By contrast, increases in the numbers of general medical practitioners, general dental practitioners, health visitors, midwives and home nurses were fairly small.

Yet 5.7 per cent of the GNP does not seem an excessive amount to spend on all our services for prevention, cure, palliation and support. France spends 5.9 per cent of its GNP on health and disease, West Germany 8.3 per cent and the U.S.A. 7.4 per cent.

One may perhaps query the proportions, as indicated later, asking for instance whether we really need over 29,000 hospital doctors (including 10,510 of full consultant status) as against only 25,000 general practitioners, or whether it is justifiable to have more than thirty times as many hospital nurses for treatment as health visitors for health promotion and disease prevention; but on over-all costs the figure of 5.7 per cent of GNP is impressively low.

Some writers have argued that there would be more efficient use of the services if people in need of care had either to pay directly or to insure personally, as in many other countries. Even if the cost per head were lower in countries like the U.S.A. in which 62 per cent of health and disease expenditure is from private sources, the argument would be a tenuous one, because an alternative possible explanation would be that some people were not getting services that they needed, because they either lacked the money to pay or grudged paying. However, whether because of or in spite of absence of direct payment, Britain's health and disease services cost proportionately less than those of other industrialized countries.

Too cheap? The strong argument against any suggestion that Britain's preventive and curative services are run on a shoestring is that study of vital statistics shows that, in terms of survival at various ages, Britain is the fourth healthiest of all countries, surpassed only by Sweden, Norway and in some points Holland.

Yet, when Britain spends in relation to gross national product less than five-sixths of what the U.S.A. expends on health and less than three-quarters of what West Germany spends, there is obviously a case for maintaining that Britain is trying to provide its services too cheaply. Exponents of this view rely mainly on two indications.

Firstly, doctors are relatively very well paid among the various health professionals in Britain, but barely sufficient young men and women from Britain qualify as doctors and practise in this country to maintain the services. There are some unfilled vacancies both in hospital and in general practice; and of the doctors working in this country in 1972 exactly one-third had been born outside the United Kingdom and the Republic of Ireland. In other words, even in the best paid of the health professions we are relying to a considerable extent on workers from less highly developed countries.

Secondly, when we turn to nurses, who – even after the Halsbury Report of 1974 – are very badly paid in relation to their professional qualifications and heavy responsibilities, and whose professional standing is perhaps lower than in any developed country except France, the situation is vastly worse. No fewer than three aspects have to be considered. (1) Despite the enormous reliance on students and persons from overseas (mentioned later) virtually every hospital and every community has unfilled nursing vacancies, often numerous. (2) In many hospitals a majority of the qualified nurses are from overseas. The services are kept going by nurses (and to a lesser extent by doctors) who enter Britain from under-developed countries, take their professional training here and then consolidate by working in Britain for a few years before returning home. Clearly, as developing countries establish their own schools of nursing this source of recruitment will dry up, as indeed it is already beginning to do. (3) Even with roughly half of the qualified staff being persons from overseas, the nursing service manages to continue without an even more massive number of unfilled vacancies only by misusing student nurses as 'pairs of hands'. Of the 350,000 'nurses' recorded in the official statistics, 75,000 (or almost a quarter) are unqualified students, roughly 50,000 of them student nurses seeking the registered qualification and 25,000 aspiring to the lower qualification of enrolled nurse. Few people would be happy to think that in a serious illness requiring nursing for 168 hours a week a quarter of their nurses would be unqualified students and half the remainder persons from foreign countries, with limited knowledge of British customs and sometimes communication difficulties. Moreover, if student nurses ever receive the status of students – as has already happened with student teachers and student social workers, and as is already recommended in the official Briggs Report and as is probably necessary if recruitment to nursing is to be improved – a very large number of extra staff will be required.

Those who claim, with considerable evidence as indicated above, that Britain is running its health and disease services on the cheap also use various subsidiary arguments. They point out that members of paramedical professions (e.g., speech therapists and chiropodists) are paid less than persons in non-health professions of comparable training and responsibility. They maintain that nurses have long professional preparation, heavy responsibilities and many unpleasant tasks, that some highly qualified nurses (such as tutors and health visitors) have professional preparation comparable with that of doctors and more extensive than that of secondary school teachers, and that nurses are badly underpaid simply because they were initially a purely female profession. Not least, they point out that insufficient recruitment of students is aggravated by the fact that, after qualification, both doctors and nurses can gain – even allowing for differences in the cost of living – considerably higher remuneration by emigrating to other English-speaking countries.

Wrong priorities? Many people argue that the main defect of Britain's health and disease services is a distortion of priorities. There are increasingly vociferous suggestions that it is wrong to devote 58 per cent of health expenditure to treatment and palliation in our 510,000 hospital beds and 11 per cent to supportive services like old people's homes and domestic helps, but less than 3 per cent to all services aiming at promotion of health and reduction of disease.

Various writers have pointed out that, if a health visitor in an entire year prevents six serious domestic accidents that would otherwise have each required four weeks in hospital at £120 a week, she has saved the country considerably more than her whole year's salary; that the same applies in respect of a health visitor or dietitian whose guidance saves four people from attacks of coronary thrombosis which would otherwise have meant that they averaged six weeks in hospital; and that the worker who prevents the birth of a single highly deformed child saves the country many thousands of pounds. In particular, emphasis has been laid on the proved success of health education in eradicating many infections, making 'dirt' diseases rare, reducing nutritional disorders, decreasing home and traffic accidents, diminishing many physical and emotional diseases of children and preventing the conception of many unwanted children; and it has been indicated that substantial increase in health visitors and other health educators would pay enormous dividends both in happiness and in saving of staff and money through reduction in the number of people requiring treatment or support.

The difficulty, of course, is that prevented diseases simply become forgotten, whereas existing conditions that have not been prevented manifestly call for sympathy and support.

The outlook. In the last dozen years there has been a gradual but nevertheless fairly steady trend in official circles to accept that health services have been run too cheaply – to give a measure of priority to the building of hospitals and health centres, to offer slightly larger salary increases to nurses and paramedical workers than to members of most professions, and to show concern about staff shortages and inadequate recruitment. Simultaneously there have been movements towards a reassessment of priorities – official circulars advocating a 50 per cent increase in the number of Britain's health visitors, the opening of additional schools of health visiting, emphasis on the general medical practitioner as opposed to his hospital colleague, and increasing recognition of the importance of health education. The 1974 integration of all health and disease services under the same management perhaps caused a temporary pause, because any major reorganization produces some initial confusion, but should in due course accelerate all these trends.

Couéism. See AUTO-SUGGESTION.

cough. A sudden noisy expulsion of air from the lungs. Its purpose is protection, to expel any inhaled foreign matter or secretions that are produced in response to infection. A cough that is accompanied by the production of phlegm is achieving this purpose and generally should be encouraged, while one that produces nothing is a dry cough resulting from laryngeal irritation rather than the presence of undesirable substances on the lining of the larynx, trachea or bronchial tubes.

Cough is a prominent symptom of any disorder of the lungs, particularly infections such as bronchits or tuberculosis. The linings of the tubes respond to infection by increased production of mucus which is swept upwards from the smallest bronchial tubes into the windpipe and then into the larynx. Presence of this mucus in the larger tubes, particularly the larynx, stimulates the cough. In this the pressure in the chest is suddenly increased while part of the throat, the glottis, remains closed and then suddenly opens so that air moves very rapidly through the upper part of the airway carrying mucus and other debris with it. Such coughing is desirable in the acute stage of any chest infection.

Any irritation of the larynx can produce coughing. This occurs most commonly with colds and infections of the upper respiratory tract and, of course, smoking. The coughing thus produced is usually of a dry barking nature and, if severe (as can occur in whooping cough) is best suppressed. Suppression of the cough reflex is produced by various drugs such as codeine and morphia. Most proprietary cough mixtures contain such substances or their derivatives in addition to demulcents (soothing substances that reduce the congestion of inflamed membranes).

The early morning 'smoker's cough' is one of the earliest features of chronic bronchitis and is a sign that the linings of the respiratory passages have been damaged. Smoke irritates the lining cells so that excess mucus is produced. This is not cleared from the tubes during the night because the cough reflex is slightly depressed in sleep. The accumulated mucus is cleared by coughing on awakening, and the frequent repeated coughing may contribute to the degenerative processes that occur in chronic bronchitis.

The plugging of small tubes by mucus causes air to be trapped in the small air sacs (alveoli) of the lung. Coughing increases the pressure inside the chest and because air cannot be expelled from blocked alveoli, they become stretched and the membranes between adjacent alveoli break down, thus making fewer but larger air sacs which are less efficient for the gaseous exchange upon which life depends. See EMPHYSEMA.

counter-irritation. The relief of pain or symptoms in one locality by inducing irritation in another. This was the reasoning behind the application of mustard plasters to the chest in pneumonia: it was believed that the application of such an irritant to the skin would cause congestion there, redirecting the excess blood flow and fluid from the lung to the site of new irritation. Counter-irritants are still in use, particularly as rubs and liniments for the relief of muscular pain. However, the massage and the belief in their efficacy are more likely to contribute to symptom relief than the constituents of such an application.

cowpox. A mild disease in which vesicles appear on the udders of cows and which may be transmitted to the hands of milkers. Cowpox, alternatively known as vaccinia, is caused by a virus closely resembling that of smallpox, and indeed it is probably the same virus, altered by passage through generations of cows. At any rate, the virus produces antibodies which protect against smallpox, and this is the basis of VACCINATION against that disease.

coxalgia. Pain in the hip. Any disturbance of the alignment of the hip joint usually results in pain; the commonest causes are arthritis and fractures of the hip joint, particularly fracture of the neck of the thigh bone or femur.

cracked lips. Painful fissures that are found in the lips as a result of exposure to cold, windy or dry atmospheres. The skin of the lips is very thin and has a plentiful blood supply, so evaporation constantly occurs. There are oil-producing glands in the lips to provide lubrication, but they need to be kept moist as excessive drying causes cracking. Ordinarily licking the lips provides adequate moisture, but in conditions producing rapid evaporation cracking may occur. This is prevented by the application of vaseline or some cosmetic face cream.

cracked nipple. See NIPPLE.

cramp. A painful spasm of the muscles. There are essentially three main varieties.

1. Cramp can arise from excessive loss of salt under conditions of great heat. Ships' stokers, for example, not infrequently suffer from cramp in the calves, arms and abdomen, sometimes accompanied by fall in blood pressure and by vomiting. Treatment consists of rest, plus restoration of salt balance by adequate salt in drinks and soups. Salt tablets, useful in some other conditions, should be avoided here because they are not always absorbed.

2. Bathers' cramp is thought to be due to the effects of cold on the nervous system. Simultaneous immersion of the whole body is said to be less likely to create cramp than is gradually walking into deeper water. Since cramp may prevent movement of the affected limbs and so cause drowning, sea-bathing, especially in cold weather, should be undertaken only in the company of swimmers who can use life-saving methods if one of them develops cramp, and never immediately after a meal.

3. Ordinary cramp, most frequently occasioned by sitting or lying with pressure on nerves, but occasionally produced by muscular stretching which again puts pressure on nerves. Brisk rubbing of the affected part generally ends the spasm and relieves the pain.

cranial nerves. The twelve pairs of nerves which arise in the BRAIN (in the case of motor fibres conveying impulses outwards) or terminate there (in the case of sensory fibres).

cranium. The part of the skull enclosing the brain.

crepitus. This term has two meanings:

1. The grating sound heard when the broken ends of a bone are moved and scrape on each other. The sound indicates a fracture, but fracture may be present without the sound being audible.

2. The term is also applied – more usually as 'crepitations' – to a bubbling sound heard through a stethoscope when there is moisture in the lungs or respiratory tubes.

cretinism. A condition resulting from under-functioning of the thyroid gland, which is one of the ENDOCRINE glands, before birth or in early infancy. If it remains untreated growth is stunted, the face looks prematurely aged, the skin is thickened and coarse, the hair is scanty, the abdomen is protuberant, development of the sexual organs is delayed and the victim is mentally retarded. The condition occurs in areas of severe iodine deficiency (with the thyroid gland unable to function properly through lack of iodine) and less frequently as a hereditary disorder. In districts where simple goitre is prevalent, indicating deficiency of iodine, cretinism can often be prevented by administration of iodine during pregnancy.

Where cretinism is diagnosed very early and treatment with thyroxine is instituted to replace the inadequate functioning of the thyroid, the outlook both physically and mentally is very good, but the treatment has to continue for life. Where treatment is not started until the child is 4 or 5 years old much improvement is possible but there is little chance of full recovery from the handicap imposed by several years of faulty skeletal and mental development.

croup. A general name for a harsh, stifling cough and strained, noisy breathing, occurring in children and caused by any inflammation or spasm of the larynx.

The term is still sometimes used for a very serious but infrequent inflammation of the larynx, trachea and bronchi, affecting mostly children under 2 years, thought to be due to an unidentified virus, and generally requiring full dosage of antibiotics and nursing in an oxygen tent. In the past the name was also used for the spasm found in some cases of severe rickets (laryngismus stridulus) and sometimes for the laryngeal form of diphtheria and for the inflammation accompaying some other infections and some allergic conditions.

cryptorchism. See TESTICLE, UNDESCENDED.

culture and health. A person's state of health and well-being depends primarily on three sets of factors – his genetic inheritance; the psycho-social, personal and enviromental influences affecting him in his early formative years; and the similar influences currently or recently affecting him. To some extent the two latter groups can be summed up as the culture patterns of his early years and of the present. To give examples of the effects of early culture patterns: a child who is brought up by parents who normally overeat and amid brothers and sisters who overeat is likely later in life to suffer from diseases associated with obesity; and a child reared in a cohesive, stable, affectionate family has a less than average chance of becoming a delinquent.

Often early and current patterns are similar: the boy born into a particular socio-economic group with, say, no interest in reading, often remains in that group and usually marries a girl from the same group. In such cases it is a little difficult to differentiate early and current cultural influences. However, the effect of current or recent patterns can be seen where a person transfers into a completely new social atmosphere, for example, the youth who moves from a remote rural area in which every major action is undertaken in the glare of local publicity and in which the opinions of the parson, the teacher and the doctor carry much weight, to the bright lights, temptations, increased pressures and relative anonymity of a large city. His risk of alcoholism, drug addiction and venereal disease is clearly increased, and so is his risk of depression and conditions associated with loneliness.

It is often said that the main cultural changes in Western Europe and America in this century are reduction of gross poverty, greater affluence, greater material ambition with more chance of gratifying it, and greater pressure of life – with, in consequence, a decrease in the diseases of poverty and a rise in diseases associated with affluence and greater mental stress. A change of possibly equal importance is the gradual transition from a community of physically active people, who walked to work and earned their living by manual labour, to a community of passive people, who are carried from home to job, earn their living by sitting at a desk or bench, and spend their increasing leisure watching television – so that we have an increase in diseases associated with inadequate muscular activity.

curare. A South American Indian arrow poison extracted from various plants and causing rapid paralysis of muscles. For use in hunting the poison had the advantage that after the animal died, from paralysis of the respiratory muscles, the wounded portion could be cut away and the rest of the flesh safely eaten.

Death from curare poisoning can often be prevented by applying artificial respiration until the effects of the poison wear off.

An alkaloid derived from curare is sometimes used during surgical operations to relax muscles. The muscles used in breathing are, of course, similarly relaxed, but the breathing can be regulated artificially for the necessary hour or so.

curettage. Scraping the interior wall of the uterus with a spoonlike instrument called a curette. The operation is performed in three sets of circumstances: (1) along with dilatation of the cervix in women who are having difficulty in conceiving a child; (2) after a miscarriage, to remove any remaining fragments of membrane; and (3) in some cases of chronic inflammation of the uterus.

curvature of the spine. Viewed from the side the spine has four normal curves: (1) the cervical curve in the neck, convex forwards; (2) the thoracic curve, convex backwards; (3) the lumbar curve, convex forwards; and (4) the pelvic curve, convex backwards. The two backward curves are present before birth and are sometimes termed primary curves. The cervical curve develops as the child begins to control movements of the head, and the lumbar curve appears later, as the child begins to walk.

Abnormal curvatures of the backbone may arise as exaggerations of normal curves or by the formation of new curves.

Kyphosis is the term applied to the exaggeration of the thoracic curve known in severe cases as 'hunchback' and in mild cases as 'round shoulders'. It often arises from faulty posture, or from the peering forward

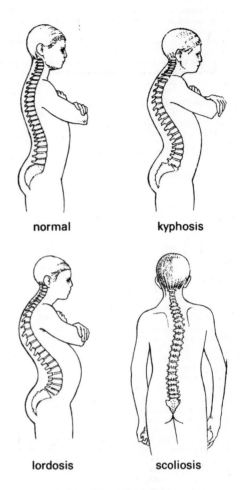

normal   kyphosis

lordosis   scoliosis

Curvature of the spine

associated with bad sight, and severe varieties are sometimes the result of rickets. Disease or injury to the spine (e.g., tuberculosis or fracture dislocation) may also cause it. Treatment varies with the cause.

Lordosis or abnormal 'hollow back' occurs from severe muscle weakness and in congenital dislocation of the hip. Owing to the combined weight of the foetus and of the liquid surrounding it, some temporary lordosis occurs in pregnancy. Treatment is not necessary unless symptoms develop.

Scoliosis is sideways or lateral curvature of the spine; there are various types: (1) congenital scoliosis, seen in babies and due to defective vertebral development; (2) rickety scoliosis due to the effects of rickets, in which the bones are softened by vitamin deprivation; (3) compensatory scoliosis due to asymmetry of the legs, usually resulting from disease or injury; (4) paralytic scoliosis from paralysis of the trunk muscles on one side, often a sequel of infantile paralysis; and (5) postural scoliosis –

the commonest type, occurring in children and delicate adolescents from bad posture at desks, sometimes in those who ride side-saddle, and in workers who have predominately to use one leg at their trade.

In the early stages the spine can be seen to straighten when the patient hangs by his arms and at this stage treatment is by exercises and, sometimes, traction, which pulls the spine straight by the use of weights. Later on the curvature of the spine becomes fixed and the person may require a supportive spinal jacket.

cuticle. The epidermis or outer layer of the skin. This layer, which does not contain blood vessels, is thick and horny on the palms and soles but thinner elsewhere. The term is applied more specifically to the layer of skin which grows round the bases of the nails.

cuts. Among domestic accidents serious enough to receive medical treatment cuts rank second only to falls. There is, however, a curious age difference: both cuts and falls are commonest among children, especially children under seven years, but in adults cuts are most frequent before middle age while falls occur mainly in middle-aged or elderly persons.

Treatment. Even where the cut has been created by a clean instrument a break in the skin provides a possible entrance for bacteria and should therefore be taken seriously. In general the wound should be cleansed with warm, boiled water, gently dried, and swabbed with a mild disinfectant (e.g., tincture of iodine), after which a gauze or lint dressing should be firmly bandaged on and left undisturbed for some days. If, however, the wound throbs or surrounding parts become inflamed, indicating that germs have penetrated to the tissues, medical aid should be promptly sought and antibiotics given.

cyanides. The salts of prussic acid, the most rapidly acting of all poisons. They are used in industry and for fumigation. The inhaled fumes of prussic acid kill almost instantaneously, while swallowed cyanides kill within minutes. In cases of poisoning an emetic should be given to induce vomiting, artificial respiration applied and medical aid summoned at once. A victim who survives for the first half hour is likely to recover.

cyanocobalamine. The chemical name for VITAMIN B12.

cyanosis. The bluish coloration of the skin which arises from inadequate oxygenation of the blood. It may be due to insufficient intake of oxygen from the lungs (as in pneumonia or suffocation) or to stagnation or inadequate circulation of the blood (as in various diseases of the heart). Localized cyanosis of the lips occurs in debilitated and rheumatic persons in

cold weather, and localized cyanosis of the fingers occurs in Raynaud's disease.

Treatment depends on the cause, and in addition the administration of oxygen is usually necessary in severe cases.

cyst. An abnormal swelling containing fluid. Cysts are found most frequently in the skin (usually from blocked sweat glands) and in the ovaries (in which they may grow to enormous sizes unless removed).

cystic fibrosis. A very serious hereditary condition (alternatively called fibrocystic disease of the pancreas) characterized by pathological changes in the pancreas, lungs, intestines and most mucous-secreting glands. The disease is inherited as a Mendelian recessive which means, in GENETIC terms, that both parents carry the genes but do not show signs of the disease.

Clinical features which appear in the early weeks of life include failure to thrive (because of absence of pancreatic juices to digest food), distended abdomen (a characteristic of all forms of malnutrition), diarrhoea with offensive stools (from failure to digest fat) and a cough which often heralds broncho-pneumonia. Diagnosis may be confirmed by examination of stools for fat and absence of pancreatic juices, or by examination of sweat for increased salt content.

A high protein diet with vitamin supplements is useful; pancreatic extract may partially replace the absent hormones; extra salt is required because of the high salt loss, and antibiotics are needed for the respiratory condition. Despite treatment a high proportion of patients die.

cystitis. Inflammation of the bladder, usually due to bacterial infection. The condition is commoner in women because of their shorter urethras, but also occurs in men, especially where enlargement of the prostate causes narrowing of the urethra and some retention of urine. Symptoms include pain in the lower abdomen, frequency of urination and a scalding sensation on passing urine. Treatment includes rest, mild alkalis especially sodium citrate, and usually sulphonamides or antibiotics.

Occasionally an acute attack which has been inadequately treated passes into a chronic cystitis with persisting frequency of urination, feeling of weight in the lower abdomen and a danger of the infection ascending to the kidneys. Treatment depends on the particular germ concerned.

cystoscope. An instrument for viewing the interior of the bladder. It consists of a narrow tube containing a sort of telescope, with an electric light at the end and an appropriate mirror in which the highly illuminated bladder surface is reflected.

D

dactylitis. Inflammation of a finger or toe. The term is used mostly for (1) inflammation of tubercular origin and commencing in the bone, and (2) inflammation in cases of congenital syphilis. Apart from treatment of the actual inflammation attention is required for the underlying disease.

dandruff. A scaly condition of the scalp in which small flakes of dead skin form and are shed. See HAIR.

dangerous drugs. In ordinary speech the term is generally used for the so-called 'hard' drugs, i.e., those that are definitely liable to lead to addiction, in particular (1) morphia, (2) some of its derivatives, such as heroin, and (3) cocaine.

Legally, however, dangerous drugs are those specified by legislation in a particular country. In the U.K., for instance, a Dangerous Drugs Act includes various drugs other than those mentioned above, e.g., Indian hemp (cannabis), restricts possession of these drugs to certain 'authorized persons' such as medical practitioners, requires that the drugs be kept under lock and key with an exact record maintained of their use, and specifies requirements for medical prescriptions containing these drugs. In a few countries the prescription of heroin, the most addictive of all drugs but also the most efficient pain killer, is illegal. See DRUGS and ADDICTION.

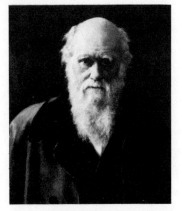

Charles Darwin

Darwin, Charles Robert. The main expounder of EVOLUTION by natural selection, Charles Darwin (1809-1882) has had perhaps greater influence on human thinking than any other scientist, with the possible exception of Freud.

After starting but not completing a medical course at Edinburgh and 'wasting' (his own expression) three years at Cambridge studying with a view to becoming a clergyman, Darwin sailed on the *Beagle* as volunteer naturalist without pay. During the five year voyage to South Sea islands, South America and Australia he amassed much zoological knowledge and began to realize that in any species variations favourable to it would tend to be preserved and unfavourable ones to be destroyed.

His first book, *Zoology of the Voyage of the Beagle* (1840) brought him into contact with Sir Charles Lyell, Professor of Geology at Oxford, and Lyell encouraged him to continue his studies of inbreeding and to publish his views.

In 1858 Darwin received from A. R. Wallace (1823-1913) an unpublished document reaching independently conclusions identical with his own, and he published Wallace's essay roughly simultaneously with his own great work, *The Origin of Species* (1859).

The French naturalist, LAMARCK, had popularized the idea that when living organisms adjusted to their environment the resulting physical and intellectual changes were passed on to succeeding generations. Challenging this belief that acquired characteristics could be inherited Darwin amassed massive and conclusive evidence from geological record, geographical distribution, comparative anatomy and selective breeding. Coherently and logically he showed that organisms had evolved, and were still evolving, by the preservation and summation of successive slight variations which favoured survival.

The first edition of *The Origin of Species* was sold out in a single day and the evolution controversy was on. The great evolution controversy raged through the rest of the nineteenth century, but Darwin gained powerful support from August Weismann (1834-1914) of Freiburg, the father of modern genetics, who pointed out that genetic material is separated from the rest of the body before birth and remains separated. The germ-cells act only as determinants for specific character-istics, and if an acquired characteristic is to be transmitted it must first be translated into a determinant. This could come about only by some accidental mutation of genes or by beneficial individual variations gradually gaining ascendancy.

Although nowadays thought obvious, these views were not popular with non-scientific philosophers and writers. People from Samuel Butler to George Bernard Shaw tried to insist – non-scientifically – that the efforts and successes of one generation could influence the next. Weismann was a particular target for Shavian ridicule in *Back To Methuselah*. It has, however, become clear that the Lamarckian theory could lead only to increasing randomness and diversity, but that natural selection on the Darwin concept ensures an ever-improving adaptation by an organism to the environment.

Darwin's main book is still regarded as the leading work on natural philosophy in the history of mankind. He also published several other important books, including 'The Variation of Animals and Plants (1868) and The Descent of Man (1871).

day dreaming. A form of thinking in which free rein is given to the imagination. Day dreaming is unrelated to constructive planning and is essentially the elaboration of fantasies, often of a wish fulfilment nature, with the dreamer as hero or, less often, as suffering martyr. Fantasy life is strong in most young children, dwindles in older children and increases again in adolescence before reducing once more during the twenties. Excessive day dreaming sometimes indicates the beginning of withdrawal from the problems of real life, as in early schizophrenia.

day hospital. An institution which provides treatment for patients who are able to live at home. It is differentiated from an out patients clinic by the fact that the patient attends for a substantial part of each day. The service varies, according to the type of patient, from active medical treatment, often including physiotherapy and occupational therapy, to merely providing a meeting place for persons with chronic disease.

As contrasted with care in the patient's own home, a day hospital gives a period of relief to overburdened relatives and can offer treatment facilities not normally available at home. As contrasted with an ordinary hospital, it gives the patient some continuation of home life and saves the cost of night staff.

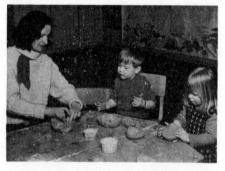

A day nursery

day nursery. A form of day care for pre-school children. Unlike a nursery school it is open for sufficiently long hours to enable the mother to undertake a full day's work and it has no lower age limit for acceptance of children. The matron is usually a qualified nurse and there are specified standards of staffing and accommodation.

For unsupported women who have to earn a living, and in times of illness and family stress, nurseries perform a valuable function, and they often improve the nutrition, physical development and habits of children from problem families. There is some evidence, however, that under normal circumstances a young child's emotional development and capacity for forming future bonds of affection make better progress if he does not have the trauma of daily separation from his mother. Hence for children under 2½ years day nurseries are regarded as definitely a second best choice.

DDT. Diclor-diphenyl-tetrachlorethane, a white crystalline powder, almost insoluble in water but easily soluble in oils. As an insecticide it is harmless to mammals but lethal to mosquitoes, house flies, bluebottles, fleas and lice. A 5 per cent spray destroys mosquitoes, house flies and their larvae and the solution if sprayed on walls and windows remains effective for several weeks.

For lice and fleas a 5 per cent DDT dust can be applied from a compression gun, enabling large numbers of people to be disinfected without the necessity of removing their clothes. This advantage may appear trivial when one is considering a single infected family, but is enormous when a typhus outbreak makes necessary the disinfection of thousands of potentially infected persons.

deaf aids. See HEARING AIDS

deaf mutism. A condition in which a person is unable to hear and therefore has not learned to speak articulately. In most cases the deafness is of hereditary origin although it can also occur through the mother suffering from German measles during early pregnancy or from various conditions occurring soon after birth. If a baby does not respond to sounds within the first three months the advice of a doctor or health visitor should be sought, because there may be some disease of the ear which can be corrected with treatment.

Hereditary deafness on the other hand is incurable, but the child should be sent to a special school where he will be taught to speak by lip reading and by the sense of touch. Training a completely deaf child to speak sufficiently clearly to convey his meaning is an arduous task but the results are worthwhile.

deafness. Complete or partial absence of hearing can result from any impairment of the chain of communication from the outer EAR to the brain.

1. Outer ear. The skin of the outer ear secretes wax from modified sweat glands. Entry of water during washing causes the wax to swell, blocking the passage, and this is by far the commonest cause of temporary deafness. It is easily cured: the wax should be softened by inserting a few drops of oil and, a day later, gently syringed out.

2. Middle ear. (1) Infection (otitis media) causes deafness and usually earache. Most cases respond to suitable antibiotics. (2) Inflammation of the Eustachian tube, which often occurs in conditions like the common cold, disturbs the middle ear and may cause temporary diminution of hearing. (3) Blockage of the Eustachian tubes by large adenoids may have a similar but more lasting effect. Treatment consists of surgical removal of the adenoids. (4) Otosclerosis, or formation of excess bone in the middle ear, ultimately creates complete deafness. It is a condition of unknown cause, tending to occur in relatively young adults; surgical reconstruction – the

operation of fenestration – has been highly successful in some cases.

3. Inner ear and auditory nerve. (1) The commonest cause of deafness from birth is a hereditary defect, causing DEAF MUTISM. (2) Maternal rubella (German measles) and possibly other virus diseases during pregnancy can also cause deafness from birth. (3) Continual exposure to loud noise, as in the case of boilermakers and riveters, damages the auditory nerve. (4) Various poisons and drugs can affect the nerve. (5) As life advances the efficiency of the nerve decreases.

In general disorders of the outer and middle ear can be successfully treated while disorders of the inner ear and nerve are as yet incurable. Where deafness is incurable the patient may be given a HEARING AID, but in nerve deafness it may be ineffective.

Deafness in children. Suspected cases are normally tested with a pure tone audiometer which emits a note of any chosen frequency (pitch) and volume (loudness), so that the child's ability to hear high and low notes can be ascertained; this investigation is generally undertaken by an audiologist. For educational purposes children with defective hearing are placed in three groups: (1) those with deafness so slight that it need merely be kept under observation but will not interfere with their education; (2) those who need special facilities (ranging from special places in class to hearing aids and special classes) but can be taught as hearing children; and (3) those whose hearing is so defective that they must be educated as deaf children, e.g., by lip reading.

Impaired hearing in the elderly. Insensitivity to high notes is the main symptom. This increasing loss of sensitivity is in considerable part a normal process: most children can hear the high-pitched cry of a bat, but few people over 25 years can hear it. Many elderly people can hear low-pitched voices but have difficulty with high-pitched voices and particular difficulty in distinguishing consonants which are higher pitched than most vowels.

The handicap of deafness. It is often said that to be deaf from birth is a greater handicap than to be blind, but that in later life loss of hearing is perhaps a less serious occurrence than loss of sight. Both are obviously grave disabilities. Yet hearing and sighted people tend to react differently to the two handicaps: the blind man is offered sympathy, understanding and help; the deaf man is too often the subject of ridicule, and becomes isolated socially because of the comparative difficulty of communicating with him.

death. If we defer for later consideration the rare cases in which the circulation of the blood is maintained through the use of an artificial respirator, death can be defined as the process which takes place when the circulation finally ceases and breathing stops. Breathing alone may cease for a number of minutes and be restored by artificial respiration. Cessation of heart action may arise during anaesthesia and in other circumstances but cardiac action can often be restored by massaging the heart. However, the outside limit for such cessation of the circulation is probably about four minutes. Any longer interruption of the circulation usually leads to irreparable damage of the brain.

Death can be ascertained by listening for the heart beat (or seeking to feel the pulse) and by holding a mirror over the mouth and nostrils and noting whether it becomes hazy with exhaled breath.

Under normal climatic circumstances the body cools at a definite rate after death, and this enables the time of death to be ascertained with some precision. Rigidity of the muscles (rigor mortis) sets in within a few hours while bruise-like marks on the parts lying lowest and post mortem lividity set in later. Also, if the time of the last meal is known, a study of the degree of digestion of the food in the stomach provides useful information.

As every reader of detective fiction knows, it can be important in cases of suspected murder to establish the approximate hour of death, and the happenings mentioned above generally enable the time to be fixed within an hour if the body is examined soon after death, or within a few hours if it is examined later.

In recent years, however, problems have arisen that involve not simply the hour of death but the minute. The first of these problems relates to the transplant of organs. If one patient is likely to die soon unless he receives a transplant of an organ (e.g., heart) to replace his damaged one, and if another patient who is willing to act as a donor in the event of his death is dying (e.g., from a traffic accident), it is clearly vital for the well-being and even the life of the intended recipient that the organ be removed and the transplant started as soon after the death of the other patient as is practicable; but the idea of over-early presumption of death of the donor is ethically completely repugnant. In general, however, the donor is in hospital and under observation when death occurs, and it is possible to begin the transplant only minutes after death has taken place. It is sometimes suggested that surgeons (anxious to save the life of one patient, especially if he is a person of national importance or great wealth, and knowing that the other patient is beyond all hope of even temporary recovery) may be over-keen to assume that death has actually taken place; but the suggestion really implies criminal activity not just by one surgeon but by the entire team of doctors and nurses concerned with the transplant.

The second problem concerns patients whose circulation has been maintained by the use of a mechanical respirator. In the ordinary case, where a person dies at home or in the street or in hospital without a respirator in position, no problem arises: even if a respirator were immediately available it takes a little time to connect it up and start it, and as indicated above death is absolute within about four minutes of the cessation of circulation. A problem can arise, however, with a patient who has been linked to a mechanical respirator because of his failing circulation. If the patient's own circulation fails to recover, the circulation can be maintained artifically for hours or even days after the brain has become permanently inactive, and there exist a full range of neurological tests to establish whether the brain has ceased to have any activity. From a strictly medical aspect, although the use of the respirator may be continued for a few additional hours for absolute certainty, there is no point in continuing artificial circulation after the brain has become permanently inactive. There is, however, an unsolved legal problem: if a person is attacked and almost killed, is taken to hospital, has failing circulation maintained by a respirator, fails to recover, and finally has the respirator disconnected after indications of brain death, can the death be deemed murder or can it be argued – on the old definition of death occurring with cessation of blood circulation – that the immediate cause of death was the switching off of the respirator? No court decision has yet been given, at least in Britain, but most lawyers hold that death in such circumstances would be regarded as murder, the disconnecting of the respirator being merely a recognition that death had occurred.

death certificate. A document, stating the cause of death and giving various other particulars, required in most countries before burial or cremation, and of which a copy is often required for the claiming of life insurance or (in countries with such schemes) the claiming of death grants and pensions for dependents. The document is completed by the physician who attended the patient in his last illness and saw him after death and is passed, usually by the undertaker, to the appropriate authority, e.g., in the U.K. to the registrar of births, deaths and marriages.

Where no doctor has been attending during the final illness, or where the doctor is uncertain of the cause of death, the doctor who certifies that death has occurred has to comply with certain legal requirements (e.g., notification of the coroner in England and Wales) and in circumstances of suspicion or uncertainty a post mortem examination may be ordered.

Death records should – and in fact do – provide important information about the diseases from which people in a district die and the ages and occupation groups affected by particular diseases. There are, however, various sources of error. In particular (1) the age or occupation of the deceased person may be mis-stated, inadvertently or advertently, by his relatives; (2) the physician's diagnosis of the cause of death may be faulty – it has been reckoned that errors occur in about 10 per cent of cases in teaching hospitals in the U.K. and the U.S.A. and presumably in greater number in deaths recorded by general practitioners; and (3) in certain circumstances, e.g., suicide or venereal disease, the doctor may desire to shield the feelings of the relatives of the diseased person. A further source of difficulty in the past was vague recording of the cause of death, but virtually all countries now use the International List of Causes of Death with 189 headings classified into 14 main groups.

debility. A vague term used popularly to describe a low state of health, a lack of vitality and an inability to withstand the normal stresses and demands of life. It is common in severe malnutrition, after convalescence from various acute illnesses and in conditions of severe nervous strain. Treatment varies with the cause.

decompression disease. A condition, characterized mainly by pains in the limbs and sometimes by changes in bones and joints, caused by excessive retention of nitrogen in the blood as a result of over-rapid return to normal atmospheric pressure after breathing under high pressure. It occurs therefore in diving, tunnel construction, and anywhere a caisson or diving bell is used, and is alternatively called the bends or caisson disease.

The severity of symptoms varies with the working pressure, the length of exposure, and the rapidity of return to normal pressure. Effects are due to the fact that the nitrogen in air is soluble in the fluids and tissues of the body, and especially in the fat. This solubility varies directly with the pressure and, when pressure is released, nitrogen bubbles form in the tissues. These bubbles are most liable to occur in the white matter of the nervous system, causing paralysis, and in the joints to produce pain and disability.

The condition can be avoided completely by slow decompression, and approved diving technique provides a code of rules specifying the stages and pauses necessary in raising a diver from various depths after various times of exposure. When cases actually occur through carelessness or accident, the victims must be immediately re-compressed and then decompressed slowly in accordance with the code of practice.

In recent years undersea oil developments have focused new attention on the problems of decompression. To mention one example, if a deep-sea diver sustains an injury, the doctor treating him may have to enter a chamber under high pressure and may thereafter have to spend the next forty-eight to seventy-two hours undergoing gradual reduction of pressure to normal, with consequent unavailability for other patients.

defective vision. See EYESIGHT.

defence mechanism. A term used to indicate measures adopted unconsciously or involuntarily as a protection against an emotionally painful subject. For example, a father unwilling to face the fact that his child is mentally subnormal may react by refusing to use the offered diagnostic services or by expressing hostility to doctors and nurses; in so acting he is behaving quite honestly because his conscious mind does not appreciate that he is unwilling to accept a diagnosis of mental handicap.

deficiency diseases. Strictly, a deficiency disease is an illness arising from prolonged inadequacy of any essential constituent of the DIET, e.g., shortage of first class protein, calcium or iodine. Increasingly, however, the term is becoming restricted to illnesses occasioned by the diet containing less than the required minimum of one of the VITAMINS, while more general deficiency is termed MALNUTRITION.

The main deficiency diseases are:

1. From inadequacy of fat-soluble vitamin A. Night blindness, xerophthalmia and hyperkeratosis, a thickening of the outer lining of the respiratory system and of the skin.

2. From inadequacy of fat-soluble vitamin D (in the absence of enough sunshine to synthesize the vitamin). Rickets in the growing child, and osteomalacia in adults, especially pregnant women.

3. From inadequacy of fat-soluble vitamin E. Sterility, proved in rats fed on a deficient diet but not definitely established in humans.

4. From inadequacy of fat-soluble vitamin K. Spontaneous haemorrhage, a result of low prothrombin content of the blood; haemorrhagic disease of the new-born.

5. From inadequacy of water-soluble vitamin B₁. Beriberi and infantile beriberi.

6. From inadequacy of water-soluble compounds collectively termed vitamin B₂. Pellagra, which is due to deficiency of nicotinic acid (sometimes called the pelagra-preventing factor), and seborrhoeic dermatitis, especially of the skin of the nose, mouth, scrotum or vulva. This is due to deficiency of riboflavine, but a similar condition can arise from deficiency of pyridoxone, sometimes called vitamin B₆.

7. From inadequacy of water-soluble vitamin B₁₂. Pernicious anaemia. Juvenile pernicious anaemia, a similar condition of hereditary origin and anaemia following operations to the stomach.

8. From inadequacy of water-soluble vitamin C. Scurvy and infantile scurvy, which broadly resembles the adult form.

9. From inadequacy of water-soluble vitamin P (if indeed this exists separately from vitamin C). Spontaneous haemmorrhages and delayed healing of wounds.

10. Certain other conditions, e.g., failure of a child to grow and increased susceptibility to infections, are associated with deficiencies of almost any of the vitamins, with A and C perhaps most heavily involved.

All the diseases mentioned above are preventable by an adequate and properly balanced diet, and, unless identified in terminal phases or after irreversible damage has occurred, can be cured by administration of the appropriate vitamin. Three final points should, however, be noted. (1) In severe illness the digestive system may be incapable of absorbing large quantities of the required vitamin, so that it may have to be administered otherwise than by mouth. (2) Over-dosage with vitamins D, A and B₁ can occur and can produce toxic symptoms. (3) Some of the vitamins are effective only in the presence of adequate quantities of other substances, e.g., ample vitamin D without sufficient calcium will not prevent or cure rickets, so that the mere administration of vitamins will not compensate for a poor diet.

Deficiency diseases are still very prevalent in underdeveloped countries. In highly developed countries they were until fairly recently second only to infections as causes of illness, and their virtual eradication is one of the greatest triumphs of the preventive services. The conditions should still be looked for in the very young, the very old, the very poor and persons with unusual dietetic habits.

deformities. By far the commonest deformities are those present at birth which are inherited. Examples include – hare lip, cleft palate, spina bifida (unclosed spinal canal), imperfect genital organs, club foot and dislocation of the hip. Prevention in these circumstances is largely a matter of studying the GENETICS of a family with a deformed child to assess the chance of that particular couple producing another. After this assessment the decision must rest with the parents or prospective parents.

Other deformities present at birth are due to illness or some other abnormal condition of the mother during pregnancy. A seriously malnourished mother has an increased chance of producing a deformed child, as has a mother suffering from syphilis or various other diseases. Prevention of this group of deformities is normally possible with adequate antenatal care.

Yet a third group of deformities present at birth are caused by the taking of drugs which affect the foetus. Thalidomide, an apparently harmless tranquillizer, previously tested on animals and human volunteers (not including expectant mothers) was widely used in several countries and resulted in the birth of babies with absent or shortened arms or legs.

Because of the frequency of deformities present at birth, every baby should be carefully examined during the first weeks of life, so that corrective treatment can be started where necessary.

There is absolutely no truth in the common superstition that deformities which arise before birth are the result of the mother suffering from some emotional shock or seeing some distressing sight.

Deformities arising subsequent to birth are the result of diseases or injuries of bones, joints or nerves, e.g., those occasioned by the faulty union of broken bones that have been badly set, or the knock knees, bowed legs, deformed chest and narrowed pelvis associated with rickets, or the round shoulders associated with persistent bad posture.

dehydration. Depletion of WATER arising from inadequate replacement of fluid loss from the body.

In temperate climates adults excrete about 3 litres (5 pints) of water daily, in urine, breath, perspiration and faeces; and a considerable amount of salt is lost along with the water. In warm climates the loss of water and salt is correspondingly greater. Since the body fluids and tissues consist largely of water, the body needs an equivalent intake, including of course the water contained in food, e.g., potatoes are slightly more than one-half water.

Dehydration occurs (1) in persons deprived of adequate fresh-water intake, as when stranded in a desert or adrift at sea; (2) in conditions associated with prolonged and profuse perspiration not balanced by water intake, e.g., various fevers (especially if the victim is delirious or otherwise unable to drink) and working in very hot weather with water not readily available; and (3) in conditions associated with excessive urination (e.g., after large doses of diuretics) excessive passing of watery motions (e.g., cholera and dysentery) and occasionally excessive vomiting.

The symptoms include extreme thirst, fatigue, giddiness and ultimately delirium, coma, and death. A human being can survive only about three days without any water.

The remedy where available is obvious – adequate intake of water and (especially in cases associated with heavy perspiration) of salt: most forms of heat exhaustion are more the result of salt deficiency than of water deficiency.

Persons with high temperatures should be given ample cool drinks of water, fruit juice and other liquids. If the patient can eat solid food the necessary salt may be more acceptable when sprinkled on food than if added to drinks.

Where there are symptoms of dehydration and the patient is unable to drink, the injection of sterile water by a doctor or nurse may well save his life, and if there is any possibility of salt depletion as well as water depletion the injected fluid should contain a teaspoonful of salt per tumblerful of water.

déjà vu. Literally 'already seen.' The technical term for the feeling that one has already experienced a situation identical with the present one. The phenomenon is common and its explanation is disputed. One theory is that the two eyes on occasion focus separately, so that impulses from the second eye seem familiar to the brain when they reach it.

delinquency. Although often loosely applied to youthful aberrations in general, delinquency in the U.K. is strictly conduct in a person between the ages of 8 and 17 years that is so at variance with the accepted pattern that the offender has been dealt with by a court, perhaps for committing an offence, or for persistent truancy or even as being beyond parental control.

Useful information for investigating the causes and prevention of delinquency is very hard to obtain – because delinquency is a legal rather than a scientific term and has no precise and uniform definition, because standards of unacceptable conduct change from time to time and vary from place to place, because offenders who are brought to court and thereafter classed as delinquents are only such of the offenders as are caught, and because most classifications of delinquents relate to the type of offence, e.g., minor theft, damage to property, sex offences, etc. In any study of causes, the actual type of offence may be very unimportant: for instance, one boy may steal because he is feeble-minded and lacks moral sense, a second may have been taught to steal by his parents or his companions, a third may have felt rejected first by his family and then by society and may steal as a form of revenge, and a fourth may be starved of affection and may seek to buy affection and admiration by demonstrating his prowess or by distributing stolen gifts.

On the whole, however, it can be said that delinquents tend to come from large rather than small families, that many of them are from broken homes or affectionless homes with parents of a cold, punitive type, that they are largely – but by no means wholly – from the lower and more impoverished socio-economic classes, that they often have histories of truancy and bad reputations at school, and that often other members of their families have been in trouble with the law.

One classification is into delinquency of gradual or sudden onset. In the former group (numerically by far the larger) personality or behaviour difficulties have appeared from the toddler stage; the child has been troublesome and naughty at home and in school; the difficulties have increased – not decreased – as he becomes older; and he steadily becomes more and more offensive to the community. This type can be subdivided into at least four subtypes, although in some measure these types overlap.

1. Predatory, i.e., aggressive and acquisitive, stealing or destroying. Possible causal factors include poor home conditions, parental neglect or indifference, lack of moral training and lack of opportunity for wholesome recreation.

2. Neurotic, e.g., the girl who commits sexual offences through an inordinate desire for affection. Possible causal factors include a broken home, a lack of affection at home,

parental disharmony, and over-strictness and domination at home and school.

3. Inadequate personality. The child becomes delinquent essentially because he cannot do even reasonably well either in school subjects or in games. All the causes mentioned in (1) and (2) above may operate, but an additional cause is over-ambitious parents who are never satisfied with the child's achievement.

4. Psychotic type, which is very rare.

Secondly (and much less commonly) there is delinquency of sudden onset, the previously 'good' child who kicks over the traces in adolescence. Here again it is possible to divide into subtypes.

1. Genuine delinquency. This is caused sometimes by over-strict discipline and repression. Instead of external discipline being gradually replaced by self-discipline, the child has to conform too closely to over-strict rules for too long, and finally reacts against dominating parents or teachers by 'sowing his wild oats'. Or it may be the result of over-forcing: the child finds that he cannot measure up to the standards expected, he becomes frustrated, feels a failure and uses delinquency as an outlet. Again this sudden, genuine delinquency may be the result of boredom at school, in the child who is much brighter or much duller than his classmates.

2. Apparent delinquency. Here the endocrine imbalance at adolescence, increased freedom and lack of maturity may combine to produce an apparent delinquency which is simply an exaggeration of normal high spirits.

Victor Hugo said, 'Society stands in the dock with every criminal'. In most cases of delinquency over-strict or affectionless or over-ambitious or bickering or separated parents are probably the main cause, though economic and environmental factors also play a part.

delirium. A disturbance of the brain, occasioned by injury, fever or poisoning, and characterized by incoherent talk, confusion, delusions and poorly regulated muscular actions. The name comes from the Latin *deliro* meaning 'I rave'.

Low delirium, associated with extreme exhaustion, consists mainly of rambling talk in which past events are jumbled together and present surroundings are ignored.

Raving delirium, associated with acute fevers, includes wild delusions and violent activity of the muscles.

Commonly known as DTs, DELIRIUM TREMENS usually occurs a few days after a period of heavy drinking.

delirium tremens. A disordered state of mind, usually including terrifying hallucinations, affecting heavy drinkers and occurring mostly after an unusually heavy bout of drinking or after injury or sudden illness following heavy intake of alcohol. Symptoms include hallucinations of the eyes (e.g., pink elephants) and of the skin (e.g., sensations of snakes or spiders crawling over it), intense anxiety and fear, restlessness and complete sleeplessness. Although recovery is usual, in about one case in twenty the condition is fatal. Immediate treatment consists of rest in bed (not always easily accepted by the patient) and the giving of adequate fluids with addition of glucose and vitamin B_1. Subsequent treatment is that of ALCOHOLISM.

It used to be believed that one of the causes

of delirium tremens (commonly known as DTs) was sudden withdrawal of alcohol but this view is nowadays regarded as quite unproved.

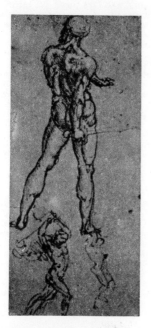

Drawings by Leonardo da Vinci showing the deltoid muscle in action

deltoid. The larger triangular muscle covering the shoulder. The apex of the triangle is on the outer side of the humerus, and the base is a broad attachment to the clavicle and scapula. The deltoid is the main muscle used in raising the arm sideways. It is named after the Greek letter delta, which in capital form, is written in the shape of a triangle.

delusion. An unshakeable false belief. It is easy to define a delusion as a belief that continues when logic and experience have proved it false, but there is no clear demarcation between mild delusion and simple error. For example, a man whose employer repeatedly passes him without a greeting has the delusion that the employer dislikes him, whereas the employer may really be short-sighted or preoccupied.

Most delusions are harmless unless they render a person's conduct antisocial but (apart from being pointers to mental illness) some delusions are dangerous. Thus a sufferer from paranoia who thinks he is being persecuted may decide to kill some of his persecuters. In paranoia such delusions of persecution are common, in schizophrenia the victim tends to live in an unreal dream world and in some forms of psychoses delusions of grandeur occur. Delusions, like HALLUCINATIONS, can occur in mentally normal people who are extremely exhausted or under great emotional strain.

dementia. Serious disorder or impairment of mental capacity, usually accompanied by disturbances in emotion and behaviour. In most cases the onset is gradual, with recently acquired memories soonest lost, decreasing ability to reason and to judge, and increasing display of emotion, e.g., tears or violent anger over trivial matters.

Senile or pre-senile dementia – a tendency to become dotards in old age – is in part familial (seen in successive generations of a family) in part occasioned by sudden stresses (like death of a spouse or loss of occupation) and in part due to arteriosclerosis and insufficient blood supply to the brain.

Dementia of cerebral arterial disease, mainly due to arteriosclerosis of the blood vessels of the brain, is very similar, as is the dementia of cerebral syphilis (dementia paralytica) and the dementia sometimes found in cases of cerebral tumour.

Dementia praecox is a synonym for SCHIZOPHRENIA.

A person suffering from dementia needs help. Complete cure is rare, but tranquillizers and other drugs can do much to lessen the symptoms and to improve the patient's sense of well-being. Occupational therapy can also be useful. Where the sufferer is treated at home his relatives have to seek to cultivate patience and tolerance of irrational behaviour and emotional outbursts; but it has to be remembered that the necessity to exercise continuing understanding, tolerance and patience for months or years places the relatives under considerable mental strain.

demography. The study of population structure or changes, e.g., high or low birth rates, changing infant mortality rates, the proportions in different age-groups or different occupational or social groups, or the relative numbers of persons born in the area and of incomers. Demographic studies, by pin-pointing groups particularly liable to – or pariculary free from – a disease, can often help to determine the causes of a condition or the appropriate techniques for its prevention.

dengue fever. A tropical disease caused by a virus transmitted by a mosquito. The symptoms are severe joint pains, backache, headache and fever with later a rash rather like that of measles. A curious feature of the disease is its so-called 'saddle back' nature: symptoms last for two or three days, remission for three or four days, and a second phase of symptoms (and rash) for about three days, followed by recovery. There is no specific treatment, although aspirin and paracetamol relieve the pain.

dental caries. Tooth decay, the commonest disease of highly developed countries and the main cause of toothache. See TEETH.

dentine. The hard, enamel-like exterior surface of the teeth.

dentist. A practitioner of the science of preventing and treating diseases of the teeth. Dental surgeon is an alternative and synonymous term.

An Egyptian papyrus of about 1500 B.C. describes the filling of cavities and the supporting of loose teeth with wire; and dentistry of a sort was certainly practised by surgeons of Greece and Rome. In the Renaissance era some surgeons showed interest in dentistry, e.g., Ambrose Paré in France and in Italy Fabricius drilled and cleaned cavities before filling them; and the earliest known sets of removable dentures are attributed to Fauchard (1678-1761) who published a book on dentistry. Such workers were exceptions however. In general doctors ignored diseases of the teeth, there was no dental profession, false teeth were made by jewellers or other persons with manual dexterity, and the itinerant tooth-puller – qualified only by apprenticeship if qualified at all – was the normal practitioner of dentistry.

The mid-nineteenth century saw the sudden emergence of dentistry as a profession. The first standard textbook, *Dental Physiology and Surgery*, was published by Dr (later Sir) John Tomes in 1848, and regular courses began to be given on the physiology and diseases of the teeth (e.g., in Edinburgh by Dr John Smith in 1856) with professional examinations for intending dentists introduced first in America and then in Britain (under the Dentists Act of 1878). However more than another forty years were to pass before it became impossible for a dentist to start to practise in Britain after qualifying merely by apprenticeship.

Dentistry is now a full profession, completely separate from medicine, and with its own specialists, such as those in orthodontics (correction of deformities of the teeth). At the 1974 integration of health services in Britain there were some 12,000 dentists working in the National Health Service as general dental practitioners and in many cases also treating patients privately; there were about 2,000 Local Health Authority dentists dealing with the treatment – and to some extent the prevention – of dental defects in expectant mothers, pre-school children and school pupils; in addition a small number worked in hospitals or purely in private practice – a grand total of about 18,000 dentists in Britain. Co-operation between doctors and dentists is already very good, but perhaps the next big advance in dentistry will be emphasis on its hitherto neglected preventive aspects, involving collaboration between dentists on the one hand and health education officers and health visitors on the other.

dentition. The kind, number and arrangement of TEETH. See also DEVELOPMENT.

dentures. Artificial or false teeth may be partial, replacing only a number of teeth, or complete, replacing all the teeth in a jaw. Their provision is essential to allow a person who has lost teeth to chew properly, and they also prevent the face of such a person from developing a sunk-in appearance.

After dentures have been inserted soft foods may have to be eaten for a couple of days until the patient becomes used to the dentures. A return visit to the dentist is often necessary as false teeth may press at one or two places and require adjustment. It is important to wear the dentures on the day before visiting the dentist, so that he can see the reddened areas and thus identify the exact points of pressure. Speech may be slightly indistinct for the first two or three days after starting to wear dentures.

The care of artificial teeth includes rinsing or brushing them after meals and placing them overnight in water containing salt or denture cleaner.

deodorants. Chemical substances which remove or mitigate objectionable smells. Some, such as eucalyptus, oil of cloves or turpentine simply mask the unpleasant odour. Others, such as hydrogen peroxide and potassium permanganate act by giving up oxygen, converting objectionable substances into acceptable ones. Some deodorants such as carbolic acid and creosote are also disinfectants and are used to purify water closets, drains, etc. In general the best method of removing body odour is frequent use of soap and water.

deoxyribonucleic acid. Commonly referred to as DNA; details will be found in the articles on RNA and on CELL.

depilation. Removal of superfluous hair from the body. Various chemicals are quite effective (e.g., a barium sulphide paste, containing one part barium sulphide, three parts zinc oxide and four parts starch), but the hair grows again in a few weeks. Electrolysis, or destruction of the hair root by electricity, is more permanently effective, but it is a slow and expensive process, since only a few hairs are removed at a sitting.

As an alternative to the removal of hair it can be made almost invisible by bleaching every few weeks with hydrogen peroxide.

depression. A lowering of spirits greater in duration and in degree than one would expect in the particular person under the circumstances present. Ordinary grief and mental suffering after bereavement is not depression, nor is the subdued mood of the person of a normally melancholy temperament. Again, we all have fluctuations of mood, and to be dejected for a day without obvious cause is not depression. Depression as an illness implies a considerable and persisting change of mood, out of all proportion to the factors that may have triggered it off.

A depressed person has a bleak and pessimistic attitude to the future, is uninterested in activities that he previously enjoyed, often complains of various physical symptoms for which no organic cause can be found, and may either lose interest in food or compulsively over-eat. In extreme cases suicide may be contemplated or attempted.

Depression occurs most commonly at critical or unsettled periods of life – in adolescence, after childbirth, at the menopause or at retirement from work. It is also common, but usually fairly transient, after certain illnesses such as severe influenza.

Simple reassurance and exhortation are useless: a depressed person can no more 'pull himself together' than can a person with a hormone deficiency produce more of the hormone. Until about twenty years ago there were essentially only two forms of treatment: (1) If the depression was considered to be of neurotic origin (i.e., to be caused by psychological difficulties below the level of consciousness) psychotherapy was undertaken to bring the problems to the conscious understanding of the patient so that he could then deal with them. (2) If the depression was deemed to be part of a psychosis (as in manic-depressive illness where periods of depression alternate with periods of of elation and over-activity) electric shock therapy was given followed by rest, good nursing, occupational therapy and sedatives as required.

The introduction of isoniazid for tuberculosis in 1952 was followed by curious zest in many patients and led to the realization that isoniazid and similar drugs increased the concentration of the hormone noradrenaline in the brain and relieved depression. This led in turn to the discovery that drugs like reserpine (used for the treatment of anxiety which is in some ways the reverse of depression) stimulate the formation of an enzyme, monoamine-oxidase, which destroys noradrenaline and can, if it is in excess, cause depression; drugs like isoniazid inhibit production of the enzyme and relieve depression.

The monoamine-oxidase inhibitors, generally abbreviated to MAO-inhibitors, are now widely used for the treatment of depression, as are certain other anti-depressant drugs (e.g., imipramine) which tend to increase the supply of noradrenaline. Four points should, however, be noted. – (1) Neither MAO-inhibitors nor other anti-depressant drugs are helpful unless there is a deficiency of noradrenaline to correct; the neurotic type of depression is unaffected by these drugs and still requires psychotherapy. (2) The drugs take about a week to produce effects, and the patient should therefore be warned not to discontinue them as useless. (3) For reasons not yet known patients respond differently to the various drugs, so that it may be necessary to try one drug for a week or so and then another. (4) The drugs do not cure depression; they merely temporarily correct a chemical deficiency. If the depression of psychotic type recurs, electric shock therapy may be needed to provide prolonged relief.

Derbyshire neck. A name for simple GOITRE which is fairly common in that part of England in consequence of a deficiency of iodine in the water.

dermal. Pertaining to the deeper layer of the skin, as contrasted with 'cutaneous' which refers to the superficial layer.

dermatitis. Alternatively known as eczema, this is an inflammation of the skin. It may occur in any part of the body, and takes the form of reddening of skin, the development of blisters and, if the condition becomes chronic, a thickening of the skin. External irritants are a common cause. Workers in certain trades – gardeners, bakers, french polishers and others who handle potentially irritating substances – often suffer from dermatitis on exposed parts of the body; but many people handle these substances without ill-effect, and in affected people the dermatitis often persists long after contact with the irritant has ceased. In other words, dermatitis depends on the existence both of an internal factor leading to the sensitivity and of contact with an irritant. There is also probably a strong emotional factor.

Local treatment consists mainly of the application of soothing ointments. General treatment involves either separation of the person from the irritant or an attempt at desensitization by gradually increasing injections of the offending irritant.

The term dermatitis probably covers several diseases that are not yet clearly differentiated but that are mostly related to ALLERGY. One attempt at classification is into the following types: atopic dermatitis, a patchy inflammation with itching disproportionate to the amount or severity of the inflammation; contact dermatitis, where the inflammation is on the part exposed to the particular irritant; seborrhoeic dermatitis, essentially scaly spots especially on the scalp; and sunlight dermatitis,

from exposure to more sunshine than the particular skin can stand.

dermographia. See SKIN WRITING.

desquamation. The shedding of superficial layers of the skin. This may occur after some local injury such as sunburn or in the healing of a slight burn from other causes.

The skin rashes which occur in a variety of infective fevers or as a result of sensitivity to certain drugs are an indication of general toxic damage to the skin which eventually sheds its injured cells either in a powdery fashion or as large flakes.

The desquamation which follows scarlet fever is a particularly well known example of this.

Desquamation is also the principal feature of the primary skin disease pityriasis or dermatitis exfoliativa.

development. Human development begins when a female germ-cell or ovum is fertilized by a male germ-cell or spermatozoon and proceeds by stages until the full adult status is achieved. The first 40 weeks of this progression are the period of intra-uterine development during which the fertilized ovum gradually grows from a single cell no more than 0.1 mm. in diameter to the fully-formed infant with an average length of 50 cm. (20 in.) and an average weight of 3.4 kg. (7.5 lb.).

At birth. The infant has the appearance of a miniature adult but its head is relatively larger than in the adult and the face (owing to the small size of the jaws, nasal cavity and air sinuses) forms only one-eighth of the size of the head compared with one-half in maturity. Its abdomen is also relatively larger because of the increased relative size of the liver. Its skeleton is also different since most of its 'bones' are still mainly cartilaginous; the skull bones in particular are only partially ossified and are incompletely joined together so that gaps may be felt in the skull. These gaps are known as fontanelles and the largest is the anterior fontanelle easily located in the centre of the crown of the head. It gradually diminishes in size and will generally be completely closed by 18 months.

Physical growth. The child continues to grow and to increase in size and weight from birth until about 18 years of age but the progress is not uniform. Broadly a child reaches a weight of 9 to 11 kg. (20 to 24 lbs.) by 1 year, doubles that weight by 5 years and then increases by 1.5 to 2.5 kg. (4 to 6 lb.) each year until the growth spurt at around 11 years in girls and 12 years in boys, with larger increases for the next few years. Ideally an adult should neither gain nor lose weight after the age of about 25 years, although most of us gain a little in middle age. See HEIGHT AND WEIGHT.

Tables of heights and weights of children are much used but of fairly limited value. Firstly, the tables represent averages, not optimum weights: in the first half of this century malnutrition was common in Britain (as it still is in most developing countries) so that tables of average weights were distorted by considerable numbers of undernourished children; and today an appreciable number of children are above their optimum weight, so that modern tables are distorted in the opposite direction.

Secondly, a table of average heights and weights must show three variables, not two,

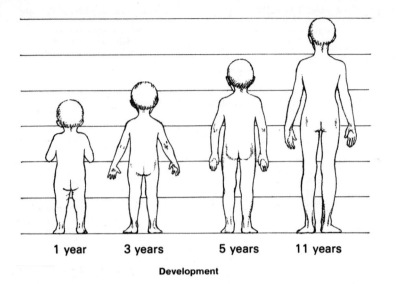

1 year   3 years   5 years   11 years

Development

with the third variable – age – acquiring increasing importance as the child grows older; thus we can perhaps say that an average child of either sex measuring 106 cm. (42 in.) weighs around 19 kg. (42 lb.) irrespective of whether he or she is a fairly tall child of 5 years or a small child of 7 years; but while tall girls of 7 years measuring 134 cm. (53 in.) might average 30.3 kg. (67 lb.), small girls of 12 years measuring the same 134 cm. would average about 32.6 kg. (72 lb). The average weights of 11 year old and 17 year old girls both of 152 cm. (60 in.) show a still more marked difference, the younger child weighing 45 kg. (100 lb.) while the older child is 4.5 kg. (10 lb.) heavier.

Thirdly, average weights, even when adjusted for height and age, have little meaning when one is considering an individual child: the big-boned son of large parents may be both taller and heavier than the average and yet be undernourished; and the child of small frame and slender bones may be adequately nourished although below the normal for his age and height. The important question is not how the child compares with a rather artificial average, but how he compares with his past performance. Is his weight gain balancing his height increase, or too little, or too much?

Dentition. Two sets of teeth are developed during growth. The first, temporary, or milk teeth totalling twenty, appear as follows:

2 lower central incisors	6 to 8 months
4 upper incisors	8 to 10 months
2 lower lateral incisors	12 to 14 months
2 upper front molars	12 to 14 months
2 lower front molars	12 to 14 months
4 canines	18 to 20 months
4 posterior molars	2 years to 2½ years

These times are subject to considerable variation. The temporary teeth are then followed by the permanent dentition (32 teeth).

4 first molars	6 years
4 central incisors	7 years
4 lateral incisors	8 years
4 anterior pre-molars	9 years
4 posterior pre-molars	10 years
4 canines	11 to 12 years
4 second molars	12 to 15 years
4 third molars	17 to 25 years

Puberty and sexual development. Puberty is the age at which reproductive organs begin to become functionally active and ushers in the period of adolescence.

In girls this may be between 10 and 14 years of age but extremes in either direction are not unusual. In boys it is slightly later. There is said to be a tendency at present for puberty to occur at earlier ages, the average onset falling by two months every decade. Possibly this is a temporary trend due to better general standards of nutrition.

The changes of puberty are brought about by the fact that the sex glands, the ovaries in girls and the testes in boys, have become mature. The internal secretions which these produce stimulate the development of secondary sex-characteristics. In girls there is pubic hair, breast development and the onset of menstruation; in boys the external sex-organs enlarge, there is growth of body and facial hair, the larynx and vocal cords enlarge and the voice 'breaks'. In both sexes, psychological changes occur. Boys become more aggressive, adventurous and addicted to active pursuits. Girls usually become more appealing and seductive. Both tend to cast off the former associates of their own sex and form friendships with members of the opposite sex.

Mental development. Intellectual capacity depends on a combination of basic inherited intelligence and its enhancement by experience. Mental development during the formative years is therefore influenced to a considerable extent by the opportunities for

Children - Heights and Weights at Various Ages (Median 50 per cent of population)

Age (years)	BOYS Height in cm. (in.)	BOYS Weight in kg. (lb.)	GIRLS Height in cm. (in.)	GIRLS Weight in kg. (lb.)
1	73.6 to 76.9 (29.0 to 30.3)	9.5 to 10.8 (20.9 to 23.8)	72.3 to 75.9 (28.5 to 29.9)	9.0 to 10.4 (19.8 to 23.0)
2	85.8 to 89.4 (33.8 to 35.2)	11.9 to 13.5 (26.3 to 29.7)	84.5 to 88.9 (33.3 to 35.0)	11.5 to 13.2 (25.3 to 29.2)
3	93.9 to 98.5 (37.0 to 38.8)	13.7 to 15.6 (30.3 to 34.5)	93.4 to 98.0 (36.8 to 38.6)	13.4 to 15.7 (29.6 to 34.6)
4	100.8 to 106.4 (39.7 to 41.9)	15.4 to 17.7 (34.0 to 39.0)	100.3 to 105.6 (39.5 to 41.6)	15.2 to 18.0 (33.5 to 39.6)
5	107.1 to 113.2 (42.2 to 44.6)	17.5 to 20.5 (38.6 to 45.3)	106.4 to 112.2 (41.9 to 44.2)	17.2 to 20.2 (38.0 to 44.5)
6	114.0 to 120.9 (44.9 to 47.6)	20.1 to 23.6 (44.4 to 52.1)	113.2 to 119.3 (44.6 to 47.0)	19.4 to 22.8 (42.9 to 50.2)
7	120.3 to 127.5 (47.4 to 50.2)	22.5 to 26.6 (49.7 to 58.7)	119.1 to 125.9 (46.9 to 49.6)	21.8 to 25.5 (48.1 to 56.3)
8	126.4 to 134.1 (49.8 to 52.8)	25.1 to 29.7 (55.5 to 65.5)	124.7 to 131.5 (49.1 to 51.8)	24.1 to 28.7 (53.1 to 63.3)
9	131.5 to 139.7 (51.8 to 55.0)	27.7 to 32.7 (61.1 to 72.3)	129.7 to 137.1 (51.1 to 54.0)	26.2 to 32.0 (57.9 to 70.5)
10	136.3 to 144.2 (53.7 to 56.8)	30.0 to 36.1 (66.3 to 79.6)	134.6 to 142.4 (53.0 to 56.1)	28.5 to 35.9 (62.8 to 79.1)
11	140.4 to 149.0 (55.3 to 58.7)	32.5 to 39.5 (71.6 to 87.2)	140.2 to 149.0 (55.2 to 58.7)	31.7 to 40.4 (69.9 to 89.1)
12	145.2 to 153.4 (57.2 to 60.4)	35.2 to 43.5 (77.5 to 96.0)	145.7 to 156.4 (57.4 to 61.6)	35.4 to 44.8 (78.0 to 98.8)
13	149.6 to 160.7 (58.9 to 63.3)	38.0 to 48.9 (83.7 to 107.9)	152.6 to 161.5 (60.1 to 63.6)	40.5 to 50.3 (89.4 to 111.0)
14	156.4 to 168.4 (61.6 to 66.3)	43.3 to 55.8 (95.5 to 123.1)	156.2 to 163.5 (61.5 to 64.4)	45.3 to 54.3 (99.8 to 119.7)
15	162.3 to 172.9 (63.9 to 68.1)	49.0 to 61.2 (108.2 to 135.0)	157.7 to 164.8 (62.1 to 64.9)	47.7 to 56.2 (105.1 to 123.9)
16	167.1 to 176.5 (65.8 to 69.5)	53.9 to 65.5 (118.7 to 144.4)	158.4 to 165.6 (62.4 to 65.2)	49.2 to 57.7 (108.4 to 127.2)

contact with and participation in the realities of the outside world.

At birth an infant responds to external stimuli in a primitive protective fashion by reflex actions. As the functional capacity of his brain develops, external stimuli are received with increasing discrimination of their significance and produce increasingly purposeful and accurate responses. The rate and extent of progress are thus affected very much by the opportunities for gaining experience; see INFANCY, PSYCHOLOGY OF.

In the very young child these are provided by contact with his mother and by being talked to and played with. As he grows he becomes influenced successively by his home surroundings, by his brothers and sisters, by his play with other children and still later by his schools, his teachers and his work and by all the other opportunities which daily life affords.

The progress of the child under 5 years of age

is now generally assessed by a consideration of his success in reaching certain 'milestones' of development. These are based on criteria related to (1) posture and large movements (2) vision and fine movements (3) hearing and speech (4) social behaviour and play.

Basic intelligence can be tested by standard intelligence tests. These permit the determination of an Intelligence Quotient which is calculated as one hundred times the mental age divided by the chronological age.

Full mental development however must aim at something more than mere ability to achieve a respectable score in standard tests of intelligence. The emphasis in modern education is towards the enhancement of creative ability. Learning by rote is no longer sufficient for the demands of modern life, and the stimuli provided by music making, dancing, claywork, picturemaking, constructional equipment and 'projects' are designed to provide the more comprehensive experience which is now required to foster the development of the abilities and competence necessary for success in an increasingly competitive and challenging environment. See also BACKWARDNESS IN CHILDREN.

dextrocardia. An unusual condition, probably always congenital, in which the position of the heart and associated blood vessels is the mirror-image of the normal, so that the heart lies slighty to the right (not the left) of the centre of the chest. As a rule the condition – diagnosed only accidentally on radiological or clinical examination – causes no harmful effects.

diabetes insipidus. A disturbance of the water-balancing mechanism of the body characterized by an enormous output of low specific gravity urine and a correspondingly great thirst for water. 'Insipidus' means 'tasteless' and marks the distinction from the ordinary type of diabetes (d. mellitus) in which the urine contains sugar and tastes sweet.

Diabetes insipidus is due to a deficient secretion of hormones by the posterior lobe of the pituitary, which is one of the ENDOCRINE GLANDS, and requires to be treated by replacement of the deficient hormone either by nasal insufflation or by injection. The treatment continues for life.

diabetes mellitus. An endocrine disease producing chronic disorder of the digestion and usage of starches and sugars. The pancreas contains special tissue known as the Islets of Langerhans which are ENDOCRINE GLANDS and produce insulin, which passes straight into the blood stream. An insufficiency of insulin damages the ability of the body to store and utilize glucose so that it remains in the blood (hyperglycaemia) and there is a loss of sugar in the urine (glycosuria). The disease is characterized by thirst, increased urinary output, emaciation and a tendency to coma.

Diabetes is an important and interesting disease. Its incidence in the community is increasing and is probably now about 1.5 per cent; about half of the cases go unrecognized until the symptoms become sufficiently noticeable to make the patient seek advice, often because of a complication such as impaired eyesight. It occurs in both sexes and at any age but it is more common after middle age.

There is an undoubted hereditary factor and diabetic tendency is inherited as a Mendelian recessive according to the laws of genetics. This is the probable explanation for its higher incidence in some communities such as Jews and certain Indian castes, where inter-marriage is common.

Apart from genetic considerations, obesity, over-eating and worry are regarded as contributory factors. The importance of the latter is well recognized and in America it has been said, and not entirely as a joke, that the incidence of diabetes varies inversely with the share prices on Wall Street!

The hereditary nature of the disease and its increasing incidence give rise to speculation as to what may happen in future generations. Before there was effective treatment about 70 per cent of adult cases died within ten years and the outlook was even worse for children. Nowadays most diabetics can be well-controlled and although their longevity is still somewhat below that of the general population most of them can be enabled to lead a fairly normal life. The implications of this are obvious.

Diabetic coma and other complications. In severe untreated diabetes the inability of the body to store and utilize sugar means that it has to derive its energy needs from other sources. Use of protein leads to tissue wasting and the abnormal use of fat causes the accumulation of poisonous subtances in the blood and these produce diabetic coma.

Other complications of diabetes are increased susceptibility to infections, neuritis, cataract and retinitis, gastric and renal disorder, myocarditis, and vascular disease sometimes causing gangrene of the extremities.

Treatment. Mild diabetics may often be controlled by dietary measures alone. The aim is to give a balanced but adequate diet and restrict carbohydrate foods to the minimum. If sugar loss in the urine cannot be prevented by this means, it will be necessary to give a suitable dose of insulin by injection. The development of slow-release types of insulin has reduced the number of injections required to one or two per day.

The discovery and subsequent commercial preparation of insulin by Banting and Best in 1921 is one of the great triumphs of scientific medicine. Until about 1954 insulin was the only effective treatment for diabetes but since then certain drugs have become available which may be taken by mouth. The first of these were compounds of sulphonylurea which acted by stimulating remnants of functioning pancreatic tissue to produce more insulin.

Others drugs have subsequently been developed. Their mode of action is less well understood but they appear to increase the activity on cells of any insulin still being produced by the pancreas. These drugs are mainly of use in certain cases of mild diabetes of late onset. Their success is dependent on the continued presence of at least some functioning insulin-producing tissue.

Insulin coma (Hypoglycaemia). Overdosage of insulin, or delay in taking food after an injection, or excessive exercise, may lead to a serious fall in blood sugar with symptoms of weakness, muscular tremors, drowsiness and ultimately coma. The swallowing of sugar leads to rapid recovery and well-instructed diabetics who are taking insulin will be made aware of the condition and the appropriate emergency action. In other circumstances the differentiation between diabetic coma and insulin coma may be difficult.

'Renal diabetes'. Not all cases of glycosuria are due to diabetes mellitus. In certain individuals the kidney has a lowered 'leak-point' for the elimination of sugar so that sugar appears in the urine even with a normal blood sugar level.

This is an individual idiosyncrasy; it causes no symptoms and requires no treatment. It is sometimes referred to as diabetes innocens.

Community surveys. Since there are at least as many unrecognized diabetics as those which have been diagnosed, and since the treatment is fully understood and very successful, there is great scope for organized measures of detection. Populations can be asked to provide urine samples which are simply and easily tested for glycosuria. Those who show a positive reaction are then given further tests to differentiate between renal glycosuria and true diabetes; the patient eats a known amount of glucose and the urine is tested every half hour to see how the body is dealing with it.

diagnosis. The term is used in two senses. Primarily it refers to the procedure, partly an art but increasingly a science, which a physician employs to assess the symptoms and signs presented by a patient and to identify the disease from which he is suffering. It can also refer to the actual disease as, for instance, in answer to the question 'What is the diagnosis?'

Diagnosis as a procedure is fundamental to the effective practice of medicine and surgery and on its accuracy depends the best hope of rational and effective treatment.

Before the advent of supplementary aids to diagnosis a physician had to depend on what he could learn by questioning the patient and on the signs which he could recognize during the actual examination.

The interrogation or case-history is of great importance and should cover general matters such as age, occupation, marital status, family history, personal history (environment and habits) and previous health. This is then supplemented by more detailed enquiry regarding the actual symptoms. The nature and scope of these further questions will be governed by a preliminary and provisional assessment of which particular system of the body is at fault.

Even before proceeding to physical examination the skilled diagnostician will have taken note of the general appearance, demeanour and behaviour of his patient since these may often afford valuable clues. Complexion, attitude (standing or in bed), voice, restlessness, development, nutrition and gait should all be noted.

In the physical examination much can be learned by a systematic visual survey supplemented by careful feeling with an educated sense of touch. A sharp tap on the surface of the body elicits a sound which is either resonant or dull according to the nature or condition of the underlying structures. This is known as percussion, and by this means the borders of organs can be mapped out and an opinion formed as to their condition. Auscultation is the procedure by which the physician listens to what is going on within the body and this can afford helpful information about the state of the heart and its valves, of the lungs and sometimes also of the digestive tract. Originally this was done by directly applying an ear to the part being examined.

In relation to the nervous system physical examination entails an assessment of the patient's special senses, touch, taste, sight, hearing, balance and co-ordination, together with an examination of both voluntary and reflex movements.

Aids to diagnosis. So far the procedures described have been dependent entirely on the physician making use of his own unaided senses guided by experience and knowledge. The development of more precise diagnosis has followed the development of ever more sophisticated items of equipment.

The first of these was the clinical thermometer, since elevation of the body temperature is an important indication of fever due to some infection. Direct auscultation was a difficult and unsatisfactory procedure until Laennec's invention of the stethoscope (1819), which transmitted sound to the doctor's ears from a sound-piece which could be applied to the body. Blood pressure estimations were made possible by the invention of the sphygmomanometer and availability of small battery-operated light sources led to the development of various instruments which extended the scope of examination of the eyes and body orifices. The variety, complexity, capacity and performance of such instruments continues to extend.

Perhaps the greatest single advance was the discovery of x-rays by Roentgen in 1895 and x-ray apparatus of increasing power and capabilities, assisted by the use of appropriate contrast media, now facilitates the examination of almost every part of the body. Electrocardiographs and electroencephalographs record the electrical activity of heart and brain and provide a visual 'trace' which records their functional condition. Other appliances are used to measure respiratory capacity and metabolism and even radio-isotopes and ultra-sound are used for other types of investigation.

Laboratory aids. Laboratory investigations are dependent on the work of the bacteriologist, the histologist, and the biochemist who deal respectively with the presence or effects of bacteria and other invaders, the changes in tissue brought about by disease, and abnormalities of body chemistry.

The information provided by appropriate tests is often essential, not only to confirm a tentative diagnosis but to assess the progress of treatment and its likelihood of success.

Community diagnosis. The procedures previously outlined have been concerned with the management of an individual patient but many diseases may be present in latent form before they give rise to symptoms. Pre-diagnostic screening of sections of the population holds prospects of detecting latent conditions before they give rise to actual disease so that appropriate early treatment can be instituted.

The first great successes of such a concept were the mass radiography campaigns of the detection of tuberculosis, but screening procedures are now used for a variety of other diseases such as diabetes and carcinoma of the uterine cervix, and more elaborate forms of 'health-check' are being pioneered or being employed in the care of selected groups with special risks.

One important advance with great potentialities would be the development of a simple routine test for latent cancer of any site and there are prospects that a practicable routine procedure for this purpose will be developed eventually.

diaphoretics. Drugs which increase the amount of perspiration; they can act either on the central nervous system or on the blood vessels in the skin. Diaphoretics are given either to bring down a feverish temperature by increased evaporation of sweat, or to compensate for failing urinary secretion. However, better drugs are now available for both purposes and specific use of traditional diaphoretics has greatly declined.

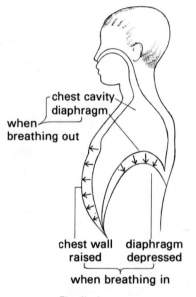

The diaphragm

diaphragm. The dome shaped musculo-fibrous partition which separates the abdominal cavity below from the cavities of the chest above. The diaphragm is the principal muscle of RESPIRATION. It is attached below to the lumbar vertebrae, sternum and lower ribs.

Occasionally, part of the diaphragm is congenitally deficient or weak allowing some of the abdominal contents to protrude into the lower part of the chest cavity. This is known as a diaphragmatic or hiatus hernia which requires surgical treatment if it gives rise to serious symptoms.

diaphysis. See EPIPHYSIS.

diarrhoea. A disorder of bowel function characterized by the frequent evacuation of loose, fluid or semi-fluid stools. Severe cases may be accompanied by the passage of blood and mucus or by tenesmus which is a painful and ineffectual straining in the attempt to pass stools.

Causes. Diarrhoea is a common type of illness at all ages (in fact INFANTILE DIARRHOEA is a significant cause of death during the first year) and its possible causes are both numerous and diverse. Normally the entry of food into an empty stomach produces a reflex which results in the pelvic colon being emptied once a day after breakfast but an over-active reflex may cause loose stools after every meal. This is post-prandial or lienteric diarrhoea, and in a somewhat similar fashion a sudden fright or emotional stress may cause nervous diarrhoea.

Apart from infections the commonest cause of diarrhoea is excess or unsuitable food, such as eating unripe fruit, which irritates the intestine chemically or mechanically.

If there is a lack of hydrochloric acid in the stomach (achlorhydria) insufficiently digested food may be passed on from there to the intestine to set up irritation both mechanically and by fermentation. Excessive use of laxatives is another possibility, and many poisonous substances may irritate the bowel.

Diarrhoea also often accompanies disease of the bowel or of its associated digestive glands. Chronic peritonitis, tuberculosis, mucous and ulcerative colitis, cancer and pancreatic and biliary insufficiency are examples.

It may occur too in general diseases of the heart, lungs or liver where there is interference with the general venous or portal circulation, or in kidney disease with uraemia where toxins usually excreted in the urine pass through the bowel and upset its normal function.

Infection, however, is by far the commonest cause and the agents responsible include viruses, the organisms causing dysentery (both bacillary and amoebic), food poisoning, typhoid fever, and cholera.

Accurate diagnosis depends on bacteriological, chemical and microscopic examination of the stool with perhaps the aid of x-ray or examination of the bowel if organic disease is suspected.

Treatment. This largely depends upon the cause but attacks of acute diarrhoea should be regarded as infective until proved otherwise and precautions taken to protect other persons.

The routine treatment of simple cases of diarrhoea suspected of being infective is usually based on a kaolin or chalk mixture which absorbs toxins and allays intestinal irritation, and on the administration of antibiotics. Since there is fluid loss in the stools adequate fluids should be given. Sweetened drinks such as barley water with 1 teaspoonful of salt added to every litre (2 pints) are useful.

In severe diarrhoea a danger is dehydration from excessive loss of fluid and this is especially so in infants who rapidly collapse from this cause. The same is true of cases of cholera. Because of the extreme diarrhoea fluid replacement by mouth is usually ineffectual and intravenous infusions of a suitable solution will be required.

diastole. See SYSTOLE.

diathesis. A particular constitution or functional response of the body which makes a person more than usually susceptible to certain diseases.

The term has in the past been applied rather indiscriminately as an explanation for the development of a wide range of diseases. Modern opinion is less dogmatic but on the basis of clinical experience there is perhaps some justification for the following:

Tuberculous diathesis characterized by fair skin and hair, long eyelashes, 'peaches-and-cream' complexion, long narrow chest and slender configuration. Rheumatic diathesis: fair skin and red hair. Exudative diathesis: infantile eczema followed by asthma in later life. Gouty diathesis: hereditary predisposition to gout. Gastric diathesis: hyper motile stomach with excessive secretion of hydrochloric acid; alert over-anxious type with lantern-jaw and deeply-lined facial features.

diet. An individual's customary daily intake of FOOD and drink.

The body requires food for several purposes: as fuel for the production of body-heat and muscular energy, as raw material for the growth, replacement, and repair of tissue, and as a source of the mineral salts, vitamins, and liquid necessary for the vital processes of the cells.

Since foods differ in composition they provide for these needs to different extents, so that a person requires not only an adequate total amount of food but a proper balance of the basic nutrients.

Proteins. These are needed for growth and repair of tissues. An adult of average size requires about 90 g. (3 oz.) of protein daily, of which at least half should be of animal origin. As explained under PROTEIN no vegetable protein contains all the essential amino-acids, so a complete vegetarian needs about 150 g. (5 oz.) of well mixed plant proteins. In proportion to size children need two or three times as much protein as adults, with at least 60 per cent of animal origin (including, of course, protein from milk, eggs, cheese and fish as well as meat).

No foods consists wholly, or even mainly, of protein. Most cheeses, the foods of highest protein content, are roughly one-third protein, one-third fat, and one-third water. An egg is about 12 per cent protein, so that a hen's egg weighing 50 g. provides 6 g. of protein. Lean bacon and lean beef are about 25 per cent protein. Milk is about 3.5 per cent protein, so 300 g. (10 oz.) of milk provide about 10 g. of animal protein. In an affluent society we can get three-quarters of our daily requirements of animal protein from a breakfast egg, a generous helping (60 g.) of bacon and about 300 g. of milk during the day, and a fairly small helping of meat, fish or cheese later in the day will complete our requirements. Alternatively, if we prefer a cereal breakfast 160 g. of meat (5½ oz.) and the same amount of milk will meet our needs.

As for plant protein, bread is about 6.5 per cent protein, potatoes about 2.2 per cent, broad beans and dried peas approximately 20 per cent protein (although not wholly absorbed in digestion) and most vegetables and fruits contain a little protein.

In affluent communities protein deficiency is rare. Apart from a few food cranks, people who can afford sufficient animal protein usually have plenty of protein in their diet. Excess protein is less likely to cause obesity than is excess of other foods, because the unrequired protein is largely excreted, in cases of great excess causing diarrhoea. Poor people in developed countries often have diets inadequate in animal protein and are sometimes unaware of the importance and relative cheapness (in some countries at least) of milk, cheese and eggs. In underdeveloped countries insufficiency of protein is a widespread, major nutritional problem.

Fats. Although it is sometimes said that the average adult in a temperate climate needs about 90 g. of FAT daily – or about the same as his protein requirement – there is little scientific evidence of minimum need, except that the diet requires to contain sufficient fat to supply adequate quantities of the fat-soluble vitamins. Butter and margarine are about 80 per cent fat, and other rich sources are meat fat, fatty fish and cheese. The burning up of fat takes place only in the presence of sufficient carbohydrate, and consumption of fat to an amount disproportionate to carbohydrate leads to indigestion. On the other hand persons living in extremely cold climates appear to be able to consume enormous amounts of fats.

Apart from being needed for their vitamin content, fats are required to prevent the diet from becoming too bulky. Not only does an ounce of fat provide more Calories than an ounce of protein and an ounce of carbohydrate together, but most protein foods and starchy foods contain very considerable amounts of water. A fat-free diet of 3,000 Calories daily would involve enormous meals.

In recent years it has been suggested that too much animal fat (e.g., from butter, cheese and meat fat) raises the blood cholesterol level and may predispose to coronary thrombosis, and that about half of the total intake of fat should be obtained from vegetable oils.

Excess deposition of fat in parts of the body is generally caused not by over-eating of fats but by over-eating of carbohydrates. The body stores excess of sugar, or of starch which is converted to sugar, as fat.

Carbohydrates. These are the starches and sugars, all eventually broken down by digestion to glucose and then stored mainly in the liver and muscles as the polysaccharide glycogen. When required, glycogen is reconstituted as glucose and oxidized to provide muscular energy and heat.

Sugar is of course entirely carbohydrate except for a trace of moisture; flour varies from 70 to 75 per cent carbohydrate; potatoes are approximately 20 per cent carbohydrate; the proportion in fruits varies from nearly 20 per cent in bananas to just under 3 per cent in tomatoes; and in common vegetables the proportion ranges from 10 per cent in carrots to about 5 per cent in turnips.

Excessive carbohydrate is converted into fat in the body and stored as fat in the tissues. During periods in which food intake is insufficient, to balance energy requirements the fat stores are reconverted into carbohydrate and then utilized for energy.

In developed countries 50 to 70 per cent of the total Calories are usually derived from carbohydrates; and the carbohydrate foods consumed in greatest quantities include wheat, corn, rice, barley, potatoes and other vegetables and fruits. Increased usage of cane and beet sugar, white flour and polished rice produces risk of obesity and also risk of nutritional hazards from decreased intake of minerals and vitamins.

If the common dietetic danger of the poor is protein deficiency, that of those not on the

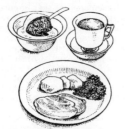

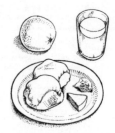

MEAL 1 (containing 740 calories)
70g. (2.5 oz.) roast beef
170g. (6 oz.) boiled potatoes
110g. (4 oz.) cabbage
85g. (3 oz.) raisin suet pudding
55g. (2 oz.) custard sauce
0.25 litres (0.5 pt.) tea
(food values on chart shown ▮▮▮)

MEAL 2 (containing 790 Calories)
100g. (3.5 oz.) bread or rolls
15g. (0.5 oz.) butter
55g. (2 oz.) cheese
0.25 litres (0.5 pt.) milk
an orange
(food values on chart shown ▨▨)

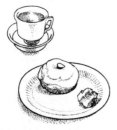

MEAL 3 (containing 436 Calories)
100g. (3.5 oz.) bun
15g. (0.5 oz.) butter
0.25 litres (0.5 pt.) tea
(food values on chart shown ▧▧)

protein	1 2 3	
calcium	1 2 3	
vitamin **A**	1 2 3	
thiamin	1 2 3	
riboflavin	1 2 3	
vitamin **C**	1 2 3	
vitamin **D**	1 2 3	nil

Diet: three meals, showing the food values of each

poverty line is carbohydrate excess leading to obesity.

Vitamins. These comprise certain organic substances necessary for normal metabolism and variously present in many foodstuffs. They do not form a chemically related class of compounds and they range from the relatively simple ascorbic acid (vitamin c) to much more complicated molecules.

An adult requires about five thousand international units of vitamin A daily, about 1.5 mg. of aneurin (vitamin B_1), approximately 2 mg. of riboflavine and 15 mg. of nicotinic acid (components of the vitamin B_2 complex), about 55 mg. of ascorbic acid (vitamin c) and about 100 international units of vitamin D. Vitamin excess can occur with vitamins A and D. Vitamin deficiency is, even in developed countries, still relatively common in children and old people. See VITAMINS.

Minerals. The body requires a variety of MINERAL SALTS. Sodium, potassium, magnesium, and phosphorus are present in adequate amounts in any ordinary diet and need no special attention. There may, however, be deficiencies of calcium, iron, or iodine. Calcium is required for bones and teeth; children should have at least 1 g. per day and the best source is milk. Iron is essential for the synthesis of haemoglobin and insufficiency leads to anaemia. The daily requirement is 15 to 20 mg. and the best sources are meat, eggs and certain vegetables, especially spinach. Iodine is needed for the production of thyroid hormone and deficiency leads to goitre. Sea foods are the chief natural source but many brands of ordinary table salt contain added sodium iodine (1 in 100,000) and provide for the small daily requirement of 15 micrograms.

Other 'trace-elements' needed are cobalt, manganese and copper but they are rarely lacking from human diets although some are of importance in animal husbandry. Special interest also attaches to the element fluorine, lack of which reduces the resistance of tooth enamel to decay.

Roughage or fibre. The indigestible residues of diet are mainly fibrous material derived from vegetable food. Until recently little attention has been paid to the role of ROUGHAGE in the diet but it is becoming clear that it is important in maintaining the bulk and plasticity of faeces and that modern low-residue diets are a main cause of constipation which in turn is associated with varicose veins, haemorrhoids, and various diseases of the colon.

Amount of food. Heat production and muscular activity are forms of energy derived by the body from the METABOLISM or 'burning' of its food, and the amount of food eaten must be sufficient to provide for an individual's energy requirements.

The energy value of any foodstuff is measured in CALORIES which are units of heat. A person at rest in a normal environment expends a certain amount of energy merely to maintain his temperature, circulation, respiration and other vital functions. This basic demand for fuel is his basal metabolism, quite easily measured physiologically by recording oxygen consumption.

The basal metabolism of the average man calls for about 1100 Calories per day but in addition provision must be made for the energy expended daily in his normal life. This varies widely according to environmental temperature and the amount of exercise taken.

Heat is an expensive form of energy – more so than exercise. Eskimos and polar explorers need a large Calorie intake. This can be illustrated by the fact that 1000 watts of electrical energy used by a one-bar electric fire is equivalent to more than 1 horse-power.

The average total Calorie requirement in various circumstances can be stated approximately as follows: sedentary life: 2,200 Calories; light work 2,300 to 2,900 Calories; moderate work 3,000 to 3,500 Calories; heavy work 3,600 to 6,000 Calories.

It should be noted that it is not necessary to have a large, elaborately-prepared meal to ensure the best food value, as is clearly demonstrated by the example on p. 132 of three possible meals, showing the Calorie content and the important food values of each.

Energy balance. The laws of the conservation of energy demand that an organism must obtain an amount of energy, in utilizable form, equal to the amount which it expends.

Animals, including man, carry a body reserve of energy in the form of fat, stored mainly in the subcutaneous tissues where it also provides thermal insulation, mechanical protection and a cosmetic function. This store is both large and variable. An average male may have 16 per cent of his body weight as fat and this represents a reserve of perhaps 100,000 Calories, very adequate in relation to his daily turnover of (say) 3,000 Calories, but an obese person may be 65 per cent fat which is grossly excessive. Fluctuations in the daily intake-output balance are compensated for by this reserve.

However since adults may eat as much as half-a-ton of food per year some mechanism is required to ensure that small daily excesses do not build up to an impossible extent. This is dependent on appetite, at least partially indicative of the body's need for food, and controlled by centres in the mid-brain. The effectiveness of this control can be affected by over-indulgence in attractive foods or by using food as a solace for psychological stresses. In these circumstances obesity results and there is also evidence that over-feeding in infancy

increases the number and capacity of fat cells so that they store fat more readily in adult life.

Civilization leads to an increased intake of readily available food and to reduced energy output as we replace internal production of heat by a controlled environment (e.g., central heating) and substitute transport and machinery for walking and manual labour.

All these are factors which tend to increase obesity – perhaps the major dietary problem of the age.

diets, special. The treatment of various diseases may sometimes be influenced beneficially by dietary adjustments designed to add or exclude certain factors. Diets specifically so prescribed are known as special diets and although many may only reflect a current fashion or the personal fad of a particular physician there are at least some basic regimes based on recognized physiological principles.

Light or milk diet. Commonly prescribed for any invalid or convalescent or in the treatment of gastric or duodenal ulceration, gastritis, or other disorders of the gastro-intestinal tract. The basic constituent is usually milk with the addition of easily digested foods, such as eggs, chicken, fish, potatoes and so on. Milk diets or modified milk diets given at short intervals are frequently used in the treatment of acute gastric ulcer with the intention of continuously neutralizing gastric juice and are sometimes associated with the names of Sippy, Meulengracht or Witt.

In general, foods with indigestible residues, spices and fried dishes are excluded. Supplements of vitamins and minerals should be added.

Salt-free diet. It is difficult to exclude salt entirely but low salt diets are recommended for kidney disease and hypertension. Bacon, ham, salted butter, cheese and bread should be avoided, and no salt used in cooking or at table.

Low-protein diet. Some varieties of chronic kidney disease lead to nitrogen retention, the forerunner of uraemia. Nitrogen is derived from protein and so meat, fish, eggs, milk and cheese are restricted.

High-protein diet. In kidney disease with marked albuminuria, excessive protein loss occurs and this is compensated for by allowing up to 0.5 kg. (1 lb.) per day of meat or fish. It is also desirable to reduce fats and therefore eggs and full cream milk are unsuitable. This regime is known as Epstein's diet.

Extra protein is also indicated in certain liver diseases and during recovery from wasting conditions.

Low-carbohydrate diet. Used in the reduction of obesity; bread, cakes, confectionery, sugar, potatoes and cereals are eliminated or reduced in this diet.

High-fat or ketogenic diet. Formerly this diet was used in treatment of epilepsy. It had been noted that epileptics had fewer fits if they were starved and became acidotic and since excess fats cause acidosis due to incomplete metabolism producing ketone bodies, such a ketogenic diet enjoyed a vogue as a means of treatment. It is now largely out-moded by modern anti-convulsant drugs.

Since acid substances appeared in the urine it was also used for treatment of urinary infections, but again better methods are now available.

Low-fat diet. Recommended for gall stones and other disorders of liver and gall bladder as well as for arteriosclerosis, in which fatty deposits collect on the artery walls. Butter, cheese, milk, fatty and fried foods are excluded. In arteriosclerosis it is particularly desirable to exclude the saturated fats of animal origin.

Gluten-free diet. In abdominal disease patients cannot digest gluten, a protein found mainly in wheat products. Gluten-free bread (from which the gluten part of the cereal has been removed) is obtainable and other carbohydrates such as rice and tapioca are permissible.

Diabetic diet. Diabetic patients require restriction of carbohydrate intake. A specific regime requires to be worked out for individual patients.

High-calcium diet. Pregnant and nursing mothers require to double their intake of calcium, and this is best supplied in the form of additional milk and cheese. See also VEGETARIAN DIET.

digestion. The process by which the alimentary tract breaks down the elements of food and prepares them for absorption into the blood stream so that they may be utilized by the body in its vital functions; see METABOLISM. Digestion combines both mechanical action – chewing, swallowing and movement by the stomach and intestines – and chemical action by ferments and similar substances.

The constituents of FOOD requiring digestion are proteins, carbohydrates and fats: the parts of the DIGESTIVE SYSTEM concerned in dealing with them in varying degrees are the mouth, stomach and small intestine.

Proteins. Protein molecules consist of linked chains of amino-acids. In the stomach, hydrochloric acid and pepsin break protein down into proteoses and peptones, and another ferment, rennin, coagulates milk for subsequent attack by pepsin. Further protein digestion occurs in the small intestine where the ferment trypsin breaks down the proteoses and peptones from the stomach into successively smaller groups of amino-acids (polypeptids and peptids), and finally, by the action of erepsin, into individual amino-acids suitable for assimilation. Trypsin and amylopsin are secreted in the pancreatic juice; erepsin is present in the intestinal secretion.

Absorption of the amino-acids occurs mainly in the small intestine, where they pass into the body through fine projections known as villi.

Carbohydrates. These are the starches and sugars. The ferment ptyalin in the saliva acts upon starches converting them to the disaccharide maltose. Further digestion of starches and sugars then occurs in the small intestine where the pancreatic ferment amylopsin and the intestinal ferments sucrase, maltase and lactase finally convert them to glucose ready for absorption.

Some absorption of simple sugars takes place in the stomach, which is the reason why sugar is given when energy is required quickly, the only food rapidly absorbed being alcohol. Most carbohydrates, however, are – like proteins – absorbed in the small intestine.

Fats. Fats are almost entirely dealt with by the small intestine. A ferment lipase, acting upon fats, is secreted by the stomach but, except in infants, its action is weak. In the intestine fats are emulsified by bile and then

split by the pancreatic ferment lipase. The products of fat digestion are fatty acids and glycerin. These are absorbed by the epithelial cells of the intestine and reconstituted as neutral fats. Only a small fraction of these synthesized fats passes directly into the portal blood stream. The rest is taken up by the lymphatic system and then reaches the main blood stream via the main lymphatic channel (thoracic duct) which discharges into the venous system at the junction of the left subclavian and left internal jugular veins.

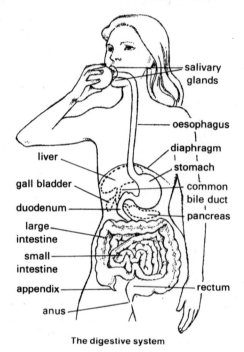

The digestive system

digestive system. In order to maintain life and provide for all its vital activities the body requires FOOD but it cannot utilize the ordinary substances of a normal diet until these are broken down into simpler elements capable of absorption into the blood stream for subsequent distribution to the tissues. The process by which food is thus broken down is known as DIGESTION, and this process, as well as absorption, is carried out by the digestive system, a term which comprehensively includes the several parts of the food canal together with associated organs such as the salivary glands, pancreas and liver.

The first part of the system is the mouth equipped with jaws and teeth. Teeth are of two basic types: incisors or cutting tools serving to bite off convenient portions of food, and molars designed to grind it down into smaller particles. The teeth are set in the upper and lower jaws which are fixed and moveable respectively so that the grinding action can take place by muscular action.

Food taken into the mouth is said to be ingested and the function of the mouth, jaws and teeth is to chew small quantities of food and, in breaking it down, to mix it with saliva, a digestive ferment supplied by three pairs of salivary glands known as the parotid, sub-maxillary and sublingual glands. Saliva also assists in the formation of the food into a slippery mass or bolus of a size suitable for swallowing (deglutition).

When prepared in this way the bolus enters the pharynx which is a cavity common to both the air- and food-passages and which provides arrangements for ensuring that the food does not get into the larynx but instead correctly enters the oesophagus or gullet, a muscular tube traversing the chest in its downward passage to the stomach.

In the stomach, which acts as a reservoir, food is delayed for some four hours while it undergoes preliminary digestion. The stomach walls contain cells which provide hydrochloric acid and the ferments rennin, pepsin and lipase.

The lower opening of the stomach is controlled by a muscular ring or sphincter known as the pylorus. Food released from the stomach next traverses the small intestine, a convoluted musculo-membranous tube some 6 m. (20 ft.) in length. The intestine is lined with mucous membrane which is not smooth but composed of innumerable fine projections known as villi disposed like the pile of a piece of velvet.

The intestine secretes a digestive fluid, the succus entericus, produced by glands whose mouths open into the intestinal lumen at the bases of the villi.

The parts of the small intestine are known successively as duodenum, jejunum and ileum and in the upper duodenum is an opening, the ampulla of Vater, which represents the junction of the common bile-duct with the pancreatic duct and through which bile from the liver and pancreatic juice from the pancreas enter the intestine. Bile serves to emulsify fats and pancreatic juice provides certain ferments; together they help to complete digestion initiated in the stomach.

Food is moved along the intestine by waves of muscular contraction – peristalsis – and ultimately reaches the lower end of the ileum. From there it passes by the ileo-caecal valve into the caecum and thence to the large intestine. The material reaching the large intestine is food which has been fully digested and stripped of its nutriments by absorption in the small intestine.

The large intestine, which comprises successively the ascending, transverse and descending colon and finally the rectum is some 1.5 m. (5 ft.) in length. It absorbs water from the fluid material reaching it from above and forms waste matter into a semi-solid state suitable for evacuation through the anus as faeces.

The functioning of the digestive tract as a whole is under both nervous control from the sympathetic and autonomic nervous systems, and chemical control by the hormones, (gastrin, secretin, cholecystokinin, and entero-gastrone) secreted by ductless glands in the walls of the stomach and small intestine.

Diseases. Diseases affecting the tract from the mouth to the anus may include those due to general causes such as infections and malignant change, but some conditions are peculiar to the stomach and intestines.

Of these the commonest is ulceration which may be either gastric or duodenal. In this condition the lining of these organs is itself locally digested by the digestive ferments, which produces ulceration. This is particularly apt to occur in tense and nervous persons and is recognized as a typical psychosomatic disease. The ulceration may cause haemorrhage or perforation and then requires emergency treatment. Chronic gastritis results usually from over-eating or over-indulgence in alcohol.

The colon is subject to two types of chronic disease: simple colitis usually caused by excessive dependence on laxatives, and ulcerative colitis, mainly affecting the lower end of the colon. In the latter there is abdominal pain and often severe diarrhoea with the evacuation of blood and mucus. A potential risk is perforation which requires emergency treatment.

digitalis. A drug, originally obtained from the powdered leaf of the foxglove, with a specific action on heart muscle: slowing its rate of contraction and increasing the strength of contractions. Curiously its earliest recorded uses were quite ineffective for the treatment of tuberculosis, not very effective for the production of vomiting and later (in 1785) moderately effective for increasing the flow of urine. In the nineteenth century its effect on heart muscle became recognized and it was thereafter widely used in cases of failing circulation.

It was, and to some extent still is, given in the form of a tincture, i.e., essentially a solution of the powder in alcohol, and it is valuable in various heart diseases, especially auricular fibrillation. To a considerable degree, however, it is now replaced by drugs derived from it, such as digitalin in which the exact strength is more easily measured and the derived drug is usually given by injection.

Digitalis is not useful in all forms of heart disease: where the heart muscle is exhausted to give digitalis is equivalent to whipping a tired horse. Also the drug is not easily destroyed or excreted by the body and therefore can have a cumulative action. So it should be used only under strict medical supervision.

Poisoning or overdosage is suggested by failure of appetite, going on to nausea and vomiting, and by some irregularities of the pulse. Unless there is considerable vomiting an emetic may help, followed by strong tea or coffee, but the most important measure is temporarily stopping the doses of digitalis.

diphtheria. An infectious disease caused by the diphtheria bacillus (*Corynebacterium diphtheria*) and characterized by inflammation of the fauces or larynx with a typical fibrinous exudate ('wash-leather' exudate) and often by severe general symptoms produced by the effect of toxins on the heart muscle and the peripheral nerves.

It was formerly a common endemic disease of children usually causing a long, serious, and tedious illness which often ended in death, but since about 1940 a generàl policy of active immunization has resulted in its virtual eradication from all countries with an adequate health service.

Laryngeal diphtheria causes special difficulties because of obstruction to respiration and may require tracheotomy. Otherwise the treatment is by complete bed rest and the administration of diphtheria anti-toxin and penicillin.

Active immunization involves a course of usually three suitably-spaced injections of diphtheria toxoid starting at about 4 months of age. Further 'booster' doses are usually given at school entry and again at about 9 years of age. Diphtheria toxoid is a component of 'triple antigen' which provides simultaneous protection against diphtheria, whooping cough and tetanus.

The Schick test is a skin test for susceptibility to diphtheria but it is now seldom used. If injection with a small amount of diphtheria toxin produces a limited area of redness it constitutes a positive reaction indicating the need for protection by active immunization.

The carrier state is common in diphtheria epidemics and such people must be sought for and isolated. The bacillus is also occasionally found in unusual situations e.g., in rhinitis, conjunctivitis, or in infected wounds.

diplopia. A disorder of vision in which the patient sees single objects as double.

Each eye forms a separate image on its own retina and for these images to become fused in accurate binocular vision the visual axes of both eyes must be truly directed at the object or 'point of fixation'.

If any of the muscles moving the eyeballs are paralysed, weakened, or uncoordinated, this will not be achieved and the patient then 'sees' two objects.

This is binocular diplopia and the double vision disappears on closing one eye.

In monocular diplopia, which is much less common, two images are formed on the retina of one eye and this can result from irregular refraction, early cataract, dislocated lens or the congenital condition of double pupil.

dipsomania. An intermittent craving for alcohol which is then taken in excess to the point of severe intoxication. It is a compulsion neurosis usually related to conditions of mental stress or depression. The frequency of attacks varies with circumstances.

A chronic alcoholic has come to be dependent on alcohol as a drug of addiction but the dipsomaniac between bouts may appear to be quite normal. Nevertheless the condition is an indication of a manic-depressive personality, and proper psychiatric supervision is desirable.

disabling diseases. Almost any chronic disease can produce some measure of disablement. In a child disablement is some condition which precludes his education in a normal school. An adult of employable age is disabled if, on account of injury, disease or congenital deformity, he is substantially handicapped in obtaining or keeping employment. After pensionable age a severely disabled person is someone who by reason of physical or mental disability requires continual supervision and attention.

A broad classification is as follows: (1) disease of the heart and circulation; (2) diseases of the lungs and respiratory system; (3) diseases of digestion and assimilation; (4) diseases of the nervous system such as epilepsy, and disseminated sclerosis; (5) mental deficiency and mental illness; (6) diseases and injuries of the skeletal and locomotory system such as osteo-arthritis or loss of limbs; (7)

endocrine disorders, and obesity; (8) chronic nephritis; (9) defects of the special senses, especially blindness, partial sightedness and deafness.

discharging ears. See EAR.

disease. The World Health Organization in its constitution defines health as 'a state of complete physical mental and social well-being, and not merely the absence of disease or infirmity'. To regard disease as merely the opposite of health raises a philosophical conflict because it is absurd to assert that all are diseased who do not conform to the World Health Organization ideal.

We must therefore recognize that between health and disease there exists an intermediate state in which individuals may fall short of what is a desirable ideal but nevertheless are free from pain and disability and not unduly impeded in the normal activities of their lives. Many factors and conditions operate to maintain this intermediate borderland, and their correction lies perhaps more in the field of health education than in that of clinical medicine. In expecting to eliminate them entirely we may be no better than Horace's yokel waiting for the river to flow away.

While any attempt to define disease as absence of full health would clearly be too wide it is almost equally easy to err in the direction of being too narrow.

A statement that disease is a condition of the body (or of some part or organ) in which its functions are disturbed or deranged, would really limit disease to conditions which result from such things as infections, toxins, degenerative processes and accidents, and which are detectable by the doctor or laboratory scientist. It takes no account of conditions of inferior health of which both clinician and patient may be unaware and which may be undetectable by any laboratory investigation; it also overlooks diminution in physiological reserves, and the reaction of the body to the stresses of modern life. Above all it omits any reference to 'social illness' which is really a psychological rather than physical disorder. The mental make-up of the individual is apparently healthy but he reacts in a fashion which is at variance with the accepted pattern of society; such persons provide the delinquents, the problem children and the problem parents, the neurotics, hypo-chondriacs and escapists.

The struggle against disease. Disease of some kind or other is a universal experience of mankind. Although its variety, nature, and incidence vary from country to country a broad but sometimes an overlapping classification is possible into (1) inherited disorders, (2) infections, (3) nutritional disorders, (4) diseases due to environmental factors, (5) conditions due to violence, (6) degenerations and (7) mental illness.

Measures against disease can be taken at two levels. Clinical medicine sets out to treat the individual patient who already is diseased. Community medicine or public health, on a more rational basis, seeks to eradicate the causes of disease. In underdeveloped countries with their huge populations, their vast burden of ill-health and their scanty medical facilities, only community action holds any prospect of effective action; and even in highly developed countries it is generally true that prevention is cheaper than cure, as well as pleasanter.

The first essential in disease control is accurate information about its causes and incidence. Great progress has been made thereby, especially in the control of infections and infectious disease. The procedures are clear-cut and relatively cheap and easy to apply. Smallpox has been almost eradicated from the world by vaccination, and programmes aiming at the control of diseases spread by insect carriers (such as malaria, yellow fever, and plague) can be assured of spectacular success.

Much could also be achieved by a determined attack on nutritional inadequacies. Probably a third of the world population is still under-nourished on a Calorie basis and more than half has less than enough daily protein in its diet. The supply of sufficient food for all is, however, more difficult to achieve because of the economic implications.

The ecological problem. In nature the survival of any species is the result of its successful struggle with its environment and multiplication depends fundamentally on food gathering; under good conditions numbers grow very rapidly until they are reduced by disasters such as disease or famine.

By his superior intellectual powers man has to some extent begun to emerge from this primary biological cycle: he has shaken off his jungle competitors, he has multiplied his food resources by changing from a hunting to an agricultural economy, and he has begun to win the war against disease. All this progress makes for unlimited expansion of populations. Man has invested human life with sanctity and elevated the importance of the individual, but the facts of ecology are not set aside thereby: the operation of its laws are only postponed. Biological regulations of population will be inexorable unless forestalled by human wisdom, forethought and constructive action.

disinfection. The destruction by artificial means of disease-producing organisms and particularly those liberated by, or removed from, the body and environment of an infectious patient. Disinfection implies something less than sterilization (the extinction of all life) but more than antisepsis (the prevention or retardation of bacterial growth).

Disinfectants include liquid or gaseous chemicals and the physical effects of heat, as hot air or steam. Air and sunlight dry and oxidize bacteria and destroy them by ultra-violet light, and the purifying influence of plain soap and water is also of disinfectant value in relation to many diseases not calling for more drastic measures.

The measures which may be taken to disinfect the sick room and its furnishings at the conclusion of a case are now regarded as comparatively unimportant, except perhaps in smallpox, and ritual fumigation, spraying and steam sterilization of mattresses has largely been given up in recognition that only the patient presents any real danger. However, there should be an immediate disinfection of discharges and excreta and of inanimate objects as soon as they are infected during the course of an illness.

Disinfection by heat. Swabs and dressings should be burned. Most textiles except blankets can be boiled, which kills non-sporing organisms immediately; if maintained for one hour it kills most spores. Steam disinfection requires a special pressure chamber.

Liquid disinfectants. The standard solutions employed are 5 per cent carbolic acid, 2 per cent cresol ('lysol'), 5 per cent chlorinated lime, or one of the proprietary disinfectants. Formalin solution (1 per cent) is used in sprays.

Gaseous disinfectants. Sulphur dioxide produced by burning 'sulphur candles' has been abandoned as ineffective against bacteria. Formaldehyde gas is now standard, liberated by heat-vaporization of solid formaldehyde or by the action of potassium permanganate on formalin (a 40 per cent solution of formaldehyde). Fumigator outfits are available for either method.

The following represents an effective code of practice:

1. Nasal discharges etc. – received on paper handkerchiefs subsequently burned.

2. Sputum – received into container with 5 per cent carbolic acid; paper sputum containers which can be burned are available.

3. Faeces and vomit – mixed with 5 per cent carbolic, 2 per cent cresol, or 5 per cent chlorinated lime and allowed to stand 2 hours before disposal to drains.

4. Urine – mixed with equal volume of similar disinfectant solutions and allowed to stand for two hours before disposal.

5. Textiles – soaked in 2 per cent cresol for twelve hours before being boiled and washed. If boiled before soaking any discharges will cause staining. Blankets and most synthetic fabrics should not be boiled.

6. Cutlery, crockery etc. – kept for individual use: sterilized by boiling; food residues burned.

7. Nursing equipment – boiled or treated with above disinfectant solutions: thermometers, toothbrush etc., kept in 2 per cent proprietary disinfectant.

8. Hands – 5 per cent commercial preparation for two minutes.

9. Person – protected by overalls kept in sick room; use of mask if appropriate.

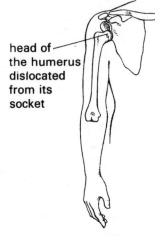

head of the humerus dislocated from its socket

Dislocated shoulder

dislocations. A dislocation is a displacement or separation of the bony surfaces which form a joint.

It is accompanied by rupture of the supporting ligaments and of the joint capsule. Subluxation is a partial dislocation.

Dislocations commonly occur in the joints at the ends of the long bones when indirect violence levers the joint beyond its normal range (traumatic dislocation), but a joint may become displaced through bone disease (pathological dislocation), or be unstable at birth through developmental abnormality especially in the hip joint (congenital dislocation).

The knee cap, jaw, and shoulder are quite often liable to dislocate through muscular action alone, without any external violence.

Dislocations usually occur in active mature adults. The bones of the elderly will fracture rather than dislocate and in young children a separation of the growing end of the bone is more likely to occur.

Signs of dislocation. There is usually deformity, loss of function, rigidity, and swelling with pain both at the site of injury and referred down the limb through pressure on nerves by the displaced structures. This may also produce numbness.

Treatment. Traumatic dislocations are restored (or 'reduced') by manipulation, usually under a general anaesthetic. Some dislocations, especially of shoulder and jaw, are very liable to recur and in many such instances the patient may become quite adept at reducing them himself.

In congenital dislocation of the hip, reduction is obtained by moving the leg from its natural position, and rotating it. This posture is maintained by some form of splintage until the joint surfaces develop sufficiently to ensure stability.

disseminated   sclerosis. See MULTIPLE SCLEROSIS.

distension. The swelling and enlargement of a body cavity or of a hollow organ by its retained and accumulating contents.

Abdominal distension may be due to ascites (i.e. free fluid which accumulates in the abdominal cavity) or to the accumulation of gastro-intestinal fluid and gas within the stomach and bowel, usually as the result of digestive disorder, infective processes or obstruction.

Distension of the bladder occurs when there is obstruction to its outflow as from stricture of the urethra or prostatic enlargement.

diuretic. Any drug which increases the quantity of urine excreted by the kidneys. Diuretics act either on the circulation to increase blood flow through the kidney, or directly on the renal cells to increase their action.

The most important of the former group is digitalis which regulates the rate and rhythm of heart action, and reinforces ventricular contraction.

Of the numerous old-style drugs reputed to act directly on the kidney probably only caffeine and potassium citrate are now of much importance. The place of the others has been taken by new synthetic compounds of much greater effectiveness most of which act by interfering with enzyme control of the kidney tubules so that more fluid is excreted.

Prolonged use of powerful diuretics leads to potassium depletion in the body and this requires correction.

Diuretics are given to relieve oedema – the accumulation of fluid in the tissue spaces of the body – usually resulting from chronic cardiac or renal disease.

diverticulitis. Inflammation of a diverticulum which is a small protrusion of mucous membrane bulging out through a weak part of the bowel wall.

The condition where diverticula are present is diverticulosis and tends to occur in older persons with a long history of constipation. The diverticula are usually numerous and they become filled with stagnant faecal matter which may cause infection and inflammation of the surrounding tissue. When this occurs symptoms are produced very similar to those of acute appendicitis but on the left side of the lower abdomen.

Acute diverticulitis may proceed to abscess formation or peritonitis and requires prompt surgical treatment.

Chronic diverticulitis requires investigation to exclude the possibility of other conditions. X-ray examination following a barium enema will show evidence of the pocket-like diverticula. If the condition is extensive, of long standing and perhaps giving rise to symptoms of obstruction it is often best dealt with by removing the affected area of bowel.

divorce. A formal breaking of the legal tie of marriage by a decree of an appropriate court or other authority.

Clearly divorce must be seen as a corollary of marriage. No question of divorce can arise until a primitive community has evolved the idea of the long-term union of a man and a woman as desirable for perpetuation of the race and as a practical expedient to meet the problems of daily life; and the attitude of any community to divorce obviously depends to a large measure on the degree of importance that it attaches to marital stability.

In the Greek, Roman and Hebrew civilizations economics and other practical considerations tended to play larger parts than did romance or religion in the initiation of marriages and in their continuation or termination. Divorce was easy for the dissatisfied man though it might involve surrendering a dowry. For the dissatisfied woman it was less easy unless she could convince her husband that a parting would be advantageous to them both. That is broadly the position in many Eastern countries today.

The Western Church made both marriage and divorce more difficult because of the idea that sex was inherently sinful. Marriage became a sacrament and, under the influence of St. Augustine, theoretically indissoluble. However in practice incompatible couples could not be compelled to live together and it was difficult to prevent a separated person from taking another partner. So ecclesiastical lawyers became adept at finding reasons for declaring that a marriage had been invalid from the beginning, e.g., because the couple were discovered to be distantly related or because there had been some fault in the marriage ceremony. The view of the Catholic Church, however, still remains that a valid marriage can be dissolved only by the death of one partner and that the remarriage of a divorced person during the life of the former partner is sinful and not a true marriage.

In many countries divorce became a practical possibility when jurisdiction in matrimonial matters was transferred from ecclesiastical to civil courts in the nineteenth or early twentieth century, e.g., in Britain after the Matrimonial Causes Act of 1857. While the exact grounds on which divorce is permissible vary from country to country the general trend in legislation has been able to move away from the idea of proving 'guilt' (such as adultery, cruelty or desertion) towards that of simply establishing that a marriage has irretrievably broken down.

Because of changes in the grounds for divorce and because of decreases in the costs of obtaining a divorce the proportion of marriages ending in dissolution is increasing in many countries. The rising divorce rate is sometimes quoted as an indication of increased permissiveness or of lowered moral standards. It is not really such an indication. Indications can reasonably be sought in such things as the number of extramarital conceptions or the number of cases of venereal diseases, but the main explanation of the increasing divorce rate is that in many western countries divorce is now available to an incompatible couple without proving 'guilt' (which may not exist) and at much lower cost than in the past.

In considering divorced persons and their children health workers and social workers often tend to lump together all divorced, separated and widowed persons, and to discuss, for instance, simply the problems of ONE-PARENT FAMILIES. For many purposes this aggregation of different groups is satisfactory enough: a large number of the needs and difficulties of a woman with a young child and no husband are the same, whether she is a widow, a divorcee or an unmarried mother. However certain differences between the groups should be noted. The widowed person looks back to a happy married life and feels grief for the dead partner: the divorced person often looks back to a long period of disharmony and bickering, and, if religious and contemplating remarriage, sometimes finds her instincts and emotions in conflict with her beliefs; the unmarried mother has no recollections of happy or unhappy married life. The widowed or divorced person has to learn to tackle many tasks formerly undertaken by the partner; the unmarried mother has no such problems. The children not only look back to entirely different home atmospheres but in the case of a divorce may also have conflicting loyalties.

Couples who find themselves in continuing disharmony often seek to delay divorce until the children are 'old enough to stand it'. Where a couple who have lost affection for each other can contrive to live in the same house without bickering, having their separate interests and going their separate ways but showing the same courtesy and toleration that they would give to strangers with whom they happened to be sharing lodgings, the delay is probably beneficial to the children. On the other hand, if the domestic situation is one of constant stress and frequent quarrels, the delay may well be harmful to the children. In at least some cases, however, a couple who earlier had enough mutual affection and community of interest to marry may have temporarily irritated each other, so that an agreed short period of separation – e.g., for six weeks with the question of permanence considered after the trial period – may remove the need or desire for divorce.

dizziness. A feeling of unsteadiness in relation to the surroundings; 'giddiness' is an alternative term but 'vertigo' more properly denotes a sensation of spinning.

Dizziness results from two distinct groups of causes. The function of nerve cells in the brain can be disturbed by disorders of the circulation, toxins of various kinds, and conditions affecting intracranial tension. Examples of these are high blood pressure; disease of the heart valves; heart failure; low blood pressure such as occurs in certain diseases of the endocrine glands; in acute infections and in anaemia, cachexia and malnutrition; toxins such as alcohol and carbon monoxide; brain tumours and other intracranial conditions such as epilepsy. The brief giddiness when standing up suddenly or after a very hot bath are due to temporary changes in the blood supply to the brain.

The second group is related to the balancing mechanism or vestibule contained in the inner ear which may be damaged by infection or by some vascular disorder. Symptoms produced in this way are usually known as Ménière's disease often characterized by true vertigo. Disorders leading to double vision may cause similar feelings of instability because of the lack of co-ordination between visual and balancing sensations. The giddiness of travel sickness is probably due to vestibular effects.

Giddiness in a young person is generally of small significance. It is related to fainting which commonly results from an unduly sensitive vaso-motor mechanism. In older persons it requires investigation to discover the underlying cause.

DNA. See RNA and CELL.

doctor. The word originally means 'teacher', which is ironic since most modern medical practitioners regard their function as that of diagnosing and treating illness after the patient has made a layman's assessment of sickness and has decided to consult a doctor, and since teaching about emotional and physical health and prevention of disease is increasingly regarded as the province of such professionals as health education officers and health visitors.

In Britain 'doctor' has two completely separate meanings: (1) A person possessing a higher or postgraduate degree from a university, e.g., as a doctor of science, doctor of philosophy or doctor of medicine. Only a minority of medical practitioners are doctors in this sense. (2) As a courtesy title, any medical practitioner who holds a bachelor's degree in medicine and surgery from a university or a similar licence from a recognized college. The picture is further confused by the fact that, while a clinical medical consultant, a community medicine specialist and a general medical practitioner are called 'doctor' irrespective of whether they possess a higher qualification in medicine, a surgeon – who must hold a medical practitioner's bachelor's degree or college licence – is traditionally addressed as 'Mister'; and still further confused by the fact that in some countries (e.g., West Germany) a doctorate is awarded to a person who completes a primary degree, whether in arts, science, medicine, divinity or some other discipline.

This article considers only doctors in the sense of medical practitioners.

Differentiation between priest (or witch-doctor), scientist, medical practitioner, nurse and wise woman occurred very gradually during the dawn of civilization: an individual, perhaps prevented by deformity from becoming a warrior or a tiller of the soil, became the tribal expert in omens, spiritual matters, removal of arrows and care of the sick. Although Imhotep (about 2900 B.C.) is traditionally regarded as the 'father' of medicine, the early medical papyri of ancient Egypt are largely devoted to spells and incantations, and later Egyptian papyri show little if any advance. Egyptian medicine in fact failed to progress.

Aesculapius, founder of Greek medicine, remains largely legendary, although one surviving fragment suggests that his sons were skilled respectively in medicine and surgery – the first indication of a separation between branches of medicine.

The writings attributed to Hippocrates of Cos (about 460 to 370 B.C.) are perhaps the product of a number of early Greek physicians, but he – or they – introduced some principles of diagnosis, scientific case-histories (including some that ended with the death of the patient), consideration of public health or community medicine (e.g., the treatise *Airs, Waters, Places*) and consideration of surgical procedures (e.g., descriptions of fractures and of head injuries). Medicine had become separated from other studies and the whole of medicine – internal medicine, surgery, public health, paediatrics and so on – was still a unity. Although the leading experts of the Roman civilization (like Galen) and of the Arabic civilization (like Rhazes and Avicenna) were primarily physiologists and physicians they took the whole of medical science as their province.

In the middle ages medicine to some extent regressed, with all learning in the hands of the priesthood, but a re-separation began earlier than is sometimes realized: the University of Bologna started to award medical qualifications in the thirteenth century, and Chaucer's Doctor of Physick in the fourteenth century was manifestly not a clergyman.

Around the end of the sixteenth century, when William Harvey (perhaps the greatest name in British medicine) was studying at Padua and when Queen Elizabeth (on discovering a wax image of herself with pins in it) was turning not to her physician but to her astrologer, or a few years later when Harvey was being elected a Fellow of the recently formed Royal College of Physicians and James I was writing his diatribe against witchcraft, there begins to emerge a fourfold picture of people who might nowadays be regarded as practitioners of medicine.

(1) Medical practitioners who held a degree or licence obtained after taking a recognized course and passing specific examinations. (2) Practitioners qualified only by apprenticeship and hard to differentiate from bone-setters and other non-medical workers. (3) Surgeons (barbers) who practised blood-letting and carried out various operations but were denied professional recognition by their medical colleagues. The status of the surgeon began to rise in the later seventeenth century when several Chairs of Surgery were established in France. (4) Apothecaries, the ancestors of the modern pharmacists, who not only dispensed medicines but often prescribed them and were in fact the family doctors of the poor.

Apart from sporadic treatises public health was virtually ignored. Its resuscitation can perhaps be considered as beginning with the publication in Germany of the first of P. J. Frank's volumes (1779) on medical policy.

Surgeons gained acceptance to the medical fraternity and apothecaries lost out. In the nineteenth century medicine advanced enormously and all practitioners – whether physicians ('internists' in America), surgeons, obstetricians or practitioners of public health (later renamed 'community medicine') – were required to hold a primary degree or licence from a recognized institution. It was made illegal for a person to call himself a medical practitioner or a 'doctor' with medical implication unless he was recorded on a national medical register as possessing an appropriate qualification.

With enormous advances not only in medicine but also in the sciences on which it depends (e.g., physiology, psychology, sociology and genetics) the last eighty years have inevitably been the era of medical specialization. By 1974 there were in Britain approximately 30,000 hospital doctors (about 11,000 full consultants in specialities and 19,000 junior doctors the majority of whom were trying to specialize); about 2,500 community doctors (rather under 1,000 full consultants and over 1,500 junior doctors) and about 25,000 medical practitioners, together with smaller numbers in occupational health services and in the Forces. In some countries, such as Sweden and the Western States of America, the ratio of specialists to generalists was even higher. There is some gain in such specialization, for the specialist inevitably knows more about the particular disease; but there is also some loss, for the generalist or personal doctor knows or should know more about the problems, difficulties and attitudes of his patient.

domiciliary. Pertaining to a person's home. A domiciliary visit implies that the doctor, health visitor or nurse travels to the person's house, as contrasted with the person travelling to hospital or clinic.

dominant. The term is frequently used in the sense of influential or ruling: for instance, 'In that family the wife is the dominant partner'.

In GENETICS the word is used specifically in respect of one gene (dominant) over-ruling another (recessive). To give an example, for determination of colour of eyes the gene for 'brown' is dominant and that for 'blue' recessive. Thus if one parent contributes a gene for brown eyes and the other a gene for blue eyes, the child will carry the two genes and will have brown eyes because the one gene over-rules the other. If that child in due course marries another person of similar genetic make-up in respect of colour of eyes, on average one quarter of their children will be brown eyed and carry two genes for brown, one half will be brown eyed but carry a recessive gene for blue, and one quarter will be blue eyed, having inherited the recessive gene from both parents.

dose. The quantity of a medicine to be taken at one time. The official or standard dose, as set out in the pharmacopoeia, is usually given as a range, e.g., 50 to 100 mg. Within this range lie the doses suitable for most adults. The right dose for a particular adult depends partly on size and body-weight and partly on individual tolerance or susceptibility. Where a patient's reaction to a medicine is unknown – because the patient is new to the doctor or because the drug is new to the patient – it is generally considered good practice to start with a dose near the lower end of the range and subsequently increase if necessary.

For a child the dose of any medicine is always less than for an adult, but the broad rule of proportion – e.g., a child of one-quarter the weight of his father requires a quarter of the adult dose – has many exceptions. For instance the dose of morphia for a child is considerably less than in proportion to weight.

double personality. A disordered state of mind in which the patient appears alternately to lead two lives with neither personality being aware of the memories and experiences of the other.

In the majority of cases it is a hysterical phenomenon. Hysterical persons over-react to any situation either to fulfil subconscious wishes or to evade difficulties.

A later stage of this behaviour is the development of hysterical 'fugue' or flight from reality, which is a narrowing rather than a clouding of consciousness, with dissociation of existing memory.

The patient can thus live out some fantasy or more commonly simply pass into a state of amnesia where he does not know who or where he is.

Double personality is in fact only a fragmentation of a single personality with different aspects predominating from time to time. In extreme cases it can be extended to the condition of MULTIPLE PERSONALITY.

double vision. See DIPLOPIA.

Down's syndrome. See MONGOLISM.

drains. In building construction, drains are the underground pipes usually made of jointed, glazed-stoneware sections, which convey water-borne excreta, house waste-water, and rainfall from the fixtures of a house to the public sewer or to other facilities for their ultimate disposal, such as a cess-pit. In legal terms drain is that part of the underground drainage system within the property on which the building stands.

Fixtures within the building are equipped with water seals or 'traps' usually of S- or P-shaped construction to prevent the reflux of air from the drain into the house.

The requirements of an efficient house drain are (1) that it should be aligned in as straight a course as possible or with easy curves, (2) that it should have access openings at suitable points and distances, (3) that it should be laid on a solid bed, (4) that it should have a sufficient gradient related to its diameter, (5) that all branch connections should be made obliquely in the direction of flow, (6) that its interior should be smooth and (7) that it should be disconnected from the soil pipe (which carries waste material down from the house) by an efficient intercepting or disconnecting ventilating trap.

A drainage system is usually tested either by a hydraulic test where the system is filled with water and observed for leaks or by the 'smoke test' in which the pipes are filled with smoke from a special generator, and escapes are sought by sight or smell.

Surgical drains. In a medical context, 'drain' is a piece of rubber tubing, corrugated rubber, gauze-wick or other device inserted into a wound to facilitate the discharge of fluid or pus and so helps to promote healing.

dreams. Sequences of thought, fancy, and imagery occurring during sleep and impinging on consciousness to a variable degree.

In common with many other animals, human physiology provides for a daily cycle of being awake and being asleep. The depth of intensity of the state of sleep fluctuates considerably. A relatively simple way of measuring this is to subject a sleeper to a progressively louder sound until he awakes but a great deal more about the inner nature of sleep has been learned through the introduction of the electro-encephalograph. This is an instrument which, by means of electrodes attached to the skull, records the electrical activity of the brain. The tracings thus produced show a wave-pattern which varies with the level of consciousness and cerebral activity. It has been demonstrated that dreams occur during light sleep when the subject is still unconscious of the outside world but yet sufficiently aware to appreciate and remember temporarily his dreaming impressions. A person wakened from light sleep will often be able to recall his dream; suddenly roused from deep sleep he will usually have nothing to report.

All the experimental evidence suggests that everyone has dreams but that not everyone can recall them. Moreover it is a matter of common experience how quickly a dream is forgotten unless special steps are taken to preserve it, either by rehearsing it in full consciousness or by writing it down.

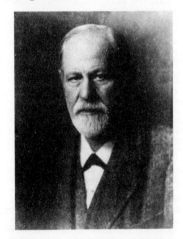

Sigmund Freud, author of *The Interpretation of Dreams*

Significance of dreams. Sigmund Freud (1856-1939) said that 'the interpretation of dreams is the royal road to a knowledge of the unconscious activities of the mind', and he elaborated this thesis in his very important work, *The Interpretation of Dreams,* which he published in 1900. Freud was a positivist, committed to the belief that everything must have a cause, and he therefore maintained that dreams could not be as irrational as they often seemed. Instead he regarded them as symbolic of personal matters arousing strong emotion; lesser symbols which the mind substituted for inner conflicts which would otherwise disturb and interfere with sleep.

In his work as a psychoanalyst he used the analysis of dreams as a tool to explore the emotional life of his patients. His preoccupation with sexuality as the force motivating all abnormal psychological activity was such that he would tolerate no dissent. As a result the birth of psychoanalysis and acceptance of its tenets and techniques was marred by his quarrels with his associates, Adler and Jung, who regarded dreams as an unconscious attempt to achieve a success and perfection which real life denied.

Nevertheless, despite these basic divergencies of view, the study of dreams remains as a useful and important part of psychoanalytic practice.

dropsy. The accumulation of fluid in the tissue spaces and body cavities. Dropsy is not a separate disease but only a symptom of a variety of serious conditions affecting the heart, kidneys or liver.

The fluid is serum from the blood stream and its effusion into the skin and superficial tissues produces a swollen appearance known as anasarca.

The swelling from heart disease tends to occur in dependent parts; in kidney disease its distribution is determined more by relative tissue laxity. The affected areas 'pit on pressure'; i.e., pressure by an examining finger leaves a depression which disappears only slowly. Accumulation of fluid in the abdomen cavity is ascites; in the chest cavity it is known as hydrothorax.

Dropsy in heart disease is due to failing circulation; in kidney disease to diminished elimination of fluid associated with salt retention and protein depletion; in the liver disease, which produces ascites rather than tissue oedema, there is usually obstruction to venous blood-flow in the portal circulation resulting from cirrhosis of the liver or malignant disease.

Treatment. The first essential is accurate. diagnosis to determine the cause of the dropsy.

Drugs to increase the flow of urine will assist in the elimination of surplus tissue fluid and a salt-free diet is usually prescribed. Fluid in the chest and abdomen may be removed by suction.

Otherwise treatment requires to be directed to underlying causes, but dropsy is always of serious significance and any measure may give only temporary relief from the symptom.

drowning. Drowning is asphyxia caused by the mouth and nose being submerged in fluid and the consequent exclusion of air from the lungs. For emergency treatment see ARTIFICIAL RESPIRATION, Schafer's method.

Although most drowning accidents occur through falls into deep water, it is not essential that a person should get into shallow streams and inebriates stumble into ditches with equally disastrous results.

Moreover, individuals tend to panic in shallow water. They scream and struggle using up the air in their lungs, and with gasping inspirations inhale water as well as air. In a potentially dangerous situation a victim should try to remain calm, keep his mouth shut, breathe through his nose and endeavour to keep his head above water by treading water or doing a 'dog-paddle'.

These measures will at least improve the chances of successful rescue but every child should be taught to swim and have confidence in water from an early age.

A person who drowns in deep water usually sinks and it may be some days before the gases of decomposition provide sufficient flotation to bring the body to the surface. If a body is found floating medico-legal problems arise. Did the person actually drown or did he die from other causes and fall or be thrown in?

To answer this question post mortem examination is required but the proverb that 'Drowning men clutch at straws' has some foundation in fact, and a corpse with clenched hands holding fragments of seaweed or grass and earth from river banks will probably have died from drowning.

An interesting point is that it is more dangerous to fall into fresh water than into the sea; fresh water in the lungs causes tissue damage and breakdown of red blood cells.

drowsiness. A state of failing or impaired consciousness in which a person readily tends to fall asleep.

Drowsiness may be the normal preliminary stage of ordinary sleep, particularly likely to occur after excessive fatigue when circulatory exhaustion, depletion of fuel reserves, and delayed elimination of the waste products of muscular activity, combine to lower nervous activity. It is also common in old age.

It may also be a symptom of any disease which impairs the circulation of adequately-oxygenated blood to the brain or causes deficient elimination of toxins as in heart disease or kidney disease with uraemia.

Many drugs produce drowsiness. Hypnotic drugs are given to induce sleep and the production of drowsiness is the first stage towards achieving the desired result. Tranquillizers on the other hand are given to reduce cerebral activity and anxiety while preserving normal awareness, and drowsiness is an unwanted side-effect. Attempts to overcome this dilemma have resulted in the great variety of formulations now being marketed.

There is however, less obvious risk of drowsiness with many modern drugs given for quite different purposes; medicines given for heart disease, high blood pressure, troublesome cough, thyroid over-activity, diabetes, epilepsy, migraine, motion sickness and hay-fever are examples. Care is required when patients taking them have to drive road vehicles or work at tasks requiring care and alertness.

drug addiction. See ADDICTION.

drug rashes. Skin eruptions of diverse type produced by the toxic effects of drugs on the skin. The old style of medical practice used many substances which were liable to cause rashes; prominent amongst these were metals such as arsenic, gold, silver, antimony, and mercury, and organic substances such as turpentine, copaiba and other oleo-resins all of which have largely fallen into disuse. Nevertheless many of the newer drugs also produce similar effects.

In most cases drug rashes are not precisely typical of any particular drug and may take any form, such as red patches, small haemorrhages in the skin or itchy weals. They can easily be confused with various infectious diseases but consideration of the history, the anomalous distribution, their variability, and the occurrence of weals should avoid mistakes. Rashes of these types occur with a wide variety of common drugs – aspirin, salicylates, barbiturates, sulphonamides, belladonna, coumarin, phenothiazine, penicillin and other antibiotics – to name only a few.

Some drugs on the other hand produce specific rashes with characteristics which can be recognized. Bromides, iodides, antipyrine, and phenolphthalein are the most common of these.

A third group of substances produce skin effects in a rather different way. Protein-containing substances such as vaccines and sera may produce an allergic skin reaction usually in the form of itchy swellings.

The treatment of drug rashes is to stop the drug and allay skin irritation with some suitable soothing lotion.

drugs. Any substances used in medicine for the treatment of disease or the alleviation of symptoms.

The study of drugs and their action upon living cells and tissues is known as pharmacology, a branch of knowledge which only began to achieve its present stature as a science during the present century. Before then, the drugs in general use included a very wide range of substances, both inorganic and organic, most of which were either useless or dangerous and whose claim to be 'good' for certain diseases was generally based entirely on chance happenings, rather than understanding.

Although the remedies available to the prescriber had moved on from the 'scale of dragon, tooth of wolf, gall of goat and slips of yew' type of medication it perhaps still justified Bernard Shaw's gibe that medical science was a branch of witchcraft, or Voltaire's dictum that a physician was someone who poured drugs of which he knew little into a body of which he knew less. Nevertheless there were a few effective drugs, notably quinine and iron, and extracts of certain plants which contained powerful alkaloids such as digitalis, morphine and atropine.

The advent of the organic chemist and developments in medicine and related sciences have resulted not only in the availability of an enormous range of completely new specific remedies but in the facilities to determine their mode of action and their effectiveness as therapeutic agents.

The credit for initiating this new approach should perhaps go to Paul Ehrlich (1854-1915) who conceived the idea of 'magic bullets' – drugs aimed at the real causes of disease – and whose work resulted in the production (1907) of the drug '606' or salvarsan, specific against syphilis. The next great steps forward were the discovery of penicillin by Sir Alexander Fleming in 1928 (but not exploited until 1942) from which has stemmed a large range of other antibiotics, and the elaboration of the sulphonamide group of drugs from their parent azo-dye Prontosil (1935). Together these have revolutionized the treatment of infectious diseases.

These drugs, however, like Ehrlich's bullets, were still only directed against infections. The goal of the present day pharmacologist is to produce drugs which can correct the abnormalities of body function by influencing the activities of cells and enzyme systems. This group can be taken to include not only the vitamins, hormones and biological products creating immunity, but the enormous range of new drugs used to influence the nervous system, to improve the coronary circulation and reduce blood pressure, to alter kidney function, to suppress inflammation and allergy, to allay pain, and destroy malignant tissue.

The classification of drugs in the broadest terms is thus (1) those replacing or reinforcing normal tissue constituents (2) those interfering with normal biological processes to produce some desired effect (3) agents capable of destroying invaders.

Hazards of drugs. The very potency and wide distribution of many new and powerful drugs has produced accompanying risks. Many may produce undesirable and dangerous side-effects or lead to ADDICTION. The well known thalidomide tragedy illustrates the completely unexpected effects which can result unless new products are exhaustively tested and controlled. Lastly, there is the danger of accidental or deliberate poisoning.

It is now more essential than ever that any drug should be taken in strict accordance with qualified instructions and that all medicines should be safeguarded from improper use or accidental ingestion.

drunkenness. A state of habitual intemperance in which the excessive consumption of ALCOHOL leads to chronic intoxication.

ductless glands. Glands which produce chemical substances to control various bodily processes but which have no secretory duct or tube. They are known also as ENDOCRINE GLANDS and the special substances or hormones which they produce pass directly into the blood stream.

ductus arteriosus. A blood vessel in unborn children joining the pulmonary artery to the aorta so that blood circulates without passing through the lungs, which are, of course, not yet functioning. The oxygen supply for the infant's blood is drawn from the mother's blood in the placenta.

After birth the ductus normally closes. An unclosed or patent ductus arteriosus is a fairly common variety of congenital heart disease but is easily treated by tying a ligature round the vessel.

dumbness. The state of being without the power of speech.

It is essential to differentiate between the child who has never spoken and the individual previously able to speak who has become dumb. In the latter the causes are either diseases affecting the speech centres in the brain – APHASIA – or disabilities affecting the mechanism of voice production – APHONIA.

The dumb child is a more complex problem. Speech is not an inborn ability; it is a skill which has to be learned by imitation, and if a child does not learn to speak by the usual time there is either failure to hear or inability of the centres in the brain to appreciate and reproduce what is heard. DEAFNESS is thus of two kinds: (1) where the fault lies in the ear or its connections with the brain; (2) where the fault is in the brain centres. If the degree of hearing loss or brain-damage is considerable the child will be dumb or fail to acquire acceptable speech.

Dumbness in a child may therefore be due to (1) defects of the mechanism of hearing, (2) mental deficiency, and (3) aphasia due to brain damage. The speciality of audiology seeks to investigate the relative importance of these factors in the patient in order to make a decision about treatment and education.

duodenal ulcer. An ulcer of the small intestine, characterized by pain, sensation of fullness and tenderness in the pit of the stomach, the symptoms usually arising some two to four hours after a meal and being temporarily relieved by taking food. The immediate cause is excess quantity or undue acidity of secreted juices which in effect begin to digest the lining of the duodenum. Hence treatment involves alkaline drugs to combat excessive acidity, atropine or a similar drug to reduce activity and spasm of the stomach and duodenum, mild sedatives to improve physical and mental rest, avoidance of smoking or alcohol before meals (since these stimulate the flow of juices), and regular, well-chewed meals. Treatment generally starts with a very bland diet consisting mainly of milk, custard and junket, but progresses rapidly to a fairly normal diet with, however, permanent avoidance of highly indigestible foods. Surgical treatment is very seldom needed, and the very strict dietetic regime of the past is nowadays regarded as being needed for only a very few weeks.

Duodenal and gastric ulcer produce very similar symptoms and respond to much the same treatment, so clinical workers have tended to class them together; but they are widely different in respect of relative frequency in men and women and in rich and poor people, in probable causes and indeed in most of the features studied by epidemiologists.

Duodenal ulcer is four times commoner in men while gastric is about equally common in the two sexes; duodenal is more frequent in the more affluent social groups while gastric is rather commoner in the poor; and duodenal is on the increase whereas gastric is not. While both are similar to the extent that the mucous membrane is irritated and eroded by over-acid secreted juices, the underlying causes of duodenal ulcer appear to include an over-active, ambitious or worrying personality while gastric ulcer is associated more with nutritional factors.

While regular and well-chewed meals and avoidance of smoking before meals may contribute to the prevention of duodenal ulcer, the main preventive measure is clearly attention to personality development in the early formative years, including attempts to avoid excessive ambition without removing all desire for progress and attempts to create reasonable sense of security without inducing smugness and total incapacity for worry.

dura mater. The outermost of the three membranous layers which enclose the brain and spinal cord. It is tough and fibrous.

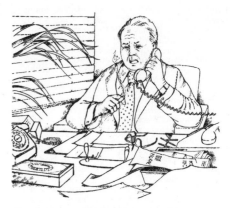

Circumstances predisposing to duodenal ulcer

dust. Dust is any dry powdery material of a particle size small enough to remain suspended in (or be wafted by) the air.

Its importance in relation to medicine lies in the varieties of lung disease which it can produce when inhaled with air. Disease of this kind is known by the general name of pneumoconiosis of which there are many examples related to different trades and industrial processes.

Dusts may be either inorganic or organic and the distinction is of importance in relation to the type of disease which they produce.

Inorganic dusts. Of these the most damaging is undoubtedly silica in various forms. Typical industrial processes involving silica are sand-blasting, flint and pebble crushing, manufacture of refractory bricks and materials, pottery manufacture, grinding of metals, manufacture of scouring powders and abrasive soaps, quarrying, tunnelling and mining of all kinds.

It used to be thought that the disease condition silicosis was produced by damage from the sharp edged 'sandy' particles but by some classic experiments it was eventually shown that silica (silicon dioxide) forms silicic acid in the tissues and that it is this that causes damage to the lung.

Another important factor is particle size; anything smaller than five-thousandths of a millimetre becomes increasingly hazardous.

Other common inorganic dust diseases are anthracosis of coal-miners, siderosis found in knife grinders and metal polishers and asbestosis affecting asbestos workers. Although each has some special features all are essentially due to silica in some form. Asbestosis carries a special risk of eventually inducing malignancy.

Organic dusts. A wide variety of trades produce organic dusts which although less harmful than silica may produce chronic respiratory disease of a bronchitic rather than pulmonary character. Byssinosis is related to the cotton industry and bagassosis to the conversion of spent sugar cane into insulating board.

Organic dusts also carry other hazards such as anthrax from wool-sorting and tetanus from jute processing. Mycosis of the lung may arise from malting or from the handling of mouldy straw.

Chemical dusts. Inhalation of these cause various types of poisoning. Compounds of chromium, lead, arsenic, zinc manganese, cadmium and nickel are the chief offenders.

House dust. In conclusion reference must be made to house dust which may cause illness in quite a different way. Compounded as it is of finely divided particles derived from textiles, feathers, hair and fur of pets, and even the dried and broken down tissues of the house mite, it contains allergens which may provoke attacks of asthma in susceptible subjects.

See also ASPERGILLOSIS.

dwarfism. A condition in which an individual animal or plant fails to grow to normal height having regard to its age and species.

The causation of human dwarfism is complex. Some races of mankind such as the pygmies are typically all very small although otherwise perfectly formed. Their stature is determined by their normal genetic inheritance and this is known as primordial dwarfism. Similarly small parents of all races tend to have small children.

Other varieties of dwarfism are due to disease or organic abnormality of some kind and these causes may be divided into (1) disorders of the endocrine glands, (2) various general diseases, and (3) genetic abnormalities.

Endocrine abnormality. Growth hormone is an internal secretion produced by the pituitary gland. Deficiency leads to the condition of infantilism, in which the individual is not deformed but is abnormally small for his age. The typical pituitary type dwarf is often not much more than 60 cm. (2 ft.) tall but is otherwise intelligent and well-formed. This is the Tom Thumb or circus-freak kind of dwarf, but another variety of pituitary abnormality can produce Fröhlich's syndrome or dystrophia adiposo-genitalis in which fatness and defective sexual development are the main features rather than extreme diminutiveness.

Deficiency of thyroid secretion produces the thyroid dwarf or cretin who is mentally retarded, slow and apathetic, as well as being of small stature.

Other diseases. Retarded or deficient growth is seen in a variety of conditions which influence nutrition and development. Examples are rickets, coeliac disease, pancreatic disease and vitamin deficiency.

Genetic abnormalities. Best known of these is achondroplasia. In the achondroplasic dwarf the arms and legs are short in relation to the body ('human dachshund'). The condition is inherited as a Mendelian dominant, as is another rare disease, osteogenesis imperfecta, where there is both diminished stature and fragility of the bones.

In glycogen-storage or von Gierke's disease which is inherited as a recessive characteristic there is excessive storage of glycogen and failure to bring it into the blood as required, so that the blood-sugar remains low and growth and development are retarded.

Treatment. For pituitary dwarfism, anterior pituitary growth-hormone may be given by injection but the results are not particularly impressive. Cretins respond well to the administration of thyroxin although their mental retardation may not be improved. The treatment of vitamin deficiencies is

straightforward. Little can be done to influence the other congenital and genetic conditions.

dysentery. Infection of the large intestine, characterized by severe diarrhoea, abdominal pain, painful desire to pass a motion and the presence of blood and mucous in motions.

1. Amoebic dysentery. This type is common in the tropics, caused by infection by a single-celled organism, *Entamoeba histolytica,* which usually reaches the victim from food or water contaminated from the excreta of a previous victim. Hence prevention is essentially a matter of proper sanitary facilities and personal hygiene especially by all food handlers. Typical symptoms are as indicated above, but some people have amoebic dysentery for long periods almost without symptoms. Emetine is still regarded as the drug of choice, though some of the newer antibiotics (e.g., paromomycin) are also claimed to be useful. The very fact that new drugs are being tried indicates that the existing treatments are not always fully effective.

2. Bacillary dysentery. Much commoner and occurring in all climates, the bacillary type is caused by infection by bacteria of the genus *Shigella.* The types most frequently seen are, in descending order of severity: the Shiga variety, common in the Far East, often associated with violent diarrhoea and dehydration, even to the extent of being confused with cholera; the milder Flexner variety which can nevertheless cause severe illness; and the relatively mild Sonne variety which usually results in two or three days of slight illness. Many other varieties exist. Transmission is normally by contaminated food or water, so prevention involves essentially the same measures as for prevention of amoebic dysentery. Soluble drugs which are absorbed from the gut to the blood-stream (and so useful in many infections) are useless here. Treatment is by insoluble sulphonamides or insoluble antibiotics.

Bacillary dysentery, even of Sonne type, is serious in young babies. Diarrhoea occurring in a nursery or children's hospital should be regarded as dysentery until a definite diagnosis has been made.

dyslexia. An inability to read properly owing to a disorder of the brain causing letters to be confused (e.g., d and b) or the order of letters in a word to be altered (e.g., 'cat' read as 'tac'). Dyslexic children may be of normal intelligence, so that treatment, although difficult, is well worth attempting.

Until the last few years dyslexia usually remained undiagnosed and untreated, but diagnostic tests have now been developed and specially equipped teachers have had some success in treating the condition.

dysmenorrhoea. Pain during menstruation. Primary dysmenorrhoea is pain of this nature affecting girls from the start of their periods. The pain may be due to spasm of the uterus, congestion of the uterus, defective balance of hormones or emotional factors. In many cases the pain is relieved by drugs that relax spasm or by hormone treatment, including contraceptive pills. Secondary dysmenorrhoea is pain of this nature occurring in women who have previously had painless periods. It may be due to a number of gynaecological conditions and, if persisting, requires special investigation.

dyspareunia. Painful coitus. In males the common causes are inflammation and tightness of the foreskin, both easily treated. In women the condition may be due to a well-developed hymen, to inflammation of the vagina or to shrinkage of the vagina after the menopause, but in many cases it is the result of an involuntary contraction of the muscles immediately before coitus, i.e., an expression of unconscious aversion to sex. Medical examination should exclude or deal with physical causes. If none are found, a great deal of tact and patience is required to remove the underlying emotional causes which may be rooted in earlier unpleasant experiences.

dyspepsia. Discomfort after eating and difficulty in digesting food; see INDIGESTION.

dysphagia. Difficulty in swallowing. It may arise from any painful condition of the throat, such as tonsillitis or quinsy; from paralysis of the muscles of swallowing, in certain nervous diseases; from pressure of tumours in the vicinity of the throat; and occasionally from hysteria. Treatment depends on the cause.

dyspnoea. Undue BREATHLESSNESS and abnormal awareness of the effort of breathing.

E

ear. The organ of hearing and balance; it is divided into three parts.

1. The outer ear consists of the pinna (large and movable in many animals to help to collect and locate sounds) and the sound canal, or external auditory meatus, which passes inwards and forwards to end at the ear-drum. Sound waves travel along the meatus and vibrate the ear-drum.

2. The middle ear is a small cavity in the temporal bone, separated from the external meatus by the tympanic membrane or ear-drum. The cavity is bridged by three tiny bones – malleus, incus and stapes (otherwise called the hammer, the anvil and the stirrup) – which pass vibrations from the drum to the inner ear. At the back the cavity has an incomplete wall, with the hole leading to the mastoid antrum, and in front of that there is a communication with the Eustachian tube leading to the back of the nose.

3. The inner ear consists of several cavities in the petrous part of the temporal bone. The cavities are collectively called the labyrinth and consist of (1) a central part called the vestibule with which all other parts communicate, (2) three semicircular canals all at right angles to each other, and (3) the cochlea, a spiral tube twisted on itself and resembling a snail-shell.

Movement of fluid within the three semicircular canals is responsible for the sense of balance. Inside the cochlea is the organ of Corti which is the true organ of hearing. The cochlea is filled with fluid and contains hair-bearing cells linked up with the auditory nerve, which carries impulses of hearing to the brain. Vibrations received by the ear-drum are transmitted by the three bones in the middle ear, the last of which, the stapes, closes the small hole between the middle and inner ear. Thus the vibrations of these bones set up waves in the cochlear fluid and these stimulate the hair-cells. Here they are altered into electric currents which pass along nerve fibres to the brain.

Earache. Causes of this unpleasant symptom include:

1. Changes in atmospheric pressure (e.g., in an aeroplane) when a blockage of the Eustachian tube, as occurs in a head cold, makes it difficult to equalize the internal and external pressure on the eardrum.

2. Wax in the meatus (see below) especially in association with changes in atmospheric pressure.

3. A foreign body in the meatus. This is fairly rare in adults, though an insect has been known to fly in and be unable to get out, but not uncommon in children. A foreign body can often be floated out in a few drops of oil, a much less dangerous procedure than seeking to extract it with tweezers.

4. A boil in the meatus. An appropriate antibiotic may help, and warmth – e.g., application of a comfortably warm rubber hot-water bottle – may temporarily ease the pain.

5. Inflammation or increased pressure in the middle ear known as otitis media; see below. This cause is very dangerous, since the infection may spread to the mastoid and thence to the meninges, causing meningitis. Hence, unless the cause of earache is obvious, a painful ear should warrant immediate medical attention.

Wax in the ears. Wax is a normal secretion of glands on the external ear canal. In some people wax accumulates and may obstruct the passage, causing temporary deafness, especially if water enters the ear during washing and makes the wax swell. The wax should be softened by introducing a few drops of slightly warmed olive or almond oil, and a day later very gently syringed out with warm water. Gentleness in syringing is essential, because excessive force may injure the ear drum. Various commercial preparations are said to be useful in breaking up wax or preventing its accumulation.

Otitis media or discharging ears. Children are particularly susceptible to inflammation of the middle ear (otitis media) occurring usually as a complication of upper respiratory tract infection or of specific diseases such as measles and scarlet fever. Enlarged and unhealthy adenoids are often present and infection reaches the middle ear by the Eustachian tube.

In non-suppurative otitis there is pain, temperature and discharge of pus into the middle ear and on examination the eardrum (tympanic membrane) is reddened and may be distended. In pre-antibiotic days the pus accumulated until it escaped in one of three

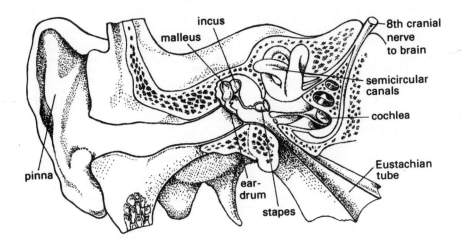

Anatomy of the ear

ways – by spontaneous perforation of the eardrum, by surgical puncture of the eardrum or by seeping inwards to cause inflammation of the mastoid bone and sometimes meningitis.

In chronic otitis the drum becomes perforated but, instead of the acute condition then clearing up, the discharge of pus continues for many months, and hearing usually becomes impaired.

The best treatment is an early administration of antibiotics to combat the infection, but in some cases it may be necessary to puncture the eardrum (paracentesis or myringotomy) to allow drainage of the pus. The ruptured eardrum with purulent discharge requires painstaking daily cleansing with cotton wool mops and the installation of antiseptic drops – spirit or hydrogen peroxide being commonly employed.

Other conditions. The middle ear is subject to abnormal deposit of bone cells (otosclerosis) and the inner ear may be the site of diseases both of balance and of hearing, e.g., Ménière's disease, causing HEAD NOISES, and DEAFNESS.

ecchymosis. The technical term for bleeding under the skin. A typical example is a bruise.

eclampsia. An acute but fortunately relatively uncommon infection of the blood, occurring during pregnancy, labour, or the puerperium, and characterized by convulsions and coma. The cause is unknown, but the condition occurs more in cold than in warm countries, more in cities than in rural areas and more in first than in later pregnancies.

Early symptoms include flashes of light, dizziness, headache and vomiting, and the urine has a high content of albumin. In the early stages rest, restriction of protein foods and the use of drinks to flush the kidneys are advocated. Where fits are actually occurring the patient should be given sedatives and placed in a quiet and darkened room under the care of a special nurse.

economics and health. Although a detailed study of the complex inter-relationships between economics and health is beyond the scope of this book a few illustrative points are given below.

1. Health and disease services are a very major industry in any developed country. Irrespective of whether these services are provided on a basis of direct payment of the supplier by the user, or through insurance schemes, or wholly or mainly by a state service, the total cost of provisions for health promotion, disease prevention, diagnosis, treatment, rehabilitation and after-care varies in advanced countries from 6 to 9 per cent of their national gross product: in other words between one-sixteenth and one-eleventh of the national income is spent on health and disease. The bulk of that expenditure consists of the remuneration of people – doctors, dentists, nurses, health visitors, physiotherapists, chiropodists, staffs of biochemical and bacteriological laboratories, staffs of x-ray departments, administrative and clerical workers, ambulance drivers, porters, cooks, domestics, and so on. Broadly, in developed countries something like 3 per cent (or a shade more) of all adults of working age are employed in the health and disease services; and, as will be apparent from the first ten groups listed above, quite a high proportion of the persons so employed are necessarily highly qualified professionals. So the health and disease services are not only a considerable drain on a nation's manpower but a very serious drain on the educated portion of that manpower.

2. The amount of work lost through spells of illness is very large indeed. In the U.K., for instance, it is reckoned at over three hundred million working days annually, or about fifty times as much as the average annual loss through industrial disputes. In other words on the official figures, an average adult in the U.K., if normally working on a basis of a five-day week for forty-eight weeks a year, actually works on 226 days and is off work through illness on 14 days, losing 6 per cent of his total

working time through sickness. These official figures, however, are actually an underestimate because they cover only illness of persons still normally employed or eligible for employment. To the figures have to be added the work losses through men and women who have retired early because of lasting illness or disability.

3. In most of the developed countries the total numbers of persons employed in hospitals and other institutions are rising almost every year – partly because nurses and other health professionals formerly worked for very long hours but have to some extent shared in the general tendency towards reduction of working time, but largely because of increased survival of the elderly who have both more spells of illness and longer spells than younger adults. To illustrate the last point it may be mentioned that a U.K. table produced by the government actuary gives the average annual loss of work of employed males as just under one week at 20 to 24 years and as over seven weeks at 60 to 64 years.

4. The situation in respect of the amount of work loss over a series of years is complicated. Firstly, advances in treatment mean that people who would have died in an earlier period survive but often have a long illness and a longer convalescence. Secondly, these advances quite often shorten the duration of illnesses. Thirdly, advances in health education and disease-prevention help to reduce the total amount of illness. Fourthly, to a considerable extent the reduction in the advanced countries of infections and diseases associated with malnutrition is balanced by increases in the so-called 'self-induced' diseases, associated with such factors as over-eating, over-smoking, inadequate exercise and mental or physical stress. Not least, as a society becomes more affluent people's tolerance of minor illnesses appears to decrease, so that they will stay off work and seek treatment for a condition which an earlier generation would have suffered in silence. At any rate, in many of the advanced countries the amount of work loss through sickness is, in proportion to total adult population, still undergoing a gradual increase.

5. In some of the developed countries the idea is gaining currency that it is not possible to continue indefinitely the gradual increase in the proportion of persons, and particularly of persons of intelligence, employed in the health and disease services, and also that a loss of about one-sixteenth of the nation's working time through illness severely limits productive work. In connection with the second point it should be noted that the existence of a pool of available unemployed persons does not greatly help except in unskilled work: if a skilled worker has an illness expected to be of fairly short duration it is seldom possible to find a temporary replacement. So, on economic grounds, increasing attention is beginning to be paid to health education and prevention of disease. This holds not only in countries in which the direct cost of sickness falls mainly on the state but also in countries relying largely on private insurance schemes: the insurance companies find that education on health reduces their costs.

6. In developing countries the disease picture is entirely different. Infections and diseases of malnutrition are still very prevalent (although in some the transition to diseases of affluence is remarkably rapid) and qualified doctors and nurses are in very short supply. There are therefore two notable trends. Firstly, to a much greater extent than in the advanced countries there is a tendency to concentrate on prevention of diseases and the simpler aspects of health education. Secondly, and in part conflicting with that tendency, there is sometimes a belief that improvements in agricultural methods, advances in mechanization and improvements in housing may produce larger dividends than the same amount of expenditure on things directly related to health and disease.

ECT. Electrical convulsive therapy. The treatment of certain forms of mental illness was introduced by von Meduna in 1933 (using drugs), and by Cerletti and Bini in 1937 (using electrical current). The electrical method has completely superseded the drug method for these particular conditions. The treatment, which is essentially stimulation of a convulsion of about one minute's duration several times weekly by passing a current through two electrodes placed on the forehead, is beneficial in many cases of depressive illness (but not for corresponding cases of manic conditions) and has also some slight value in schizophrenia.

ectopic pregnancy. A pregnancy in which the embryo begins to develop elsewhere than in the uterus. Normally the ovum and sperm unite in one of the Fallopian tubes and the fertilized egg passes along to the uterus. In an ectopic pregnancy the fertilized egg becomes lodged in the tube or, much more rarely, in the ovary. Causes are normally grouped under two headings (1) those of congenital origin e.g., if the tube is unusually long or twisted or if there are indentations in the wall of the tube, and (2) acquired causes – damage to tube from previous disease.

The main symptoms are bleeding and pain, and differentiation from miscarriage is not easy. Since the condition is dangerous to the mother and since there is no chance of the embryo surviving, the normal treatment is removal of the tube and embryo by abdominal operation. Because the woman has a second tube, she can have further pregnancies.

eczema. See DERMATITIS.

effort syndrome. Also called disordered action of the heart (DAH) and soldier's heart. A neurotic state in which the individual complains of heart pains, palpitations and breathlessness, and has a loss of energy and an unwillingness to work; yet examination of the heart reveals no abnormality. Essentially the condition is an anxiety state and usually requires psychotherapy.

effusion. Leakage of fluid into one of the cavities of the body. The term is also sometimes used for the pouring out of fluid to the exterior.

ego. The conscious mind. Sigmund Freud (1856-1939), the founder of psychoanalysis and perhaps the greatest of all psychologists, divided the mind into the super-ego (which has analogies to conscience), the ego (or personal consciousness) and the id (or primitive impulses).

ejaculatio praecox. Premature ejaculation of semen before coitus or early in coitus.

In some cases there is a lack of the normal control, so that in extreme cases the mere idea of a sexual situation can cause ejaculation. In other cases there is an extreme sensitivity of the urethra, and the ejaculation is not merely premature but sometimes painful instead of pleasurable.

The condition is a cause of a considerable amount of marital unhappiness but is seldom treated, because (1) the man generally feels shy and embarrassed and so hesitates to consult his doctor; (2) the wife who could often help by patience and reassurance is herself emotionally involved and distressed; and (3) the doctor, if consulted, is often perplexed since psychosexual problems are far removed from the illnesses that constitute the bulk of a general practitioner's work. A restoration of self-confidence is almost certainly the main necessity in treatment. To this end alcohol – by removing inhibitions and creating temporary confidence – often helps, but if neither counselling directed to restoring confidence nor the boosting of confidence by spirits helps, the advice of a psychiatrist may be required.

elbow. The hinged joint formed by the humerus (the bone of the upper arm), the ulna and the radius. The point of the elbow is the olecranon process of the ulna. The 'funny bone' is the point at which the ulnar nerve passes over the lower end of the humerus just under the skin.

There is a bursa, i.e., a small sac containing fluid, on the point of the elbow and this may become inflamed from constant pressure as from leaning on a table.

Injuries. The elbow joint is subject to sprains and dislocations, and the component bones may be fractured. Dislocations, the commonest serious injury, are usually backwards, while bending the elbow too far can tear ligaments and force a sprain. Frequent minor jarring of the joint produces the pain and stiffness described as tennis elbow, a condition involving either strain of the muscle on the outer side of the elbow joint or inflammation of the bursa lying beneath that muscle. Without treatment, other than some inevitable restriction of movement of the elbow, the symptoms disappear in about five or six months. Adequate rest of the muscle may shorten the duration appreciably, and an injection of hydrocortisone into the painful spot produces rapid alleviation of the pain.

X-ray examination is usually desirable to check whether sudden pain is caused by dislocation or fracture, so that the proper treatment can be undertaken. For other conditions the best treatment is rest.

Electra complex. Named by Freud after Electra's devotion to Agamemnon in the Greek legend, the Electra complex is excessive love by a daughter for her father, i.e., the female equivalent of the Oepidus complex.

To some extent the attraction of a child to the parent of the opposite sex is a natural phenomenon created by the equally natural phenomenon of the parent being more attracted to the child of the other sex. The expectant mother (more often than her husband) hopes that the baby will be a boy; the mother finds in the son whom she has reared the desirable qualities that originally attracted her to her husband; the daughter becomes the apple of her father's eye; and the child naturally responds to the parent that shows the greater interest and sympathy.

It is important that parents should try to show equal interest in – and sympathy with –

children of both sexes. In extreme cases, excessive attraction of a child to the parent of the opposite sex can not only make it difficult for that child to find a marriage partner but can also lead to repression and psychoneurosis.

electric shock. A person touching a 'live' electric wire and receiving a shock may be unable to let go, or may fall to the ground unconscious and with breathing stopped. If the victim is still in contact, the rescuer should turn off the current if practicable; or, failing that, should use insulating material, such as a dry stick or a piece of rubber, to remove the victim from the wire. If breathing has stopped, artificial respiration should be carried out.

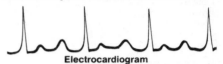

Electrocardiogram

electrocardiogram. A tracing (usually known as an ECG), made by an electrocardiograph, of the electrical changes in the heart muscles. The electrodes of the electrocardiograph, which is essentially a sensitive galvanometer, are normally fastened on both arms and on a leg, with sometimes a fourth electrode placed over the heart. They detect the impulses produced by the heart as it beats and they produce a record of these impulses as a tracing on paper. The procedure in no way hurts the patient.

Examination of the tracing reveals disturbances of rhythm, damage to heart muscle and imbalance between the two sides of the heart with remarkable precision.

The procedure is sometimes used in ordinary, thorough medical examination, but is more often employed where there is a suspicion of some cardiac abnormality, and is regularly used to check progress and recovery after a heart attack.

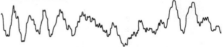

Electroencephalogram

electroencephalogram. A record, made by an electroencephalograph (or EEG), of electrical changes in the brain. By placing the electrodes on different parts of the scalp the discharges from various portions of the brain can be studied.

Electroencephalograms are now used routinely for the diagnosis of minor varieties of epilepsy (which were formerly difficult to differentiate from other conditions) and they are also valuable for the recognition of certain other disorders of the brain. There is, however, some variation in the tracings obtained from normal individuals, with about one-eighth of ordinary persons having 'abnormal' electroencephalograms. Hence an EEG, while a useful aid to diagnosis, cannot be used in isolation.

electrolysis. Chemical destruction of tissue by passage of electrical currents. The procedure is sometimes used to destroy birth marks, warts and the roots of superfluous hair.

elephantiasis. Gross enlargement of parts of the body (the legs below the knee being most often involved, with the scrotum, breasts and arms sometimes affected) due to obstruction of the lymphatic vessels by a parasitic worm, filaria. The embryos of the worms are conveyed to the body by the bite of an infected mosquito. Diethylcarbamazine is the only effective drug but sometimes causes allergic reactions which can be avoided or modified by the use of antihistamine preparations.

The term elephantiasis is also sometimes applied to an enlargement of the leg that may arise from inflammation and partial blockage of lymph glands after childbirth. See WHITELEG.

emaciation. Extreme loss of flesh and wasting of the body. Causes include: (1) various severe disorders, e.g., cancer, chronic nephritis and tuberculosis, (2) starvation, (3) dehydration, i.e., extreme loss of fluid, as in cholera or in severe dysentery, (4) terminal stages of a few rare organic diseases of the nervous system, or (5) anorexia nervosa and hysterical refusal of food.

Progressive loss of weight is always an indication for medical investigation.

embolism. Blockage of an artery by an embolus, e.g., a fragment of a diseased heart valve, a fragment of a blood clot, a foreign body or an air-bubble. The effects of an embolism depend on the size and position of the vessel blocked. If the vessel is small and there is an alternative channel of circulation, the effects may be minimal. If the blockage is in an artery of the brain the embolism may cause paralysis of one side of the body (hemiplegia), if in the retinal artery it may cause blindness of one eye, and if in a coronary artery it may cause sudden death.

In some circumstances surgical removal of an embolus is practicable.

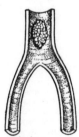 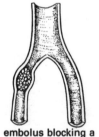

embolus   embolus blocking a
travelling along narrow vessel and
the blood vessel preventing blood flow

Embolism

embrocations and liniments. Preparations that are rubbed into the skin for the treatment of muscle strains, joint sprains and injured ligaments, to encourage the dispersal of inflammatory nodules as in fibrositis. Soap liniment is a simple alcoholic solution of soap and camphor, suitable for most mild cases. Camphorated soap liniment is a stronger preparation containing a little ammonia as a stimulant. Camphorated oil is a much favoured application for the chest and back of children.

Various other liniments are also in common use.

Most liniments are poisonous if taken internally. They should therefore be kept in a safe place, along with other poisons, and should not be applied to broken skin.

embryo. The unborn offspring from the time of union of the ovum and the sperm to the time, about two months later, when its form has become recognizably human. After that time the term 'foetus' is used.

The ovum is fertilized in the Fallopian tube and the resultant embryo is just large enough to be visible to the naked eye; it travels down the Fallopian tube to the uterus, implants itself in the uterine wall and divides and re-divides into a cluster of cells. The outer cells in due course form the placenta (from which the embryo draws nourishment from the mother) and the chorion, or outer membrane, enveloping the embryo. The inner cells form the amnion, or inner protective membrane, and the embryo proper.

Growth of the embryo proper occurs in three separate layers. The ectoderm or outer bone layer forms an outer wrapping and curls over to create an inner tube (the neural tube). The skin is later formed from the outer wrapping and the nervous system from the inner tube. The endoderm or inner growth layer later forms the digestive system and the lungs; and the mesoderm, or middle growth layer, forms the heart, muscles and bones.

As the embryo grows it essentially re-enacts human EVOLUTION. At about three weeks it has gill-slits, occurring in the same position as the gills of a fish; by a few weeks later it is definitely mammalian; and by eight or nine weeks it is identifiable as human in its structure.

By that age the embryo is about 4 cm. (1.5 in.) long, has a relatively enormous head of about 2 cm. (0.75 in.) and very rudimentary limbs. It has lost its tail and its heart has begun to pump blood through the system.

By about 16 weeks the foetus is roughly 10 cm. (4 in.) long and weighs approximately 100 g. (3.5 oz.), and by 24 weeks it has reached 20 cm. (8 in.) and 600 g. (21 oz.) and has some chance of survival if born prematurely. However, in English law it is not considered viable until 28 weeks.

embryology. The study of the growth and development of the EMBRYO and the FOETUS. The science began with Aristotle's investigation of developing chicks in the fourth century B.C. but made little progress until after the advent of the microscope in the seventeenth century.

Broadly, embryology has three uses. It increases knowledge of the course of evolution, since the early stages of any embryo recapitulate these stages in its remote ancestors; it helps understanding of the anatomy and physiology of man and animals; and it throws some light on how congenital defects arise.

emetic. A substance given to induce vomiting. This may be needed in cases of narcotic and irritant poisoning but should never be used in corrosive poisoning, i.e., in poisoning by strong acids and alkalis. An easily prepared emetic is a tablespoonful of mustard to half a tumblerful of water or two tablespoonfuls of salt to the same amount of water.

emotion. The state of consciousness in which such sensations as joy, love, anger and hate are experienced.

In an early classification William McDougall (1871-1938) related instincts and emotions in partnerships of 'feeling' and 'action'. For instance, the emotion of fear is related to the instinct for escape or self-preservation; anger is related to our instinct for combat or aggression, and amusement to laughter. In this way he related fourteen separate emotions with instincts, but some psychologists maintain that this is an over-simplification. They assert that these 'emotions' are merely primary feelings, that an emotion implies both a feeling and an impulse to act, and that there also exist blended emotions (e.g., hearing a noise when alone in a house a person may feel both fear, with impulse to seek safety, and curiosity, with impulse to investigate).

Whatever the exact definition accepted, the emotions give colour and vitality to life. They govern our behaviour to a greater extent than does reason and they enable us when strongly moved to perform feats of physical and mental endurance which would be impossible in the absence of emotion. The completely unemotional person tends to lack drive and to be unattracted to others.

Emotions, however, are considerably modified by upbringing. We learn, for example, not to hit someone when we are angry, and a soldier learns not to run away when afraid. For the proper development of character, the emotions, which have free expression in a baby, must come increasingly under the general control of persisting sentiments. In a healthy mind there should be a reasonable balance between, on the one hand, expression of emotion and, on the other, conformity not only to the patterns imposed by training and associates but also to the sentiments created in the formative years. Full indulgence in such emotions as rage and lust with their characteristic actions can produce conflict with others and with the law, but to give free rein to the feeling without the action can harm the individual, e.g., the man who masks his barely controlled fury may have a dangerous rise in blood pressure or develop indigestion. On the other hand, excessive repression of emotions can contribute very materially to the production of PSYCHOSOMATIC DISEASE and also of NEUROSIS.

In the rearing of children the fostering of emotional health is particularly important, and there are four points to be especially noted.

1. For the child's emotional development he needs a sense of security, an awareness of continuing parental affection and a reasonably permissive atmosphere with only such rules and restrictions as are essential for his safety or for the well-being of the household.

2. Battles of wills should be avoided. Parental victory carries with it dangers of resentment and repression of feelings in the child and certainly does not help his emotional development; child victory is even more dangerous, leading to the 'spoiled' child who later has to learn with difficulty that a hard world will not conform to his wishes. It is better to distract the child, or ignore him, during an emotional crisis, and at an unemotional period to seek to discuss the situation in an attempt to work out a solution satisfactory to both parent and child.

3. The child (an imitator from infancy) should be made aware of his parents' love of fair-play, justice, beauty etc., and gradually brought to see that most human situations involve the feelings and desires of more than one person.

4. Complete supression of emotion should not be encouraged. The 'stiff upper lip' policy of the past can perhaps be correlated with the fact that one British adult in every nine receives treatment during his life for a disorder of emotional origin.

emphysema. A condition in which the fine air-cells of the lungs are distended and their dividing walls destroyed, so that less space remains available for the exchange of oxygen and carbon dioxide. Emphysema occurs as a result of the physical stress of frequent coughing, in chronic bronchitis and sometimes in asthma, or as a result of years of blowing wind musical instruments. It causes the chest to become enlarged and barrel-shaped, is associated with breathlessness, and may ultimately damage the heart.

Since lung tissues cannot be replaced, treatment consists essentially of dealing with the causal disease before the emphysema has developed. In existing emphysema residence in a warm, dry climate is often beneficial, breathing exercises may help and the patient should be given a portable oxygen inhaler to use at need.

empyema. A condition in which pus is present in the chest cavity, between the two layers of pleura. Before the era of antibiotics it was not uncommon as a complication of pneumonia, and it can also arise from wounds of the chest.

Symptoms are pain, breathlessness and swinging temperature. Treatment consists of removal of pus through a hollow needle inserted through the chest wall, followed by injection of penicillin solution. During convalescence breathing exercises are useful to promote expansion of the lung and to prevent adhesions.

encephalitis. Inflammation of the brain. It occurs (1) as a rare complication of almost all of the acute infectious diseases, (2) through virus infection, as in ENCEPHALITIS LETHARGICA, or rabies, (3) following wounds of the skull, (4) from spread of inflammation from the ear or nose, and (5) very infrequently as a complication of vaccination against smallpox.

Symptoms include headache, irritability, fever and vomiting, followed by convulsions and drowsiness. Sulphonamides and antibiotics are the drugs of choice.

encephalitis lethargica. An inflammation of the brain, caused by a virus, and characterized by headache, high temperature, double vision and disturbance of sleep rhythm – drowsiness by day and irritability at night. Complete recovery is unusual, the majority of victims being left with disturbance of muscular co-ordination (post-encephalitic parkinsonism).

There was a widespread outbreak in many countries from 1917 to 1923, but since then the disease has disappeared.

The condition is sometimes known as 'sleepy sickness' and should not be confused with SLEEPING SICKNESS, a tropical disease caused by a trypanosome transmitted by the bite of a tsetse fly.

endemic. Persistently present. The term is used to indicate diseases always present in a population, in contrast to epidemics: e.g., bronchitis is endemic in Britain, whereas at intervals there is an epidemic of influenza.

endocarditis. Inflammation of the lining of the HEART, particularly that of the valves. It can occur as a complication of rheumatic fever (rheumatic endocarditis) or from bacterial infection (bacterial endocarditis). The heart valve becomes deformed, so that it does not close fully when the heart contracts. Apart from damage to the circulation there is a danger of a fragment of a deformed valve being carried in the blood-stream and producing an EMBOLISM.

Bacterial endocarditis responds well to antibiotics. Rheumatic endocarditis may largely subside after the rheumatic fever is cured, but in some cases the valves are so badly damaged as to warrant surgical repair.

endocrine glands. The endocrine glands are ductless glands which pump the hormones or 'chemical messengers' of the body directly into the blood-stream. These messengers are as important as the brain and nervous system: for instance growth, menstruation and the changes that occur during pregnancy are in no way under the control of the brain, but are regulated by hormone secretion from the endocrine glands.

Study of these glands and the hormones they produce has widely affected scientific opinion about the functioning of mind and body, and has given increased understanding of human behaviour. Anomalies of development, idiosyncracies of personality and some mental disorders have been found to be related to variations in the activity of the glands.

Analysis of the exact functions of the various glands is difficult because (1) several of the glands produce more than one hormone, e.g., the pituitary secretes at least eight; (2) several glands may be involved in a single function, e.g., growth depends largely on a hormone from the pituitary but partly on hormones from the thyroid and the sex glands; (3) there are complex relationships between the nervous and chemical functions of the body, e.g., the conscious emotion of rage stimulates the secretion of adrenaline by the suprarenal glands; and (4) the effect produced by a hormone depends not only on the amount of hormone secreted but also on the responsiveness of the organ or tissue, e.g., the same amount of secreted hormone may create excess, or normal amounts, or sparcity of facial hair.

The individual glands are; pituitary, thyroid, parathyroid, adrenal (or suprarenal), thymus, islets of Langerhans in the pancreas, male testes and female ovaries. After a brief historical sketch these are described separately, but their interconnections should be remembered, e.g., a pituitary hormone stimulates the thyroid to produce more thyroxine and an excess of thyroxine lowers pituitary secretion.

History. Roger of Palermo in the twelfth century treated simple goitre (thyroid deficiency) with burnt seaweed, rich in iodine which the thyroid needs for its work; Parry (1825) and Graves (1835) established the functions of the thyroid; and Kendall (1915) discovered its hormone, thyroxine. Addison

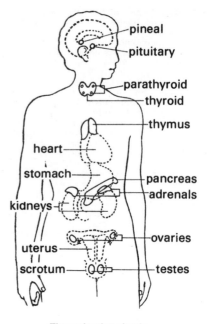

The endocrine glands

(1849) described the effects of suprarenal failure. Bartolin of Copenhagen found an association between pancreatic disease and diabetes about 1670, and Banting and Best (1921) isolated the hormone insulin. Collip (1925) isolated a parathyroid hormone. Butenadt and Ruzicka separately isolated sex hormones about 1939. Diseases associated with defects of the pituitary were suggested by Cushing and others in the nineteenth century, but the complete story of the pituitary is not yet fully known.

Pituitary. The pituitary, a two-lobed gland about the size of a pea, lies at the base of the skull, beneath the central part of the brain and resting on a depression of the spenoid bone. Despite its small size the pituitary produces various hormones which in part control the other endocrine glands, so that it is often called 'the conductor of the endocrine orchestra'.

The front lobe of the pituitary secretes at least six hormones. These include a growth hormone which controls the growth of the skeleton, a thyroid-stimulating hormone, adrenocorticotrophin (ACTH), which controls the activity of the cortex of the adrenal glands, gonadotrophic hormones which regulate the activity of the ovaries and testes, and prolactin which is responsible for the secretion of milk in the nursing mother.

The rear lobe of the pituitary releases two hormones – vasopressin, which causes constriction of small arteries and also acts on the kidney, regulating water absorption and hence the amount of urine, and oxytocin, which stimulates the muscles of the uterus causing it to contract during labour.

The secretory activities of the pituitary itself are regulated partly by messages from the portion of the brain that appears to control emotions (hypothalamus) and partly by 'feed-back' from the hormones secreted by the other endocrine glands.

Thyroid. The thyroid gland in the front of the neck consists of two lobes (roughly 5 cm. long and 3 cm. wide which is very approximately 2 in. by 1 in.) on each side of the windpipe and connected by a narrow isthmus. It manufactures two hormones, thyroxine and tri-iodothyronine. These secretions regulate the rate at which the body uses energy, e.g., speeding up the heart rate and the respiratory rate by extra secretion where necessary.

Parathyroid. These are four tiny glands (about 6 mm. by 2 mm.) lying behind the thyroid. Hormones secreted by these glands control the level of calcium and phosphorus in the blood by regulating the excretion of phosphates by the kidneys and by mobilizing calcium from its stores in the bones.

Adrenal or suprarenal. These are two bean-sized glands situated above the kidneys. The outer shell of each gland is called the cortex and produces several steroid hormones, one of which (aldosterone) regulates the levels of sodium and potassium in the blood and urine, while another (cortisol or hydrocortisone) permits the formation of glucose from protein – with excess leading to hyperglycaemia, and insufficiency causing hypoglycaemia. Other hormones from the cortex (androgens) are responsible for the development at adolescence of the scrotum, penis, prostate and larynx and for the growth of facial hair; and in both sexes they stimulate sexual activity.

The inner core or medulla of the suprarenals secretes two hormones, adrenaline and noradrenaline. Adrenaline combats the metabolic consequences of stress: that is to say, it raises the level of blood sugar by mobilizing glucose from stores in the liver, dilates the bronchioles to allow greater intake of oxygen and speeds up the heart rate. Noradrenaline constricts the peripheral blood-vessels, reserving blood for the parts that are more important in fighting. In short, the suprarenal hormones prepare the body for 'fight or flight'.

Thymus. A two-lobed gland lying behind the breast bone and extending into the neck. It grows until puberty and thereafter shrinks away to practically nothing. The function of its secretion is imperfectly understood but it is concerned with the production of lymphocytes and of antibodies to infection and there is some evidence that it is also concerned with growth and development.

The islets of Langerhans. While the pancreas is a gland with a duct, carrying digestive juices to the small intestine, small portions of tissue embedded in the pancreas have entirely separate functions. They secrete insulin which is responsible for the level of blood-sugar for the utilization of sugar in the tissue and so for the production of energy.

The ovaries. Besides producing ova (eggs), the ovaries secrete various hormones including oestrogen and progesterone. These are responsible for the growth and development of the uterus and vagina at puberty, for the menstrual cycle and for the changes that take place in the uterus during pregnancy. Progesterone is thought to be the cause of fluid retention, weight gain and psychological change in pregnancy.

The testes. Besides producing spermatozoa, the testes secrete a hormone testosterone. It is responsible for the maturation of the spermatozoa and for the development and maintenance of masculine characteristics.

Additionally the stomach secretes hormones needed for digestion and the kidney produces a hormone which regulates the production of red blood corpuscles.

Diseases of endocrine glands. Only the main diseases can be mentioned here.

Tumour or syphilitic disease of the pituitary may result in either increased or decreased secretion, and may affect both lobes or only one. Increased secretion in a child causes giantism, resulting in a weakly giant of seven to eight feet tall and, in an adult, acromegaly. Decreased secretion causes stunting of skeletal development, depression of sexual function, mental retardation and increase of fat tissue. The 'fat boy' of Dickens was probably a case of under-activity of the pituitary. Diseases of under-activity go under various names, e.g., Simmond's disease, diabetes insipidus and Brissaud's disease, according to which symptoms predominate. Headaches and disturbances of vision, especially of colour vision, are common in diseases of the pituitary but have many other causes.

Thyroid over-activity without excessive secretion occurs from lack of iodine in food and water and creates simple goitre. Deficiency of thyroid secretion – from congenital causes, from tumours or from extreme lack of iodine – in childhood causes cretinism, and in adults myxoedema. Excessive activity of the thyroid causes hyperthyroidism or Graves' disease.

Over-activity of the parathyroids (most commonly caused by a benign tumour) leads either to renal calculus, from excess calcium in the blood and hence formation of a 'stone' in the kidney, or to signs of calcium excess in the blood, namely weight loss, lack of appetite, nausea, drowsiness and weakness. Tetany, still ascribed to parathyroid deficiency in some text-books, can actually be caused by such deficiency – which, however, practically never occurs except in rare circumstances of the parathyroids being damaged during an operation on the thyroid. It is far more often due to malabsorption of calcium or lack of vitamin D.

If adrenals are over-active it causes Cushing's syndrome, characterized by obesity, high blood pressure and absence of menstruation. Depending on the part of the gland most affected it can also cause masculinization of women, with increased facial hair and enlargement of the clitoris in the genital region, and in males it can lead to precocious puberty. Deficiency causes the progressive muscular weakness and skin pigmentation known as Addison's disease.

An enlarged thymus can cause pressure on the trachea which results in breathing difficulties; this is usually found in children who are fat, anaemic and lethargic (see STATUS LYMPHATICUS). Treatment is by irradiation of the thymus gland with x-rays.

Insufficiency of insulin production by the islets of Langerhans in the pancreas leads to the condition of diabetes mellitus.

Deficiency of the secretions of the ovary leads to absence of menstruation, lack of development of the female characteristics at puberty, and infertility. Decrease of ovarian activity in middle age is the main cause of menopause. Similarly, deficiency of testosterone from the testes may lead to failure to manufacture spermatozoa and hence to infertility or sterility, and also to failure of the development of the masculine characteristics at puberty.

endometritis. Inflammation of the mucus membrane lining the inside of the uterus. In the acute form the main features are abdominal pain, raised temperature and often a semi-purulent discharge from the uterus. The chronic form is characterized by pain both in the back and in the lower abdomen, and by a blood-stained discharge. The causes are numerous and treatment varies according to the cause. Hormones are often required, but some cases need operative treatment.

enema. Injection of liquid into the rectum to clear the bowel, to dispel persistent wind or, in some cases, to introduce fluid or nutrient (although a nutrient enema is usually called a rectal injection or RECTAL FEEDING). An enema is normally given before any major surgical operation.

A barium enema, containing a suspension of barium sulphate, is used in x-ray examination of the rectum and large intestine. Since the barium sulphate is opaque to x-rays, the bowel shows up clearly and any ulcers or tumours can be identified.

enteric. Literally, pertaining to the intestine. The term is used mainly for the group of infectious diseases including typhoid and paratyphoid fever.

enteric fever. A general name used to describe both TYPHOID FEVER and a milder disease of shorter incubation period, paratyphoid fever.

enteritis. Inflammation of the intestines, usually manifested by diarrhoea and abdominal pain. Causes include bacterial infection, virus infestation, chill, indigestible food, certain poisons, a grossly excessive meal and a heavy consumption of alcohol. If the condition is severe, bacteriological and biochemical examination of the motions is desirable. In mild cases an aperient should be given to remove any possible irritant, the patient should be rested in bed with only liquid diet for two or three days and an astringent such as chalk and catechu may be given.

enterostomy. A surgical operation by which an artificial opening is made in the intestine, usually to by-pass an obstruction created by a tumour or an ulcer. If the opening is made in the large intestine (colon) it is called a colostomy.

enuresis. See BED-WETTING.

environment and health. Until this century environment was usually regarded as the aggregate of surrounding physical conditions, e.g., air, water, housing, food, clothes and heating. Nowadays the term is increasingly employed to include also emotional, social and cultural influences, such as congenial or antagonistic associates and the availability or otherwise of reading matter. The three cardinal factors affecting health are genetic inheritance and past and present physical and psycho-social environment. Physically, emotionally and intellectually we cannot grow beyond our inherited potential, but growth can be stunted by faulty environment. Thus the son of tall parents may fail to reach even average height if deprived of adequate food and exercise; and the intellectually bright child reared in a home that lacks books and magazines is clearly at a profound disadvantage.

Childhood environment is of tremendous importance. For instance, a child brought up in an area where the water has an inadequacy of fluoride, in a household where excessive sweet-eating is normal and with parents who do not encourage tooth-brushing is likely to become an adult with decayed or missing teeth; and a child who is dominated and given no opportunity to make his own explorations and form his own decisions is unlikely to develop into an adult with mature personality. An adult with good heredity and good childhood environment has considerable resistance to adverse environmental factors; but the healthiest lungs will ultimately deteriorate from continued atmospheric pollution, and few of us could live for years in slum conditions and on a bare subsistence income without both physical and mental deterioration.

The influence of environment on health is so profound that only a few points can be selected for mention here.

Climate. There is a vast difference between a hot dry climate (e.g., the Sahara or the Kalihari) where low humidity permits rapid absorption of perspiration and so renders exercise practicable, and a steamy hot climate of high humidity (e.g., West Africa or the Amazon basin). In general, however, hot climates are associated with lethargic and indolent inhabitants, with extreme activity of – and therefore liability to diseases of – the skin and digestive organs. There is a prevalence of bacterial and parasitic diseases (such as malaria, yellow fever and typhoid) and relative infrequency of respiratory diseases. Cold climates are associated with hardy, vigorous inhabitants, with fewer infectious diseases but with higher incidence of respiratory and kidney diseases.

Temperate climates (including those from the Mediterranean to Britain and including the northern states of the U.S.A. and the south of Canada) have to some extent the best of both worlds; most scientific inventions and advances in literature, art and music have emanated from temperate zones. However, better sanitation, sewerage and water-supplies, improved prevention and treatment of infections and systems of artificial heating and cooling of buildings and of increasing or decreasing humidity are steadily making the hotter and colder parts of the world more tolerable to people from temperate regions.

Apart from the basic classification into hot, temperate and cold, climate is often sub-classified into sea-board, inland low, mountain and dry. Sea-board and ocean climates have denser air, more moisture and – apart from large centres of population – fewer bacteria; a sea-side holiday is traditionally regarded as best for the jaded town-dweller. Inland low climates have greater than average variation between summer and winter temperatures and are often termed 'relaxing'. Mountain climates, with slightly rarer air, are invigorating for the young but unsuitable for persons with diseases of the heart or kidneys. Dry or desert climates, often very warm by day but cold by night, are said to be useful for persons suffering from rheumatism, kidney diseases and asthma.

Rural and industrial communities. Peasant societies in countries with under-developed economic systems are usually based on subsistence agriculture and nutrition is often poor, especially in winter and spring. Sewerage systems are frequently inadequate or non-existent, infections are very common and medical and nursing services are generally very limited with the result that mortality in infancy and childhood is high, and survival into old age is relatively rare. Manifestly, however, most of the effects on health are not the direct result of the environment but of inability – as yet – to control it.

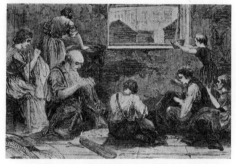

A slum environment detrimental to health: 'Room occupied by a military tailor and his family at no. 10, Hollybush Place' – from the *Illustrated London News,* 24 October 1863.

Industrial societies have an elaborate division of labour (including specialization within the various branches of medicine and nursing), an advanced technology and a highly developed social system. At the time of the industrial revolution and the rapid expansion of cities, health in these cities was far worse than in many rural communities: jerry-built houses, gross over-crowding, inadequate sanitary facilities and absence of measures either to prevent or to treat diseases took an enormous toll of human lives. Nowadays, however, most industrial societies have better nutrition, better environmental hygiene, better housing, better health services, lower child mortality and greater survival into old age than have rural communities. On the other hand, the industrial societies also have higher incidence of mental disorders and of diseases occasioned by stress and by accumulation of population.

The change from a predominantly rural to a mainly urban population in countries like Britain and some of the states of the U.S.A. has vastly altered the disease pattern. For instance, both in the U.K. and in the U.S.A., accidents – home, traffic and industrial – are now the highest cause of death between the ages of 1 year and 45 years. Again, diseases that were uncommon in the past, such as coronary thrombosis, lung cancer and peptic ulcer, have become the modern epidemics of urban populations.

Some effects of scientific advances. We all tend to think of the scientific revolution as having affected health advantageously by providing greater variety of food, better housing and better services for the prevention and treatment of illness, and disadvantageously by creating risk of damage from such substances as lead, mercury, DDT and strontium-90, and by the sheer accumulation of houses, factories and vehicles giving rise to problems of air-pollution, noise-pollution and even waste-disposal. Yet perhaps the biggest effects are on mental life. A young couple, moving to where work is plentiful, set up house far from the parents and associates of either; their dwelling is in a dormitory suburb which is almost deserted by day; they travel miles to factory or office to join workers from a variety of similar dormitory suburbs; they make their purchases at supermarkets; and they have none of the companionship and community life of residents in a village or small, self-supporting town.

As transport becomes easier and as industries become less dependent on the proximity of coal mines or steel works, some planners envisage a gradual return to the 'small town' community – not the dormitory suburb but the self-supporting town, with its own industries, factories, offices and social life. Meantime, we increasingly face the problem of the person who lives in a city or dormitory suburb without recognized and accepted membership of any group, and with consequential effects on emotional and mental health.

A healthy environment. Writers of sixty years ago would probably have defined a healthy environment as comprising a climate tolerable to the individuals concerned, unpolluted air, pure water, adequate sanitation, clean food of reasonable variety, fit houses with proper heating and ventilation systems and perhaps reasonable access to facilities for sport and recreation. Certainly all these are needful but there are less easily stated needs – such as a modicum of privacy, reasonable proximity of friends or relatives and active, participating membership of some form of group.

Yet many human beings have a resilience that enables them to remain healthy despite adverse environmental factors. Examples are the villagers who appear to have developed an immunity to the contaminated water that they drink, the vagrant who seems none the worse for sleeping in a house long condemned as beyond repair, and the solitary who remains healthy despite the absence of human companionship.

See KEEPING FIT.

enzyme. A highly specific catalyst produced by living cells within the body and promoting chemical changes, especially those in which complex substances are broken down into forms which the body can use. Examples are ptyalin (secreted by the salivary glands) which initiates the breakdown of starches to sugars; lactase (in gastic juice) which reduces lactose, the sugar in milk, to the simpler glucose; pepsin (also in gastric juice) which acts on protein; and tsypsin (secreted by the pancreas) which also acts on protein.

The enzymes – probably thousands in number – are in most cases essential to life. Certain poisons operate by inactivating enzymes, e.g., cyanides block the action of the particular enzyme that controls the release of oxygen from the red blood corpuscles.

Several hereditary diseases are due to

enzyme deficiency. For example, the amino-acid, phenylalanine, is normally converted to a simpler amino-acid, tyrosine, under the influence of a particular enzyme, but where this enzyme is deficient or absent phenylalanine accumulates, producing the disease of phenylketonuria, which shows itself in brain damage and mental deficiency. In this condition, mental deficiency can be prevented if, following very early diagnosis, the affected baby is given a diet virtually free from phenylalanine. Again, another enzyme converts tyrosine to thyroid hormone, and a congenital absence of the enzyme is the underlying cause of cretinism.

Various enzymes are themselves activated by co-enzymes. For instance, the enzyme which causes blood to clot is at all times present in the blood but is activated only when a co-enzyme is liberated at the site of an injury.

In recent years the relationship between vitamins and enzymes has become appreciated. Most – and perhaps all – vitamins act as co-enzymes. Hence the underlying mechanism of most deficiency diseases is not simply the absence of the vitamin but the failure of an enzyme to act because of the absence of the appropriate co-enzyme.

eosinophil. A variety of white blood corpuscle containing large granules which are readily stained with the red acidic dye, eosin. Normally about 2 or 3 per cent white blood corpuscles are eosinophils. An increase to above 4 per cent suggests the presence of – (1) certain intestinal parasites, or (2) some allergic conditions, especially asthma, or (3) various skin diseases, such as psoriasis, or (4) Hodgkins' disease or, very rarely, (5) a form of leukaemia. Although of some diagnostic importance especially if found repeated or continuing when a second drop of blood is examined a few days after the first, an increase in the number of eosinophils must be interpreted with a certain amount of caution. To give one example, if blood from a person suffering from scarlet fever is examined at different days after the appearance of the rash, the eosinophil count will be found to be increased at one stage and decreased at another.

ephedrine. An alkaloid originally derived from the Chinese plant *ma huang*. It has effects broadly resembling those of adrenalin and has the advantage that it can be taken by mouth. In many cases of asthma it eases the breathing by widening the bronchial tubes and bronchioles, but a few asthmatics find it unhelpful. It is useful in many cases of hay fever, is often included in drops or sprays to relieve nasal congestion, and is sometimes employed in eye-drops to dilate the pupil before eye examinations.

epidemic. An outbreak of disease simultaneously affecting large numbers of people. The term has undergone three changes of meaning during the last half century.

It was originally applied simply to outbreaks of infectious disease, whether spread by direct contact, by inhaling infected droplets from breath or sneezing, by drinking infected water, by eating infected food or by other methods of transmission. Epidemics affecting a number of countries were termed pandemics. The smallpox pandemic of A.D. 165-180 killed Marcus Aurelius and did much to destroy the Roman Empire, the plague of 1346-51, known as the BLACK DEATH, destroyed about one-third of the world's population, and the influenza pandemic of 1918-19 killed more people than the First World War.

We still have pandemics of influenza, and Asia suffers – and Europe suffered – from epidemics (or sometimes pandemics) of smallpox, plague, typhus and cholera. Epidemiologists contrasted 'epidemic' (abnormal prevalence) with 'endemic' (persistent prevalence) and even tried to restrict 'epidemic' to a prevalence exceeding 1 per cent of the population.

Vaccination and immunization, and education of the public about their desirability, provided individual protection against many infections and, when the majority were rendered immune, reduced the likelihood of spread to the unimmunized minority; and general public health measures further reduced the frequency of most infections. By the 1950s most developed countries no longer had epidemics, in the old sense of the term, excepting influenza and the common cold (which is endemic rather than epidemic). Consequently 'epidemic' began to be used for any considerable outbreak of an infectious disease, without any restiction to a particular degree of prevalence.

With the realization that the same epidemiological investigatory procedures as for infections could be used to study the causes of non-infectious diseases, and that similar health education methods could be employed for their reduction and control, 'epidemic' has in recent years come to mean simply 'widely prevalent', with the old distinction from 'endemic' lost. Thus we nowadays speak of bronchitis, coronary thrombosis, rheumatism, cancer and home and road accidents as the modern epidemics.

epidemiology. The science that studies the prevalence of a disease in the community, the groups affected and the groups spared, the methods of spread, and the effects.

Because infections were initially easier to investigate, epidemiology was until this century applied mostly to infections, but its contribution to non-infectious diseases is already considerable.

Essentially while the clinician is concerned with the treatment of sick persons, the epidemiologist is concerned with disease and absence of disease in the community. Indeed the persons who escape are just as important to the epidemiologist as are those who develop the disease. To give a single example, pellagra, in certain countries then common among the poor and in prisons, was regarded as an infectious disease. The fact that certain people in frequent contact with the disease – prison warders – did not contract it gave an epidemiologist the clue that it was not infectious but related to diet; and, long before any of the vitamins of the B complex were identified, pellagra – which is caused by deficiency of nicotinic acid and riboflavine – was established as a deficiency disease, preventable or curable by alteration of the diet.

A clinical doctor alone is badly placed for finding the causes or method of spread of a disease. If he covers the entire field of medicine (like the general practitioner of the U.K.) he sees only a few cases of each of a multitude of diseases: for example, if the association between grief or bereavement and predisposition to tuberculosis was not yet known and if a general practitioner came to suspect it, he would in an average practice encounter about one new case of tuberculosis each year and would therefore have little chance of confirming his theory. If the clinical doctor is specialized, he sees many cases of the particular disease but usually has little knowledge of the home conditions or working circumstances of his patients, and in particular no knowledge of how many persons with similar home conditions or similar working circumstances do not develop the disease.

It is unlikely that clinical doctors alone would have differentiated typhoid and paratyphoid fever: clinically paratyphoid is almost identical with mild typhoid, although the incubation periods and methods of spread are different. Clinicians for long grouped gastric and duodenal ulcer together as 'peptic ulcer' with similar symptoms and similar immediate treatment, but they affect different socio-economic groups and both prevention and long-term treatment are clearly different. It is very unlikely that a specialist in cancer would have noted that, with some lifelong non-smokers among his lung cancer cases, there were a higher proportion of heavy cigarette smokers among his patients than in the community. With a disease that has many causes, such as coronary thrombosis, it is particularly unlikely that doctors who specialized in treatment of the condition would have appreciated that they had an over-average proportion of patients who were overweight, or heavy consumers of animal fats, or heavy cigarette smokers, or under prolonged emotional stress.

Clearly epidemiology can contribute enormously to ascertainment of the causes, and therefore of the means of prevention, of many diseases, and to working out the particular age, sex and occupation groups to which preventive techniques for particular conditions can most usefully be directed. Clearly, too, epidemiologists, clinicians and backroom laboratory workers should work together to elucidate the causes, methods of spread and means of prevention of diseases.

There are, however, two main difficulties. First, in all countries John Citizen sees the need for a highly skilled physician or surgeon who will treat his disease or that of his neighbour, but is much less aware of the need for equally highly skilled epidemiologists whose work may render that treatment unnecessary. Secondly, in appointments to the numerically small profession of epidemiologists there is a tendency to think exclusively of a medical background, with its inevitably clinical orientation. From their different types of expertise it is likely that a doctor, a health visitor, a social worker and a statistician, each given advanced training in epidemiology, would – other factors being equal – do work of more value than would four doctors, all with similar background, given the same advanced training in epidemiological methods.

There is also a further difficulty. The epidemiologist may discover the groups most susceptible and the conditions under which they are most at risk, e.g., that falls in the home are frequent in the elderly and middle aged, that they are commoner in women than in men, that they are commoner in the widowed or separated than in married or single persons, that they are associated with the ends of periods of maximum activity and that they are more frequent at times of emotional upset; but the epidemiologist is not as a rule trained to communicate his findings meaningfully to the persons at greatest risk.

Unless the epidemiologist on the one hand and the health education officer, health visitor or other worker with skill in communicating and persuading can collaborate, many of the findings of epidemiology will fail to improve the health of the community. To take two simple examples, epidemiological studies have proved beyond a shadow of doubt that the risks of damage from whooping cough vaccination are less than one-thousandth part the risks from whooping cough and can be further reduced by excluding the tiny proportion of children unsuitable for vaccination, and epidemiological investigations over a quarter of a century have established beyond a shadow of doubt that removal of fluoride deficiency where it exists in drinking water can enormously reduce dental disease without creating any disease whatsoever; but – because the epidemiological findings have not been suitably communicated to the public – a goodly number of parents still hesitate to have their children protected against whooping cough and many communities still resist the addition of fluoride to water deficient in it.

epidermis. The outer layer of the SKIN.

epididymis. A curved structure attached to the testicle, consisting of a twisted tube leading to the duct which conveys the sperms from the testicle.

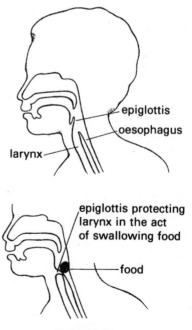

The epiglottis

epiglottis. A yellowish, leaf-shaped flap of fibro-cartilage situated at the back of the throat, behind the root of the tongue. During the act of swallowing the epiglottis is pressed against the opening to the larynx thus closing it, with the result that food enters the oesophagus. The not uncommon experience of choking during swallowing is a result of the epiglottis acting imperfectly or belatedly, so that particles of food enter the larynx and trachea.

epilepsy. An ill-defined but common group of disorders characterized by recurrent convulsive seizures and affecting about one in every two hundred of the population.

Epileptic fits are a symptom of brain damage. Causes include hereditary defect, foetal injuries and disturbances of development, birth injuries, cerebral infections and head injuries, but in many cases no cause can be identified. In most cases the first seizures occur in childhood or adolescence, the condition is not progressive, and the person has a normal span of life.

In the severest form (grand mal) the fit is often preceded by an aura or warning such as flashes of light or ringing in the ears. This warning is usually the same for any one patient and may enable him to lie down in a safe place. With or without the aura the patient loses consciousness, becomes rigid with muscles contracted and teeth clenched for some seconds, and thereafter has violent jerkings of the limbs and facial muscles, passing in a minute or so to a comatose stage. The immediate treatment of a fit is to turn the patient on his side (lest he vomits and blocks his respiratory passages) and to place a spoon or similar object in his mouth (to prevent the tongue from being bitten).

A milder form (petit mal) is characterized by momentary loss of consciousness without convulsions; and a third form (psycho-motor seizures) is marked by restlessness and confused movements.

Various drugs (e.g., phenobarbitone and primidone) are useful for controlling the fits, and an epileptic can lead a reasonably normal life except for such activities as ladder climbing, swimming and car driving.

Over the centuries epilepsy has been the subject of a vast amount of superstition. The Greeks regarded it as indicating 'possession' by a god, an idea which Hippocrates tried to debunk in his treatise, *On the Sacred Disease.* The Romans and early Christians still clung to the idea that 'the falling sickness' was divinely inspired. In mediaeval and early modern times epilepsy was often thought to indicate either insanity or mental deficiency. Even today it is perhaps desirable to state clearly that an epileptic is a normal person except during his fits, and that the only barriers to his physical and intellectual activity are those in which a fit would harm himself or other people.

See also CATAPLEXY.

epiphysis. Bone formed from a secondary centre of calcification. Most bones are originally formed of cartilage and later calcified. The part in which the process of calcification – technically termed ossification – first starts is called the primary centre (e.g., in the shaft of a long bone) and the portion calcified from that centre is known as the diaphysis. Ossification starts later at secondary centres (e.g., in the head of a long bone) and the portion calcified from a secondary centre is called the epiphysis.

Ultimately the epiphysis and diaphysis join and (because cartilage can grow but bone normally cannot) the growth of the bone ceases. The age of a child at death can sometimes be determined by examination of the diaphysis and epiphysis of several bones, since for any one bone the junction of the two tends to occur at a fairly constant age.

epistaxis. See NOSE BLEEDING.

epithelioma. The term used for CANCER of the surface cells (epithelium) of the skin or a mucous membrane. An epithelioma may appear as a wart, fissure or nodule. It grows fairly slowly but presently ulcerates, forming an ulcer irregular in shape and with hard floor and margins.

epulis. A benign (non-malignant) tumour on the gum, usually near a tooth socket. A minor operation suffices for its removal.

erection. The rigid state of the penis when filled with blood. Under physical or emotional stimulation (which affects the parasympathetic nerves) the muscles round the veins contract and prevent blood from leaving, so that, as more blood arrives from the arteries the organ becomes engorged, elongates and grows hard and erect.

Inability to have an erection (impotence) is usually a result of psychological difficulties and does not imply sterility. Conversely a man who is sterile, e.g., after vasectomy, can still have erections. Painful and involuntary erection is called priapism.

ergosterol. A substance which, when irradiated with ultra-violet rays, is converted to calciferol, i.e., vitamin D.

ergot. A drug, originally made from a fungus which grows on rye, which stimulates contraction of the uterus and is therefore used at the end of labour. Excess, as from eating infected rye bread over a period, causes poisoning, starting with itching and inflammation of the skin and going on to loss of sensation in the fingers and toes and, in severe cases, to gangrene; this is known as St. Anthony's Fire.

The drug contains several different alkaloids and these are now generally used in pure form. Thus ergometrine is employed to stimulate uterine contractions, and ergotamine is used to relieve migraine. The alkaloids of ergot are compounds of lysergic acid and are therefore related to the hallucinogen LSD.

eructation. See BELCHING.

erysipelas. Literally 'red skin'. A painful infection of the skin caused by streptococci, the same bacteria as cause scarlet fever.

The disease may appear anywhere but occurs most frequently on the face. The affected patch of skin is hot, dark red, painful, tender, rather shiny and with a definite raised edge. The disease spreads by extension of the edge, while blebs sometimes appear in the older portion. General symptoms include rise of temperature, headache and vomiting. Until the advent of sulphonamides and antibiotics erysipelas was considered a very dangerous disease, but it is nowadays easily controlled. The condition, however, is highly contagious, so that care is required in nursing.

In mediaeval times the disease was known as

St. Anthony's Fire, and was confused with a different disease caused by ergot poisoning.

erythema. Abnormal reddening of the skin. Generalized reddening with raised temperature may indicate the beginning of an acute fever, e.g., scarlet fever or measles, while localized erythema with raised temperature suggests either early erysipelas or inflammation of a cut or wound. Erythema without rise in temperature is most commonly the result of an ALLERGY but is sometimes of toxic origin. A small irritable patch on the skin follows the bite of a midge or the sting of a nettle. A hot bath may produce a temporary generalized erythema, a blow may cause a localized erythema, and a blush is an erythema of emotional origin.

Pending investigation of the cause calamine lotion or a dusting powder may help.

erythrocyte. A red blood corpuscle. The colour is due to haemoglobin which carries oxygen from the lungs to the tissues.

erythrocyte sedimentation rate. The rate at which red blood corpuscles in a tube containing citrated blood fall out of suspension and settle at the bottom of the tube. A rapid sedimentation rate suggests the presence of active infection. However, the rate is also increased during pregnancy and in some forms of cancer.

The test (often known by its initials as the ESR) is useful to determine the presence of early infection or of late infection that has not yet cleared.

ethmoid. A light spongy bone situated at the roof of the nose, and wedged between the sockets for the eyes. The thin perpendicular central plate of the ethmoid forms the upper part of the nasal septum. The name ethmoid, meaning 'like a sieve', refers to the large number of holes in the bone; through these holes pass branches of the olfactory nerves, carrying sensations of smell to the brain.

eugenics. The science of the improvement of the human race by selective breeding. Essentially attempts to improve the mental and physical qualities of future generations fall into two groups – positive eugenics, or encouragement of the reproduction of desirable stock, and negative eugenics, or limitation of the reproduction of persons of undesirable stock.

An early example of positive eugenics was perhaps the mediaeval French *droit de seigneur,* whereby the feudal superior was entitled to spend the first night with the newly married bride; and in many countries the ruling group fathered large numbers of illegitimate offspring. Clearly, however, these happenings were eugenic only if there was reason to assume that the offspring of a nobleman and his selected mistresses would on average be superior to the children of those of lower station.

Scientific positive eugenics was impracticable until we had the genetic knowledge of today. It is still impracticable unless a community can select the qualities that it deems most desirable, e.g., intelligence, beauty, physical strength or compassion, and it would still to some extent be vitiated by chance inheritance of recessive characteristics. Apart from recessive inheritance from several generations back we could breed for one quality but combination of qualities would still

be a matter of chance: the son of a brilliant but physically unattractive father and a beautiful but unintellectual mother might well inherit his father's appearance and his mother's brain. Also we have to remember chance mutation: a Stratford butcher of no unusual ancestry and his wife, also of no unusual stock, created William Shakespeare.

Negative eugenics – reduction of the numbers of those who are likely to become degenerates, criminals, mental defectives or carriers of serious genetic defects – is perhaps seen in the ancient Greek practice of destroying deformed or puny babies, a practice still employed by many tribes. The idea of sterilizing feeble-minded persons and persistent criminals gained considerable popularity in the early years of this century, but subsequently fell into disrepute because it was employed in some countries (e.g., Germany under Hitler) both with inadequate knowledge of genetic inheritance and with political and racial implications.

Looking ahead, we have to realize several points: (1) Increased knowledge of genetics enables us to forecast with reasonable accuracy the degree of probability of any two parents producing a child suffering from serious hereditary defect (e.g., spina bifida, Huntington's chorea, deaf-mutism and schizophrenia). (2) Improved antenatal and child health services greatly increase the likelihood of survival of children with such defects. (3) Oral contraceptives, male vasectomy and female tying of tubes make it possible for those who should not reproduce to enjoy normal sex lives. (4) Increased educational and occupational opportunities make it increasingly likely that the more intelligent citizens will be literate and will be members of occupational groups in which family limitation is normally practised. That is to say that unless there is widespread health education about family planning there is a real danger of a decreasing number of children of intelligent parents but no corresponding decrease in the number of children of less intelligent parents. (5) Genetic counselling, facilities for family spacing and, where necessary, family avoidance (coupled with health education on both) could drastically reduce the numbers of children born with serious hereditary defects.

Few informed workers would advocate obligatory sterilization of those who are likely to produce children with serious genetic defects; but an increasing number would suggest that the undesirability of procreation should be made known to such people and that facilities for contraception and sterilization should be made freely available.

Apart from the obvious desirability of reducing the numbers suffering from serious hereditary disease, the effect of family allowances has to be considered. These allowances obviously mean more to the poor than to the wealthy. The case for their continuation is that they improve the nutrition and general environment of the child born into a poor home. The case for their abolition is that better educational and occupational opportunity implies that the poorest groups, to whom family allowances mean most, are increasingly of inferior mental or physical stock.

euphoria. Abnormal elation. A feeling of well-being unrelated to actual circumstances. Alcohol and certain anti-depressant drugs produce this sensation of comfort which is undoubtedly useful in certain abnormal circumstances but is at most times dangerous in that it divorces people from problems requiring to be solved. In this connection it should be remembered that alcohol and drugs are not the only creators of euphoria: Karl Marx called religion 'the opiate of the masses'; a declaration of war produces a remarkable enthusiasm, national pride and feeling of participation and partnership; and, at individual level, a young man whose proposal of marriage has just been accepted may well be in a state of euphoria.

Eustachian tubes. The two narrow passages between the cavity behind the eardrums and the back of the nose. They were first fully described by Eustachius in Rome in 1562 but were actually mentioned by Alcmacon some two thousand years earlier.

euthanasia. The securing of painless death, especially to a person suffering from incurable disease.

Advocates of euthanasia point out that we put incurably diseased animals to death and claim that human beings have at least an equal right to be spared suffering. Such advocates say that a temporary decision by a patient under emotional stress could be prevented by a legal requirement for him to request euthanasia twice at a specified distance of time, and that a requirement for two doctors to be involved would safeguard the patient against the persuasion of inheriting relatives.

Organized religion is opposed to euthanasia on essentially the same grounds as its opposition to suicide; and most doctors have so far taken the view that, while they should relieve pain and suffering, their function is to preserve life, not to end it.

evaluation of health education. Most health services seek to cure disease, so their success or failure is easily measured. Most forms of education seek to impart knowledge, which can be subjected to examination, but HEALTH EDUCATION aims to change attitudes, habits and behaviour, and its success is therefore much harder to measure.

Specific health education campaigns with short-term objectives are fairly easy to evaluate. To mention three examples: if we seek to persuade parents to have their children immunized against a particular disease, we can in due course calculate the number and percentage of children protected; if we try to collect unused pills which children might swallow in the belief that they were sweets, we can reckon the numbers handed in, or can even ascertain a year later whether there has been a reduction in poisoning among young children; and if we try to encourage family planning, we can not only count attendances at family planning clinics but can - in a year or so - note any changes in the birth rate either in the community as a whole or in specific sections of it.

General health education for the improvement of emotional and physical health is extremely difficult to evaluate. One difficulty is that its effects are mostly long-term. For example, education directed towards the prevention of obesity in children and adolescents may show its success mainly in a reduction of coronary thrombosis, chronic bronchitis and arthritis thirty or forty years later; and education of young parents or prospective parents about the dangers in child management of inconsistency, over-strictness and over-licence may show its effects twelve or twenty years later in the incidence of delinquency, illegitimacy and other signs of adolescent rebellion. Another difficulty is that, while a laboratory experiment or a trial of a drug in hospital can be conducted under controlled conditions, people who are offered health education live in a changing community. Thus the effects of health education about diet in year 1 may be affected by changing prices or availability of certain foods in year 2, by changing financial circumstances of the persons educated in year 3, or by altering cultural patterns in year 4. Similarly the apparent prevalence of delinquency may be affected by the altering attitudes of magistrates or by increase or decrease in the number of policemen.

Health education is perhaps the most important and most potentially valuable of all the health services, but its evaluation involves not simply measurement but also assessment of sociological and cultural factors. To take a simple example: an educational campaign by British health vistors or American public health nurses as to the main causes of home accidents could probably be evaluated by measuring the change in the numbers receiving medical treatment for such accidents (though even this measurement would imply that a base-line was produced by ascertainment of numbers before the campaign started) but evaluation of a similar campaign on road accidents would have to take account not only of changing numbers receiving treatment but also of increase in the number of vehicles on the roads and of any improvements in the roads.

In many cases assessment of the success or failure of a health education project has to be made on incidental side effects. Because we are unable to measure this year the long-term effects on a group being voluntarily educated, we have to fall back on the simple criterion of whether they are continuing to attend; or because any effects of a particular poster will not show statistically for years, we have to judge its value by finding to what extent its message is remembered a month after it is withdrawn. Essentially we have to bear in mind that health education is an art as well as a science, and that an art is not wholly susceptible to scientific measurement.

evolution. The derivation of different species from a common ancestor and the process of gradual change over the generations. Two illustrative examples are that the six thousand different, true-breeding species of apple-trees today have been developed, mostly in the last three hundred years, from the single type of apple-tree known to the Romans two thousand years ago; and that the apple-tree and the rose-bush, vastly different though they are, are judged by experts to have developed from the same ancestor.

From Aristotle onwards some scientists advanced the idea of more complex species evolving from simpler forms of life, and the concept of evolution appears in the writings of such philosophers as Bacon, Descartes and

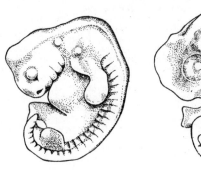

human   chicken   fish

Evolution: embryonic evidence

Kant. Yet it was not until the simultaneous appearance in 1859 of the work of Darwin and Wallace that the concept really became scientifically based, although Lamarck's suggestion that acquired characteristics could be inherited – itself later largely disproved – helped to prepare people for the acceptance of a thoroughly scientific theory of evolution.

Darwin started with the obvious facts of variation under domestication, e.g., the deliberate production of better varieties of wheat or the breeding of cart horses or race horses to suit our particular needs. He went on to consider natural selection or survival of the fittest. Essentially Darwin pointed out four things:

1. In any species variations from the normal pattern occur frequently.

2. Some of these variations are hereditarily contained in subsequent generations.

3. Plants and animals (including man) compete for space and food. So there occurs a process of natural selection whereby possessors of disadvantageous variations are eliminated – in one generation or in many – while possessors of advantageous variations continue to flourish.

4. Isolation of new departures (e.g., by a geographical change cutting off an island or a peninsula) facilitate the breeding together of those with the new features, thus stabilizing those new features that are advantageous.

He carried his explanation of slow and slight successive modifications and tendency for possessors of advantageous modifications to survive into all species without exception, pointing out for example the identical number of bones in the arm of man, the wing of a bat, the fin of a porpoise and the leg of a horse, and pointing out that the embryo of a mammal has at one stage branchial slits like the gills of a fish.

Since the poetical idea of a single divine creation of all species, propounded by priests at the very dawn of civilization, was regarded by many people as literal and sacred truth, violent controversy was inevitable. How could a religious man of that era accept that the cat and the tiger had a common ancestor when God had created both entire? How in particular could he believe that man and monkeys were related and that all mammals were descended from

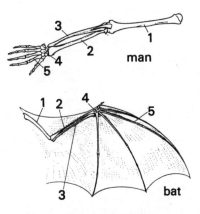

Evolution: skeletal evidence

amphibia? On the other hand, how could a thinker deny evolution when it was manifestly still occurring? And how, without evolution, could he explain that a human embryo at a fairly late stage was indistinguishable from that of an ape, and at earlier stages had characteristics of an amphibian and a fish?

The nineteenth century struggle between the *Book of Genesis* and the *Origin of Species* is now essentially a thing of the past. Benjamin Disraeli was perhaps the last outstanding person to declare himself 'on the side of the angels'; and nearly a century after Disraeli's death (in 1881) it would be a very bold man who would seek to challenge the evidence of evolution.

Following the rediscovery of Mendel's work and subsequent advances in the science of genetics we now understand the remarkable process of the halving of male and female chromosomes to produce ova and sperms. We appreciate that changes occur by spontaneous or accidental mutation of genes or by the occasional 'crossing over' of two adjacent chromosomes. We realize that most changes are unfavourable and decrease the likelihood of survival of descendants but that occasionally changes are favourable and confer advantages that can be transmitted to the off-spring. In other words, what Darwin merely observed we can now explain.

Again, with anthropological discoveries of bones to some extent intermediate between those of anthropoid apes and of man, the idea that man came into existence completely human – like Aphrodite rising from the waves – has become untenable.

Yet again, evolution of relatively long-lived creatures is slow: it took three-quarters of a century for the one existing type of Australian love-bird to give rise to the many different colours and shapes of the budgerigars of today. By using short-lived creatures, such as various types of flies, we can study over a period of a few years the evolutionary changes taking place in hundreds of successive generations.

To forecast the future evolution of *Homo sapiens* is a dangerous exercise but perhaps four suggestions can be offered, although they point in different directions:

1. In an increasingly mechanized and automated world cerebral development may well become more important than physical development. People who inherit high intellectual capacities may be more likely to secure mates and to provide for children in times of food shortage or other emergency than people who inherit strong teeth or powerful arms. It may well be that in another ten thousand years there will be a race of intellectual supermen with large cranial capacities and puny muscles.

2. Improved treatment of persons with inherited handicaps and disabilities may in large measure neutralize the effects of natural selection and survival of the fittest. Unless better treatment and more humane care are accompanied by successful genetic guidance there may be a deterioration of human stock both mentally and physically.

3. If contraceptive techniques are more accepted by the intelligent and provident than by the unintelligent and feckless there may well be a gradual degeneration of human stock. This could be the case unless there is intensive health education of the public about the advantages of family spacing and family limitation and perhaps financial measures to render large families unattractive.

4. In our present state of civilization anything in the nature of selective breeding is unthinkable. There would be endless dispute as to whether we should seek to breed for mathematical ability, literary creativity, honesty, compassion, beauty, physique or other qualities; and even within each category there would be dispute as to its most desirable qualities. Manifestly any attempt to introduce selective breeding would be acceptable only to the favoured groups and absolutely unacceptable to the overwhelming majority of the people.

excretion. The elimination of waste matter from the body. The working of the human machine depends on the maintenance of its energy supply and this requires the intake of sufficient fuel, i.e., food. The digestive system breaks down the raw fuel into sources of energy and waste products. Solid waste materials are excreted through the bowel, and liquid waste is excreted partly through the kidneys and partly in perspiration. Carbon dioxide and some water vapour are also excreted in the breath.

Efficient excretion is as essential to the body as is good ventilation to a house. Many minor and some major maladies are results of impaired excretion.

exercise. Physical exercise is essential for the growth and muscular development of children, and in adults is necessary for the proper functioning of the digestive, respiratory and excretory organs. Adequate regular exercise develops the muscles and maintains muscle tone, improves posture, deepens breathing and stimulates the circulation. Additionally it produces a sensation of well-being and appears to improve mental activity.

The type and amount of exercise needed varies with the individual's age, state of health, diet and other factors. In general exercise should not aim at the development of abnormal strength and endurance: big muscles have to be fed, and extra work is therefore thrown on the digestive system and the heart.

Babies not yet walking should be given special daily periods for free kicking, unencumbered by clothing, but usually young children after babyhood provide their own exercise, although attention may be needed for those children who are prevented by physical disability from indulging in vigorous games. In older children and adolescents physical training and organized games are important, and those of academic disposition who grudge time spent on sport should bear in mind the Roman aim, 'a healthy mind in a healthy body'. Doctors of the first quarter of this century, who very readily debarred children with any disorders of the circulatory or respiratory systems from participation in gymnastics or active games bear considerable responsibility for the extent of illness in persons now around retiring age.

For those of sedentary occupation (becoming a majority in the era of automation) there are perhaps two points at which exercise is in special danger of being sharply reduced. The first is at the change from a learner (in school, college or university) with normal participation in organized games to an earner who has to find his own recreations and leisure activities. The second is at the period, which often coincides with promotion and increased preoccupation with work, when the middle-aged person begins to feel unfit for the strenuous pastimes of his youth. With a little care both risks can be avoided.

In middle and later life walking and golf are excellent forms of exercise, as is cycling and, in moderation, swimming. Considerable additional exercise can be secured by fairly minor changes of habits, e.g., walking to the second nearest bus stop (instead of the nearest) and in the office using stairs rather than the lift. Exercise should be regular, not spasmodic. Persons who have long discontinued strenuous activities should think of moderate ones and should be hesitant about re-starting violent activities: while somebody who has played tennis for many years may well continue at 60, to take up tennis again at that age, after having discontinued all vigorous activity at 46, is merely to put a heavy and unanticipated strain on the heart and indeed on the whole body.

Men and women who are becoming overweight often try to counteract a sagging waist-

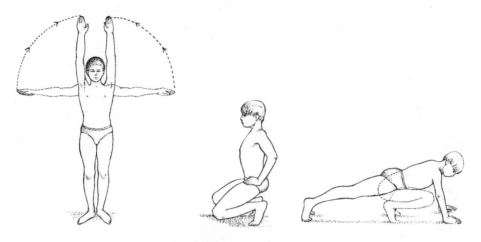

Three different exercises

line by increased exercise. The exercise, if reasonably moderate and regular, may be good for them in other ways but it tends to stimulate the appetite, and one has to walk many miles to use up the energy provided by a single additional slice of bread. Exercise is not a cure for obesity, a recipe for longevity or a means of preventing the ailment of old age; but regular, moderate exercise is usually beneficial.

Exercise, suited to a person's age and very gradually increased in persons of previously sedentary life, tends to be pleasant and therefore easily continued. By contrast, specific exercises – again adapted to age and physical condition – tend to be dull and to require much personal discipline for continuation. A person who considers himself in need of special exercises is perhaps as well to consult an expert about his needs, but it is a little difficult to suggest what expert to consult.

For example, in the U.K. (1) a health visitor can sometimes give very useful advice but in other cases may be preoccupied with the emotional and physical health of children and the health and well-being of the elderly; (2) a physiotherapist can sometimes give excellent guidance but in other cases has concentrated for years on the rehabilitation of persons recovering from serious diseases or injuries; (3) a general medical practitioner can sometimes be extremely helpful but in other cases is concerned almost exclusively with the diagnosis and treatment of illness; and (4) a gymnast can sometimes give very useful guidance but in other cases is preoccupied with the advanced training of athletes.

Three simple examples are given here:

1. To strengthen the muscles of the arms and shoulders, stretch the arms sharply to the sides and then swing them in an arc up above the head and down again.

2. To strengthen the leg and thigh muscles, start from a standing position and first rise onto the toes; from there bend the knees until the buttocks almost touch the heels and then slowly resume the standing position.

3. To strengthen the abdominal muscles, crouch with the weight on the hands which are placed rather more than the shoulder-width apart palms down on the ground; from there shoot the legs backwards till the body and legs are straight.

See also KEEPING FIT.

exophthalmic goitre. A condition in which the eyeballs protrude, giving a staring appearance, and the person is nervous and over-excitable. The cause is over-activity of the thyroid gland. See GOITRE.

expectation of life. If we could follow 100,000 children from birth, recording deaths until the oldest survivor died, we could construct a complete table from which we could find the average expectation of life at birth (by adding up all the years lived and dividing by 100,000) or the average expectation of life at any particular age (by adding all the years subsequently lived and dividing by the survivors at that age). The table would be completely accurate for children born around 1875 but would not have much current practical value.

However, by using details of recorded births and deaths and census information about the age and sex distribution of the population, we can construct a similar life table which is accurate in respect of the past but merely assumes for the future a continuation of present trends: e.g., if we consider as an example the age of 65 years, we know exactly what proportion of children born 65 years ago have survived to that age, but we can only guess that their subsequent pattern of survival will resemble that of people who are already beyond that age. Such a life table is obviously essential for insurance companies to calculate, for instance, what annuity should be offered to a woman of 68 in return for a fixed sum, and what annuity should be offered if she postpones the purchase until she is 73. A life table also has important national uses: e.g., to reckon how many pensioners we can expect to have in ten years' time or how many additional pensioners we would have if we reduced the pensionable age by one year.

In England and Wales the expectation of life at birth in the period 1838-1844 was approximately 40 years for males and 42 years for females. Since then it has risen to over 71 for males and about 75 for females. This does not, of course, mean that the average reader of this note can expect to die at 71 or 75. Since roughly 2 per cent of children die during the first twelve months, a child who has successfully reached his first birthday has a longer expectation of life than has a newborn infant; and with each year of survival the average total expectation of life increases. For example, people of 80 can on average expect to live about another five years, but those who have survived to 90 can on average look forward to nearly another two years.

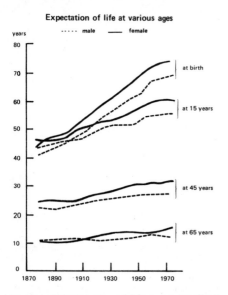

Expectation of life at various ages

Increased expectation of life is an excellent measure of the degree of improvement in social conditions, nutrition and preventive and curative health services; and average expectation of life (at birth or at some specified age) can be utilized to compare different cities or different countries.

In highly developed countries the longer survival of females, traditionally the stronger sex, is in large measure related to the first 65 years of life. More boy children than girl children die and more young men than young women succumb to disease or injury, so that, although slightly more boys are born than girls, women outnumber men in developed countries from about the age of 40/45. In middle life proportionately more men than women die, so that by 65 years there is a considerable preponderance of women. In respect of the survivors, however, there is little difference in the remaining expectation of life: where a husband and wife of the same age have passed 75 years it is statistically almost an even chance as to which will outlive the other.

An individual's expectation of life depends on his heredity (there are definitely long-lived and short-lived families), his childhood experience (e.g., whether he was half-starved, grossly overweight or reasonably nourished), his occupation, his present state of health and

various other factors. What life tables measure is not the extent of probable survival of any one person but the average survival of all persons of a particular age.

Increased expectation of life has been a feature of this century, rather than of last century: for example, in England and Wales from 1840 to 1880 the expectation at birth in males rose by only one year, from 40 to 41, as contrasted with the very large increase from 1940 to 1970. Major components in the twentieth century rise have been improved antenatal and obstetric services, better child health services, the conquest of many infectious diseases, better nutrition and better housing. As further improvements take place in the prevention and cure of diseases that are still prevalent, it seems likely that the expectation of life will continue to increase; but such increase, however welcome, will create problems. The rise in the ratio of pensioners to persons of working age has hitherto been balanced by a fall in the birth-rate and therefore a reduction in the number of dependent children, but in another dozen years we may have to face the situation of having a considerably increased number of pensioners and simultaneously of having fewer young entrants to the working group.

expectorant. Any drug which aids the expulsion of phlegm or sputum (spit) from the bronchial tubes. Essentially expectorants – of which ipecacuanha, squills and senega are examples – do two things. They increase the flow of mucous and so make the expulsion of phlegm easier, and they stimulate the cough centre in the brain.

expiration. Breathing out.

exposure to cold. Prolonged exposure to cold, insufficient to cause frost bite, results in HYPOTHERMIA which may end in death. Less severe cold (with which a healthy person's body's temperature regulating mechanism can normally cope) can cause local effects. For instance, elderly people with little fat in their skin may develop an itchy rash on legs or arms; this is most marked on exposure to sharp changes of temperature, such as undressing in a cold bedroom or sitting close to a fire after enduring cold external temperature. In susceptible persons cold causes the bluish-red, itchy swellings known as chilblains. Another example is where the feet have been long immersed in cold water: the numbness and cramp known as trench foot may develop.

In all cases gradual warming is the most important feature in treatment. Prevention includes adequate wrapping up before going outside in cold weather, reasonable heating of bedrooms and bathrooms and avoidance of alcohol for an hour or so before exposure to cold, because alcohol dilates the blood vessels of the skin and increases heat loss.

In contrast with alcohol, anything that narrows the superficial blood vessels and so decreases heat loss reduces the harmful effects of cold. A tale is told of Avicenna, the greatest physician and scientist of the Persian-Arab civilization. Having incurred the anger of a potentate he was sentenced to spend a night outdoors in the bitter Persian winter. He contrived to give himself a large dose of opium shortly before the night of exposure; by that means he slowed his circulation and lessened his heat loss, and so survived.

extension. The movement of straightening a joint or of treating a damaged arm or leg by a steady pull to prevent the muscles from contracting.

extrovert. A person primarily interested in things outside himself, fond of company, sociable and out-going. The term was devised by Carl Jung (1875-1961) as a contrast to the isolated, inward looking, self-centred INTROVERT. Both terms are still in common use, and probably most people can legitimately be described as being to some extent either extroverted or introverted.

The distinction is, however, much less clean-cut that Jung imagined and it is probably incorrect to classify any person simply as an extrovert or an introvert. A person may, for example, be lively and outgoing at home and the 'life of the party' on social occasions, but quiet and self-centred at work. Another may be an active, forceful leader at work but quiet and subdued on social occasions. Yet another may be sociable and lively at most times but apparently introverted this month because of some domestic worry or personal illness while yet another may be shy with strangers but out-going with established friends.

eye. The eye may be regarded as a camera in which the light rays from an object are concentrated by a contractable diaphragm (the iris), focused by the lens, and received as an inverted image on the retina.

The spherical eyeball is protected by the eyelids and moved by six muscles – the superior, inferior, internal and external rectus muscles and the superior and inferior oblique muscles; these six are supplied by the third, fourth and sixth cranial nerves.

The eyeball has three coverings. (1) The sclera, or tough outer coat, forms the white of the eye and is continuous in front with a transparent, window-like membrane, the cornea. (2) The choroid, or middle coat, is a pigmented membrane which in front becomes the iris, the coloured diaphragm in front of the lens. The central opening in the iris is called the pupil. (3) The retina, or inner coat, contains the terminations of the optic nerve which are light-sensitive. There are two types of cells – the 'cones', with which we see in bright light, and the 'rods' which are used in dim light.

From front to back the eyeball therefore has: (1) the transparent cornea; (2) an anterior chamber between cornea and iris; (3) the coloured iris with a central hole, the pupil; (4) a posterior chamber between iris and lens; (5) the lens; and (6) a large rear portion extending from lens to retina and filled with a jelly-like fluid, the vitreous body.

The cornea acts as a transparent window, protecting the structures behind it. The iris controls the amount of light entering the eye. The lens focuses rays of light to produce a clear image on the retina in the function known as accommodation. When an individual is trying to view a distant object, the lens is only slightly convex and rays of light coming from the object are focused on the retina. To allow a nearer object to be seen clearly the lens is pulled into a more globular shape by the small ciliary muscle: in other words it 'accommodates' by becoming a lens of higher power, so that the diverging rays from the object are still brought to a focus on the retina. As people grow older the lens gradually loses its elasticity, so that

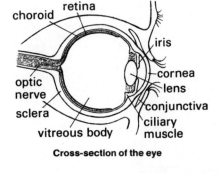

Cross-section of the eye

from the age of about 40 or 45 years a person may need the aid of glasses for reading, sewing, or fine work. This natural loss of accommodation is called presbyopia. Defects of EYESIGHT can usually be corrected with glasses. Lastly the retina receives the images and transmits them along the optic nerve to the visual area of the brain.

Since the eyes are, of necessity, a short distance apart, the images which they receive must differ from each other. However, the difference is so slight that the two images can be 'fused' into one by the visual centre of the brain, and this blending of the two images received in binocular vision gives rise to the three-dimensional aspect of sight known as stereopsis.

Eyestrain. Prevention of eyestrain should begin in childhood. The child's bed should not face the window, the sun should not shine directly into the baby's eyes, and toys should be reasonably large. If there is any suspicion of short-sight the child's eyes should be examined and appropriate glasses regularly worn. Ideally, since children are liable to falls and other accidents, the lenses should be plastic, not glass.

In early school life teachers, health visitors and parents should be on the lookout for signs of eyestrain, such as rubbing of the eyes, frequent blinking and reddened eyelids; and attention should be paid to natural and artificial lighting in school and at home, with testing of the child's vision undertaken as a routine every year.

Eyestrain can also occur during years of prolonged study and at various later periods. Good lighting is an essential preventive measure, as is occasional testing of vision and the prescription of glasses where required.

Diseases. Short-sight (myopia), long-sight (hypermetropia) and uneven curvature (astigmatism) are considered under EYESIGHT. Other disorders of the eye include CONJUNCTIVITIS, where the conjunctiva is infected, the eyeball becomes red and the lids become sticky; CATARACT, in which the substance of the lens grows hard and opaque, preventing light from reaching the retina; GLAUCOMA in which the pressure of the fluids within the eye becomes gradually greater so that the retina is damaged; detachment of the retina, a condition – resulting from ageing or violence – in which the retina becomes detached from the inner surface of the eyeball;

retinitis, an infection of the retina; and, commonest of all, SQUINT.

Watering eye. Persistent overflow of tears on to the face implies either over-secretion of tears or, more usually, blockage of the tear-ducts which would normally convey the secreted moisture to the nose. The condition is annoying and unsightly. Treatment varies with the cause, e.g., an astringent lotion may help to reduce excessive tear-secretion, a foreign body in the duct may be removed, and gentle syringing may help where the lachrymal sac is distended with mucus and pus.

Injuries. The commonest injuries affecting the eye are black eye and presence of a foreign body.

A black eye is simply a condition of bruising, caused by violence, and is best treated by immediate application of a cold, damp cloth. There is no additional merit in the old-fashioned remedy of application of a piece of raw beef-steak.

A foreign body in the eye may be removed by repeated blinking or by pulling one eyelid over the other. If these measures are unsuccessful the upper lid may be rolled upwards, or the lower lid rolled downwards, over a pencil or knitting-needle, and the foreign object gently removed by application of the moistened corner of a clean handkerchief.

Injuries other than an obvious black eye and a removable foreign body call for medical aid. Such a condition might be a corneal abrasion, when the surface layer of cells is irritated or damaged; this will heal over rapidly (in about a day) with no scarring if it is not infected. However, if the substance of the cornea beneath the surface layer is damaged healing may take many months because the blood supply to the cornea is minimal. Such damage is found in corneal ulceration which may occur as a result of infection following injury, or infection by itself, as can happen with shingles of the face. If the damage is severe, scarring of the cornea will occur with consequent impairment of vision. Such a scarred cornea can be removed and replaced with a graft from a donor and, because of the limited blood supply, rejection of the grafted cornea does not occur.

eyelids, diseases of. Common diseases of the eyelids include the following.

1. Cyst. A hard swelling of the gland of an eyelash, usually of the lower lid. It is painless but disfiguring. It usually requires removal.

2. Drooping eyelid (ptosis). This result of weakness of the muscle that raises the upper lid may be congenital, may arise after disease damaging the nerve which controls it (e.g., shingles) or may occur as a senile condition. Treatment depends on the cause but often involves a small operation to enlist the aid of another muscle.

3. Ectropion. A condition in which the margin of the lower lid is turned outwards, so that the eye cannot be fully closed. Ectropion arises from contraction of scars (e.g., from ulcers or burns) or as a senile condition. A slight operation is often necessary for remedy.

4. Entropion. A turning inwards of the margin of a lid. The causes are similar to those of ectropion. A common treatment is to increase the normal 'pull' of the skin by removing a small piece of skin.

5. Ingrowing eyelash. A lid margin is displaced inwards and the lash irritates the conjunctiva causing pain and watering of the eye. The offending eyelashes can be removed with special forceps.

6. Stye. Suppurative inflammation of one of the glands at the margin of a lid. In very early stages an antibiotic may abort the stye. Where a hard, painful swelling has developed, hot antiseptic compresses may help to bring about pus formation, after which the abscess either bursts or can be opened by incision with a small knife.

7. Blepharitis. A crusty scaling of the lid margins fairly common in children; it may be associated with dandruff of the scalp and is often found in situations of poor general health.

Temporary episodes of muscular twitching of the eyelids (myokimia) can occur during periods of fatigue or general ill health; they are generally unimportant.

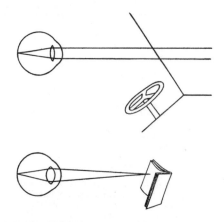

Whether driving a car or reading a book, the lens of the normal eye can adjust the focus to see clearly.

eyesight. The optical principle to be kept in mind in considering eyesight is that rays of light entering a denser medium are bent out of their course. Thus light passing from air into the eye is first deflected by the cornea and again by the lens; the more curved the lens of the eyes, the greater is the bending that takes place.

As indicated under EYE, the eye is like a small camera with a shutter, a lens and a screen.

A normal or emmetropic eye is in perfect focus for objects at a distance of more than one metre. Rays from such objects reach the retina without any additional curving of the lens. Nearer objects are brought into focus by an appropriate degree of bulging of the lens, achieved without conscious effort, known as accommodation. An object very close to the eye cannot be brought into focus because the capacity of the lens to increase its curvature is limited.

The common departures from normal vision – excluding diseases of the eye – are hyper-metropia (or long-sight), myopia (or short-sight) astigmatism (or uneven curvature), which are all errors of refraction, and presbyopia.

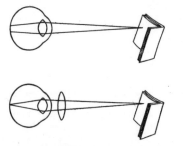

The long-sighted person requires a convex spectacle lens to help bring the light from a near object to a focus point on the retina.

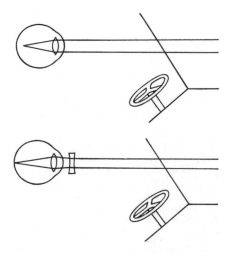

The short-sighted person needs a concave lens to help bring the light from distant objects to a focus.

Hypermetropia. The hypermetropic eye is either shorter from front to back than the normal eye or has a lens with less than the normal curvature. Either of these deviations from normality implies that, if no bending of the lens occurred, rays from a distant object would be brought to a focus not on the retina but on an imaginary point beyond it, so that the image produced on the retina would be blurred. Actually in the hypermetropic eye the lens fattens sufficiently to bring distant objects to a correct focus, so that the long-sighted person can see distant objects clearly. For nearer objects (for which a normal eye would need bulging of the lens) the hypermetropic eye needs greater accommodation so that for objects fairly near the eye there is a blurring because the lens is already bulging to capacity. Hence a long-sighted person can see distant objects (and can, for example, drive a car without spectacles) but cannot bring near objects to a focus (e.g., read a book). Correction of long-sightedness is by convex glasses which bend rays inwards and in effect do some of the work of the lens.

Myopia. The myopic eye is abnormally long from front to back or has a lens with more curvature than normal before any accommodation takes place. Hence rays from a distance come to a focus at a point in front of the retina and then spread out, producing blurring. Nearer objects can be brought to focus on the retina with less bulging of the lens than in the normal eye. Hence the short-sighted eye can clearly see near objects (e.g., a book held at average distance) but to focus distant objects requires the help of concave glasses which in effect balance the excessive curvature of the lens.

Presbyopia. From the age 40 years presbyopia begins to develop, that is to say, the elasticity of the lens begins to decrease. Hence the normal eye begins to require a convex glass for near objects, 'reading glasses', and another glass which is only mildy convex as 'distant glasses'. Such persons can usefully obtain bi-focal lenses, in which the upper segment corrects distant vision and the lower segment corrects near vision. Bifocal glasses save the person from having to switch from one pair of spectacles to another, e.g., a teacher who desires repeatedly to transfer his gaze from book to class and back again. Some such people find bifocal glasses a great advantage, but others find it very difficult to become accustomed to wearing glasses with the upper and lower parts of completely different focusing power. To lessen the sharp change from an upper segment for distant vision and a lower segment for near vision, attempts have been made in recent years to introduce an intermediate zone: tri-focal glasses.

The myopic eye, which previously needed a concave glass to counteract excessive curvature of the lens, requires a progressively weaker glass as presbyopia develops, then perhaps no glass for a period, and finally, when the ageing process has more than balanced the short-sightedness, a mildly convex glass.

Astigmatism. In the astigmatic eye the cornea at the front is not curved uniformly. Hence, unless the abnormality is balanced by a glass appropriately curved, the whole of an image cannot simultaneously come into focus. In regular astigmatism, the directions of greatest and least curvature are at right angles and a suitable cylindrical lens will readily correct the difference in refraction in the two axes. In irregular astigmatism, usually due to previous corneal ulceration, refractive power varies irregularly and is usually impossible to correct effectively with traditional spectacles, although if there is no scarring of the corneal surface, contact lenses can be very successful. Astigmatism can, of course, exist simultaneously with myopia or hypermetropia.

Finally, it should be mentioned that not all defects of vision can be cured by suitable glasses. Glasses can ensure that appropriate images are focused on the retina; but if the retina is detached or if the optic nerve is damaged, glasses will not restore vision.

F

facial nerve. The seventh cranial nerve carries impulses to the muscles of facial expression. It emerges from the base of the brain and passes through a small hole in the mastoid bone to emerge just below the opening of the ear. The nerve is liable to be damaged in inflammatory conditions of the ear and in mastoid operations.

facial paralysis. Paralysis or weakness of one side of the face due to damage of the FACIAL NERVE on that side. The paralysis does not affect sensation but creates a lop-sided appearance with the mouth drawn towards the unaffected side. It may arise following any damage to the nerve, as in head injury, infection (particularly in the ear, close to which the nerve passes on its course to the face) or exposure to intense cold. The palsy often recovers quite spontaneously.

facial spasm. A one-sided disturbance of the facial nerve causing twitching of the muscles of the face. Mild cases are best left untreated, although tranquillizers and sedatives sometimes help, or at least make the twitching more bearable. In serious cases cutting of some branches of the facial nerve can be considered but the operation produces a permanent facial paralysis and should therefore not be lightly undertaken.

facies. The appearance of the face as a clue to diagnosis. The facial appearance in grave illness, the Hippocratic facies, was described by Hippocrates; indicating probable approaching death, it is drawn, pinched and livid. The cardiac facies, seen in cases of valvular disease of the heart, shows bright purple cheeks and lips with the rest of the face sallow. The typhoid facies, seen in various debilitating illnesses, has a vacant, bewildered expression.

faeces. Faeces (from the Latin *faex,* dregs) is the technical name used for the motions or STOOLS discharged from the bowel.

failure. The dictionary definition of failure is 'a falling-short or cessation,' and in a medical context the word may be used in either sense. Thus death may result from cardiac failure, but a diagnosis of 'heart failure' or 'kidney failure' (perhaps prefixed by 'chronic'), is often merely a convenient way of saying that the particular organ at a particular moment is inadequate to meet the demands made upon it.

It may, or may not, be possible to restore the failing action of an organ, either by reducing the demands made upon it (as, for instance, by rest and dietary measures), or by more active therapeutic procedures designed to improve function.

fainting. Temporary loss of consciousness through deficient blood supply to the brain.

Some persons faint easily from such causes as strong emotion, an over-heated atmosphere or the sight of blood. Other causes of fainting include a blow on the abdomen or on the head, acute pain, sudden change of posture (e.g.,

getting very quickly out of bed), and abnormal exertion.

If warning symptoms – such as dizziness and dimming of vision – appear, the faint can sometimes be prevented by getting the person to improve the blood supply to the brain by lowering his head; this is best done by bending forward with head between knees. Where fainting has occurred, clothing round the neck should be loosened, the head kept low and smelling salts, if available, held to the nostrils.

Sal volatile may be given in the preliminary dizzy stage and after the return of consciousness, but not during the unconscious phase.

While prolonged unconsciousness (over three minutes) or repeated fainting requires medical investigation, most occurrences of fainting are followed by immediate recovery even without treatment. After regaining consciousness, whether after treatment or spontaneously, the person should lie or sit quietly for about a quarter of an hour.

falling sickness. An old term for EPILEPSY.

Fallopian tube. The oviduct or tube which leads from each of the two ovaries to the uterus, and through which the unfertilized ova travel. Occasionally a fertilized ovum travels back into the tube and begins to develop there (ectopic pregnancy).

When a woman has had the number of children that she desires, she may elect to have the small operation of tying the fallopian tubes. This operation, by stopping ova from reaching the uterus, renders her permanently infertile. Other methods of BIRTH CONTROL are not permanent.

family planning. Deliberate restriction of children born to the number desired and to the times at which their births are desired. See BIRTH CONTROL.

Faradism. Use of an interrupted electrical current to cause contraction of a muscle when the current is passing (as contrasted with Galvanism where contraction occurs only when a current is made and broken'). Faradism is used to treat various forms of paralysis and muscle weakness.

fascia. A sheet of fibrous tissue. Fasciae are found in all parts of the body and vary in thickness and strength from the loose open-work structure of fibro-areolar tissue (superficial fascia) to well-defined anatomical entities which are dense, tough, and tendinous (deep fascia). In some areas, a particular condensation of the deep fascia may be called an aponeurosis.

Fasciae connect the skin to the underlying structures, provide capsules for muscles, organs, blood-vessels and nerves, and subdivide muscle-groups. Some fascial sheets are themselves under muscular control so that

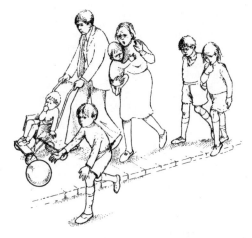

The benefits of family planning

they can tense or relax to conform with adjacent muscle-movements.

They are also of importance in suppuration and haemorrhage since pus or effused blood may flow along fascial planes to emerge at points remote from the actual lesion.

fasting. Deliberate abstension from food. A fasting person generally does take water as he would otherwise die in about three days. Assuming that he has water, he lives essentially on his own tissues. The glycogen (sugar) stored in the liver is first utilized, and thereafter fat and protein are mobilized from the tissues.

In a healthy and well-nourished person a fast of two or three days may be harmless, and in certain diseases it is even beneficial, although it is accompanied by hunger-pangs and a feeling of weakness. In prolonged fasting the hunger-pangs disappear but the fasting becomes dangerous. A fasting person would die of starvation in about a month but might well develop deficiency diseases or infection (through lowered resistance) in less than a month. After prolonged fasting the return to food should be gradual, with no heavy meal during the first thirty-six hours.

Intermittent fasting, e.g., complete abstension for one day each week, or partial fasting for a few weeks, is on the whole commendable for well-nourished adults.

fat. A type of FOOD, and one of the essential constituents of the DIET but digested only in the presence of carbohydrates. For equal weights fats supply more than twice the energy of proteins and carbohydrates. In addition to providing sources of energy in concentrated form, animal fats (e.g., butter, which is about 80 per cent fat, cheese, cream and the fat of meat) carry the fat-soluble vitamins A and D, but certain vegetable oils differ from animal fats in not containing fat-soluble vitamins, unless these are artificially added.

Fats are derived from both animal and vegetable sources and are combinations of fatty acids and glycerin. At ordinary temperatures they may be either solid like lard, or fluid, like olive oil. They differ also in their molecular structure. If their carbon atoms are uniformly linked by single bonds they are said to be 'saturated fats'; if there are one or more double bonds they are 'unsaturated' or 'poly-unsaturated fats'. Saturated fats are derived from animal sources and the other kinds are of vegetable origin. In recent years it has been suggested that too much animal fat (e.g., from butter, cheese and meat fat) raises the blood cholesterol level and may predispose the individual to coronary thrombosis, and that about half of the total intake of fat should be obtained from vegetable oils.

It is difficult to envisage a state which is solely fat deficiency although low fat diet has the disadvantage that it would result in a diminished intake of fat-soluble vitamins. In addition to being an energy source, fatty compounds are integral components of the structure of the cell.

fatigue. Weariness, normally occurring after prolonged physical or mental effort, and acting as a signal that the person suffering from it needs rest, change of activity, or medical treatment.

Study of fatigue in apparently normal persons is of great value in industry. For instance, during the 1939-45 war factory working hours were increased to raise output, but the output actually fell because of fatigue and the hours had to be shortened again. Similarly industrial psychologists have established that a short break in mid-morning and mid-afternoon lessens fatigue and improves the quality and quantity of work. Fatigue is increased by bad working conditions, such as excessive heat, poor illumination or unsatisfactory ventilation.

While fatigue is usually a sign of working too hard or too long or at unusual tasks, with the remedy obvious, abnormal fatigue without any of these causes may indicate that the person is suffering from an undiagnosed illness, such as diabetes or anaemia; or that he is under sustained emotional stress either at work or domestically; or that he has become bored and dissatisfied and requires a change of occupation, a good holiday or an interesting hobby.

Fatigue is usually easy to diagnose. Its manifestations include quickened pulse and respiration, perspiration and lowered body temperature, frequent yawning, impaired muscular co-ordination as revealed for example in handwriting, a feeling of tiredness, a reduced power of concentration and span of attention, weakened memory, impaired judgment, irritability, and increased liability to accidents.

Physical fatigue can be measured in various ways, e.g., by the time taken to perform a particular piece of manual work or by use of an instrument called the ergograph .which demonstrates among other things the economy of movement of an alert worker doing a familiar job and the increase in unnecessary movements as fatigue increases. An easy way to measure intellectual fatigue is to reckon the time taken to add up various columns of figures.

Unless the cause is obvious, medical examination for possible undetected disease is desirable, and, if that is negative, attention to the emotional state including both manifest and hidden worries and conflicts.

In general a fatigued person needs REST and change of activity; and the persons hardest to treat are those in posts of responsibility who, while making errors of judgment because of exhaustion, often genuinely believe that the business or department would collapse if they took a fortnight off. Tonics and 'pick-me-ups' though much advertised, are not of much value. Where immediate continuation of the activity is essential, as with a tired soldier during a battle, benzidrene will postpone fatigue for many hours. So to a lesser extent will strong coffee. Both of these, however, merely delay the onset of fatigue, and the subsequent physical and emotional exhaustion is all the greater. In fatigue of emotional origin tranquillizers may help, although generally the background condition requires treatment.

Where abnormal fatigue is found in children one should think of over-pressure either in school or at home, unsatisfactory environmental conditions again either in school or at home, anaemia, nutrition insufficient for rapid growth, insufficient recreation and unidentified defects of vision or hearing.

fattening. A deliberate attempt to gain weight, as opposed to slimming. The young girl whose face begins to look 'pinched' and whose body loses its natural curves and the older woman with haggard appearance, dry and sallow skin and folds of loose skin on face and neck, often set out to eat more food in an attempt to gain weight. In many cases a good nourishing diet and a moderately restful life – including mental as well as physical rest – will produce the desired result.

Three sets of conditions should however be noted. (1) Excessive thinness, often coupled with excessive physical and mental activity, may be the result of an over-active thyroid gland, and a good diet will not correct that over-activity. (2) Loss of weight may be the first symptom of various diseases, such as tuberculosis and cancer. (3) Increasing or persistent thinness may be the result of worry, either in consequence of abnormal emotional or stress factors or as a result of the person having a worrying personality.

In general, therefore, a person who is steadily losing weight is well-advised to consult a doctor. Treatment – sometimes surgical – is clearly needed in glandular upset, and may be life-saving in cases of undetected serious disease; in abnormal emotional stress tranquillizers may help, although what is really needed is modification of the factors involved; and the person of worrying personality, with its causes rooted in childhood, may need considerable psychological help.

Where fattening is attempted without medical aid a few points are worth noting. Physical and mental REST are important and since the person's appetite has probably been small, the increase in food should be fairly gradual, because otherwise there is danger of nausea and indigestion, especially if the new diet contains large amounts of fat. Carbohydrate foods are particularly valuable for weight gain, e.g., plenty of sugar in tea and coffee, and abundance of cakes and scones. Milk should not be forgotten as an easily digested source of extra calories.

fatty degeneration. Cellular damage accompanied by the appearance of fat-droplets within the cells. In most organs the fat has come from the affected tissue, but in the liver, which has a specific role in fat-metabolism, the visible fat which overfills the cells has been transported from elsewhere and accumulates because the liver-cells have become unable to deal with it.

There are various causes of fatty degeneration. It occurs as a result of deficient oxidation, as in anaemia, or from actual interference with local blood-supply, for instance to the heart muscle; from cell-poisons such as phosphorus, chloroform, and bacterial toxins; and from nerve injuries which tend to produce degeneration in the fatty myelin envelope of nerve-fibres on the far side of the injury and in the associated muscle-fibres.

fauces. The fairly narrow opening between the mouth and the throat, with the soft palate above and the root of the tongue below. On each side there are two folds, the pillars of the fauces, in which the tonsils are imbedded. When the tonsils are swollen the fauces may be narrowed to such an extent that swallowing becomes difficult.

favus. A skin disease, caused by a fungus, mainly affecting the scalp and sometimes the nails. Yellow cup-like crusts form and adhere together. When they drop off the portion of scalp is hairless and scarred. Infection is by direct contact with a person or a cat suffering from the condition. Treatment consists of removing the crusts and applying an appropriate antiseptic ointment. Where this does not suffice, exposure to x-rays may be necessary.

fear. Fear of things or situations that are known by experience to be dangerous is a normal human reaction, leading to the person taking special care, or avoiding the danger, or preparing to fight. Fear of the unknown is also in considerable part normal, although it is in some measure created or exaggerated by parental over-protection of children.

Both of these types of fear can to some extent be reduced in various ways. Calm consideration of the reasonably worst expectation can be helpful: it frequently appears that the worst that can be expected to happen is far less than the person in mental apprehension had vaguely anticipated. Another possibility is to discuss the fear with a trusted friend who can bring a rational and unemotional outlook to bear on the situation. Yet another is to steel oneself to tackle the source of fear, as in deliberately setting out to drive a car shortly after a terrifying skid.

In many cases, however, fear is a projection of hidden emotional conflict and cannot be fully dispelled until the conflict is resolved. Pathological fears and PHOBIAS are forms of NEUROSIS.

There appears to be little relationship between physical and moral fear. The man who will unhesitatingly tackle an unknown intruder may be afraid to express an unpopular opinion, and vice versa. Moreover, physical cowards who succeed in temporarily repressing their fears sometimes perform remarkable acts of bravery.

Fear of pain and fear of disease affect patients or prospective patients in two opposite ways. In some cases these fears cause a person to seek medical examination, but in many cases it is these very fears that make a person hesitate to seek expert advice.

Practitioners of health education are virtually unanimous in holding that an appeal to fear, e.g., by showing pictures of diseased lungs in a drive against cigarette smoking, does not achieve much long-term success.

febrile. Having a raised temperature.

fecundity. See FERTILITY.

feeble-mindedness. A term of differing meaning in Britain and America. In the U.K. the term, which is now falling into disuse, was employed to cover the lesser degrees of mental handicap. Taking the intelligence quotient as a very rough measure of ability, one could say that about 50 per cent of people are 'average' (with IQ 90 to 110), about 22 per cent 'superior' (110 to 130), about 22 per cent 'dull' (70 to 130) and about 3 per cent each in the gifted and mentally handicapped groups.

The last-mentioned group was divided ascendingly into idiots, incapable of guarding themselves against common physical dangers (IQ under 25), imbeciles, incapable of managing themselves or their affairs (IQ 25 to 50) and the feeble-minded (U.K.) or the morons (U.S.A.) who require care, protection and control for their own protection or for the protection of others (IQ 50 to 70). In the U.S.A. the term feeble-minded is employed for the entire category of mentally handicapped persons, i.e., for the whole 3 per cent of the population who are intellectually lower than 'dull'.

femoral vessels. The main artery and vein of the thigh. The femoral artery passes from the abdomen in the middle of the groin where it can be felt pulsating and, if the thigh is moved slightly outwards, can be compressed against the head of the femur to stop bleeding. The artery passes down the inner side of the thigh and in the lower third passes behind to become the popliteal artery at the back of the knee. The femoral vein corresponds with the artery and drains blood from the leg. One of its tributaries is the long saphenous vein which is often varicose and liable to phlebitis.

femur. The thigh bone, the longest and strongest bone in the body. Its head articulates with a cavity in the hip bone called the acetabulum, forming the hip joint; below the

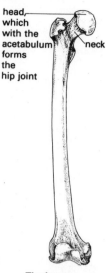

head, which with the acetabulum forms the hip joint

neck

The femur

head is a narrowed part, the neck, and where the neck joins the shaft there is a protuberance, the great trochanter. The lower end consists of two bulges or condyles which articulate with the tibia and the patella in the formation of the knee joint. Fractures of the femur are not uncommon: displacement, pain and inability to move the limb are general features but beyond these the signs vary according to the part of the bone fractured.

Fracture of the neck of the femur is commonest in elderly people, especially elderly women. It used to be regarded as always being the result of indirect violence, e.g., landing heavily on the foot after missing a step on the stair. Increasingly however experts are beginning to question that explanation (though it is certainly true in some cases). If the hormone changes after the menopause are followed by a diet poor in calcium the bone may become thin, especially at the neck, and incapable of supporting the weight of the body, which is often increasing about this time. So in at least some cases the situation is not that a woman falls and breaks her leg but that the leg breaks and causes the fall.

fenestration. An operation, for relief of deafness due to otosclerosis, a hardening of the bones of the ear, involving the making of an artificial opening into the inner ear. The operation had a considerable vogue for a number of years but is being increasingly superseded by newer operations that claim better results.

fertility. The ability to procreate children.

While fertility in women begins to decrease about the age of thirty and of course disappears at the menopause, and while fertility in men also decreases although much more slowly, most couples can produce as many children as they desire; and indeed the modern stress on family planning and birth control is testimony to the fact that most couples need assistance to keep them from having more children than they desire.

When one thinks of nature's provision for the maintenance of most species, e.g., the enormous numbers of sperms and ova produced by fishes, it is hardly surprising that the main human problem today is over-fertility. Consider a hypothetical community of ten men and ten women at three points in time and assume that one man and one woman were infertile and that one of each sex did not marry or beget children. (1) At the dawn of monogamy, about 2,400 years ago, about three-fifths of all offspring died before becoming adult. So, to maintain the community at twenty adults, the eight marrying couples would need to produce fifty children, or an average of six to seven per couple. (2) By early Victorian times improvements in nutrition, environmental conditions and health care had resulted in about two-thirds of babies surviving to adult life. So, to maintain the community at twenty adults, the eight marrying couples would require to produce thirty children, or almost four per couple. (3) Today, vaccines and antibiotics, antenatal and child health care, improved prevention and treatment of illnesses, and so on, have made death in infancy and childhood a rarity. So to maintain the community, the eight married couples have to produce about twenty children, or an average of 2.5 per couple. Yet human beings and their hormones have changed very little in the short space of 2,400 years, and without some form of natural or artificial family limitation the average couple would still produce the six to seven children that were needed by their ancestors in the past.

About one-tenth of marriages, however, are infertile although the partners desire to produce a family. Some of the causes of such infertility are:

1. Ignorance of sexual techniques, e.g., premature ejaculation by the man, or inadvertent avoidance by the couple of the days midway between the menstrual periods when the woman is most likely to conceive.

2. Physical ill-health, temporarily reducing the fertility of one of the couple.

3. Male infertility, which should not be confused with impotence. One not uncommon cause is orchitis occurring as a complication of mumps. Examination of the number and motility of the sperms in the seminal fluid will determine whether the man is the infertile partner, but male infertility is on the whole more difficult to treat than female infertility.

4. Female infertility due to a deficiency of hormones (which can often be remedied) or to various gynaecological conditions (for which there is often treatment) or to neurosis (which can usually be cured).

5. Sexual incompatibility, where both partners are fertile but, for reasons not yet fully understood, there appears to exist an antagonism between the sperms and ova of the particular partners.

Investigation of both partners at a sub-fertility clinic is desirable where a couple are more than two years without a wanted child. In many cases the condition can be cured, although it must be appreciated that some are as yet incurable, and in these cases alternatives have to be considered, e.g., artificial insemination of the woman with the husband's semen, or adoption.

In view of the age-old and still prevalent belief that in a childless marriage it is always the woman who is barren, it is perhaps desirable to state that in over one-third of investigated childless marriages the infertility is in the male.

Fecundity, i.e., abnormal fertility with a tendency to multiple births, is largely an inherited trait: twins occur about once in every eighty births and triplets about once in every seven thousand births, but the chances are appreciably higher in families with a history of multiple births in grandparents, parents or brothers and sisters. Apart from the hereditary element, it should be noted that some synthetic drugs employed to treat infertility occasionally lead to multiple births, even including quadruplets and quintuplets.

fester. To generate pus. The term is not much employed in medicine but is in popular use for any inflammation with formation of pus, as in an abscess, boil or ulcer. The term is also used metaphorically in the sense of allowing resentment to rankle.

fetishism. A fetish is an inanimate object which is regarded with awe or reverence, or creates sexual satisfaction on the part of a person who handles, destroys or steals it. Fetishism is the belief in or use of fetishes, and is thus a form of sexual PERVERSION.

In religious fetishism the object, e.g., the idol, the alleged fragment of Christ's cross or the bone of a saint, becomes gradually invested with the miracle-working or divine attributes of what it represents, until at last the idol-worshipper is not praying to his deity but concentrating all his hopes and fears on the idol.

In erotic fetishism certain articles of attire or objects used by the beloved person – or even by any member of the opposite sex – come to arouse the emotions of sexual pleasure, even sometimes to the point of orgasm, and attraction to the article or object is often to the exclusion of normal sexuality. Fetishism, it is said, often starts with a part of the body, such as the hair, hand, foot or leg, and is transferred by association of ideas to the hat, gloves, shoes or petticoat.

Fetishism is predominately a male sexual deviation, and some psychiatrists claim that it does not occur in women.

Where fetishism is confined to secreting a handkerchief or a lock of hair and using it as a love-object, it probably does little harm, although it may prevent normal sexual intercourse and procreation of children; but where it involves the stealing or destruction of articles of attire, such as women's underwear hanging on a clothes line, it clearly requires psychiatric treatment. Such treatment is often successful.

fever. Otherwise known as pyrexia, this is strictly any condition in which the bodily temperature is increased materially above the normal. In many diseases the rise of temperature is the result of a separate condition, e.g., high temperature may occur after exposure to great heat, after swallowing various drugs, and in severe nervous shock. Normally, however, the term is reserved for a number of specific infectious diseases which produce pyrexia as one of their main characteristics.

Symptoms. The start of a fever is often marked by rigor or shivering, pallor, or in children convulsions, accompanied by a general feeling of illness, headache, backache and often sickness. After the chilly stage, which lasts for minutes or hours, the temperature rises rapidly, the skin feels hot and dry (although in a few fevers such as rheumatic fever and malaria profuse perspiration is a feature), characteristic rashes may appear, the tongue becomes furred and dry, appetite is poor, thirst is considerable, the pulse is rapid (although there are some exceptions), respiration is accelerated, urine is diminished and highly coloured, and headache, sleeplessness and delirium are common.

Classification. Continued fever is the term used when the high temperature persists, technically with variations of less than 1.5 °F., until it falls, usually suddenly 'by crisis' as in lobar pneumonia, scarlet fever, measles and typhoid. Remittent fever is the name employed when the temperature varies, being high at one part of the day and normal or subnormal at another, as in bronchopneumonia and pulmonary tuberculosis. In intermittent fever, as in malaria, the high temperature occurs regularly only once a day, or once every two days, or once every three days.

Specific fevers. This term is sometimes used to differentiate from other causes of high temperature the particular fevers that are (1) caused by specific micro-organisms, and (2) infectious, i.e., transmissible from person to person. Other characteristics are that they run a fairly defined course and that an attack tends to confer an immunity which may be long-lasting (as after smallpox) or of short duration (as after influenza).

Most specific fevers have fairly consistent incubation periods during which the invading organisms multiply until numerous enough to produce symptoms. For instance, the incubation periods of both scarlet fever and diphtheria are one to four days, that of measles is ten to fourteen days and that of rubella is twelve to twenty-one days. A very few fevers have variable incubation periods: e.g., while the incubation period of typhoid is normally around fourteen days, it can be as short as seven or as long as thirty days, depending on the quantity of organisms swallowed and on various other factors.

Many fevers have a characteristic rash, such as minute red spots on a flushed background in scarlet fever, the slightly coarser spots of rubella and the more blotchy rash of measles; but in some, such as whooping cough and mumps, there is no rash, and in some others (such as typhoid and cerebrospinal meningitis) the rash is not always seen.

Treatment. Ascertainment of the exact cause and its treatment is highly important. Apart from such therapy skilled nursing plays the major role. In particular rest is essential (including, for example, in diphtheria not allowing the patient to subject his heart to the strain of raising his head from the pillow); warm baths stimulate the skin and excretory organs and so facilitate heat loss; tepid sponging is useful when the temperature passes above 104 °F., and should aim at reducing it to 100 to 101 °F. but not lower; frequent changes of clothes may be necessary if there is much sweating; dehydration must be avoided; by drinking quantities of fluids; regular turning of the patient decreases the

chance of lung involvement; the mouth and teeth should be carefully cleaned periodically; bed-sores should be prevented by scrupulous cleanliness and thorough drying, and in long fevers by hardening the pressure areas of skin with methylated spirits; and the nurse must constantly bear in mind that in most fevers the patient is infectious and his discharges and bed-linen are infectious.

Prevention. Measures include: health education to encourage routine immunization against many formerly common fevers (e.g., diphtheria, poliomyelitis, whooping cough, measles and rubella), and to encourage immunization in special circumstances against various other fevers (e.g., smallpox, cholera, typhoid and typhus); hygienic measures to prevent diseases spread by faulty hygiene (e.g., typhoid and cholera); destruction of insects and their breeding grounds in areas liable to insect-borne infections (e.g., malaria and yellow fever); and, where infection occurs, strict isolation of patients, exclusion of visitors, recording names and addresses of all contacts (including members of the medical, nursing, paramedical and domestic staff), surveillance or quarantine of all contacts and investigation of the source of the outbreak, together with many other measures as appropriate, such as boiling of all water where a water-borne outbreak is suspected.

The reduction of food-borne specific fevers by personal and environmental hygiene, and the virtual eradication of many droplet-borne specific fevers by immunization and vaccination, together with education of the public about these measures, have been among the greatest triumphs of preventive medicine or indeed of all medical science. For instance, as late as 1943 there were over a million cases of diphtheria in Europe, and in 1941 – the year in which diphtheria immunization started on a large scale in Scotland with deliberate education of the public about it – there were in that country over 10,000 cases and 519 deaths, as compared with a total of under 20 cases in each recent year.

fibrillation. The involuntary, uncoordinated action of individual muscle fibres, which alternately contract and relax in a rapid irregular fashion so that tremors occur and the normal muscular movements are impaired and weakened. It particularly affects heart-muscle (ventricular or AURICULAR FIBRILLATION) and is the result of degenerative disease. It is characterized by an extremely irregular pulse and greatly-reduced cardiac output.

Fibrillary twitching of muscles normally under voluntary control is a sign of several degenerative nervous diseases, such as Parkinson's disease. Effects are usually first seen in the smaller muscles of hands, forearm, and face.

Transient episodes of muscular twitching sometimes occur in the eyelids and around the orbits. This is called myokimia. It is generally unimportant and is related to fatigue or debility.

fibrositis. Alternatively called muscular rheumatism, this is a condition, probably rheumatic, but affecting not joints but soft tissues, characterized by pain and tenderness at localized 'trigger-points' and by muscular stiffness. Muscular strain, mental stress, chill and even dietetic errors are suggested as causes, with American experts particularly emphasizing the mental factors and calling the condition psychogenic rheumatism. Yet against the psychological factor is the fact that the condition occurs twice as frequently in outdoor as in indoor workers. According to the part of the body affected the disease may be called lumbago, sciatica, intercostal neuralgia or rheumatic headache.

Treatment involves rest, analgesics to relieve the pain, and application of heat until the muscular spasm is relieved. Thereafter normal activity can be resumed.

fibula. The long slender bone on the outer side of the leg. It is attached to the broader and thicker tibia at both ends, enters into the structure of the ankle joint at the lower end but takes no part in the formation of the knee joint.

Fractures of the fibula alone are not uncommon, usually caused by direct violence. Because the tibia acts as a splint they generally produce no displacement, although pain is produced by pressing the bone below or above the fracture. Fractures of both tibia and fibula are also not uncommon and may be due either to direct violence, such as a blow on the leg, or to indirect violence, which would fracture the fibula by, for instance, jumping from a height and landing heavily on the heels.

filariasis. Infection with certain tiny worms (filaria) transmitted from the blood of an infected person to another person by several species of mosquito. The incubation period is remarkably long, usually eight to twelve months. After developing, the worms block lymphatic vessels, causing painful and tender swellings, and subsequently the enormous swellings known as elephantiasis.

Diethylcarbamizine is the most effective drug so far, but it sometimes causes acute allergic reactions and it does not always secure a complete cure. Prevention includes anti-mosquito measures in endemic areas, e.g., draining of stagnant water in which mosquitoes may breed, screening of sleeping places and use of insect repellents. Essentially filiarisis is a disease likely to respond not so much to treatment as to education of the public about its transmission and about methods of insect control.

fingerprints. The outermost layer of the skin is the epidermis or cuticle and everywhere it is marked by a network of linear furrows of varying size and arrangement. On the finger-tips these lines are fine but very distinct and regular forming a succession of more or less parallel curves caused by the large size and peculiar arrangement of the sensory cells deep in the skin. The resultant pattern of these skin furrows is unique to each individual, even in identical twins, and does not change throughout life. They can thus be used to ensure positive identification.

Finger-prints are a record of such patterns made by smearing the finger-tips with ink and then taking a 'rolled' impression on white paper or card. Prints are also unavoidably left on any smooth article which has been handled because the natural skin-secretion leaves a similarily-patterned trace which can be 'developed' by dusting with powder and then photographed for permanent evidence.

The uniqueness and permanence of individual finger-prints has long been recognized since they were adopted in China and Japan as a means of signing or certifying documents from very early times. They were also used by the Indian Civil Service in the nineteenth century to prevent impersonation in court proceedings, but credit for the development of an organized finger-print identification system really belongs to Francis Galton (1822-1911) an English scientist and mathematician who published his monograph, *Finger-Prints*, in 1892, and to Sir Edward Henry, a Chief Commissioner of the Metropolitan Police who improved on Galton's system of classification.

In practical terms, classification is all-important, because on it depends the ability to store recorded prints in a systematic manner so that they can be retrieved for comparison when required. Any finger-print left at the scene of a crime by a known criminal whose prints are on record can very rapidly be matched and similar evidence may be used to convict first-time offenders taken into custody on suspicion and finger-printed after arrest.

Classification is based on the characteristics of each print and on how these characteristics relate to the ten digits. Individual prints are of four main types: (1) arches, in which the epidermal ridges run from side-to-side without any backward turn; (2) loops, which make a backward turn without any spiralling and which may be further differentiated by whether their downward slope is towards the outer or inner side of the limb; (3) whorls, which make a spiral turn through at least one complete circle; and (4) composites, which show two or more of the other features. Numerical values are assigned to the various types and to the finger on which they appear and on the basis of these findings a formula is worked out to determine where a set of prints should be filed for future reference. In matching prints further refinements may be employed such as counting the number of ridges from the core to the outer edge of a print.

Somewhat similar to finger-prints are palm- and sole-prints which also present individual patterns. Some maternity hospitals now record foot-prints of new-born babies to guard against them getting mixed up and discharged with the wrong mother. Unusual prints are also features in some genetically determined diseases such as mongolism.

fingers. The five separate members forming the extremities of the hand. In man, apes and monkeys the fingers have the unusual characteristic that the thumb and the other fingers can be brought together for grasping. From the thumb inwards the others are named the index, the middle, the ring and the little finger, and each has three small bones (the phalanges). The knuckle joints are formed by the first phalanges and the metacarpal bones. Fingers have great range of movement and are very richly supplied with nerves and nerve-endings; at their tips the sense of touch is particularly acute.

The fingers are subject to all the diseases of skin and bone, but are particularly liable to abscess, especially at the root of the nail, and to injury and septic inflammation. Chilblains are among the commonest affections of the fingers, and spasm of the fingers may arise in tetany and in writer's cramp. Scabies commonly makes its first appearance on the skin between the fingers.

FIRST AID

People do not usually have heart-attacks or accidents involving serious bleeding or poisoning, gassing or apparent drowning immediately outside a hospital gate or in close proximity to a doctor or nurse. Again and again in accidents and sudden illnesses the victims endure very considerable needless pain and suffering, and some of them needlessly die, simply because the persons present do not have the knowledge to undertake emergency resuscitation, to control bleeding, to cope with poisoning or to treat shock.

It is therefore important that every intelligent adult should acquire a reasonable working knowledge of first aid - the efficient rendering of immediate assistance to a person who has suddenly become ill as a result of disease or accident - because that intelligent adult may well be the only person available to offer prompt help in an emergency. Thirty hours of theoretical and practical instruction (three hours a week for as short a period as ten weeks) may easily make the difference between the death and the life of a relative or a friend in a subsequent emergency.

Yet it is almost equally important to emphasize that a person who has gained a working knowledge of first aid should not attempt to do too much. Where the illness or accident has occurred far from available skilled help the efforts of the first-aider may easily be life-saving; but where such skilled help is available within minutes the first-aider should content himself with doing what is immediately necessary and should appreciate that, while he has spent thirty or forty hours in learning to cope, the doctor or nurse has had years of full-time professional preparation.

Commonsense judgment is always required. To get the airways clear, to attempt mouth-to-mouth resuscitation if breathing has stopped, to control serious bleeding, to begin heart massage if the heart has stopped, and to treat poisoning if the source is known are always useful and sometimes life-saving; but to try to act as a professional by using treatment that goes beyond the limits of first aid and to delay the summoning of skilled help means that the first aider is accepting a responsibility that he is wholly untrained to bear. In other words, there is a considerable difference between the type and extent of first aid usefully attempted in accident or illness on a lonely mountain and the type and extent in a situation where an ambulance or a doctor may be expected to arrive within a few minutes.

There are many excellent small books on first aid, such as those published by the British Red Cross and the St. John's and St. Andrew's Ambulance Associations, but neither these books nor the even briefer guide given below are a substitute for practical training. Information about courses can be obtained from any local branch of an ambulance association or from the nearest ambulance station.

The short outline that follows begins with a few general principles and then discusses individual matters, such as the stopping of bleeding and the restoration of breathing. Clearly the seven general points and their order of priority have to be considered in the light of the particular situation.

Some general principles

1. Keep cool. A quiet, calm demeanour allays excitement and inspires the patient with confidence if he is conscious.

2. Protect the patient from obvious physical dangers. In some cases, e.g., fire or serious gas leak, this may involve moving him.

3. Clear a space, both to give the victim air and to give yourself room for action.

4. Unless the injury appears trivial send for a doctor with such information as is immediately available, not forgetting the exact place at which the patient is. Information such as 'Probable fracture of femur following bicycle accident' or 'unconscious and said to be a diabetic' may help a doctor to assess priorities between two urgent calls and may also help him to decide what apparatus and instruments to bring.

5. Quickly observe both the surroundings and the patient. A weapon or a bottle that contained poison or alcohol can disappear easily but its existence may be important both for early diagnosis and for criminal proceedings. Also note the victim's posture, position, expression and position of injuries.

6. Give immediate first aid.
There are several things which you should check and act on straight away.
Airways. Check that the air-passage is open so that the patient can breathe. Clear the mouth and nostrils of any blood or vomited material, and if vomiting or bleeding in mouth or nose is continuing turn the patient's head to the side so that the material can leak out without obstructing breathing. Loosen tight collar, belt or corset. In an epileptic fit try to insert a hard, smooth, unbreakable object (e.g., a lead pencil) between the teeth to prevent the patient from biting his tongue.
Bleeding. Keep the patient's head low and if practicable raise the bleeding part. If there is appreciable bleeding stop it by direct pressure of the fingers on the wound. Types of bleeding are considered later, but essentially in a case of a smooth trickle of purplish blood there may be time to get a sterile dressing if available or even a clean handkerchief, or to wash dirty fingers; but where bright red blood is spurting out there is no time for such measures.
Breathing. If the patient is not breathing attempt mouth-to-mouth or mouth-to-nose resuscitation; but in a case of apparent drowning another form of artifical respiration may be better.
Circulation. If the pulse cannot be felt (at the wrist or just in front of the ear) start massage of the heart.
Fainting. Keep the head low and make sure that the air-passages are clear.
Fractures. Run your hand gently along the limbs to detect a possible fracture. If there is one, avoid all rough movement and if possible immobilize the fracture before moving the patient at all. An immediate commonsense decision must be made between avoiding worsening of the fracture and protecting the patient: for instance in a burning building or a car likely to go on fire the person must be moved at all costs.
Shock. Virtually every serious injury produces a considerable amount of shock. Unless there is some reason for moving the patient or altering his position, leave him lying recumbent but protect him from cold by covering him with a blanket or coat. If he is unconscious or has an abdominal injury, give nothing by mouth. If he is conscious and collapsed and has

no apparent injury of the digestive tract, let him sip a cup of hot tea or coffee. Do not give alcohol, because while it is helpful in some emergencies it is definitely harmful in others. Keep the patient comfortably warm. Sudden serious illness or injury is terrifying to the victim, so, if he is conscious, remember the importance of reassurance: the patient may well think he is about to die and may be vastly helped by such remark as 'I think you have had a mild heart attack but are already beginning to recover. Just try to rest easy until the doctor arrives'.

7. Examine the patient and give less immediate first aid. If he is conscious he may be able to supply useful information, and in some cases of serious disease or injury he may lapse into unconsciousness before skilled help arrives. If a limb is injured, remove the clothing from the uninjured side first and then if necessary rip down the seam on the injured side; and in re-applying the clothing for warmth replace it first on the injured side. If he is unconscious, look for wounds, swellings or depressions of the skull; and notice whether the pupils are contracted or dilated, whether they are equal in size and whether they contract on the admission of light. If the doctor has not yet arrived, examine the jaw, ribs and spine, looking for irregularities, grating sound on touch, or tender spots; and look generally for wounds of the body.

Bright red spurting blood means bleeding from an artery and its prompt arrest is essential. Darker, smoothly flowing blood means haemorrhage from a vein and is usually much easier to stop. Pallor, rapidity of pulse, gasping or sighing respirations, cold and clammy skin and other signs of severe collapse and shock suggest haemorrhage - internal bleeding if no blood is visible. Fracture is suggested by loss of function, tenderness, unnatural mobility of the part, swelling and deformity. Unconsciousness with flushed, congested face, may be due to cerebral haemorrhage (stroke), a specific fever, or drunkenness. Powerlessness of the arm and leg on the same side, in the absence of fractures, suggests cerebral haemorrhage or cerebral thrombosis. Unconsciousness with dilated pupils may mean belladonna (nightshade) poisoning or pressure on the brain or - if the pupils react to light - severe shock. Contracted pupils may be due to morphia poisoning but have some other possible causes. Bleeding from the ear or nose after a head injury generally means a fractured skull. The coughing up of bright red frothy blood suggests lung injury or lung disease, while the vomiting of dark blood suggests damage to the stomach.

Sudden vomiting may be the result of dietetic indiscretion, food poisoning, excess alcohol, gastric ulcer, abdominal obstruction, some diseases of the kidneys and some diseases of the brain. Also it may follow a blow on the abdomen; it may be a symptom of pregnancy; and in a child it may herald the onset of a fever, e.g., scarlet fever or measles.

Fainting may be caused by terror, emotional shock of any nature, severe pain, external bleeding, internal bleeding, extreme heat, physical or mental exhaustion, or various diseases that interfere with the blood supply to the brain.

Severe pain in the region of the heart and stomach is likely to be related to the stomach in persons under 40 years and likely to be related to the heart in persons above the age of 50. Severe pain on the right side of the lower abdomen may well be appendicitis.

Procedures

The above paragraphs give only a few of the commoner manifestations of sudden illness or injury, and the first aider should remember that detailed diagnosis is not his function. His function is to give such immediate aid as will be helpful (and sometimes life-saving) and to supply such information as will facilitate diagnosis and treatment.

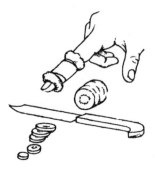

Bleeding. The three types of external bleeding are described under HAEMORRHAGE but are here summarized. Capillary bleeding is a steady reddish ooze from cut tissues; venous bleeding is a steady purple stream; and arterial bleeding is bright red and spurting. Although bleeding is a very common emergency and one which calls for prompt and effective treatment, it is really only arterial haemorrhage which presents the first aider with much difficulty.

For any appreciable bleeding it is useful to keep the head low (to allow adequate flow of blood to the brain) and to raise the affected part. For capillary or venous haemorrhage a dressing and a cotton-wool pad secured by a firm bandage will generally achieve all that is required. Ruptured varicose veins of the leg, however, will bleed heavily as long as the patient is upright: in that case it is essential to get the patient to lie down and to raise the leg, so as to reverse the pressure of blood.

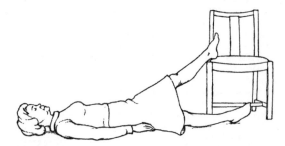

When a large artery is severed a great deal of blood escapes in a short time, and even a small artery can soon pump out the litre or so of blood whose loss can endanger life. The obvious immediate method of controlling arterial bleeding is by direct firm pressure on the wound (or on the wound and on the side of it nearer to the heart). Fingers are available for this pressure, and there is no time to wash them or to secure a sterile dressing to place between the fingers and the wound. Certainly dirty fingers can cause infection, but infections can be treated; whereas if the bleeding is not stopped quickly the patient will die.

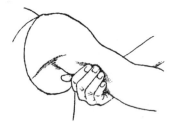

As soon as is reasonably practicable the fingers can be replaced by a sterile dressing and pad above the dressing, secured by a firm bandage. If the bleeding does not stop, the dressing and pad should be reinforced by towels or other soft material, again secured by a firm bandage.

An alternative method for wounds in the region of the groin, armpit, knee or elbow is forced flexion. A pad is placed in the bend of the joint and the joint is then fully bent and secured in the bent position by a firm bandage.

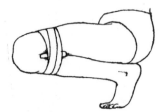

Many manuals on first aid stress the importance of pressure points at which (nearer the heart than the wound) an artery can be compressed against an underlying bone. Some of these pressure points are described and illustrated below:

Scalp area.   The temporal artery can be compressed just in front of the ear opening and the occipital artery about 2cm. behind the ear.

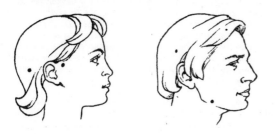

Face.   The facial artery can be compressed where it crosses the border of the lower jaw about 2 to 3cm. in front of the angle of the jaw.

Head and neck.   The common carotid artery can be reached in the neck alongside the windpipe and about 3cm. above the shoulder blade, but its compression requires considerable expertise.

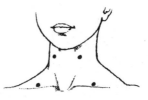

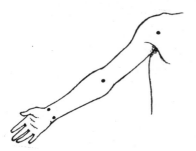

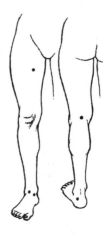

Arm.   The brachial artery can be compressed against the shaft of the humerus about half way down the upper arm, and the axillary artery can (less easily) be pressed against the head of the humerus at the top of the armpit.

Leg.   With great pressure usually involving two hands the femoral artery can be pressed against the brim of the pelvis near the middle of the groin.

These pressure points have been mentioned because they are emphasized in most books on first aid. They can be useful to a person who has received considerable training in first aid; but a person with little knowledge of first aid is more likely to stop arterial bleeding by firm pressure on the wound, followed by a firm pad and bandage, than by groping for a pressure point.

A TOURNIQUET is suitable only for use on the arms and legs and then only if other methods fail. It may be improvised from a narrow folded triangular bandage or any similar strip of material, tied round the limb and twisted by any form of short rod. It has to be placed between the wound and the heart, tightened only enough to control the bleeding and not left on continuously for more than 25 to 30 minutes at a time.

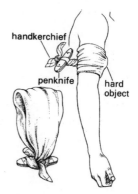

handkerchief

penknife   hard
                           object

In arterial bleeding to stop or reduce the bleeding is a matter of life and death. It is also important to send for medical help as quickly as possible, and to be alert for - and ready to treat - stopping of the heart (see p.189) and signs of severe shock (see p.186).

See also BANDAGES AND BANDAGING.

Burns and scalds. Irrespective of whether these are caused by fire, electricity, boiling liquids or chemicals, the essentials of treatment are to separate the casualty from the danger, to bathe the damaged part freely in cold water in order to reduce pain and heat, and thereafter to apply a sterile non-adherent dressing and to cover the dressing with available soft materials, such as cotton-wool and a bandage. (See BANDAGES AND BANDAGING.)

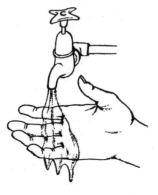

The application of greasy substances (such as butter) was at one time recommended, but these substances probably do more harm than good. Similarly cold tea, because of its tannic acid content, was much advocated but it is doubtful whether it is more useful than plentiful cold water.

In severe burns and scalds dangers to be watched for - and treated if they arise - include stopping of breathing, stopping of the heart and serious shock (see p.188,189,186).

See also BURNS AND SCALDS for more information.

Choking. The various causes of choking are indicated in the article on that subject. Where choking is due to a foreign body (e.g., a lump of food) in the throat it is often possible to remove the object by the fingers.

Failing this, the object may be dislodged by a couple of hard slaps on the upper part of the back between the shoulders. Clearly the dislodging will be easier if the object can simply fall out. So a young child before the slaps can be held up by the legs with the head downwards, and an older child can be placed over an adult's knee with, again, the head downwards.

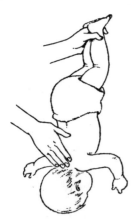

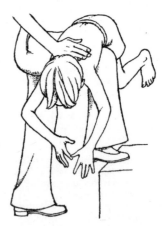

After the object is removed it is essential to ensure that the airway is clear, so that the person can breathe. If breathing has actually stopped, artificial respiration will be required (see p.188).

Drowning accidents. It is useful to remember as a preliminary that every child should be taught not only to swim but also to float: a person who is able to float and to tread water is seldom in immediate danger. (See also DROWNING.)

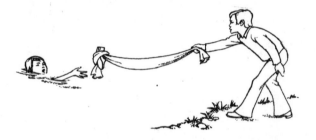

Rescuing the person.   Anything that floats (e.g., a branch of a tree) can be thrown to the victim to make it easier for him to float, and similarly anything that floats (e.g., a pair of trousers knotted at the ankles and filling with air as the rescuer enters the water) will give the rescuer additional buoyancy.

To make a life-line from the shore or bank a rope or belt or large towel is useful, and it can be thrown more accurately if the end is weighted with a shoe or a small piece of wood (but not with something so heavy that it may cause injury to the person in difficulty). The 'human chain' method of rescue, useful in strong currents, involves several rescuers facing in opposite directions, clasping hands wrist to wrist and stretching from shore to victim. It is important that the rescuer on the shore is a strong person and is firmly stationed on solid ground.

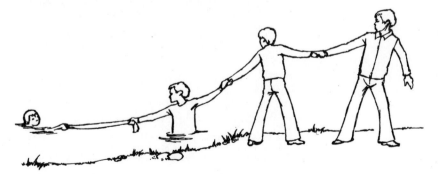

A swimmer proposing to effect a rescue should use his strength reasonably. There is little point in reaching the drowning person a couple of seconds earlier than would have normally been anticipated if, as a result of his burst of speed, the swimmer lacks the strength to tow the victim to land.

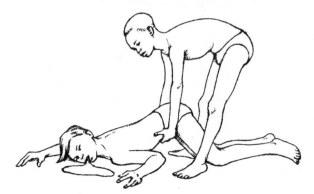

Treatment of the apparently drowned.   If the person has stopped breathing the first essential is to make an attempt to expel water from the lungs by placing the patient face downwards, raising the lower part of his body and allowing water to run out through the mouth and nose. Thereafter artificial respiration has to be started. The rhythmical compression of the chest according to Schafer's method is perhaps the most desirable here: it also helps to expel water and leaves the drowned person in the best position for getting rid of the water; see page 189.

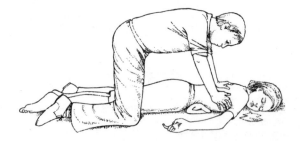

The mouth-to-mouth (kiss of life) method is very effective once the air passages are reasonably clear but cannot be expected to succeed with a seriously waterlogged patient.

If the ordinary respiration does not restart, artificial respiration should be continued for half an hour before hope of recovery is abandoned.

When the patient is breathing, either never having stopped or having restarted in response to artificial respiration, it has to be realized that he may well be in a condition of shock, and shock has to be treated (see p.186).

Electric shock.   If the victim is still in contact with a high tension wire it is unwise to attempt to rescue him. However callous it may seem the best action is to notify an expert and await his arrival.

If the victim is still in contact with ordinary domestic electric current, disconnect it by turning off the appropriate switch or jerking the plug from its socket, or, if both of these are impossible, try to push the victim away from the wire using insulating material, e.g., a dry walking stick. Do not attempt to cut live wires.

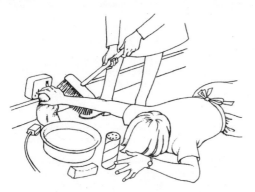
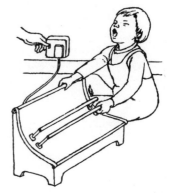

After the victim is no longer in contact with the wire, treat as for burns, and if breathing has stopped apply artificial respiration (see p.188).

Fractures.   Often the victim, if conscious, will be able to tell you that he heard or felt the bone snap and that he now has pain and tenderness at the site of the break and cannot move the limb. In any case the limb looks deformed in shape and often appears shorter than the opposite limb, and in the case of fracture of a flat bone (e.g., in the skull) there may be either a depression or an elevation. While abnormal mobility and a grating sensation when the broken ends are moved against each other are commonly stated as additional evidence of fracture, the first aid worker is strongly advised not to look for these signs: excessive examination can easily convert a simple break into a compound fracture.

Where a fracture is suspected the immediate aims should be (1) to prevent further damage by rough handling or needless movement, (2) to treat shock (see p.186) which is often considerable, and (3) to secure prompt medical attention. In general the patient should not be moved unless he is in a position of danger; and if it is necessary to move him the injured limb should first be fixed in as good a position as the circumstances allow. For this purpose a splint should be improvised out of any available suitable material, e.g., walking sticks, umbrellas or boards. A splint should be rigid enough to immobilize the broken bone, long enough to reach from beyond the joint above the break to beyond the joint below it, and preferably wider than the limb. If practicable the splint should be padded with cotton-wool or similar material. It should be firmly fastened by bandages or strips of clothing (e.g., neckties or braces) and should prevent movement without obstructing the circulation or causing pain.

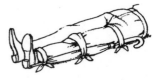

In measuring the length and breadth of the required splint there is no need to use the injured limb and possibly cause pain. Any measurement can be done on the opposite limb. It is very difficult for one person to apply a splint. Ideally three are needed: one to hold the upper part of the broken limb, one to pull very gently on the lower part, and one to apply and fix the splint. The knots of bandages, straps or tapes - preferably reef-knots - should be over the splint, not over the bone.

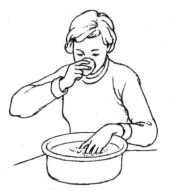

When the splinted patient is being moved to a stretcher or to a vehicle one person should have the sole duty of supporting the injured limb with both hands.

Much that has been said above also applies to a fractured spine or pelvis, but the danger of moving the patient is greater, so that if possible he should be left lying until a doctor arrives. As mentioned at the beginning of this note, there is likely to be a considerable degree of shock and it is important to treat it.

Frostbite. The condition is diagnosed by the affected part (usually toes, fingers, tip of ears or tip of nose) becoming very white and hard. The best treatment is to bathe the part gently with cold water, delaying the use of warm water until the part has thawed.

The old treatment of rubbing the frozen part with snow is no longer advocated. The rubbing can damage the tissues.

Poisoning. Many substances, harmless or even beneficial when taken in appropriate quantities, are poisonous when consumed in considerable excess. Aspirin tablets and iron tablets are examples. So three commonsense measures are: (1) to keep all medicines, tablets, cleansing fluids, disinfectants and so on completely out of reach of young children and to explain their dangers to older children; (2) to ensure every potentially poisonous substance in the house is clearly labelled - both to lessen the chance of anybody consuming it by mistake and to ensure that if some is swallowed the nature of the substance is immediately known;

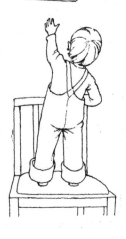

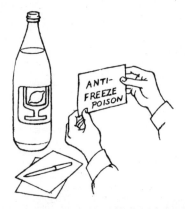

and (3) in no circumstances to extract something from the medicine cupboard and swallow it in the dark - since two containers of similar shape can easily become interchanged in position.

On the other hand it is worth remembering that, apart from cases of deliberate suicide, death from poisoning is an extreme rarity. Apart from strong acids and strong alkalis the overwhelming majority of substances found in an ordinary house or garden are less serious in their effects than is sometimes imagined.

Where the poisonous substance is unknown. If it has been swallowed an immediate drink of milk will dilute it and so make it less harmful. If it has been inhaled fresh air will probably help and artificial respiration may be needed if the breathing shows signs of stopping. If it has got into the eyes the

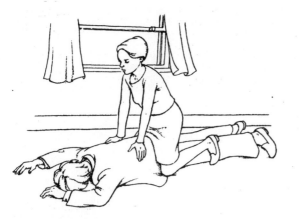

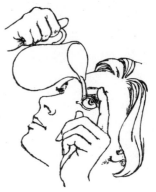

lids should be held well apart and the eyes bathed with a gentle stream of warm - but not hot - water. If it is on the skin, thorough washing with soap and water is likely to remove it. Clearly decision about whether to seek immediate medical aid is difficult if the poison is not known. One has to be guided largely by the condition of the patient.

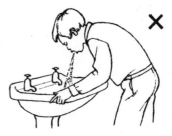

Where the poisonous substance is known. It is manifestly not possible to list every possible poison in a single article, but acids, alkalis and petroleum products are generally recognized as such, and, for these, vomiting would be positively harmful as it would bring the substance back into the throat. For any other substance deemed to be poisonous or probably poisonous, a fairly sound procedure is to give a drink of milk and then try to induce vomiting.

Poisons may be divided into five groups. The following three groups are the main ones for which vomiting is definitely harmful: (1) If the poison is a corrosive acid (e.g., sulphuric or nitric) do not on any account induce vomiting; give milk or milk of magnesia or very soft white of egg in large quantities and seek immediate medical aid. (2) If the poison is a strong alkali (including some floor strippers and oven cleaners) again do not on any account induce vomiting: give large amounts of milk or water, followed by diluted vinegar or lemon juice, and seek immediate medical help. (3) For petrol products (including lighter fluid and turpentine) again do not try to induce vomiting: give large quantities of milk, attend to the breathing and seek immediate medical aid.

In the remaining two groups an attempt to induce vomiting should be made: (4) For many moderate, non-corrosive poisons (e.g., alcohol, antifreeze, hair dyes, household antiseptics and methylated spirits) try to induce vomiting with syrup of ipecac if available or by pushing a finger to the back of the throat. After vomiting has occurred, check with hospital or doctor as to whether any further treatment is necessary. (5) For the vast majority of non-corrosive poisons (e.g., arsenic, boracic acid, camphor, carbon tetrachloride, iron tablets, marking ink, moth balls, naphthalene, most of the poisonous plants, most sleeping tablets and strychnine) try to induce vomiting and - without even awaiting its occurrence - bring the doctor to the patient or the patient to the doctor.

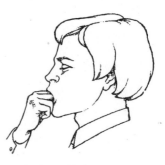

If the patient has to be taken to a doctor or to a hospital, it is important that the substance (if known) and the approximate amount consumed are notified to the person dealing with the patient; or, failing fuller information, the partially empty container can be taken along with the patient. The doctor is placed under a very severe handicap if he is merely told that the person has swallowed some unspecified poisonous material.

Shock. To a greater or lesser degree shock occurs in all serious injuries and in many cases of sudden, severe illness. The face becomes pale, the skin cold and clammy, the pulse weak, the breathing shallow, the eyes sunken and the pupils dilated.

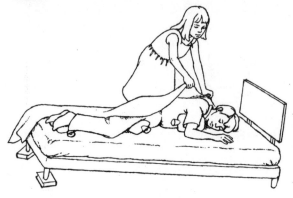

Immediate treatment is to keep the patient lying down, if practicable indoors and in bed, and with the head preferably a shade lower than the feet so as to allow easy flow of blood to the brain; keep the patient comfortably warm, e.g., by placing warm - but not overwarm - water bottles at the feet, armpits and groin. If the person is lying on a bed or a sofa it is fairly easy to raise the foot slightly by using bricks or other solid materials. If there is a possibility of a water-bottle being too hot a blanket can usefully be placed between the bottle and the patient's skin.

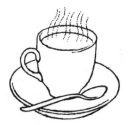

If the patient is conscious he will require reassurance and he should be encouraged to sip hot sweetened tea or coffee unless the shock is due to abdominal injury.

Occasionally in severe shock breathing becomes difficult and artificial respiration may be needed.

Wounds. Where the skin is broken there are three essentials of first aid treatment - to stop the bleeding, to cleanse the wound and to combat shock. Bleeding is discussed on page 178 and shock in the preceding paragraph. For cleansing a wound it is best to start by bathing it with warm, boiled water, then to swab with any available mild disinfectant in appropriate dilution (using boiled water as the diluting agent), and finally to cover the wound with any available sterile dressing or with a piece of wet linen that has been boiled.

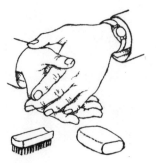

While the stopping of serious bleeding (see page 178) is an essential first priority, the vast majority of wounds and cuts do not involve arteries or large veins. Where blood is merely oozing out or slowly trickling out the person proposing to apply first aid should, where practicable, thoroughly wash his hands before starting treatment.

If the implement that made the cut is liable to have been contaminated by garden or field soil or by street dust or stable refuse, a doctor should be consulted because the patient may require anti-tetanus serum. In other cases there is no need for a doctor unless the wound is large enough to require stitching or unless the wound becomes inflamed and throbbing, indicating that it has become infected.

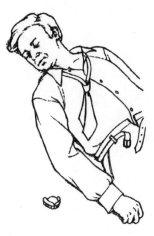

Unconsciousness. Irrespective of the cause five essential measures in dealing with an unconscious patient are: (1) to stop serious bleeding if there is any (see p.178); (2) to maintain a clear airway, involving turning the head to the side so that saliva or blood can trickle out, removing dentures and loosening clothing at neck and waist; (3) to ensure that breathing continues, using mouth-to-mouth respiration if breathing stops (see p.188); (4) to keep the patient lying down with no unnecessary movement; and (5) to keep him warm (e.g., by covering with blankets) except in unconsciousness due to heat-stroke. A sixth general point is a negative one: no attempt should be made to give an unconscious person anything by mouth.

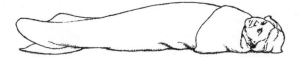

Beyond these points treatment varies with the cause and a competent first aid worker should attempt to make a provisional diagnosis, both because of possible additions to the immediate treatment and because of possible aid to the doctor when he arrives.

The main causes are: (1) injury: concussion, shock, bleeding, electrocution, and heat-stroke; (2) diseases of the nervous system: apoplexy (stroke), epilepsy, and hysteria; (3) poisoning: alcohol, opiates, hypnotics, other drugs and chemicals; (4) toxaemia: diabetes and uraemia; (5) lack of oxygen to the brain: fainting and heart disease; and (6) asphyxia: gas poisoning, drowning, choking and strangulation.

Information from a friend of the unconscious person may be helpful: for instance the friend may be able to state that the person is subject to epileptic fits (in which case it will be useful to separate the clenched jaws by an improvised wedge) or suffers from diabetes or from kidney disease. Information about the mode of onset is useful: in apoplexy the unconsciousness is usually sudden whereas in diabetic coma it is usually gradual. Inspection of the patient provides many clues: a head injury is often obvious; a flushed face and noisy breathing suggest apoplexy; foaming at the mouth suggests epilepsy. To smell the breath is often helpful: in uraemic coma (kidney disease) the breath smells like urine, in diabetic coma it smells like apples, and in unconsciousness due to alcohol the smell is characteristic (but if the first aider is not the person first on the scene he should check that an odour of alcohol is not a result of a misguided attempt to help the patient by pouring whisky into his mouth). In opium or morphine poisoning the pupils are contracted, whereas in most forms of unconsciousness they are not. In heat-stroke the skin may feel hot (and the patient should not be kept warm).

In all cases of unconsciousness except a faint with recovery of consciousness within three minutes medical aid should be sought immediately.

General.

The eleven occurrences so far discussed - bleeding, burns and scalds, choking, drowning, electric shock, fractures, frostbite, poisoning, shock, wounds and unconsciousness - are the emergencies most likely to be encountered; but five important matters have still to be considered - what to do if breathing stops, what to do if the heart stops, how to move the patient if movement is necessary, how to reduce some hazards, and what sort of medicine chest can reasonably be provided in an ordinary house.

Artificial respiration.   If breathing stops the patient will die or suffer irreparable damage within minutes unless oxygen is pumped into his lungs until such time as natural breathing returns. Even where some breathing continues but is clearly difficult - with the face becoming blue and the veins of the neck enlarged - artificial respiration is needed.

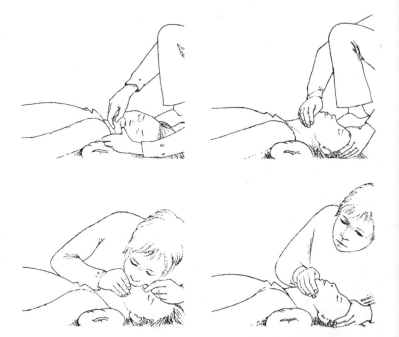

Kiss of life.   Except for drowning cases the mouth-to-mouth method is generally best as well as easiest. After separating the patient from the cause and ensuring that the airway is clear (including removing dentures and loosening tight clothing), lay the patient on his back, kneel beside his head, use one hand to press the lower jaw upwards and forwards (so that the head is tilted back thus providing a straighter airway) and the other to close his nostrils, pinching them between thumb and forefinger. Take a deep breath, place your lips firmly round the patient's mouth and breathe out into the patient's mouth. If you are doing it correctly you should see the patient's chest beginning to rise as the lungs fill. If the chest fails to rise, check that you have closed the nostrils and check that your mouth is firmly round the patient's mouth. If the chest is duly rising, remove your mouth and take another deep breath while the chest is falling. Then reapply the mouth and breathe into the patient. Aim at about ten to twelve breaths a minute, and every three minutes desist for a single breath in and out, to see whether natural breathing has been resumed. If it is not resumed, continue for half an hour before abandoning the attempt.

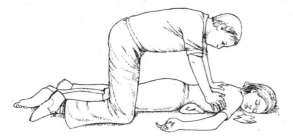

Schafer's method.   In drowning accidents this is better because it facilitates the escape of water and mucus from the air passages. Clear the airway, place the patient on his stomach with the head turned to one side, kneel across his buttocks or on one side of his back facing the head, place your hands over the lowest ribs on the back one on each side, quite slowly throw the weight of your body on the hands (thus pressing the back of the chest downwards), then slowly raise your body to remove the pressure but leaving the hands in position, and repeat this double movement about twelve times a minute. If there is no evidence of resumption of natural breathing, continue for a full hour before abandoning hope.

After breathing has been restored, whether by mouth-to-mouth or by Schafer's method, remember to treat the patient for shock (p. 186).

Stimulation of the heart.   Even if the patient is breathing his brain will be damaged unless oxygen reaches it.

The pulse is more easily felt in front of the ear than at the wrist.

If the circulation stops and the pulse cannot be felt, start by separating the patient from the cause, clearing the airway and trying half a dozen breaths of mouth-to-mouth respiration (see p. 188). In most cases this re-establishes the heart beat.

If no heart beat can be detected, begin massage of the heart. Place the patient on his back, kneel beside his chest, place the palm of one hand on the lower end of the sternum (breastbone), cover the one hand with the other, with arms straight rock forwards over the patient until your shoulders are vertically above your hands (thus pressing downwards), rock backwards releasing the pressure, and repeat the double movement about sixty times a minute for an adult. For a child less pressure is needed: place one hand on the lower part of the sternum and the other on the ground; and aim at between eighty and ninety double movements per minute. In both cases pause occasionally to see if the natural heart beat has been restored, but in the absence of restoration continue the massage for at least half an hour.

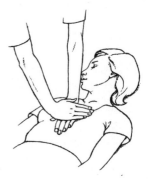

A highly skilled person can sometimes manage to combine heart stimulation and mouth-to-mouth respiration. If both breathing and circulation have stopped and if the only person available cannot manage both techniques, he is probably wiser to concentrate on respiration: as indicated above, a few breaths will often restart the heart, but a restarting of the heart will not re-establish breathing.

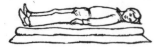

Moving the patient. The broad general rule is 'don't'. Needless movement may increase bleeding, may make a fracture worse and may do other damage; but clearly there are circumstances in which a patient has to be moved for his own safety.

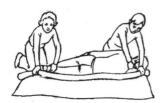

Where removal for a few yards is necessary (e.g., from the road to the pavement) the sound procedure is to attend to serious bleeding, to clear airways, to hold any fractured limb to minimize its movement and to move the patient as gently as is possible.

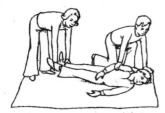

In extreme emergency (e.g., an adult overcome by smoke in a burning house) the easiest way to move a heavy person quickly is to pull his hands over your shoulders and crawl out, dragging him behind you. An alternative which leaves your hands free is to tie his wrists with a belt and loop his arms over your neck.

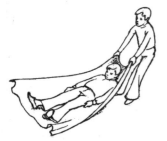

Reduction of hazards. Excepting the degenerative conditions of old age most diseases and injuries are in large measure preventable. Much of this entire book is devoted to prevention, and it is manifestly impossible in a single short section to deal with matters like the prevention of infections or the prevention of coronary thrombosis, even though these have their first aid aspects. All that will be attempted here is to pick out five sets of common hazards and to offer a few hints about their reduction.

Home accidents. Check the safety of gas and electrical appliances. Attend to the safety of the kitchen, the most dangerous room in the house. Keep sharp implements, matches, medicines and cleansing liquids out of reach of the toddler. Avoid placing articles where you could trip over them if you have occasion to rise during the night. Beware of polished floors and of inadequately lit stairs. Don't smoke in bed. Remember that all these points apply to your holiday cottage or temporary residence just as much as to your permanent home. See also ACCIDENTS.

Motor accidents. Check the efficiency of brakes, etc., from time to time. Concentrate when driving. Keep a reasonable distance behind the next vehicle in case it stops suddenly. Take special care at cross-roads, crossings and bends and on roads made slippery by ice or sudden rain after a drought: change down when in doubt. Make a habit of using your driving mirror and of giving your signals in plenty of time. See also ACCIDENTS.

Hiking accidents. Learn in advance about anticipated weather conditions and about your intended route. Leave information about your route and your expected time of return. Learn the rudiments of first aid. Dress sensibly and remember the importance of carrying matches, a knife and a whistle. If hill-walking always take a map, compass and emergency rations as well. Remember that weather conditions can rapidly turn fierce in mountains even in summer, so take spare clothing and waterproofs. Preferably hike with a companion, not alone. When forced to walk on the road keep to the side facing on-coming traffic.

Sunbathing hazards.   In warm climates use a sunburn preventive cream; sunbathe sparingly for the first few days until you are used to the climate, trying as a start ten minutes a day if you are more than four hundred miles nearer the equator than in your home and five minutes a day if you are more than seven hundred miles nearer the equator; and until used to the climate do not sunbathe between the hours of 10.30 a.m. and 3.30 p.m. Remember that when the sun is partially obscured by light cloud the danger of sunburn is increased, not decreased.

Bathing accidents.   Don't swim in an unfamiliar place and don't let your child swim in such a place without learning about currents. To swim alone is always dangerous. If you get into difficulties, try to float and don't panic. When swimming or bathing in a warm sea, beware of stings by a Portuguese man-of-war or a jellyfish: if bitten, place dry sand over the part, gently scrape it off, avoid rubbing, apply methylated spirits as soon as practicable, and if badly stung seek medical aid.

Medicine chest for the family.   Sudden illnesses and injuries occur in every household, and a medicine chest - containing first aid materials and household remedies - is an obvious necessity. A chest with a lock is in general undesirable, because if the key is left in position the chest can be opened by a child, and if the key is removed it tends to be momentarily lost at the very time access is urgent.

Ideally it should be a small wall cabinet, well out of reach of young children but easily opened by any adult. Such a cabinet should be used for storing any medicines currently prescribed for a member of the family, simple home remedies such as aspirin and antiseptics, dressings and other basic first aid requirements. It should not be used to store other items. Any medicine remaining at the end of a prescribed course of treatment should be removed and destroyed, as should any medicine which has been kept for a long period. The medicine chest should be kept closed except when an item is being removed or replaced.

The following articles might be regarded as a useful list of contents of the medicine chest:
> adhesive plaster dressings for minor cuts and wounds; absorbent gauze dressings for minor burns; cleansing tissues; cotton wool; narrow bandages (2 cm.); wide bandages (5 cm.); safety pins; dressing scissors; soluble aspirin; junior aspirin; calamine lotion; antihistamine cream; a mild laxative; sal volatile or brandy; tincture of iodine.

Probably no two doctors would agree on the exact contents of a medicine chest and much depends on available space, but the above is a reasonable list.

fistula. An abnormal channel or passage connecting two hollow organs (e.g., recto-vaginal fistula) or connecting a hollow organ with the body surface (e.g., anal fistula). In most cases a fistula develops from an abscess, fissure or operational wound, but occasionally fistulas arise from deep-seated disease of the bones or joints, and some fistulas are congenital. A fistula is easily infected and is often extremely painful. Treatment varies with the situation and the cause, but often involves surgery.

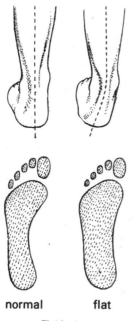

normal   flat

Flat foot

flat foot. A condition in which the arch of the instep is lower than normal so that in standing or walking the whole of the sole rests on the ground. Some of the main causes are (1) hereditary weakness of the tendon running from the back of the heel up the leg; (2) excessive weight, especially if coupled with standing for long periods; (3) badly fitting shoes; (4) certain acute and debilitating illnesses; (5) occasionally, pregnancy; and (6) very occasionally, accidental injury as in jumping from a height.

Prevention by well-fitting shoes and the adoption and maintenance of good posture is important, and in the early stages of the condition exercises and manipulation can help greatly.

In advanced stages it is necessary to differentiate between flexible flat foot in which the bones can be brought back into their normal position and rigid flat foot in which return to normal position is no longer possible. In the former case, which is often characterized by pain, manipulation, arch supports and special shoes are often valuable. In the case of rigid flat foot where changes have occurred in

the bones and joints, there is deformity but seldom pain, and arch supports merely cause discomfort; it is best to leave the condition untreated.

flatulence. Uncomfortable accumulation of gas in the stomach or intestine, relieved by the passage of the gas through the mouth or anus. In some cases flatulence is caused by the swallowing of the air during the gulping of food or drink, and in others it is essentially due to anxiety and the air is swallowed in unsuccessful attempts to belch. For further details see AEROPHAGY.

In another sizeable group of cases the flatulence is a result of excessive fermentation of food in the stomach, either because the digestive juices of the particular person are poor in ferments or because the muscular wall of the stomach is flabby so that the food is not firmly held. In the gas production type the patient may learn by observation that certain foods produce flatulence and so learn to avoid them. The foods vary slightly from person to person, but cabbage, cucumbers, melons and nuts are common causes. Flatulence is also sometimes an indication of the presence of gall-stones.

As a rule half a teaspoonful of bicarbonate of soda in a cup of warm water will relieve the immediate symptoms.

fleas. Wingless, blood-sucking insects that live as parasites on man and other animals. They have powerful back legs which enable them to jump several feet to a new host, carrying disease from the infected person or animal previously bitten to the one on whom they next alight.

There are several hundred varieties of fleas. The common man-inhabiting flea, *Pulex irritans,* causes unpleasant and itching bites but has seldom been incriminated in the spread of serious diseases although the possibility must be recognized. The rat flea, *Xenopsylla cheopis,* can feed on man as well as on rats and is the means of transmission of the bacterium of plague from rat to rat, from rat to man and from man to man.

A partially developed flea can lie dormant in dust for several months.

Measures of control include strict cleanliness in the home, the use of DDT and other insecticides in infested houses, suppression of rats and vermin by known methods of destruction, special attention to destruction of rats on ships arriving from infected ports and rat-proofing of ships so that rats cannot board them. In any area deemed to be at risk from plague, examination of the corpses of dead rats is useful, because plague in rats tends to occur before plague in human beings.

flexion. The movement of bending a joint.

flies. This is a general term for two-winged insects with jaws adapted for piercing and sucking. Some well known varieties are the house-fly (*Musca domestica*), the tsetse fly (transmitter of sleeping sickness), mosquitoes (some of which transmit malaria and yellow fever), gnats, etc. In Britain, although gnats are abundant and some forms of mosquito exist, the insect usually implied by the term is *Musca domestica* which, unlike the majority of flies, is capable only of sucking, not piercing.

Despite its lack of biting capacity the house-fly is a dangerous pest, because it can pick up from the excrement and sputum of persons and

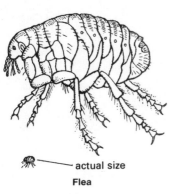

 ———— actual size

Flea

animals the bacilli of typhoid, dysentery, poliomyelitis, cholera and possibly tuberculosis. It carries the organisms on its hairy legs and abdomen and in its alimentary canal and infects food on which it lands or on which it feeds.

Flies breed in all forms of refuse and excreta so long as they are warm and moist. Much of the reduction of the fly population in recent decades has been due to the replacement of middens by proper sewerage systems. Measures for fly control include the treating of manure heaps with suitable disinfectants such as strong solutions of borax, the keeping of all refuse in closely covered bins, the killing of adult flies with DDT (although DDT-resistant flies are now appearing), the use of other insecticides, and the covering of all food – especially food that will not subsequently be cooked – to prevent contamination.

floating kidney. A condition, sometimes related to rapid loss of abdominal fat, in which (as in MOVEABLE KIDNEY) there is an abnormal amount of mobility of the kidney. Usually there are no symptoms and the condition is discovered by accident, but if the mobility is such as to cause kinking of the duct connecting the kidney and the bladder (the ureter) there may be bouts of severe pain. Apart from that possibility, the condition is often blamed for vague abdominal discomfort and persistent indigestion. Abdominal massage and the wearing of a suitable belt may help.

floating ribs. The ribs are long curved bones springing from the spine and sweeping round to be attached to the breast bone, or sternum, in front. However, the two lowest ribs on each side are not attached to the sternum and are therefore sometimes described as 'floating'. An interesting but unimportant developmental abnormality is that in a small minority of persons these ribs are in fact attached to the sternum, so that these individuals have no floating ribs.

flooding. Excessive bleeding during menstruation. The technical term is menorrhagia. Since the blood loss varies appreciably from woman to woman, flooding is best defined as appreciably greater loss than the particular woman normally has. Common causes include anaemia, raised blood pressure, ovarian cysts or tumours, hormonal disorders and severe anxiety. Flooding also sometimes occurs in the periods immediately before the menopause. Treatment varies according to the cause but in general serious flooding warrants medical investigation. See also METORRHAGIA.

fluke worm. Flat, bilaterally symmetrical worms with a very complicated developmental history. The schistosomes are mentioned elsewhere: see BILHARZIASIS. Another parasitic variety, the liver fluke, is here briefly described. It is a leaf-shaped worm, about 2.5 cm. (1 in.) long and roughly half as wide. The fluke lives in the bile ducts of a sheep and causes the serious and usually fatal disease of liver rot. The eggs, passed out with the excreta of the sheep, develop in damp spots into free-swimming, conical shaped miracidia. If these reach an available water snail they enter its tissues and

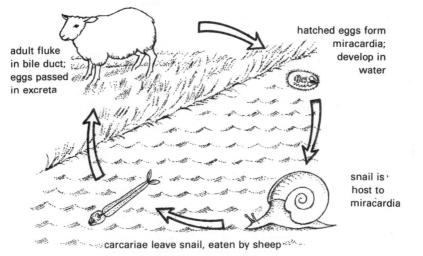

adult fluke in bile duct; eggs passed in excreta

hatched eggs form miracardia; develop in water

snail is host to miracardia

carcariae leave snail, eaten by sheep

Life cycle of the fluke worm

develop there, ultimately becoming cercariae which leave the snail, settle on blades of grass, and may be eaten by a sheep or occasionally by man. The clinical features of infection in the human are rather vague – high temperature, impaired appetite, abdominal pain and loss of weight. Diagnosis can be confirmed by a blood test. Many drugs are tried, but emetine hydrochloride probably gives the best results.

fluoridation of water. Artificial addition of fluoride to water supplies which show a deficiency of this mineral.

The fluoride content of water varies from about 0.1 parts per million to over 6 p.p.m. Prolonged studies of communities drinking water naturally high or low in fluoride (including 903 separate high fluoride communities in the U.S.A. alone) have shown several features.

1. The incidence of tooth decay decreases steadily as the fluoride level rises up to about 1 part per million; broadly the amount of dental decay in persons normally drinking water of 1 p.p.m. or above is only a shade over half of the amount in persons drinking water with less than 0.6 p.p.m.

2. There is no further decrease in tooth decay where the fluoride content is above 1 p.p.m.

3. Concentrations of above 5 p.p.m. produce harmless mottling of the enamel of teeth – dental fluorosis.

4. No toxic effects (e.g., on bones or arteries) have been demonstrated where the fluoride level is below 5 p.p.m. In particular analysis of deaths and diseases in communities drinking water of high and low fluoride content provides no shadow of evidence that consumption of water of high fluoride content (i.e., 1 to 5 p.p.m.) improves health except dental health and no shadow of evidence that consumption of water of low fluoride content has any effect except on dental health.

Virtually all dentists, doctors, health visitors, nurses and other health workers agree that a concentration of up to 1 p.p.m. (or perhaps a shade lower in tropical climates where more water is drunk) is beneficial to dental health, that higher concentrations confer no proved benefit, and that the kidney can deal adequately with concentrations up to at least 5 p.p.m.

For over thirty years artificial rectification of fluoride deficiency has been a controversial and emotive subject. Fluoride up to the desired limit, usually 1 p.p.m., can be added very simply and with absolute guarantees against over-dosage. Advocates of artificial fluoridation point out (1) that the taste of the water is so little altered that few if any people can tell whether they are drinking rectified or deficient water; (2) that the cost of rectification is trivial by comparison with the saving on dental treatment; (3) that fluoridation reduces the emotional and physical trauma of toothache and of dental treatment; (4) that artificial fluoridation has been adopted in many communities (e.g., in more than two-thirds of the major cities of the U.S.A.) , with absolutely no evidence of any harmful effects on the health of the people; (5) that claims that fluoridation is dangerous or harmful have been supported neither by scientific evidence nor by courts of law; (6) that opponents of fluoridation frequently shift their ground, arguing today that it causes one effect and tomorrow that it causes a completely different effect; and (7) that the professions with expertise in health matters are overwhelmingly in favour of fluoridation.

Opponents of fluoridation have perhaps lost the part of their battle relating to danger: it is difficult to maintain that fluoridation is dangerous when, without evidence of damage of health, many communities have drunk water naturally high in fluoride for centuries and other communities have consumed artificially fluoridated water for three decades. The opponents contend, with more effect, that artificial addition of fluoride is mass medication and a dangerous precedent which might be followed by the addition of other drugs, that it is wrong that adults with dentures or already damaged teeth should be forced to consume a substance that will do them no good, and that there are other methods – fluoride rinses, fluoride tablets and fluoride toothpastes – available for those who would benefit from extra fluoride.

In general topical applications, fluoride tablets, etc., are much less effective, although undoubtedly of some value, and very much more costly. Perhaps we have to come back to a basic question: are pre-school children, school pupils, adolescents and young adults who live in an area with water deficient in fluoride to endure the pain and discomfort of preventable tooth decay, and is the community to pay directly or indirectly for much treatment that would otherwise have been needless, or are the middle-aged and elderly to submit to drinking water to which there has been added a substance that will in no way benefit them?

There is, however, another point which may influence that question. In recent years there has been growing evidence of the association between soft water and high incidence of certain diseases of the heart. There is no suggestion that deficiency of fluoride is a factor, but if in due course we have to add perhaps calcium or magnesium to soft water for the benefit of the middle-aged and elderly, it will become increasingly difficult to resist the addition of fluoride for the benefit of the young.

fluorine. A chemical with many properties resembling those of chlorine, required in the human body as an ingredient of bones and teeth, present in many substances (e.g. fish, tea and beer) in small quantities and present to a varying extent in all natural water supplies. It occurs mostly in the form of its sodium and potassium salts (fluorides), and, like many other substances essential in small quantities for life, is toxic if taken in large doses.

flushing. See BLUSHING.

foetus. The term is sometimes used non-specifically for the unborn offspring of mammals while in the mother's uterus, i.e., from conception to birth. Many writers, however, try to differentiate the embryo and the foetus. Where such distinction is made, the embryo is the early developing mass of cells, from the union of ovum and sperm up to the stage where the developing creature is recognizably human in form; and the foetus is the unborn child from the age of about 8 weeks.

At 8 weeks the human foetus is about 4 cm. long, the head is proportionately very large, the limbs are perceptible and the heart is pumping

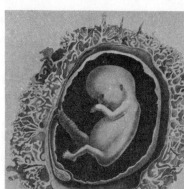

blood through the body and out to the placenta. Growth is fairly slow at first. By 16 weeks the foetus is about 10 cm. long and weighs 100 g. By 24 weeks it is about 20 cm., weighs around 650 g. and has a faint chance of survival if then born. At 28 weeks it is considered viable under English law, although a child born at this stage is dangerously premature and can survive only with very expert nursing. Most of the intra-uterine increase in weight occurs during the last ten weeks of pregnancy.

folic acid. A VITAMIN of the B group, found in liver, milk, spinach, yeast and various other foodstuffs. Deficiency causes the formerly fatal disease of PERNICIOUS ANAEMIA.

folie à deux. A curious condition in which a person, usually suffering from paranoid delusions of persecution or injustice, persuades a wife, sister or other closely associated person of the justice of the complaints, so that the second person comes to have the same delusions. If the two persons can be separated for any appreciable time, the person who has been 'infected' usually recovers completely.

fomentations. See POULTICES.

fomites. A term used to designate articles of clothing, bedding, toys, food utensils and so forth which have been in contact with a person suffering from an infectious disease and are therefore liable to spread the disease. See DISINFECTION.

fontanelles. Soft areas on a baby's head where the skull bones have not yet fused. In the new-born baby there are normally six fontanelles. Of these the largest, the anterior fontanelle, is a diamond-shaped aperture on the top of the head, about 2.5 cm. in diameter, and normally remaining unclosed until about 15 to 20

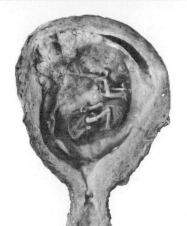

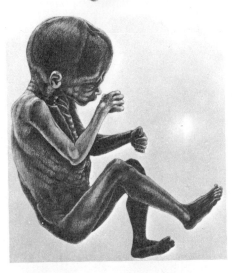

Foetus at 8 weeks, 12 weeks and 28 weeks

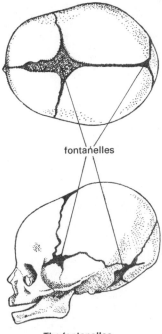

fontanelles

The fontanelles

months. The second largest, the posterior fontanelle, nearer the back of the head, normally closes before 12 months, as do the others which are situated at the temples and behind the ears.

The presence of these soft areas makes obvious the importance of protecting a baby's head from injury.

Continued presence of an unclosed fontanelle after the age of 24 months is suggestive either of rickets or of some other state of defective development.

food. The term is sometimes used for solid nourishment as differentiated from drink, but is normally employed for anything – solid or liquid – of nutritional value and passing into the digestive system.

Food is essential for various reasons. Firstly, the average adult at complete rest requires about 1,000 Calories a day for basal metabolism, i.e., to balance the energy used by the body in maintaining warmth, keeping the heart beating and lungs breathing, and so on. Secondly, additional food is needed to balance the energy used in all forms of activity – the amount of such energy varying from about 40 Calories per hour when relaxing about the house to as much as 600 an hour when engaged in very strenuous athletic activity. Thirdly, food, and in particular protein, is needed for growth and for repair of worn tissues: hence a growing child needs proportionately more food than an adult and an adolescent requires more Calories than an adult of the same size and sex engaged in the same activities.

The energy requirement is measured in Calories, one Calorie being the amount of heat needed to raise 1,000 g. of water through 1 °C. A gramme of protein or carbohydrate when completely absorbed and digested yields 4.1 Calories and a gramme of fat yields 9.3 Calories. Taking average sizes, a child of 2 years needs 1,300 Calories daily, a child of 5 years requires 1,700, a boy of 15 years needs about 2,800 and a girl of 15 about 2,300, a man of sedentary occupation requires about 2,500 and a woman of sedentary occupation about 2,100, while a man doing heavy manual work requires well over 3,000. Roughly, an adolescent needs 300 Calories a day more than an adult doing similar work, a pregnant woman needs an additional 200 and a woman breast-feeding her baby requires an additional 500.

The foods required by the body may be of animal or VEGETABLE origin; they are PROTEINS, FATS, CARBOHYDRATES, MINERAL SALTS and VITAMINS, together with WATER and ROUGHAGE. General insufficiency of food (MALNUTRITION), finally resulting in death from starvation, is rare in developed countries, although common enough in underdeveloped countries especially when crop failure creates famine conditions.

Proteins. The only foods containing absorbable nitrogen and sulphur, proteins are essential for replacement of worn out cells and tissues and in children for growth.

Fats. These are the most concentrated sources of energy and so are required in considerable amounts for very strenuous work and in very cold climates.

Carbohydrates. Sugars and starches are the most readily available sources of energy and therefore essential for children and others who use energy quickly. They are the body's main source of energy, they are required for the complete digestion of fat, and they are in general the cheapest forms of food.

Mineral salts. The body requires small but calculable amounts of various minerals, e.g., calcium, phosphorus, sodium, potassium, chlorine, sulphur and magnesium, and even smaller amounts of such minerals as iron, iodine, copper, cobalt, fluorine, manganese, selenium and zinc.

Vitamins. These are the 'trace substances', discovered during the last half century, essential for growth and health.

Water. Water is essential for the functioning of the body. About two-thirds of the body weight is water, and there is constant loss by respiration, perspiration and excretion. About two or three litres are required daily, the amount varying mainly with the external temperature.

Roughage. If the bowel is to excrete waste products it needs sufficient material on which to function. Most of the unabsorbed and apparently valueless food material, which is nevertheless essential for bowel action, comes from the cellulose of vegetables.

Food may be adequate enough when purchased but may be damaged by cooking: in particular the water-soluble vitamins may be removed or destroyed by cooking in water. The food, still adequate in Calories and in individual constituents, may be so cooked or so served as to be unattractive to the nose or the eye, so that, even if it is completely eaten, digestion is slowed down and the food is not fully utilized. Not least, food properly cooked and attractively served may be inadequate if there are factors interfering with chewing (e.g., lack of teeth) or interfering with the ingestion of the food (e.g., peptic ulcer or gastro-enteritis) or interfering with its absorption (e.g., diseases of the gall-bladder, liver or pancreas).

Fortification of food is the addition of necessary minerals and vitamins that have been removed by processing, or, in the case of synthetic foodstuffs, that are found in the naturally occurring substance for which the synthetic is a substitute. The major products so treated are flour (to which are added B vitamins, iron and calcium) and margarine (which is fortified by the addition of vitamins A and D).

The reverse process to fortification is adulteration of food in which the nutritive content of food products is diminished by their dilution, as can occur with milk, or the addition of cheaper, bulk-increasing substances, as can occur with flour.

In developed countries protein deficiency and vitamin deficiencies are rare and mineral deficiencies even rarer; the commonest error in the developed countries, and particularly in the affluent sections of the population, is carbohydrate excess, i.e., the creation of obesity from over-eating sugars and starches. It is also claimed by some experts that developed countries make wasteful use of food resources by feeding vegetables (mainly carbohydrate) to cattle and sheep for conversion into smaller quantities of protein; however, this claim is disputed by others who point out that much of the vegetable matter not converted by animals into protein returns to the soil as manure, and also that a hillside

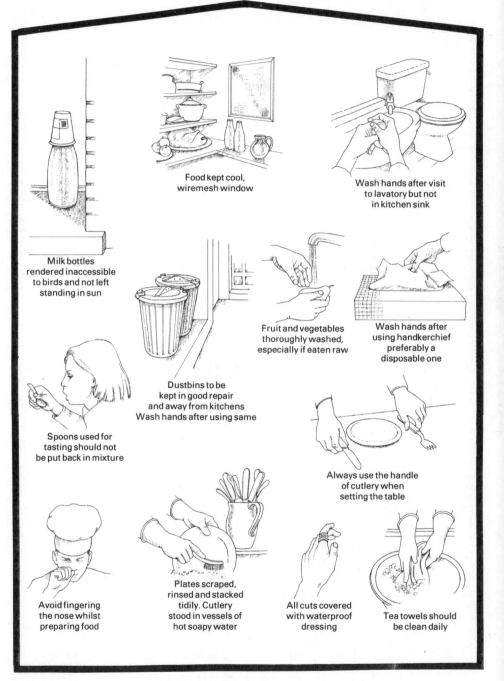

Milk bottles rendered inaccessible to birds and not left standing in sun

Food kept cool, wiremesh window

Wash hands after visit to lavatory but not in kitchen sink

Fruit and vegetables thoroughly washed, especially if eaten raw

Wash hands after using handkerchief preferably a disposable one

Dustbins to be kept in good repair and away from kitchens Wash hands after using same

Spoons used for tasting should not be put back in mixture

Always use the handle of cutlery when setting the table

Avoid fingering the nose whilst preparing food

Plates scraped, rinsed and stacked tidily. Cutlery stood in vessels of hot soapy water

All cuts covered with waterproof dressing

Tea towels should be clean daily

Prevention of food poisoning in the home

which will feed sheep or goats will not grow vegetables suitable for human use. See also DIET.

food legislation. A complex mosaic of laws, regulations and by-laws designed (1) to prevent adulteration of food; (2) to ensure that all food sold is of the substance, nature and quality demanded; and (3) to safeguard the cleanliness of food.

During the last century food adulteration was common: as late as 1875 in England one-fifth of food samples sent to public analysts were found to be adulterated. Crude adulteration (e.g., addition of water to milk or sand to brown sugar) has been stamped out by adequate sampling and sharp penalties, and is now almost unknown. What occasionally occurs nowadays is 'sophistication', i.e., artificial improvement of the appearance, colour, taste or keeping qualities by the addition of chemicals. An example is the addition of anti-oxidants to prevent fats from becoming rancid.

While sophistication is not necessarily entirely a bad thing, most developed countries restrict the use of preservatives and colouring agents to specified amounts of listed substances and also require that foods to which preservatives or colouring agents have been added shall be appropriately labelled.

Similarly most developed countries have elaborate regulations about the exact content of many foods. For instance, in the United Kingdom flour must contain 1.65 mg. iron and 0.24 mg. thiamine per 100 g., and milk must have not less than 3 per cent fat and 8.5 per cent milk solids other than fat.

For cleanliness and protection from bacteria the requirements at the 'wholesale' end are gradually approximating to the very strict regulations of the Scandinavian countries, e.g., in respect of examination of all meat at slaughterhouses, handling of fish in ports and conditions under which milk is produced. At the 'retail' end, however, despite the efforts of public health inspectors, Britain's hygienic standards for handled food tend to lag behind those of Scandinavia and of the most advanced of the states of the U.S.A., and in some countries of Southern Europe the standards are still rather primitive and elementary.

food poisoning. An acute illness characterized by vomiting, diarrhoea or both, and by pain in the abdomen; it is usually caused by eating food contaminated by bacteria.

The disease is notifiable in many countries but is probably much commoner than is indicated by notifications. Many mild cases clear up without the victim having consulted a doctor, and in some cases that come to medical notice the infecting organism cannot be found and the disease cannot be differentiated from other conditions causing diarrhoea and abdominal upset. Yet, taking England and Wales as an example, 6,910 cases were notified in a recent year and 48 of them died.

Food poisoning should always be suspected if several people who have eaten the same food develop abdominal symptoms roughly simultaneously. In the most frequent type, poisoning by bacteria of the salmonella group, symptoms begin between twelve and thirty-six hours after eating the contaminated food, the time period varying with the number of organisms swallowed, the general health of the person and several other factors. In poisoning by staphylococci the symptoms begin between one and six hours later, and in the rare but serious botulism they appear in twelve to twenty-four hours.

Treatment includes rest in bed, abundant water or fruit juice to drink (to prevent dehydration) and in severe cases an appropriate antibiotic. If any of the suspected food remains available portions of it should be sent to a bacteriological laboratory to try to establish the source and to save other people from becoming infected.

Bacterial food poisoning occurs in three main ways. (1) The bacteria or their toxins may be present in the animals or fowls which are subsequently served as meat or poultry products. (2) Cooked food may be contaminated by bacteria on the hands, cloths or utensils. (3) If food is kept warm for a long time after cooking, a few bacteria that have survived cooking or that have reached the food subsequently have time to multiply.

The hygiene of livestock, poultry and abattoirs is beyond the scope of this book, but much food poisoning could be prevented by scrupulous personal hygiene by all food handlers (e.g., thorough hand-washing after using the lavatory or blowing the nose), cooking food thoroughly (remembering that the temperature should be high enough to kill organisms in the middle of the joint or bird – frozen chickens should always be thawed out for twenty-four hours before cooking) and storing uneaten cooked food under conditions both of coolness and cleanness.

Non-bacterial food poisoning can occur from the eating of poisonous fruits or berries, or from the eating of unwashed fruit recently sprayed with poisonous pesticides.

food preservation. See PRESERVATION OF FOOD.

food values. The approximate or exact dietetic values of measured amounts of different foods.

Fifty years ago, when values were considered essentially in terms of Calories, protein, fat and carbohydrate, the construction of tables of food values was relatively easy, and many books published around 1930 contained such tables. Increased knowledge of trace elements and of their measurement, the discovery of the various vitamins and the evolution of methods of estimating these vitamins quantitatively have enormously complicated the whole question of food values.

Where a table of half a century ago would contain four columns for a particular food, with perhaps a fifth column for remarks about trace elements, the tables of today are highly complicated. Here are four examples: (1) A breakfast cup of milk contains 165 Calories, 9 g. of protein, 9 g. of fat, 12 g. of carbohydrate, 288 mg. of calcium, 0.2 mg. of iron, 390 international units of vitamin A, 0.09 mg. of thiamine and 3 mg. of ascorbic acid. (2) A piece of cheddar cheese weighing 30 g. (about 1 oz.) contains 115 Calories, 7 g. of protein, 9 g. of fat, 200 mg. of calcium, 0.3 mg. of iron, 400 international units of vitamin A and 0.01 mg. of thiamine. (3) An average hen's egg contains 75 Calories, 6 g. each of protein and fat, 26 mg. of calcium, 1.3 mg. of iron, 550 international units of vitamin A and 0.05 mg. of thiamine. (4) A boiled potato of 6 cm. (2½ inches) diameter yields 105 Calories, 3 g. of protein, 24 g. of carbohydrate, 14 mg. of calcium, 0.9 mg. of

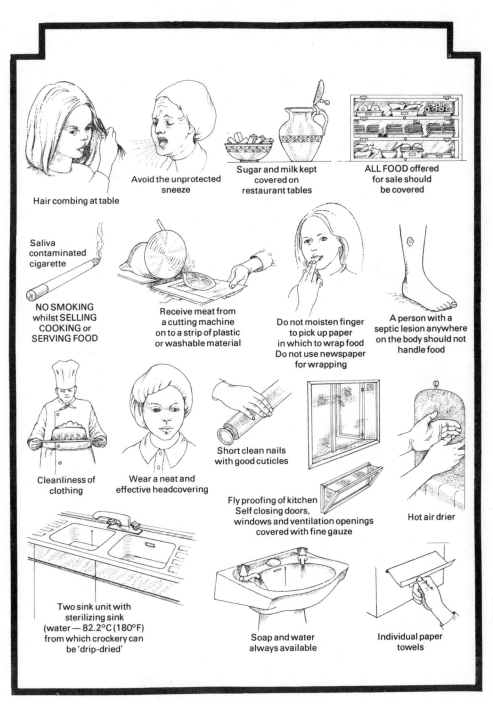

Hair combing at table

Avoid the unprotected sneeze

Sugar and milk kept covered on restaurant tables

ALL FOOD offered for sale should be covered

Saliva contaminated cigarette

NO SMOKING whilst SELLING COOKING or SERVING FOOD

Receive meat from a cutting machine on to a strip of plastic or washable material

Do not moisten finger to pick up paper in which to wrap food Do not use newspaper for wrapping

A person with a septic lesion anywhere on the body should not handle food

Cleanliness of clothing

Wear a neat and effective headcovering

Short clean nails with good cuticles

Fly proofing of kitchen Self closing doors, windows and ventilation openings covered with fine gauze

Hot air drier

Two sink unit with sterilizing sink (water — 82.2°C (180°F) from which crockery can be 'drip-dried'

Soap and water always available

Individual paper towels

Prevention of food poisoning in a restaurant

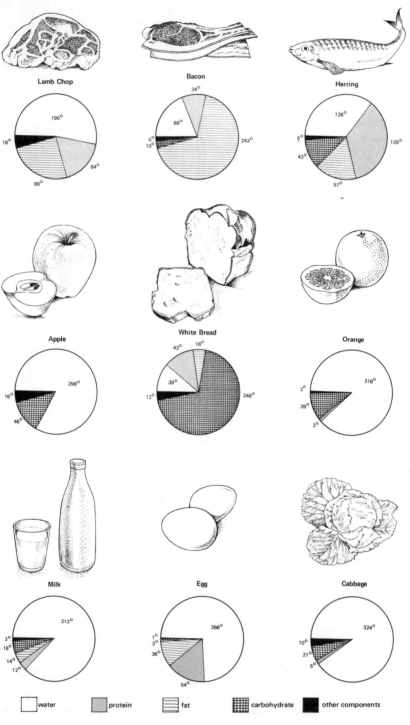

Lamb Chop

Bacon

Herring

Apple

White Bread

Orange

Milk

Egg

Cabbage

water protein fat carbohydrate other components

Food values

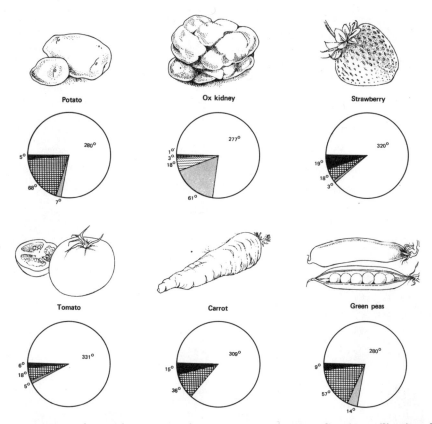

Potato   Ox kidney   Strawberry

Tomato   Carrot   Green peas

iron, 20 international units of vitamin A and 17 mg. of vitamin C. In these four examples vitamins and trace elements present in very minute quantities have been omitted for simplicity.

As set down the examples look highly scientific, but in reality they vary with (1) domestic measures – breakfast cups are not uniform, (2) size of individual food articles – an egg may be larger or smaller than average, and measuring the diameter of every potato would be a weary task, (3) growth conditions – not all potatoes contain exactly the same proportion of calcium, or of vitamin A, (4) conditions before use – the milk may lose part of its vitamin C through sitting in bright sunlight, and (5) cooking – some of the vitamin C in the potato may be destroyed.

Tables of food values are therefore highly complicated. They are very useful to nutritionists and dieticians and sometimes useful to doctors and health visitors; but they have become too complex and subject to too many modifications to be useful to most members of the public.

foot. The portion of the lower limb situated below the ankle-joint. The foot consists of twenty-six bones forming a series of arches and some thirty-three joints, bound together by many strong ligaments. From back to the front of the foot the bones can be considered in three groups: (1) the seven tarsal bones, strong and compact, and so jointed that the foot can be

rotated in any direction; (2) the five metatarsals, long bones running between the tarsals and the phalanges or toe-bones; and (3) the fourteen phalanges, two for the great toe and three for each of the other toes.

The foot is arched longwise so that in standing only the outer edge touches the ground, and in walking the weight is normally taken partly by this weight-bearing arch and partly by the ball of the great toe. There is also a second arch running crosswise at the ball of the foot.

Strain of the foot with pain and ultimate deformity may arise from badly fitting shoes with insufficient room for the toes or with inability for the foot to alter shape as the weight of the body shifts. Other causes include overweight and persistently bad posture.

Since the foot bears the entire weight of the body and of any additional burden carried, e.g., twenty stone in the case of a twelve stone man carrying a sack with a hundredweight of coal, diseases and disabilities are not uncommon. See CLAWFOOT, CLUBFOOT, CORNS, FLAT FOOT, GOUT.

footwear. A general term for boots, shoes, sandals, slippers, etc.

In Britain fully 50 per cent of persons over middle age have foot trouble, traceable in the main to badly fitting footwear, and backache and other disturbances can also frequently be a result of foot trouble. All too often shoes are bought as articles of fashion without any consideration of their ultimate effect on the user's feet.

Firstly, new shoes should feel comfortable: if uncomfortable at the beginning they are likely to become more – not less – uncomfortable as time passes. Secondly, since there is much free movement from the ball of the foot forwards, the front part of the shoe should not only allow each toe to lie perfectly straight without side pressure but should permit some movement of the toes. Thirdly, since there is little movement behind the ball of the foot, there should be a reasonably close fit in this part. Fourthly, there should be a cut-in at the back to fix the shoe in position. Fifthly, high heels create an excessive incline from the heel to the ball and so force the toes forwards, restricting their movement; they also may cause weakening (through disuse) of the muscles at the back of the leg, and are, therefore, to be avoided.

Feet vary greatly and footwear – especially for children – should be chosen with care and with adequate time for trial of different types. Sufficient attention to boots and shoes in the first thirty years of life can save much discomfort and disability in middle and old age.

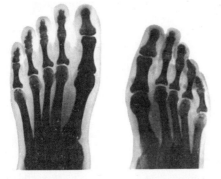

Footwear: the two feet of the same person, the left one in a well-fitting shoe and the right one crowded into a shoe that is too small

foreign body. Any substance which penetrates an individual's body, either through an opening such as the mouth, or through the skin. A particle of dust in the eye is a foreign body and so is mud in a cut. There is usually a defensive process put into action to counteract the presence of a foreign body – in the two examples given the eye 'weeps' to wash out the dust and the white blood cells gather to engulf the bacteria in the mud.

forensic medicine. The branch of medicine concerned with the law, the proper application of justice and medico-legal problems.

Where the clinical expert looks at a wound, fracture, injury or case of poisoning and asks himself, 'How best can I treat it?', and where the community physician asks himself 'How can I aim to reduce the likelihood of a similar occurrence?', the forensic expert asks himself exactly how and when it occurred and whether it was the result of accident, self-inflicted injury or external violence.

That medical skill could contribute to the evenness of justice was recognized in France and Germany in the eighteenth century; the first chair in forensic medicine in Britain was established at Edinburgh University in 1806 and within the next sixty years the subject became everywhere an established part of the medical curriculum.

Inevitably much of forensic medicine is unspectacular – involving, for example, knowledge of the laws relating to the granting of death certificates and of the laws regulating the sale of poisons. However, a couple of examples may demonstrate a more dramatic role:

1. A youth complains that he has today been cruelly beaten with a whip. An examination of the bruises reveals that they are two days old and were caused by a non-pliable object such as a stick. Clearly his accusation is false.

2. A man has been shot. Estimation of the cooling of the body suggests that death occurred between 10 p.m. and midnight; examination of the stomach contents and their extent of digestion indicates that he died about four hours after a meal known to have been eaten at 7 p.m.; a blood stain at the broken window, where the assassin inadvertently damaged his finger, proves to be of group AB rhesus positive; and the bullet is from a .25 revolver with identifiable characteristics as shown by marks on the bullet. Clearly these various points enormously assist the police in their task.

Problems of identification, post-mortem changes, the examination of blood and hair, differentiation of accident and suicide and murder, identification of types of wound, and medico-legal aspects of insanity are subjects that fall within the scope of forensic medicine.

There is really no difference between forensic medicine and medical jurisprudence, but the former term is normally used when doctors or medical students are studying law as it impinges on medicine, whereas medical jurisprudence is generally employed when lawyers or law students are studying medicine as it impinges on law.

foreskin. The prepuce, a fold of skin covering the head of the penis. It can normally be retracted. Tightness of the foreskin (phimosis) is a not uncommon inherited condition, leading in extreme cases to difficulty in passing urine, and sometimes to bed-wetting and to inflammation of the skin lining the head of the penis. Slight degrees of phimosis often respond to artificial retraction and in due course disappear, but failure to respond should be followed by the very trivial operation of circumcision. This operation is sometimes performed for religious – quite apart from medical – reasons.

forgetfulness. Although often used as a synonym for AMNESIA, forgetfulness normally implies difficulty in recalling a few inter-related associations whereas amnesia implies the blocking off of a large number of these associations. Returning from a wedding I find that I cannot describe the bride's dress while my wife cannot remember a joke made at the reception: these are examples of normal forgetfulness. On the way home I sustain a head injury and cannot recall the entire wedding: that is amnesia, in this particular case retrograde amnesia.

Some forgetfulness of past events and experiences is essential if memory of the past is to serve as a guide in the present. We must be able to select important or relevant happenings for recall without being cluttered by unimportant and irrelevant details: we must be able to remember that a no. 24 bus will take us to our friend's new house without also recollecting that the number of the bus ticket was A 41258.

In the elderly it is common to have an impaired memory for recent events, as compared with clearer recollection of significant earlier events; this is probably explicable by the events being less vigorously noted – because of thickened arteries or cerebral anaemia or simply because as life experience extends fewer current events seem important.

Forgetfulness is in considerable part a defence mechanism: we forget the disagreeable appointment scheduled for today or we repress from our conscious memory the unpleasant experience of last month. Freud considers that most forgetfulness is the result of such unconscious repression, and points out that repressed memories reach consciousness in distorted forms, e.g., in dreams and in slips of the tongue. Some forgetfulness, however, is explicable simply in terms of lack of interest: in the example in the first paragraph I would probably have remembered the bride's dress if I had expected to be asked about it, but my mind dismissed it as being of no long-term interest to me. A child, fired by his teacher's enthusiasm, remembers the causes of a historical event; his neighbour, bored and uninterested, forgets them in an hour.

A good or bad memory is in large part innate. No amount of training is likely to give most of us the memory of a Napoleon or a Macaulay. To some extent, however, forgetfulness can be decreased in several ways. (1) By conscious or subconscious realization that a particular experience is important to us: a lawyer will develop a remarkable ability to recall legal precedents while remaining unable to recollect the names of the flowers in his garden. (2) By forming connecting links with information already in the mind: because Mendel's genetic experiments were ignored until long after his death I had difficulty in 'placing' him chronologically until I appreciated – by chance – that he was born in the same year as Pasteur (1822). (3) By mechanical methods: e.g., tying a knot in a handkerchief as a reminder of an engagement or deliberately repeating a name several times to impress it on the memory. (4) As a very temporary measure, by the use of artificial linkages, such as mnemonics – useful where the information is required for only a few weeks but of little use for the permanent retention of information.

fracture. A break in a bone. Fractures may be caused by direct violence, as when the skull is fractured by a blow on the head; by indirect violence, as when a fall on the outstretched hand causes a fracture of the wrist; and occasionally by muscular action, as when sudden spasm of the thigh muscles causes fracture of the patella. In old people a spontaneous fracture may very occasionally occur without injury: in such a case the person does not 'fall and break his leg' but rather 'breaks his leg and therefore falls'.

A simple fracture has no external wound communicating with the surface. A compound fracture has such a wound. A simple or compound fracture may be complete (dividing the bone into two parts) or incomplete, common in children (where the break does not extend right across the bone); and it may be comminuted, where the bone is broken into several pieces, or impacted, where one end of a broken bone is driven into the other.

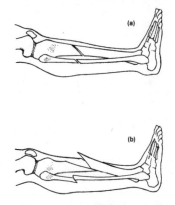

Diagram of (a) a simple fracture, and (b) a compound fracture of the leg

There is pain and tenderness near the site of the fracture, loss of movement in the limb or unnatural mobility, deformity (i.e., alteration of the shape and outline of the fractured bone), shortening of the affected limb, and crepitus (i.e., a grating sound when the broken parts rub together).

Whatever the type of fracture it is likely to require an x-ray to determine the exact nature of the break and amount of displacement, careful manipulation by a doctor to place the broken bones in complete alignment, and splinting in the position of best alignment.

Where a fracture is suspected or diagnosed the immediate aims should be to prevent further damage, to reduce pain, to guard against shock and to secure prompt medical attention. In general the victim should not be moved unless he is in a position of danger, and if he has to be moved a splint – e.g., an umbrella, walking stick or board covered with any available soft material – should be placed from above the joint above to below the joint below the fracture and tied with bandages or slings to reduce movement.

fraternal twins. See TWINS.

freckles. Localized deposits of brownish colouring matter in the superficial layers of the skin, arising after exposure to the sun's rays. Freckles are peculiar to northern races and found particularly in persons with fair or red hair. They can be regarded as nature's attempt to provide a sunshade for the tissues underneath.

Freckles are harmless and in general not unattractive, but where prevention is desired it involves the wearing of broad-brimmed hats and the use of sun-screening creams. Where existing freckles are deemed disfiguring they can be very slowly modified by the use of various soothing lotions and by avoidance of exposure to the sun. Attempts to remove freckles by peeling agents are dangerous, may cause dermatitis, and should be deprecated.

fresh air. Everybody 'knows' that fresh air is important to health.

Air is drawn into the lungs and expelled from them about seventeen times a minute, and the blood takes up oxygen from the air and discharges carbon dioxide into it.

It used to be thought that the ill-effects of air that was not fresh were mainly due to insufficient oxygen or excessive carbon dioxide, but even if ventilation is very limited the air provides enough oxygen for breathing and does not accumulate enough carbon dioxide to be harmful. The oxygen content at high altitudes is appreciably less than in stuffy rooms, yet people soon become accustomed to high altitudes. Carbon dioxide is harmless up to a concentration of about 5 per cent in the atmosphere, whereas the content in a very stuffy room is usually a fraction of 1 per cent.

Air movement is particularly important. The air that surrounds the body becomes warm, moist and incapable of soaking up more water vapour. Hence, if the air is stagnant, the body cannot lose water vapour, from breath or from perspiration. Thus in the Black Hole of Calcutta, where 146 persons were confined overnight in a room of 18 by 14 by 10 feet, and 123 died, the two small windows were sufficient to supply all the oxygen needed and to remove the excess of carbon dioxide. The deaths occurred as a result of stagnation of air, high temperature and high humidity.

Sunshine in moderation is beneficial, as is exercise which is most easily taken in the open air; but for the adequate ventilation of rooms we have to consider mainly the creation of air movement to a degree sufficient to keep the air moving and to remove unpleasant odours without creating a draught. We also have to consider the achieving and maintaining of a comfortable temperature. These things are important, rather than the freshness of the air. At a temperature of 65 °F. an air current of 2 feet per second produces a comfortable flow of air while a velocity of over 3 feet per second creates an uncomfortable draught.

The nineteenth century vogue for fresh air – as opposed to sufficient air exchange to keep down the humidity and avoid the accumulation of unpleasant odours – was fundamentally based on misconceptions.

Freud. Sigmund Freud (1856-1939) was the founder of psycho-analysis and is perhaps the most outstanding figure in the entire history of psychology and psychiatry.

He is often described as the discoverer of the unconscious, but he made no such claim; Schopenhauer and Hartmann had suggested the existence of unconscious mental activity about the time Freud was born. What Freud did was essentially to explore the hitherto unknown territory of the unconscious, to indicate the strength and complexity of unconscious motivation, to devise methods of investigating the unconscious, and to cure neurotic and some other disorders by bringing their causes to the surface.

A physician and a distinguished neurologist before he became interested in psychology, Freud started with cases of neuroses, and found that – first under hypnosis and later by using techniques of free association – patients could be gradually led to bring to consciousness long forgotten experiences which were responsible for their present illnesses. The method worked. It rendered the psychoneuroses curable.

Even more importantly, it led Freud to a concept of unconscious motivation. Essentially he divided the mind into the superego (which has analogies with conscience), the ego (or conscious mind, including things of which we are at present conscious and things that can easily be brought to consciousness), and the id (the vast unconscious portion in which lie many forgotten experiences and repressed desires which motivate many of our actions). A mechanism which he termed the censor prevents the appearance in the ego of ideas and desires incompatible with a person's general ethical and other codes of what is acceptable; but the ideas and desires emerge in distorted or hidden form – as symbols or substitutes, as trivial accidents or 'slips of the tongue' and in dreams – and they constitute the motivation for many of a person's actions.

Because Freud used 'sex' in a very wide sense, including virtually the whole of our desires for pleasure and affection, and regarded it as the mainspring of human behaviour, his views throughout most of his life were regarded as highly controversial. Himself a highly moral man, he was accused of being a destroyer of moral values and of being obsessed with sex, and his ideas, such as those of a male child's love for his mother and jealousy of his father, were easily distorted by his adversaries. Indeed as late as 1963 two eminent British psychiatrists, while admitting his genius and penetrating insight, described him as 'the most controversial figure in the history of medical psychology'.

Time, however, has been on Freud's side. His discoveries of unconscious motivation and of methods of exploring the unconscious rank among the greatest of human achievements; and his work has rendered possible the successful treatment of psychoneurotic and psychosomatic diseases and also of the psychological element in many organic diseases. While no pioneer can hope to be completely accurate in the exploring and mapping of a vast and previously unknown territory, most modern psychiatrists accept something like 90 per cent of Freud's teaching as beyond dispute.

Friedreich's ataxia. A hereditary disease transmitted through either sex and characterized by progressive loss of co-ordinated movement as a result of degeneration of the nerve columns in the spine and cerebellum.

Awkwardness of gait and a tendency to stumble are early signs and often appear before the age of 6 years. As the disease progresses the gait becomes more irregular and clumsy, the patient walks with feet wide apart, and he begins to reel from side to side when walking. Later similar lack of co-ordination appears in arm movements. The disease, while progressive, does not appreciably shorten life. There is as yet no specific treatment.

frigidity. Inability to derive pleasure from sexual intercourse, commoner in women than in men. It may arise through both partners being ignorant of sexual matters, as where the husband reaches his climax too hurriedly and with insufficient preliminary sex-play, leaving the wife unsatisfied and coming to regard intercourse with distaste. Perhaps more often it has its origin in conscious or unconscious faulty attitudes to sex: because of inadequate or erroneous sex education intercourse is associated with ideas of sins, dirtiness or fear. Again, it may be due to a physical cause which renders intercourse painful, or to sheer fatigue.

In general there is a difference between the attitudes of the sexes: the woman is more affected by 'atmosphere' in sex relations and needs to be brought gradually to the stage where she desires intercourse; whereas the man has a more physical and more rapid desire. Given mutual love and respect, and a willingness to learn sex manners, many couples can themselves overcome frigidity. If they fail, they should first seek medical help lest there is any physical cause, and in the absence of a physical cause should seek the aid of a psychotherapist. Psychotherapy is usually needed if the woman has a persisting view of sex as sinful or dirty.

A marriage in which one partner has normal sexual desires and the other is frigid is unlikely to be successful. So it is important that a couple in these circumstances should study sex manners and should, if necessary, seek medical and psychiatric aid.

fringe medicine. Systems of treatment that fall outside the scope of orthodox medicine. Examples are ACUPUNCTURE, chiropraxis, HOMEOPATHY, naturopathy and OSTEOPATHY.

Acupuncture, discussed in a separate article, has not achieved success in Europe or America despite considerable success in China. Chiropraxis, or manipulation of bones, has considerable prestige in the U.S.A. where there are 25,000 practising chiropractors, but is almost unknown in Britain. Homeopathy, treatment by minute doses of drugs, appears to be in a phase of decline in most countries. Naturopathy, or treatment by diet, seems to vary enormously with individual practitioners – from a vegetarian diet to the use only of foods grown without the aid of fertilizers. Osteopathy, treatment – like chiropraxis – by manipulation of bones, is the most popular form of fringe medicine in Britain (there is a school for osteopaths in London, although only a fraction of all practising osteopaths have attended that school), and osteopaths appear to have abandoned the idea that they can treat all diseases and have begun to concentrate on diseases and disorders of bones, joints and muscles.

It is unlikely that any system of treatment for which thousands of persons are willing to pay has absolutely no merits. The marked hostility of the medical profession to the various forms of fringe medicine is based on three main points:

1. Very few homeopaths, naturopaths, etc. have had any long, rigorous training with periodical examinations, practical and theoretical. A qualified doctor can use any form of treatment, including fringe methods, but doctors – after lengthy study of anatomy, physiology and pathology – object to diagnosis and treatment being undertaken by people who have had much less training or no training at all.

2. Orthodox practitioners maintain that the causes of diseases are numerous and that no one form of treatment (e.g., exercises, diet, drugs or surgical operation) will suffice for a mass of entirely different diseases. They allege that practitioners of fringe medicine seem willing to treat almost any disease by the one method.

3. Orthodox doctors claim that the results of new treatments attempted by them are subjected to rigorous scientific testing, including, for example, the 'double-blind' method. In this system patients matched for age and sex are respectively given the old or the new drug, while the doctor responsible for assessing the patients' progress is left unaware of which drug was given to any one patient; treatments by practitioners of fringe medicine, they say, are not subjected to any such rigorous testing.

On the other hand, persons who have not been cured by orthodox medicine often visit chiropractors, homeopaths or osteopaths, and some of them are cured or improved. Fringe practitioners would claim that they are getting the 'difficult' cases, the 'simple' one having been cured by orthodox doctors. Traditional physicians while not denying that fringe practitioners tend to get their own failures suggest that a good proportion of illnesses are psychological in origin, and that the cure or alleviation depends more on the confidence inspired by the fringe practitioner than on the method of treatment employed. In response, the unorthodox worker would doubtless ask why – if the inspiring of confidence is all that is needed – it should be regarded as their monopoly: why should the orthodox doctor, presumably no less capable of inspiring confidence, attribute his cures to method (not confidence) but attribute the cures of some of his failures to confidence (not method)?

frontal sinuses. Two air cavities in the frontal bone of the skull, situated above the eyes and connected with the nose. They may become infected from the nose, causing headache and a feeling of fullness. Occasionally pus may form in them, sometimes necessitating an operation for its removal.

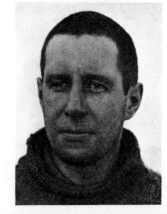

Frostbite: Captain Oates, one of the members of Scott's Antarctic Expedition which reached the South Pole on January 17th, 1912. Rendered lame by frostbite on the return journey, he deliberately walked out into the blizzard to die rather than delay his companions and reduce their chance of survival

frostbite. Injury to the skin and underlying tissues through exposure to intense cold and consequent constriction of peripheral blood vessels.

Frostbite arises most commonly in the toes, fingers, ears and nose. The affected part becomes dead white and hard. On recovery it can become painfully inflamed, with blisters which rupture, producing ulcers and sometimes even gangrene.

Prevention is largely by taking adequate precautions, including the wearing of sufficient warm, suitable clothing (loose enough to allow free circulation of blood) and avoidance of exposure to cold in persons with poor circulation. It is important to remember in connection with prevention that frostbite is not related to the temperature (32 °F. or 0 °C.) at which water freezes; the colder the atmosphere the greater the risk of frostbite, but cases have occurred considerably above 32 °F.

Treatment involves very gentle warmth – in a comfortable room but not close to a fire or stove, and bathing of the affected parts with cold water. The old remedy of massaging with snow is now discredited: the rubbing is more likely to harm the tissues than to benefit them.

frozen shoulder. Pain and stiffness due to inflammation of the BURSA in the shoulder joint. Spontaneous recovery tends to occur in three or four months but can sometimes be hastened by injection of procaine (a local anaesthetic allied to cocaine) either alone or mixed with a hydrocortisone (a cortocosteroid).

fugue. A disturbance or restriction of consciousness, predominantly occurring in hysterical illness.

The patient continues to act in a purposeful manner but retains no conscious remembrance of having done so, and may disclaim any knowledge of his identity or whereabouts. A hysterical fugue with such amnesia, or loss of memory, represents a subconscious attempt to escape from some predicament. (The term derives from the Latin *fuga*, meaning 'flight'.)

See also AUTOMATISM and DOUBLE PERSONALITY.

fundus. The bottom of a structure from the Latin word for 'base'. The plural is fundi. Anatomically, the term mainly refers to the rounded part of a hollow organ furthest from its opening and it is most commonly used in relation to the uterus, bladder, and the upper portion of the stomach. The spherical rear part of the eyeball to which the retina is attached is known as the fundus oculi, and a dome of bone in the middle-ear which separates the jugular vein from the tympanic cavity is the fundus tympani.

fungus. A low form of vegetable life, of the botanical class thallophytes, distinguished mainly by absence of chlorophyl. Fungi are parasitic on living plants or animals. Yeast, moulds, mushrooms and toadstools are fungus growths. Acthinomycosis, ringworm, favus and asperillosis are fungus diseases affecting man.

Fungi are medically important in at least four ways: (1) certain toadstools are highly poisonous; (2) some moulds cause infection, just as bacteria do; (3) some fungi cause allergic reactions; (4) some are highly important for the obtaining of drugs, e.g., yeast (essential for production of alcohol) is an excellent source of the B vitamins, and moulds are the source of pencillin and other antibiotics.

'funny bone'. In its path from the armpit to the wrist the ulnar nerve at the elbow lies close to the skin and also just over the swollen end of the humerus. So a very minor injury can temporarily compress the nerve between an external hard object and the bone, producing a tingling sensation popularly known as 'striking the funny bone', and of course giving rise to puns in consequence of the name of the bone passively involved.

furred tongue. A condition in which the tongue is covered by a whitish-brown layer consisting of cast-off surface cells, food debris and bacteria. Causes include constipation, digestive disorders and some fevers. The condition itself is of little significance.

furunculosis. The technical term for 'suffering from BOILS'.

G

gait. The way a person walks often gives a clue to his psychological make-up or current emotional state, e.g., depressed people tend to walk slowly with bowed head and bent shoulders, and elated people with vigorous and springing step. Yet many trivial causes, such as a blister on the heel or the need to hurry for a bus can temporarily alter the gait.

In infants congenital dislocation of the hip, if missed earlier, may be suspected from a waddling gait. In children faulty gait may indicate bad posture, which can be corrected by suitable exercises, or early disease of the hip joint; and a jerky gait is observed in chorea. In adults a reeling gait suggests over-indulgence in alcohol or disease of the cerebellum; a 'broad base' gait with feet well apart is found in locomotor ataxia; a high-stepping gait is common in neuritis of the legs; and a shuffling gait occurs in paralysis agitans and after a stroke.

It should of course be remembered that an unusual gait may simply be a mannerism.

Galen. A Greek physician and biologist of the second century A.D. whose prolific writings dominated medical thinking for the next 1,500 years. Galen's observations were extremely astute: for example, he described the muscles of the eyelids and traced the course of the spinal nerves. Much that he wrote on hygiene and dietetics was sound. His clinical methods were good: they were essentially those of Hippocrates five centuries earlier but set out without the latter's compassion and humility.

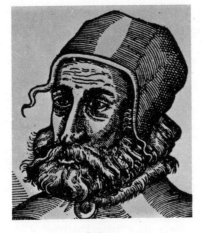

Galen

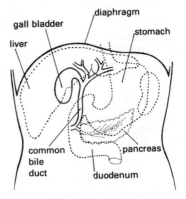

The gall-bladder

His lists of drugs were comprehensive if a bit uncritical. His great defect was that, often with insufficient data, he evolved many theories, inevitably sometimes wrong.

Had he had successors who would experiment, verify and where necessary contradict, Galen would have made a priceless contribution to medical science. Unfortunately his observations (mostly right) and theories (sometimes wrong) – in garbled Latin translations, later translated into Syriac and Arabic and at the Renaissance re-translated into Latin – were accepted as the final authority for well over a thousand years, so that much of the achievement of the sixteenth and seventeenth century anatomists and physiologists consisted of freeing medical thinking from the domination of Galen.

Yet Galen should not be under-rated. We owe to him most of the preservation, classification and systematization of the Greek contribution to medical knowledge, and this far outweighs a few faulty and dogmatically expressed theories.

gall. Another name for BILE, the bitter-tasting liquid that is secreted from the liver into the gall bladder, from which it trickles into the intestine, where it helps to digest fats.

gall-bladder. A pear-shaped muscular bag situated on the under-surface of the liver. It acts as a receptacle for the BILE secreted by the liver. From the gall-bladder bile travels along the cystic duct and common bile duct to reach the duodenum.

For inflammation of the gall-bladder, see CHOLECYSTITIS.

gallstones. Solid, pebble-like masses formed in the gall-bladder. There are three main varieties – multiple faceted stones composed of calcium and bile pigment, single stones of cholesterol, and pure granules of bile pigment.

The causes are not fully understood, but include chronic inflammation of the gall-bladder (causing albumen to be added to the bile, with precipitation of calcium, and formation either of a stone of calcium and bile pigment or of a nucleus round which cholesterol crystallizes). Other probable causes include excess of cholesterol in the diet and stagnation of bile.

Gallstones occur mostly between the ages of 30 and 60 years, are found in 20 per cent of women and 7 per cent of men, and are particularly associated with child-bearing, sedentary occupation and obesity.

Stones may exist for years and cause no trouble, or cause only occasional mild discomfort, heart-burn and flatulence. If a stone passes down the cystic and common bile ducts, which lead from the gall-bladder to the duodenum, and becomes lodged, there is intense pain (often tranferred to the right shoulder), collapse, vomiting, high fever and rigor, with – through blockage of the duct – jaundice appearing in due course. The condition is at first liable to be mistaken for a perforated peptic ulcer or acute appendicitis.

Prevention is largely by early recognition and treatment of CHOLECYSTITIS, and by attention to diet. During an attack the pain may be controlled by injection of morphia and atropine, and various drugs may be used to aid the passing or the dissolving of the stone. If the stone is duly passed, it has to be considered whether it was an isolated event or is likely to be repeated, and x-ray examination may provide useful information on this point. If stones are numerous and attempts to dissolve them unsuccessful, surgical treatment will be required – the gall-bladder being either opened and drained or else removed.

Galvanism. Use of a constant electrical current which causes muscular contraction only when it is made and broken (unlike FARADISM which uses alternating current), Galvanism is employed in the diagnosis of muscle and nerve injuries, and also in the treatment of neuritis, arthritis and synovitis.

gammaglobulin. The plasma or fluid part of the blood is a sticky solution composed mainly of two types of protein, albumin and globulin. The globulin component, produced by the lymphatic system, can be separated by chemical means and further fractionated. When this is done it is found that antibodies to infection are particularly associated with the so-called 'gamma' fraction (IG). Gamma-globulin or human immuno-globulin is now prepared from 'pooled' human sera and is available for the prevention and treatment of certain infections. By using sera from persons known to have natural or induced immunity to specific diseases it is also possible to produce hyper-immuno-globulin, as for instance, vaccinial immuno-globulin. Certain persons have a genetically determined deficiency of gammaglobulin and suffer from hypogamma-globulinaemia.

Gammaglobulin is given by injection usually in doses of 0.02 to 0.05 ml. per kg. body weight and may be used in a variety of infections – particularly those transmitted by viruses.

Viral hepatitis occurs as two types, infective hepatitis (virus A) and serum hepatitis (virus B). The first is generally a mild illness with jaundice, often occurring in sporadic outbreaks. Gammaglobulin given within one week of exposure is useful in controlling spread of infection in institutions and other closed communities. It is however, ineffective in the second more serious condition which is contracted from contact with infected blood (Australia antigen) as in dialysis units.

When ordinary measles occurs in institutions, gammaglobulin can be used to protect specially susceptible infants (such as those suffering from cystic fibrosis, tuberculosis, heart disease, asthma, etc.), but prior active immunization by measles vaccine is preferable. German measles (rubella) carries a risk of foetal damage if a non-immune mother is exposed to infection during the first three months of pregnancy, and it is usual to give gammaglobulin as a preventive measure although the real effectiveness of this is still debatable.

In the control of smallpox, protection can be practically guaranteed by vaccination within seven days of exposure. There is however risk in vaccinating pregnant women and patients suffering from leukaemia, eczema and hypogammaglobulinaemia or undergoing cortico-steroid therapy. The risk can be minimized by the simultaneous administration of vaccinial immuno-globulin and of methisazone, an anti-viral drug.

Tetanus should always be prevented by prior active immunization but in an actual case the use of human tetanus-immuno-globulin will avoid the serious serum reactions sometimes associated with the injection of ordinary anti-tetanic serum prepared from horse-serum.

In whooping cough, active immunization by pertussis vaccine after contact is too late to be effective but a brief passive immunity may be conferred by administration of gammaglobulin and is worth considering for susceptible children in institutional outbreaks.

There are also other tropical or rarer diseases in which gammaglobulin is useful. These include various forms of viral encephalitis such as equine encephalitis and Rift Valley fever.

ganglion. A swelling or cyst containing a jelly-like substance and developing as a round, hard mass on a tendon sheath or joint capsule. The back of the wrist is the commonest site. A ganglion is painless and harmless but, if unsightly, can easily be removed surgically. The seventeenth century method of squashing a ganglion with a heavy object – often the family Bible – was crude but reasonably effective.

The term is also used for a 'junction' in the nervous system, where nerve fibres connect with each other.

gangrene. Mortification; death of the tissue in one part of the body.

Dry gangrene is essentially due to loss of blood supply to the part affected. For instance, old people with hardened and thickened arteries may develop gangrene of the toes and this may spread to the foot. Causes include any interference with the blood supply, e.g., blockage of an artery, injury to an artery, or extreme spasm of an artery in severe cases of Raynaud's disease. Diabetes and chronic nephritis favour the development of gangrene which may also occur following frost-bite, burns, crushing injuries and ergot poisoning.

The dead part becomes hard, dry, wrinkled and (from diffusion of disintegrated haemoglobin) dark brown in colour, with a sharp line of demarcation from adjacent living tissue. Attempts to preserve the circulation and close attention to the feet and hands of those at risk may prevent gangrene. Where it occurs surgical removal of the dead tissue is usually necessary.

Gas gangrene is a complication of severe wounds in which tissue is crushed. Bacteria, mostly *Clostridia welshii*, breed in the damaged tissue which first becomes reddish, then greenish-yellow and finally black, while bubbles of gas appear between the muscle fibres. Apart from pain, swelling and discoloration, the symptoms are those of acute toxaemia. Antibiotics and drainage of the wound help, especially if used early, but in many cases amputation is necessary to preserve life.

gargle. The process of applying a cleansing or antiseptic solution to the back of the throat. It consists of taking a very small mouthful of the liquid, throwing back the head and making the liquid bubble in the throat without swallowing it. Gargles are quite useful in cases of tonsillitis and pharyngitis. Two simple gargles are: (1) crystals of potassium permanganate in warm water in sufficient amount to turn the water faintly pink (not red which would be so strong that it would damage the tissues); and (2) salt (half a teaspoonful to a tumbler) in warm water.

Although gargles are of some use, their value has been overrated in the past. In general, throat infections need treatment with appropriate antibiotics or sulphonamides; and for a mildly inflamed throat rest from speaking and smoking is far more important than the use of a gargle.

gas poisoning. See CARBON MONOXIDE.

gastric ulcer. An ulcer is an eroded open sore on the surface of the skin or a mucous membrane. A gastric ulcer is such a sore occurring in the wall of the stomach.

The stomach contains highly acid gastric juice which digests the protein of food but does not normally affect the living tissue of the stomach wall, because that wall is protected by gastric mucus. However, about 20 per cent of people have a short and over-active stomach, a higher than normal concentration of acid gastric juice, and a deficient secretion of the protective mucus. In such persons any minor injury of the stomach wall (e.g., from a sharp swallowed substance or even from hard and insufficiently chewed food) is likely to be extended by the action of gastric juice on the damaged area, so causing an ulcer.

The main symptom is pain in the region of the lower end of the breast bone, recurring regularly about half to one-and-a-half hours after food, and usually relieved by an alkaline drink or tablet. Other features are tenderness over the pit of the stomach and sometimes vomiting of blood-stained stomach contents. For accurate diagnosis a TEST-MEAL is often required (to determine the chemical characteristics of the gastric secretion) and an x-ray after a barium meal (to render the stomach temporarily opaque to the rays).

Treatment is based on rest, an easily digested diet, and the giving of antacids to neutralize excess acid and of other drugs to diminish secretion of acid and to reduce the movements of the stomach.

Gastric and DUODENAL ULCER are very similar clinically and sometimes classed together as peptic ulcer, though there are some differences in symptoms, e.g., while the pain of a gastric ulcer comes on fairly soon after a meal and is not relieved by eating more food, the pain of a duodenal ulcer comes on about two hours after eating and is temporarily relieved by further eating. There are, however, considerable differences in the groups of people who suffer from each type and in the underlying causes: gastric ulcer is a disease of the poor more than of the rich; emotional stress and worry, while playing some part in the production of gastric ulcer, play a far more important part in duodenal ulcer; and faulty dietetic habits – e.g., meals at very irregular intervals – are very important in causing gastric ulcer but relatively unimportant in the other condition.

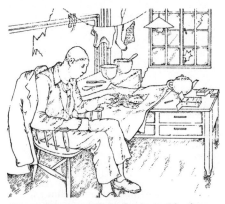

Circumstances predisposing to gastric ulcer

gastritis. Acute gastritis usually follows ingestion of unsuitable or grossly excessive food or large amounts of alcohol. An intense form occurs after the swallowing of some poisons. Symptoms include headache, discomfort in the upper abdomen, nausea and sometimes vomiting. Initially the diagnosis is difficult: typhoid often has a similar onset; cancer of the stomach is also similar although there is more pain and a wasted appearance; and gastric ulcer is not dissimilar although the pain has more relation to meals. After diagnosis has been made treatment consists of giving a laxative, withholding food for a day or so and giving a mild alkali.

Chronic gastritis occurs as a sequel to repeated acute gastritis; following prolonged excess of alcohol, condiments, tea or tobacco; or in association with various severe diseases, such as chronic nephritis and diabetes. Symptoms include poor appetite, diffused pain after food, bouts of headache and vomiting, especially in the morning. After serious diseases have been excluded, treatment is on the same lines as for GASTRIC ULCER.

gastro-enteritis. Inflammation both of the stomach and of the intestines. The condition is characterized by diarrhoea and vomiting, high temperature, and signs of dehydration. In severe cases and especially in young children treatment of the dehydration is essential, so frequent drinks should be taken.

There are four groups of causes: (1) infections such as cholera and dysentery; (2) defects of metabolism or absorption e.g., indigestion following excess starches, diarrhoea following too much protein, and various conditions (such as coeliac disease) resulting from inability to digest fat; (3) emotional and nervous conditions, e.g., nervous diarrhoea; (4) various other causes, such as allergies or tumours of the colon.

Severe cases and outbreaks affecting more than one person are best regarded as due to infection until the contrary is proved. Pending diagnosis the patient should be given no solid food for a day or so but encouraged to drink sufficient water. Antibiotics and other drugs should not be given until the cause has been established, because they may mask the cause.

general paralysis of the insane (GPI). A chronic progressive disease of the brain occurring ten to fifteen years after the contraction of SYPHILIS that has been inadequately treated or left untreated.

The condition often first appears as a lack of emotional control, followed by a deterioration of judgment and reasoning, persistent absence of energy, and failure of accomplishment. In the absence of effective treatment character changes follow, the sufferer often becoming erotic, obscene, immoral or extravagant. Delusions of grandeur may appear: starting with boastfulness and apparent megalomania, the victim comes to believe that he has limitless wealth and amazing capabilities. After some months he gradually loses virtually all memory and judgment, his speech becomes incoherent and his grandiose manner changes to a childish complacency. Finally he passes into a stage of complete helplessness, with loss of control of bladder and bowels.

Prevention depends either on prevention of syphilis or on its early and adequate treatment. Because syphilis is now fairly rare in developed countries and inadequately treated syphilis is even more rare, GPI has almost disappeared.

Until about 1910 GPI was regarded as incurable. Thereafter Ehrlich's arsenical preparations checked many cases of the disease, but they have more recently been replaced by large doses of penicillin. If given early enough treatment can stop the progress of the disease, but it cannot replace any cerebral tissue that has already been damaged.

general practitioner. A doctor who undertakes diagnosis and treatment without limitation of the age or sex of his patients and without restriction of the types of illness handled.

While the clinical consultant or specialist limits himself to certain varieties of illness (e.g., the cardiologist deals only with heart conditions and the psychiatrist only with mental disorders) or to certain portions of the community (as in the case of the paediatrician or the gynaecologist), and while the community physician or public health doctor studies the health and sickness of the people as a whole, the general practitioner seeks to provide primary medical care for all individuals who have accepted him as their personal physician.

The term 'family doctor', sometimes used as a synonym, expresses the broad meaning but is less accurate because (1) persons working far from their families may need a general practitioner but can hardly be said to have a family doctor, (2) members of a family may elect to enroll with different practitioners, and (3) in the group practice that is becoming increasingly common – and is necessary to enable doctors to have freedom from emergency calls when not on duty – a family, even if enrolled with one practice, may in three successive episodes of illness be treated by three different members of the practice.

The family doctor beloved of fiction, who knew his patients well from their birth onwards and advised on many personal and social problems as well as on health, perhaps existed – and to some extent still exists – in rural areas, but in towns was largely a figment of the imagination of those wealthy enough to pay for private treatment. A doctor with 2,100 patients (if he worked for forty-five hours a week, exclusive of travelling time, for forty-six weeks a year) would have an average of one hour a year to devote to each; and, apart from persons who change their doctor without moving to another town, an average British town each year loses by migration about 5 per cent of its citizens and gains roughly the same number of newcomers.

Although the general practitioner cannot claim the clinical expertise of the specialist or the preventive and epidemiological expertise of the community physician, he should not therefore be considered of lesser importance. He has chosen to exercise his skills over a wider range and in less detail, and he is in many ways the key medical figure who calls in appropriate clinical or community specialists at need.

Until 1948 most doctors in Britain – whether trained by apprenticeship, as was common until last century, or equipped by university courses – started their careers in general practice, with those who had a flair for a clinical speciality or for community medicine subsequently seeking to specialize. The life of the single-handed practitioner of the early 1900s was interesting but hard. He had to try to remain reasonably knowledgeable of the whole field of medicine, and because, when insurance schemes were non-existent or only beginning to develop, he depended for income mainly on private patients, he could hardly take a night off without risking the untreated suffering of a genuine emergency or the financial loss inherent in one of his patients calling in another doctor.

Three main changes occurred in the 1950s and 1960s. Firstly with the advent of National Health Insurance, private (or 'paying') patients steadily became rarer. This removed the practitioner's 'vested interest' in illness: previously, if he cured a private patient too quickly, his income fell. The swing to insured patients also shifted the emphasis from home visits to treatment in the consulting room: the doctor expected patients who were well enough to visit him, saving his time and enabling him to use diagnostic tools not easily transported. Secondly, as mentioned later, single-handed practice was increasingly replaced by group practice. And thirdly, there was a steady trend to early specialization, so that many surgical and medical specialists or community physicians today have had little or no experience of general practice. This trend perhaps made for consultants more expert in their selected field, but the fact that many of the best medical undergraduates opted for immediate specialization has perhaps reacted adversely on the reputation of general practitioners at a time when medical knowledge is advancing more rapidly than ever before. It is very easy for a young consultant, with excellent knowledge of a limited branch, to feel contempt for – and even inadvertently to reveal that contempt for – the practitioner's ignorance, utterly forgetting the breadth of the latter's professional territory.

Internationally, two opposed trends can perhaps be noted. (1) In some states of the U.S.A., and to a limited extent in Scandinavia, the idea has gained currency that nobody can become or remain reasonably expert over the entire field of medicine, and that it is therefore better that the patient should make a layman's diagnosis – 'My child needs a paediatrician' or 'My symptoms suggest that I should see a heart specialist' – and then consult directly the appropriate specialist, with excellent results if the layman chooses correctly, but sometimes resulting in an unfortunate transfer from specialist to specialist if the choice is wrong. (2) In Britain and in some other countries increasing stress has been laid on the primary care doctor. He has been supported by easier access to radiological and biochemical diagnostic facilities; and he has been further supported by an association with HEALTH VISITORS (selected nurses with further training in psychology, sociology and health teaching) who often have knowledge of the stresses and prejudices of individual families and are experts in the unobtrusive altering of attitudes and habits.

Nearly half of the 55,000 doctors in Britain are general practitioners. They are paid a fee calculated on the number of patients on their list, with the fee slightly increased for persons of pensionable age (because of greater liability to illness) and with additional payments permitted for some services (e.g., supervision during pregnancy and childbirth). A person is free to choose his own practitioner and to change that practitioner at any time; and a practitioner can refuse to have a patient on his list, either because the list is full or because he considers the particular patient unreasonable.

Some private practice still exists in Britain. A patient who thinks he will get better service by paying for it directly may consult any practitioner privately, with the single exception that a practitioner cannot accept as a private patient somebody for whom he is already receiving a fee from the National Health Service.

In the past, a retiring practitioner sold his practice, often to the highest bidder. The sale of practices in Britain has been forbidden since 1948 (with a pension scheme provided in lieu) and practice vacancies are now filled largely on merit but with consideration of the wishes of the non-retiring members of the practice.

The current tendency in Britain is very much towards group practice, where perhaps six doctors, five health visitors, four district nurses and a receptionist accept responsibility for a 'panel' of 14,000 patients or prospective patients. There are advantages to the professionals, for instance a doctor can know that he is liable for night calls on only one night out of six and that when he takes a holiday his patients are in the hands of trusted colleagues, not of untried 'locums'. Also there are advantages to the patients such as the better equipment that a multiple practice can provide, the knowledge that a doctor is always available who has access to the patient's records, and the knowledge that the doctor who attends in an emergency is not exhausted because of his previous night's sleep having been disturbed by another emergency call. Where single or double-doctor practices remain, two or three practices often enter into deputizing arrangements whereby evening or night calls are transferred to the particular doctor on duty. These group-practice and deputizing trends are undoubtedly beneficial on the whole, but implicit in them is the final abandonment of the idea of a 'family doctor' with intimate knowledge of his patients and available whenever they need him.

genes. Minute particles inside the cells which pass on all the physical and mental characteristics that a person inherits, e.g., blood group, colour of eyes, colour of hair, mathematical ability, linguistic ability, etc. Large numbers of genes, far too small to be visible under a high-powered microscope, are located in a line down each of the chromosomes. See GENETICS.

genetic guidance. Counselling of married couples, or preferably of persons contemplating matrimony, as to their degree of risk of producing a child seriously handicapped by hereditary disease. Essentially such guidance is based on two factors: detailed study of pedigree and microscopic examination of the chromosomes of body cells.

Where a family has a history of hereditary disease inherited as a dominant gene (see GENETICS), as in Huntington's chorea or congenital dwarfism (achondroplasia), the ascertainment of risk is easy: the son or daughter of a sufferer has a 50 per cent chance of inheriting and transmitting the disease, but the nephew or niece of a sufferer, provided the parents were unaffected, will not transmit the disease. Where there is a family history of disease inherited as a recessive gene, as in cystic fibrosis or deaf mutism, the ascertainment of risk is more difficult, because the disease may miss a generation or a couple of generations and then reappear. Where several genes are involved, as in spina bifida and schizophrenia, the full skills of a geneticist are needed to estimate the risk of producing a damaged child.

Most of the highly developed countries have genetic clinics to which persons of suspicious family history or couples who have produced a handicapped child can be referred. Essentially these clinics perform three functions: (1) they reassure many couples who wrongly think themselves at risk because of the illness of a relative of one of them; (2) in cases of bad heredity they can advise married couples or couples contemplating marriage of their degree of risk of producing a seriously damaged child; and (3) in the case of a pregnant woman they can sometimes determine whether the foetus is seriously damaged, although in this case the investigation is pointless unless the woman is prepared to have the pregnancy terminated if necessary.

Since improvement in maternal and child health services enables a higher proportion of handicapped children to survive, and since in some hereditary diseases (e.g., Huntington's chorea and schizophrenia) even a direct transmitter may reach child-bearing age before showing any signs of the disease, genetic clinics are clearly very important, but it should be appreciated that they cannot stand on their own. For their success there also has to be a well-developed service (such as health visitors in the U.K.) to reassure many people who falsely suspect that they may be transmitters of hereditary disease (and who might otherwise swamp the clinics) and to persuade others who may be at risk that it is desirable for them to attend genetic clinics.

Assessment at a clinic is not the end of the story. The geneticist's job is essentially to say, 'If you produce a child there is a 10 per cent chance that it will suffer from a particular disease'. Thereafter there must be people – health visitors, general practitioners, social workers – prepared to discuss with the couple the seriousness or otherwise of the possible disease, the degree of risk in relation to that seriousness, the means of having a full sex life without producing children (contraceptives, tying of female tubes, male vasectomy) and the methods of compensating for natural desire to have children (e.g., adoption).

In developed countries, just as the biggest health advance of the first forty years of this century was almost certainly improvement in child health, exemplified for instance by the dramatic fall in the baby death rate, and just as the biggest advance of the last forty years has probably been reduction of infections by immunization and education of the public about its desirability, some workers have suggested that the largest advance in the next forty years is likely to be reduction of hereditary diseases by genetic guidance and the accompanying educating and counselling services.

genetics. The study of the factors which determine the transmission of inherited characteristics from parents to offspring. An individual's total make-up is not entirely determined by genetic factors, since heredity and environment go together to mould the human being.

The narrower field of medical genetics is concerned primarily with the transmission of hereditary diseases. These are becoming of greater relative importance both because many non-genetic conditions can now be successfully prevented or treated and because facilities for effective treatment result in many more children with congenital defects surviving to adult life.

Biological inheritance. It is now necessary to consider the mechanism of biological inheritance. The old name for this was Mendelism because the broad principles of heredity were originally worked out by an Austrian monk, Gregor Mendel, between about 1850 and 1860, and later verified in 1900 by independent workers.

Mendel experimented with ordinary pea-plants and identified paired characteristics in which they varied. As an example he found that if he interbred plants with red flowers all the offspring had red flowers too. If he bred red-flowered plants with white-flowered plants all the hybrid offspring had red flowers and he concluded that redness was a dominant characteristic, and that whiteness was recessive. If he then interbred the red/white hybrids he obtained both red flowers and white flowers in the proportion of three to one, but of the three reds one was a pure red which would continue to breed true and the other two were red/white hybrids. This became known as the Mendelian ratio and on the basis of this he formulated two laws. These were the law of segregation (that paired characteristics were inherited one from each parent) and the law of independence (that paired characteristics were inherited independently). The second is now known not to be wholly true because 'linkage' can occur unless the separate characteristics are carried on separate chromosomes.

The four possibilities in inheritance

Father's paired genes [1][2] × [3][4]   Mother's paired genes
Offspring [1][3]   [1][4] [2][3]   [2][4]   Average 25% each

Inheritance of dominant Gene
e.g. achondroplasia (six possible matings)

1. Parents both true dwarfs   [1][2] × [3][4]
   Offspring all true dwarfs   [1][3] [1][4]   [2][3] [2][4]

2. Parents one true and one apparent dwarf (carrying a normal gene)   [1][2] × [3][4]
   Offspring 50% true dwarfs and 50% apparent dwarfs.   [1][3] [1][4]   [2][3] [2][4]

3. Parents both apparent dwarfs   [1][2] × [3][4]
   Offspring 25% true dwarfs, 50% apparent and 25% normal.   [1][3] [1][4]   [2][3] [2][4]

4. Parents true dwarf and normal   [1][2] × [3][4]
   Offspring all apparent dwarfs   [1][3] [1][4]   [2][3] [2][4]

5. Parents an apparent dwarf and a normal   [1][2] × [3][4]
   Offspring 50% apparent dwarfs and 50% normal.   [1][3] [1][4]   [2][3] [2][4]

6. Parents both normal   [1][2] × [3][4]
   Offspring all normal   [1][3] [1][4]   [2][3] [2][4]

Inheritance of recessive genes, e.g., cystic fibrosis, is shown by the same diagram but reading ▢ as normal and ▢ as affected, so that individuals with ▢ ▢ are apparently normal, but carrying the affected recessive gene.

Chromosomes and genes. The next step came with the growing elucidation of cell-structure. The cell-nucleus contains chromatin, made up from protein, ribonucleic acid (RNA) and deoxyribonucleic acid (DNA). In the resting phase chromatin appears as a network of nuclear material but when the cell is about to divide the chromatin becomes defined into rod-shaped bodies called chromosomes. In man there are forty-six of these, arranged in twenty-three sets of similar pairs (diploid chromosomes), one member of each pair having been derived from father and mother respectively. As cell and nuclear division proceed each chromosome splits longitudinally and separates (mitosis) to form a new but identical chromosome. Collectively these are again reconstituted as two sets of twenty-three and shared between the two daughter cells.

An important exception to this general rule occurs in the ovum and sperm (gametes). Since these unite to form the zygote the union would produce twice the proper number of chromosomes, so during maturation they undergo a process called meiosis and their individual chromosomes are reduced to twenty-three. Twenty-two of these are autosomes and similar in both sexes but the remaining chromosome is known as the sex-chromosome and occurs in two forms, X and Y. All female gametes contain an X chromosome; male gametes have either an X or a Y. Accordingly when they join to form an embryo or zygote the sex-chromosome pair resulting may be either XX in which case the child will be female, or XY resulting in a male. See also CHROMOSOME.

Finally a word about the structure of DNA, which appears in the chromosome as a long complex molecule like a double thread or tiny twisted rope-ladder with its steps made up of the bases adenine, thymine, cytosine and guanine. The order in which these bases occur along the ladder form the genetic code. If the DNA becomes disarranged as by chemical agents or radiation a mutation results. Most mutations are harmful but natural selection tends to retain favourable ones and reject the unfavourable.

The genes are the units of inheritance, also bi-parental in origin, and they occupy corresponding positions on the chromosomes. As already mentioned a gene occasionally alters by spontaneous or induced mutation and it can then be present in two or more forms known as alleles. If an individual inherits from each parent the same allelic form of a particular gene he is said to be homozygous for that gene position; if different alleles are present he is heterozygous. When a particular allele gives rise to an obvious physical characteristic in a heterozygote it is said to be dominant but if the characteristic only appears in the homozygote it is recessive. In addition to their function in determining sex the sex-chromosomes carry other genes affecting other characteristics and hence the inheritance of such genes is sex-linked but, since the human Y chromosome is much smaller than the X-chromosome, linkage is mainly to X.

It can now be explained how the foregoing considerations work out in practice.

Dominant inheritance. While the Y-chromosome of a father can pass only to his sons and his X-chromosome only to his daughters all the other autosomes of both parents pass equally to sons and daughters. When two unequal genes (alleles) meet in a pair the stronger prevails and is said to be dominant. Pigmentation for instance is dominant to albinism which is an undesirable trait. In general, dominant genes are related to normal or beneficial characteristics, but the rule is by no means invariable; achondroplasia, short, webbed or additional fingers and toes, Huntington's chorea, diabetes insipidus and some eye defects, all relatively common, are due to dominant inheritance and will appear in heterozygotes. On the average, affected persons married to normals will have affected and normal children in equal proportions. Normal children of the union marrying normals will have only normal offspring.

Recessive inheritance. The effects of a recessive gene are seen only in homozygotes, where both parents carry the gene and contribute an affected chromosome to the offspring. Albinism is recessive to pigmentation and so two apparently normal persons may marry but if each is a heterozygous carrier of albinism there is a one in four chance of an albino offspring (Mendelian ratio). There are many recessively inherited diseases but most of them are individually uncommon. The chances of marrying someone with the same harmful gene are low but marriage with a close relative obviously increases the risk and similarly the effects of modern treatment in securing the survival to adult life of patients with such conditions as cystic fibrosis and phenylketonuria also have implications for the future. Amongst other recessive conditions are amaurotic familial idiocy, Friedrich's ataxia, Ménière's disease, deaf mutism and osteosclerosis.

Because these conditions continue to be carried by apparently normal heterozygotes they may reappear after missing a generation or two.

Sex-linked inheritance. The classic example is HAEMOPHILIA in which the male victim carries the gene in his one x-chromosome. So far all sex-linked diseases have proved to be x-linked and nearly all are recessive. Thus in haemophilia an affected male cannot transmit the disease to his sons, whose x-chromosome must have come from the mother, but his daughters will be heterozygous (one x from mother and another x with the weak gene from the father) and they will be able to transmit the condition to the next generation. Muscular dystrophy (Duchenne type) is inherited similarily.

Mixed inheritance. Some conditions do not quite follow these rules precisely, probably because of segmental interchange between chromosomes and hence may occur either as dominant, recessive, or sex-linked types. This is true of congenital deafness, other types of muscular dystrophy, and retinitis pigmentosa. Pyloric stenosis, spina bifida, hare-lip and cleft palate, congenital dislocation of the hip, congenital heart disease, diabetes, schizophrenia, manic-depressive psychosis and spondylitis also show evidence of a partial or complex inheritance.

Chromosome abnormalities. The abnormality may be of number or of structure where chromosomal breaks have led to loss or rearrangement of chromosomal material. The best known condition is mongolism or Down's syndrome where there is an extra no. 21 chromosome making a total of forty-seven in all. Hence the name 'trisomy 21'.

Genetic counselling. Persons with a family history of inherited disease or who have already had an abnormal child are naturally concerned to know what are the risks of the condition arising or recurring in their family. Genetic Advisory Centres are now available in most main hospital centres, and the family doctor if he cannot resolve the problem himself can make arrangements for consultation in order that appropriate advice may be given. This will be based on a careful analysis of the family pedigree and on chromosome studies. In some instances enzyme tests are available to determine whether prospective mothers are in fact carriers of an x-linked recessive gene. Marriages between blood relations carry an increased risk of the emergence of a recessive characteristic and advice should be sought.

It is also possible to demonstrate chromosomal abnormalities and determine sex before birth by examination of amniotic cells. A pregnancy could thus legitimately be terminated if it were found that the child would be a mongol or if the child was a male and the mother was a carrier for a serious x-linked condition in which there is a one in two risk of a son being affected but no risk to a daughter. Additionally ultrasonic techniques may be used for the early identification of conditions such as spina bifida.

The logical extension of genetic counselling is eugenics where positive steps are taken to discourage or prohibit marriages with a genetic risk or even to sterilize defectives. Even if this were tolerated or approved by society the problem would not be solved because on the basis of our present knowledge it is impossible to detect all the heterozygotes with some transmissible defect which may reappear in later generations.

Nevertheless, GENETIC GUIDANCE, with the object of persuading known carriers of serious hereditary conditions to avoid producing children, could vastly improve the health of the community. It also has an important negative aspect: many people who wrongly suspect that they may be carriers of hereditary disease could learn that their fears are groundless.

genitals. Those parts of the REPRODUCTIVE SYSTEM which are on the body surface.

genu valgum. See KNOCK KNEE.

geography and disease. Where disease is related to climate, to urbanization or industrialization, to the pollution that tends to accompany these processes or to changes in plant or animal life, the terms 'medical geography' and 'epidemiology' have become remarkably similar in meaning. At the simplest end of the scale, we are more likely to develop frost-bite in northern Canada and heat-stroke in the Amazon valley than vice versa, we will not suffer from snake-bite in a country that has no poisonous snakes and our chance of typhoid is vastly greater if water supplies are liable to pollution from sewage. Looking at more complex points, a map of Britain with differential shading for areas with high, moderate and low incidence of chronic bronchitis is startlingly like one shaded for densities of population, while a description of soft- and hard-water areas shows a great resemblance to that of areas with respectively high and low incidence of cardiovascular disease.

However, diseases which are genetically determined have little connection with geography: the genes responsible for spina bifida, schizophrenia or haemophilia can be transmitted whether their donor lives in the tropics or the arctic, in a city or in a remote area. To the extent, again, that disease is a result of disharmony within the social group, geography plays an insignificant part, although the bewildered adolescent and the handicapped adult may fit more easily into the relatively simple patterns of an agricultural community than into the competitiveness and aggressiveness of city life. It is important to state these points, because some geographers – ignoring hereditary disease (probably the biggest problem currently facing health workers), and ignoring the frequency and complexity of disorders of psycho-social origin – would almost seem to be seeking to transfer the study of epidemiology from community physicians and medical statisticians to their own sphere of influence.

The connection between geography and disease is important, and geographers can undoubtedly contribute to the advance of epidemiological knowledge, but we must also remember that by no means all diseases have geographical associations.

geriatrics. The branch of medicine concerned with the health and diseases of those who are AGEING. While similar concern with diseases of children (paediatrics) began to emerge as a speciality towards the end of the last century, the rise of geriatrics is very much a feature of the last two or three decades.

Old people differ from younger adults in many respects. For instance their recovery from any illness tends to be slower but, because of risk of joint stiffening, they often have to be got out of bed at an earlier stage of the illness. Again, while younger adults, when ill, generally have a single disease, old people may well suffer from a number of simultaneous diseases and disabilities, with each condition reacting on others. To take another example, if a young adult has normal appetite and an adequate and well-balanced diet, we can usually forget about deficiency diseases; but in respect of the nutrition of an old person we have to consider such points as: (1) the food available (having regard to the relative poverty of many old persons), (2) the foods actually used (having regard to likes and dislikes acquired over many years and also to possible chewing difficulties), and (3) digestive and absorptive capacities (which may make it desirable that a pensioner with an apparently well-balanced diet should nevertheless receive vitamin supplements).

As the conquest of infections and the reduction of many of the hazards of younger life have dramatically increased the proportion of people surviving into old age, geriatrics has not only become established as a legitimate speciality but has tended to become subdivided into clinical geriatrics (the study of physical diseases at the upper end of life), psycho-geriatrics (the similar study of mental and psycho-social diseases), and gerontology (the investigation of the ageing process and of its medico-social and preventive aspects).

germ. A germ or micro-organism is a minute living creature which cannot usually be seen without a microscope. The term is mostly reserved for micro-organisms which cause disease (pathogens) but can be used also for harmless micro-organisms and for micro-organisms that are actively useful, such as the mould from which we derive penicillin or the yeast used in baking. Germs include BACTERIA, VIRUSES and RICKETTSIA. Bacteria can be seen through an ordinary microscope; examples are those organisms that cause typhoid, bacillary dysentery and diphtheria. Viruses are much smaller and can be seen only by using an electron microscope; examples are the microbes that cause smallpox, chicken pox and influenza. Rickettsia are to some extent intermediate. An example is the organism that causes typhus.

Yeasts and moulds are included under the term 'germs', and so usually are somewhat larger single-celled organisms, PROTOZOA, such as the germ which causes amoebic dysentery.

Germs enter the body in three main ways: by inhalation of air particles carrying them, by swallowing of food containing them, or by penetration of the skin or access through an open wound.

In many cases bacterial and rickettsial diseases can now be prevented by immunization, or treated by antibiotics. Both prevention and treatment of virus infections is more difficult: vaccines have been devised for only a minority of these infections, and many virus diseases are resistant to antibiotics.

German measles. Otherwise known as rubella, this is a mild, infectious, feverish disease, caused by a virus. There is a rash which is less coarse than that of measles, mild catarrhal symptoms and enlargement of the glands behind the ears. The incubation period is about eighteen days and the duration of illness is about three days, and one attack results in permanent immunity.

Although a trifling illness, rubella is of considerable importance if it occurs during early pregnancy because of the risk of viral damage to the developing foetus. In 1940 there was a particularly widespread Australian epidemic and in the following year Dr Norman Gregg drew attention to an unusual incidence of congenital cataract in babies born to mothers who had been affected. Subsequent research has confirmed that rubella during the first three months of pregnancy may cause other defects, including deafness, mental deficiency and congenital heart disease, and that it may sometimes produce miscarriage.

In order to prevent this situation arising some countries are attempting to eradicate rubella completely by immunizing all children (of both sexes), while other countries, including Britain, are trying to prevent the occurrence of the disease during pregnancy by offering immunization to all girls aged about 13 years, and in some cases by also offering immunization to young women, not yet pregnant, who have neither had rubella earlier nor been immunized against it.

If, despite the availability of immunization, a woman develops rubella during the first three months of pregnancy, the question of abortion should be considered. It should be noted that rubella later in pregnancy causes no risk to the child, and that rubella in early pregnancy –

whether followed by a therapeutic abortion or by the birth of a deformed or a healthy child – carries no risk to subsequent children.

gestation. The period during which the unborn child develops within the uterus, i.e., from conception (the union of the ovum and the sperm after intercourse) to birth. In the human female it averages 266 days, although 6 days longer and 6 days shorter are both considered to fall within the limits of normality.

giardiasis. Infestation of the bowel by a pear-shaped microscopic parasite, *Giardia lamblia.* Infection, just as in typhoid and paratyphoid, comes from consuming food or drink contaminated by the excreta of sufferers, so the condition could be eliminated by proper sewerage and good personal hygiene.

In highly developed countries the disease is rare but by no means unknown, but in some countries infestation is so common in apparently healthy children that some experts question whether the parasite really does any harm. In at least a proportion of cases, however, it causes diarrhoea and abdominal discomfort with the passing of motions containing excessive fat, perhaps because the parasites line the mucous membrane of the intestine and hinder the proper absorption of fat. Tablets of mepacrine hydrochloride (100 mg. daily for a week) usually effect a complete cure.

giddiness. See DIZZINESS.

gigantism. See ACROMEGALY AND GIGANTISM.

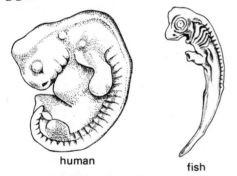

human

fish

The human embryo (left) passes through a stage of development with gills not unlike those of the fish embryo (right).

gills. Part of the respiratory system of fish and other aquatic animals, the gills are multiple clefts in the sides of the 'neck', forming passages between the mouth and the exterior. In 'breathing' by means of gills a fish takes in water by mouth and forces it out in an intermittent stream through the gill-clefts. The exchange of gases occurs as the water passes over the blood-filled lining membrane which is usually arranged in numerous folds to enlarge the surface area.

In the course of evolution, land animals developed from aquatic animals. They acquired lungs adapted to air so that their gills gradually disappeared, although some animals still exist with both systems. The evidence for this evolutionary change can still be seen in the early human embryo because five rudimentary gills, called the branchial arches, persist until

about the sixth week of intra-uterine life. These have pouches within and clefts without, and represent primitive gill-clefts.

Very occasionally the development is faulty and these 'gills' do not entirely disappear and this may give rise to a branchial fistula, with a communication between the pharynx and the surface of the neck, or to a branchial cyst. Both conditions have a tendency to malignant change and should be treated surgically without undue delay.

gingivitis. See GUMS.

glanders. A dangerous infectious disease, caused by a bacillus, occurring mainly in horses but occasionally communicated to persons in close contact with horses. In man the condition usually starts with an outbreak of spots on the nose, there is a semipurulent nasal discharge, and symptoms of pneumonia and general fever follow. If untreated the disease is fatal in about 90 per cent of cases.

For treatment a combination of streptomycin and a sulphonamide is usually advised. With such treatment the survival rate is certainly far above the 10 per cent for untreated cases, but, because the disease is so rare, it is difficult to establish a definite survival rate.

glands. Organs which manufacture and release substances necessary for the working of the body. There are two broad types, those with ducts which carry their secretions, and those that pass their secretions directly into the bloodstream.

Examples of glands with ducts include the various salivary glands required for digestion, and the sweat glands needed for release of perspiration. Glands without ducts secrete hormones or chemical messengers; these are the ENDOCRINE GLANDS, such as the pituitary and the thyroid.

Additionally, the term 'glands' is used for lymph glands or nodes which are interposed in the course of lymphatic vessels and through which the lymph is filtered. Apart from arresting inert or harmful substances (including bacteria) lymph glands manufacture lymphocytes which are important for the destruction of bacteria.

Inflammation of glands has, consequently, two separate meanings. Firstly, it applies to swelling of organs of secretion: e.g., in tonsillitis and scarlet fever the neck glands are enlarged, and swelling of glands behind the ears is an indication of a doubtful rash being that of German measles. Secondly, the term applies to the lymph nodes, as when infection of the gland spreads up the lymphatic vessels to produce reddening of small glands near the elbow and swelling of glands in the armpit.

glandular fever. An acute infection characterized by fever, sore throat, swelling of cervical and other lymph glands, and enlargement of the spleen. The symptoms last for about a month, and diagnosis – formerly rather difficult – can nowadays be made by blood-test.

The cause and mode of transmission are not yet understood, although it is thought that the spread is from the nose and throat of infected persons. The normal treatment consists simply of rest and light diet, and spontaneous recovery occurs in four or five weeks. Many drugs have been tried but none have been shown to shorten the disease, although antibiotics are useful if complications occur, such as tonsillitis.

Probably many cases have remained undiagnosed in the past. Now that we have an accurate means of identifying suspected cases we may hope to learn more about the cause and method of spread. So far, however, we are largely working in ignorance: for instance, authorities in the U.S.A. regard the disease as too common to justify isolation, whereas in Britain isolation is recommended for confirmed cases.

glaucoma. A disease of the eye caused by increased pressure of fluid within the eyeball. If untreated the increasing pressure damages the optic nerve and retina, and causes blindness. The cause is thought to be obstruction in the drainage of fluid from the eyeball. Very occasionally the condition occurs in infants through a developmental abnormality, but usually the disease appears only above the age of 50 years.

Acute glaucoma may start with severe pain in the eye, disturbance or blurring of vision, and sickness. Chronic glaucoma comes on gradually, with little pain but steady deterioration of vision; there are attacks of 'mist before the eyes' and the seeing of rainbow rings round a distant light.

Early diagnosis is important because of the danger to sight in untreated cases. Indeed the risk of glaucoma is one reason why it is advised that persons over 50 should have their eyes examined every two years. Pressure can be estimated by the specialist's finger or by an instrument called a tonometer.

In early cases treatment with suitable drugs is often effective. Where drugs fail, a small operation may create an outflow canal for the excessive fluid. Once the retina and optic nerve have been damaged, medical or surgical treatment may prevent a worsening of the condition but cannot undo the damage already done.

glioma. A tumour of the tissue connecting and enfolding the substance of the brain (neuroglia). The commonest intracranial tumour of adults, glioma may occur in the cerebrum or less often in the cerebellum or pons. While symptoms vary with the site, frequent ones are headache, mental changes such as stupor and dullness (especially in tumours of the frontal lobes), vomiting (especially in tumours of the cerebellum and pons), visual disturbances and vertigo. Unlike a cancer a glioma does not spread by secondaries to other parts of the body; but because of its situation it may be highly dangerous. Whether it can be operated on depends on its size and position.

glossitis. Inflammation of the TONGUE.

glottis. The entrance to the main air-way from the throat (pharynx) to the voice-box (larynx). It alters in width according to the movement of the vocal cords, opening for breathing but narrowing for speaking or singing.

Oedema of the glottis – usually the result of an allergy that causes the swelling and inflammation – is a serious condition requiring urgent medical attention.

glucose. A simple form of sugar found in ripe fruits and in honey, and tasting less sweet than cane-sugar (sucrose).

While starches have to be converted to sugars by intestinal juices before being absorbed, and while even sucrose requires chemical action in the intestine, glucose can be directly and immediately absorbed and so can provide a very quick source of energy. The energy is created during the combustion of glucose and oxygen to water and carbon dioxide.

Where nourishment is needed very quickly glucose has an advantage over all other foods, and where a patient has to be fed through a vein a solution of glucose is essential; but apart from these circumstances glucose has no special advantages.

If sugar is excreted from the body in the urine, the condition is known as GLYCOSURIA, and is investigated by the glucose tolerance test.

glycosuria. The presence of sugar in the urine. This is normally an indication of the existence of DIABETES MELLITUS. However, glycosuria also occurs in certain other circumstances. (1) A few people have a lowered kidney threshold for the transfer of sugar to the urine. (2) Many people temporarily have sugar in the urine after a very large, carbohydrate meal. (3) Temporary glycosuria can occur after severe emotional shock. (4) It is also found in some diseases of the nervous system.

Glycosuria should therefore not be regarded as establishing that a person has diabetes, but merely as justifying the use of a glucose tolerance test. In this test the patient eats a specified and known amount of glucose and his blood and urine are examined at half-hourly intervals to ascertain how the body is dealing with the glucose.

gnat. A general term employed to describe all forms of small, biting flies, such as midges and MOSQUITOES.

goitre. A persisting enlargement of the thyroid gland. If not associated with general symptoms of disturbed thyroid function it is a simple goitre commonly seen in adolescent girls and young women.

The thyroid is an endocrine gland producing the hormone thyroxin, a complex organic compound containing iodine. In the tissues this acts as a catalyst to increase the rate of oxidation and so influences metabolism.

The symptomatology of the various types of goitre depends on whether the gland produces excess thyroxin (hyperthyroidism), or too little (hypothyroidism).

Endemic goitre. Certain parts of the world have been notorious for a high incidence of very large goitres. 'Derbyshire neck' was well-known and some parts of Switzerland had a similar reputation. This proved to be due to a deficiency of iodine in water and soil. The use of iodized table salt (1 part sodium iodide to 100,000 parts sodium chloride) has now virtually eliminated endemic goitre.

Hypothyroidism. Under-production of thyroxin leads either to cretinism or myxoedema. In cretinism thyroxin deficiency begins during foetal life and unless treated early a child so affected is dwarfish, apathetic, somnolent, and usually seriously mentally deficient.

In the adult, thyroid deficiency causes myxoedema, a condition marked by a lowered basal metabolism with resultant intolerance of cold, and by mental slowness, loss of hair, and thickening of the skin and subcutaneous tissues.

Hyperthyroidism. This condition, sometimes known as Graves' disease, is commoner in women than in men, usually occurs between the ages of 15 and 50 years, and tends to have a hereditary element. Precipitating factors include sudden severe fright or shock, prolonged worry and overwork, and tumours of the gland.

Symptoms include tiredness, nervousness, tenseness, anxiety, tremors of the hands, rapid pulse, excessive perspiration, and in some severe cases emaciation and protrusion of the eyes. The last named symptom accounts for the alternative name, exophthalmic goitre.

There are essentially three possibilities for treatment. (1) Rest in bed, absence of excitement, a good diet, elimination of any septic foci and use of antithyroid drugs. This is certainly the method of first choice for younger patients. (2) The use of radio-iodine to lessen the activity of the gland. (3) Thyroidectomy – surgical removal of part of the gland.

General. Apart from metabolic effects, goitres may cause other symptoms merely from their presence. Large goitres may extend behind the breast bone (retro-sternal goitre) to compress the trachea and cause difficulty with breathing and secondary effects such as bronchitis and emphysema. The laryngeal nerves in the neck may be affected causing hoarseness and loss of speech.

The thyroid gland may also be the seat of local tumour growth either cancerous or of a non-malignant type, where the growth produces a localized swelling with signs of hyperthyroidism.

Another condition causing fibrous changes in the thyroid gland and looking like a goitre is known as Hashimoto's disease.

gold treatment. Preparations of gold have been advocated as treatment for certain diseases.

In 1923 Mollgaard, a Danish veterinarian, introduced a gold preparation, Sanocrysin, for use in the treatment of pulmonary tuberculosis. Its reputation rested on the fact that very weak solutions of gold salts inhibited the growth of tubercle bacilli in culture but the evidence that it did this in the body was doubtful. Nowadays much better anti-tuberculous drugs are available.

Gold salts were next used for the treatment of rheumatoid arthritis (1930) and still have their advocates. The usual preparation is sodium aurothiomalate (Myocrisin) given by injection either as a watery or oily solution. It probably acts by providing a general stimulus to the body's immunity mechanisms.

Although opinion has been somewhat divided about the efficacy of gold therapy, the results of recent controlled trials by the Arthritis and Rheumatism Council have been in its favour. What is certain, however, is that gold salts are very toxic, and readily cause severe damage to the liver, kidney and the blood-forming elements in the bone marrow. Gold therapy requires very careful control and should be discontinued on the appearance of skin rashes, albuminuria, jaundice, or on any reduction in the white blood-cell count (leucopaenia).

gonadotropic hormones. Internal secretions affecting the gonads or sex-glands. Two such hormones are produced by the front lobe of the pituitary gland.

In the female they are responsible for the initiation of sexual development and the subsequent control of the production and maturation of the egg-cells, with their enclosing follicles, which in turn produce the sex-hormones oestrin and progestin. These are related respectively to sexual activity and to the changes in the uterus which lead either to menstruation or to preparation for pregnancy should a ripe ovum become fertilized.

Similarly, in the male they initiate the sexual development which occurs at puberty and continue to stimulate the formation of sperms and the production of male sex-hormone.

gonads. The reproductive glands of the body comprising the ovaries in women and the testes (or testicles) in men.

The ovaries produce the female gametes or ova and the testes the male gametes or spermatozoa which unite in the process of fertilization.

gonorrhoea. The commonest of the venereal diseases, caused by infection of the urethra and genital tract by the gonococcus (*Neisseria gonorrhoea*).

The disease is almost always acquired by sexual intercourse with an infected person. Two other possible sources of infection are (1) of the eyes of babies during passage through the birth canals of infected mothers (opthalmia neonatorum), and (2) of female children through contamination with infected material, e.g., a lavatory used only minutes before by an infected person.

Symptoms appear between two and ten days after infection. In the male there is slight tingling of the urethra, followed in a day or two by a little pain on passing urine and by a purulent discharge from the urethra; but apart from these mild symptoms the patient usually does not feel ill. In the female the same symptoms occur but are often even milder and are completely absent in about one-third of cases. There is thus a faint possibility in a man and quite a chance in a woman that the disease will remain unrecognized in its early stages.

Apart from the fact that the person with unrecognized gonorrhoea can unknowingly infect a sexual partner, untreated gonorrhoea can produce serious results. In the male the condition may become chronic and cause stricture of the urethra, inflammation of the prostate gland, or infection spreading to other parts of the genito-urinary system. Similarly, in the female upward spread may involve the cervix, uterus, Fallopian tubes and ovaries with a risk of permanent sterility.

In both sexes the blood stream may spread the organism more widely to cause arthritis or heart complications.

Since the introduction of penicillin the treatment of acute gonorrhoea has become both rapid and effective. In all developed countries venereal disease clinics are accessible and well-publicized in all areas, and immediate advice should be sought when suspicious symptoms arise.

For preventive and social aspects see VENEREAL DISEASES.

gout. A disease in which there is an increase of uric acid in the blood. This results from a failure of the body-chemistry to deal with purines, which are substances produced during the digestion of protein, and which also occur naturally in certain foodstuffs. Examples are xanthine, caffein and theobromine found in tea and coffee; malt, as in beer, is also a source of xanthine.

In gout, deposits of sodium urate occur in the body tissues and especially in the cartilage of joints, to cause symptoms of acute or chronic arthritis. The cartilage of the ear is another common site, and urinary stones also occur. The deposits of sodium urate are sometimes visible as nodules called tophi.

Gout tends to be hereditary and is traditionally associated with over-indulgence in rich foods and wines, but it is relatively common in men over 30 even in the absence of such excesses.

Acute gout responds to treatment with colchicine, an alkaloid derived from the autumn crocus (*Colchicum autumnale*); and anti-inflammatory drugs such as phenylbutazone, with or without steroids, are often now used as well.

For long term treatment the aim is to prevent recurrence by lowering the uric acid blood level either by increasing the rate of uric acid excretion (cinchopen group of drugs) or diminishing its production (allopurinols). Cinchophen is toxic and its administration requires care and supervision. The diet should be adjusted to be as simple as possible with ample fluid, and purine-containing items should be restricted or eliminated.

grafting. The surgical implantation of portions of skin or bone to repair defects resulting from injury.

Skin-grafting is mainly required after extensive burns and there are several procedures. In the commonest method a strip of epidermis (the outer layer of the skin) is shaved off the thigh or upper arm and transferred to the new situation. This is relatively easy if the dermis beneath the skin graft duly grows, but if the regrowing dermis contracts, an unsightly scar may be produced.

Alternatively, a flap of skin (including dermis as well as epidermis) may be detached at one end from its original part of the body, placed in the cleaned gap, but left with the other end of the flap attached to the original part until there is a firm growth in the new situation. This method gives better cosmetic results, but for a face wound it may necessitate an arm being bound near the face for an appreciable time.

Bone-grafting is used in repair of fractures or for joint fixation. Suitable strips of bone are cut, usually from the tibia in the lower leg, and implanted to provide a scaffolding for new bone growth.

Modern organ TRANSPLANT is also a form of grafting but it is essentially the grafting of tissues or organs from one individual to another. The difficulties are of an entirely different scale of magnitude and the procedure is complicated by the body's reaction to tissues which are not its own.

granulation tissue. In a clean cut where the skin edges can be brought together, the separated tissues soon re-establish their continuity and this is known as 'healing by first intention'. If tissue is missing, as in lacerated wounds or ulcers, a vascular mass of soft tissue gradually grows from the base of the wound to fill up the deficiency and ultimately develops the epithelial form of the outer skin layer or is covered by skin. This is granulation tissue, bright red in colour and bleeding readily when touched. It contains many fibrous-tissues cells (fibroblasts) and wounds thus healing by 'granulation' or by 'second intention' produce scarring, puckering and sometimes troublesome contractures as the fibrous tissue retracts.

granuloma inguinale. A venereal disease, not uncommon in some tropical countries, characterized by ulcers in the genital region; it is in general curable by an appropriate antibiotic.

gravel. Small concretions composed of mineral salts originating in the kidney or bladder and usually causing some pain and bleeding when intermittently passed with the urine. Gravel differs from stone or CALCULUS in the urinary tract only in the size of the concretions.

Graves' disease. See GOITRE.

greenstick fracture. A fracture occurring in the long bones of children generally under the age of 12. Since the 'bone' is still cartilaginous and only partially ossified it breaks incompletely in the manner of a green twig. The bending stresses produce a fracture of the convex side of the bend and a longitudinal split of the shaft.

griping. A common term for abdominal COLIC - an intermittent type of spasmodic pain produced by excessive intestinal contractions. It is mostly used in relation to infants in whom such symptoms may reflect an unsuitable diet or an unskilful nursing technique which encourages flatulence.

Abdominal colic also occurs in more serious conditions such as enteritis, intussusception or volvulus. If it persists or recurs, or if the infant appears to be seriously affected, advice should be sought without delay.

groin. The junction of the lower abdomen and thigh on each side is marked by an oblique fold, which, with the immediately adjacent and underlying parts, is known as the groin or inguinal region.

Near the surface, the area contains lymph glands and it overlies the upper attachments of the thigh muscles on the front of the leg which swing the leg inwards. Within it runs the inguinal canal traversed in the male by the spermatic cord and by the round ligament of the uterus in the female. The large blood vessels of the leg lie below the canal.

Conditions affecting the groin are related to these structures. Local sepsis may cause enlargement and inflammation of glands (see BUBO); inguinal or femoral HERNIA may occur; in boys an undescended testis may remain in the canal. It is a common site for fungoid skin disease, favoured, especially in the obese, by moist skin surfaces rubbing together.

Pain may be a symptom of strain of the muscles, and penetrating wounds give concern because of the proximity of large blood vessels and the peritoneal cavity containing the abdominal organs.

group psychotherapy. A method of treating neurotic illnesses by assembling a small group of patients under the leadership of a psychotherapist or psychiatrist who guides and encourages them in free and frank general discussion about their individual and common problems. The members of the group become more aware of the deeper causes of their neurotic behaviour and are helped to conquer their emotional difficulties by a clearer understanding of how these are caused and by

Grafting: skin from the abdomen taken via the wrist to a site on the cheek

the mutual support which they individually receive from each other.

Group psychotherapy may be used both as an adjunct to individual psychoanalysis, or, in the view of some psychiatrists as a more effective substitute.

The underlying principles of group psychotherapy are also employed (not necessarily with professional supervision and leadership) in the support of people with a variety of personality problems, such as alcoholism, gambling, smoking and drug taking. Associations, such as Alcoholics Anonymous, exist to encourage such activities and undoubtedly achieve good results.

Since the success of group psychotherapy depends on the participants being able to talk freely and make confident personal relationships amongst themselves, it is important that groups should not be too large. Five to ten persons is regarded as the optimal size.

growing pains. Limb and joint pains in young children were formerly regarded as an almost normal accompaniment of growth but rheumatic infection in childhood is often an insidious disease which may ultimately cause serious damage, especially to the heart. So such pains should not be ignored, especially if there are other suggestive symptoms such as recurrent sore throat, pallor, fatigue, loss of appetite, failure to develop healthily, or jerky movements.

'Growing pains' should be investigated. This will usually entail electrocardiographs and blood tests. One simple test is to note the pulse-rate when asleep; it may not show the normal slowing-down. If suspicions of rheumatic infection are confirmed, long-term penicillin may be advised as a preventive measure.

Other causes of pain in childhood are often related to some orthopaedic defect – flat feet or weak ankles – especially if the pain occurs towards the end of the day or after over-fatigue, or during rapid growth.

These conditions need appropriate treatment with attention to footwear. Muscular tone can be improved by exercises, massage and improved general nutrition.

growth. The word has several meanings. In phrases like 'growth in the breast' it is used as an alternative to tumour; in phrases like 'the child's mental and physical growth' it means development; but when we speak of 'growth of cells' or 'population growth' we are talking principally of increase in size. The present article concerns the latter meaning.

Biological growth. In many organisms the increase in size from conception to adult status is of astronomical proportions. For instance, a full-grown man is thousands of millions times larger than the fertilized ovum from which he originated. Even so, the adult body is not complete and permanent, except in form, because there is a constant interchange as cells waste away and are replaced. Similarly, with a part of the body such as the skull, it is clear that it cannot grow in a simple way of just adding cell to cell. It must increase in size by additions on the exterior and removals on the interior in order to maintain its shape.

Even as simple increase in size biological growth must be considered as two processes. One of these is the formation of inert matter to produce an end-product, an accretion, or a crop. Obvious examples are the hair, the nails and the outer layers of the skin; less obvious are accumulations of fat and glycogen; still less obvious are the blood cells, both red and white corpuscles, which are manufactured from cells in the bone-marrow and cast out into the blood-stream. In health the cells that manufacture corpuscles are never found in the blood; they stay in the bone-marrow and maintain their numbers by cell-division.

Cell-division is the other type of biological growth. It is multiplicative and always associated with the activity of nucleo-protein whereby two strands of nucleic acid replace a single ancestor in continuous succession. Outside the body, as in tissue culture, cells grow like this indefinitely if food is provided and waste-matter removed. What is still not certain is whether this is their normal behaviour or whether their unnatural environment has caused some change in their metabolism. Whatever the reason there must be some difference to account for their behaviour, because land animals do not grow indefinitely and something must determine this. It may in fact be only the geometry of size in relation to design. Weight-bearing capabilities impose an effective limit on size and undoubtedly contributed to the evolutionary disappearance of the very large animals of prehistoric times. Aquatic animals, because they are supported in water, are not subject to the same limitations and so we have whales ten times as heavy as the largest elephant (10 tons) and many fish which continue to grow throughout their life. Another interesting point is that growth is not necessarily irreversible; the absence of a skeleton allows some simple animals to reduce in size when food is short.

Biological growth is best studied by graphs plotting size (or for technical reasons the logarithm of size) against age. Broadly the curve starts off slowly as cells adapt to their environment, then accelerates rapidly but at diminishing rate and finally levels off. In other words, the rate of multiplication of cells falls progressively, as if living matter steadily lost its ability to maintain its early reproductive rate. This has been expressed as Minot's Paradox which says that organisms age fastest in their youth.

Population growth. Although there is a record of a Russian mother reputed to have had sixty-nine children (including seven sets of triplets!) a more reasonable figure for human fecundity, or maxium reproductive capacity, is probably about twenty.

Fertility however means the average number of children born to the mothers of a given population and it is this which determines what will happen to the size of a population.

In projections of population growth it is only the numbers of females which are of importance. If the women of the present generation produce an average of one female child each who survive to become the possible mothers of the future, the net reproductive rate is 1.0 and the population will remain static. The calculation of this rate from the recorded births has of course to take account of current mortality trends.

If the net reproductive rate is greater than one the population can be expected to grow. When populations grow they grow exponentially; that is to say they continually double in unit-time if fertility and mortality are constant. The length of the time-unit depends on the net reproductive rate; if it is 2.0 the population will double in a generation. This is the problem of the less well-developed countries with average families of six, and hence about three girl-children per mother.

However, in the past infant and child mortality were such that by no means all girls survived to reproductive ages, so despite large families population increased by under 50 per cent in each generation. With improvements in health services and medical care this figure is rapidly rising and short of cataclysm nothing can avert the difficulties which will be created when great sections of world population double in the next generation. Fertility is of course very sensitive to economic conditions and to cultural practices, and may be changed radically by the wider use of contraception; but the likely size of populations thirty years hence is already set by the numbers of children now alive.

growth in childhood. Amongst mammals the state of development of their offspring at birth varies very widely. At one end of the scale we have young animals like colts, calves or lambs who can stand up and move independently as soon as they are born and at the other end helpless blind kittens and still-foetal marsupials, like young kangaroos, who require to be sheltered in a maternal pouch.

The human infant is something of a compromise between the advantages of being born in a state of developmental advancement and the disadvantage of the birth-hazards imposed by his relatively large brain and head. At birth he is uncommonly helpless and dependent but his sensory system is well-developed and he is well-equipped to demand the attention which his senses tell him that he needs.

On average the new-born infant weighs about 3.4 kg. (7.5 lb.) and a relatively large proportion of this is fat. During the first nine months weight growth is rapid – a useful rule-of-thumb is that birth weight should double in six months and treble in a year. Most of this weight gain is still skeletal growth and fat, but at about a year old there is a shift in emphasis from fat to muscle as the child learns to move independently and begins to walk, and this happens again at about 5 years as activity increases still more.

After one year of age the rate of growth is much less: although birth weight trebled in the first year it does not treble again until the child is 9; however, from 10 onwards children begin to enter into the period of puberty, a new phase of accelerated growth with increased metabolic activity, increased food uptake, and a corresponding increase of tissue-mass. The weight gain in the six years from the age of 10 to 16 is approximately the same as in the nine years from 1 to 10.

Although children at birth weigh on average about 3.4 kg. and are about 50 cm. (20 in.) long there are wide variations even allowing for the fact that girls tend to be slightly smaller. Basically, size and weight depend on two factors – the size of the parents and the length of the development in the uterus before birth.

Growth after birth depends very much on nutrition. If this is good, departures from the average are likely to be due to inherited characteristics, but malnourished, sick, or debilitated children show major delays in both growth and development. In underdeveloped countries where there is total calorie and protein deprivation, a child of 6 may only be as large as one of 4 from countries where nutrition is adequate. Over-nutrition and under-exercise however produce opposite effects and there is some evidence that growth rate is related inversely to length of life.

Since at least the year 1800 people have been growing bigger and maturing earlier. This has been due to improved nutrition with adequate calories, protein and vitamins on the one hand, and on the other, reduced energy expenditure from warmer homes, better clothing and no child-labour. The energy thus saved is spared to be available for growth. Another testimony to better early nutrition is the lowering of the age of onset of menstruation, which has fallen from 15 to 13 or less.

Although it has been shown that many factors can effect growth there have been attempts to arrive at some formula by which ultimate stature can be predicted. As a general rule it can be said that the length of male infants at birth is about 27 per cent of their adult stature. The corresponding figure for females is 30 per cent. Girls reach 90 per cent of their final height by 12 and boys by 14. Another way of estimating is to determine 'skeletal age' as opposed to chronological age. This can be done by x-raying the hand to examine the stage of ossification – that is, the change from cartilage to bone; the pattern of ossification is very regular in relation to stages of development.

Over-nutrition is perhaps the chief danger of the present generation in developed countries. Fat children tend to grow up to be fat adults with reduced life-expectancy, and children over-large and over-mature for their age by comparison with their contemporaries tend to develop psychological difficulties.

gullet. See OESOPHAGUS.

gumboil. An abscess occurring within the expanded margins of the upper and lower jaws containing the teeth and covered by the gums.

The abscess is usually associated with the fang of a decayed tooth and infection makes its way down the pulp-canal and through the opening at the end of the root to infect the tooth-socket. Suppuration ensues with swelling and pain, and pus ultimately tracks through the bony socket and overlying gum or between the tooth and the wall of the socket.

Treatment is by hot mouth-washes to hasten suppuration and evacuation of pus, and by the administration of analgesics and an antibiotic. Surgical incision may be required when the abscess shows signs of 'pointing' (i.e., coming to the point at which the surface breaks) but sometimes the associated tooth will have to be extracted. Dental treatment is needed in any event. With proper care of the teeth and regular visits to the dentist, gumboils should seldom if ever occur.

gumma. A painless inflammatory swelling occurring in the tertiary or late stages of SYPHILIS and resulting from tissue reaction to the continued presence of the infecting organism, the thread-like *Treporema pallidum*.

gums. The layer of tissue (gingiva) which covers the tooth-bearing margins of the jaws. Gum-tissue consists of a dense fibrous layer connected to the underlying bone and covered on its surface by vascular membranes. Extensions of the gums, known as papillae, occupy the spaces between the necks of the teeth and prevent lodgement of food-debris.

Diseases. Inflammation of the gums is known as gingivitis; the gums become congested and often bleed, either when food is being chewed or when the teeth are being brushed. There is also some tenderness, so that solid food tends to be swallowed without chewing, creating risk of indigestion. At a late stage the gum margins may shrink away from the teeth, leaving the necks of the teeth exposed.

Apart from occurring in certain serious diseases (e.g., scurvy) and certain acute poisonings (e.g., by mercury) gingivitis starts gradually through defects of dental hygiene, allowing food debris to collect and to form breeding grounds for bacteria. Care of the gums, by regular brushing, massage and the removal of debris before it destroys gum-tissue by pressure can help to prevent gingivitis. Treatment involves removal of all debris (usually by a dentist), mouth washes and daily massage of the gums with the finger.

Advancing age may cause the gums to recede, allowing infection to reach the sockets and loosen the teeth.

gynaecology. The branch of medicine which deals with diseases peculiar to women and in particular those involving the genito-urinary tract and the hormonal control of the reproductive system. Doctors practising gynaecology are known as gynaecologists but the speciality is nearly always combined with obstetrics which deals with pregnancy and childbirth.

Gynaecologists also concern themselves with problems of contraception and the investigation and treatment of sub-fertility and sterility.

H

habit. A fixed or constant routine practice established by constant repetition.

Most habits are physical actions of one kind or another forming a response acquired by deliberate or unconscious learning, but mental reactions and the formation of thoughts and ideas may be similarly conditioned. Once established, habits are remarkably stable; they tend to become automatic or easily elicited, and they are difficult to break.

The importance of habit as a mainspring of conduct was first pointed out in a systematic way by William James (1842-1910), the American psychologist and philosopher (and brother of Henry James, the novelist). He was of course only emphasizing the tenets of universal experience enshrined in traditional sayings such as 'Practise makes perfect' and 'Train up the child in the way he should go; when he is old he will not depart therefrom'.

In his classic work *The Principles of Psychology* he stated, in a wider and more philosophical vein, 'Habit is the enormous flywheel of society and its most precious conservative agent. It alone is what keeps us all within the bounds of ordinance. . . .'

The effect of habit is to simplify the movements required to achieve a desired result, to make them more accurate, and to minimize fatigue; indeed a purpose of all education is to make useful actions automatic and habitual. The acquisition of a new habit or the breaking of an old one requires motivation, repetition and resolution to persist. After the age of 30 it becomes increasingly difficult to alter a person's character and behaviour.

'You cannot teach an old dog new tricks'. The same principles hold good in the inculcation of new ideas, and the psychological techniques of influencing the young by the constant repetition of exhortations (usually under conditions where members of a group reinforce each other) are the methods of the more unscrupulous political leaders.

Health education. In any developed country elaborate measures are now taken to protect people from every conceivable hazard in their environment. There remain malign influences which only individuals themselves can overcome – obesity, alcoholism, smoking, uncleanliness, carelessness and disregard for others, to name only a few.

The task of those undertaking HEALTH EDUCATION is to apply to the community at large the principles of habit formation and habit alteration in relation to patterns of conduct which will best serve the purposes of better health for all.

habit spasm. See TIC.

haematemesis. Vomiting of blood. The bleeding usually comes from a chronic ulcer of the stomach or duodenum and may be very considerable. Other causes are carcinoma of the stomach and varicose veins at the lower end of the oesophagus (usually associated with liver disease). Susceptible persons may develop gastric bleeding after taking aspirin, and rarer causes include a form of anaemia and a form of purpura.

In contrast with blood from the respiratory tract (haemoptysis), vomited blood is usually brownish rather than red owing to alteration by the gastric juice; it is acid in reaction because it is mixed with stomach contents; and it is vomited rather than coughed up.

The treatment is complete rest and sedation with transfusions of saline, plasma, or whole blood if necessary. Fluid by mouth is avoided for two 'or three days followed by gradual return to a suitable light diet. Cases of recurrent haematemesis may require an operation.

haematoma. An accumulation of blood which has leaked into the tissues usually resulting from violence without an external wound, as in blows from a blunt instrument or falls on a hard surface. Milder injuries, which have broken the blood vessels but caused less damage to the tissues, result in BRUISES, when the blood is diffused and does not accumulate.

Head injuries may be seriously complicated by a haematoma within the skull.

A haematoma sometimes occurs after surgical operations when failure to secure complete stoppage of bleeding allows further bleeding within the operation site.

The area over a haematoma is swollen, tender, discoloured and fluctuant to touch. Small haematomatas generally disperse and absorb spontaneously; if large they will require to be drained.

haematuria. The presence of blood in the urine due to haemorrhage in the urinary tract. The appearance of the urine may range from deep-red to faint pink depending on the amount of bleeding, or red-cells may only be detectable microscopically.

Although haematuria may occur in a variety of general medical conditions, it is more usually due to some local abnormality affecting the urinary tract. Stones in kidney or bladder, infections (including tuberculosis), malignant growths and prostatic enlargement are the commonest causes. In 'essential haematuria' no obvious cause can be found and the bleeding probably proceeds from some congenital weakness in the kidney.

Haematuria always calls for investigation, and treatment will be for the condition which is causing the bleeding.

haemoglobin. The oxygen-carrying pigment of the red blood corpuscles. It is a complex organic compound composed of a protein globin combined with haematin, which is a compound of iron and porphyrin (the latter being one of a class of coloured substances widely distributed in nature, as in plant chlorophyll and the pigments of feathers).

Haemoglobin is thus made up of globin-porphyrin-iron. It forms a loose compound with oxygen-oxyhaemoglobin – which readily gives up oxygen on tissue demand to become reduced haemoglobin.

Aerated blood from the lungs, passing along the arteries, contains oxyhaemoglobin and is bright red. It returns from the body by the veins, stripped of its oxygen, and then has the bluish-red colour of reduced haemoglobin.

Assessment of anaemia measures the amount of haemoglobin in blood. The normal figure is 14.8 grammes per 100 ml. of blood.

Some hereditary abnormalities in the haemoglobin molecule are related to certain rare blood diseases such as sickle-cell anaemia and thalassaemia.

haemolysis. A breakdown of the membranes of red blood corpuscles so that their contained haemoglobin is liberated into the plasma. It is caused by osmosis when the pressure of the corpuscles and the plasma is unbalanced, so that plasma diffuses into the corpuscles which swell and ultimately rupture.

Haemolysis occurs in certain hereditary and acquired types of anaemia (the hereditary acholuric jaundice being perhaps the best known), in destruction of red blood cells by parasites (as in malaria) and in some allergic conditions.

haemophilia. A disease in which blood clotting is abnormally delayed. It is a sex-linked inherited condition which affects only males (see GENETICS). However, the genetic defect is carried on the mother's X chromosome so that an affected male cannot pass the defect to his sons with the result that the occurrence of cases in a family always skips a generation.

Haemophiliacs bleed excessively from trivial wounds and may bleed internally into muscles and joints with resultant disability. Care should be taken to avoid any injury.

Blood clotting is a complex process primarily initiated by the ferment thromboplastin liberated from damaged areas, from the plasma, and from the plasma platelets which adhere to injured tissues.

In haemophilia there is absence of this 'clotting-factor' or anti-haemophilic factor (AHF). In Christmas disease (named after the patient first described) there is absence of other related factors – thromboplastin component

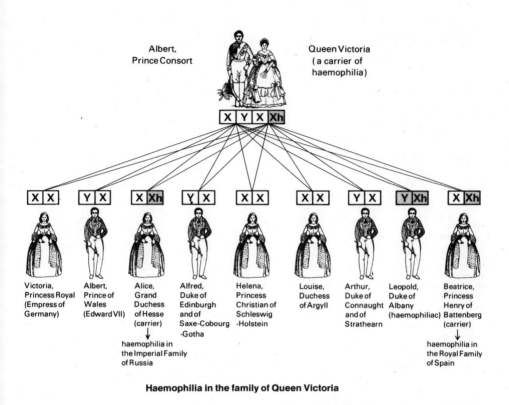

Albert,
Prince Consort

Queen Victoria
(a carrier of
haemophilia)

X Y X Xh

| X X | Y X | X Xh | Y X | X X | X X | Y X | Y Xh | X Xh |

Victoria,
Princess Royal
(Empress of
Germany)

Albert,
Prince of
Wales
(Edward VII)

Alice,
Grand
Duchess
of Hesse
(carrier)

↓
haemophilia in
the Imperial Family
of Russia

Alfred,
Duke of
Edinburgh
and of
Saxe-Cobourg
-Gotha

Helena,
Princess
Christian of
Schleswig
-Holstein

Louise,
Duchess
of Argyll

Arthur,
Duke of
Connaught
and of
Strathearn

Leopold,
Duke of
Albany
(haemophiliac)

Beatrice,
Princess
Henry of
Battenberg
(carrier)

↓
haemophilia in
the Royal Family
of Spain

Haemophilia in the family of Queen Victoria

(PTC) or plasma thromboplastin antecedent (PTA).

Certain hospitals are designated as haemophilia centres and sufferers should register locally because minor injuries and operations require special measures such as plasma transfusion and administration of concentrated AHF.

haemoptysis. The spitting of blood from structures below the larynx, especially the lungs. The blood is bright, frothy and alkaline, whereas in haematemesis (vomiting of blood from the stomach) the blood is dark or brownish and acid. Causes of haemoptysis include pulmonary tuberculosis, cancer of the lung or bronchus, chronic venous congestion as in mitral stenosis, bronchiectasis, various parasitic diseases, scurvy, and occasionally smallpox and measles. Treatment varies with the cause.

Confusion with bleeding from the nose, nasopharynx or spongy gums (sometimes termed spurious haemoptysis) is unlikely.

haemorrhage. The formal term for bleeding, defined as any escape of blood from the blood-vessels. For immediate treatment see FIRST AID.

Bleeding from various sites is given special names: (1) from the lungs and air-passage, haemoptysis; (2) from stomach or duodenum via mouth, haematemesis; (3) from bowel, melaena; (4) from urinary tract, haematuria;

(5) from the nose, epistaxis; (6) abnormal uterine bleeding, metrorrhagia.

Primary haemorrhage is the immediate result of injury to a blood-vessel and its characteristics vary according to the type of vessel: (1) arterial, which is bright red and pulsating; (2) venous, which is dark-blue or purple and in a steady stream; (3) capillary, which is a steady reddish ooze from cut tissues where no large vessel is involved.

Reactionary haemorrhage is the recurrence of bleeding from a wound within twenty-four hours of initial stopping. It may be due to slipping of an insecure ligature or to the restoration of normal blood pressure which displaces the clots.

Secondary haemorrhage is recurrence of bleeding after a period of twenty-four hours without bleeding. This happens when infection in the wound weakens the walls of blood vessels, which give way under pressure. It usually occurs eight to ten days after injury.

If blood escapes through a wound in the skin it is said to be external haemorrhage, but if it escapes into the tissues under undamaged skin it is said to be extravasated and the result is a bruise or a haematoma. If blood escapes from damaged vessels into the body cavities, the result is a concealed or internal haemorrhage; this may be difficult to diagnose except by the general signs of haemorrhage.

Features. The local signs of external

haemorrhage are obvious. In cases of internal haemorrhage, pain, tenderness and dullness on percussion over body cavities may provide the doctor with an indication of the site of any haemorrhage when general symptoms arouse suspicion of its occurrence.

The general signs of severe haemorrhage are those of shock and collapse owing to diminished blood volume so that less blood reaches the brain. The patient is restless, feels faint and looks pale; the skin is blanched, cold, and clammy; the respiration is in rapid gasps and distressed; there is apprehension and complaint of thirst, and the pulse is rapid, weak and easily compressible. If the haemorrhage is not controlled unconsciousness and death soon supervene.

Children and old persons bear loss of blood badly but while the former rapidly recover from the effects, recuperation is slow in the aged.

The body's reactions to haemorrhage are clotting of the blood, contraction and retraction of the walls of cut vessels and the fall of blood pressure which occurs after severe haemorrhage.

Treatment. The active treatment of haemorrhage is by immediate arrest of the bleeding at the point of severance of the vessel. In venous and capillary bleeding local pressure usually suffices. In arterial bleeding pressure should be applied to a 'pressure point' between the wound and the heart. These are points at which the arteries are close to a bone so that the pressure is more effective in reducing blood-flow. Alternatively the wound may require to be explored and the cut ends secured by ligature. Application of a tourniquet is a temporary expedient only: it will cause gangrene of a limb if left on too long.

Styptics, applications which contract the blood vessels or hasten clotting time, are sometimes useful for capillary bleeding, and elevation of a limb combined with local pressure will always stop venous bleeding.

The general symptoms of haemorrhage should be treated by warmth, fluids, elevation of the foot of the bed, cardiac stimulants and in severe cases transfusion of plasma or whole blood.

haemorrhoid. See PILE.

Hahnemann. A German physician, Christian Frederic Samuel Hahnemann (1755-1843), was the founder of HOMEOPATHY.

hair. A single hair is a filamentous outgrowth on the surface of the body derived from the cells forming the skin; hair, collectively, is an aggregation of such filaments covering the scalp and some other parts of the body.

Hairs are found on nearly every part of the body-surface except the palms and soles but they vary very much in length, thickness and colour. A hair consists of a root implanted in the skin and a shaft or projecting part. The root is lodged in a skin depression called a hair-follicle and at its base it is expanded as the hair-bulb which contains the hair-papilla or growing point supplied with blood vessels and nerve fibres. This is continuous with the cells of the dermis or true skin.

Opening into the follicle, near its outer end, are the ducts of one or more sebaceous glands to provide an oily dressing for the hair so as to maintain its lustre and waterproof qualities. Straight hairs are round or oval in cross section

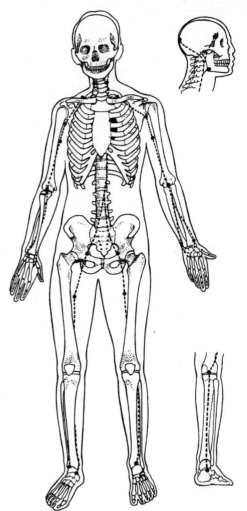

Haemorrhage: the skeleton, principal arteries and pressure points

and grow from straight follicles. They are generally stronger than curly hairs which are flattened and owe their curliness to a curve in the follicle.

Care. One of our poets spoke of 'live hair that is shining and free' and his conception is expressive of the aesthetic ideal which hair-care seeks to achieve. Hair, despite the poet, is a dead structure, but if it is kept clean, untangled and not deprived of its natural oils it will remain glistening and mobile and give an appearance of healthy vitality.

The routine of normal care for the hair is simple. It should include a weekly shampoo and thorough combing and brushing every day. The natural oily dressing of the hair is provided by the sebaceous glands around the hair-follicles and brushing stimulates the scalp and glandular activity and helps to disperse the secretion along the hair. Harsh soaps should be avoided since they dissolve the sebaceous material and leave the hair dull and lustreless. Proprietary shampoos are less apt to do this and if the hair is exceptionally 'dry' application of olive oil, lanolin, vaseline, or special dressings which mimic the natural secretion will ensure an attractive sheen.

Permanent waving is carried out by forming the hair round rollers and applying heat or chemicals so that it retains the required curvatures. The chemicals may effect sensitive skins and the risk of this should be ascertained beforehand by testing a small area. Hair dyes require similar precautions.

In certain circumstances hair requires more particular attention. The scalp hair may harbour the head-louse (*Pediculus capitis*) a well-known parasite. The female lays eggs called nits which adhere to the hairs at their roots. This infestation (pediculosis) is particularly likely to be found in school children or even in adults, especially if they have elaborate coiffures which they are reluctant to disturb unduly. A search of the scalp will disclose nits and the hair should then be treated with an insecticidal shampoo and thoroughly fine-tooth combed to get rid of nits.

Dandruff is an accumulation of fine flakes of the dead superficial layers of the skin of the scalp. It may be occasioned by deficiency or excess of normal sweat secretion or there may be a low-grade superficial infection of the sweat glands (seborrhoea). The scalp should be washed several times a week using a detergent shampoo. Preparations containing 1 per cent cetrimide are available and are of service in true seborrhoea because of their anti-infective properties.

Superfluous hair. Hair grows on most parts of the body. If it is so profuse, long, or dark at any site as not to conform with fashion or conventional appearance it is known as superfluous hair. Women in particular are distressed by the growth of obvious facial hair, by hairy legs, or by the occurrence of isolated long hairs on the face or neck.

Various methods are employed to eradicate superfluous hair or to minimize its anti-cosmetic effect. Bleaching with hydrogen peroxide will make it less obvious, commercially produced chemical or wax depilatories will remove it temporarily, or some areas can be shaved. Isolated single hairs can be pulled out by tweezers and because of resultant damage to the hair-papilla take longer to grow again than if cut.

Electrolysis will destroy unwanted hair permanently but is impracticable except for limited use and it requires expert use to avoid scarring.

halibut oil. A liquid fat obtained from the liver of the halibut. It contains vitamin A and vitamin D and is a much richer source of both than cod-liver oil. Since fish-oils are not very palatable it is advantageous to be able to give the required dosage of vitamins in a smaller bulk of oil.

Commercial preparations are available in vials with a dropping-pipette or as three minim capsules which are the equivalent of four teaspoonfuls of cod-liver oil. The recommended daily dosage is for infants eight to ten drops, and for adults one or two capsules.

hallitosis. See BREATH, OFFENSIVE.

hallucination. Something perceived or appreciated by the senses which has no basis in reality. Hallucinations may thus be sensations of seeing, hearing, smelling or touching and they are most commonly experienced by patients with mental disease or persons under the influence of drugs. They may also be provoked by extreme fatigue or by emotional stress.

A peculiar example affecting the proprioceptive senses (i.e., awareness, of the body and its position in space) is the so-called 'phantom limb', a condition in which a patient who has lost a limb experiences sensations which persuade him that the amputated member is still there.

Hallucination must be distinguished from DELUSION in which there is a false belief rather than a false sensation.

hallucinogen. A drug which alters mental and emotional processes, producing visual or auditory hallucinations. The commonest are (1) cannabis (marihuana or hashish), a mild and probably non-addictive hallucinogen with a long history of ritual use in certain religious cults; (2) mescaline, which produces stronger dreams or ecstatic states; and (3) LSD, which produces a state of mental disorientation thought to resemble that of schizophrenia.

None of the hallucinogens has much medical application and the unauthorized possession of any of them is illegal in Britain; but while at the one extreme LSD is generally recognized as highly dangerous, at the other extreme cannabis is judged by many experts to do no more harm than tobacco or alcohol.

hallux valgus. See TOE.

hammer toe. See TOE.

hamstring muscles. A group of muscles at the back of the thigh which are attached by tendons to the bones of the lower leg. These muscles by contracting bend the knee, and they also take part in straightening the hip.

hand. Apart from his superior brain capacity man owes his success in evolutionary terms largely to the design of his hand which provides a thumb which is capable of reaching across to the fingers, so that grasping is strengthened and precise manipulation is made possible. This ability is common to the higher mammals, known as primates, which include man and the apes, monkeys and lemurs.

The skeleton of the hand consists of the wrist (or carpus), made up of eight small bones articulating with each other and with the bones of the forearm; the palm (or metacarpus) consisting of five elongated bones known as metacarpals; and the five fingers or digits, which each contain three phalanges – except in the thumb, which has only two.

The movements of the hand and fingers are produced mainly by muscles situated in the forearm whose power is transmitted by long tendons running in tendon-sheaths to their points of attachment. There are also palm muscles concerned with movements of the thumb and little finger and with the spreading of the other digits.

On the palmar surface the skin of the hand is thick and dense and firmly attached to the underlying tissues. It shows characteristic markings especially over the tips of the fingers where the highly individual patterns provide the basis for the science of identification by FINGERPRINTS. The extremities of the fingers are protected by the nails which have evolved from claws originally intended as weapons, tools or grasping equipment.

Inspection of the nails can be a useful diagnostic procedure since they may show 'clubbing' in severe respiratory or cardiac disease or other abnormalities of shape, colour, or texture. Examination of the hand as a whole may often be equally informative. Its general position, the condition of the skin, the presence of rheumatic nodules, twitching of small muscles, and general tremor, can all provide clues for the acute observer.

Diseases. As a universal tool, the hand is particularly exposed to injury – burns, cuts, penetrating wounds, impact, crushing, dislocation and peculiar damage such as having skin stripped off by machinery.

Burns and cuts present no special features and are treated on routine principles. Bleeding from cuts is generally profuse, and they should be carefully sutured especially on the palm, where an irregular painful scar may cause later disability. Special attention should be given to antisepsis since deep infections can be troublesome. In the palm infection can spread in the tissue spaces and into tendon-sheaths to cause a painful abscess and later disability if the tendons become fixed by scar-tissue.

A whitlow is an acute septic inflammation of the deep tissues in a finger, often developing at the side of the base of a nail. The cause is infection by bacteria, usually through a prick with a dirty pin or other sharp object. The main symptoms are throbbing pain, swelling and redness; and if the condition remains untreated there is danger of the infection spreading over the hand and extending up the arm. In cases treated early hot fomentations or kaolin poultices often suffice. In more severe cases an appropriate antibiotic or sulphonamide may be required, and sometimes an incision is needed to allow pus to escape.

Fractures are common in crush and impact injuries. Any of the palm or finger bones may be broken and are best healed in plaster of Paris with traction if necessary to secure good position. Bennett's fracture is a fracture of the base of the thumb – a common injury in boxing. It is difficult to reduce satisfactorily, and may cause arthritis later. 'Mallet-finger' results from cutting the tendon on the top of a finger, so that the finger cannot be straightened at the last joint. If not recognized at the time of injury and appropriately treated, an operation may be required.

Dupuytren's contracture is a permanent bending towards the palm of the little finger and sometimes also of the ring and middle fingers. This is due to contraction of the tissues of the palm often caused by repeated irritation as from pressure of tools on the palm and hence seen in various tradesmen.

handicapped persons. People with appreciable and lasting physical or mental disability. Although the general meaning is clear enough the exact definition varies from country to country and even from district to district. There are at least three reasons for this variation.

1. There is no universal acceptance of what degree of disability is appreciable enough to be designated a handicap. For instance, in the U.K. there are about five-million persons who have some pain and limitation of movement from osteoarthritis or rheumatoid arthritis: are all of them handicapped, or only the 150,000 who are housebound, or does the boundary lie somewhere between minor pain and stiffness and inability to go beyond the house? Again, a blind person clearly has a serious handicap but may be perfectly capable of earning a living; a person with full vision in one eye and blind in the other is incapacitated from certain jobs but is obviously not a handicapped person, but at exactly what point in partial sightedness is the term applicable?

2. There is no general agreement as to how lasting a condition must be before the person is graded as handicapped. Probably in all countries a person with a serious inherited disability, e.g., spina bifida or phenylketonuria, would be deemed handicapped, although in some cases of spina bifida surgical operations can remove the handicap and in most cases of phenylketonuria early and continued dietetic treatment can convert the person to a normal individual. In most of the advanced countries a person with a paralysed limb following a stroke would not be classified as handicapped until after treatment and rehabilitation had failed to restore the limb to functioning capacity: but experts differ as to how long these measures should be continued before being regarded as having failed.

3. Handicapped persons are often divided into handicapped children and handicapped adults, but exact meanings differ. In the U.K., for example, a handicapped child is between the age of birth and 16 years, and there are fairly specific criteria for the borders of the various types – blind, partially sighted, deaf, partially deaf, educationally subnormal, maladjusted, physically handicapped, and so on; but neither the age range nor the criteria are identical with those in other countries; and in Britain itself large regional differences in the proportions of children with handicaps of different types (e.g., a variation in educationally subnormal children from under five per thousand children in the south-east to over nine per thousand in Wales) suggest that standards of assessment are far from uniform. For handicapped adults criteria are usually much less clearly defined and the term is sometimes used to cover all handicapped persons other than children, and at other times employed merely for handicapped persons of working age. Clearly for estimating things like the amount of need for help it is desirable to include all adults, but for considering the need for sheltered workshops or special training only persons below pensionable age need be counted.

Because of such differences, international comparisons are not of much value, but as a rough indication of prevalence it may be mentioned that in the U.K. about a million people (almost 2 per cent of the population) are on disability registers, and the numbers are growing slightly each year – partly because of the greater survival of handicapped infants and partly because of general prolongation of life and the frequency of handicap in the very old.

Services for handicapped children, e.g., open-air day or residential schools for delicate children, are not further considered in this article.

For handicapped adults most of the advanced countries have some residential provisions, such as hostels for the infirm elderly, occupation centres for the mentally handicapped and special centres for some varieties of physically handicapped persons. The latter may be long-term centres or short-term resettlement centres which seek to help the individual (e.g., after a long illness in hospital) to become able to cope with a domestic environment or to resume some form of remunerative employment.

By reason of sheer numbers, however, the vast majority of handicapped adults must live in their own homes. Where the handicap is severe and they are living alone they are often struggling desperately to keep going and to maintain their independence against progressively disabling disease, and in great need of help which may range from assistance with the heavier aspects of housework to personal help over such things as dressing and washing. Where the handicapped person lives with a relative he may have more physical help and more companionship but if there is no external aid the strain on the relative is enormous.

Available services vary from country to country but those of the U.K. may be outlined as illustrative. Britain, apart from Northern Ireland, has separated its health services and social services, and there are really four components.

1. Ascertainment of handicap and of changes from time to time needed in the nature and amount of help is inevitably done mainly by health workers, in particular health visitors, home nurses and general medical practitioners. The health visitors also give guidance on many problems of physical and emotional health; the home nurses undertake any skilled nursing required; and the doctors are concerned both with medical treatment at home and with questions of temporary or permanent admission to a geriatric hospital.

2. Financial aid is provided from national funds at specified rates, and from national funds also come certain expensive items of equipment.

3. Personal services, other than preventive and remedial medical and nursing treatment, are the reponsibility of the social work department of the local authority. These services may include practical assistance with housework (e.g., the supplying of a part-time home help), a mobile meals service, provision of social centres and appropriate recreational facilities (and transport to them), provision of library and wireless facilities, assistance with adaptations to the house (e.g., a widened door to the toilet to permit access of a wheel chair), provision of suitable appliances, assistance with home employment and with the marketing of goods produced, provision of subsidized or free holidays, and admission to old people's homes or appropriate centres.

4. Voluntary bodies play important roles supplying visitors to reduce the loneliness of the handicapped and producing many appropriate gadgets for their use, and in some cases providing residential homes or special centres. However, since the registered handicapped are equivalent to almost 2 per cent of the entire population, or equal to about 3 per cent of the total population of working age, and since there are an even greater number of elderly persons who need some help but are not registered as handicapped, the services are necessarily thinly spread. This applies whether we think of geriatric hospitals (with shortage of nurses), of old people's homes and special centres (with difficulty of providing enough staff without excessive burden on the ratepayers), of health visitors (in short supply and with important duties to the young in addition to ascertainment, advice and guidance for the handicapped and the elderly), of home nurses, of social workers, of home helps or of any other workers.

There is no easy solution to the vast problem of catering for the needs of the steadily increasing number of handicapped persons. Clearly in the health field there is a spectrum of health and disease services — fostering of good health, prevention of disease, diagnosis of illness or defect, treatment, rehabilitation, and supportive care of the physically or mentally handicapped. If decisions are left mainly to health workers they may feel that public money is more usefully devoted to the prevention of handicaps (e.g., reducing diseases of hereditary origin, removing the main causes of stroke and coronary thrombosis, vaccinating against diseases like poliomyelitis and preventing the known causes of osteoarthritis) or to the treatment and rehabilitation of such persons as can be restored to full working capacity than to helping those who are incurable. In other words, they may seek to concentrate scarce resources on the provision of more health education officers and health visitors, or more hospital nurses and physiotherapists. Yet in common humanity we cannot let the handicapped drag out the remainder of their lives with minimum subsistence and minimal help. On the other hand, where social services and health services are separated they compete for scarce funds (and if social services get the bulk on humanitarian grounds there is an unending increase in the numbers of handicapped persons). There is also constant argument between health workers and social workers about whether a person who can no longer manage at home is more suitable for a short-staffed geriatric hospital or for a short-staffed old people's home; social workers are dependent on health workers both for diagnosis of the original handicap and its extent and for information about changes in the medical condition perhaps necessitating more help; and health visitors and other health workers, after recommending perhaps an additional home help session per week for a deteriorating client or a bath grip for a person who has difficulty in getting out of a bath, feel frustrated when their recommendation is 'checked' by a social worker of short training and with very little health knowledge, and even more frustrated when the duly corroborated recommendation fails to produce prompt action.

Whether health services and social services are better combined or separate is arguable, but it is clear that, as the number of handicapped persons increases, the solution is threefold: such increase as the national economy can stand in health workers concerned with the prevention of handicap; such increase as the economy can stand in paid workers for support of the handicapped (e.g., home helps); and extensive use of voluntary workers, particularly persons in the first decade of retirement, themselves still physically and mentally fit and prepared to act as part-time unskilled assistants both to health workers and to social workers.

hand-washing and food sanitation. Bacterial food poisoning and other infections such as dysentery are due to micro-organisms derived from the intestinal tracts of persons who may or may not show signs of disease. Some are also of direct animal origin and appear in raw foodstuffs, particularly meat and poultry.

Such organisms are thus very apt to be spread to other persons, especially by food-handlers who do not thoroughly wash their hands after visiting the toilet, or who handle raw meat and then proceed to prepare other food. Staphylococcal food poisoning may also be passed on by hands contaminated by discharges from skin diseases, superficial injuries, boils or infections of the nose, throat and ear.

All toilets should therefore be equipped with wash-hand basins and with hot water, soap, nail-brush and individual arrangements for hand-drying – paper towels or hot air. Food-handlers should be impressed with the need to use these facilities, and the advice is equally applicable in the home.

Steps should also be taken to minimize opportunities for hand contamination – no smoking; do not touch mouth, nose, hair, etc. at work; wash hands after using handkerchief; handle food with fork, tongs, etc.

hangover. A colloquial term for the unpleasant after-effects of over-indulgence in alcohol (or more rarely in food). The symptoms include a dull headache and sensation of dazedness, a general feeling of discomfort and sometimes dizziness. Many remedies have been advocated, e.g., strong black coffee to improve alertness, various bitters and sauces to stimulate gastric juice and biliary secretions, and – on doubtful physiological grounds – a further small quantity of alcohol ('a hair of the dog that bit you').

The value of all of these is uncertain, though persons who occasionally over-indulge usually have their own specific. Broadly alcohol is burned up in the normal body at a rate of about 10 per cent per hour. So a person whose blood content is 240 ml. (or three times the legal limit for driving in the U.K.) can expect it to fall to roughly 216 ml. in an hour, 195 in two hours, 85 in ten hours and 68 in twelve hours, with the side-effects passing off as the alcohol is used up.

However, these figures are very approximate and subject to many variations. For instance, alcohol consumed on an empty stomach gets into the blood more rapidly and is burned up rather more quickly, while a glass of milk shortly before drinking delays the passage of alcohol into the blood and consequently may delay its destruction.

In general a hangover is an indication that a person has exceeded his limits of toleration and should in future keep within these limits. Many points, however, are still unexplained. For example, a whisky drinker who knows his normal capacity may develop a hangover after consuming a quantity of sherry containing considerably less alcohol than he can normally take in whisky. Again some workers have claimed that a person who takes alcohol to about his limit of toleration is more likely to have a hangover if he smokes heavily while drinking than if he does not smoke in that period.

hare-lip and cleft palate. Hare-lip may appear only as a slight notching of the red margin of the upper lip on one or both sides or may be present as a complete fissure running into one or both nostrils. In cleft palate there is a gap along the mid-line of the roof of the mouth and this too may vary from a split in the uvula and soft palate at the back of the mouth to a complete division of the hard plate so that there is a passage between mouth and nose. Both defects are congenital malformations and are usually inherited.

In severe cases a child is unable to suck. There is risk of choking and infection through fluid getting into the air-passages, and feeds need to be carefully given by pipette or tube.

Repair of the mouth and lip requires plastic surgery. Hare-lip can be dealt with in the first few months but cleft palate treatment is usually postponed until about 1½ years of age. A series of operations and the co-operation of a dental surgeon may be required, and the results of treatment are generally excellent. Later on, even after successful repair, speech difficulties may need help from a speech therapist.

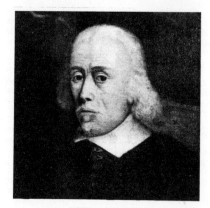

William Harvey

Harvey, William. Probably the most famous of British physicians and often called the 'father of English physiology'. He lived from 1578 to 1657.

His primary discovery, that of the circulation of the blood, is sometimes impugned on the ground that it was in part anticipated hundreds of years earlier by an Arab physician, Ibn-an-Nafis (1210-1288) and more fully anticipated by Michael Servetus (1500-1553). Servetus's book was destroyed when he was burned at the stake but three copies have survived and it is not impossible that Harvey saw a copy. The supreme importance of Harvey's discovery is not, however, its originality, but the fact that his book – De Motu Cordis (1628) – was so well reasoned and so adequately supported by a mass of carefully recorded experiments that it overturned the venerated doctrines of Galen and convinced most of Harvey's contemporaries within his own lifetime.

A later publication which Harvey himself deemed more important was *De Generatione Animalium* (1651) in which he denied the long-existing theory of spontaneous generation which suggested that living organisms could develop from non-living material, e.g., flies from a rubbish heap. In opposition to this theory Harvey inferred that every creature begins as an egg produced by a member of the same species, even if the egg is too small to be visible.

Apart from his writing Harvey was the leading practising physician of his time and was one of the first Englishmen to study the nature of disease by post mortem examination.

hashish. An Arabian name for preparations of CANNABIS made from the plant Indian hemp (*Cannabis indica*). The dried leaves and stalks are smoked or made into beverages or confections and taken as a drug for their intoxicating effect.

The 'hashish-eaters' (*hashashin* in Arabic) were members of an eleventh century military and religious order in Syria who fortified themselves for secret murders by taking hashish – hence the word 'assassin'.

hay fever. An acute attack of nasal catarrh resembling a common cold. There is usually profuse watery nasal discharge, sneezing and conjunctivitis and there may also be asthmatic symptoms. It is an allergic response, primarily to pollen, but other allergens cause similar symptoms. True hay fever recurs every summer when pollens are in the air. The Meteorological Office provides information about pollen counts, and risk increases when the index rises over thirty.

Treatment. In an acute attack antihistamines and ephedrine are usually prescribed. The relatively new drug sodium cromoglycate is also useful.

Persons who suffer repeatedly may be skin-tested with various allergens in an attempt to identify the one responsible for their recurrent attacks. Once this is ascertained a course of de-sensitizing injections may prove helpful.

In the pollen season sufferers should avoid districts where the pollen count is high. The wearing of a mask has been recommended but this is hardly a measure compatible with normal activities.

headaches. Headache is a symptom of many conditions ranging from serious organic disease of the brain in which the cause is clear to the less well-defined type of pain which accompanies conditions of worry, anxiety and strain, and which is to be regarded as of psychosomatic origin.

It is convenient to consider first headaches which originate from causes outside the skull. Very often these headaches are localized and arise from fibrositis affecting either the related nerves carrying sensations or from the muscles of the scalp and neck. Massage and local treatment may prove helpful. In the same category are headaches caused by inflammatory conditions affecting the teeth, the nose and its sinuses, the eye or the ear, in all of which treatment must be directed to the primary cause. Eye-strain caused by a need for spectacles also requires consideration, especially in young persons.

Within the skull, the brain itself is insensitive to pain but the sheaths surrounding it are supplied by sensitive nerves.

General disorders, including indigestion, constipation, nephritis, uraemia, and jaundice can give rise to headaches and they also occur as an almost inevitable symptom of fever.

Diseases within the brain will of course tend to cause headaches – these include meningitis, encephalitis, brain abscess, cerebral syphilis and such conditions as tumours or haemorrhage, which press on the brain.

In the same way disturbances of the blood supply to the brain due to blood pressure problems, anaemia or decompression disease will also result in headaches.

Alcohol is perhaps the commonest drug causing headaches but overdoses of many potentially poisonous substances, and some particular drugs which interfere with the function of haemoglobin, may also be responsible.

'Tension' headaches are a common complaint in nervous individuals under strain. Since migraine, a particular type of very sudden headache, is now generally regarded as being due to spasm of blood vessels supplying the brain, it is likely that nervous or tension headaches are produced in a somewhat similar fashion.

With such diverse causes it is clear that no single line of treatment can be recommended for headaches. In most cases the traditional analgesic based on a combination of aspirin, phenacetin and caffein will produce some relief of symptoms but more basic causes must be sought for and eliminated or relieved so far as proves possible.

head injuries. These arise from either direct violence, such as a blow on the head, or indirect violence, as in a fall on the feet or a blow on the chin, which cause jarring to the head.

Scalp lacerations bleed profusely but generally heal well after cleaning-up and careful suturing.

Blows to the head may cause concussion in which there is no gross damage but brain-function is temporarily disturbed by pressure effects producing symptoms of shock; there may be unconsciousness, nausea, giddiness and mental confusion. Any case with concussion demands careful subsequent observation to ensure that there is not also contusion of the brain with haemorrhage or an actual skull fracture.

Fractures vary in type. A direct blow with some weapon may produce a depressed fracture of 'pond' or 'gutter' conformation with a corresponding portion of the skull driven inwards to compress the brain. Blows with a blunt instrument, or indirect violence from falls on the feet or a blow on the chin, tend to produce linear fractures. The danger of these, especially when involving the base of the skull, is damage to blood-vessels which results in intra-cranial haemorrhage. Depressed fractures and intra-cranial pressure from haemorrhage require surgical treatment.

In general, head injuries need expert assessment and even the less serious benefit from prolonged rest. Even with the best care there may be troublesome after-effects from severe injuries such as epileptic seizures and psychological disturbance.

Most head injuries occur in industry and traffic accidents. Risks can be reduced by safety precautions – re-inforced headgear, seat belts and crash helmets.

head noises. The experience of persistent recurring noises in the head is known as tinnitus. The term does not include impressions of such sounds as voices, bells or musical sequences. These are hallucinations, often accompanying mental disease, and a patient with tinnitus, which is much more a 'ringing in the ears', should be reassured that it has no psychiatric significance.

Many people over 65 with tinnitus also have presbyacusis or senile deafness. Noisy occupations, arteriosclerosis, and various diseases affecting the ear, or the nerve carrying the sensations of hearing, or even the brain itself, may make the patient experience continuous high-pitched noise.

Ménière's disease was described by Prosper Ménière (1799-1861), physician to the Imperial Institute for Deaf-Mutes in Paris. Its features are fluctuating deafness, tinnitus and vertigo. Although its primary cause is unknown, abnormalities in the ear (particularly of the cochlear and vestibular lymph-spaces) have been demonstrated. The disease occurs usually after 50, more often in women, and sounds heard may be distorted as well as lessened. High tones are sharpened and low tones flattened giving a 'Punch-and-Judy' quality to voices.

In presbyacusis noises are generally continuous and high-pitched; in Ménière's disease they tend to be intermittent and to be heard as low-pitch humming, roaring or banging.

Some other conditions also produce head noises – wax in the ear, otitis media, tic of ear-drum muscle, intra-cranial aneurysm, high and low blood-pressure and also certain drugs such as salicylates and quinine.

Tinnitus is notoriously difficult to treat effectively but patients usually learn to adapt to it.

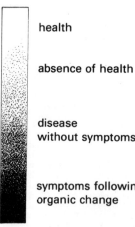

health

absence of health

disease
without symptoms

symptoms following
organic change

There is no clear boundary between health and disease

health. A state of physical, emotional, mental and social well-being, in which the body is functioning harmoniously and efficiently and the person is reasonably in tune with his environment and with most of his associates. In recent years there has been a tendency in some quarters to extend the meaning to include both health and disease (as in 'Mental Health Act' which deals with mental disease), but health – alertness and vigorousness of mind and body and capacity for enjoying life – is so much more than absence of disease that the linking of health and disease is to be deprecated. There are many people who are persistently tired, dull, apathetic and incapable of enjoying life but are nevertheless not suffering from any diagnosible illness.

The old idea that physical or mental absence of health is a punishment inflicted by an angry deity or a test imposed to purify the spirit has gradually given place to the realization that a person's health and well-being (or alternatively his absence of health) depends essentially on three sets of factors – his inherited characteristics and proneness to (or resistance to) various diseases; the physical, emotional, social and mental effects of his early years (with almost certainly the formative pre-school period most important of all, and the school and immediate post-school years next in importance); and the emotional, social and physical effects of his current and recent environment – in the widest sense of that word – including, for example, his diet, exercise and housing conditions, his work satisfaction or stress or frustration, and his matrimonial and family relationships.

1. Heredity. Apart from various serious defects being inherited (e.g., spina bifida, cleft palate, schizophrenia) HEREDITY can create an increased or a decreased liability to many diseases, e.g., persons of blood group A are more than normally liable to cancer of the stomach and uterus, and some families have a natural tendency to longevity while others usually die relatively early. Again, much of one's intelligence is a matter of inherited potential, although no intelligence can develop to its full inherited capacity in the absence of appropriate stimuli, such as suitable toys, books, associates and, not least, encouragement. Similarly, stature is basically inherited but requires adequate food, fresh air and exercise: adult Australians of today are in general taller than British adults because the former have mostly grown to their potential while many of the latter have been stunted.

2. Effects of early years. A young child malnourished to the extent of developing manifest rickets will carry the bony deformity for life, and a person undernourished in the formative years will never develop to his full anatomical and physiological potential. As an illustration of the last point, until the era of allegedly equal opportunity brought to universities persons from all types of background, it was well known that university graduates were on average considerably taller than labourers, because many of the latter had been undernourished as children. Similarly, the youngster reared in a house that lacks books and magazines and in a family that despises book-learning is unlikely to become a keen reader. The under-exercised sedentary child is later liable to the diseases associated with lack of exercise. The youth who has been deprived of parental love may have difficulty in ever forming bonds of affection.

The effects of past – as opposed to current – social and environmental circumstances can to some extent be seen by studying the disease patterns in countries that move quickly from primitive conditions to affluence, advanced economic levels, good provision of health services and an approximation to Western culture. Before the change the main killing conditions are infectious and parasitic diseases, diseases of malnutrition and diseases arising out of poverty, squalor and ignorance. In the early years after the change these diseases still take a considerable toll. It is only after the new conditions have existed for a considerable number of years that these diseases gradually disappear and begin to be replaced by our Western pattern of the so-called 'diseases of affluence' – many of which are largely caused by eating too much, smoking too much, drinking too much, striving too hard, breathing polluted air and misusing leisure.

3. Current or recent aspects. While predisposition to certain diseases or considerable resistance to them is largely a matter of nature (heredity) or nurture (earlier conditions and influences) current or recent conditions commonly trigger off disease. Thus the elderly man develops a heart attack by frequently sprinting for a bus, the lonely and introverted widow acquires senile delusions from lack of companionship (and perhaps also from inadequate diet), the person who gourmandizes at Christmas has a bilious attack, and the adolescent who slims vigorously to get rid of 'puppy fat' has an increased liability to tuberculosis.

Improvement of health. All these factors have to be considered in respect of improvement of health which can in turn be discussed under three main headings: cure or palliation of disease, prevention of disease and promotion of health.

1. Treatment of disease or injury. Despite emphasis on disease prevention and health promotion by a few early physicians, treatment clearly comes first historically and of course remains very important today. Yet it has obvious limitations. In the first place it is useless where the lack of health first shows itself in sudden death, e.g., where the man who has for years eaten too much animal fat, smoked forty cigarettes a day, taken little exercise and worried constantly about his work or about marital problems, but has never been so ill as to consult a doctor, dies from a coronary thrombosis. In the second place, treatment is inevitably often far less than complete restoration of function, e.g., where an undiagnosed diabetic develops diabetic gangrene necessitating amputation of the foot. Thirdly, treatment is often slow, e.g., it may take many months of skilled medical and nursing care to restore to health the person who has a (preventable) traffic or domestic accident or the person who develops tuberculosis or poliomyelitis. And fourthly, because of the amount of medical, nursing and paramedical time involved, treatment is very costly, whether the cost falls on the state or on the individual.

A criticism increasingly levelled at health and disease services in Britain is that about 70 per cent of the total money for health and disease is devoted to hospitals (for the treatment of persons already seriously ill) and about 23 per cent to general practitioners and home nurses (both concerned mainly with conditions that receive professional attention only after the victim has made a layman's decision that he is ill).

2. Prevention of illness and injury. The importance of prevention is becoming increasingly recognized. It had a massive triumph in decreasing deaths of children in the first few decades of this century: following the creation of maternity services and child welfare clinics, the establishment of a profession of health visitors and general improvements in sanitation and hygiene, the infant death rate in England and Wales fell from 129 per thousand births in 1911 to 91 in 1917. Following the expansion of the health visiting service in the years after the First World War it fell further to 59 per thousand births by 1934, years before the improvements in treatment created by the introduction of antibiotics and sulphonamides. An equally massive advance in the middle years of the century was the virtual elimination of many serious infections (e.g., diphtheria and poliomyelitis) by immunization and education of the public about its desirability.

Yet prevention of serious hereditary conditions (by discouraging persons likely to convey them from producing families) is still in its infancy, and attention is only beginning to be devoted to the prevention of diseases of later life (such as coronary thrombosis and stroke) and of diseases due to emotional and social factors. Indeed, perhaps the very improvements in treatment in recent years (e.g., antibiotics and corticosteroids) have temporarily masked the crucial importance of prevention.

3. Promotion of health. Manifestly the fostering of good health has an overlap with the prevention of disease. In Britain the beneficial effects can perhaps clearly be seen in respect of the improved health of children since the creation of home visiting by health visitors, the setting up of child health clinics (formerly called child welfare clinics) and the provision of welfare foods: children are taller and heavier and suffer from fewer diseases than in the past. On the emotional side, counselling of parents on child management (including, for example, the need to give the child an assured base of security and love from which to start exploring his 'world', and the dangers of over-strictness, over-indulgence and inconsistency) has already begun to improve the mental health of the young and to promote the development of personalities fit to cope with the normal stresses of life.

Yet, apart from health promotion for pre-school children, most of the vast field of promotion of health remains as a future task for health workers. In respect of family spacing and family limitation we have devoted too little time to advising the woman (not a carrier of hereditary disease) about the dangers – to her children as well as herself – of having so many children in rapid succession that she cannot give them adequate personal attention. In at least some areas the School Health Service has been more concerned with the important task of finding and remedying defects than with the even more important job of improving emotional and physical health. Often children leave school without having been taught even the elements of human relations. Adolescents and adults have in the main been left without counselling on the maintenance and improvement of health; and the young elderly (persons nearing retirement age) who could remain in good health for many years have in general been neglected until their health deteriorated to the stage of illness.

Perhaps the most hopeful sign for the future in the U.K. is the expressed intention of the Government, despite financial stringency, to train and appoint more health education officers and more health visitors. After all, a 1 per cent reduction in treatment services could give us at the same cost something like a 25 per cent increase in preventive and promotive staff, with enormous benefit to the health of the people.

See also CAUSES OF DISEASE, HEALTH EDUCATION, INDICES OF HEALTH CARE, MEASUREMENT OF HEALTH, and KEEPING FIT.

health education. Education aiming at improving or maintaining the physical and mental health of persons and of the community, preventing or reducing disease, decreasing the likelihood of relapses or recurrences, and promoting the efficient use of the health services.

Historically, health education has several beginnings which foreshadow the modern division into individual teaching, group teaching and use of mass media. Attempts to instruct the public by written material on the conservation of health began in classical times and books on this subject multiplied after printing facilitated their production. An example is William Buchan's *Domestic Medicine* (1769) which covered hygiene and such aspects of prevention as were then known, as well as medical treatment, and went through nineteen editions.

An obvious off-shoot of printed health instruction for adults was the introduction of the idea that schools should be concerned with more than mere literacy, and health books designed for children were published, often – in the fashion of the nineteenth century – with what strikes us today as a curious omission of all reference to the reproductive system. W. A. Alcock (1798-1859) in America was a pioneer both of the idea that schools should play a part in health education and also in the production of health guides for children.

Since only a minority of people were sufficiently educated (or sufficiently interested) to study fairly massive books on health, the idea of popular lectures inevitably followed. These started in several countries in the eighteenth century, and perhaps reached their peak in Edinburgh during the period from 1923 to 1930 when William Robertson was Medical Officer of Health of that city. Roughly simultaneously – and probably much more important – the creation of a profession of HEALTH VISITORS in Britain (initiated in 1862 but emerging as a full profession as late as 1919) provided a method of one-to-one discussion of health problems in the homes of the people, and of teaching small groups in antenatal and child health clinics. This was paralleled in other developed countries by the introduction of similar public health nurses with educative functions.

One-to-one discussion in the home and the formation of small discussion groups in clinics together contributed greatly to the fact that both maternal mortality and infant mortality were halved in the period from 1915 to 1940.

The dramatic reduction of nutritional diseases and of the so-called 'dirt' diseases (like scabies, impetigo and ringworm) in the middle years of this century, and the public acceptance of immunization against various infections, can also be attributed to this development. In connection with immunization it is worth noting that smallpox vaccination was made legally obligatory in the nineteenth century (without health education) and in large measure failed, while protection against diphtheria, poliomyelitis and other infections this century relied on health education (without legal compulsion) and succeeded.

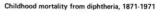

Childhood mortality from diphtheria, 1871-1971

England and Wales

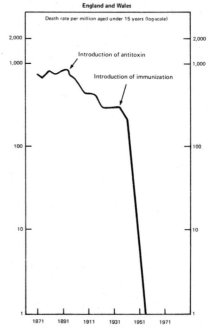

In some areas individual counselling and group discussion, supplemented by exhibitions and use of newspaper articles and radio talks, also achieved striking success in reducing accidents in the home and in creating a climate of acceptance that family spacing and family limitation were desirable. Simultaneously, sound radio, television and other mass media proved extremely effective in creating interest as a prelude to individual and group teaching and in stimulating short-term action (such as attendance at a mass radiography unit) although they appeared initially to be less effective in creating lasting changes of attitude and behaviour.

In the third quarter of this century education for health – perhaps led in America by the State of California and in Britain by such cities as Aberdeen and Croydon – expanded greatly and also changed enormously. The old idea was formal instruction by a knowledgeable and respected lecturer; the new concept is subtle and unobtrusive attempts to help people to achieve for themselves habits and behaviour likely to foster good health and unlikely to lead to emotional or physical illness. The old idea was that the lecturer did the talking; the new concept is of discussion, with the learner often doing more speaking than the 'instructor' and with the learner formulating his own decisions. The old idea was that health education was simple and could be undertaken by any articulate person with adequate knowledge of health and disease; the new concept is that education for health is highly complex and that its practitioners are unlikely to succeed unless they possess, in addition to articulacy and health knowledge, insight into the culture patterns, social pressures, prejudices and beliefs of the persons taught. Except in the minds of a few enthusiasts the old idea was of health education as a useful 'frill' to be added to medical and nursing treatment where time permitted; the new concept of education for health is that it is one of the most important tasks of the health services and perhaps the only way of reducing the ever-increasing mass of unprevented preventable disease.

The main professional sources of health education include the following: (1) Health visitors, whose post-nursing education (in health teaching, psychology and elements of sociology) and whose unrivalled tradition of access to homes without the presence of emotionally disturbing factors such as illness or social emergency, place them in an ideal position for one-to-one teaching and for the formation and counselling of small groups. (2) General medical practitioners who, although primarily concerned with diagnosis and treatment, can make a large contribution. (3) Midwives, whose contact with their patient, though brief, is intimate. (4) Other health professionals, such as physiotherapists, home nurses, hospital nurses, community physicians, hospital doctors, etc. (5) Environmental health officers (formerly called sanitary inspectors) especially on prevention of food-borne diseases. (6) Social workers, although their primary skill and main function is in a different sphere. (7) School teachers, especially in respect of younger children, although for the health education of older children teachers have the limitation already indicated for social workers. (8) Writers and other publicists, although to some extent they – like teachers and social workers – can only act as relayers of information initially provided by health professionals. (9) Health education officers who act as co-ordinators of health education and advisers on audio-visual aids and resource material.

This last group is sometimes confused with health visitors but the distinction is clear: a health visitor is a nurse who has been selected on academic and personal qualities for further education in health teaching and medico-social counselling, and he or she plays an enormous part in the health education of individuals and small groups; a health education officer (often with the background of a health visitor or school teacher) has had additional training both in group discussion and in such subjects as the effective use of libraries, the selection of teaching aids and the evaluation of health education projects. The one is a practitioner, the other is qualified to practise but is mainly a co-ordinator.

Health education in the home is probably of basic importance, for three reasons: because problems can be seen there, because the client is relaxed, and because the formation of any discussion group presupposes that potential attenders are already motivated to seek further education. Health education of persons initially motivated at home (e.g., prospective parents and parents of pre-school children) is increasingly a feature of doctors' consulting rooms, child health clinics and health centres. Health education in schools is developing apace, with some doubt as to the exact boundary between the non-expert who knows the child (the teacher) and the expert with less knowledge of the child (the health visitor or medical officer). In factories and offices, health education is beginning to develop, especially in the form of pre-retirement classes; and some long-stay hospitals have made a useful start in health teaching of patients and their visitors.

In Britain the Central Council for Health Education (in England and Wales) and the Scottish Council for Health Education provide frequent courses to refresh and improve the knowledge of health visitors, midwives, doctors, teachers and others; and the same Central Council and the Scottish Health Education Unit initiate mass campaigns on specific subjects, using all available media, including television, radio, newspaper articles and advertisements, leaflets, posters and health exhibitions.

The general value of health education is beyond question: a health visitor who in an entire year prevents four serious accidents that would otherwise have required six weeks each of hospital treatment saves more than her year's salary; a health education officer who prevents a single case of serious hereditary disease that would otherwise have required many years of institutional care saves the community far more than a year's salary. Education for health has already vastly improved the health of children and mothers. It is, however, a legitimate criticism of health education as hitherto practised that – with the exception of prevention of home accidents, a few pre-retirement classes and occasional and rather unsuccessful campaigns against cigarette smoking by adults – it has tended to stop at the age of 35 or 40 years. On the whole, the prevention of diseases of maturity by health education is still a thing of the future. So is the teaching of the public about the need to seek medical advice quickly when they really require it, and about the need to avoid wasting professional time and resources on trivialities.

The present climate of opinion in Britain (and in most developed countries) is strongly favourable to health education. The Health Ministries have called both for larger establishments of health visitors and for the provision of additional training schools for selected nurses aspiring to that qualification in universities and polytechnics. Health Boards have been encouraged to appoint chief area health officers, with medical, nursing and dental consultant advisers, and to appoint adequate staffs of health education officers. The funds at the disposal of central health education bodies have increased rapidly.

The general development of health education is, beyond question, a success story of such magnitude that beside it most medical achievements pale into insignificance. However to demonstrate its success in any one aspect is never easy: if, for example, we succeeded in favourably influencing women who are beginning to develop 'middle-aged spread', or men who, because of excessive ambition or undue worry about their jobs, are having little mental or physical relaxation and are smoking excessively, any resulting decrease in diseases associated respectively with obesity, stress and cigarette smoking will not appear for some years. As is perhaps true of all forms of education, we can appreciate its general value but on many particular aspects have to accept – or reject – on a commonsense basis, although scientific evaluation is desirable whenever practicable.

See also EVALUATION OF HEALTH EDUCATION, PREVENTABLE DISEASES and PREVENTIVE MEDICINE.

health screening. The aim of health screening is the systematic examination of various sections of the population in order to detect hidden defects and if possible to initiate appropriate measures to correct them, or at least to lessen their affect. In relation to the infant, toddler and schoolchild the problem is a simple one (given the necessary resources) because there are already organized arrangements for the supervision of all children up to school-leaving age. Great progress has therefore been made in the early detection of abnormalities such as congenital dislocation of the hip, phenylketonuria, and any defects of sight and hearing, and also in carrying out general developmental assessment as a guide to educational placement and general supervision during the formative years.

With the adult population the problem is more difficult. It is generally accepted that there exists a vast amount of hidden disease which has not progressed to the point at which the patient goes to the doctor. It is logical that steps should be taken to examine populations systematically to detect abnormalities and to institute appropriate treatment. However, this simple proposition is hedged with difficulties. In the first place the ethical position is different from the one in which a patient consults a doctor. In the latter case he expects no more than that the doctor will do his best, but if the doctor proclaims that he will detect and arrange to treat a certain condition there is some risk of criticism and perhaps legal action if he fails. He has therefore to make sure that his procedures are reliable, that they offer prospects of changing the natural course of disease for the better, that treatment facilities are available, and also that his tests are simple, acceptable to the patients and not outrageously expensive on a cost-benefit assessment.

Screening procedures for the adult population vary considerably. They may be offered to the public at large or within defined age-limits; they may be applied to selected groups of a particular practice or clinic; or they may be a project for the better care of a specific group of employees. The screening may be aimed at a single disease or it may be a 'blunderbuss' procedure covering many different diseases.

The earliest example of the single disease approach was the development of Mass Miniature Radiography pioneered by de Abreu of Brazil about 1936 and since widely adopted. It had great success in detecting large numbers of unsuspected cases of pulmonary tuberculosis and has played a significant part in accelerating the decline of that disease. Diabetic surveys are also testing for a single disease.

However, most screening campaigns now concern themselves with a search for a variety of pathological conditions. Even 'Well-Women Clinics', primarily established to look for early signs of cancer in the cervix, normally extend their work to include at least other gynaecological conditions, breast disease and the checking of urine samples.

Multiple screening. There is as yet no absolute agreement as to what tests are most profitable to include. Modern techniques have made possible the inclusion of many tests the practical value of which is still debatable.

The usual programme includes a selection of the following: (1) Height, weight, and skin-fold thickness, indicative of general nutrition and obesity. (2) Chest radiology, revealing abnormalities of heart and lungs. (3) Blood samples, for the detection of anaemia and of any abnormalities in the chemical content of the blood. (4) Urine samples, for indications of diabetes or nephritis. (5) Heart and lung function such as electrocardiographs, blood pressure estimations, and respiratory capacity. (6) Special senses, that is tests of vision, colour blindness, ocular tension (for glaucoma), and hearing. (7) Personal and family history, by questionnaire. (8) Personality assessment, by questionnaire, designed to elicit indications of mental instability. (9) Uterus, with cervical cytology, testing for cancer. (10) Breasts, giving instruction in the technique of self-examination for early detection of cancer.

Screening of older persons. It is probably wise not to include pensioners deliberately in general screening surveys. Older persons have their particular problems and need a more personal approach. An individual and sympathetic but none the less systematic scheme provides an opportunity for assessing and explaining any abnormalities and also for exploring the more practical difficulties which affect the health of the elderly, e.g., household composition problems of retirement or bereavement, domestic and social help, meals, special diet and medication, ability to shop, cook and housekeep, financial problems, and worries from mental or physical difficulties.

Industrial health checks. Many firms now realize that facilities for health supervision are a matter of common prudence and help towards good staff relations. They are applied both to executives and to work-people. It is equally important that the sales director should not have a coronary infarct in the middle of an export drive, as that those on the shop floor should not be prematurely incapacitated by industrial disease. Many such diseases are in fact already covered statutorily by the Factory Acts.

General. There is no doubt that screening programmes are gaining in popular support and they can already claim substantial successes especially when directed against a single disease where the problem is well-defined and the prospects of successful intervention are good.

However, a very large question mark still hangs over the large-scale multiple procedures. The difficulty is not in organizing and carrying out such a programme but in interpreting the results and being able to act upon them effectively. It may even be a disservice to a patient to uncover signs of departure from normal which one cannot influence beneficially.

health services. In different countries there are all sorts of different health and disease services. In some developing countries there is less than one doctor per hundred-thousand people, and in some advanced countries more than one doctor for every thousand of the population. In some countries there are hardly any qualified nurses and the nursing care of patients even in hospital is fundamentally left to the unskilled efforts of their relatives, while in other countries there are university degrees in nursing and post-graduate qualifications in its specialized branches. In some countries maintenance of good health is deemed a priority, while in others little is attempted except treatment of such sick people as can afford to pay fees or can secure charitable services. Also there is every conceivable variation from absolutely no state aid or intervention to all health workers being salaried.

Because Britain's National Health Service (1948) and revised National Health Service (1974), while not necessarily better than those of Sweden, Finland and parts of Russia, have attracted world-wide attention among English-speaking races, a brief outline may be useful.

Position up to 1948. There was enormous regional variation, e.g., in the Scottish Highlands the general practitioner was often paid for undertaking certain preventive – public health – functions and such very limited health visiting as was attempted was undertaken by district nurses without qualification in health teaching or health counselling. Very broadly, however, the health and disease services might be thus summarized.

1. Services for promotion of health and prevention of disease, in so far as they were developed, were administered by local authorities and were co-ordinated and directed by a salaried doctor called the MEDICAL OFFICER OF HEALTH. The services included such things as antenatal clinics, domiciliary midwifery, maternity hospitals, visiting of mothers and children at home by HEALTH VISITORS, child health clinics, school health services, such immunization services as then existed, supervision of the purity of water and food, and port health services. The public health medical officers, health visitors, sanitary inspectors, domiciliary midwives, etc. employed in these services were full-time salaried officers, and the services while conforming to nationally specified minima varied enormously according to the wealth or poverty of the particular local authority and according to its willingness or reluctance to spend money on services.

2. Treatment of illness at home fell into two groups. The upper and middle classes employed general medical practitioners to visit them at home on a fee-for-service basis, while the less affluent were increasingly covered by insurance, the GP receiving a small fixed annual payment for each insured person and the patient being expected if at all possible to visit the practitioner's consulting room. In many cases, however, insurance covered only the wage-earner, so that if wife or child fell ill the family had either to find the fee or to find a doctor generous enough to treat the poor without charge. Inevitably a wealthy area would have many doctors and an impoverished area would be under-doctored.

Nursing services for patients ill in their own homes were available from district nurses employed by voluntary agencies, financed to some extent by charity and to some extent by regular contributions from potential users, but availability depended largely on the wealth and generosity of the particular district; and the more affluent in need of nursing skills tended to employ nurses privately.

3. Hospitals had originally been established by charitable organizations and benefactors, but by 1948 the 'voluntary' hospitals (allegedly maintained through charitable donations) were increasingly requiring and receiving financial grants towards their upkeep, and, because of the inadequacy of these hospitals, local authorities had, starting with infectious diseases and tuberculosis sanatoria, built and staffed a multitude of general and mental hospitals, until more than two-thirds of hospital beds were under the jurisdiction of local authorities.

There was much jealousy between voluntary and local authority hospitals, e.g., if out of two hospitals in the same town one provided a brain surgery unit sufficient to meet the town's needs, the other was perhaps more likely to devote any available money to providing a rival brain surgery unit than to modernizing its kitchen or building a modern nurses' home. In voluntary and local authority hospitals nurses and paramedical staff were salaried; in local authority hospitals doctors in general were salaried; in voluntary hospitals junior doctors were given free board and in general no salary (years of poverty being a prelude to the high earnings of consultants) and senior doctors gave their services free, making their livelihood from private patients usually treated in nursing homes.

As insurance schemes multiplied, since few people with ordinary incomes could afford doctors' fees in sudden illness or desired to rely on uncertain charity, as war and post-war financial stringency reduced the number of people who could pay consultants' fees and nursing home charges, and as voluntary hospitals came to require increasing grants from national funds, a reorganization of the services became almost inevitable.

The National Health Service of 1948. The health and disease services were reorganized in three branches, with the cost of the second and third branches (and in part the first branch) falling on national funds, partially on a newly instituted national health insurance and partly on ordinary revenue (e.g., income tax).

1. Services for promotion of health and prevention of disease continued to be salaried services administered by local authorities and headed by medical officers of health, with the functions of health visitors considerably extended and with home nurses coming under the jurisdiction of local authorities.

2. The general practitioner service, administered by bodies called Executive Councils, became fundamentally a service under which the patient was entitled to treatment without direct charge (although some exceptions like prescription charges were introduced later) and the GP received a fixed

sum for each person on his list, although a GP remained free to enter into arrangements to treat on a fee-for-service basis persons not on his list.

3. All hospitals, whether previously voluntary or previously local authority, were placed under the control of nominated hospital boards. Hospital staff other than senior doctors and senior dentists were salaried, including junior doctors so that aspiring consultants no longer had to endure years of poverty. Consultant doctors and dentists could opt to be either full-time and salaried (as about half of them were) or paid for a number of theoretically calculated sessions and entitled to undertake private work.

In general the health of the people, as measured for instance by average age at death or by infant mortality rates, improved enormously although there were some initial complaints that some people sought 'free' medical treatment for trivia. Defects, however, became apparent. To take some examples at random: there was no co-ordinated planning, e.g., the development of heart transplant operations might occupy the full time of five doctors and seventeen nurses on a single patient, and it was no concern of the hospital boards that prevention of the births of children born with severe handicaps through maternal rubella or prevention of coronary thrombosis in the middle-aged was being thwarted by sheer shortage of health visitors and public health medical officers; similarly, when renal dialysis saved the lives of patients who would otherwise have died, it was no concern of the hospital authorities that the local authorities had to find the money for expensive adaptations of the patients' houses and thereafter to provide supportive services. Again, as the health visitor's post-qualification training improved and as the general practitioner's income ceased to depend on the amount of illness it became increasingly obvious that two experts could collaborate and reinforce each other, but the GP was in a separate service, largely unaware of what was being attempted by preventive workers on the one hand or by hospital doctors and nurses on the other.

Local authority services varied greatly. In some towns and counties diseases susceptible to immunization and diseases of malnutrition were virtually eradicated, there were dramatic reductions in road and home accidents and much success in the education of the public in the maintenance of emotional and physical health; in other areas the elected councillors pleased their electors by keeping down the rates and excused their lack of development of preventive services by the fact that public health doctors and health visitors were scarce.

Yet again nursing, and to some extent also other health professions, began to rise to full professional status with its own expertise and priorities, but both in hospitals and in local authority services there was tremendous medical domination; there was, for instance, a reluctance to accept that health visitors (with at least four and a half years of professional education) might undertake developmental screening of infants just as capably as public health doctors at about twice the remuneration, an unwillingness to believe that dietitians could function without being 'supervised' by a doctor, a contentment with a situation in which all the highly paid posts in a department were filled by doctors and perhaps a single dentist, while the administrative and teaching heads of health visiting, midwifery, nursing and other large services were paid less than a trainee consultant.

Perhaps the biggest defect of all was that more than 60 per cent of the available money was spent on curative and palliative services in hospital and most of the remainder on curative, palliative and supportive domiciliary services, with very little expended on promotion of mental and physical health, health education and prevention of disease.

The National Health Service of 1974. Various tentative experiments took place. For instance, in Oxford (with many other towns and counties following) general practitioners and health visitors, although still paid by executive councils and local authorities respectively, began to work in close association; in Aberdeen the medical officer of health gave up his dictatorial powers and formed an administrative group (including the chief nursing officer and the chief health education officer) to advise the local authority on matters of policy; various hospitals employed general practitioners on a part-time basis; liaison health visitors appeared in many hospitals; and in some cases joint appointments were made of doctors or nurses working partly in hospital and partly in the local authority services.

Finally, the social work services having already been separated off and left with local authorities, in 1974 the strictly environmental services (i.e., those of the former sanitary inspectors) were left with local authorities and all other health services – whether hospital or otherwise, and whether curative, palliative, educative, preventive or supportive – were placed under nominated health boards, with each board having an executive group of chief officers: a medical officer, a nursing officer, a secretary or administrator, and a finance officer, with the chief dental officer and the chief pharmacist attending meetings of the executive group when their services were under discussion.

Many difficulties remained and still remain. The tradition of spending nearly all the available money on treatment and palliation will not easily disappear. The variation in methods of payment remains, with about half the clinical consultants spending part of their time on private work, with general practitioners remunerated by annual fee for each person on their list (including a larger fee for each elderly person) and also fees for certain items of service (such as vaccinating a child), with some workers, e.g., general dental practitioners, paid entirely on items of service and with most members of the various health professions salaried. This variation could have unfortunate results, e.g., some dental officers might resent the efforts of health education officers and health visitors as tending to reduce the amount of dental treatment needed, and some general medical practitioners might prefer that they themselves should immunize 50 per cent of children and provide family planning services for 30 per cent of women (with due payments for items of service) rather than that clinic services with salaried staff should raise the immunization level to 90 per cent and the family planning figure to 60 per cent.

Not least, the rigid separation of health needs and social needs may make for difficulties, with the health visitors – selected nurses with subsequent full-time training both in health teaching and in social science – uneasily poised between the Health Board and the Social Work Department, employed by the former but often knowing more about the social needs and problems of their clients than do the less numerous and in most cases less highly trained workers of the Social Work Department. This difficulty may arise too in the case of home nurses who in the past recommended appliances for the handicapped (such as wheel chairs and walking aids) but now find that the issue of such appliances is controlled by the Social Work Department.

Similarly the separation of environmental health officers from other health workers may create difficulties. It seems inevitable that in any major outbreak of food-borne disease the former sanitary inspectors will need the help of the Health Board's epidemiologists for investigation, of its health education officers for urgent education of the community, and probably of its health visitors for eliciting information from cases and contacts about foods eaten and their sources.

Yet, despite these and other difficulties, the integration of curative and preventive health services should substantially assist forward planning. For the first time each area and district has an interdisciplinary group studying all the health services and responsible to a single board. Many changes may well be needed in the future, but the 1974 integration represents a vast step forward, and it is interesting and perhaps significant that the infant death rate for England and Wales in 1976 was considerably lower than ever before.

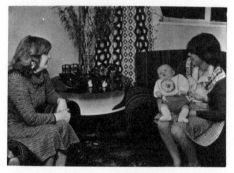

A health visitor with her clients

health visitor. A qualified nurse, with additional training in psychology, sociology and health teaching, whose primary functions are the health education and medico-social counselling of individuals and families. Although in some ways resembling the public health nurse of Scandinavian countries the health visitor is really a unique product of the U.K., subsequently introduced into some other countries, e.g., South Africa.

Although several towns in the U.K. and at least one in the U.S.A. employed nurses earlier

to teach parents hygiene and child care, health visiting is generally said to have originated in Salford and Manchester in 1862, partly because these adjacent towns first used the name 'health visitor' and partly because the success of the experiment in these towns led to rapid imitation in many other districts. In the next hundred years or so, while the numbers of health visitors increased fairly steadily, there were many changes in their required background, their specialist training and their functions. Essentially in the 1870s the health visitor was a 'respectable working woman' with no training or merely in-service training and concerned only with the simplest aspects of child health. By the early 1900s she had one of a mixture of backgrounds – a few health visitors were doctors, many were nurses, some were female sanitary inspectors and some (from 1907) had taken courses specially devised to equip them for the job – but her scope in maternal and child health had widened, and in 1917 the Board of Health for England and Wales described her as 'the most important element in any scheme for maternity and child welfare.'

In 1919 regulations both in England and in Scotland required that future entrants to health visiting be (1) registered nurses with subsequent special training, or (2) university graduates with a different subsequent special training, or (3) persons with two years (later two and a half years) of special training. The second and third of these categories ultimately died out, because local authorities found that the nursing background produced the best results, and in due course a midwifery qualification was added to entry requirements. Health visiting had now become a recognized profession, but still dealt only with mothers, pre-school (and in some districts school) children, and cases involving infection. By the 1940s, however, health visitors had contributed greatly to the reduction of infant deaths (in England and Wales from 154 per thousand births in 1900 to 50 in 1939, well before the era of sulphonamides and antibiotics) and the general improvement of child health, the diminution of many nutritional diseases and of such 'dirt' diseases as ringworm and impetigo, the reduction of child deaths from burns and scalds, and to public acceptance of diphtheria immunization.

The twenty-six years from 1948 to 1974 saw a revolution in the health visitor's functions, status and professional preparation: a change from 'mother and baby nurse' to family health counsellor; from authoritarian adviser on diet and hygiene to the person employing sociological insight and psychological skill to create unobtrusively attitudes and behaviour conducive to good emotional and physical health; and from the assistant reporting to a doctor to the professional, collaborating on a basis of equality with doctors, social workers and school teachers.

Preliminary entrance requirements came to include not merely qualification as a registered nurse and some training in midwifery or obstetrics but also academic and personality standards beyond those needed for entry to nursing. The special full-time course after acceptance as a student was extended to a calendar year and was placed in the hands of lecturers (formerly called tutors) who had supplemented experience as practising health visitors by a further year's advanced training in educational psychology, teaching techniques for adults and other subjects; and the health visitor course was reorganized to include substantially more psychology, sociology and teaching theory and practice. This last was achieved largely through the efforts of the Council for the Education and Training of Health Visitors, established under an Act of 1962, and incidentally the only body dealing on a U.K. basis with any branch of nursing. As early as 1951 an official report had drawn attention to the health visitor's important roles in maintaining the health of old people, in general health education of the public, and in the promotion of mental hygiene. By the time of the integration of hospital and local authority health services (1974) she had an accepted place in health-promotion and disease-prevention in all age-groups, from prospective parents to old age pensioners, and – in addition to home visits which are essential both for identifying problems and for establishing and maintaining rapport – an accepted role in the health education of groups of adults and of children. Despite national shortages of numbers, the health visitor became increasingly regarded as the main family counsellor on matters of physical, emotional and social health, performing broadly the same functions in the field of prevention as did the general medical practitioner in the field of illness.

Three further developments were: (1) the introduction of men into health visiting, starting in Aberdeen in 1961 and accepted nationally in 1972; (2) the association of health visitors with general practitioners, not as one profession assisting the other but with the two workers exercising their different skills on the same group of clients or patients, and thereby minimizing duplicate visiting and reducing the possibility of contradictory advice; and (3) the appearance of specialist health visitors who could act in particular fields as consultants to their colleagues. Perhaps almost equally important was the appointment in many areas of registered or enrolled nurses as assistants to health visitors, to relieve them of tasks not requiring their full skill.

It is indicative of the importance that Britain attaches to health visitors that in the extreme financial stringency of 1976, when virtually all forms of public expenditure were being reduced or at least held stationary, the central government departments both in England and Wales and in Scotland advised area health boards to arrange for increases in their numbers of health visitors. Implicit in that advice, of course, was a recognition that, by preventing cases of various deseases, health visitors could decrease the total volume of illness and therefore its cost.

The health visitor is an essential and indispensable member of the team providing a health advisory service to families and individuals, and his or her main functions have been thus summarized by the Council for the Education and Training of Health Vistors:

1. Prevention of mental, physical and emotional ill-health, and alleviation of the consequences of such ill-health.
2. Early detection of ill-health and surveillance of high risk groups.

3. Recognition and identification of need, and mobilization of appropriate resources.
4. Health teaching.
5. Provision of care – including support during periods of stress, and advice and guidance in case of illness as well as in the care and management of children.

A recent joint report of the Royal College of General Practitioners and the Council for the Education and Training of Health Visitors stresses the need for most health visitors to be attached to general practices and the importance of general practitioners and health visitors recognizing each others' independent professional status, different priorities and individual responsibility and initiative. The report expressly indicates, however, that not all health visitors can be practice-attached: there must also be specialist health visitors who act as consultants to their colleagues.

The latest development in health visitor preparation is an interesting attempt to shorten total duration of training for suitable candidates – by providing a course of four and a half years which leads to a university degree (with or without honours), qualification as a state registered nurse, and a health visitor's certificate.

Largely because of under-payment and poor promotion avenues in the past, health visitors are in very short supply, although numbers are increasing. A recent official circular advocates one per 3,000 population (a figure already achieved by a few districts that recognized early the importance of improving health and reducing preventable disease), but many areas have less than one per 4,500, or less than two-thirds of the number really needed. Yet if a serious attempt is to be made to reduce disease by the education and unobtrusive counselling of the people in matters pertaining to emotional, physical and mental health, the health visitor is from her background, her training and her tradition of access to the homes of the people, almost certainly the key to success.

In extremely remote areas it is customary for geographical reasons to employ the same person as health visitor (on health education and counselling) and district nurse (on treatment). This saves travelling time but means that a person with the higher qualification of a health visitor has to devote part of her time to work requiring only a very short post-registration training; and at busy periods education for health and prevention of disease tend to be pushed aside by the demands of treatment.

hearing aids. For the elderly, unsophisticated, and non-mobile patient the old-fashioned ear-trumpet is still very good. It is simple to use, costs nothing to run, and is free from background noise.

However, the ordinary person with irreversible hearing loss seeks an aid which will be inconspicuous in use but will still make sound louder and speech more intelligible. Modern aids are therefore electro-magnetic devices consisting basically of microphone, amplifier, and receiver. Miniaturization of electrical components and the replacement of valves by transistors has enabled smaller and smaller aids to be developed with increased flexibility to match different needs.

The heart of a hearing aid is the amplifier. Its

degree of amplification is known as gain, usually of the order of 60 decibels at a frequency (pitch) of 1,000 Hertz. With an input of 65 dB, which is the average strength of ordinary conversation, an output of 125 dB will result. Since the maximum the receiver can handle is only a little more than this it does not help to shout: only distortion will result. Amplifiers can be designed to be more efficient on certain frequencies since those above 1,000 Hertz are more important for speech. All aids have a control for volume which may operate automatically and some have also a tone-control. Microphones do not pick up sound uniformly over the whole possible range of pitch: the smaller they are the more restricted their range, but fortunately high tones are least likely to be lost.

Selection. Before choosing a hearing aid the type of DEAFNESS should first be investigated. It is important to discover the amount of hearing conveyed in the normal way by air-conduction through the outer ear to stimulate the normal process of hearing, compared with the amount of hearing being conveyed by bone-conduction. A tuning-fork vibrated first while not quite touching the head and then while touching the skull will show the difference. According to the result the patient will benefit most either from a hearing aid which is inserted into the ear to amplify air-conducted sound, or from an aid placed behind the ear to help bone-conduction. In nerve deafness neither may be effective.

Types. There is a range of styles of aid, each designed for specific uses.

1. Body-worn – microphone and amplifier worn on the body. There is a cord to the ear-mould with single or Y-cord to both ears. National Health Service 'Medresco' aids are of this type, and there are various models – adult, child, and 'special' with more gain but limited frequency. Commercial aids are legion.

2. Post-aural aids – contained in a case which fits behind the ear. A National Health Service model is becoming available.

3. Spectacle aids – components housed in an enlarged side-piece of a spectacle frame and sound conveyed by a tube or vibrator.

4. In-the-ear-aids – generally have poor gain and limited frequency and are subject to 'squeal' (acoustic feed-back) because of the proximity of the receiver to the microphone.

5. Non-wearable aids – used in schools and for speech training. There is an amplifier and headphones, either single, or multiple for groups of children. The perimeter of the class-room is wired and individual hearing-aids have a pick-up coil so that children can move about freely in the class-room. A variation of this is the use of a VHF radio-transmitter by the teacher.

heart. A hollow muscular organ designed as a pump whose purpose is to circulate blood to all parts of the body. In shape it is conical with base uppermost and apex pointing downwards. It is situated centrally in the chest, behind the breast-bone and in close relation to the lungs with one-third of its bulk to the right, and two-thirds to the left of the mid-line. It is enclosed within a fibrous sac known as the pericardium and weighs about 480 to 560 g. (17 to 20 oz.) in males and rather less in females.

Internally it is divided by muscular partitions into four chambers – the right and left atria (or auricles) above, and the right and left ventricles

below; the right and left halves of the heart are completely separated and not in communication. However, the atria and ventricles of each side are connected through openings, each guarded by a non-return valve. The right valve is the tricuspid valve; on the left side is the bicuspid or mitral valve.

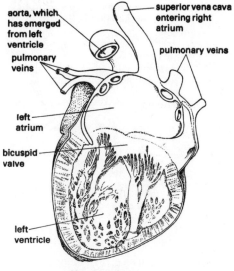

Heart: anatomy

The heart is composed almost entirely of a special type of muscle referred to generally as the myocardium, a term which also differentiates it from its delicate lining membrane, the endocardium (which also covers the valves), and its external sheath, the pericardium. The muscular walls of the atria are relatively thin compared with those of the ventricles and the left ventricle wall is about twice as thick as that of the right, since its work in propelling blood through the whole body is much greater than the work of the right ventricle, which is merely circulating blood through the lungs.

The blood supply to the heart itself comes from the right and left coronary arteries, branches of the aorta (the arterial trunk leaving the left ventricle). Narrowing or blockage of these arteries reduces or cuts off blood to the heart-muscle and causes myocardial ischaemia – the so-called 'heart-attack'.

Cardiac action is as follows: venous or deoxygenated blood returns from the body by the superior and inferior venae cavae to the right atrium, passes to the right ventricle and is pumped through the pulmonary arteries to the lungs. After oxygenation there it returns to the left atrium by the pulmonary veins, passes to the left ventricle and is propelled through the aorta and so to the rest of the arterial system, supplying oxygenated blood to the whole body.

Rate and force of cardiac contraction are controlled by the 'pacemaker', an area of specialized tissue at the base of the heart which is sensitive to chemical and nervous stimuli. Impulses arising in the pacemaker are propagated by a band of specialized muscle-

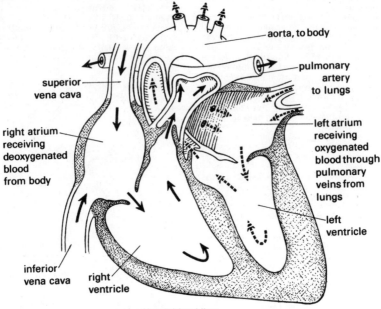

aorta, to body

pulmonary
artery
to lungs

superior
vena cava

left atrium
receiving
oxygenated
blood through
pulmonary
veins from
lungs

right atrium
receiving
deoxygenated
blood
from body

left
ventricle

inferior
vena cava

right
ventricle

Heart: blood flow

fibre (the bundle of His) to the atria and ventricles so that their contractions are regulated and co-ordinated.

The blood output of the heart is about 3 to 5 litres per minute but can rise to ten times as much during violent exercise.

The action of the heart in circulating the blood was first described by William Harvey (1578-1657) in 1628. Before then, unconvincing explanations advanced by Galen (A.D. 131-201) had held unchallenged sway.

Diseases. More than one-third of all deaths occur from various types of heart disease, which are the result of pathological processes affecting either the heart-muscle (myo-cardium), its lining membrane (endocardium), or its outer covering and enclosing sac (pericardium). Before describing these in detail, mention must be made of congenital heart disease which is an important cause of disability in infants and children but quite unrelated to the other conditions.

1. Congenital heart disease. Embryologically the primitive heart is a single continuous tube consisting of an atrial part, a ventricular part, and the aortic bulb. In the course of development each of these divides and eventually forms the right atrium, ventricle, and pulmonary artery and the left atrium, ventricle, and aorta.

If this process goes wrong congenital abnormalities result, such as defects in the wall dividing the right and the left sides of the heart, narrowing of either the pulmonary artery or the aorta, or persistence of certain structures which are needed in foetal life to draw oxygen from the mother's blood, because of course the unborn child cannot use its own lungs. It has been realized that the defects may be due to adverse influences during intra-uterine life,

notably the occurrence of German measles (rubella) in the mother. Rubella vaccination of adolescent girls is therefore a very important preventive measure; and advances in heart-surgery have been conspicuously successful in dealing with many such abnormalities and restoring normal life-expectancy.

2. Diseases affecting the myocardium. Acute myocarditis occurs mainly from (1) a complication of specific fevers such as diphtheria and typhoid fever, (2) rheumatic fever, (3) blood disorders such as uraemia and acidosis, and (4) sudden interruption of the blood supply to the heart muscle as by thrombosis or embolism.

Chronic myocarditis on the other hand is predominantly the result of vascular disease resulting from raised blood-pressure causing arteriosclerosis, from degeneration of vessel walls as in arteriosclerosis and syphilis, and from the general atrophy which accompanies old age. Angina is essentially severe pain due to shortage of blood to the heart muscle.

3. Diseases affecting the endocardium. Acute endocarditis occurs from invasion by bacteria, e.g., during rheumatic fever. The heart valves are particularly affected, becoming either narrowed (stenosis) so that the blood flow through them is diminished, or unable to close fully (incompetence) so that some of the blood flows backwards when the valve is supposedly closed. Both stenosis and incompetence lessen the efficiency of the heart as a pump. Chronic endocarditis occurs following acute endocarditis, or as a sequel to very prolonged physical strain, syphilis and some other diseases. Both in acute and in chronic endocarditis the commonest conditions are mitral incompetence, mitral stenosis and aortic

incompetence. Many cases of these can now be treated successfully by heart surgery.

4. Hypertensive heart disease. High blood pressure occurs either as an isolated condition – 'essential hypertension' – or as a secondary effect in other diseases. Death-rates were rising rapidly until about 1950; since essential hypertension is regarded as a stress disease this may have been due to the increased strains of modern life. From 1950 the rates have shown a modest decline and this period coincides with the introduction of hypotensive drugs. As a preventive measure it seems reasonable to advocate systematic search for cases of seriously elevated blood pressure so that affected individuals may be treated and helped to live less stressful lives.

5. Arteriosclerotic heart disease. This is the main cause of the blood supply to the heart muscles being insufficient and accounts for most cardiac deaths in men of middle-age and beyond. The recorded rates continue to rise steeply. There is no known single cause: rather there is a 'web of causation' which includes many risk factors. It has been demonstrated that if a man's age, blood pressure, serum cholesterol level, body bulk, physical activity, and smoking habits are all known, the risk of his having a coronary attack can be predicted with considerable accuracy.

Obesity, inertia, and raised fat levels in the blood, are all related to over-eating and are susceptible to dietary restriction and the substitution of unsaturated fats for those of animal origin. Machinery has lessened the need for activity at work and leisure pursuits are becoming more sedentary – spectator sports and television. The statistical association incriminating cigarette smoking is impressive; its effects are probably due to action on the sympathetic nervous system.

Coronary artery disease thus provides great opportunities for health education: avoid stress, eat less, reduce animal fats, stop smoking, and take more exercise – things easy to advocate but difficult to advocate successfully to a man who does not yet feel ill, thinks himself only mildly overweight and smokes heavily because of stresses beyond his control.

6. Diseases affecting the pericardium. Inflammation of the pericardium most usually accompanies the conditions producing endocarditis but it occasionally occurs in pneumonia, in tuberculosis, in terminal illness generally, and as a complication of trauma to the chest. Its importance lies in its disabling effect on cardiac action either from fibrinous exudation or from fluid effusion.

7. Disorders of cardiac rhythm. These affect the functional efficiency of the heart and result from damage to the 'pacemaker' and conducting mechanism brought about by almost any of the diseases described above.

8. Heart-block. This occurs when disease or degeneration of the 'pacemaker' causes partial or complete arrest of the impulses governing the heart beat. The ventricles then contract more or less independently and pulse-rate may fall to 20 or 30 beats per minute. Severe cases may have fainting or convulsive attacks from cerebral anoxia (Stokes-Adams syndrome), which is a condition in which insufficient oxygen reaches the brain.

Some patients are now treated by the implantation of an 'artificial pacemaker', which is electrical. See also HEART, DISORDERED ACTION, HEART FAILURE and HEART SURGERY.

heartburn. A peculiar burning sensation felt behind the lower part of the breast-bone, and often accompanied by flatulence and belching. It is common in chronic indigestion and is presumed to be due to irritation of the lower end of the oesophagus by the stomach contents. Antacids usually afford relief but heartburn is not specifically due to the action of gastric hydrochloric acid since it may occur in achlorhydria.

heart, disordered action. This condition, sometimes referred to briefly as DAH, is also known as soldier's heart, effort syndrome and neuro-circulatory asthenia. It occurs mainly in adolescence and early adult life when poorly-developed individuals are abruptly subjected to unaccustomed physical exertion, as in military training.

The symptoms are breathlessness, palpitation, chest pain, and sometimes nervousness and fainting, related to physical exertion but often persisting at rest. The pulse-rate is increased and makes an exaggerated response to effort. Treatment is by rest, sedation and a more gradual training regime.

heart failure. A very general term, indicating inability of the heart to maintain an efficient circulation, so that an individual gradually finds that he cannot undertake customary physical exertion without symptoms of distress.

Basically failure develops from heart-muscle (myocardial) insufficiency or from some interference with the stimuli which cause its rhythmical contraction (see HEART). Lessened contraction or slowing rate of contraction causes less blood to be pushed through. Heart-muscle may be weakened by toxaemia or by interference with its blood supply, but insufficiency may also develop when the heart is called on for more work than it is capable of performing. This happens when there is excessive resistance in either the pulmonary or systemic circulation or when narrowed or leaking valves impair the heart's mechanical efficiency as a pump. For a time these difficulties are met by compensatory changes, the heart increasing in size and muscularity to pump more forcibly, but eventually compensation fails.

Slower or irregular contractions of heart muscle occur as the result of toxaemia, in poisoning by certain drugs, in endocrine disorders, particularly thyrotoxicosis, and in myocarditis and myocardial degeneration. Clinically cardiac failure is regarded either as acute or chronic.

Acute heart failure. The most common cause is coronary artery thrombosis, leading to cardiac infarction. The symptoms are severe pain in the cardiac area, often radiating down the left arm, with palpitation, severe breathlessness and collapse, leading in extreme instances to unconsciousness and death. Although the onset may be unexpected it is likely that gradual diminution of cardiac reserve will have been noted before the actual attack. Other causes of sudden failure are toxaemia from infections, notably diphtheria, sudden changes in rhythm as in fibrillation or heart-block, and less usual incidents such as pulmonary artery embolism.

Cases of acute heart failure need complete rest and expert care, and most general hospitals now deal with such patients in intensive-care units where the cardiac action can be monitored and immediate steps taken to institute appropriate treatment.

Chronic cardiac failure. The main causes of more gradual failure of the heart are (1) myocardial insufficiency from disease of the blood vessels, (2) disturbances of rhythm, (3) increased pressure in pulmonary circulation due to chronic bronchitis, emphysema and pulmonary fibrosis, (4) increased pressure in systemic circulation due mainly to arteriosclerosis or chronic nephritis, and (5) mechanical effects such as adherent pericardium or the presence of mediastinal tumours. The salient features are increasing breathlessness on exertion, palpitation, and oedema of dependent parts, especially legs and ankles. Water-logging of tissues may develop and with right-sided heart failure there is often a troublesome cough and profuse, watery sputum. Impaired circulation also effects other systems to produce indigestion, sleeplessness, restlessness, impaired memory, diminished urinary output, and albuminuria.

Treatment is based on rest, light diet, cardiac tonics such as digitalis, the administration of diuretics, and sedation as indicated.

heart murmur. An abnormal sound heard on listening to the heart with a stethoscope.

Since many children have in the past been needlessly debarred from taking part in athletic activities because a general practitioner heard a murmur, it is important to stress that murmurs of no significance are much commoner than murmurs of significance.

Soft murmurs while the heart contracts (systolic murmurs) can be heard in many apparently healthy hearts. Observation over many decades of persons with such murmurs has revealed no evidence of heart disease, and post mortem examination of such persons after their death from unrelated causes has shown healthy hearts. Again, a soft, blowing murmur is common in anaemia, in several fevers and in various other illnesses, and tends to disappear when the condition is cured.

However, certain murmurs occurring at the various valves of the heart indicate disease of the particular valve. Broadly these are of two types: stenosis (narrowing or shrinkage) where the valve is unable to resist the pressure of blood in a contracting chamber of the heart; and incompetence (leaking) where the valve cannot efficiently close and so permits a back-flow of blood during the phase of relaxation.

heart surgery. Despite the increasing competence of general surgery in every other field, the difficulties of cardiac surgery still loomed large as late as 1930 and the prospects of any really fruitful progress seemed dim. The operative problems facing the would-be heart surgeon were much more daunting than those of his colleagues in other fields because a functioning circulation was essential to life and the heart could not just be shut-off, stopped, and emptied of blood while the operator repaired its defects.

The earliest operations were therefore those which could be done entirely from outside the heart or at least by some rapid procedure which, although allowing limited access to its interior, would interrupt its action for only a brief period. Such operations rectifying minor congenital abnormalities or enlarging a narrowed valve in mitral disease, were undertaken with encouraging success.

Since those early beginnings there have been great advances. The surgeon's need was for more time and this was met by the development of heart-lung machines which could maintain the circulation while the heart was stopped and bypassed. Some use was also made of the principle of hypothermia: lowering body-temperature reduces tissue-demand for oxygen and gives the surgeon perhaps eight minutes to work instead of four but obviously this was not the real answer.

Although efficient and reliable heart-lung machines were the key to real progress this has not been achieved without help from other specialities, and especially in the fields of anaesthetics, blood-transfusion and pharmacology (for anticoagulant drugs). Above all, the ability to undertake cardiac operations on a more or less routine basis meant that it was necessary to know exactly what defect was present in order to plan procedures and give some sort of assessment of the likely results of treatment. Thus diagnostic tests had to be developed to a greater degree; and it has turned out that the use of x-ray diagnosis has supplied the answer.

A considerable range of operations is now undertaken. Commonest are repairs of congenital defects, repair or replacement of valves, and procedures to replace narrowed or diseased sections of the blood vessels supplying the heart muscle.

Even more dramatic have been recent developments in heart TRANSPLANT using healthy hearts from cases of sudden accidental death. The surgical problems of transplant operations have been overcome, but the factors still preventing reliable results are those of tissue-rejection. The most satisfying successes of cardiac surgery have been in dealing with congenital heart disease. Perhaps 75 per cent of 'blue babies' (i.e., those with a hole in the central wall of the heart that allows the blood to mix between the two sides) can now be saved who would otherwise have died for certain; and older children with lesser defects can in most cases be assured of growing up to lead a normal life. Valve operations on well-chosen adult cases also give encouraging results.

heat. The effect of heat on matter is to increase the activity of molecules and hence their energy; thus energy and heat are interchangeable.

Body temperature is maintained at a constant figure of 37 C. (98.4 F.) by a temperature-regulating centre in the mid-brain. Heat production results from the metabolism of food and from muscular activity, and heat-loss occurs mainly from the body surface by radiation and convection and particularly by the evaporation of sweat which has a cooling effect.

If heat-loss exceeds heat-production the body attempts to correct this by shivering in order to produce more heat from additional muscular activity. If this fails the condition of hypothermia will ensue. In a climate with high temperatures and high humidity heat-loss is insufficient and the body temperature will rise to produce hyperpyrexia. This may result in

MEN

Height in cm. (in.)	Weight in kg. (lb.) at ages shown		
	20 YEARS	25 YEARS	30 YEARS
149 (59)	45.7 - 50.7 - 57.0 (101 - 112 - 126)	47.5 - 53.0 - 59.3 (105 - 117 - 131)	49.3 - 54.8 - 61.6 (109 - 121 - 136)
152 (60)	46.6 - 51.6 - 58.0 (103 - 114 - 128)	48.4 - 53.9 - 60.7 (107 - 119 - 134)	50.2 - 55.7 - 62.5 (111 - 123 - 138)
154 (61)	47.5 - 53.0 - 59.3 (105 - 117 - 131)	49.3 - 54.8 - 61.6 (109 - 121 - 136)	51.1 - 56.6 - 63.4 (113 - 125 - 140)
157 (62)	48.9 - 54.3 - 61.6 (108 - 120 - 135)	50.7 - 56.1 - 62.9 (112 - 124 - 139)	52.1 - 58.0 - 65.2 (115 - 128 - 144)
160 (63)	50.2 - 55.7 - 62.5 (111 - 123 - 138)	52.1 - 58.0 - 65.2 (115 - 128 - 144)	53.4 - 59.3 - 66.6 (118 - 131 - 147)
162 (64)	51.6 - 57.5 - 64.8 (114 - 127 - 143)	53.9 - 59.8 - 67.0 (119 - 132 - 148)	55.2 - 61.1 - 68.8 (122 - 135 - 152)
165 (65)	53.4 - 59.3 - 66.6 (118 - 131 - 147)	55.7 - 61.6 - 69.3 (123 - 136 - 153)	56.6 - 62.9 - 70.7 (125 - 139 - 156)
167 (66)	55.2 - 61.1 - 68.8 (122 - 135 - 152)	57.0 - 63.4 - 71.1 (126 - 140 - 157)	58.4 - 64.8 - 72.9 (129 - 143 - 161)
170 (67)	56.6 - 62.9 - 70.7 (125 - 139 - 156)	58.9 - 65.2 - 73.4 (130 - 144 - 162)	59.8 - 66.6 - 74.7 (132 - 147 - 165)
172 (68)	58.4 - 64.8 - 72.9 (129 - 143 - 161)	60.2 - 67.0 - 75.2 (133 - 148 - 166)	61.6 - 68.4 - 77.0 (136 - 151 - 170)
175 (69)	59.8 - 66.6 - 74.7 (132 - 147 - 165)	62.0 - 68.8 - 77.5 (137 - 152 - 171)	63.8 - 70.7 - 79.3 (141 - 156 - 175)
177 (70)	61.6 - 68.4 - 77.0 (136 - 151 - 170)	63.8 - 71.1 - 79.7 (141 - 157 - 176)	65.7 - 72.9 - 82.0 (145 - 161 - 181)
180 (71)	63.8 - 70.7 - 79.3 (141 - 156 - 175)	66.1 - 73.4 - 82.4 (146 - 162 - 182)	67.9 - 75.6 - 85.2 (150 - 167 - 188)
182 (72)	65.7 - 72.9 - 82.0 (145 - 161 - 181)	68.4 - 76.1 - 85.6 (151 - 168 - 189)	70.7 - 78.4 - 87.9 (156 - 173 - 194)
185 (73)	67.9 - 75.2 - 84.3 (150 - 166 - 186)	71.1 - 78.8 - 88.3 (157 - 174 - 195)	72.9 - 81.1 - 91.1 (161 - 179 - 201)
187 (74)	69.7 - 77.5 - 87.0 (154 - 171 - 192)	72.9 - 81.1 - 91.1 (161 - 179 - 201)	75.6 - 83.8 - 94.3 (167 - 185 - 208)

Table of ideal weights at various heights and ages; three weights are given in each instance, and refer to small, medium and large builds. All weights given are for unclothed persons.

heat-exhaustion, HEAT-STROKE, or muscular cramps due to excessive loss of salt in perspiration.

In medicine heat is also used therapeutically. Poultices or heating-pads induce hyperaemia or increased blood flow and relax muscle spasm. This increases cell activity, stimulates repair and healing, and relieves pain and

WOMEN

Height in cm. (in.)	Weight in kg. (lb.) at ages shown		
	20 YEARS	25 YEARS	30 YEARS
142 (56)	43.0 - 47.5 - 53.0 (95 - 105 - 117)	43.9 - 48.9 - 55.2 (97 - 108 - 122)	45.3 - 50.2 - 56.6 (100 - 111 - 125)
144 (57)	43.5 - 48.4 - 53.9 (96 - 107 - 119)	44.9 - 49.8 - 56.1 (99 - 110 - 124)	46.2 - 51.1 - 57.5 (102 - 113 - 127)
147 (58)	44.4 - 49.3 - 55.7 (98 - 109 - 123)	45.7 - 50.7 - 57.0 (101 - 112 - 126)	47.1 - 52.1 - 58.4 (104 - 115 - 129)
149 (59)	45.3 - 50.2 - 56.6 (100 - 111 - 125)	46.4 - 51.2 - 58.0 (103 - 114 - 128)	47.5 - 53.0 - 59.8 (105 - 117 - 132)
152 (60)	46.6 - 51.6 - 58.0 (103 - 114 - 128)	47.1 - 52.5 - 59.3 (104 - 116 - 131)	48.4 - 53.9 - 60.7 (107 - 119 - 134)
154 (61)	47.5 - 53.0 - 59.8 (105 - 117 - 132)	48.4 - 53.9 - 60.7 (107 - 119 - 134)	49.8 - 55.2 - 62.0 (110 - 122 - 137)
157 (62)	48.9 - 54.3 - 61.1 (108 - 120 - 135)	50.2 - 55.7 - 62.5 (111 - 123 - 138)	51.1 - 56.6 - 63.8 (113 - 125 - 141)
160 (63)	50.2 - 55.7 - 62.5 (111 - 123 - 138)	51.1 - 57.0 - 64.3 (113 - 126 - 142)	52.5 - 58.4 - 65.7 (116 - 129 - 145)
162 (64)	51.1 - 57.0 - 64.3 (113 - 126 - 142)	52.5 - 58.4 - 65.7 (116 - 129 - 145)	53.9 - 59.8 - 67.5 (119 - 132 - 149)
165 (65)	53.0 - 58.9 - 66.1 (117 - 130 - 146)	54.3 - 60.2 - 67.5 (120 - 133 - 149)	55.7 - 61.6 - 69.3 (123 - 136 - 153)
167 (66)	54.8 - 60.7 - 68.4 (121 - 134 - 151)	55.7 - 62.0 - 69.7 (123 - 136 - 154)	57.0 - 63.4 - 71.6 (126 - 140 - 158)
170 (67)	56.1 - 62.5 - 70.2 (124 - 138 - 155)	57.5 - 63.8 - 71.6 (127 - 141 - 158)	58.9 - 65.2 - 73.4 (130 - 144 - 162)
172 (68)	57.5 - 63.8 - 72.0 (127 - 141 - 159)	59.3 - 65.7 - 73.8 (131 - 145 - 163)	60.2 - 67.0 - 75.6 (133 - 148 - 167)
175 (69)	59.3 - 65.7 - 73.8 (131 - 145 - 163)	60.7 - 67.5 - 75.6 (134 - 149 - 167)	61.6 - 68.4 - 77.0 (136 - 151 - 170)
177 (70)	60.7 - 67.5 - 76.1 (134 - 149 - 168)	62.0 - 68.8 - 77.5 (137 - 152 - 171)	63.4 - 70.2 - 78.8 (140 - 155 - 174)
180 (71)	62.9 - 69.7 - 78.4 (139 - 154 - 173)	63.4 - 70.7 - 79.7 (140 - 156 - 176)	64.8 - 72.0 - 81.1 (143 - 159 - 179)

Table of ideal weights at various heights and ages; three weights are given in each instance, and refer to small, medium and large builds. All weights given are for unclothed persons.

tension. General application as by an electric-blanket or hot-air cage are used to counteract shock. If continued they will cause increased perspiration (diaphoresis) and this is sometimes used to assist in the elimination of waste-products as in kidney disease.

heatstroke. A state of general collapse brought about by exposure to excessive heat. It is synonymous with sunstroke but exposure to the sun is not essential. A better term is heat hyperpyrexia which emphasizes the essential feature of a markedly raised body temperature.

The condition mainly occurs in tropical climates when the shade temperature reaches about 43 °C. (110 °F.). Exercise and high atmospheric humidity increase the risk. Symptoms are usually sudden in onset with malaise, headache, restlessness, nausea and vomiting. The body temperature may rise to 43.3 °C. (110 °F.) or more with mental excitement, delirium, convulsions and, sometimes, coma and death.

Prompt and adequate treatment is required, with cold sponging and ice-packs to lower body temperature, and the replacement of fluid and salt. Recovery may be followed by signs of heart strain and mental disturbance. Later re-exposure to heat may induce further attacks more readily than before.

height and weight. Variation occurs in all biological phenomena and in any population it is a matter of everyday observation that individuals differ widely in bulk and stature. Considerable variation in height and weight is quite compatible with normality. There are many reasons why this is so: no population is at all homogeneous; it is made up of a variety of racial types, and individuals are also affected by their personal heredity. Apart from these genetic considerations bodily development is markedly influenced by nutrition, exercise and disease during the period of growth. In adult life fluctuations of weight should be investigated.

Tables which purport to show ideal heights and weights have to be employed with these considerations in mind but they are sufficiently representative to indicate whether a person is seriously under- or over-weight. Those given on the previous pages relate to adults; for children's tables, see DEVELOPMENT.

For adults of both sexes, three weights are given for each height related to small, medium or large build. All weights given are for unclothed persons. The weights shown for age 30 should ideally be maintained throughout life although some authorities are prepared to accept a further rise of roughly 0.5 kg. (1 lb.) per year until the age of 45 as still being within acceptable limits.

The arithmetical mean of a particular set of observations is obtained by adding up all the individual measurements and then dividing by their total number. This is not a particularly useful statistic because it tells nothing of the range of variation nor of the frequency with which particular values occur. If instead a large number of measurements of a particular characteristic are plotted on a graph according to their size and frequency, the result is a bell-shaped curve known as the normal distribution curve which serves to illustrate both the extent and numerical importance of any deviations from the average.

Attempts have been made to devise formulae as a substitute for tables. Two useful rules of this kind for adults are (1) ideal weight in kg. = height in cm. minus 100 or, alternatively, (2) ideal weight in kg. = height in cm. multiplied by chest measurement in cm. divided by 240.

heliotherapy. The treatment of certain

Inches converted into centimeters (to nearest 0.5 cm.)					
in.	cm.	in.	cm.	in.	cm.
15	38.0	37	94.0	59	149.5
16	40.5	38	96.5	60	152.5
17	43.0	39	99.0	61	155.0
18	45.5	40	101.5	62	157.5
19	48.0	41	104.0	63	160.0
20	51.0	42	106.5	64	162.5
21	53.5	43	109.0	65	165.0
22	56.0	44	111.5	66	167.5
23	58.5	45	114.0	67	170.0
24	61.0	46	117.0	68	172.5
25	63.5	47	119.5	69	175.0
26	66.0	48	122.0	70	178.0
27	68.5	49	124.5	71	180.5
28	71.0	50	127.0	72	183.0
29	73.5	51	129.5	73	185.5
30	76.0	52	132.0	74	188.0
31	78.5	53	134.5	75	190.5
32	81.0	54	137.0	76	193.0
33	84.0	55	139.5	77	195.5
34	86.5	56	142.0	78	198.0
35	89.0	57	144.5		
36	91.5	58	147.0		

diseases, particularly rickets and tuberculosis of bones and joints, by exposure of the body to direct sunlight. See SUNLIGHT TREATMENT.

hemicrania. See MIGRAINE.

hemiplegia. Paralysis affecting one side of the body. Nerve-fibres controlling voluntary movements of face, arm and leg originate from either side of the cerebral cortex of the brain, cross over to the opposite side in the brain-stem, before continuing on their way to the muscles.

Any disease, such as haemorrhage, thrombosis, embolism or other organic disease such as tumour which results in damage to only one side of the brain thus causes paralysis of varying extent on the opposite side of the body.

Because speech centres are situated in the left of the brain, loss of speech facility (aphasia) is associated only with right hemiplegia but impaired muscular action may cause speech difficulties (dysphasia) irrespective of the side involved.

hemp. The plant *Cannabis sativa* from which the drug CANNABIS is prepared.

heparin. A complex organic substance, secreted by connective tissue cells, which acts as an anticoagulant of the blood (i.e., it reduces blood-clotting). This it achieves mainly by inhibiting the conversion of pro-thrombin to thrombin. It is prepared commercially from cattle lung and is injected into the vein in conditions where it is desirable to reduce the tendency of the blood to clot, such as in cases of thrombosis. The effect of a single dose lasts for about two hours but a 'sustained-release' preparation is also available.

hepatitis. Inflammation of the liver. Although this may be a complication of various infections or result from poisoning by certain drugs, the most common cause is a virus infection and two distinct types are recognized.

1. Acute infective hepatitis tends to occur in local outbreaks and is probably a food-borne

infection. An attack usually starts with the appearance of jaundice and bile-coloured urine, followed by symptoms of toxaemia – loss of appetite, headache and fever. The jaundice may take some weeks to clear up and convalescence may be prolonged.

2. Serum hepatitis is due to a specific virus known as SH or 'Australia' antigen. Cases result from contact with infected blood. The disease may be serious and is a hazard in blood transfusion, in renal dialysis, and in transplant surgery, and since it may also be communicated by improperly sterilized syringes and other instruments it often affects drug addicts and may occur after tattooing.

Gammaglobulin is used both for the prevention and treatment of infective hepatitis. It is particularly important that cases of hepatitis should avoid alcohol for at least a year after an attack because of its toxic effect on liver cells already weakened by the disease.

heredity and environment. heredity is the organic relationship between parents and offspring which leads to the transmission of characteristics and diseases from earlier ancestors. The study of the factors which determine this transmission is known as GENETICS. Human inheritance is bi-parental (derived partly from the father and partly from the mother), and it is a matter of common knowledge and experience that obvious traits of parents, such as skin and eye colour, curly hair, and shape of nose, reappear in their children.

These are examples of biological inheritance the content of which is determined at the time of conception when an egg-cell and sperm-cell unite to produce a fertilized ovum or zygote. At early stages of development the human embryo looks exactly like that of any other mammal but it contains within itself a biological code of instructions which determines its future conformation and characteristics.

Heredity is of course only partly responsible for an individual's total make-up because development after birth is universally influenced by every conceivable environmental factor – and even before birth, as witness the thalidomide disaster. The sum of these influences is the cultural inheritance.

No two persons are exactly alike. Identical twins arise from a single ovum and share a common biological inheritance but although they may look alike they may develop quite differently in different environments. This is the fundamental difference between inherited and acquired characteristics. A parent with six toes, which is quite a common deformity, has a good chance of producing a child with six toes too, but a parent who accidentally loses a toe will never have a four-toed child.

The inheritance of mental traits is no different from the inheritance of physical characteristics. The capacity to learn is inborn just as is ability for music, or mathematics, or any special skill. Exploitation of such capacities depends on environmental opportunities.

In relation to disease the same situation is found. Many diseases are now known to be due to abnormalities present in the biological inheritance – haemophilia and colour-blindness are familiar examples – and similarly there may be inborn characteristics which only become manifest after interaction with the

environment, as an increased susceptibility to develop specific diseases.

Although heredity is a complex subject the basic laws are now well understood and they have practical applications in the production of improved breeds of plants and animals and also in GENETIC GUIDANCE.

hermaphroditism. The combination of essential male and female structures and functions in one individual. Although this is normal in flowering plants and in lower animals of such types as worms, molluscs, snails and polyps, it is a very rare abnormality in mammals, and in man very few examples of true hermaphroditism have ever been recorded.

In the cases of 'sex change' which are occasionally seen the condition is really pseudo-hermaphroditism. Either ovaries or testes are present as usual but malformation or imperfect development of the external sexual organs leads to a child being regarded as of the opposite sex to its real hormone condition. Difficulties then arise at puberty or in later life when the error becomes apparent. In the past the best advice that could be given was that doubtful cases should be brought up as boys until proved otherwise but it is now possible to determine genetic sex positively by chromosome examination and specialist advice should be sought immediately.

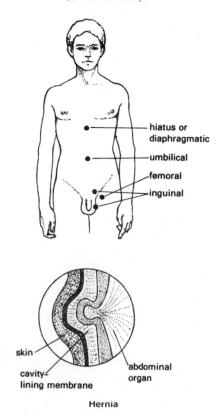

Hernia

hernia. The protrusion of some organ or part of an organ through a weak spot in the wall of its containing cavity, the protrusion remaining covered by the lining membrane of the cavity and by the overlying soft tissues and skin.

Hernia is most frequently seen in the lower abdomen (where it is popularly called 'rupture') and appears as a swelling in the groin. In inguinal hernia a portion of bowel passes down the inguinal canal in the pelvis and in men may reach the scrotum. Femoral hernia occupies the femoral canal alongside the main blood vessels to the leg. Both these types may be controlled by the wearing of a TRUSS. Other abdominal hernias include umbilical hernia (through the umbilicus), incisional or ventral hernia (through a weak abdominal scar) and hiatus or diaphragmatic hernia in which congenital or acquired weakness of the diaphragm allows abdominal contents to bulge into the chest cavity.

So long as a hernia can be returned to the abdomen by external manipulation it is 'reducible' and can generally be controlled by a truss. If adhesions form it becomes irreducible, and is then more likely to become a potential danger as the section of the intestine concerned may become obstructed or strangulated by the wall through which it has protruded. Both of these situations will necessitate an emergency operation.

Trusses are rather unsatisfactory because although they have relieved the situation, they have not corrected it; most hernias can be satisfactorily repaired by a relatively simple and effective operation at negligible risk.

heroin. Di-acetyl morphine, a powerful alkaloid derived from opium. Although less depressant of the respiratory centre than morphine it is perhaps the most dangerous drug of ADDICTION. Its use is now restricted and (in the U.K., by the Misuse of Drugs Act, 1971) may be prescribed for addicts only in special centres.

In underworld jargon it goes by various names such as 'boy', 'horse', 'jack', 'schmee' and 'schmeck' or 'smack'.

herpes. A superficial skin infection due to the virus *Herpes simplex* and not to be confused with herpes zoster, more commonly known as SHINGLES. A crop of small watery blisters usually occurs on the face around the margins of the nose and mouth; these dry up and form crusts which separate in about a week. It is frequently seen in association with the common cold (cold sore) or with more serious infective illnesses such as pneumonia.

No treatment is really required. The lesions may be dabbed with spirit and kept dry.

herpes zoster. See SHINGLES

hiccough (hiccup). A troublesome symptom produced by repeated sudden spasms of the diaphragm with simultaneous closure of the glottis.

Usually transitory and unimportant, it is often produced by taking food or drink too rapidly with sudden distension of the stomach. Expedients such as holding the breath, sucking an ice-cube, or holding a hot-water bottle over the stomach soon bring relief.

In a more prolonged form it occurs as a symptom of serious disease of stomach or bowel (because of irritation to the diaphragm), and it may complicate the after-treatment of operations on the upper abdomen. It is also common in uraemia and cirrhosis of the liver, and occurs in encephalitis lethargica. Hiccough from such causes exhausts the patient and is very difficult to treat without resorting to powerful sedation.

high blood pressure. See BLOOD PRESSURE.

hip. The joint between the pelvis and the upper end of each femur, or thigh bone. The rounded head of the femur fits into a cup-shaped cavity (acetabulum) on the pelvis and this ball-and-socket design ensures that it is both freely movable and strong enough to withstand the stresses imposed by weight-bearing, walking, running, and jumping. It is further supported by ligaments and the overlying thigh muscles.

Injuries. Dislocation of the joint may occur as may fracture of the narrow neck of bone between the rounded head and the shaft of the femur.

Diseases. (1) Tuberculous arthritis, formerly common in children, is now less often seen since milk became largely free from bovine tuberculosis; (2) Perthes' disease, an obscure degenerative process, affects the femoral head during growth and occurs mainly in boys; (3) osteo-arthritis, a degenerative joint disease, is found in older persons.

Congenital dislocation. It has been recognized since the time of Hippocrates that some new-born infants have hip-joints which are either dislocated or easily dislocatable because the socket (acetabulum) on the pelvis is too shallow to retain the head of the femur.

The cause is unknown. The incidence is about 1.25 cases per 1,000 births and females are three times more commonly affected than males. The condition can be recognized in new-born infants within their first week of life with a high degree of certainty by a manipulative test. If it is not recognized and treated promptly the patient develops a characteristic 'dipping' gait and is liable to osteo-arthritic changes and further crippling.

Treatment is simple: the hips are placed in full abduction, the legs splayed at 90 from the line of the body. Splints or plaster may be used but in many cases the application of specially bulky 'nappies' will suffice to maintain the required position. With prompt diagnosis, splinting is seldom needed for longer than twelve weeks and follow-up of cases has shown uniform success. If the diagnosis is missed subsequent treatment is much more difficult, troublesome and prolonged, and not always so effective.

The virtual eradication of this condition is one of the unappreciated triumphs of preventive medicine and testing for the condition should be a routine of every doctor, health visitor or nurse with responsibility for the care of a new-born infant.

Hippocrates. Hippocrates of Cos (about 460-370 B.C.) is traditionally regarded as the 'father of medicine'. Egyptian physicians and early Greeks, like the semi-legendary Aesculapius, were essentially witch-doctors who effected their 'cures' largely by spells and incantations and recorded no failures. Hippocrates, however, employed rational methods of treatment and described more failures than successes. His *On the Prognostics* gives a magnificent description of the signs of approaching death. His *Epidemics* contain the first scientific case-histories – forty-two in number, of which twenty-five ended fatally – and constitute essentially the beginning of clinical medicine. His essay *On the Sacred Disease* denies the supernatural origin of epilepsy. His *Airs, Places, Waters* is the first treatise on public health and medical geography. His *Aphorisms* have been described as 'the essence of the therapeutics and ethics of medicine'.

Many of his aphorisms have a startlingly modern note, e.g., 'fat people tend to die earlier than slender people', and 'consumption is commonest between the ages of 18 and 35'; but perhaps his first and best known aphorism may be quoted in full: 'Life is short and the art is long; the occasion fleeting; experience fallacious and judgment difficult. The physician must not only be prepared to do what is right personally but must also make the patient, the attendants and the surroundings co-operate'.

Some modern iconoclasts deny that Hippocrates ever existed. Yet somebody changed the face of medicine, and people who were alive during his lifetime – such as Plato – mention Hippocrates by name. Certainly he did not write all the seventy books attributed to him: some are manifestly written in a later century, and some may well be the work of his colleagues and contemporaries, or of his students. Yet when all removals of possibly later work are made, his finest books reveal a man of startlingly original observation, humane attitude and scientific enquiry, a man who emancipated medicine from priest-ridden magic and founded the science and art of clinical medicine, a man who set a standard of honesty (for instance, in recording his failures) for all future physicians to follow, and a man who gave medicine its ethical basis. After twenty-four centuries he still stands as probably the person who has made the greatest contribution to medicine.

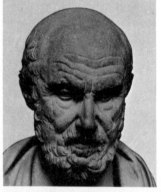

Hippocrates

Hippocratic oath. The oath, attributed to Hippocrates but in all probability of earlier origin, traditionally taken by doctors when they qualify, but presumably initially taken by students on admission to the medical school at Cos. The oath makes seven pledges: (1) that the doctor will hold those who taught him as dear to him as his own parents; (2) that he will impart knowledge of medicine only to his own sons, his teachers' sons and recognized students; (3) that he will treat patients to the best of his ability and judgment; (4) that he will

not perform surgical operations but will leave them to persons specializing in that line; (5) that he will not have sexual relations with patients or members of their households; (6) that he will not give poison and will not give a woman a pessary to cause abortion; and (7) that he will keep to himself all information obtained. These things he swears by Apollo, Aesculapius, Hygeia and Panacea; the latter two, goddesses of health and healing respectively, are daughters of Apollo in Greek mythology.

The prohibition on operative surgery at first appears strange since surgery did not become a separate speciality until many hundreds of years after the time of Hippocrates and since the Hippocratic writings themselves contain detailed instruction on various surgical procedures. Probably the intention was merely to debar the young, inexperienced doctor from attempting on his own procedures for which he as yet lacked the requisite experience.

histamine. A substance produced in all body tissues by the breakdown of the amino-acid, histidine. Its main action is to enlarge small blood vessels and so increase the blood supply to the tissues. Abnormally large quantities of histamine, or of closely related substances, are produced in conditions of allergy, in shock, and in certain injuries. Excess histamine is the principal cause both of inflammation and of allergic symptoms. Drugs which reduce the action of histamine are called ANTIHISTAMINES.

histology. The study of bodily tissues under the microscope. This investigation of the structure of the cells in tissues and organs has contributed enormously to our knowledge of physiology, and therefore of pathology. The tissues to be studied are prepared by cutting very thin slices (or 'sections') and staining them with dyes which are taken up by the various structures within the cells so that they show up more clearly.

An average human cell has a diameter of about 0.02 mm. (or one-thousandth of an inch) and can therefore be easily examined under the high power lens of a standard microscope which magnifies objects about 1,000 times. For more elaborate study of detail the electron microscope provides magnification up to about 250,000 times – sufficient to render a large molecule visible.

histoplasmosis. A disease of the lungs – also known as Darling's disease and cave disease – caused by infection with *Histoplasma capsulatum,* a fungus found in the dried excreta of bats and various birds. The disease has an acute form with symptoms resembling those of influenza, and a more severe chronic form which resembles tuberculosis of the lungs and spleen. The condition is almost unknown in Britain but not uncommon in the U.S.A.

Prevention would seem to lie mainly in avoidance of air-borne spores in caves, old silos, etc. Most cases recover without special treatment, but where this is not so, antifungal antibiotics are worth trying.

hives. An allergic reaction to foods (especially strawberries, shellfish, eggs and chocolate) or less commonly to antibiotics or to pollen, causing reddish, itching, circular weals. Prevention is difficult and involves identifying the cause so that the patient may try to avoid it. Calamine lotion or a paste of bicarbonate of soda applied to the itchy skin may help, but in severe cases antihistamine drugs are desirable.

hoarseness. A rough, grating or 'husky' tone of voice. When air is forced through the larynx and between the vocal cords a sound is produced which is then modified by movements of the palate, tongue, mouth and lips to form intelligible speech. The pitch and tonal quality of the basic sound is determined by the tension and position of the vocal cords.

Inflammatory conditions and tumours affecting the larynx and vocal cords interfere with this mechanism and the vocal cords themselves may become paralysed from damage to their nerve supply. Any of these conditions may affect the character of the voice.

Persistent hoarseness calls for examination of the larynx to determine the precise cause.

Hodgkin's disease. A condition, also known as lymphadenoma, in which there is a painless progressive enlargement of lymph glands near the body surface, and ultimately of lymphoid tissue throughout the body. It can occur at any age but most commonly in males under 40.

The initial stages are followed by the development of general symptoms of anaemia, lassitude, breathlessness, and loss of weight, and the occurrence of a characteristic fluctuating fever (Pel-Ebstein fever). There is often itching and the skin may become sallow or pigmented.

The disease was formerly always fatal, few cases surviving for more than five years, but modern treatment either by radiotherapy alone or combined with courses of cytotoxic drugs (i.e., drugs which prevent cells from reproducing, so that the enlargement of the lymphoid tissue is halted) has considerably improved the prospects of at least securing some measure of remission for considerable periods.

holly berries. The fruit of the holly tree occurring as clusters of bright red or scarlet berries. The common garden holly is *Ilex aquifolia* but other species of *Ilex* have a worldwide distribution. Children should not be allowed to eat the attractive berries. They are mildly poisonous and will cause abdominal pain, headache, vomiting and purging. The active ingredient is ilicin.

If vomiting does not occur spontaneously, an emetic (e.g., a tablespoon of mustard in a glass of water) should be given to induce it, followed later by a laxative. The berries are so bitter to taste and are usually rejected so promptly, that it is unlikely that any serious harm will result.

home nursing. The increasing urbanization of the community brought about by the Industrial Revolution led to the recognition of the need for some kind of organized nursing service which would be able to come to the help of persons lying ill at home. Various pioneer ventures were started both in London and Liverpool but the beginnings of a more comprehensive district service arose from a gift of money made to Queen Victoria in 1887 by the Women of Britain on the occasion of her Jubilee. By the direction of the Queen this was utilized to establish the Queen Victoria Jubilee Institute which later became the Queen's Institute of District Nursing. The work of this organization was gradually extended by the development of local voluntary associations until eventually the whole country had some sort of home-nursing service affiliated to the Queen's Institute, and the Queen's Nurse became a familiar figure in practically every community.

In 1948 in the U.K. the National Health Service Act recognized the importance of home nursing as an essential element in any comprehensive system of health care and local health authorities were required to provide a service for this purpose. Although this has now led to the virtual disappearance of local voluntary associations, the Queen's Institute remains in being and continues to fulfil an important role in education and training. Most local health authorities now provide nurses of various grades in relation to the tasks to be undertaken and a sensible innovation of recent years has been the recruitment of male nurses.

The demand for home nursing is likely to increase. With better housing and more effective general practitioner treatment many patients can be cared for quite suitably at home and there are often positive advantages in doing so. Other factors increasing the need for home nursing are the present pressures on hospital beds for the elderly, the trend towards early discharge from hospital, and the recognition that unnecessary or prolonged hospitalization of children inflicts psychological trauma.

However, no service, however comprehensive, can provide for the continuous help and supervision that some patients inevitably require and everyone likely to be faced with the task of caring for a sick or ailing relative at home should endeavour to acquire some basic knowledge of the skills needed to provide for a patient's comfort and happiness. Many simple manuals are readily available and in many areas the British Red Cross Society and other organizations provide classes of instruction.

Practical comments and advice on home nursing are given in the article on NURSING but some essentials are summarized here. The sick-room should be bright, airy and uncluttered and an attempt should be made to maintain the patient's interests by flowers, books, newspapers, or a portable radio and by not leaving him alone too long. The bed should be convenient for nursing purposes, preferably single and not too low. Two people are better than one for bed-making purposes. A drawsheet and mackintosh should be provided and a back-rest and foot-support will add to comfort. For bed-ridden or partially bed-ridden patients a bed-pan and urinal will be required or a bedside commode, and also a basin for washing and toilet purposes. Some cases will require a sick bowl or sputum-receiver and a clinical thermometer with container.

Immobile patients are very liable to develop BED SORES. These should be guarded against by changes of posture, by protection of pressure points, and by the use of spirit to dry and toughen the skin.

Special precautions are necessary in relation to cases of infectious illness. These are dealt with in the article on DISINFECTION.

homeopathy. A system of medical treatment based on the proposition, 'similia similibus curentur' (let likes be treated by likes).

Systematic medical practice dates from Hippocrates (c. 400 B.C.) who stressed the healing power of Nature and the duty of a physician to be Nature's intermediary and assistant. This philosophy was reversed by Galen (A.D. 131-201) who conceived that the aim of treatment was to fight and destroy disease, and to subdue Nature rather than support her. Slavish adherence to Galen's ideas became systematized as allopathy and produced such confused precepts and fantastic methods – bleeding, purgation and the use of potentially poisonous drugs – that Hermann Boerhaave (1668-1738), Professor of Medicine at Leyden, was once constrained to say that it would have been better for mankind had physicians never existed.

Into this scene in 1755 was born Christian Frederic Samuel Hahnemann, son of a Meissen porcelain-painter, who graduated as Doctor of Medicine from the University of Erlangen in 1799, married an apothecary's daughter and set up practice in Dessau. He grew dissatisfied with the methods of the day, threw up his practice, and instead supported himself by translating scientific works into German. Working on Cullen's *Materia Medica* he was attracted by an account of Peruvian Bark and its fever-dispelling powers. Trying this on himself he found that it induced an intermittent fever. He tried other experiments and reached the conclusion that the effects of every true drug were specifically related to the disease which it could cure.

He fostered this doctrine against great opposition and finally became Professor of Medicine in Leipzig (1812) where he taught the system of medicine which he called homeopathy. Not least he had to contend with the opposition of the apothecaries since he advocated the use of single drugs and those only in minute quantities.

Basically medical treatment concerns itself with diet, physical measures, and pharmaceutical remedies. It was in relation to the last that allopathy and homeopathy parted company. The allopaths advocated strong medicines to relieve symptoms: the homeopaths attached less importance to suppression of symptoms than to the support of natural healing by minute doses of drugs directly affecting diseased cells and organs. Their procedure was to test a drug on a healthy body; to equate the symptoms produced with similar symptoms occurring in disease; and to give the selected drug in such small doses that it could produce no injurious effect. An example will make this clear: arsenic causes watery diarrhoea and so was recommended for cholera.

The homeopaths, however, maintained that curative doses must be minute (one part in ten thousand to one part in a million, or even greater dilutions) so that the amount of drug actually received was so infinitesimal that it was difficult to believe that it could be of much effect.

Nevertheless, homeopathy continued to attract adherents and by 1870 or so had won a measure of grudging acceptance. Homeopathic hospitals and practitioners became established in many centres and especially in America where by 1900 one-quarter of the practitioners were said to be homeopaths.

Although homeopathy is still practised, it is in decline. In its time it exercised a powerful influence on medical practice by reviving interest in the rational use of drugs. The methods suggested by Hahnemann for study of their actions laid the foundations of pharmacology. The huge doses of the allopaths are no more. They have gradually been eliminated from orthodox medical practice and been replaced by newer drugs whose use is based on a scientific approach to their development and use. For this at least some credit must be accorded to Samuel Hahnemann.

homicidal mania. Mental disease which leads to the killing or attempted killing of another individual.

In manic-depressive psychosis the patient alternates between extremes of depression and excitement. In the manic phase he may become quarrelsome, aggressive and intolerant of restraint and may strike out in an irresponsible fashion at those who seek to restrain him.

In schizophrenia and paranoia any homicidal act may be of a more deliberate and calculated character. Such a patient may suffer from delusions of persecution or a perverse interpretation of the actions of other persons, with the result that he may attempt to kill people whom he falsely imagines to be seeking to injure him.

homosexuality. A sexual attraction between persons of the same sex either with or without sexual activity of a physical nature. Homosexuality between women is known as lesbianism and the prostitution or seduction of boys by adult males is pederasty.

Homosexuality can sometimes be a problem in boarding schools but this is no more than an adolescent exploratory phase of development which has been termed 'puppy pruriency'. It occurs also under circumstances where the sexes are segregated under abnormal conditions as in prisons, reformatories, at sea, or in the armed forces. One researcher working with college students found that as many as 60 per cent admitted to some homosexual experience.

These examples, however, do not represent true homosexuality, because there is no real change in personality and homosexual attitudes and activities are outgrown or abandoned when opportunities with the other sex become available. Nevertheless in such segregated communities, when discipline is poor and standards low, the opportunities for the seduction of young people by older confirmed homosexuals are obvious and call for vigilance on the part of those who are responsible for the conduct of such schools and institutions.

Various theories have been advanced as to the cause of homosexuality. It clearly cannot be regarded as a form of degeneracy, since many homosexuals are gifted and artistic. It has not been proved to be due to genetic or endocrine causes although recent work based on improved biochemical techniques suggests that these may possibly account for some cases.

Psychological influences are probably more important: Freud contended that it arose from over-attachment to the mother, especially in circumstances where the father had proved an unsatisfactory parent or had died, with the result that the child's personality tended to become excessively feminine. The fact that some homosexuals have responded to treatment by psychological methods lends weight to this view.

Homosexuals vary in type. Some may be exclusively so motivated; some may be bisexual and seek heterosexual relationships as well; some are transvestists who take pleasure in dressing as women; and some are trans-sexualists, playing either an active or passive role with another male.

The attitude of society to homosexuality is variable and undecided. Lesbianism has always been ignored by the law. In male homosexuality importuning and especially seduction of youth is generally condemned. On the other hand the law in the U.K. has recently been changed so that homosexual acts in private between consenting males over 21 are no longer crimes. Whether this is right or wrong is a matter for argument. No enlightened person would deny that the homosexual temperament should receive understanding and sympathy. Though changing social attitudes now encourage much more open discussion of the social and moral issues involved, and though more people can accept homosexual relationships as 'different' rather than 'perverted', homosexuality is still regarded by many with fear and intolerance and can still be exploited as a vice (for example in cases of blackmail).

hookworm disease. Anaemia arising from infection with hookworms, which are of two main types: *Ankylostoma*, prevalent in Egypt and the Middle East, and *Necator* (slightly smaller), common in Central and South America. An alternative name for the disease is ankylostomiasis.

The hookworm's eggs, passed with the faeces of a victim, hatch in warm, damp earth. The hatched embryo penetrates the skin of feet or legs in contact with the contaminated soil, and travels by the blood stream to the lungs and ultimately to the intestine, where the now adult worm 'hooks' itself in and sucks blood.

The symptoms are simply those of severe anaemia, and diagnosis is made by examination of the faeces, in which eggs can be seen under a microscope.

Treatment is with drugs which dislodge the hookworm and the anaemia also requires attention.

hormones. The 'chemical messengers' produced by the ENDOCRINE GLANDS such as the pituitary and the thyroid. Hormones play a vital part in many of the activities of the body.

hospitals. Institutions for the care and treatment of the sick have passed through several historical phases.

Starting with the temples of Aesculapius and the dressing-stations attached to army camps, the hospitals of the Ancient World attained at their best a surprisingly modern appearance in such respects as ventilation, drainage, water-supplies and provision of numerous small wards; and these were surpassed by the Arab civilization at its zenith. Baghdad in the tenth century, for instance, had sixty hospitals with separate wards for different ailments and with nurses of both sexes. However limited medical knowledge might then be, these hospitals aimed at treatment and cure.

From the close of the Dark Ages Europe began to develop shelters for the sick and the poor, at first attached to monasteries and later largely separate from monasteries but depending either on them or on public charity. These 'infirmaries' were refuges for the infirm and the disabled, rather than centres of treatment. They consisted of large wards in which patients lay crowded together, irrespective of their diseases, with scant attention to hygiene – St. Thomas's in London had no water closets in the late eighteenth century – and with staff of minimal numbers, untrained, badly fed and poorly paid. Yet these institutions, and the pest-houses established by towns to isolate victims of major epidemics, were the direct ancestors of modern hospitals. Gradually treatment facilities developed, but hospitals were for the destitute or for persons too infectious to be treated at home.

The nineteenth century saw the arrival of anaesthesia, antisepsis and later asepsis, and also Florence Nightingale's sustained campaign both for nursing training and for better accommodation and equipment. Hospitals became respectable, nursing became a profession, death rates fell dramatically and cures became more frequent. To the general hospitals maintained by endowments and charity were added hospitals maintained by local authorities – fever hospitals, tuberculosis hospitals, mental hospitals and finally additional general hospitals. By the 1930s two-thirds of the hospital beds in Britain were in local authority institutions. Yet hospitals still carried the stigma of pauperism: the senior physicians and surgeons gave their services free and few patients who could afford to be treated at home or in a nursing home entered a hospital ward.

In the middle third of the twentieth century all this changed. Medical and surgical advances at unprecedented pace made the treatment of serious disorders impracticable at home or in a small nursing home: radiological, biochemical, bacteriological and other facilities could normally be made available only in a large unit. Hospitals became the normal places for the treatment of serious illness. Individual hospitals tended to become larger, providing more diagnostic and therapeutic aids but often separating the patient by long bus journeys from his visiting relatives. Hospital finance was aided by State grants, and in Britain virtually all hospitals became State-owned in 1948 with all staff paid. Progressively the hospital came to dominate medical thinking. The clinical consultant was now remunerated but inherited the tradition of hospital routine being adjusted to suit his convenience, a tradition stemming from the days when this courtesy was afforded him in return for the services he gave the hospital without charge. He became the supreme figure in medicine. In the nineteenth and early twentieth century doctors tended to start in general practice and later, if they had a flair for a particular branch, to seek to specialize; now, however, specialization has begun to start from the time that a medical student qualifies, so that in due course consultants have become more expert on particular diseases but perhaps less aware of the problems and home circumstances of people.

The last third of the century shows signs of yet other changes: one is the idea, apparently gaining ground, that money spent on health education and prevention of disease may pay bigger dividends than the same amount of money expended on providing more wards or more hospital doctors and nurses; a second is that, with the simplifications created by many new drugs, many persons who fall ill are perhaps better treated at home by persons who know their problems and surroundings than in the impersonal atmosphere of a hospital; and finally a belief that the actual or potential contributions to health of the health educator, the health visitor, the social worker and the nurse may have been undervalued in the past, while excessive emphasis was placed on the medical profession and particularly on hospital consultants. It is, however, too early to say whether the hospital will really cease to be the centre of health and disease services.

housemaid's knee. A form of bursitis in which the bursa in front of the knee-cap becomes inflamed as a result of pressure from frequent kneeling, so that the part becomes hot, swollen, tender and red. Prevention is by using a thick, soft mat when kneeling. Treatment involves rest, firm bandaging and in some cases removal of fluid by a needle and syringe.

housing and health. Bad housing is undoubtedly very detrimental to health. To give a few examples: (1) An overcrowded or badly ventilated house favours the spread of communicable diseases, such as tuberculosis. (2) Food hygiene is more likely to be defective in a house that has inadequate washing or sanitary facilities. (3) A damp, poorly heated house is manifestly harmful to persons suffering from rheumatism or liable to bronchitis. (4) A house with bad lighting, uneven steps or twisted stairs has more than average likelihood of being the scene of a home accident. (5) A house with a difficult stair or a very steep access road puts a strain on an occupant with a disease of the heart or lungs. (6) A house that is very difficult to run – e.g., too small for the occupants, with minimal cooking facilities, with poor lighting and with very little storage space – has a profound effect on morale: the association of slum areas with high child mortality, filth, faulty diets, alcoholism, violence, truancy, delinquency and petty crime is not solely because the most deprived persons tend to gravitate to the worst houses but also because prolonged residence in very defective accommodation often gradually reduces the standards of the occupants.

Yet the relationship between housing and health is highly complex, and good housing does not necessarily lead to improved health. Unquestionably the replacement of slums by well-constructed houses with reasonable facilities and built in well-planned housing estates tends in general to improve both mental and physical health, but several adverse factors may operate in individual cases. (1) If rent, rates and heating are more costly than in the previous house and if travelling to work involves increased bus fares, the rehoused family may be under severe financial strain. (2) Rehousing some miles away from the previous home may involve separation from relatives and friends, and so create problems of loneliness as well as the acute difficulties of elderly people who formerly received physical aid from younger relatives. (3) A family with 'slum habits', rehoused in a good neighbourhood, may be shunned by neighbours, increasing the problems of isolation. (4) Some characteristics acquired in the poorer environment may persist for a generation: the often quoted use of the bath as a storage receptacle occurs in only about five per cent of rehoused slum dwellers, but ten years after rehousing the incidence of

delinquency is almost as high in the transferred children as in those not rehoused. (5) Some of those who made a terrific effort to maintain standards under bad conditions progress on rehousing to the extreme of tidiness and cleanness, forgetting the useful maxim that a house should be clean enough to be healthy but untidy enough to be comfortable.

Some of the basic requirements for a house are as follows. It should afford adequate protection against damp and cold, and in hot climates also against heat. It should have good ventilation and sufficient air space. It should have good natural and artificial lighting. It needs reasonable heating facilities. It needs appropriate washing and sanitary facilities. It should have adequate cooking facilities and accommodation for food storage. There should be an adequate system of refuse disposal. The house should afford reasonable privacy to the occupants. It should be situated not too far from shops, main roads and recreational spaces.

One of the difficulties confronting housing authorities is the determination of priorities. It seems inhumane to refuse rehousing to an elderly slum-dweller with a bad heart and four flights of stairs to climb, or to victims of rheumatism and bronchitis living in damp houses, or to a very large family living in conditions of gross overcrowding. Yet there are seldom enough fit houses for all such persons. Moreover, always to give such people priority over healthy young couples in the process of starting their families is undesirable on a long-term basis in that – until the problem of unfit housing is completely solved – otherwise healthy children (and their parents) are being forced to spend their most important formative years in a slum environment.

Many other problems arise, e.g., should the housing authorities treat married and cohabiting couples equally or endanger the health of children in the second group, and should they provide houses for unmarried women and their children or again endanger the health of the young? Still further problems arise in connection with the needs of the disabled and of the growing army of elderly persons.

humerus. The bone of the upper arm. It forms, with the glenoid cavity of the scapula, a ball and socket JOINT which is capable of a wide range of movement but easily dislocated. At the lower end it forms a hinge joint with the ulna.

hunger. The sensation of desire for food. It arises strongly in the early stages of fasting or starvation but is lost in later stages. Hunger pains, which disappear after eating, occur when a meal is delayed beyond its normal time and are also a symptom of gastric ulcer.

Hunter, John. Scottish surgeon and physiologist (1728-1793) who practised in London and has been described as 'the biologic Titan of his time'. Largely self-educated – at the age of 17 years he could neither read nor write (he may have been a victim of dyslexia) – and described by his contemporaries as uncouth and ungrammatical, he nevertheless provided by dissection and experiment an antidote to the sterile theorizing of the era. His museum has served as the mould from which all subsequent museums of natural history have been fashioned. He gave the first satisfactory description of inflammation, elucidated the

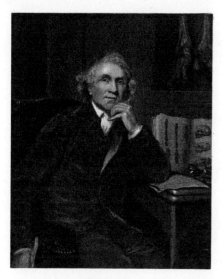

John Hunter

pathology of appendicitis and made a brilliant study of venereal disease.

Huntington's chorea. A hereditary disease – named after the American physician, George Huntington (1850-1916) – characterized by disordered and involuntary muscular movements and by progressive mental deterioration. There is as yet no cure, though sedatives and tranquillizers help to relieve the symptoms.

The disease usually appears at 35 to 50 years, by which time the individual will probably have completed his family; by the Mendelian laws of GENETICS about half of his children are likely to carry the gene and to transmit it to their offspring who will in turn have their children before they show signs of the disease. The disease could be eliminated by successful GENETIC GUIDANCE.

hydatid disease. A disease due to a tapeworm (*Taenia echinococcus*) conveyed to people and sheep from infected dogs. The eggs are passed in the faeces of the dogs and are eaten by sheep in which hydatid cysts form. Humans become infected by handling the dogs or eating food contaminated by their excreta. The embryo worms develop in the stomach and pass by blood-vessels to the liver (or occasionally the kidney or brain) where they form cysts which produce symptoms by pressure. Treatment is by surgical removal.

hydrocele. A collection of fluid in a sac-like cavity, most commonly the scrotum. The condition, which sometimes follows an injury and is sometimes congenital, usually appears gradually in middle-aged men as a smooth, uniform, pear-shaped, painless swelling which may cause a dragging sensation from the weight of the fluid. The inherited form also occurs in children. The usual treatment is periodical 'tapping', i.e. drawing off the fluid through the outer layer of tissue.

hydrocephalus. The term means 'water on the brain' The condition is characterized by abnormal enlargement of the head through accumulation of cerebrospinal fluid in the cavities of the brain. The accumulation results either from excessive secretion of cerebrospinal fluid or from blocking of the opening through which it normally escapes from the brain cavities into the sub-arachnoid space surrounding the brain and spinal cord. In most cases intelligence is defective, and convulsions may occur.

The condition is mostly seen in association with SPINA BIFIDA, but occasionally occurs as a complication of meningitis or brain tumour.

Mild cases may clear spontaneously. More severe cases can be treated by an operation in which a tube is introduced behind the ear and into a vein in the neck, so that the excess fluid is carried by the tube from the brain to the blood stream. In a severe untreated case there is progressive destruction of brain tissue with consequent deterioration of cerebral functioning.

hydrochloric acid. A strong corrosive acid which in dilute form is a normal constituent of gastric juice and is used in the process of digestion. Excessive hydrochloric acid in the stomach – technically known as hyperchlorhydria – is an important factor in causing gastric ulcers.

In a case of hydrochloric acid poisoning an alkali, such as baking soda or milk of magnesia, should be given as soon as possible, followed by milk or white of egg. Emetics to induce vomiting must not be used. See FIRST AID.

hydrocyanic acid. See PRUSSIC ACID.

hydrophobia. An alternative name for RABIES.

hydrotherapy. Treatment of disease by means of water.

In the past there was extensive use in medical practice not merely of hot baths at 37 to 45 °C. (100 to 112 °F.) (relaxing surface blood vessels and increasing the activity of sweat glands), tepid baths at 33 to 36 °C. (92 to 97 °F.) (lowering the temperature in fever) and cold baths at 10 to 24 °C. (50 to 75 °F.) (constricting surface blood vessels and lessening the activity of sweat glands) but also of sulphur baths (allegedly beneficial in rheumatism), effervescing or carbonic acid baths (claimed as valuable in certain heart diseases), alkaline baths (said to relieve the itching in jaundice), peat or mud baths (favoured in obesity and in many inflammatory conditions) and even paraffin wax baths (for inflammation of the hand or foot). Most of these are nowadays regarded sceptically.

Hydrotherapy today is virtually restricted to the use of swimming baths in the rehabilitation of patients suffering from partial paralysis or severe arthritis; because the water partially supports the weight of the body, movement is easier than in air.

hydrothorax. Accumulation of watery fluid in the pleural cavity between the layers of pleura, the tissue which surrounds the lungs. Inflammatory causes of active pleural effusion include tuberculosis (still by far the commonest cause) and occasionally pneumonia and lung abscess. Passive accumulation of fluid from the blood also occurs as a late symptom in cardiac failure, some varieties of nephritis and certain forms of cancer. The fluid is removed by the simple operation of 'tapping', but in the active forms treatment of the underlying cause is also essential.

hygiene. Hygiene (from the Greek *hygieia*, meaning health or wholesomeness) is essentially the science of maintaining or improving health, although the term is sometimes restricted (wrongly) to purely physical aspects of health.

Environmental hygiene, or the creation and maintenance of an environment compatible with good health, includes such matters as establishing water supplies and safeguarding their purity, setting up proper systems of sewage disposal and preventing the contamination of water or food by sewage, ensuring that infectious persons are segregated in isolation hospitals, building and maintaining fit houses, ensuring that at each stage from the grower or manufacturer to the householder food is clean and not contaminated by germs, protecting the public from noxious vapours, maintaining the purity of the air and providing reasonable protection against excessive noise.

Three points should perhaps be noted in respect of highly developed countries. Firstly, both increase of population and the accumulation of large numbers of persons in towns initially aggravate problems of environmental hygiene. Secondly, aggregation of large numbers renders practicable measures that would be too costly in a scattered rural population, so that ultimately the cities tend to have higher standards than the districts of low population (it is in the latter that the fly menace persists, that there are no facilities for pasteurization of milk and that the small shopkeeper has too few customers to enable him to afford proper refrigeration). Thirdly, as soon as the majority of voters become convinced that a particular hygienic measure is desirable and become prepared to pay for it (either by increased rates for something installed by the community or by increased prices to recoup the shopkeeper for his expenditure) the particular measure can be enforced by law. Hence, on a reasonably long-term basis, environmental hygiene should not only improve but should need a steadily diminishing number of enforcement officers. This is already the case in Sweden, which is regarded as leading the world in environmental hygiene and which now has a very small number of public health inspectors.

Personal hygiene includes such items as ensuring that persons in each age-group have adequate amounts not just of total calories but of proteins, mineral salts and vitamins; ensuring that each person drinks sufficient fluid, both for temperature regulation and for removal of waste products; prevention of obesity, not just in the middle-aged and elderly (in whom the results appear) but also in children and adolescents; provision of facilities for exercise and encouragement of people to take exercise appropriate to their age and state of health. It also means inducing people to wear clothing that will protect against heat loss but will also allow free movement; making people aware of the need for adequate rest and sleep – with sleep needs varying from the infant's 14 hours to the old person's 6 or 7 hours; and encouraging the development of leisure interests and recreations.

The aspect of personal hygiene usually implied in the popular usage of the word means making people aware of the importance of washing their hands after using the lavatory and before handling food; encouraging people to have regular baths for the removal of the solid constituents of sweat and of oily sebum, with cleansing of the genitalia, toes and armpits particularly important. Personal hygiene is a matter of persuasion and education, not legal enforcement. Health teaching in school is clearly important, but some habits and attitudes are best inculcated before school entry, and some aspects are perhaps best taught after leaving school.

Mental hygiene includes at its lowest level the development of affection and of consideration for others and the instillation of codes of behaviour that respect the desires and needs of other people. At a higher level it involves knowledge of elementary psychology, in order, for example, to avoid entering into argument with somebody who is clearly in a temper; awareness of the customs and traditions of persons of different background, race or religion; insight into the long-term and short-term effects of habits and behaviour on mental and physical health; and some awareness of many factors of importance in modern life – of which genetics, contraceptive facilities, economic stresses, problems of bereavement and social services are examples. In Britain perhaps the biggest contribution to the improvement of mental hygiene has been the creation of health visitors – selected qualified nurses with subsequent training in psychology, sociology and health education – who, although originally advisers on the personal hygiene of children, have increasingly become family counsellors on all matters of personal and emotional health.

hymen. The membrane that partially closes the entrance to the vagina in women. Although it is normally ruptured on the first occasion of intercourse, its intact presence is not absolute evidence of virginity and its rupture is not evidence of absence of virginity. It can occasionally be ruptured during violent exercise and can – very occasionally – remain intact after intercourse.

hyperaemia. The congestion of blood which occurs in any part of the body that has become inflamed, and which causes the reddening and heat of inflammation. Hyperaemia may be induced artificially as a COUNTER-IRRITATION by for example applying a mustard plaster to the skin.

hyperaesthesia. Excessive sensitiveness of any of the senses but especially of the skin, so that, for example, a tap may be felt as a sharp blow. Hyperaesthesia is common in hysteria, occurs in some diseases of the spinal cord and is sometimes noted in women during their menstrual periods or at the menopause.

hyperemesis gravidarum. Excessive vomiting in pregnancy, usually beginning as an exaggeration of morning sickness. There are two overlapping types: (1) the neurotic variety – with retching and vomiting at all hours and a risk of dehydration; and (2) the toxic variety – where, in addition, the patient looks toxic (with muddy skin and sunken eyes) and the scanty urine contains albumin. Diagnosis cannot be certain until investigations have confirmed that such conditions as gastric ulcer and strangulated hernia are not present. The cause is not yet fully understood. Treatment involves rest and quiet, good nursing, and in some cases antihistamine drugs and tranquillizers. In the toxic variety the pregnancy may have to be artificially terminated.

hyperglycaemia. A condition characterized by excess sugar (glucose) in the blood, usually occurring because the pancreas is not producing an adequate amount of insulin. Hyperglycaemia is the basic feature of diabetes mellitus and may be corrected in mild cases by strict adherence to a diet low in carbohydrates and in more serious cases by a combination of suitable diet and of regular injections of insulin (or in some persons by administration of an alternative drug by mouth.)

The blood of a normal person contains 0.09 to 0.12 per cent of glucose after he has fasted for some hours, and after a meal containing a large amount of carbohydrate the percentage rises to about 0.15. Glucose begins to appear in the urine when the blood level is about 0.17 per cent, but in some people traces appear at a blood level of 0.15 or even 0.14, so that these people excrete glucose in their urine (glycosuria) after meals although they do not suffer from diabetes.

In an untreated case of diabetes the blood glucose may be of the nature of 0.3 to 0.6 per cent.

hyperidrosis. Excessive sweating, often accompanied by an unpleasant odour. Generalized excessive perspiration occurs from heat, exertion, fear, feverish and toxic states, and also in hyperthyroidism and some diseases of the central nervous system. Fat people are liable to it in conditions of heat or exertion, and it is more a condition of adolescents and young adults than of older persons. The localized forms are common in nervous or highly emotional people, in sufferers from exophthalmic goitre and in heavy drinkers; these tend to affect the feet, hands, arm-pits, genital region or face.

Frequent washing is essential and application of a dusting powder of zinc and salicylic acid is useful, but it is also necessary to investigate the cause and treat it, and also to seek to relieve any associated anxiety or feeling of guilt.

hypermetropia. A defect of EYESIGHT, commonly known as 'long sight' with which there is usually difficulty in reading or sewing.

hyperpiesis. High BLOOD PRESSURE.

hyperpyrexia. Bodily temperature substantially above the normal 37 °C. (98.4 °F.). Some experts try to restrict the term to temperature of 40.5 °C. (105 °F.) or more. The condition occurs in many severe fevers and also in sunstroke. Apart from the rise in temperature, the skin becomes hot and dry, and the patient's condition is one of apathy followed by stupor and coma. Hyperpyrexia is most likely to occur in persons with defects of the sweat glands or after the administration of sweat-inhibiting drugs such as atropine. Treatment includes spraying the body with cold water.

hypertension. High BLOOD PRESSURE.

hyperthyroidism. See GOITRE.

hypertrophy. Increased growth of tissue mainly by multiplication of its cells. It may occur (1) from hormone stimulation, as in the growth of the breasts and uterus during pregnancy; (2) from frequent exercise, as in the muscles of athletes; or (3) as a compensatory mechanism, as when the heart enlarges to pump blood more vigorously into narrowed arteries.

Hypertrophy should be differentiated from TUMOUR (neoplasm). In hypertrophy the cells are increased in number but are completely normal.

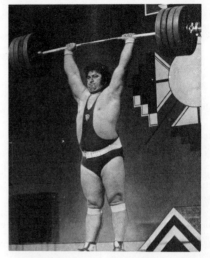

The hypertrophy of a weightlifter

hypnosis. A special form of sleep or trance induced by an operator who suggests the idea of sleep in various ways, e.g., by getting the patient to look at a bright object and by monotonously repeating a phrase. Hypnosis is not effective unless two conditions are satisfied: (1) that the patient is willing to co-operate, and (2) that the operator can hold the patient's complete attention. With a skilled operator about 80 per cent of willing persons can be hypnotized.

Hypnosis can be used to enable a patient to recover long-forgotten memories which, long repressed into the unconscious, may nevertheless be the causes of diseases, such as psychoneurosis. Hypnosis is therefore of considerable value in establishing the cause of neurotic diseases, thus permitting rational treatment.

A hypnotized person can also be given instructions which, after awakening, he will follow – provided they are compatible with his general codes of behaviour – without realizing that they have been implanted in his mind. For instance, hypnosis can be used to help a person who desires to stop smoking but lacks the will-power to do so. Again, in the absence of anaesthetics, operations have been painlessly performed under hypnosis: but with anaesthetics virtually 100 per cent effective no surgeon would willingly rely on a procedure with a failure rate of one in five.

Although very valuable for reviving repressed memories and for giving curative suggestions, hypnosis can be abused. A generous person might be induced to give money on awakening to an apparently desirable cause, and an unmarried girl already thinking about sexual relations with her lover might be persuaded to lose her virginity. Hence patients should consult only hypnotists of known integrity and should preferably be accompanied by reliable friends. Moreover, in unskilled hands hypnotism can do considerable emotional damage; and, while it can cure a particular symptom – e.g., a stammer – it does not treat the underlying cause of the symptom.

Despite the suggestion by many writers of fiction, there is absolutely no evidence that hypnotic subjects will, after hypnosis, obey instructions which are repugnant to them, e.g., that a person of normal standards could be hypnotically persuaded to commit a serious crime.

An early practising hypnotist and the first to bring the procedure to wide notice was the Austrian physician Anton Mesmer (1734-1815), and the term mesmerism is sometimes used as a synonym for hypnosis.

hypnotic. A drug which promotes sleep but does not relieve pain. Hypnotics should be differentiated from NARCOTICS (such as morphia) which relieve pain and induce sleep, ANODYNES (such as aspirin) which reduce pain without causing drowsiness and TRANQUILLIZERS, which relieve anxiety.

The barbiturates are by far the most commonly used hypnotics. Other sleep-stimulating drugs include chloral hydrate, paraldehyde, bromides and nitrazepam (Mogadon). Every known hypnotic has some potential unfortunate side-effect, e.g., the barbiturates are mildly habit-forming and are also thought to repress dreaming which some experts deem to be necessary for mental health.

hypochondria. Abnormal preoccupation with one's real or imaginary ailments. Concern with health is normal, especially in persons suffering from illness or disability, but the hypochondriac makes his ailments the absolute centre of his thoughts, and if a mild symptom which he regards as an indication of serious disease is satisfactorily explained, he promptly finds another symptom to worry about.

The condition should be differentiated from MALINGERING and HYSTERIA. The malingerer alleges illness that he does not have; the hysteric produces illness in himself; the hypochondriac generally goes to work, discusses his symptoms with anybody who will listen, consults a series of different doctors, studies medical textbooks and spends a relatively happy life considering new methods of investigation or of treatment. There is often a deep underlying cause of hypochondria, e.g., it may be a defence mechanism in work failure or marital failure or a self-punishment for imaginary guilt. So extreme cases need skilled psychological investigation.

hypodermic injection. A method of giving drugs in solution by injecting them under the skin, using a syringe and a hollow needle. The method is sometimes employed for quick action but is more often used for drugs which, if swallowed, would be destroyed in the digestive tract. The injection is normally made in a part of the body where the skin is loose and where blood-vessels can be avoided. The outer and upper part of the arm and the buttock are the usual sites.

hypoglycaemia. Deficiency of sugar in the blood (below the 0.09 to 0.12 per cent level in the blood of a normal person who has not eaten for some hours). Since all carbohydrate absorbed from the diet is converted into glucose, stored as glycogen in the liver and muscles, and immediately available for release to provide energy, deficiency of sugar in the blood is relatively rare. Essentially it occurs in three sets of circumstances: (1) where there is over-activity of the insulin forming tissue of the pancreas (an extreme rarity, in contrast to the frequent under-activity that causes the hyperglycaemia of diabetes); (2) in severe disease of the liver where that organ is unable to store glycogen (again an extreme rarity); and (3) in cases of excessive dosage of insulin to diabetic patients. The body's need for insulin varies from time to time with the amount secreted by a healthy pancreas adjusting to the need. In the diabetic the need similarly varies, so that what was a correct dose of insulin yesterday may be an excessive dose under the different bodily circumstances of today.

Early evidences of hypoglycaemia – nearly always due to insulin dosage disproportionate to the immediate circumstances – include general uneasiness, chilliness, hunger and perspiration; and if untreated the patient may lose consciousness and ultimately die. Treatment at the early stage consists of the immediate eating of sugar. All diabetic patients should be instructed to carry a lump of sugar at all times and to recognize the symptoms which should lead to the immediate eating of sugar.

Where a diabetic patient develops coma the attending doctor has to make a swift decision. A diabetic (hyperglycaemic) coma may be caused by a missed insulin injection, the onset is usually slow, the skin is dry, the blood pressure is reduced, respiration is deep and slow, the breath may smell of acetone and the urine will contain ketones. Heavy dosage of insulin and replacement of water and salt deficiency are essential for the preservation of life. In hypoglycaemic coma there may have been a missed meal or unusual exertion, the onset is rapid, the skin is moist, the blood pressure is normal or raised, respiration is rapid and shallow, the breath has no smell of acetone and the urine has no ketones although it may contain sugar. An intravenous injection of a glucose solution may save life. Clearly a mistake, resulting in the giving of glucose to a patient in hyperglycaemic coma or in the giving of insulin to a patient in hypoglycaemic coma, is likely to cost a life.

hypothalamus. A part of the brain situated in the floor of the portion of the brain, connected by nerve fibres with most other parts of the nervous system. It has functions that include regulation of the sympathetic and parasympathetic nervous systems, to some extent regulation of the emotions, regulation of the body temperature and control of the pituitary gland which in turn influences the other endocrine glands.

The enormous role of the hypothalamus is only in the process of becoming appreciated. While the cerebral hemispheres are pre-eminent for intellectual functions, it appears that the hypothalamus is the centre concerned with excitement, elation and depression, the link between the central nervous systems and the autonomic nervous system and the link between the nervous systems and the endocrine glands.

hypothermia. Chilling of the body, technically after the temperature falls below 35 °C. (95

F.); see COLD, EFFECTS OF. This is a common and serious condition in old people because (1) the body's heat-regulating mechanism often becomes inefficient in the elderly; (2) many old people live in grossly underheated accommodation, e.g., in a recent study three-quarters of old people had morning temperatures in their living rooms below the recommended minimum of 18.3 °C. (65 °F.) and one-tenth had morning temperatures below 12 °C. (53.6 °F.); and (3) many old people are relatively insensitive to cold and unaware of the need for more warmth or more clothing.

Hypothermia can lead, without symptoms of discomfort, to drowsiness, slumber and death. Apart from sometimes causing death directly it is probably a factor in the increased death rate of old people in winter from such diseases as pneumonia and bronchitis. Prevention is partly a matter of lessening poverty and partly of educating old people about the need for a proper DIET, CLOTHING and household warmth. Since elderly persons spend at least one-third of their time in bed and since the bedrooms are usually colder than living rooms, the invention of a cheap and absolutely safe electric blanket and the persuasion of old people to use it would contribute materially to the reduction of the condition.

For some operations on the brain or heart a measure of hypothermia is deliberately employed to lessen oxygen requirements; the patient is restored to a normal bodily temperature as soon as the operation is over.

hypothyroidism. See CRETINISM.

hysterectomy. Surgical removal of the uterus. The operation is required in cases of fibroid tumours of the uterus and cancer of the uterus, and sometimes in cases of excessive menstruation not relieved by the simpler method of curettage, i.e., scraping the lining of the uterus.

If the vagina and ovaries are left in position, hysterectomy does not remove either sexual desire or ability to have intercourse, although of course it makes conception and childbirth impossible. A woman contemplating the operation should ascertain whether the surgeon proposes to remove only the uterus or also the ovaries. As normally undertaken the operation leaves a faint vertical or horizontal scar on the abdomen, and necessitates ten to fourteen days in hospital with avoidance of heavy work for a further six to eight weeks.

hysteria. A psychoneurosis, in which signs of physical and mental illness are produced by the unconscious action of the mind. Essentially the sufferer from hysteria is one whose personality has failed to meet the full responsibilities of life; a person who unconsciously produces his symptoms partly as an expression of frustration and helplessness (and in effect a cry for help), partly as a means of escape from an intolerable situation, and partly as a compromise between an unconscious wish and its conscious inhibition or repression.

Hysteria can take the form of almost any illness, producing for example blindness, dumbness, deafness, tremors or paralysis. By far the commonest variety consists of outbursts of uncontrolled emotion, occurring mostly in persons of a highly emotional temperament and persons with little self-control. While the typical hysteric is emotionally unstable and self-centred, hysteria can occur in very stable persons after prolonged strain and considerable suppression of emotion: it is recorded that Bismarck had a fit of uncontrollable weeping when, after a day of great strain, he learned of his victory over the Austrian forces.

In simple hysterical outbursts three forms of treatment are advocated by different schools of thought, and all three often work. (1) Allow the emotion to expend itself without interruption: 'let her have a good cry'. (2) Allay the emotion by quiet reassurance and suggestion. (3) Remove the emotion by firm handling, e.g., a sharp slap. In persisting and recurring cases intensive psychotherapy may be needed, including a search for the unconscious strivings that have given rise to the disease. If, as is often the case, the causes lie in early childhood experiences it may be very difficult for the psychotherapist to overcome them.

I

ichthyosis. A hereditary condition in which the skin is abnormally dry and scaly. It varies greatly in severity but in general causes no itching and no impairment of general health. There is as yet no specific cure, but the condition may be helped by frequent warm bathing followed by application of ointment based on petroleum jelly or application of cold cream. The affected skin should also be protected from cold.

icterus. Yellowness of the skin and mucous membranes through staining by bile pigment. It is a symptom, not a disease, and is simply a technical name for JAUNDICE.

id. A term used by psychoanalysts for the most instinctive and deeply unconscious part of the human mind, the reservoir of many hidden and repressed impulses and wishes, and the unconscious source of much human behaviour. It contrasts with the ego, the conscious and rational part of the mind, and the superego, the censor or conscience that holds in check the self-gratificatory impulses of the id. See FREUD.

identical twins. See TWINS.

idiosyncrasy. Mental attitude or behaviour peculiar to a person, or peculiar reaction by a person to a particular substance. The term is often used in the sense of allergy to some drug or food.

ilium. The main bone of the pelvis which is formed by the union of three bones at the acetabulum, the cup-shaped cavity that receives the head of the femur in the formation of the hip joint. The three are the ilium (uppermost), the pubic bone (in front) and the ischium (behind).

The ilium is a flattish, curved bone. To its outer surface are attached the muscles of the buttock, while the iliacus muscle is attached to its concave inner surface. The bone has a crest at the top, to which are attached several abdominal muscles. The crest ends in front in a prominence (the anterior iliac spine) to which the inguinal ligament is attached; and at the back it articulates with the sacrum, while below that junction is a notch through which the sciatic nerve passes down to the thigh.

illusion. A false perception arising from genuine external stimulation, such as a shadow being mistaken for a man or a noise misinterpreted as a voice. Illusion should be differentiated from delusion, where a false belief persists in defiance of reason, and from hallucination, where the false sensation occurs in the absence of any external stimulation. Since our senses are imperfect, illusions are common in normal people: if you draw two lines of identical length, and put arrows on the ends of one line and reversed arrows on the other, most observers will have the illusion that the second line is longer than the first. In normal people illusions are removed by investigation and reasoning, but in some diseases illusions tend to persist.

imagination. The ability to create images independent of previous perception.

While remembering is essentially a selective reproduction of past perceptions, as in recollecting the appearance of a house we lived in or the sound of a relative's voice, imagination, although inevitably based largely on past experiences, is much wider and freer. We may, for example, imagine a known house but with fewer or additional rooms and placed in an entirely different setting, or envisage a combination of two objects, such as a horse that can fly, or convert a reporter's brief, factual story into a novel with realistic characters and specific motivation.

At its peak imagination may produce in others the 'willing suspension of disbelief' that makes an audience view a play about Ancient Rome as events happening in the present, or makes a reader become completely enthralled by a poem about 'magic casements opening on the foam of perilous seas in faery lands forlorn'. It may produce the inspirational spark that made Priestley ask, 'are we right in thinking that when an article burns part of it is lost, or could it be that in combustion something is taken into the article from the atmosphere?'

Some try to differentiate imagination, as an extension or manipulation of the real, from fancy or fantasy, which steps outside the bounds of reality or possibility. For instance *Alice in Wonderland* is glorious fantasy, whereas the best modern science fiction displays rich imagination.

Imagination is a necessary process of mental life, a means whereby we can reach forward into the future or back into the past, and a method whereby we can grasp – however dimly – possibilities that lie ahead. When a young child says, 'I saw a lion in the garden', he is not telling a lie but beginning to use imagination.

Many people have primarily a visual imagination, fewer an auditory imagination, and perhaps still fewer a spacial imagination. Clearly poets, artists and inventors possess imagination of unusual quality. At the other end of the scale are people almost without imagination.

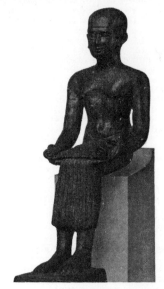

Imhotep

Imhotep. The bald prime minister and architect of the third Egyptian dynasty (around 2900 B.C.), in addition to being the designer of the Step Pyramid, is the earliest physician who has remained on record as more than a name (unlike Sekhetenanck of about six hundred years earlier).

Egyptian medicine acquired a remarkable reputation. Homer, writing perhaps a thousand years after Imhotep, sang of 'Egypt teaming with drugs, the land where each is a physician, skilful beyond all men'; Herodotus described it as a land of specialists each treating a single disease; the Bible says 'Moses was learned in all the wisdom of the Egyptians' and several times mentions Egyptian skill in healing. Yet what has survived of Egyptian medicine seems barren and non-progressive. The Egyptians knew no pathology and – despite embalming – very little anatomy, and their prescriptions sound like a witch's cauldron. They understood a few drugs – opium and castor oil are examples – but their treatment relied heavily on magic and incantations. Nevertheless Imhotep was – like the Greek Aesculapius – deified as the god of healing.

immaturity. A state of being not completely formed or developed. Any child is therefore immature. The term is normally used, however, for adults whose judgment or behaviour is childlike or for children whose attitudes and conduct resemble those of considerably younger children.

Immaturity should be clearly differentiated from mental deficiency and backwardness. Mental deficiency means appreciable intellectual impairment and of course has, as one feature, an inability to make mature judgments. Backwardness implies either a milder degree of intellectual impairment or educational retardation such as may occur from long illness or very poor home conditions. An immature person may be of low intellect (combining immaturity and backwardness), of average intellect or of high intellect (sometimes shown by obtaining degrees and higher degrees).

Immaturity is perhaps best explained by comparing an intelligent, mature man of 40 with the same person as a boy of 16. At 16 his intelligence is fully developed but we do not expect him to display fully balanced judgment, self-control, general competence, evaluation of priorities, ability to modify aggression and capacity to react normally to stresses; and we would tolerate minor abnormalities of conduct that would be intolerable in an adult. When a man frequently acts like a boy of 16 (or in more extreme cases like a child of 10) we call him immature.

Immaturity is essentially a failure of the personality to develop properly. Its causes are not yet fully understood but its prevention would seem to lie mainly in the provision throughout childhood of a healthy emotional climate – where the child knows he is loved and secure but is not mentally choked by excessive affection, where he is, in large measure, free to investigate and to learn from his own mistakes but is neither over-indulged nor dominated, and where he gradually learns self-control and self-evaluation by example and precept. In many cases an immature person is the son or daughter of an immature parent, but the explanation lies in the upbringing, not in heredity.

immunity. In ordinary speech immunity simply means the state of being protected or exempt, e.g., having once been tried and acquitted a man is immune from any other trial for that particular offence. In medicine, however, the term is applied specifically to power to resist invading germs or their toxins.

Natural immunity. The species, the race, the family or the person may have a natural immunity to a disease. Thus no human being suffers from hog cholera and less than one in a million develops the avian (or bird) variety of tuberculosis. Europeans, even if they have not had measles in childhood, are much more resistant to measles than are South Sea Islanders, and, if they develop the disease, have it in much milder form. Some families are notoriously susceptible to various infections while other families have a tradition of escaping them. Of two persons eating exactly the same infected food, one may develop the particular food-borne disease (e.g., typhoid) while the other remains healthy. While this natural immunity depends in part on general health and adequate body store of vitamin A, it appears that in each of the above examples the leucocytes (white blood corpuscles) of the particular species, race, family or person have a marked capacity to engulf or destroy invading bacteria of the relevant type and the antigens produced by the bacteria.

Again, people who have recovered from certain infections have an acquired natural immunity. Even in the era when smallpox was very common it was almost unknown for a person to have two attacks during his lifetime.

The same holds with various other infections (e.g., rubella and poliomyelitis) while, for many other infections, illness is followed by a temporary immunity lasting for some years. The mechanism is perhaps best understood by thinking back to days when no specific treatments existed. The victim of an infection in those days either died or else his body learned the art of manufacturing antibodies (to combat the invading antigens) or antitoxin (to neutralize the toxin produced by the bacteria); and today, although the body is assisted by the administration of antiserum, antitoxin or antibiotics, it still acquires during the illness the power to manufacture appropriate antibodies. This power remains – permanently or for an appreciable time – so that, if the body is again invaded by germs of the same type the antibodies promptly destroy the invaders. A fair comparison would be with the defence forces of a country: before the first attack there was no standing army, so a defence force had to be mobilized and trained with desperate urgency (although nowadays there is also foreign aid, e.g., antibiotics); if the attack has been successfully resisted, there is now a standing defence force which can deal effectively with future invaders, although it could still be overwhelmed by sudden onslaught by an invading army of quite abnormal size (as in a laboratory accident involving many millions of bacteria).

Active artificial immunity. This is the result of 'tricking' the body into producing the relevant antibodies or antitoxins. If we deliberately inject into the body very small, carefully measured doses of either (1) the original germ, weakened by many generations of growth under artificial conditions (as in immunization against tuberculosis) or (2) the organism or toxin after being inactivated by heat or an appropriate chemical (as in immunization against diphtheria), the body responds by beginning to manufacture antibodies or antitoxins, and exactly as after recovery from the disease, retains this manufacturing power, so that invaders of the particular type will be efficiently destroyed.

In most developed countries active immunization is now offered against diphtheria, tetanus and whooping cough (usually simultaneously to reduce the total number of injections); poliomyelitis (usually by mouth); measles; rubella – GERMAN MEASLES – (either to older children in the hope of eliminating the disease or to girls of about 13 years to give them maximum protection against developing the disease in pregnancy to the danger of the unborn child); tuberculosis; and, where still deemed necessary, smallpox. Similar immunization is available when needed against typhoid, paratyphoid, plague, cholera, typhus, yellow fever and several other infections. Protection against diphtheria, tetanus, whooping cough, poliomyelitis and measles should be regarded as the birthright of every young child, while protection against rubella for girls and tuberculosis for both sexes should be afforded to older children.

Many forms of immunization have tiny disadvantages. Diphtheria-whooping cough immunization is remarkably free from reactions or side-effects, but needs a reinforcing dose about three years later. Protection against typhoid and paratyphoid can cause a sharp feverish illness and the protection lasts for only two or three years. Smallpox vaccination – which has virtually eradicated the world's greatest killing infection – causes serious illness about once in a million times. Immunization against influenza is of variable efficacy because there are many strains of influenza virus: by the time an outbreak has swept through a few countries it is generally possible to produce a specific vaccine that gives high protection against that particular strain for six to nine months; but at the beginning of the next outbreak a vaccine produced against the strain that caused the previous epidemic gives a poorer – but by no means negligible – protection against the new strain.

Artificial immunization against any serious infection is really an intermediate stage: the ultimate aim is to eliminate the disease altogether. For such eradication a hundred per cent protection of the community is not essential: once the protected persons are so numerous as to make it unlikely that a case of the disease will come into contact with a susceptible person, the disease tends to die out. In the case of smallpox the disease has now been restricted to a few countries, so that the generalized vaccination of the past is now replaced by vaccination of the few travellers to these countries.

Immunization procedures have eliminated smallpox, made poliomyelitis and diphtheria extreme rarities, and are in the process of greatly reducing many other formerly common diseases. Despite the glamour of heart transplants and artificial kidneys, immunization procedures stand as one of the three main life-saving discoveries of recent centuries, the other two being the discovery and isolation of vitamins and antibiotics. It is interesting, however, to note certain differences between the three: the effect of antibiotics depends simply on administration of the right antibiotics to the persons who are ill and therefore seeking treatment; the effect of the discovery of vitamins depends in small part on their administration to the persons who are ill but mainly on education of the not-ill community; and the effect of immunization depends entirely on health education of parents as to the need for protection of apparently healthy children, with – perhaps inevitably – considerable opposition from cranks.

Passive artificial immunity. It is possible to achieve temporary protection against infection by injecting serum from a protected person or animal into a person susceptible to the particular disease. For instance, if a debilitated child is in contact with measles and not previously immunized, active immunization is useless (because the disease would develop before the body had acquired the power to produce antibodies) but injection of a few millilitres of serum (concentrated from the blood of a person who has had measles or been immunized against measles) will provide circulating antibodies that can in the immediate future destroy the virus of measles. The protection lasts only three or four weeks, until the circulating antibodies in the bloodstream become worn out; it will tide the child over the immediate danger but does not stimulate active production of antibodies. It can be life-saving in protecting an exhausted child from immediate attack, but leaves the child at normal risk if he becomes a contact a month later. A refinement of this passive and temporary immunity procedure is to give the debilitated child a smaller or slightly delayed dose of serum from an immune person: this, deliberately insufficient or too late to prevent the disease by passive immunization, will produce a very mild attack, with subsequent active acquired immunity.

Broadly, natural immunity is a phenomenon interesting to doctors, passive artificial immunity is an infrequent but useful procedure, and artificial acquired immunity is one of the biggest advances of medical science.

immunization. The process of artificially producing IMMUNITY to an infectious disease by introducing appropriate substances into the body.

Inoculation, in the sense of arm-to-arm transmission of smallpox from a mild case to an uninfected person, was started by Chinese physicians, spread through Asia and was introduced to Britain by Lady Mary Wortley Montague in 1718. This method often created immunity, sometimes caused a mild attack and very rarely led to a severe or even fatal attack. Jenner in England, having noticed that milkmaids seemed resistant to smallpox, in 1796 started VACCINATION with lymph from cows that had suffered from cow-pox: although the full explanation was not discovered for about a century and a half, the virus was the same but modified by passage through generations of cows. Although some modifications were later made, e.g., sheep lymph for calf lymph, vaccination eliminated smallpox from country after country.

After Pasteur in France and Koch in Germany had shown how germs cause infections, methods of producing immunity by weakened or killed organisms were increasingly developed, and it seems likely that almost all infectious diseases will be eradicated before the end of this century. It has to be remembered, however, that such eradication depends either on legal enforcement of immunization or on active persuasion of the people by health education. If, before a disease was completely eliminated, people stopped being immunized (because the condition was now rare) we could within a decade revert to the prevalence of fifty years ago.

It was formerly customary to differentiate vaccination and immunization. Vaccination involved the use of live but weakened organisms, as in protection against smallpox and yellow fever, while immunization involved the use of killed organisms, as in the protection against typhoid or diphtheria. The distinction is becoming blurred, however. For instance, the Salk method of protecting against poliomyelitis by injection of a killed virus is strictly immunization and the Sabin method of protecting against the same disease by administering a weakened and harmless virus by mouth is technically vaccination, but it seems absurd to use different terms for the two processes. Again, protection against tuberculosis by injection of the weakened BCG bacillus is vaccination, but it is a little difficult to find the exact name for protection against tuberculosis by injection of the vole virus, since this is a live virus that causes tuberculosis in voles but acts as an inert substance in man.

polio diphtheria tetanus
so easy to prevent

so difficult to cure
immunization protects

An immunization poster

impaction. A condition in which the broken ends of a fractured bone are driven together and firmly interlocked, so that – for healing without deformity and pain – the bone has to be reset before being allowed to knit together.

An impacted tooth is one that has grown out of line, has become firmly wedged in the gum and is unable to break fully through to the surface.

impetigo. A skin disease commonest in children, in conditions of poverty and poor hygiene. It is due to staphylococcal infection and usually shows as small blisters which become purulent and produce dirty, greenish-yellow crusts, with some inflammation of the surrounding skin. The disease appears most commonly on the face and hands, and is highly contagious (i.e., spread by direct physical contact).

Treatment consists of gently removing the crusts with lint or cotton wool soaked in soapy water, and then applying an ointment containing a suitable antibiotic. If the infection is spreading, injections of an antibiotic may also be needed. One of the triumphs of community health services – including education on personal hygiene and on nutrition – in recent decades has been a drastic reduction in impetigo and in other diseases (e.g., ringworm and scabies) associated with dirt and poverty.

impotence. Inability to perform or complete sexual intercourse. It occurs mostly in men, in whom the numerous causes include (1) congenital malformations, deformations or injuries of the penis, preventing erection and penetration; (2) disorders of the glands and nerves controlling the sex organs, including common after-effects of mumps in adolescents or young adults; (3) lessened desire and potency through old age, exhaustion, illness, drugs or alcohol; and (4) many emotional causes, as for example when a man is potent with a prostitute but not with his wife (sometimes because he is over-anxious). Impotence also occurs in women, where the causes include structural abnormalities, spasm of the muscles, revulsion created by faulty or absent sex education or fear caused by an unhappy first experience of intercourse.

Treatment varies with the cause. Rest, reassurance and understanding from the partner, with pre-intercourse 'courting' and sex play, may suffice in cases due to exhaustion, worry, slight fear or temporary illness. Medical examination may be needed in some cases, and sometimes psychological help is useful.

While alcohol in moderation may allay nervousness and decrease inhibitions, alcohol in large quantities tends to increase desire but diminish capacity for performance (as was noted by that very astute non-medical observer, William Shakespeare). Aphrodisiacs, though often used, are in general valueless.

Impotence should be differentiated from STERILITY. The impotent man may produce sperms and – by permanent or temporary cure of his impotence or by artificial insemination – become a father. The sterile person, on the other hand, may have normal sexual desires and be perfectly capable of having intercourse.

incapacity for work. One of the most difficult tasks of the physician is to determine capacity or incapacity for work. Fortunately, in about 90 per cent of allegedly sick persons it is relatively easy to decide whether they need 'treatment and rest' or 'treatment and duty'. There are, however, about 5 per cent who are so eager to work that they minimize their symptoms: in many of these the physical findings, such as pulse rate or respiratory rate, are a good guide. Another 5 per cent are 'work-shy', exaggerating or faking their symptoms, even to the extent of using a hot-water bottle to raise their apparent temperature or producing a non-existent paralysis of a limb.

Since intelligent people tend to find jobs that they enjoy, the doctor may well discover that the patient whom he suspects of being over-keen to work has an intelligence that equals or outstrips his own, so that the physician who diagnoses possible over-enthusiasm – either because the patient feels that he cannot be spared or because he is very aware of the need of his family for overtime payments – has to look very carefully for signs not under the patient's control. On the other hand, the intelligent patient, on being told of the dangers of too early return to work or of being advised of modifications during the early period of his return, is likely to co-operate. Nevertheless, it is because of intelligent work-enthusiasts that doctors as a whole acquire the reputation of being over-cautious and of prescribing three weeks convalescence when two would suffice.

The work-shy person is often of lower intelligence, so that the doctor who suspects MALINGERING can sometimes trap the suspect into admitting to an absolutely unrelated symptom; but a highly intelligent malingerer with a rudimentary knowledge of anatomy and physiology has a very good chance of deceiving his physician in respect of temporary incapacity for work. Before long-term incapacity is certified many investigations are made, and the chance of deception is much smaller.

Yet in certifying incapacity the scales are weighted in favour of the traditional over-caution: if a man is kept off work for a needless fortnight, nobody knows that it was needless; if he is permitted to resume work a week too soon and has a relapse, relatives and friends blame the doctor.

incontinence. Inability to control the reflex emptying of URINE from the bladder (urinary incontinence) or of the bladder and rectum (double incontinence). The commonest causes are: (1) loss of co-ordination in the nervous system, as in brain damage or senility, and (2) diseases of the bladder or rectum. Treatment varies with the cause, but if the patient is prepared to co-operate the condition is in large measure curable. Failing cure, incontinence pads and rubber sheeting are required.

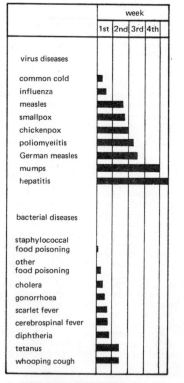

Average incubation periods

incubation period. The interval between infection and the appearance of symptoms. In this period the invading germs multiply until they are numerous enough to overwhelm the defence mechanisms of the body and produce the disease.

The common cold and influenza have short incubation periods (one to three days normally), but most other virus diseases have long incubation periods (e.g., measles, ten to fourteen days). By contrast, most bacterial infections have short incubation periods (e.g., staphylococcal food poisoning, a few hours, or diphtheria, one to four days). In general the incubation period for any infection spread from nose to nose (by breathing infected droplets) is fairly well defined for any one disease; but for food-borne infections - e.g., typhoid - the period varies with the amount of infected food consumed, or rather with the quantity of germs in it.

For diseases caused by droplet spray the incubation period is still an excellent guide. For instance, a rash which might be a rather fine measles or might be a rather coarse rubella (German measles) is likely to be rubella if the incubation period has been nearer three weeks than two, and a rubella contact who does not develop the disease within twenty-three days can be regarded as having escaped. For diseases transmitted by eating infected food the advent of refrigerators (and deep freezes) has considerably altered the picture: infected food may be kept in a refrigerator (with the germs neither killed nor multiplying) for a week, so that the period from purchase to appearance of the disease is a week longer than would have been anticipated.

Indian hemp. An alternative name for CANNABIS or hashish, smoked as a mild narcotic and sedative, producing pleasurable dreams.

indices of community health. Accurate information about community health and the influences affecting it is essential in order to plan health services intelligently and to make the best use of money and resources. It is also helpful to be able to compare the experience of one place or country with others because this may provide clues to the cause of disease or help to evaluate services and procedures.

Much of the required information can be obtained by the collection and interpretation of suitable statistics and these can be broadly classified into vital statistics, health statistics and special indices.

1. Vital statistics are the numerical facts related to or derived from vital events which are statutorily recorded (see VITAL STATISTICS). Basically these are births, marriages and deaths (including foetal deaths) together with information regarding sex, marital status, occupation, and cause of age and death. There is also an increasing tendency to require at registration further details with a social connotation.

Information of this kind, no matter how completely and accurately recorded, is still comparatively useless without accurate knowledge of the whole population and this has to be obtained periodically by means of a census. Over eighty countries now have reasonably comparable census data but the difficulties of accurate census-taking in undeveloped countries are obvious.

2. Health statistics are wider in scope than vital statistics but often less precise. They include morbidity data from hospital, public health and insurance sources; information about environmental factors - housing, sanitation, nutrition, industry, occupation, accidents and so on; and records relating to preventive services - pre-school and school health, mass-screening and special surveys.

Sample surveys are an important source of accurate data in limited fields. Individual enquiries are carried out within a selected group of manageable size in order to obtain information which will be of value generally. They may be diagnostic, seeking to demonstrate a cause and effect relationship as for instance between smoking and lung cancer, or descriptive in concept, when they attempt to illustrate for a selected group the particular characteristics which may be of significance in determining the general pattern of its health. Surveys of the nutritional and social problems of the aged are examples. These special investigations have been said to be concerned with 'the anatomy and physiology of society'.

3. Special indices or health indicators. Vital and health statistics as already described are useful in relation to the state and progress of individual communities but are of lesser value in a wider context. Crude death rates, for example, are not comparable if population structures are different. There is therefore a need for comparable health indicators both general and specific. One general indicator which has been proposed is the number of deaths before the age 50 expressed as a percentage of total deaths. Of specific indicators infant mortality is still useful if recording is complete, and an accurate figure for deaths from communicable disease is also informative, but so far there are no convincing ways of numerically assessing environmental conditions, nutrition or mental health, to name only some of the factors which are of great importance for community well-being.

indigestion. Normally the stomach carries on its work of digestion without its activity giving rise to any sensations or reasons for complaints, but a large proportion of persons do in fact experience discomfort related to the eating of food. This is loosely called indigestion or dyspepsia but it may arise from a variety of causes. The symptoms usually include one or more of the following: upper abdominal discomfort or pain; a feeling of fullness after eating; flatulence; nausea; heartburn; waterbrash; hiccough; constipation, or diarrhoea. Another common manifestation is the skin condition known as rosacea in which there is chronic congestion of the small blood vessels of the nose and central part of the face producing an unsightly reddened area.

Dyspepsia may be experienced in many abdominal conditions including chronic appendicitis, colitis, chronic gall-bladder disease, cirrhosis of the liver, and tumour, and also in general diseases such as gout, nephritis, anaemia and heart conditions, but more commonly it is related to disease specifically affecting the stomach itself.

Acute gastritis is usually due to dietary indiscretion. Over-eating, indigestible foods, hurried, imperfectly-chewed, irregular meals, excessive fats, spices, and especially alcohol, can irritate the stomach lining and upset the digestive function. Certain drugs such as aspirin are also liable to cause gastric upset. The condition usually responds quickly to simple treatment – a laxative, starvation, fluids, glucose and the giving of antacids.

Chronic gastritis may develop as a sequel to repeated attacks of acute gastritis but more often it will have been chronic from the beginning. Such cases call for fuller investigation with x-ray examination and test-meals to eliminate the presence of more serious conditions. Prolonged treatment will probably be required with careful dietetic control and suitable drugs.

Peptic ulcers of the stomach or duodenum are a particularly common cause of indigestion. Usually they are accompanied by more definite pain usually of a characteristic pattern related to the intake of food. Suspicion of such conditions also calls for full investigation and a careful regime of subsequent treatment.

Nervous dyspepsia is a condition occurring in neurasthenic patients and accompanied as a rule by other signs of anxiety and stress such as headache, backache, insomnia and loss of appetite. In these cases there is no abnormality of the stomach and treatment has to be directed towards the patient's general physical and mental health.

Intestinal carbohydrate dyspepsia is caused by a failure of starch digestion in the intestine and is characterized by excessive flatulence. Starch granules can be found microscopically in the stools. Treatment is by restriction of starches and their replacement by sugar, with the giving of diastatic ferment, available in tablet form.

Antacids are much employed in the treatment of dyspepsia. They act by neutralizing the gastric hydrochloric acid. The simplest and most readily available is sodium bicarbonate or baking-soda but its reaction rapidly evolves a large volume of carbon dioxide and may worsen the symptoms of flatulence. Calcium carbonate and magnesium carbonate neutralize hydrochloric acid more slowly over a longer period and are probably better, particularly as the latter is also a mild aperient. Aluminium hydroxide and magnesium trisilicate are also popular forms of treatment since they neutralize acid without gas formation.

Antacids of various proprietary brands are very extensively employed as self-treatment without medical advice. Their use in excess carries a risk of developing alkalosis with headache, nausea, vomiting and drowsiness – symptoms which resemble uraemia.

induction. Used in normal speech for 'introduction' or 'initiation', the term is applied in medicine to induction of labour, i.e., the artificial starting of childbirth, either (1) because of delay in the natural starting of labour (post-maturity), or (2) because the birth of a slightly premature child is desirable on account of danger to either mother or child. The old method of giving 300 mg. of quinine at four-hourly intervals for a day and then 30 ml. of castor oil is quite effective but nowadays it is usually replaced – or reinforced – by injections of pituitary hormone. In some cases rupture of the membranes is required.

industrial hygiene. The very wide-ranging science of maintaining and improving health is known as HYGIENE, and in order to safeguard and promote their health it is important that persons employed in industry should have good working conditions and be protected from any hazards resulting from industrial processess. In the U.K. the statutory provisions controlling working conditions are contained in the various Factory Acts and in a considerable body of subsidiary legislation covering special situations. These are administered by a Factory Inspectorate responsible to the Department of Employment. Local health authorities also have certain duties in relation to sanitary provisions and environmental conditions. Medical aspects of industrial employment are now supervised by an Employment Medical Advisory Service.

Every industry has its own particular problems and hazards for which particular measures are required, but certain general principles of hygiene and safety can be identified. In the first place the factory or work place should be adequate in size and suitably adapted for its purposes. It should be kept clean and be properly ventilated and lit, and there must be sufficient and proper sanitary provision. Moving machinery, process-vats and stairways must be protected. Steps should be taken to minimize the ill effects of excessive heat and noise, and there should be first aid provision. Machinery should be designed for its special purpose and where dust and gases are generated there should be arrangements for their extraction and disposal. Where poisonous materials are employed special precautions are necessary such as avoidance of direct contact, protective clothing, reduction of work hours, alternation of employment and periodic examination. Personal protection by means of suitable work clothes, helmets, goggles and gloves is desirable in many work situations.

Personnel are frequently reluctant to make use of such equipment but workers should always be instructed in the hazards of their employment and in what they can personally do to protect themselves. It should be a responsibility of management to see that all dangerous processes are constantly supervised by experienced and responsible senior staff. Similarly employees should be impressed with the need to make use of the facilities provided for their personal cleanliness so that any contamination which they acquire can be removed as soon as possible. Any symptoms of illness must be reported immediately and any injury however slight should receive early attention.

Employers are becoming increasingly conscious of the need for good industrial hygiene. It will be obvious from the foregoing that the measures to secure this fall into two categories related either to the physical equipment of the work-place or to the attitudes and conduct of the employees. Many factories now have their own efficient health organizations under the charge and direction of an industrial medical officer whose tasks will include the selection of personnel for particular work in accordance with their ability and aptitude, their instruction in the appreciation and avoidance of unnecessary industrial risk, and their regular medical supervision to detect the earliest signs of ill-effects. He will also concern himself with the sickness record of individual employees who may suffer from an excessive incidence of incapacitating illness related less specifically to their occupation but which may be indicative of occupational stress.

Finally it should be noted that in Britain general practitioners are required to notify certain prescribed industrial diseases to the Chief Inspector of Factories.

infancy, psychology of. The quality of parental care given to an infant is of vital importance for his future personality development and mental well-being. The evidence for this assertion comes from studies of children in institutions, from studying the early childhood of adolescents with psychological illness and from knowing the progress of children who are known to have been deprived in infancy. It is of course not a new discovery because many writers from Aristotle onwards have regarded a child's mind as a blank slate on which only experience can write the elements of knowledge and reason which ultimately determine personality. There is however a growing appreciation that psychological development tends to proceed by steps related to experiences which are common to every child and that personality can be profoundly affected by the manner in which those successive steps, or 'cognitive' transitions, and their individual problems are handled. It has been suggested that personality can be conceived as comprising three elements; the id or the deepest unconscious part of the mind influenced by pleasant or unpleasant experiences; the ego controlling conscious experience and interaction with the environment; and the super-ego, or conscience, concerned with moral and judicial attitudes.

The personality of the infant is determined by what happens to its id and ego, especially at these periods of cognitive transition.

Birth provides the earliest of these transitions and although not remembered consciously it must obviously provide a traumatic experience. The foetus secure in its insulated environment is suddenly and forcibly squeezed through a dark passage and cast out into the adversities of an unfriendly environment. To neutralize the damaging effects of this transition a great deal of mothering is required, with the child's senses stimulated by the feel and warmth of the parent and also by the sound of her voice. The effects of maternal neglect at this stage can often be seen in very young motherless babies whose failure to thrive requires to be treated by cuddling and by vigorous excitation of the sucking reflex. This highlights the emotional importance of breast feeding which provides solace and relief of tensions, but breast feeding is unfashionable nowadays in many societies, and the infant will accept a substitute procedure without harm providing that the maternal cuddling and nursing which is an inevitable part of breast feeding is not also abandoned.

Weaning is the next stage. Since the infant's pleasures and satisfactions are centred around the act of nursing he is disturbed if this is suddenly withdrawn. The transition should be achieved gradually and there is advantage in starting the process by the fourth month. With longer delay it is more likely that the infant will become over-dependent on his mother and that he will retain immature character traits.

Toilet training is a further important step which can produce emotional anxiety and tension in both mother and infant. Excessive zeal at too early an age will result in the child associating the procedure with discomfort and compulsion, and he also soon learns to appreciate that this is a situation which can be used as a potent weapon to secure his mother's praise, discomfiture or attention. Conflict will result either in a performing or a non-performing reaction and according to the theorists these are associated in later life with personalities which are respectively careless, wasteful and extravagant or compulsive and fastidious. Before the age of 12 months the child can be given the opportunity to perform regularly, provided that no conflict element is introduced. By the end of the first year the child will be more ready to co-operate, and conflict is less likely to arise. As in any habit-training the basic principle is to avoid showing much disappointment at failure and to praise success so that a child gradually learns to conform to a pattern of desired behaviour.

See also CHILDHOOD, PSYCHOLOGY OF and PARENT AGE AND CHILD CARE.

Comparison of human milk and cow's milk		
	Human	Cow's
Protein:		
caseinogen	0.5 to 0.7%	2.25 to 3%
lactalbumin	0.75 to 1.3%	0.75 to 1%
Fat	3 to 4%	4%
Sugar	6 to 7%	4 to 5%
Water	87 to 90%	87 to 90%
Minerals	0.3%	0.7%
Vitamins	A, B, C, D	A, B, C, D
Reaction	alkaline	acid
Temperature	body	varies
Bacteria	sterile	unknown

infant feeding. In its early months an infant depends exclusively on milk with the addition of appropriate vitamins. The natural source of this milk is its mother's breast and reference should be made to the article on BREAST FEEDING.

Nowadays breast feeding is regrettably in decline in some countries and has been replaced with BOTTLE-FEEDING so that most infants are fed 'artificially' on milk re-constituted from dried milk powder or less often from condensed milk. Expert advice on individual regimes should be obtained from the health visitor or other professional worker. An infant requires 35 ml. of milk per kg. (2.5 oz. per 1 lb.) of 'expected' body weight per day, usually divided into six feeds at three-hourly intervals until 3 months of age and five feeds at four-hourly intervals thereafter.

Weaning should be commenced at 3 to 4 months or when the child reaches 7 kg. (151 lb.) in weight, by the gradual introduction of mixed feeding – cereals, vegetables and protein supplements. Commercially prepared infant foods of this type are available and provide a safe and convenient method of extending the infant's diet.

infantile convulsions. See CONVULSIONS.

infantile diarrhoea. Diarrhoea is one of the commonest disorders of infancy and an important cause of death during the first year. It is significantly less frequent in breast-fed infants partly because of the greater risks of contamination of the bottle feeds and partly because of the difference in composition of human milk and other milk-feeds. The commonest causes are the bacteria responsible for various types of dysentery, and certain viruses.

Outbreaks of infantile diarrhoea are common in children's wards and institutions. The infectivity is very high and since infants withstand fluid loss badly there is apt to be a considerable risk of death.

Minor attacks of diarrhoea may be treated by discontinuing the usual feeds and substituting a solution of sugar (1 tablespoonful) and salt (1 teaspoonful) in 1 litre (2 pints) of boiled water, but if the condition persists, or the baby appears generally ill, medical advice should be sought without delay.

infantile paralysis. See POLIOMYELITIS.

infantilism. The persistence of childhood characteristics into later life. There is impaired physical development, delayed sexual matura-tion and often mental retardation. Diminutive stature (DWARFISM) is not synonymous with infantilism. There are three groups of causes.

1. Endocrine causes. These include thyroid deficiency producing cretins; pituitary defi-ciency producing a condition called dystrophia adiposo-genitalis (Fröhlich's syndrome) and other similar conditions; and deficiencies of the sex glands (eunuchoidal infantilism). The rare condition of progeria where infantilism is associated with premature ageing also occurs.

2. Disease of other organs. Delayed development may result from coeliac disease; from congenital disease of the kidney (renal rickets); from pancreatic insufficiency; from congenital heart disease; or from forms of mental defect.

3. Constitutional and metabolic disease. Various chronic infections such as congenital syphilis and chronic tuberculosis may retard development. Malnutrition, vitamin de-ficiencies, rickets, diabetes and a glycogen-storage disease (in which there is inability to mobilize glycogen when it is needed) are other causes.

The management of cases of infantilism depends primarily on an accurate assessment of the cause followed by appropriate treatment.

infant mortality rate. The number of deaths of infants under one year of age per thousand live births in the particular year. In underdeveloped countries and in developed countries in the past it is – or has been – very high. For instance, in England and Wales it was 151 in 1901, i.e., rather more than one baby out of every seven died before reaching its first birthday; and as late as 1911 it was 129, representing more than one death in every eight babies.

The main causes of these deaths, in highly developed countries in the past and to a large extent in underdeveloped countries today, fell into four groups: (1) developmental conditions (including birth injury, prematurity, malformations, etc); (2) respiratory diseases; (3) infantile gastro-enteritis (infantile diarrhoea); and (4) acute infectious diseases (including measles, whooping cough and tuberculosis), with malnutrition and bad housing playing appreciable parts. With improved nutrition, better housing, provision of antenatal services, better obstetrics and provision of child health services, the infant mortality rate in highly developed countries has fallen dramatically, reaching figures as low as 12 per thousand births in Sweden and Finland; and it is sometimes said, with reason, that the reduction of baby deaths represents the biggest health advance of all time. As a concrete example, the rate for Scotland fell from 129 in 1900 to 18 in the 1970s.

Because young babies are the most

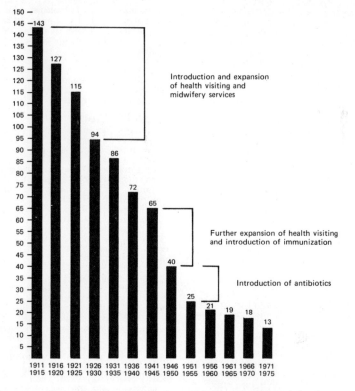

Infant death rate per thousand births in one city (Aberdeen, Scotland).

vulnerable group in the community the infant mortality rate has for many decades been regarded as the best index of the health services and social circumstances of an area, tending to be high in places with bad housing, overcrowding, maternal ignorance and poor services.

However, it is no longer a completely satisfactory index for several reasons. Firstly, although there is some overlap, infants die from two main groups of causes: most deaths during the first month are related either to hereditary factors or to factors during pregnancy and child birth, and most later deaths are related to infections and to child care after the infant is born. Secondly, with improved social and environmental conditions and provision of good advisory services (e.g., health visitors in the U.K.) deaths after the first month have become infrequent. Thirdly, there is little difference between a child that is born dead (a stillbirth) and a child that is born in such condition that it dies within the first few days.

In order to study different influences in more detail three additional indices have been introduced. These are the perinatal mortality rate, which is the total of all stillbirths and deaths under the age of 1 week expressed as a rate per thousand of all births (live and still); the neonatal death rate which is the number of deaths under 28 days per thousand live births;

and the post-neonatal death rate which is the number of deaths at 29 to 365 days per thousand live births.

Average figures for an area with good social conditions and well developed health services would be, for a thousand pregnancies, about twelve stillbirths, about eight deaths during the first seven days, about five during the next three weeks and about five during the rest of the first year.

Deaths after the first seven days are not further discussed in this article but are still frequent and important in many countries.

The factors influencing the perinatal mortality rate (i.e., stillbirths and deaths in the first seven days) have been subjected to exhaustive and detailed examination in the U.K. in the British Perinatal Mortality Survey (and to some extent by parallel surveys in some other countries). A large number of interesting points have emerged.

Many of these points naturally relate to the mother. In particular the standard of prenatal care has proved of enormous importance: if there was no prenatal care at all the perinatal mortality rate was five times as high as the general average; or, in approximate figures, while about 2 per cent of all pregnancies ended in stillbirths or early infant deaths, 10 per cent of pregnancies with no prenatal care ended with these tragedies. Perhaps because unmarried women are more reluctant to seek prenatal help than married women, the perinatal death rate was almost twice as high for illegitimate pregnancies as for the pregnancies of married women.

Again there was an interesting relationship with the mother's age: stillbirths and early infant deaths were fewest when the mother was between 20 and 30 years, slightly more frequent if she was a little under 20 or a little above 30, and appreciably commoner if she was 40 or over. The mother's height also appeared to play a part, perhaps because a tall woman usually has a large pelvis. At any rate there was a higher proportion of stillbirths and early infant deaths in small women and a lower proportion in tall women. Another factor that emerged was that first babies had a higher than average risk, second babies had the lowest risk of all, third babies came close to first babies in risk, and fourth and subsequent babies had an appreciable and steadily rising risk.

The survey also confirmed a point that public health doctors and nurses had stressed for years – namely that, despite the provision of welfare foods, the creation of antenatal clinics and the expansion of health visiting and midwifery services, the amount of risk remained highest in the least affluent and least educated groups. When the parents were divided into occupational categories, there was a steady rise in the perinatal death rate from the highest to the lowest group, with the rate twice as high in unskilled workers as in persons from professional and managerial classes. We can speculate that this finding may mean that the more intelligent parents took greater advantage of the available services (as is known, from other evidence, to be the case), or derived benefit from better food or better houses, or were genetically superior, or that all these factors operated.

The Survey also studied mortality in relation to duration of pregnancy. For women delivered at term (40 weeks) the perinatal death rate was less than half the average. At a fortnight postmature (42 weeks) it was one and a half times the average. At a fortnight premature (38 weeks) it was twice the average.

By far the worst outlook for a child was to be born prematurely to a small unmarried woman, from an unskilled occupation, aged well under 20 or substantially over 30, and receiving no prenatal care.

infant welfare. Organized and systematic arrangements for the protection and promotion of health in infancy. During the second half of the last century general mortality in several developed countries declined steadily but infant mortality showed no decrease. Advances in hygiene were concerned mainly with public sanitation and industrial conditions, much less with living standards, and not at all with milk-supply. From about 1899 milk depots were set up in various cities in Britain, France and the U.S.A. and these later developed as infant consultation centres. Infant welfare thus began by tackling the most urgent and obvious cause of illness and death, namely the feeding of infants on unsafe cow's milk. Simultaneously many towns in the U.K. began to appoint health visitors (or female sanitary inspectors as some of them were at first called) to teach and help mothers in their own homes. The value of these pioneer efforts led to the inception of statutory child welfare schemes.

Infant welfare arrangements seek to ensure that every child is given the best possible chance of survival and healthy development, but equally important is the proper supervision of pregnancy because prenatal influences have a profound effect on subsequent progress.

A comprehensive scheme for welfare therefore has three components: adequate prenatal and childbirth services; an infant consultation clinic; and organised home supervision by HEALTH VISITORS or similar public health nurses with subsequent training in health maintenance. At all stages there must also be recognition of the importance of health education for the mother as provided by mothercraft classes and individual tuition. To ensure that all these provisions are fully utilized the persistence and professional expertise of the qualified health visitor are indispensable.

Prenatal supervision aims at the detection and appropriate timely treatment of conditions likely to lessen the chances of infant survival. Amongst these are haemolytic disease of the new born (RHESUS incompatibility) and factors such as maternal conditions likely to cause premature birth. Skilled obstetrical management will reduce the possibility of injury or other problems at the time of birth.

A high proportion of infant deaths occur during the first four weeks of life. To reduce these the essentials are special facilities for premature babies, expertly controlled feeding, and strict measures to avoid infection. Routine tests are now employed to detect congenital dislocation of the hip and metabolic disorders such as phenylketonuria, but systematic examination by a doctor experienced in dealing with newly born babies is desirable to detect other indications of abnormalities.

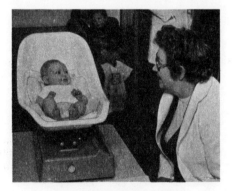

Infant welfare

In later months most infant deaths occur from infections of the respiratory or digestive systems. The influence of the child health clinic and of the health visitor are of paramount importance in educating the mother in general hygiene, feeding methods and commonsense precautions in order to minimize these and other risks. Steps are also taken to have infants immunized against various diseases in accordance with a routine schedule. Child welfare schemes are now increasingly providing for developmental assessment by systematic medical examination during the first year at 6 weeks, 6 months and 10 months of age in order to detect deviations from normal development, or defects such as deafness or poor sight which will prejudice progress.

The psycho-social aspects of child welfare and the enormous role of the HEALTH VISITOR therein are considered elsewhere.

infarct. A small portion of tissue that has died through loss of blood supply as a result of blockage of an artery by a blood clot (thrombus) or a foreign body (embolism). Infarction is rare in tissues that are supplied by a mass of small, inter-communicating arteries, because if one channel is closed the blood travels by other channels. It is relatively common in the heart (causing coronary thrombosis) and not uncommon in the brain, lungs, kidneys and intestines.

infection. The condition that arises when disease-producing micro-organisms successfully invade the body, establish themselves and multiply. The common sources of infection are discharges or excreta from the body of a person suffering from the disease or of a carrier, or, less frequently, the body of an infected animal. Droplet infection, which is spread in talking, laughing, coughing and sneezing is much the most frequent. The main paths of infection are:

1. Inhalation, in which the organism (e.g., the virus of measles or influenza) is breathed out by a patient and inhaled by the next victim, with the organisms settling on the mucous membrane of the nose, mouth or pharynx, and thereafter passing to any part of the body in which they can breed.

2. Ingestion, in which the food or water contaminated from the excreta of a case or carrier (as in typhoid and paratyphoid) is consumed, the organisms reach the digestive tract, and in due course pass to any portion of the body.

3. Inoculation, in which the organisms gain access through a wound in the skin or mucous membrane (as in tetanus) or enter through previously intact skin transmitted by the bite of an infected mosquito (as in malaria).

4. Very rarely transmission before birth, as in transmission of syphilis through the placenta or infection with gonorrhoea while the child is passing through the birth canal.

After the micro-organisms have obtained a habitation they breed, some germs doubling every half hour (so that one unopposed germ might become about 100 million in about fifteen hours) while the defence mechanisms of the body (e.g., white blood corpuscles) endeavour to kill them off. This is the INCUBATION PERIOD (fairly specific for any one disease) in which the organisms multiply before symptoms of the disease appear.

The symptoms of infection vary with the disease but often include: (1) Nervous system: headache, malaise, insomnia, drowsiness, high temperature, rigor, shivering, delirium and convulsions; (2) circulatory system: rapid pulse, irregularities of heart beat, pallor, cyanosis and coldness of extremities; (3) alimentary system: dry mouth, furred tongue, loss of appetite, thirst, nausea, vomiting, diarrhoea or constipation; (4) respiratory system: rapid respiration and sometimes breathlessness; (5) excretory system: hot dry skin (or perspiration), scanty and highly coloured urine, and diarrhoea or constipation;

and (6) muscular system: general weakness and prostration.

Until about a hundred years ago half the population of highly developed countries died as the result of infections. Developments which have enormously reduced the danger of infections include: (1) antisepsis and later asepsis which removed the likelihood of infection after surgical or gynaecological operations; (2) purity of water supplies, installation of sewerage systems and improved food hygiene, which together made food-borne and water-borne infections uncommon; (3) vaccination and immunization against an increasing number of diseases – incomparably the biggest medical development of modern times; and (4) the introduction first of sulphonamides and later of antibiotics which rendered possible the successful treatment of many infections.

infectious diseases. Diseases which result from the successful invasion of the body by living organisms. These organisms may be bacteria, viruses, rickettsia or protozoa. Invasion of the body by fungi is more usually called mycosis and the presence of more complex metazoan animals such as worms or flukes is parasitism or infestation rather than infection.

Infectious diseases are essentially preventable. The measures necessary are good hygiene, the protection of food and water supplies, the early identification, isolation and treatment of cases, the quarantining or surveillance of contacts, and the protection of individuals by specific immunological procedures where these are available. There are statutory powers for the notification and control of certain infections.

inferiority complex. A persistent feeling of guilt or unworthiness which dominates the thinking and actions of persons of inadequate or ill-balanced personality. It may occur in association with some physical disability either real or imagined or as an expression of some inner conflict with society. It may not always be obvious that a patient has feelings of inferiority as he may seek to conceal them by projecting his shortcomings on to other persons or by rationalizing them in some way, and his conduct may be aggressive rather than self-deprecatory.

It seldom helps such patients merely to tell them that such feelings are unwarranted. Rather they should be assured that there is a logical reason for their symptoms and encouraged to devote patience and thought to uncovering and bringing into the open the half-forgotten secrets of events which in the past have engendered feelings of shame or guilt.

infertility. See FERTILITY.

inflammation. The changes which occur in living tissue when it is injured (provided that the injury is not of such severity as immediately to destroy its structure and kill it). The usual signs of inflammation are swelling, pain, redness, heat and impaired function.

Inflammation may be produced by bacteria and their toxins or by trauma, injurious chemicals and the effects of physical agencies such as heat, cold, electricity, ultra-violet light, x-rays and other forms of radiation. It should be regarded as a defensive reaction of the body to repair the damage. If this is successful, resolution is said to occur, but with more

SOME COMMON INFECTIOUS DISEASES

DISEASE	INCUBATION	TRANSMISSION	PREVENTION
Anthrax	Within 7 days	To skin Inhalation Ingestion	Industrial precautions Immunization
Brucellosis (Undulant fever)	5 to 21 days or much longer	Contact in farm workers, etc. Ingestion	Work precautions Pasteurization of milk
Chickenpox	12 to 21 days	Contact - mainly Inhalation	Contact avoidance
Cholera	2 to 3 days or less	Ingestion	Hygiene Water purification Immunization
Diphtheria	2 to 7 days	Contact - mainly Inhalation	Contact avoidance Immunization
Dysentery (Bacillary)	1 to 7 days	Ingestion	Hygiene
Gonorrhoea	3 to 4 days	Contact	Propaganda against promiscuity
Influenza	1 to 3 days	Contact - mainly Inhalation	Contact avoidance Immunization
Malaria	12 to 30 days	Mosquito	Mosquito control Suppressive drugs
Measles	7 to 14 days	Contact	Contact avoidance Immunization
Meningitis (Cerebro-spinal fever)	1 to 5 days	Contact	Contact avoidance
Mumps	12 to 26 days	Contact	Contact avoidance
Paratyphoid fevers	1 to 10 days	Ingestion	Hygiene Immunization
Pneumonia	1 to 3 days but variable	Contact	Contact avoidance
Poliomyelitis (Infantile paralysis)	7 to 14 days	Contact	Immunization
Rubella (German measles)	5 to 21 days	Contact	Immunization
Salmonellosis (Food poisoning)	6 to 48 hours	Ingestion	Hygiene
Scarlet Fever	1 to 8 days	Contact	Contact avoidance
Smallpox	5 to 15 days	Contact	Vaccination
Syphilis	Usually 21 days	Contact	Propaganda against promiscuity
Tetanus	4 to 21 days	Wound infection	Immunization

DISEASE	INCUBATION	TRANSMISSION	PREVENTION
Tuberculosis	4 to 6 weeks or longer	Inhalation Ingestion	BCG vaccination
Typhoid fever	12 to 21 days	Ingestion	Hygiene Immunization
Typhus	10 to 14 days	Louse	Louse eradication Immunization
Whooping-cough (Pertussis)	7 to 18 days	Contact - mainly Inhalation	Immunization
Yellow fever	3 to 6 days	Mosquito	Mosquito control Immunization

severe injury the inflammatory processes may progress to suppuration, ulceration or gangrene before healing ultimately becomes possible, or a state of chronic inflammation may ensue.

The treatment largely depends upon the cause. The principles are to remove or neutralize or destroy the cause, to encourage blood flow to the part (hyperaemia) by the application of warmth, and to secure rest for the affected part.

In medical terminology words which mean that inflammation has occurred end in '-itis', e.g., tonsillitis.

influenza. An acute infectious disease due to the influenza virus, occurring as world-wide (pandemic) or local epidemics or as sporadic outbreaks. It has a short incubation of one to three days and the onset is usually sudden with raised temperature, headache, pains in the back and limbs, upper respiratory symptoms resembling a common cold, and a tendency to more serious inflammatory complications in the respiratory system. Recovery from the acute phase is often followed by fatigue and depression which may last for a considerable time. Five clinical types are recognized according to the incidence of main symptoms: (1) febrile, (2) respiratory, (3) malignant with severe general toxaemia, (4) gastro-intestinal, (5) nervous with headache and severe depression.

There are two main types of virus – influenza A and influenza B. The 'A' variety is usually found in the widespread winter epidemics which tend to recur every two or three years. Sporadic local outbreaks are more often the 'B' variety but its antigenic properties are variable and this makes it difficult to formulate a uniformly effective vaccine.

Vaccination is, however, a useful measure and should be offered to groups of persons at special risk, especially hospital staffs, community nurses, the elderly, and those with chronic cardiac or respiratory disease. It is also widely used in industry as a precaution against a high incidence of influenza during the winter which might disrupt work or production. On the basis of information collected by WHO, manufacturers endeavour to match their current batch of vaccine to the strains of virus most likely to be encountered at any particular time.

infra-red rays. Infra-red rays are given off by any body heated to just below redness and infra-red lamps for therapeutic purposes are basically very simple, consisting of a blackened electric bulb or a specially-shaped coil of resistance wire with a reflector. The cabinet type infra-red heat cage employs several such sources.

Infra-red rays occupy a position in the electro-magnetic spectrum just beyond the red end of the band of visible light and with waves of greater length in the range 7,700 to 4 million Angstrom units. (One AU = one ten-millionth of a millimetre.)

When absorbed by the skin infra-red rays liberate heat and cause the tissues in that area to rise in temperature, which has a sedative effect on sensory nerve-endings, produces dilatation of blood capillaries with improved circulation and induces perspiration. Heat relieves pain and muscle spasm, improved circulation helps resolution of inflammation, and perspiration aids elimination of waste-products. Because of these effects infra-red radiation is used in the treatment of neuritis, arthritis, neuralgia, fibrositis, traumatic inflammation and cellulitis and also in spastic paralysis before massage or manipulation, and in general diseases such as chronic nephritis where there is defective elimination of waste material by the kidneys.

ingrowing eyelash. This condition (trichiasis) sometimes occurs after chronic inflammatory conditions of the eyelids (blepharitis) which distort the lid margins and change the direction of growth of the eyelashes so that one or more turn inwards and rub on the eyeball to produce irritation, spasm of the eyelids and risk of damage to the cornea. The troublesome eyelash may be pulled out with forceps. If this is done repeatedly renewal of the hairs may finally cease but for a more rapid permanent cure electrolysis or removal of the roots is employed.

Occasionally a second inner row of eyelashes is found as a congenital defect (distichiasis) and this usually necessitates removal by an operation.

ingrowing toe-nail. See TOE.

inguinal region. The junction of the lower abdomen and thigh on each side is marked by an oblique fold which, with the immediately adjacent and underlying parts is known as the inguinal region or GROIN.

inhalation. Inhalation is synonymous with inspiration and is the act of drawing air or other vapour into the lungs. It is also a general descriptive term for any medicament intended to be breathed in as a vapour or powder.

This form of treatment is employed for various conditions affecting the respiratory tract. In nasal congestion, the common cold or tonsillitis, menthol, eucalyptus, or friar's balsam is added to boiling water in a jug surrounded by a towel so arranged as to form a funnel through which the patient breathes in the resultant medicated vapour. In bronchiectasis inhalation of vaporized creosote is a traditional remedy but probably only acts by inducing coughing and the expulsion of sputum.

In the treatment of asthma use is made of anti-spasmodic inhalations, usually prepared as pressurized aerosols or ultra-fine powders. Their constituents include adrenalin, ephedrine, isoprenaline, salbutamol and sodium cromoglycate.

inhibition. The blocking of any impulse or action. Inhibition occasionally has a physical basis, as when we desire to eat a food that disagrees with us but deliberately refrain because we know the consequences. More often, however, it is a result of social conditioning, e.g., we want to hit the person who has annoyed us but have learned from childhood that society disapproves of violence; or it may be a result of psychological conflict, e.g., the pupil wants to dispute the teacher's spelling of a word but refrains because of either respect or fear.

Inhibitions in moderation are conducive to the harmony of existence: a man wants to make violent love to a woman but is restrained because the place is unsuitable or because the woman is unwilling or because he is married and has feelings of guilt. In excess, however, inhibitions indicate a lack of self-confidence, a feeling of inferiority and an inadequate development of the personality.

One of the effects of alcohol is to reduce inhibitions. It can be useful in enabling a normally shy person to take his part in conversation; but the removal of inhibitions can lead to uncontrolled aggression.

Fatigue and exhaustion can increase inhibitions, so the first line of treatment of excessively inhibited persons is attention to general health. Many such persons, however, require prolonged psychological treatment.

injection. The procedure of using a syringe and needle to introduce into the body some fluid substance for therapeutic purposes.

Injections may be intradermal, i.e., given into the substance of the true skin or dermis; otherwise they may be given deep into the skin (subcutaneous), into the muscle (intra-muscular) or into the vein (intravenous), and these are variously employed in accordance with the needs of treatment or the characteristics of the material injected.

Injections may also be made into specific sites to ensure some desired local action. Examples are the induction of local anaesthesia, and the treatment of neuralgia and arthritis.

inoculation. The procedure of inducing active immunity against an infectious disease by introducing into the body a controlled dose of the causative organisms. Preparations used for this purpose are known as vaccines and the organisms they contain may be live, attenuated or killed in accordance with the need to balance considerations of safety and efficacy.

Vaccines are generally administered by subcutaneous injection using a syringe and needle but in protection against smallpox the inoculation is given intradermally through a scratch or by multiple superficial punctures. BCG vaccine is also employed intradermally. In poliomyelitis vaccination, Sabin vaccine is effective by mouth.

As indicated in VACCINATION the earliest inoculations were direct arm-to-arm transfers of material from a smallpox vesicle to the person seeking protection.

insanity. An imprecise term for MENTAL DISEASE. Its use has been largely abandoned by psychiatrists although the law still regards as insane a person who is incapable of forming moral judgements, who does not appreciate the nature and consequence of his acts, and who is incapable of managing his property and affairs.

In the early stages of mental illness the difficulty is to decide whether the patient is psychotic or suffering from neurosis – a classification which includes neurasthenia, anxiety states, obsessional states, and hysteria. Specialist advice is essential.

insect bites. See BITES AND STINGS.

insomnia. Inability to fall asleep or achieve sleep that is adequate and restful. Almost everyone complains of sleeplessness from time to time, but it can be a distressing symptom of many disease conditions and measures to secure sleep for such patients are an important part of their treatment.

The treatment of insomnia in an individual who is otherwise well requires a careful consideration of all the relevant circumstances. Sleep only occurs if there is full physical and mental relaxation and there must be no extraneous conditions preventing this. Disturbing factors such as pain, cold, heat, light and so on, should be eliminated. In the elderly the prevalence and importance of cold feet should be appreciated. Many persons complain that their thoughts are more active in bed and this may be a pointer to worries and anxieties which should be identified and assuaged. Psycho-neurotics tend to compound the effects of worrying by worrying about the dangers of not sleeping and require to be reassured that this is not deadly. Many persons exaggerate the extent of their insomnia and it is important to investigate this aspect of the problem.

Various simple measures may help to re-establish a satisfactory sleep-pattern. In elderly persons digestive processes are slower and the last meal should be taken five hours before retiral. Tea and coffee act as stimulants and should be avoided at bedtime but a warm milky drink or a small dose of whisky is useful. No great volume of fluid should be given lest rest is disturbed by need to pass urine. For the ordinary adult something light to read in bed, with the bedside-lamp within easy reach, is a good way to achieve relaxation.

Inability to sleep is very characteristic of any feverish illness particularly if accompanied by headache or the breathing problems of bronchitis or pneumonia. For these acute cases much can be done by nursing technique. Tepid sponging, bed re-making, a comfortable posture, bladder-emptying and a mild sedative are illustrative of the lines on which to proceed. In more chronic respiratory disease with a troublesome cough, the administration of a sedative cough mixture will often secure relief.

In chronic heart failure adequate rest may have quite remarkable effects in improving the efficiency of heart and circulation and sufficient sedation to secure this is generally justifiable. Similarly, sedation may be needed in uraemia, thyrotoxicosis, neurasthenia, delirium tremens, and mental disturbance.

The use of sedatives requires careful consideration. If given they should be employed in an attempt to re-establish the habit of sleep and then be gradually reduced and withdrawn. Fear of sleeplessness thereafter may be countered by having a single dose at hand to take if necessary, with the main supply held elsewhere to avoid risks of accidental overdosage. The type of sedative to be prescribed should be related to the sleep-pattern. If there is difficulty only in falling asleep a quickly-acting, quickly excreted hypnotic is best. For wakefulness later in the night a slow-acting drug is more suitable. Alcohol should not be recommended except for the elderly because of the risks of increasing dependence.

inspiration. Breathing in.

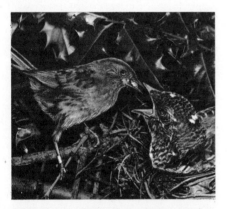

A hedge sparrow instinctively feeding a cuckoo in its nest

instinct. A purposeful and often complicated pattern of behaviour which seems to occur spontaneously rather than as the result of previous experience and learning. These behaviour patterns answer a need of a particular animal species in various environmental situations.

The word is often used incorrectly. When a person claims to have done something 'instinctively' he means that he apparently did the right thing without having considered an appropriate response. In fact he was subconsciously exploiting his own past experience of similar situations. Before a biologist will accept that some aspect of animal behaviour is instinctive he must be satisfied on certain matters which are best explained by examples.

First of all, instincts are inborn and are not improved by practice: a spider spins a perfect web first time and birds of different species build their own particular type of nest without any instruction. That no learning is involved is particularly obvious when an instinctive action occurs only once in a lifetime. For instance, eels when they reach the age of ten migrate across the Atlantic to spawn and die. The second point is that instincts are purposeful: when the cuckoo lays its eggs in the nest of the hedge-sparrow or other foster parent it ensures that its young will be fed without trouble to itself. Thirdly, instincts are automatic and inflexible: a dog before lying down on a rug will turn round as if flattening the grass; a beaver left alone in a room will destroy the furniture to build a dam.

Instinct plays a variable part in the lives of different animal species. Insects are largely dependent on it, birds less so, and mammals least of all, except in relation to maternal behaviour. Mammals tend to modify their reactions as a result of experience and so acquire personality.

Instinctive behaviour appears to be controlled by hormones – a reaction to chemical messengers in the body. This explains maternal behaviour when even a timid animal mother will fight to defend its young and why birds build nests in the spring. It explains, too, why the worker bee carries out a rigid schedule of different duties which change in invariable progression as it ages. Perhaps the most convincing proof comes from certain experiments on rats. The testes of male rats were removed and replaced by grafted ovaries. The male rats then developed female instincts, produced milk, and suckled young.

insulin. The hormone, produced by the islets of Langerhans in the pancreas, which controls the metabolism of sugar (glucose). Insufficient production of insulin is the cause of DIABETES MELLITUS which is essentially an accumulation of glucose in the blood. Excess of insulin, usually arising from over-dosage of a diabetic patient, dangerously decreases the amount of glucose in the blood (hypoglycaemia).

The hormone – postulated by Schafer in 1916 – was isolated by Banting and Best in 1922, revolutionizing the outlook for persons suffering from diabetes, and its exact molecular structure was determined by Sanger in 1958.

intelligence. The faculty of reason or the total of a person's abilities to meet and to deal with various situations. When a person is faced with an unfamiliar set of circumstances he has to decide what to do. In making his decision he either has in mind the result which he wishes to achieve or, on the basis of past experience, attempts to foresee the result of any action and regulates what he actually does in accordance with his forecast. He is in short attempting to shape the present and the future by his knowledge and experience of the past and obviously his success in dealing with a particular situation will depend not only on his native intelligence but on the relevance of his cultural background to the immediate problem.

This illustrates the difficulties which surround any attempt to define intelligence in precise terms and to devise means of assessing it. It is now generally agreed that human intelligence must be regarded as consisting of both general and special aptitudes. The standard INTELLIGENCE TESTS (as usually applied) primarily attempt to determine basic or general intelligence as shown by abilities of perception, memory, reason and so on, and to lessen or neutralize the effects of special experience or knowledge.

Many animal lovers will claim that their pets are intelligent and certainly many animals can be taught tricks and often show behaviour which has every appearance of being intelligent in that it seems to be adjusted to a particular set of circumstances. If, however, such behaviour is closely examined it will be found that it is due to past experience – an ability to learn by repetition and an ability to appreciate mistakes made in the past and to avoid them in the future. The test is really whether an animal can reason and so far this has been convincingly demonstrated only in the apes and monkeys.

intelligence tests. Everybody knows that the level of intelligence varies in different persons. We could choose from our acquaintances one whom we deem highly intelligent, one quite intelligent and one rather dull-witted. Yet our highly intelligent friend, who handles numbers so easily and spots the logical fallacy in an argument, may be a poor linguist and may lack the ability to undertake a simple household repair; and our dull-witted acquaintance may be the one who can best find his way in a strange town or the one who manages to improvise a tool for an unusual job. Clearly, even if we could devise a test independent of past experience, no one test could fully measure mental capacity.

In the eighteenth and nineteenth centuries many psychologists tried to evolve single 'scientific' tests of intelligence but inevitably failed. Then a French psychologist, Alfred Binet (1857-1911) had the idea of creating a whole series of sub-tests for children of different ages. The group of tests for any one age-group would contain items designed to test comprehension of words, understanding of numbers, recognition of shapes, memory, capacity for finding analogies, and so on; and the battery of tests for, for instance, children of 7 years would contain items that less than half of 6-year-old children could manage successfully but that more than half of 8-year-old children could do.

After trying many such tests on large numbers of children and discarding some of the tests as unsatisfactory Binet and his co-worker Simon produced in 1905 their battery of tests for establishing a child's 'mental age'. For example, think of a child who is very good when dealing with numbers but less good when dealing with shapes and spaces. He manages all the tests for 7-year-olds, all except two of the tests for 8-year-olds (failing on two involving shapes) and only two of the tests for 9-year-olds (two involving numbers). Balancing his successes in the 9-year-old group against his failures in the 8-year-old group his mental age can be stated as exactly 8 years.

However, it is long-winded to have to say, 'This bright girl has a mental age of 10 years and a chronological age of 8 years'. So the refinement was introduced of expressing the mental age as a percentage of the chronological age and calling the result the intelligence quotient (often known simply as IQ). Thus the bright girl just mentioned would have an IQ of ten-eighths multiplied by a hundred, i.e., 125; and an exactly average person would have an IQ of 100.

The tests were basically simple and performed in a short time. For example, a 3-year-old was expected to be able to point to his nose, eyes and mouth, to repeat two digits, to name well-known objects in a picture, to give his family name and to repeat a sentence of six syllables. The original Binet-Simon scale was later revised and extended, and by 1921 further revisions – notably one by two American psychologists, Terman and Merrill – were in world-wide use. The immediate international acceptance showed how great had been the need for a reasonably accurate measuring device.

Since this initial breakthrough, psychologists have produced further tests in bewildering variety. One difficulty with the Binet-Simon tests was that they used words and therefore placed illiterate children and children from homes in which there was little communication at a disadvantage. So an important step was to devise non-verbal methods of assessing illiterate children. The Collins, Drever and Wechsler Scales and the Penrose-Raven Progressive Matrices are examples of these.

Again, the tests were at first used largely for backward or handicapped children, to determine whether a child could benefit from ordinary education – see BACKWARDNESS IN CHILDREN and MENTAL DEFICIENCY - but soon came equally into use for the identification of bright children, e.g., for admission to secondary schools or later to universities and other institutions of higher learning. Naturally psychologists began to extend their activities to the testing of adults.

If tests were to be useful in the selection of the most suitable person for admission to a particular advanced course or for a post as a senior civil servant, a high ranking army officer or a managerial post in industry, it was obvious that something more than a rough assessment of general intelligence was needed. The managing editor of a large newspaper, the head of a university, a general in the armed forces and a top civil servant all need good general intelligence but require also certain different qualities or aptitudes; and, while promotion to a top post might be on displayed ability in the particular field, it would be wasteful of talent to appoint persons to important junior posts in line for promotion simply on assessment of general intelligence. So, in addition to tests for general intelligence, tests were devised for specific aptitudes, personality, imagination, patience, stability, and so forth. Some of the better known tests used for assessing perseverance, personality, imagination, association fluency and other character traits include the Dewey-Will Temperament Test, the Attitude Scale, the Mosaics Tests and the Rorshach Ink-Blot Test.

The application of such procedures gained momentum after the success of the U.S. Army Alpha Test of the Second World War and the success in Britain of similar tests to select people for wartime posts demanding particular qualities. In older children such tests provide a sound basis for VOCATIONAL GUIDANCE, and, especially in America, many business firms now carry psychological assessment to what are perhaps excessive lengths, sometimes using for their prospective employees tests which are poorly conceived and inadequately standardized.

Nevertheless, intelligence tests can do much to prevent square pegs from occupying round holes, and they will be more and more used in the future.

intercurrent. An intercurrent disease is one that occurs during the course of another disease that is already present, e.g., a person suffering from a heart attack may develop intercurrent pneumonia. While the term is applicable to any second disease developing before complete recovery from the first, by far the commonest intercurrent diseases are infections, because a person who is seriously ill has a very low resistance to any infection.

interferon. In 1956 Isaacs and Lindenmann found that embryonic cells of a chicken treated with killed influenza virus produced a substance that interfered with the growth of influenza virus in other cells. This substance, a complex protein, was appropriately named interferon, or more correctly chick-interferon. Later it was discovered that human cells when stimulated by appropriate antigens including bacteria and viruses produce human-interferon (or to be more accurate a number of allied substances known as human-interferons), and that an interferon produced by one antigen (e.g., a particular bacterium) may interfere with the growth of several different viruses and bacteria.

For relatively large germs such as bacteria the discovery is probably not very important. Sulphonamides and antibiotics can be produced more easily and at much lower cost, and appropriate ones are much more effective in destroying bacteria. Viruses, however, are in general not susceptible to either sulphonamides or antibiotics. The use of antibiotics in viral diseases (e.g., smallpox and measles) has been essentially to deal with complications, to kill off bacteria that invade tissues already weakened by the primary disease. Apart from the use of antibiotics for complications and the possibility of injecting serum obtained from the blood of a person convalescent from the particular disease or otherwise immune to it, and apart from good nursing and attention to symptoms, a viral disease has simply had to run its course.

The discovery of human interferons and of their range of action produces exciting possibilites for the treatment of diseases caused by viruses.

Additionally, just as human beings with a life-span of something like 70 to 120 years undergo alterations over thousands of years, viruses with a very brief life-span can undergo changes from year to year. So new viral diseases appear from time to time: Lassa fever and new varieties of influenza are examples. When a new disease appears it takes some months to produce a vaccine for its effective prevention, and treatment by use of serum obtained from the blood of immune persons does not become practicable until a sizeable number of people have developed immunity, either through recovering from the disease or through being immunized with a hastily prepared vaccine. In other words, until now neither treatment nor prevention has been available during the early months of an outbreak of a new viral disease. Although the obtaining of an interferon from a human donor and its purification for use on another person is at present a difficult and costly procedure, it seems likely that interferon may provide at least an emergency treatment for new viral diseases.

The long-term answer to any disease caused by a virus is to seek to eradicate it by developing a suitable vaccine and persuading susceptible people to accept vaccination: as has happened with smallpox and as is likely to happen with poliomyelitis, if enough people are rendered immune the virus cannot find human cells in which to breed and so disappears. By contrast treatment, however effective, helps only the sufferer and does not reduce the amount of disease. Furthermore, while sulphonamides and antibiotics will actively kill off bacteria, an appropriate interferon appears merely to reduce the multiplication and growth of viruses – to make it easier for the body's defences to cope with the invaders rather than to take part in the battle. Nevertheless the discovery of interferon may in course of time be ranked with the discovery of penicillin as a major contribution to man's war against disease.

international health service. Much of the stimulus for the development of national public health services arose through concern over infectious diseases and, since epidemics do not respect national frontiers, international collaboration began for the same reason. Centuries before the causes of epidemic disease were recognized countries had attempted to protect their people from imported infection by quarantine regulations, but these were often ineffective, or more honoured in their breach than in their observance, and perhaps most important of all, they were a great hindrance to commerce.

International conventions to discuss quarantine were held in Paris in 1851 and on nine subsequent occasions during the nineteenth century with little result until 1903 when proposals for a permanent international organization were finally accepted, with the knowledge that a Pan-American Sanitary Bureau had been set up in Washington in the previous year.

Following this decision there arose in Paris in 1909 *L'Office Internationale d'Hygiène Publique,* charged with the collection and distribution of information about infectious disease, especially cholera, plague and yellow fever. Over the years its interests widened.

After the First World War there was established in Geneva in 1923 the Health Organization of the League of Nations whose duty was 'to take steps in matters of international concern for the prevention and control of disease'. This was obviously a much wider remit and international health activities acquired new horizons. Not only did the Geneva office, with a branch in Singapore, produce an efficient flow of information relating to many more infections than the 'Convention' diseases (plague, cholera, yellow fever, smallpox and typhus), but it also interested itself in other topics such as standardization of sera and the control of drug trafficking. Its expert committees produced authoritative reports on many important public health subjects including malaria, cancer, nutrition, venereal disease, housing, rheumatism, heart disease and medical education, to name only a few. The Geneva and Paris offices were both casualties of the Second World War, and they were replaced first by UNRRA (United Nations Relief and Rehabilitation Organization) and then by the WORLD HEALTH ORGANIZATION (WHO) which was conceived as part of the Charter of the United Nations (San Francisco, 1945) and implemented by the adoption of its formal Constitution in an Assembly of fifty-two nations at Geneva in 1948.

Thus WHO became the sole international health organization except for the Pan-American Sanitary Bureau which later merged with it as its Regional Office for the Americas. Other Regional Offices have since been established for S-E Asia, the Eastern Mediterranean, the Western Pacific, Africa, and Europe.

The Charter of WHO has for its aim 'the attainment by all peoples of the highest possible level of health' and its activities, as required by its Constitution, go far beyond the work of previous organizations. These now include central technical responsibilities and services for epidemiology, statistics, research and standardization, and arrangements for the collection and dissemination of epidemiological information. In addition WHO provides assistance to Governments in the form of practical aid and consultant advice in relation to every kind of health problem, and it carries immeasurable promise for the future.

Its short-term campaigns have been of propaganda value aimed at getting rid of as much obvious disease as possible in the shortest possible time, but by them it seeks to demonstrate to undeveloped nations that Western methods have something to offer and so to pave the way for modern preventive medicine to supplant the folk-lore of the past. Health cannot be imposed on people; it requires their enlightened co-operation.

The technical achievements of WHO have been immense. The tasks still facing it are no less so, but perhaps its greatest impact on the world scene will yet prove to have been something more intangible. Concern for other nations and unselfish international service and co-operation foster friendship and understanding and may well do more for world peace than all the politicians.

intestine. The section of the DIGESTIVE SYSTEM which extends from the lower opening of the stomach to the anus. It comprises two distinct parts known as the small and large intestine.

Obstruction. Any condition which impedes the normal passage of intestinal contents through the small and large intestine. See BOWEL, obstruction.

Tumours. Non-malignant tumours of the intestine are rare but overgrowths of fatty or muscular tissue occur occasionally, and slightly more common are polypi or pedunculated tumours arising from the mucous membrane and its related glands. Single polypi may reach a considerable size and become a cause of intussusception but they are more often small, multiple and widespread and may arise as a sequel to chronic inflammatory disease such as intestinal tuberculosis or long-standing dysentery.

Malignant tumours practically never effect the small intestine but carcinoma of the colon is by far the commonest growth in the large intestine. It generally arises at the flexures and at narrow parts such as the upper part of the rectum and the ileo-caecal valve.

The symptoms produced are those of chronic intestinal obstruction and call for full investigation.

intoxication. In everyday usage, intoxication is taken to mean incapacity due to over-consumption of alcohol, but scientifically it is employed to describe functional impairment brought about by any poisonous substance or toxin.

Such toxins may arise from external or exogeneous causes, particularly bacterial products or drugs, or they may be endogeneous, arising within the body from metabolic faults such as uraemia or acidosis.

intra-uterine device. An appliance inserted into the cavity of the uterus to prevent conception. It was until recently thought that an IUD acted mainly by creating an obstruction, but to block the entrance to the uterus entirely is very difficult. More probably the main effect of an IUD is to irritate the muscles of the uterus so that it tends to expel any fertilized egg before it can attach itself to the uterine lining and to stimulate the uterus into producing a substance that kills the fertilized egg.

Hippocrates in his book *On The Diseases of Women* describes the converse, a tube filled with mutton fat and designed to keep the mouth of the uterus open; and until the nineteenth century there was considerable confusion as to whether devices were intended to facilitate or to prevent conception. Probably some devices, really intended to prevent unwanted pregnancy, were deliberately described as promoting conception. In America in 1846 Beers patented his stem pessary as the allegedly first device to prevent pregnancy, and the earliest really effective IUD was probably that of Richter in Germany in 1909, followed in that country by the Graefenberg Ring in 1920.

For some curious reason intra-uterine devices were little used between 1920 and 1950, but from mid-century onwards such appliances as the Zipper Ring, the Lippes Loop, the Margulies Spiral and the Birnberg Bow became popular. These are fairly small appliances which are placed in the uterus, usually by a doctor. In a small percentage of cases they are spontaneously expelled (and the woman may not know that she has lost her protective) or cause bleeding and have to be removed; but in about 96 to 97 per cent of cases they remain in position and prevent pregnancy.

In general an efficient IUD gives greater protection than vaginal methods – such as the Dutch cap and spermicidal jelly or cream – but has the limitation that it needs insertion by a doctor. To a great extent all these have been replaced by oral contraceptives, but the IUD is still useful for women (e.g., from multiproblem families) who cannot remember to take an oral contraceptive regularly.

intravenous feeding. An emergency method of giving a patient liquid nourishment – usually a saline solution with glucose added – by direct slow injection into a vein. A needle inserted into a vein is connected to an apparatus which

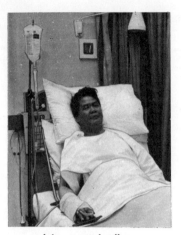

Intravenous feeding

drips in the liquid at the required rate, care being taken to ensure the absence of air which if present might block a blood vessel. The method is used if the patient is unconscious for a prolonged period, is too ill to eat or is unable to eat because of disease of the mouth, throat or stomach.

introvert. An inward-looking person concerned mainly with his own thoughts, valuing his own society, liking solitude and often enjoying reading or music. In the words of Jung, the inventor of the term, 'Introverts are taciturn, impenetrable, often shy natures who form a vivid contrast to the open, sociable or at least friendly and accessible characters (the extroverts) who are on good terms with all the world'. Morbid introversion occurs in schizophrenia and paranoia, with the personality withdrawn into itself and expended on fantasy formation.

Most people, however, are neither pure introverts nor complete extroverts but a mixture with perhaps one or the other normally predominating, as is more fully discussed in the article on EXTROVERTS.

intubation. The insertion of a tube. The term is used mainly in relation to intubation of the larynx in order to maintain a clear airway. The larynx may become obstructed in laryngeal diphtheria and other infections affecting the air-passages; in cellulitis of the neck and laryngeal carcinoma; by inflammation resulting from the inhalation of injurious vapours; and occasionally as an allergic phenomenon.

Intubation is also a necessary preliminary to specialized methods of anaesthesia.

intussusception. A condition in which a segment of bowel becomes telescoped into the part immediately below. It usually occurs in the small intestine or at the junction of the small intestine with the colon and it is the commonest cause of acute intestinal obstruction in children.

Cases usually occur between the age of 6 months and 2 years, most often in well-nourished and vigorous boys, and are probably due to disturbance of the normal digestive movements of the intestine by some irritation of the mucous membrane lining the intestine wall.

The symptoms are those of violent and persistent abdominal colic, often with the passage of blood-stained mucus, followed by signs of toxaemia and collapse. Vomiting is not usually marked until the later stages of complete obstruction.

Intussusception requires emergency surgical treatment.

iodine. A non-metallic element occurring as a greyish-black crystalline solid which on heating changes to dense violet vapour. In very small amounts, iodine is essential to the body because it is used by the thyroid gland in the manufacture of its hormone. Lack of iodine in childhood can produce physical and mental retardation (although cretinism is more commonly due to a defect of the thyroid gland itself) and deficiency in adolescent or adult life produces simple goitre, with the thyroid enlarging through excessive activity in an attempt to produce enough hormone without sufficient iodine for its manufacture.

Iodine compounds are plentiful in the sea, but in some inland areas the soil contains practically no iodine and consequently food grown in these areas is very deficient in iodine. Switzerland, the Tyrol, the Himalayas and Derbyshire are notorious for lack of iodine. Where such deficiency exists it can be easily remedied by addition of a very small quantity of iodine to table salt, and iodized salt is now in common use wherever iodine is scarce.

Iodine is only very slightly soluble in water but dissolves readily in alcohol. A solution of iodine in alcohol – tincture of iodine – is an excellent antiseptic for sterilizing intact skin but is too strong for use in wounds.

Radioactive iodine compounds are employed to treat an enlarged and overactive thyroid gland and sometimes to treat cancer of that gland.

iritis. The iris is a thin circular disc of tissue between the cornea and the lens of the eye, with a central circular aperture, the pupil.

Iritis is inflammation of the iris and may be acute or chronic. The eye appears reddened and the pupil is small and loses its natural lustre and colour. There is pain and sensitivity to light, and tears are formed. Most cases are due to bacterial or other toxaemia from local or general disease. Syphilis, gonorrhoea, tuberculosis and rheumatism are the commonest causes, less often diabetes or gout.

The basic essentials of treatment are first to ensure dilation of the pupil with atropine in order to draw it away from the lens, which lies immediately behind it, and thus prevent any adhesions developing, and second to lessen inflammatory reaction by cortico-steroids. Appropriate measures are also required to treat whatever general condition caused the iritis.

iron. A familiar metallic element with magnetic properties occurring in nature as various oxides of iron (haematite, magnetite, limonite), as sulphide of iron (pyrites, marcassite) or as iron carbonate (siderite). From these, metallic iron (pig-iron) is extracted by reduction with carbon monoxide in a blast furnace. Further treatment to eliminate impurities and to reduce and adjust its carbon content produces steel which can be alloyed with other metals to modify its properties.

Iron is of importance in medicine because it is an essential constituent of haemoglobin, the oxygen carrying pigment of the blood. It is thus an indispensable MINERAL SALT in the diet, the daily requirement being 15 to 20 mg. The best sources are meat, liver, eggs, spinach, beans, peas, and whole wheat, but milk is poor. Additional supplies of iron are required in pregnancy and while breast-feeding, and mothers should take iron tablets, usually containing ferrous sulphate. Infants may also suffer from nutritional anaemia but proprietary infant foods contain added iron.

Lack of iron in the diet results in anaemia, and for its treatment both tablet and injectable forms of iron are available. Iron preparations may cause gastro-intestinal irritation or more serious symptoms if taken in overdose.

Iron tablets should be kept secure from accidental swallowing by small children. Many cases of serious poisoning have occurred.

irradiation. The treatment of disease (e.g., cancer) by exposure of the diseased cells to x-rays, ultra-violet light or radioactive material; also the sterilization of food, medical instruments, etc. by similar methods. While irradiation is a useful weapon for certain serious conditions, it must also be remembered that it is a potentially dangerous weapon. For instance, while irradiation is useful in the treatment of certain cases of leukaemia, excessive irradiation can actually cause leukaemia – as shown in its increased incidence in survivors of the atomic bomb explosions in Japan and also in persons with anchylozing spondylitis treated by radiotherapy of the spine.

irritability. The capacity of living tissues to respond to change or stimulus. This capacity is generally described as the characteristic property of living matter. Thus a stone (non-living) responds to no stimulus: if kicked, it merely rolls until the impetus imparted to it by the foot is counteracted by the friction of the ground. By contrast a muscle responds to any stimulation of the nerve supplying it, and even a plant turns slightly towards the sun.

While ability to respond to stimulus is certainly the main feature that differentiates living from non-living matter, the criterion is less certain than was assumed in the past. The tobacco mosaic virus, for example, can remain for long periods inert and responsive to no stimulus, but can later multiply and produce its effects on the tobacco plant.

isolation. A control procedure adopted in relation to cases or carriers of highly infectious diseases who are segregated in an attempt to prevent them transmitting infection to other susceptible individuals. A limitation imposed on the movements of contacts who may be under suspicion of having contracted infection is known as QUARANTINE.

In the past most fever or isolation hospitals were constructed on the pavilion principle with large multi-bedded wards in which a number of patients with the same disease were segregated as a group. This type of construction is now obsolete and modern design is based on wards containing a number of single-bed units with complete structural separation by full-height partitions. These are usually called cubicle wards but the name is not a good one since 'cubicle' has a connotation of partitioning to less than full height.

Each chamber is separately ventilated and has its own toilet and washing facilities. They are constructed as a single row and served by an external or permanently ventilated internal corridor. In some designs mechanical ventilation or air-conditioning is also provided to minimize risks of cross infection.

Separate rooms of this kind are obviously important but do not obviate the need for separate nursing – an aseptic technique for fever nursing in which the patient and everything concerned with him is treated as infectious and the nurse wears a protective gown and mask left behind in each cubicle and carries out a 'surgical scrub' of her hands before proceeding to other patients. A similar routine carried out when cubicle isolation is not available is usually referred to as 'barrier nursing'.

Home isolation when patients are not admitted to hospital, should follow the same principles. The patient should be accommodated in a separate well-ventilated room preferably at the top of the house.

Aerial connection between sick room and the rest of the house can be restricted by a sheet over the door moistened with disinfectant and this has at least an admonitory value in reminding persons of the risks and the need for care. Separate utensils should be set aside and boiled or disinfected, and nothing should pass out of the room without disinfection. Attendants should carry out the rules of barrier nursing and visitors should be restricted or forbidden. Any who are allowed entry must adopt similar precautions of protective clothing and thorough hand-washing and disinfection.

isoniazid. A synthetic compound manufactured from isoniatinic acid and used since 1952 for the treatment of tuberculosis of the lung. It is usually given by mouth in doses of 100 mg. twice daily. The drug acts specifically against the germ which causes tuberculosis but has little if any action against other bacteria.

isotope. Two atoms are said to be isotopes if they are of the same chemical element but have different masses, i.e., a different number of electrons moving round the same proton. An isotope may occur naturally or may be created by nuclear bombardment. Thus uranium has three naturally occurring isotopes and at least ten artificially manufactured isotopes.

Radio-active isotopes can be used in medicine for three purposes: for research, e.g., to trace the movement of chemical substances in the body; for diagnosis, e.g., to facilitate x-ray investigation of a suspected lesion; and occasionally for treatment, e.g., the use of radioactive iodine to treat cancer of the thyroid gland.

itching. The skin is particularly well-supplied with sensory nerve-endings susceptible to various irritants; chronic irritation insufficient to cause actual pain is experienced as itching or pruritus.

In many cases the cause is obvious: insect bites, infestation by parasites such as the scabies mite, fungoid skin infections, eczema or other chronic skin conditions, local discharges or disorders of the blood's circulation (such as occur in chilblains or varicose veins) are commonly responsible.

In other cases there is general itching for no apparent local reason. This type of itching may occur in certain general diseases where there are circulating toxins, as in jaundice, diabetes, gout and nephritis; in certain blood diseases such as leukaemia and lymphadenoma; in old age where there is senile atrophy of the skin; from the use of certain drugs especially opium and heroin: or as a sympton in psycho-neurosis.

Treatment requires to be directed towards the precise cause. Alkaline baths and lotions may relieve general pruritus; calamine lotion, anti-histamine creams, or oily preparations containing 1 or 2 per cent phenol or camphor are useful as local applications.

Local pruritus most often affects the anus, scrotum or vulva, but may occur anywhere. Often itching starts from a transitory cause, leads to scratching and is then aggravated by the scratching. Threadworms are a common cause of anal itching, vaginal discharge may start itching of the vulva, and sweating, irritation of clothes and nervous factors are other causes. Removal of the cause is essential, extreme cleanliness of the part is useful, and the application of an alkaline lotion followed, when dry, by a fine zinc oxide dusting powder may do much to relieve the symptoms.

J

jaundice. Jaundice or icterus is not a specific disease but is a yellowish appearance of a patient occurring in various conditions and due to the deposition of the bile-pigment (bilirubin) in the skin and mucous membranes. Early indications of jaundice may be detected by inspecting the 'white' of the eyes.

Bile is a clear yellow or orange fluid secreted by the liver cells and contains mainly bile-salts and the bile pigments bilirubin and biliverdin. It passes to the intestine via the gall bladder and the bile-duct. Bile-salts are required for the digestion of fats but the bile pigments are waste products from the haemoglobin in the blood.

Jaundice thus results from excess production of the bile pigment or a failure to eliminate it so that it accumulates in the blood-stream and stains the tissue. This occurs in three groups of conditions: (1) haemolytic anaemias where there is excessive destruction of red cells, (2) disease of the liver where the liver cells are unable to transfer bilirubin to the gall bladder, and (3) obstruction of the bile-duct, preventing bile passing from the liver to the intestine.

Jaundice therefore requires detailed investigation to determine its exact cause which may be a blood disease, liver conditions such as hepatitis, cirrhosis or toxic necrosis, or bile-duct obstruction due to chronic inflammatory conditions, gall stones or neoplasm.

A transient form of jaundice occurs in a large proportion of new-born infants – icterus neonatorum. This is due to the breakdown of foetal haemoglobin which is in excess of requirements once the child begins to breathe, and to the still immature liver function. It also occurs in haemolytic disease of the newborn which is caused by the blood abnormality known as RHESUS FACTOR. Investigation of Rh factors is now a routine procedure in all antenatal clinics; it has been found that exposure of the child to ultra-violet light helps the jaundice to clear and this form of treatment is now commonly employed in maternity hospitals.

jaw. The skeletal framework of the mouth in which the teeth are set, consisting of an upper-jaw, or maxilla, which is continuous with the skull, and a movable lower jaw, or mandible.

The opposed margins are covered by the gums or gingiva and are expanded as the alveolar ridges or alveoli to provide the tooth sockets.

The mandible hinges with the skull at the temporo-mandibular joint, easily felt immediately in front of the ear, and often subject to derangement. It has cartilage rather like that in the knee-joint, and looseness of this may cause 'clicking-jaw', movements being accompanied by an audible snap. Also relatively common are unilateral or bilateral dislocations of the jaw which can usually be slipped back easily into place, even by patients themselves.

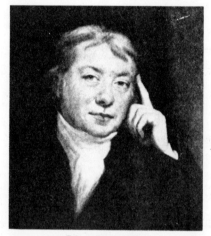

Edward Jenner

Jenner. Edward Jenner (1749-1823), medical practitioner in Gloucestershire, was the inventor of smallpox VACCINATION. Jenner, like many other doctors, originally practised the arm-to-arm method of inoculation of healthy individuals from mild cases of smallpox that had been introduced from the east by Lady Mary Wortley Montague in 1718. During his experience with this procedure he noted that persons who had suffered from the mild disease, cowpox, did not take when inoculated and also noted that it was well-known that these persons did not develop smallpox.

From these points he developed the idea that smallpox might be prevented by inoculation of persons with cowpox, which, if it proved successful, would be very much safer than inoculation from a case of smallpox. Having tested his idea by inoculating a volunteer and thereafter proving him immune to smallpox even when inoculated with material from a highly infectious patient, Jenner offered his observations to the Royal Society (which refused the paper) and himself published them in 1798. By 1901 over 100,000 persons had been vaccinated in England alone and the eradication of the commonest of the serious infections was well on its way.

jogging. Trotting or running at a slow pace. With physical work being largely superceded by sedentary work many people have become aware that they are having too little exercise and so jogging has become increasingly popular. Its big advantage is that it occupies minimal time, but its main disadvantages are first that it provides no mental, aesthetic or emotional satisfaction – unlike, say, a quick game of tennis – but is solely a means of ensuring some exercise; and second that for accelerating the heart beat and deepening the breathing it is much less efficient than shorter but more violent exercise.

Jogging has become very popular in the U.K. and to some extent the U.S.A. in the later 1970s, but as increased mechanization shortens the average working week and so provides more leisure time it seems likely that its popularity will decrease.

See KEEPING FIT.

joints. The bones of the skeleton are connected to each other in accordance with functional requirements by joints or articulations. These may be (1) immovable (synarthroses) as in the joints between the individual bones of the skull, (2) slightly movable (amphiarthroses) as between the vertebrae or the individual bones of the pelvis, or (3) freely movable (diarthroses) comprising mostly the familiar joints of the limbs and extremities. In the slightly movable joints the opposed bony surfaces are united by intervening tough and elastic fibro-cartilage but in the freely movable joints the bony surfaces are completely separated from one another and are covered by smooth and dense hyaline cartilage. Such a joint is enclosed in an articular capsule lined with synovial membrane, lubricated by synovial fluid and strengthened externally by strong fibrous bands called ligaments.

The stability of a freely movable joint is maintained (1) by the shape of the joint surfaces, (2) sometimes by internal ligaments and shaped pieces (menisci) of fibro-cartilage, (3) by the external ligaments, and (4) by the surrounding muscles and tendons. Freely movable joints may be of the ball-and-socket type, permitting movement in all directions (e.g., the hip or shoulder), or of the hinge type (e.g., the knee), or they may permit only pivot or gliding movements (e.g., the atlas vertebra).

Joint diseases. Any inflammatory condition affecting a joint or joints is loosely termed arthritis. Acute arthritis may develop as a result of bacterial infection from penetrating wounds or as a complication of other diseases

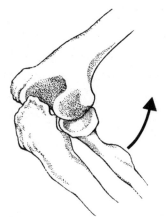

Hinged joint

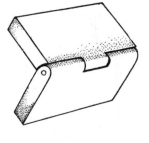

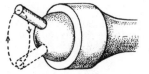

The mechanics of joints

such as rheumatic fever, gonorrhoea, pneumonia, typhoid fever, gout and dysentery. It may also be due to tuberculosis or syphilis. Haemorrhage into joints occurs in haemophilia, scurvy, other severe blood diseases and sometimes as a complication of the administration of serum. Certain diseases of the spinal cord produce degeneration of joints supplied by the affected nerves. Most of the foregoing are relatively rare but the familiar types of chronic arthritis are very common and cause widespread disability. Of these, rheumatoid arthritis occurs mainly in children or young adults, more often females, and it tends to affect the smaller peripheral joints many of which may be involved simultaneously or progressively. In juveniles the condition is called Still's disease.

Osteo-arthritis affects mainly the larger joints in older persons. Degenerative changes and over-stress damage the joint surfaces and produce pain and disability. Osteo-arthritis of

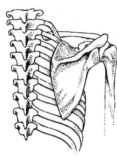
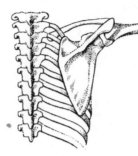
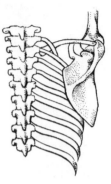

Ball and socket joint

the spine is known as spondylitis. A peculiar condition known as 'hysterical joint' is occasionally seen in neurotic subjects. A single joint, usually in a limb, appears to be fixed, very painful, and resistant to passive movement but no pathological process can be demonstrated. The disability disappears under anaesthesia and cases of this type often form the basis of so-called 'miracle cures'.

Joint injuries. Apart from penetrating wounds or contusions from direct violence these are either sprains due to tearing of the supporting ligaments or dislocations where there is displacement or separation of the bony surfaces. Both conditions are produced by forces compelling the joint to exceed its normal range of movement.

jugular vein. The right and left internal and external jugular veins are the four veins that convey blood from the head and neck to the chest.

Jung. Carl Gustav Jung (1875-1961) of Zurich became famous as the disciple and co-worker of FREUD but broke with him in 1913, not because of any difference on fundamentals but because they disagreed on certain additional concepts of Jung's. In particular, Freud had seen the libido (i.e., the individual's innate drive for pleasure and satisfaction) as primarily based on sex, whereas Jung regarded it as also including other basic drives, e.g., that connected with hunger. The majority of Jung's views, however, such as the idea that neurotic symptoms represent a retreat from life's difficulties or a retreat to the dependence of childhood, are essentially those of Freud and the psychoanalysts.

Jung's most controversial contribution to psychology is his theory of the collective racial unconscious: the idea that inherited racial experience creates part of our unconscious life, so that events outside our individual experience help to mould our actions, fantasies, dreams, symbols and mythologies. By no means all psychologists accept this idea.

He was also in large measure the co-developer (with Freud) of PSYCHOANALYSIS, with its use of the association method.

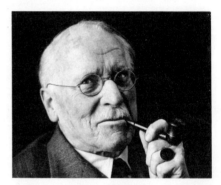

Carl Gustav Jung

His differentiation of people into extroverts and introverts has passed into everyday usage: the extrovert is out-going, concerned with external relationships and reaches the extreme in mania; the introvert is shut-in, preoccupied with inner impressions and inner subjective processes and reaches the extreme in schizophrenia. Yet in passage into everyday terms Jung's concept has been over-simplified. As Jung appreciated, external circumstances and different companions can modify our reactions, and the greater majority of normal people are neither complete extroverts nor complete introverts but simply a little nearer to one or other end of a continuous scale.

K

kala-azar. A tropical infection characterized by a very long incubation period (sometimes several months), irregular but repeated bouts of fever, progressive enlargement of the spleen and the liver, and sometimes diarrhoea and symptoms of bronchitis. The disease is caused by a tiny parasite, transmitted by the bite of the female sand-fly after it has become infected by sucking blood from an infected person or animal. Diagnosis depends on identification of the parasite in a blood specimen or in material drawn from the bone-marrow or the spleen. Antimony drugs, injected into a vein or a muscle, have become the standard treatment.

keeping fit. Since virtually all of us suffer from inherited weaknesses, faults in our upbringing or defects in our domestic or working environment, optimum physical, emotional and social health – the World Health Organization's proud claim as the legitimate birth right of every person – is probably beyond our fair expectations, although in the next century a majority of people may achieve it. Reasonably good health, however, should be within the grasp of most of us, and many diseases and disabilities are essentially self-induced.

Scores of articles in this book relate in whole or in part to the promotion of good health and the prevention or reduction of disease. All that can be done here in a single article is to bring together a few of the main points.

A fundamental difficulty about devising a regime designed to maintain or improve physical, emotional and social health is that we possess as yet very inadequate measures of health, as opposed to measures of disease. We have, for instance, no real justification for saying that an international footballer aged thirty is physically healthier than a non-athlete of the same age with no signs of present or impending disease, or that a man of seventy who still publishes articles on his particular subject is mentally healthier than a man of the same age who devotes his time to watching television and reading light novels.

However, most experts would probably agree that ten of the desirable conditions for fitness are (1) sufficient sleep; (2) adequate, well-balanced and not excessive diet; (3) reasonable but not excessive exercise; (4) either work activities or leisure activities that stimulate the brain without inducing strain; (5) interesting hobbies or recreations; (6) aims or beliefs that give some purpose to life; (7) short-term goals to provide interim satisfactions; (8) some congenial and trusted associates; (9) a satisfactory environment both at home and at work; and (10) facilities for the prompt treatment of disease or disability, and preferably for the recognition and rectification of these before they produce symptoms.

There are also desirable negative conditions of general applicability, e.g., avoidance of drugs, cigarettes and excessive quantities of alcohol; and many negative conditions that apply to persons who do not enjoy perfect health, e.g., restriction of carbohydrate intake by a diabetic and avoidance by a person with raised blood pressure of situations liable to increase the blood pressure further. The reasons for the negative conditions are fairly obvious but it may be useful to discuss the positive ones enumerated above.

Sleep. The need for adequate sleep is probably the most non-controversial of the ten selected points. The amount required varies with age, e.g., a month old baby needs about twenty hours a day, a child of 7 years needs about thirteen hours and an adolescent of 15 needs about nine hours. While these are approximate averages there are also considerable individual variations, especially in adults: many require about eight hours a night but some remain healthy on much smaller amounts.

Insufficient sleep results in fatigue, irritability, inability to concentrate and impaired general health.

Where a person finds difficulty in getting to sleep (otherwise than through pain, worry or external noise) either a gentle walk or a warm (but not over hot) bath before bedtime often helps.

The worst thing a sleepless person can do is to fret about his failure to fall asleep. By such fretting he will almost certainly ensure that he remains awake. Assuming that circumstances are compatible with slumber (e.g., reasonably warm bed, adequate fresh air without draughts, and quietness) he is better to rest quietly and to read an interesting but not too exciting book. Except under abnormal conditions (e.g., for some days after the death of a much loved relative) few people require sedatives and the immediate recourse of many non-sleepers to sedatives is a thing to be deprecated. On the other hand many middle-aged and elderly persons have used sedatives for many years without apparent harmful effect, and perhaps the opponents of sedatives have over-stated their case.

Diet. Of all the requirements for health, diet is the one that has been most extensively studied, and also the one on which the enquirer is confronted with the largest number of allegedly health-creating alternatives, e.g., lacto-vegetarian diet (including milk and eggs but no form of flesh), fully vegetarian diet, or even diet consisting of foods untouched by fire. Diet is also the thing on which there exists the largest number of religious taboos and dislikes: for instance, Jews are forbidden to eat pork, Moslems are sinning if they drink the fermented juice of the grape, Australians like a breakfast that includes steak which British people deem too strong for their first meal, and

Britons will sit down to a breakfast of bacon, eggs and kidney, but their American cousins will reject the last item as offal.

The average requirement of first and second class protein, fat, carbohydrate, mineral salts and vitamins is reasonably worked out. (See articles on these various subjects.) There are, however, many variations. To mention three: (1) size: during the British rationing of the Second World War many a man of well over average stature was appreciably undernourished through having to exist on the same rations as a person of five-sixths of his height and three-quarters of his weight; (2) stage in life: for instance a growing adolescent and an expectant mother both require slightly more food than an adult of the same size; and (3) individual variation: one person has a digestive system so efficient that he utilizes virtually every particle of food, is healthy on a minimum diet and gains weight if consuming appreciably more than the minimum, while another of identical size but with a digestive system of lower efficiency loses weight and decreases his resistance to disease when consuming a minimum diet and appears to be healthy when consuming perhaps 10 per cent more than that minimum.

For quantity a good index is provided by weight. If a person is gaining weight – a common happening in affluent Western nations except perhaps in families in which a breadwinner is unemployed – he is over-eating, unless he is thin and deliberately trying to increase his weight. If a person is losing weight, he is under-eating unless he is deliberately trying to reduce obesity.

As for quality, three points may be noted. A person who is substantially overweight is likely to be eating too much carbohydrate (e.g., sweets, cakes, bread, rice and potatoes) and possibly too much animal fat (e.g., butter). While dietary deficiencies often comprise several components of the diet together, the deficiency most commonly associated with poverty is that in first class protein: persons living near the bare subsistence level should therefore look for reasonably cheap forms of protein, e.g., in many parts of the world cheese and fish are appreciably cheaper than meat. Thirdly, in several northern countries, probably because of poor growth of many fruits and green vegetables and because of survival of traditions from an age in which transport of food was relatively much more costly than it is now, shortages of the water-soluble vitamins – c and the B group – are not uncommon.

Exercise. Exercise more violent than a particular person can stand is manifestly harmful: most of us have heard of an elderly man who had a coronary thrombosis after sprinting for a bus. Excessive exercise that creates exhaustion (as opposed to a pleasant feeling of tiredness) is also harmful: in the Second World War when the Japanese used prisoners of war for road construction the high death rate was more the result of exhaustion than of insufficient food. In reasonable amount, however, exercise keeps the muscles in trim, improves digestion by better burning up of foods, increases the rate and force of the heart beat and deepens breathing. Because highly developed nations have moved within three generations from a state of affairs in which the average person walked to his place of employment and then did manual work to a state in which he travels by bus or car and then does sedentary work, many people have far less exercise than their grandparents had.

Once we have passed beyond these simple, factual statements we are very much in the realms of controversy. At one end of the spectrum are the enthusiasts who point out that every muscle atrophies gradually if unused and stress the enormous importance of exercise or exercises, and who would in some cases even seek to restrict the term 'keeping fit' to relevant physical activity. At the other end are the sceptics who point out that the indolent tortoise and the lumbering elephant are very long-lived, that some human centenarians have had very sedentary lives and that quite a number of athletes die young. As is so often the case, the truth probably lies somewhere between the two extremes.

If, without going to the extreme of making muscular fitness the be all and end all of life, we accept the desirability of reasonable daily exercise, we are still in the realm of controversy. A few health workers maintain that for the adequate exercising of various muscles we need the carefully selected and graded exercises of a keep-fit class. Many others hold that the main benefit of a keep-fit class is social, bringing together people who have a certain similarity of interest, and that exercise can be obtained in other and perhaps to some people pleasanter ways. One school of thought favours gentle but sustained exercise, e.g., a daily four mile walk or a round of golf. Another group of workers advocate more vigorous forms of exercise, e.g., jogging. Yet another view that appears to be gaining strength is that activity should be strenuous enough to raise the pulse rate to over a hundred and that ten minutes of really vigorous activity are more beneficial than an hour of gentle exercise.

Perhaps the most important thing to be said about exercise is that adjustment should be gradual. It is a mistake for a youngster suddenly to discontinue physical activity when he leaves school and for the sedentary middle-aged man suddenly to take part in a strenuous set of tennis.

Mental stimulation. Very much the same can be said of mental as of physical exercise. Excess, either in quantity or in quality, can leave us exhausted and irritable, but a reasonable amount is essential for the well-being of the mind. Probably many of us have known an intelligent man, previously preoccupied with an interesting and mentally exacting job and rather devoid of intellectual hobbies or recreations, who rapidly deteriorated mentally after retirement, simply because of lack of stimulation.

Yet, as with physical exercise, there is wide room for controversy. Some workers maintain that we are healthiest if we use our brains to the point of pleasant tiredness. Others hold that preservation of habit is what matters: that the brain-worker will deteriorate if he ceases to use his mental faculties but that the person who slides through life with a minimum of intellectual exercise is not necessarily the worse for it. Still others think that a person becomes little more than an animated vegetable if he loses his intellectual curiosity, his aesthetic appreciation and his capacity to reason: they would say with Shakespeare's Hamlet,

> 'He that made us with such large
>   discourse,
> Looking before and after, gave us not
> That capability and godlike reason
> To fust in us unused.'

For mental fitness, as for physical fitness, the truth probably lies somewhere between the extremes, and gradual adjustment is important. The youngster who suddenly discards all non-intellectual interests and concentrates solely on his university studies or on gaining promotions in his career is courting future illness; and the elderly professional worker who at retirement gives away his books and yet acquires no alternative intellectual interest is equally making a serious mistake.

Hobbies and recreations. In the words of an old proverb, 'All work and no play makes Jack a dull boy.' It seems obvious that a brain-worker should have some pastimes or recreations involving physical exercise and that a person who works with his hands should have some recreations involving the use of mental and aesthetic capacities. Yet many of us have known people who appeared fit enough although their hobbies resembled their work – the bus conductor or gardener who as a young man occupied his leisure in playing cricket and later in life became keen on bowling, or the university lecturer who spent his spare time in writing books or playing bridge. Perhaps, too, as increased mechanization makes early retirement the rule rather than the exception, it is important that some hobbies or recreations – intellectual or physical – should be of such a nature that they can ultimately form a partial substitute for work.

Long-term aims or beliefs. It is a little difficult to see how a person leading an entirely purposeless life can be healthy. The individual who is sustained by a sincere belief in a future existence (giving him a pre-designed code of behaviour and immediate answers to many moral problems), or the humanist sustained by a passionate desire to benefit humanity, or even the person with a strong ambition for himself or for his family, is in a position of advantage: his life has some purpose. Yet we are again entering into the realm of controversy. Do people who are genuinely religious or sincere humanists or ruthlessly ambitious have any real evidence that they are healthier or happier than those who adopt the Horacian maxim of living for the day, taking the pleasures of each day as they come? As so often on problems of keeping fit, we can say vaguely that a purpose in life is probably desirable.

Short-term goals. The saint and the conqueror can perhaps sustain themselves simply by long-term aims: Alexander the Great can subdue the entire known universe and then weep that there are no more worlds to conquer. Most of us, however, are neither Joans of Arc nor Napoleons. We need the temporary and short-term satisfactions and gratifications created through the achievement of immediate aims. Examples are the ambitious person who decides to secure a promotion post within the next year (and derives great satisfaction from doing so) or the financially minded person who decides to pay off half the hire-purchase of his

television set in six months (and again is delighted at his success).

These short-term goals carry with them, of course, the danger of short-term failure: the ambitious person may not secure his promotion or the money-minded person may not manage to make his payment. Also, some people appear to go through life successfully without setting themselves any short-term objectives.

Yet the present writer feels that the few psychologists (as opposed to the mass of gymnasts and exponents of physical culture) who have studied the complex problems of keeping fit have tended to neglect or under-value the importance of short-term goals.

Congenial and trusted associates. Man is a social animal. He needs trusted friends and people with whom he can discuss his problems and his interests on level terms and knowing that his statements will not be relayed to other people. The person who moves his home, loses touch with relatives and old friends and fails to make new friends is seldom mentally healthy. Yet a minority of people seem to be able to endure a hermit-like existence without harm.

Satisfactory environment. Acceptance of the environment, domestic and working, is largely a matter of conditioning. Chaucer saw nothing unacceptable in waking up in winter in a bedroom with the temperature probably often below freezing point, and expressed no disquiet at two-fifths of the country's wealth being owned by the Church and another two-fifths by a handful of nobles. Shakespeare never heard of central heating, did not know – unless in old age – the solace or the temptations of tobacco, and saw nothing peculiar in admission to university being restricted to professed believers in a particular religion. Wordsworth was unaware of double glazing, made no adverse comment on the massacre of Peterloo and accepted as normal the employment of children of 7 years for twelve hours a day in mines or mills. Yet an average household, placed today in the slum conditions that Chaucer would have deemed good and Shakespeare acceptable, would in most cases rapidly degenerate into the multiproblem class; and an ordinary family in the social circumstances accepted by Wordsworth would probably become revolutionaries within a year.

Again there is controversy. To follow literary examples, did Dylan Thomas become an alcoholic because of his environment, and did Masefield become a teetotaller and non-smoker because of a broadly similar environment?

Perhaps, however, we can say that mental, physical and social health is difficult to maintain if a person is forced into an environment worse than that to which he or she has been accustomed.

Facilities for treatment and prevention of disease. Untreated illness is manifestly incompatible with fitness. To follow the literary examples given earlier, think of Keats dying of tuberculosis (now both curable and largely preventable) at 26 or the Brontë sisters dying in their thirties. In the U.K. and various other countries an enormous advance towards the fitness of individuals has been made by the provision of facilities for treatment without any immediate payment.

An even greater advance towards physical and mental fitness has been the provision in many countries of services to promote good health and to detect and rectify deviations from health before they produce symptoms.

The reduction of infectious diseases by immunization and health education about its desirability and by counselling on hygiene, the virtual eradication in developed countries of various nutritional diseases, and the decrease in diseases associated with dirt and destitution are examples. But, since this article started with a suggestion that the World Health Organization's aim of optimum health would not be attainable in this century, it may be appropriate to end by quoting from a 1977 report of the World Health Organization: having described mental hospitals for blacks in South Africa (with a doctor visiting each hospital once weekly) as 'a version of the Dickensian workhouse' and having pointed out that in South-East Asia there is less than one psychiatrist for every million people, the report concludes that most mental illness could be prevented by 'public education, legislation, and the provision of adequate maternal and child health services.'

keloid. An overgrowth of scar tissue, occurring at the site of the scar and extending beyond its original limits, as a raised, hard, fibrous mass. Keloids may occur following burns, cuts, abrasions and surgical operations. They are not harmful or malignant, and are in general painless, but they are often unsightly. Surgical removal of a keloid is usually unsuccessful because the same conditions that permitted the initial overgrowth of scar tissue may well cause another overgrowth. Where the keloid is unsightly, shrinkage by radium or x-rays may be required.

Kenny treatment. A method of treatment for paralytic poliomyelitis pioneered and advocated by Sister Elizabeth Kenny (1886-1952) of Brisbane, Australia, and later of the U.S.A.

In the acute stage of the disease the usual treatment of paralysed muscles is designed to secure rest and immobilization of the affected parts in a position of relaxation by means of props and supports such as sandbags, splints, pads, and slings.

Sister Kenny adopted more active procedures. Circulation was stimulated by hot packs, or by hydrotherapy in slipper or special baths, and muscle re-education was introduced as early as possible, even before cessation of pain. This was done by the nursing staff regularly moving the affected limbs, and she also laid stress on maintenance of 'impulse', the patient being encouraged to co-operate by making a conscious mental effort towards movement even when the muscles were so paralysed that no contractions could be perceived.

Some 20 per cent of initially paralysed poliomyelitis victims normally recover completely without residual paralysis. There is as yet no undeniable evidence that Kenny methods produce substantially better results, and they require much greater resources of skilled nursing and physiotherapy.

keratitis. Inflammation of the cornea of the eye. It may be the result of injury or infection or of deficiency of vitamin A. The commonest variety in the past – interstitial keratitis caused by syphilis – is now extremely rare.

Symptoms include pain, undue sensitivity to light and in advanced cases impairment of vision through scarring of the cornea. While treatment varies with the cause, antibiotics are in general useful; but any inflammation of the eye lasting for more than twenty-four hours should have medical attention, and severe inflammation demands immediate attention.

ketogenic diet. A diet in which the fat content is increased at the expense of the carbohydrate content until incomplete products of fat digestion (ketones and acetone) appear in the urine. The digestion of fat can only take place in the presence of carbohydrate and when fat is burned up in the body with insufficient carbohydrate for its combustion, one of the end products is B-oxybutyric acid which inhibits the growth of various germs. For this reason ketogenic diets were for long used in the treatment of various infections of the kidney and urinary tract. In recent decades, however, more effective treatments have been found, and ketogenic diets as a method of treatment have disappeared.

kidney. The kidneys, which are an important part of the URINARY SYSTEM, are a pair of bean-shaped organs, lying high at the back of the abdomen on each side of the spine, opposite the last thoracic and the first three lumbar vertebrae. In the adult they measure roughly 11 × 6 × 4 cm. (4.5 × 2.5 × 1.5 in.). Their main function is to filter out of the circulating blood certain waste substances – such as urea and excess water – and to excrete them through the ureters as urine, which is stored in the bladder until released.

Diseases. There are clearly two possibilities: (1) there may be deficient filtration of water (so that dropsy – usually called oedema – occurs) or of urea (so that there is danger of excess urea remaining in the blood: uraemia); or less commonly, (2) the filtering mechanism is exaggerated, so that for example, people with normal levels of sugar in the blood nevertheless have some sugar excreted in the urine and can be mistakenly thought to suffer from diabetes.

The actual diseases which can affect the kidney are so numerous that only a few can be mentioned here. It may be useful, however, to start with an exclusion. Frequency of need to pass urine, delay in starting and weakness of the stream • may be due to cystitis (inflammation of the bladder) or in men to enlargement of the prostate, but are not signs of damage to the kidney.

Congenital abnormalities include cysts of the kidney which in some cases destroy so much kidney tissue as to prevent the baby from surviving.

In circumstances in which there has been a rapid loss of abdominal fat, the normal slight mobility of the kidneys may be increased so that the condition of MOVABLE KIDNEY or, if more severe, FLOATING KIDNEY, may occur.

Suppression of urine (anuria) may result from obstruction of the ureter of one kidney by a stone when the other kidney is out of action. The symptoms – drowsiness, muscular twitchings, etc. – are essentially those of uraemia, and are followed by death unless effective treatment is undertaken.

Acute nephritis occurs most commonly in childhood and adolescence and is usually caused by bacterial infection, especially by streptococci. The disease is in large measure preventable by adequate treatment of streptococcal infections with antibiotics or sulphonamides. The signs include puffiness of the eyes and face, swelling of the legs, scanty urine of high concentration and of high colour (because it contains blood) and in most cases headache and nausea. Treatment includes rest in bed and for a considerable period a diet low in protein, salt free, and high in carbohydrate. Most patients make a complete recovery.

Chronic parenchymatous nephritis is commonest in young adults. It may follow acute nephritis or arise gradually without obvious cause. The most prominent feature is massive oedema of the face, hands, trunk and legs, with pallor (from anaemia). Since the kidney is also swollen and pale, the condition is sometimes described as 'a large pale kidney in a large pale man'. The blood pressure is slightly raised. The urine is scanty and of high concentration but does not usually contain blood. A salt-free diet is worth trying for six weeks or so, but in most cases recovery is not complete and the patient has to adjust to permanently impaired kidneys – living a regular life without excesses, and avoiding excess of salt.

Chronic interstitial nephritis or 'granular kidney' is mostly a disease of the second half of life. It often accompanies arteriosclerosis. It is made more likely by a very strenuous life, prolonged excessive indulgence in alcohol, prolonged over-eating, lead poisoning, gout and syphilis. The symptoms are rather variable but often include headache and indigestion. The urine is scanty and watery, the arteries are thickened and the blood pressure is raised. The patient should live a quiet, regular life, with a light diet and occasional doses of diuretics to induce the passing of urine.

Until recent years the long-term outlook was poor, but it has been transformed by the introduction of renal dialysis, i.e., use of a KIDNEY MACHINE to enable the body to get rid of waste products that would normally be eliminated by the kidneys. In recent years transplantation of a healthy kidney from' a donor has also saved many lives.

kidney machine. Severe kidney disease may result in kidney failure. In this case waste products, instead of being excreted in the urine, are retained in the blood stream and, as they accumulate, will ultimately cause death from uraemia. Where the kidney is too diseased to pass waste products efficiently from the blood to the urine, a machine can be utilized as a substitute kidney. The patient is connected at suitable times to the machine by tubes inserted into blood vessels of his arm or leg, so that his blood, as well as circulating round his body, goes through this machine. The circulating blood passes over a thin, plastic membrane

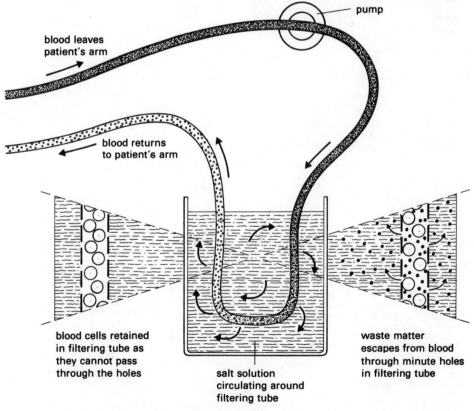

pump

blood leaves patient's arm

blood returns to patient's arm

blood cells retained in filtering tube as they cannot pass through the holes

salt solution circulating around filtering tube

waste matter escapes from blood through minute holes in filtering tube

Kidney machine

which is surrounded by a saline solution. Blood corpuscles are too big to escape through the membrane and so they duly return to the body; but waste products and excess water pass through the membrane into the surrounding solution.

Under suitable conditions a kidney machine can be installed in a patient's home, and a person with chronic kidney disease will need to spend perhaps ten hours three times a week linked to the machine but otherwise can lead a reasonably normal life.

The process of extraction of waste products through a kidney machine is technically called renal dialysis.

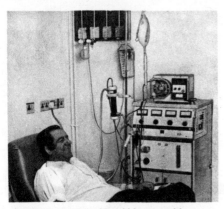

A patient connected to a kidney machine

kidney stone. An accumulation of calcium oxalate, calcium phosphate or uric acid in the collecting cavity or pelvis of the kidney. Gout and infection of the kidney are among the causes.

The stone may remain in the kidney creating no symptoms; it may remain in the kidney and cause pyelitis; it may cause attacks of renal colic, characterized by sharp pain shooting downwards from the area of the kidney; it may obstruct the ureter, rendering one kidney functionless; or it may be passed into the bladder, where it sometimes causes cystitis but is more often passed with the urine. Treatment is initially directed to flushing away the stone by large quantities of alkaline fluid, and meantime using pain-killers if necessary. If these measures fail, surgical removal may be required.

kilojoule. A unit of energy increasingly used to measure food values. A joule is the amount of heat or energy generated by a current of 1 ampere flowing for 1 second against a resistance of 1 ohm, and a kilojoule (often contracted to kJ) is 1,000 joules.

In the past the energy of food was measured in CALORIES (written with a capital C) which were, strictly, kilocalories, each being 1,000 calories. From the beginning of 1978 food manufacturers in Britain and various other countries are being encouraged to use the new units when marking food. Conversion, however, is fairly easy since 1 Calorie is equivalent to 4.2 kilojoules. Thus a person on a strict slimming diet will aim at 4,200 kJ daily, instead of 1,000 Calories.

king's evil. An old name for SCROFULA, i.e.,

tuberculosis of the lymph glands, especially those in the neck. The name was given because of the belief that the condition could be cured by the touch of the king's hand – an interesting early example of faith healing.

kiss of life. See ARTIFICIAL RESPIRATION.

kleptomania. An irresistible desire to steal without regard to personal needs. Very often the articles stolen are of no value to the stealer but perhaps have a symbolic meaning, so that by acquiring them the person relieves his mental tension. Genuine kleptomania requires treatment, usually by psychoanalysis to uncover the root of the compulsion.

True kleptomania is quite a rarity, but four other conditions are often confused with it: (1) stealing by young children who simply lack understanding of the meaning of personal property and need guidance and explanation; (2) stealing by older children as a symptom of maladjustment, often undertaken with a view to giving the stolen articles to others in the hope of gaining affection, and sometimes done in response to a 'dare'; (3) deliberate and conscious shop-lifting, where the plea of kleptomania is offered in an attempt to mitigate criminal responsibility; and (4) a senile variety which is at least partially related to absent-mindedness.

knee. The hinge JOINT formed by the rounded ends, or condyles, of the thigh bone (femur) and the head of the tibia in the lower leg. The fibula, the other bone of the lower leg, does not enter into the formation of the joint. The joint is bound by very strong ligaments. In front of it, but not really part of it, is the PATELLA or kneecap, lying in the muscle tendon.

Injury. A common accident when the knee is twisted is dislocation of one of the cartilages within the joint, so that it is partially detached and nipped between the bones, causing a 'locking' of the joint, with pain and swelling. An anaesthetic may be necessary to overcome the locking. Thereafter rest and light pressure from an elastic bandage usually suffice. If recurrences are frequent an operation for removal of the cartilage may be needed.

knee, housemaid's. Painful swelling through excess fluid round the kneecap. See HOUSEMAID'S KNEE.

knee jerk. When the leg is hanging free (e.g., crossed over the other), tapping the front just below the kneecap produces a jerking movement if the nerves from the knee to the spinal cord and from the cord to the knee are intact. The jerk is exaggerated in some diseases (e.g., disseminated sclerosis) and absent in some other diseases (e.g., locomotor ataxia and severe neuritis). Hence the knee jerk is a useful diagnostic sign.

knock knee. A deformity in which the knees are bent inwards towards each other, otherwise known as genu valgum. The commonest cause was formerly rickets but as this disease has become rare in developed countries the condition is nowadays most often associated with flat-foot.

Massage and manipulation will usually help provided the condition is identified early. In cases diagnosed later operation may be needed.

Koch. Although Pasteur, roughly twenty years before Koch, established that bacteria could cause infection, Robert Koch (1843-1910), a German physician, was in large measure the creator of the science of bacteriology. He devised methods of identifying and growing many bacteria and of demonstrating that specific germs were the causes of particular diseases. The germ responsible for tuberculosis is sometimes called Koch's bacillus.

Koplik's spots. Bluish-white spots on the mucous membrane of the inner lining of the cheek and gums, especially opposite the molar teeth. They appear only in the early stages of measles, often before the rash, and are therefore useful in the diagnosis of the disease. They were first described by an American doctor, Henry Koplik (1858-1927).

Korsakoff's syndrome. A deterioration of the nerves and brain, characterized by memory blanks, poor mental co-ordination and pathological lying, – i.e., the construction of elaborate and completely motiveless untruths; for example, a patient who has been in hospital for a fortnight gives the doctors and nurses who have been treating him a detailed description of his journey across the Atlantic yesterday. The cause is serious deficiency of the B group of vitamins, usually as a result of chronic alcoholism: excess alcohol not only lowers appetite so that insufficient of these vitamins is eaten but also inactivates them. The condition improves greatly when treated by concentrations of the appropriate vitamins.

The condition was originally termed Korsakoff's psychosis, after its discoverer, Sergei Korsakoff (1853-1900), a Russian neurologist. It is, however, not a psychosis (a specific mental illness) but rather a syndrome or group of associated symptoms.

kwashiorkor. A MALNUTRITION disease, caused by a protein deficiency, common in tropical Africa around the age of 2 to 4 years, i.e., after weaning has ended and at a time of rapid growth. Signs of the disease include a very distended abdomen (largely through water retention) and lowered resistance to infections.

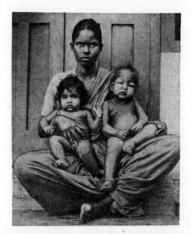

Kwashiorkor in a child recently deprived of its mother's milk by the healthy infant on the left

kyphosis. Exaggeration of the normal CURVATURE OF THE SPINE, creating if the exaggeration is mild the condition of round shoulders and if it is more severe the condition of hunch-back.

L

labour. The process at the end of pregnancy during which the muscular contractions of the uterus expel the new-born child, the membranes and amniotic fluid surrounding it, and finally the placenta through which it derived sustenance during intra-uterine life. For a detailed account see CHILDBIRTH.

Premature labour is labour occurring after viability (6 to 6½ months), so that the child is capable of survival, but before full-term. Interruption of pregnancy before viability is usually called miscarriage or abortion.

False labour is the occurrence of colicky pains towards the end of pregnancy, mimicking real labour. These usually arise from irregular contractions of other abdominal organs but are characterized by lack of rhythm, by being felt in the abdomen rather than in the back, and by the absence, when it is gently felt by the hand, of any general contraction of the uterus. Investigation may disclose constipation or an infected or distended bladder. Appropriate treatment combined with sedatives will usually allay the symptoms.

laburnum. The pods and seeds of this tree contain an alkaloid, cystisine, which is also found in broom and lupin seeds. About an hour after eating the pods or seeds a child becomes pale, dizzy and anxious, and usually suffers from vomiting and diarrhoea.

Treatment consists mainly of giving the child warmth, adequate air, reassurance, and – if vomiting or diarrhoea are severe – liquid drinks to prevent dehydration. If there is little vomiting, an emetic to induce it (e.g., salt and water) may help to remove the poison from the stomach. If there is little or no diarrhoea, a laxative may assist in the elimination of the poison from the intestine.

laceration. A wound produced by the tearing apart of tissues. Severe lacerations are typical of machinery and traffic accidents and are generally associated with considerable bruising. Such wounds are usually irregular in shape; the skin around is torn and discoloured; there may be ingrained dirt or indriven portions of clothing; pain is often slight because of nerve-fibre destruction; similarly, bleeding may be minimal because injured blood-vessels become blocked by their torn walls.

Tissue-damage and the diminished blood-supply reduces the ability to combat infections, and also means that the damaged tissues are liable to die or at least to slow delayed healing. Successful repair requires meticulous care with antiseptic cleansing, the removal of foreign matter and dead tissue, arrest of haemorrhage, assessment and repair of damage to deeper structures, and finally accurate suturing with provision for drainage. An anti-tetanus injection should also be given.

lacrimal. The eyes are continuously bathed by a watery fluid, the tears, produced by glands behind the upper eyelids, and entering the conjunctival sacs by multiple secretory ducts. Excess fluid leaves the sacs by drainage pores at the inner angles of the eyelids and is collected in a small reservoir which continues as a duct to the lower part of the nasal cavity. Lacrimal means 'pertaining to the tears', and is used to qualify the names of the successive parts of these lacrimatory arrangements as lacrimal gland, lacrimal secretion, lacrimal canals, lacrimal sac, and naso-lacrimal duct.

lactation. The period during which the mother secretes milk and the infant is suckled. See BREAST FEEDING.

Laennec. René Théophile Hyacinthe Laennec (1781-1826) was a distinguished Parisian physician, and in his capacity as head of L'Hôpital Necker was regarded as an unrivalled diagnostician. His name is still used in certain diagnostic terms, but his great claim to fame rests on his invention of the stethoscope.

From the time of Hippocrates, physicians listened to the sounds of heart and lungs by applying an ear to a patient's chest. This was the method of 'immediate auscultation' which was inconvenient, indelicate, and inefficient. In 1819 Laennec published a monograph, *De l'auscultation médiate,* in which he described a new idea. Originally he used a cardboard tube but this was later developed as a straight wooden tube, bell-shaped at one end to receive chest-sounds, and at the other end expanded to a flat, circular plate against which the physician placed his ear and listened. This procedure he called 'mediate auscultation' and it led to more accurate localization and more effective conduction of internal sounds and so revolutionized the diagnosis of heart and lung ailments. The modern binaural (i.e., using both ears) stethoscope with various types of improved chest-pieces connected to the ears by flexible rubber-tubing is now more usually employed but its development and adoption in universal medical use stems from Laennec's original ingenuity. The modern foetal stethoscope for listening to the foetus while in the mother's uterus is still very much of the old pattern.

It was an irony of fate that Laennec himself developed consumption shortly after publication of his treatise. The signs of this were confirmed by his own instrument and after some years of failing health he retired to his native Quimper to die at the early age of 45.

Lamarck. Jean Baptiste Lamarck (1744-1829) was a French naturalist who published his main work, *Philosophie Zoologique,* in 1809, the year in which Charles Darwin was born. Lamarck held that organisms evolved by adjusting to their environment and that the resulting changes were passed on to subsequent generations. This idea of the inheritance of acquired characteristics has long been regarded as disproved, but perhaps Lamarck's real contribution was to prepare people for the acceptance of EVOLUTION a generation before DARWIN.

lameness. The causes of lameness vary, from a blister or corn on the foot, or even ill-fitting or badly designed shoes, to a serious disease of the brain or spinal cord. In young children lameness may be an early sign of disease of the hip joint (e.g., tuberculous infection). In general, unless there is an obvious trivial cause, lameness requires medical investigation.

Langerhans, islets of. Clusters of cells scattered throughout the pancreas. In these cells INSULIN is produced.

laparotomy. The operation of opening the abdominal cavity either for the purpose of dealing with a diseased or damaged organ or for exploratory or diagnostic purposes.

laryngitis. Inflammation of the larynx and vocal cords resulting in dryness of the throat, hoarseness (sometimes going on to complete loss of voice), tickling cough and raised temperature.

Acute laryngitis is usually due to infection of the voice-box after it has been rendered susceptible by exposure to irritating vapours, or by exposure to cold (especially very cold air breathed through the mouth and therefore unwarmed), or by over-use of the voice. The four standard measures of treatment are rest, provision of an even temperature, cough sedatives and appropriate inhalations, such as a teaspoonful of tincture of benzoin in 0.5 litre (1 pint) of boiling water. Inhalations are very useful but the patient must remain for some hours in a warm atmosphere after each inhalation. Gargling, although often used, is of doubtful value. Generally recovery occurs within a few days, although occasionally the acute stage passes into the chronic one.

Chronic laryngitis, with similar symptoms and long-term swelling of the vocal cords, may follow an uncured acute attack, may be the result of habitual straining of the voice (clergyman's throat) or may occasionally result from excessive smoking. Uncommon causes of chronic laryngitis include tuberculosis, syphilis and cancer, so if the condition does not respond to ordinary treatment examination by a throat specialist is desirable.

larynx. The portion of the RESPIRATORY SYSTEM adapted for the production of VOICE AND SPEECH.

Lassa fever. An acute and sometimes fatal infectious disease first identified in Nigeria in 1969 and subsequently found in other countries in Central and Western Africa. The disease is caused by a virus which is carried by a particular type of African rat, but is also occasionally spread through direct personal or nursing contact with an infected person or his clothing or excretions. In general the disease occurs in countries in which the particular rat breeds. For example up to the beginning of 1977 there had been only three cases in Britain, all of them initially infected in Africa.

The incubation period is seven to ten days and the main symptoms are fever, sore throat, complete exhaustion, toxic appearance and sometimes vomiting and chest pains.

Control measures include attempts to eradicate the particular species of rat, prevention of contamination of food by such rats, and early identification and rigorous isolation of suspected cases.

Treatment consists mainly of skilled nursing with attention to symptoms, although injection of plasma obtained from the blood of recovered or convalescent cases is said to help. As yet no antibiotic useful in treatment has been discovered and no vaccine for prevention is available.

laughing gas. Another name for nitrous oxide, a colourless gas which is sometimes used for anaesthesia in dentistry. In relatively pure form it rapidly produces unconsciousness, but if administered with some air mixed with it, it gives rise to a kind of intoxication, often characterized by laughter or, less frequently, by weeping.

lavage. The washing out of any internal organ. Lavage is most commonly used for the stomach in cases of poisoning (other than corrosive poisoning) or conditions of dilatation with accumulation and fermentation of stomach contents, e.g., some cases of severe indigestion. A special rubber tube is passed through the mouth and gullet into the stomach. There is a filter funnel attached, and warmed water containing a little potassium permanganate is run into the stomach and siphoned off.

Colonic lavage is sometimes used in chronic constipation, and bladder lavage is occasionally recommended in chronic cystitis.

laxative. An 'opening medicine' alternatively known as an aperient, employed in the treatment of CONSTIPATION. In the late nineteenth and early twentieth centuries laxatives were grossly over-used owing to a then current theory that to 'clear the system' would eliminate poisons and prevent their absorption from the intestine into the blood.

In general the terms laxatives and aperient are used for mild household remedies for constipation, while stronger drugs – which can be dangerous and should only be employed under medical supervision – are called purgatives and cathartics. The distinction, however, is rather vague, because the effect of an opening drug depends not only on the particular medicine used, but on the dose, the degree of constipation, and the sensitivity of the person's intestine.

In most cases a mild laxative is preferable to a stronger one, and the dose should be the minimum to produce an easy motion.

lead poisoning. The condition resulting from absorption of lead salts by the body. Despite many precautions the condition is still not infrequent in lead workers, such as painters, glaziers, potters, plumbers and makers of electric batteries; and it is sometimes found in children who have chewed articles painted with a lead-based paint. Since most lead water-pipes have now been replaced, lead poisoning from water is becoming a thing of the past.

Acute lead poisoning from a single large dose usually starts with cramp-like abdominal pain and obstinate constipation, followed in severe cases either by intense headache, convulsions and sometimes coma (where the lead salts damage the brain) or by paralysis of the muscles which straighten out the fingers and wrists.

Chronic lead poisoning, from absorption of small amounts over a period, is commoner. Here the main symptoms are those of anaemia, (e.g., tiredness, weakness and pallor) with paralysis of wrist and fingers in due course, and sometimes with abdominal colic. A diagnostic sign, present in many but not all cases, is a blue line in the gums, not to be confused with the line sometimes seen between gums and uncleaned teeth. Where the diagnosis is in doubt, blood examination is helpful.

Prevention includes: (1) wherever practicable, substitution of non-toxic substances (e.g., plastics) for lead compounds; (2) where lead must be used the taking of appropriate steps to prevent the escape of dust and fumes; (3) personal cleanliness by workers, including the scrubbing of hands and nails before eating; (4) the use of protective clothing, including well-fitting overalls and including masks where processes are dusty; and (5) periodical medical examination of employees in lead industries.

In treatment calcium compounds (e.g., sodium calciumedetate) have largely superseded older methods, because the main effect of lead absorption is to remove calcium. Morphia may be needed for the pain, though a high calcium diet – including two pints of milk daily – will usually end the colic within two days. Laxatives are necessitated by the constipation, and where paralysis of fingers and wrist persists electrical treatment may be useful.

left-handedness. Natural dominance of the left hand. The condition, which is probably inherited, is found in about one-tenth of children.

From school desks to adult tools society has been organized for the right-handed majority. Yet attempts to force left-handed children to use their right hands sometimes result in emotional disorders or speech defects and always result in poorer performance than would have been possible with the natural hand. It is now generally accepted that a child should be allowed to use his natural hand, but since our writing is from left to right some left-handed children at first tend to reverse figures and letters, e.g., confusing 'b' and 'd', and reading 'top' for 'pot' and 'was' for 'saw'.

leg. In common usage leg means the whole lower limb sometimes including and sometimes excluding the foot. In anatomical descriptions, however, the term is restricted to the portion from the knee to the ankle, the part from knee to hip-joint being termed the thigh.

The skeleton of the leg (in the anatomical sense) is formed by the tibia or shin-bone on the inner side and the thinner fibula on the outside. The fleshy calf of the leg is formed by the gastrocnemius and soleus muscles ending in the Achilles tendon which is inserted into the heel bone.

legionnaires' disease. A new bacterial disease first recognized when an outbreak occurred at a gathering of members of the Pennsylvania State American Legion in 1976 at Philadelphia. There were 3,683 persons at the gathering, 189 developed the disease and 29 died. Retrospective study revealed that a previously unidentified outbreak in Columbia in 1965, with 89 cases and 12 deaths, was due to the same bacterium. Since 1976 there have been a few small outbreaks in the U.S.A. and one in Nottingham, England.

The disease, which has an incubation period of seven to ten days, usually starts with muscle pains, dry cough, shortness of breath and rising temperature, sometimes with rigors, and in a day or two produces signs and symptoms very similar to those of pneumonia. Oxygen treatment helps the breathing and, although not all antibiotics are effective, adequate dosage of an appropriate antibiotic usually results in rapid cure.

In an established outbreak in the future it will be easy to treat the later cases with erythromycin or tetracycline (the most effective antibiotics) but the difficulty will lie in diagnosing the early cases in time to reduce the 15 per cent risk of death, because clinically and radiologically the condition resembles an ordinary pneumonia, so that the existence of legionnaires' disease is unlikely to be suspected until several persons thought to have been suffering from pneumonia show a lack of response to normal treatment for that disease.

The method of spread is not yet certain but the majority of workers who have studied the disease believe that spread is through the air, perhaps in dust particles. The direct person-to-person spread, common in many infections, does not appear to occur.

Just as human beings alter over many generations – we differ considerably from our Anglo-Saxon and Celtic ancestors of forty generations back and enormously from the Neanderthals and Cromagnons of a thousand generations back – so germs also change, the difference being that bacteria pass through over forty generations in a day, and over a thousand in a month. Although most of the new infections that have appeared in recent years have been caused by viruses there is nothing particularly strange in a bacterium acquiring qualities dangerous to man, just as – in the opposite direction – the streptococcus that causes scarlet fever has become much less dangerous in the last fifty years.

Yet legionnaires' disease raises many questions that are not at present answerable: for instance, where does the germ exist between outbreaks, are there human or animal symptomless carriers, how exactly does the disease spread, can a rapid method of diagnosis be evolved, and are there any useful and practicable preventive measures? At least the disease serves as a reminder that scientific knowledge is very far from complete.

leisure. As the poet Cowper says,

'Absence of occupation is not rest;
A mind quite vacant is a mind distressed.'

While the play of pre-school and school children has for long been recognized as important for their physical, emotional and social development, the use of leisure by adults has been largely ignored. This is quite simply because in the era of the five and a half or six day working week of ten or twelve hours a day there was little time or energy left available for leisure activities, and only a small section of the community could be regarded as leisured. This was true even of the elderly, because there was no fixed age of retirement, in most cases no retirement pension and in general much shorter duration of life.

Mechanization has produced vast changes. In a week of 168 hours most earners work for about 40 hours, sleep for around 60 hours, spend about 20 hours in such activities as eating, washing and dressing, and have something like 48 hours – longer than their working week – available for leisure activities;

and the elderly sixth of the community, the retired, have about 88 hours a week of leisure time.

It is perhaps unfortunate that, during the decades of increasing mechanization, schools (and in large measure universities and other institutions of higher education) have concentrated more and more on equipping persons to earn a living in an appropriate occupation with little reference to leisure. As a result school leavers – freed from scholastic bonds but with no training in the use of leisure – are tending increasingly to spend their free time not in creative activity but as passive watchers of television. Similarly a good football match provides useful exercise for twenty-five people (including the referee and the linesmen) while thousands of spectators exercise only their vocal cords. In addition, a survival of puritanism has tended to encourage us to regard as 'wasted' all hours which adolescents spend on matters not pertaining to their future career.

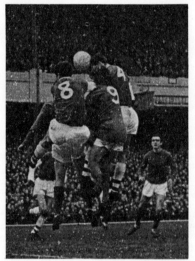

Leisure: '... thousands exercise only their vocal cords ...'

Broadly, a person employed in physical toil needs leisure interests that will keep his mind active, a brain worker needs interests that will use his muscles, and a person who sits doing routine work needs interests of both types. Personal emotional or aesthetic satisfaction is of course equally important. So any effort to stimulate a person to take up a seemingly appropriate leisure activity must take account of his inclinations and aptitudes and indeed of his entire personality; attempts to make a habitually impatient man take up fishing or to induce a woman with poor vision to start painting are clearly doomed to failure.

Suggestions are now being made that the curriculum of every pupil in school should include at least one leisure subject chosen by the pupil from a wide range; in some countries education authorities have begun to organize adult courses in such subjects; and in the U.K. local authorities are increasingly establishing leisure centres. Unfortunately in times of financial stringency leisure courses and leisure centres are often the first to suffer. However, on a fairly long-term basis such provisions as these seem likely to do much to reduce boredom and vandalism and to improve the quality of life.

For preparation for the increased leisure of retirement see RETIREMENT. See also KEEPING FIT.

lens. See EYE.

leprosy. A mildly infectious disease of prolonged incubation and very prolonged course, characterized by nodules and ulcers both in the skin and beneath its surface, and by damage to nerves. The disease is caused by a micro-organism not unlike the germ that causes tuberculosis.

Leprosy is still widespread in Asia, Africa and Central and South America with a few cases still arising in other areas, e.g., Iceland and Northern Australia. The disease is spread by close and continuous human contact, especially in unhygienic conditions; but the medieval idea of its high infectivity is quite wrong and really due to confusion with other conditions. The incubation period is usually several years, and in some cases over ten years. It is not a hereditary or a congenital disease.

Although most cases are to some extent intermediate or mixed, the two main types are here outlined.

1. The nodular type usually begins with general discomfort, bouts of fever, pains over large areas of the body, and nodular swellings, especially in the face and hands. The swollen patches become thickened and painful, and they gradually spread to become insensitive so that pain disappears. As the nose becomes involved and flattened the face assumes a so-called 'leonine' appearance. Organisms may invade the eyes, causing blindness.

2. In the tuberculoid type sharply defined patches of the skin become raised on any part of the body, the buttocks being perhaps most commonly affected. The patches expand, becoming dry, pale and devoid of sensation. Involvement of nerves often results in loss of power and loss of sensation in the fingers and toes. Ulcers may occur and the tissues of the fingers and toes may die.

If untreated, the disease may continue to progress for thirty years with or without periods of partial remission, or it may become arrested at any stage.

Oil of chaulmoogra, for many years the standard treatment and definitely useful, is nowadays increasingly being replaced by dapsone (DDS), given by mouth or by injection for a prolonged period. Additionally, antibiotics or surgical treatment may be needed for the ulcers, and special attention should be given to the eyes. Since leprosy is only mildly contagious the old idea of very strict isolation is outmoded, although it is still desirable to remove a child from a leprous parent.

Lesbianism. A sexual relationship between women, corresponding to homosexuality in men (and strictly included in the latter term). Usually the physical side of such relationships amounts to mutual masturbation.

Possible causes of Lesbianism include genetic and environmental factors, which combine to make a particular woman predominantly masculine; prolonged sexual rivalry; and disgust at the roughness of the male approach to intercourse.

The name is derived from the poetess, Sappho of Lesbos, whose surviving poems display an allegedly erotic admiration of women; but there is really no evidence that Sappho, living in an era of complete male dominance, was more than an early advocate of female emancipation.

leucocyte. A white blood corpuscle. Out of every 500 blood corpuscles about 499 are red and concerned with transport of oxygen and about 1 is white (or actually almost colourless), larger than the red cells, and concerned with defending the body against infection and engulfing invading foreign bodies. A cubic millimetre of blood normally contains about five million red blood corpuscles and nine thousand white blood corpuscles which are divisible into various types, e.g., neutrophils, eosinophils and lymphocytes.

An increase in the number of leucocytes in the blood is known as leucocytosis. A slight temporary increase occurs during digestion of food and an increase of longer duration is found in pregnancy. Normally, however, leucocytosis implies a reaction to the invasion of bacteria or other foreign bodies. It is a sign that the blood is 'on the defensive'.

Leucocytes of different types do not respond equally to any one invader. Thus eosinophils increase markedly in diseases due to animal parasites (such as various worms) and also in asthma and the early stages of scarlet fever; the number of lymphocytes rises markedly in tuberculosis; and neutrophils are increased in the majority of infections.

In any infection a leucocytosis, e.g., an increase from nine thousand to fifteen thousand per cubic millimetre, is a good sign, indicating that the white blood corpuscles are responding to the challenge. Conversely, no increase or inadequate increase in white blood corpuscles is an unfavourable sign.

leucocytosis. See LEUCOCYTE.

leucopenia. Diminution of the white blood corpuscles below the normal proportion of nine thousand per cubic millimetre of blood. Leucopenia is found in typhoid fever, measles and influenza; in some mosquito-borne infections such as malaria and kala-azar; in severe anaemias in which the red blood corpuscles are, of course, also reduced; and in some cases of exposure to x-rays or radium or atomic radiation.

leucorrhoea. Abnormal discharge of white fluid from the VAGINA.

leucotomy. An operation, also known as lobotomy, whereby an incision is made through the skull into the brain for the purpose of cutting certain nerve fibres and so removing the pathways between particular sets of stimuli and particular responses.

The operation was introduced by Moniz of Lisbon in 1936 and has been extensively used to give relief in certain serious mental disorders, especially those associated with intractable mental suffering and anxiety. It is recommended in severe cases of schizophrenia and manic-depressive psychosis which have failed to respond to other methods of treatment. Not only, however, is it quite a serious operation, but there is no guarantee that it will not also result in the destruction of useful pathways: as a result of the cutting of nerve fibres which will not regenerate there may be a blunting of some of the highest powers of the mind. In other words, the operation, while sometimes desirable, should not be undertaken lightly.

leukaemia. A disease or group of diseases characterized by grossly excessive activity of either the bone marrow (in which many leucocytes are formed) or the spleen and lymph glands (in which lymphocytes are formed), resulting in an enormous increase in the number of circulating large leucocytes or of lymphocytes.

The acute forms, which occur in children and young adults, usually start with fatigue, raised temperature, haemorrhages from mucous membranes and enlargement of the spleen and lymph glands. These acute forms show symptoms which are identical with acute septicaemia and blood tests have to be carried out to distinguish the two conditions. Acute leukaemia is fatal, usually within four months, although there are current claims for a new treatment.

Chronic myelogenous leukaemia, in which the bone marrow produces vast numbers of immature leucocytes, usually occurs in young adults. Clinical findings include gross enlargement of the spleen, pain, progressive weakness, and haemorrhages from the nose. Remissions frequently occur, sometimes lasting for several months, but the condition is always fatal, usually within four years.

Chronic lymphatic leukaemia appears more in males above middle age. Symptoms are similar, except that there is much enlargement of lymph glands and less swelling of the spleen. Remissions are frequent and lengthy and, although this form is fatal like the others, patients have been known to live for up to ten years.

While a few cases of leukaemia have been caused by ionizing radiations and especially by the explosion of atomic bombs, and while a possible hereditary element has been suggested in lymphatic leukaemia, the main factors causing it are still unknown. Most experts regard leukaemia as being essentially a cancer of the blood-forming tissues.

Blood transfusions may make the patient more comfortable, x-ray treatment of the spleen or long bones may create temporary improvement, and a vast number of drugs are alleged to be of some help; but, until more is known about the causes, all treatment merely eases the symptoms.

libido. Psychological energy; the individual's innate drive for pleasure and satisfaction.

The word is derived from the Latin word for lust, and Freud uses it as meaning fundamentally a drive for sexual gratification and for perpetuation of the species; but it has to be remembered that Freud groups together all forms of affection under this heading. Jung and other psychologists employ the term to include the drives for superiority, acknowledgement, affection, parental love, etc., as well as that for sexual gratification. As generally used in modern psychology it embraces all forms of vital energy.

Librium. A make of TRANQUILLIZER.

lice. The head louse (*Pediculus capitis*), the body louse (*Pediculus corporis*) and the crab louse (*Phthirus pubis*) are all variants of the same species. The eggs or nits are cemented to hairs or clothing and hatch in seven to fifteen

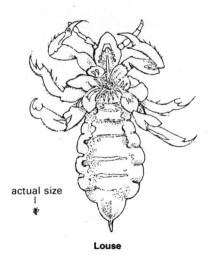

actual size

Louse

days, and the new lice become mature in about a fortnight.

Lice, traditionally associated with unclean heads or bodies, cause itching, discomfort and lack of sleep. They can also transmit the organisms of typhus fever (the dreaded 'jail fever' of the past) and relapsing fever.

Prevention is essentially by cleanliness, though it has to be remembered that a person whose personal hygiene is perfect can be infected from a less clean associate. Treatment is normally by lethane spray or by a 2 per cent emulsion of DDT rubbed on the scalp.

In outbreaks of typhus a 10 per cent DDT powder can be sprayed through the openings in the clothing, and can thus save the very considerable time that would have to be spent if thousands of contacts and suspected contacts had to undress before receiving treatment for eradication of lice.

lichen planus. An extremely itchy skin condition, with shiny, flat-topped papules particularly affecting the front of the forearms and wrists, the inner aspects of the thighs and the front of the shins. The condition is probably due to a virus. Prednisone is perhaps the most effective drug, and sedatives are also usually needed until the intense itching subsides.

life span. The maximum duration of life attainable by an appreciable number of the members of a species under current conditions.

The term should be clearly differentiated from EXPECTATION OF LIFE. The overwhelming majority of any species – indeed probably over 99 per cent in all cases – have their 'possible' lives shortened, e.g., by malnutrition or over-feeding in childhood or later, by preventable or unpreventable diseases, or by violence. The expectation of life is an average of the future prospects of individuals of any particular age, including those who have so far survived but with impaired prospects, whereas the life span is a reasonable anticipated maximum for individuals who have lived healthily through the dangers of early and middle life.

Among mammals other than man the longest living appear to be Indian elephants, quite a number of which reach the age of 60; and at least one biologist has claimed that under

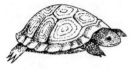

tortoise – 120 years   chimpanzee – 45 years   man – 100 years

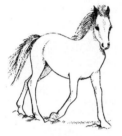   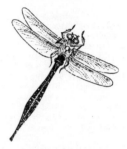

horse – 30 years   cat – 20 years   dragonfly – 7 weeks

The life span of various animals

favourable conditions Indian elephants can attain the age of 70 years. Cases of the giant tortoises of the Seychelles Islands living for more than 150 years have been recorded.

Biblical writers assessed the human life span at 70 years, despite occasional alleged exceptions like Methuselah, and this probably remained a reasonable estimate until the nineteenth century, by which time octogenerians were not infrequent. People like John Ruskin (who died at 81 in 1900) and Thomas Carlyle (who died at 86 in 1881) were merely deemed very old men, while in an earlier century they would have been regarded as phenomenally old.

In the present century improvements in the health care, social conditions and medical treatment of adults not only reduced the proportion of shortened lives but also increased the life span: by 1950, for instance, there were over 300 centenarians in England, including 153 who died in that year at ages varying from 100 to 107.

It is as yet too early to assess fully the effect on the life span of improved health care of children during this century. Already the average age at death (and those who die in infancy and childhood are included in the calculation) is approaching 70, nonagenarians are quite common and most towns of any size can boast their centenarians; but these nonagenarians and centenarians were reared long before the discovery of vitamins, vaccines and antibiotics and before modern knowledge

of the developmental and even the nutritional needs of children had been acquired.

On present indications it would seem that an individual born after 1945 and handicapped neither by nature nor by nurture might anticipate a life span of 95 to 110 years before one or other of the vital organs wears out; but these indications are questioned by some medical scientists, and we cannot have certain knowledge for another seventy years, although we already know that 5 per cent of our present population is over 75 years, including 1 per cent over 85 years.

If kidney transplants or artificial kidneys, heart transplants, etc. became common, the life span might well be extended to over 200 years, but under present conditions there is no evidence to suggest that an appreciable number of people will live beyond the age of 95 to 110. In other words, the life span today is probably about 50 per cent more than the Biblical three score and ten. By comparison, the life span of the Indian elephant would seem to be about 70, that of the horse around 30, that of the cat about 20 and that of the dog (although there is great variation between breeds) about 18.

There are, of course, complications arising out of the increase of the life span. When the average age at death was around 40 years and the life span was about 80 years it was feasible to introduce retirement on pension at 65 years for men and 60 for women, with sometimes earlier possibilities. As the average age at death approaches 70 and the life span passes 100 it becomes questionable whether the retirement of healthy persons on pension is economically practicable at 65 and 60 years.

ligament. A band of tough fibrous tissue which binds together the component bones of a joint or helps to keep an internal organ in place. Much of the strength of such joints as the knee and the ankle derives from the ligaments. When a ligament is unduly stretched or very suddenly stretched its fibres may be ruptured, causing a SPRAIN.

limb. In animals with a backbone (i.e., vertebrates) limbs are jointed structures attached to the sides of the spinal column. Human limbs are arms and legs but in all vertebrates the limb-pattern is conceived on a similar plan, even though the actual 'limb' may appear quite different or may even be a remnant indicating EVOLUTION from another creature. Fish for instance have pectoral and anal fins, birds have wings instead of arms, seals and other pinnipeds have flippers and snakes are without external remnants. The common pattern is of significance in understanding how evolution has taken place.

Each limb is of similar design. The fore-limb is attached to the spine by a pectoral (or shoulder) girdle of three bones (fused acromion-scapula and clavicle) and continues as the upper arm (one bone: humerus), the forearm (two bones: radius and ulna), the wrist (several small bones: carpus) the palm (five small straight bones: metacarpals) and five jointed digits. Similarly the rear-limb consists of the pelvic girdle (fused ilium-ischium-pubis), the thigh (one bone: femur), the leg (two bones: tibia and fibula), the ankle (several small bones: tarsus), the foot (five small straight bones: metatarsals) and five jointed digits.

In animals like lizards both fore- and hind-limbs are similarly related to the body but in man the fore-limb has rotated during development so that the elbow comes to face backwards instead of forwards like the knee. This has resulted from standing and moving on our hind legs only, and the need to use the fore-limb for other purposes than locomotion.

lipoma. A slow-growing, non-malignant tumour composed of fat. Lipomata are usually rounded and have well-marked capsules from which they can be shelled out if need be.

By far the commonest variety is the subcutaneous lipoma, occurring under the skin of the neck, shoulder, back or buttocks. It is quite painless and causes inconvenience only by its size or appearance. Less frequently lipomata occur within muscles or within the capsule of a joint. Often several lipomata develop near each other.

Small lipomata are usually best left alone. If a large lipoma causes disfiguration or creates pain through pressure, surgical treatment consists simply of opening the capsule and shelling out the fatty material. Recurrence is almost unknown.

lips, disorders of. Lip disorders, because they cause cosmetic disfigurement, are generally recognized promptly and treated vigorously.

Cleft or HARE-LIP is the most important congenital lip disorder. About two-thirds of cases are associated with cleft palate. Treatment is by surgical repair.

The commonest cause of lip swelling is a mucous cyst, resulting from blockage of a mucous gland. It should be removed by a small operation.

Chapping of the lips, with a crack in the middle of the lower lip which frequently bleeds, is a common complaint in cold weather. Treatment and prevention include the application of glycerine and bland lip protective ointments.

Herpes simplex cold sores are common, and are self-healing or responsive to simple treatments such as application of ointment or spirit, but they are liable to recur.

The lips are the commonest place, outside the genital area, for syphilitic chancre. Treatment is with penicillin in substantial and maintained dosage.

Carcinoma of the lips is commonest in old men who have followed an outdoor occupation; prolonged exposure to bright sunshine is thought to be a factor in its development. The tumour is slow-growing and generally curable by surgery or radio-therapy.

Lister. Joseph Lister (1827-1912), later Lord Lister, a son of J.J. Lister, F.R.S., the microscopist, was born at Upton, Essex and studied medicine in London and Edinburgh. He became successively Professor of Surgery in Glasgow and Edinburgh and later at King's College London (1877).

Although he made other contributions to medical knowledge, notably on coagulation of the blood and on inflammation, his great work was the introduction of ANTISEPSIS which revolutionized the practice of surgery. Wound sepsis and septicaemia delayed healing and caused high death rates after surgical operations. Various workers including Pasteur and Semmelweiss had shown that these effects were due to invasion by micro-organisms.

Lister conceived the idea of operating under the cover of chemical substances which would destroy these bacteria. The patient's skin and the operator's hands and instruments were disinfected by a solution of corrosive sublimate and the operation was conducted under a mist of carbolic acid produced as a fine spray by a steam-driven generator. The original apparatus is preserved in the museum of the Royal College of Physicians and Surgeons in Glasgow.

As a result of these methods the deaths from major operations in Lister's wards in Glasgow Royal Infirmary fell from 45 per cent (1864-66) to 15 per cent (1867-69). As Sir Joseph Lister he became President of the Royal Society in 1895 and was created a baron in 1897.

lithiasis. A condition characterized by the formation of CALCULI (stones) of any kind, especially in the bile ducts or in the urinary tract. It is generally diagnosed when symptoms arise. Treatment varies according to the site and duration of the disorder, but may include surgery.

It may also be used to describe a constitutional disposition to suffer from gout.

lithotomy. The incision of a duct or organ, particularly of the bladder, for the removal of a stone.

In the lithotomy position, commonly employed for gynaecological examination and operation and for childbirth, the woman lies on her back with legs apart and with both the hips and the knee joints well bent.

liver. The largest gland of the body lying beneath the diaphragm in the upper right of the abdomen, with an important role in the body

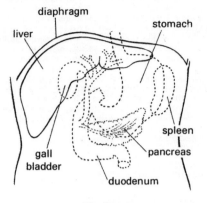

The liver

METABOLISM. It has a double blood supply, from the hepatic artery, bringing oxygenated blood from the heart via the aorta, and the portal vein, bringing blood from the stomach and intestine, rich in absorbed foods which the liver processes. It secretes BILE, destroys old red blood cells, converts most sugars into glycogen which it stores, and plays a large part in fat and protein metabolism as well. It is responsible for the control of CATABOLISM of the ammonia produced as a by-product of protein break-down in the gut.

In addition it is the body's main defence against potentially dangerous substances: many drugs (e.g., alcohol), which would otherwise accumulate in the body, are broken down to simpler non-poisonous constituents by the liver. It acts similarly in respect of the body's own hormones.

The liver of some animals is used as food.

Diseases. Because of its major role in metabolism the liver is particularly liable to blood-borne infection by diseases in other parts of the body, whilst disturbance of its own normal function by disease may have widespread serious consequences.

Infective hepatitis, caused by virus infection of the liver itself, is the commonest cause of JAUNDICE in adults. The condition gradually clears up without specific treatment, but it is usually necessary to treat the symptoms (e.g., itching of the skin).

Bacterial infection from other abdominal organs, formerly common, is now rare, due to improved diagnosis of abdominal sepsis and the widespread use of antibiotics.

Amoebic abscess, caused by the organism responsible for amoebic dysentery, is common in tropical areas with poor sanitation. Treatment is not easy but several drugs exist that act specifically against the amoeba. Hydatid disease of the liver, caused by a dog tapeworm, requires surgical removal.

Primary cancer of the liver is rare in Europeans, but common in Africa and the Far East and known to be associated with certain items of diet. Drug treatment and surgery are employed. Prevention by change of diet may be possible. The spread of cancer from the gut, lung, breast, etc. to the liver is common, and difficult to treat.

Cardiac failure, alcoholism, and other diseases of the body function have specific effects on the liver and require treatment of the original disease for their relief.

lobectomy. The surgical operation for the removal of one of the lobes of a lung. The lungs are divided into sections called lobes – three in the right lung and two in the left – and each lobe is almost completely separate with its own airway and blood vessels. Using modern methods of anaesthesia, lobectomy is now a routine procedure for the thoracic surgeon.

The operation is principally used in such conditions as bronchiectasis, chronic lung abscess, cysts of various kinds, and in carcinoma of the lung. Careful investigation of the extent of the disease is required beforehand, in order to find whether it is likely that the affected area can be completely removed.

lobotomy. Another name for LEUCOTOMY.

lockjaw. A firm closing of the jaw due to spasm of its muscles. Also known as trismus, it is usually associated with TETANUS and caused by the toxin produced by the tetanus bacteria. Treatment is directed towards maintaining respiration. Prevention is achieved by immunization with anti-tetanus toxoid.

locomotor. Pertaining to or capable of movement.

locomotor ataxia. A formerly common but now very rare disease of the spinal cord, occurring as a late complication of syphilis some five to twenty years after the original condition. An alternative name is tabes dorsalis.

The condition usually starts with sharp pains of a few seconds duration, most often in the legs. After a time the pains lengthen in duration and a numbing of sensation develops, the sufferer feeling as if he were walking on cotton wool. Later the patient's movements become poorly co-ordinated and he walks with a curious broad-based gait. Later still he may become so paralysed as to be unable to feed and dress himself. With prompt diagnosis and efficient treatment of early syphilis the condition is now an extreme rarity.

longevity. The achievement of long life, beyond 75 or 80 years of age.

The nature of the AGEING process, though the subject of increasing research, is still imperfectly understood. Nevertheless, formulae and elixirs for prolongation of life have abounded throughout history. A modern formula might well include the following items: rural residence and life-style, with physical work begun early in life and continued to a late age, a long marriage, abstinence from tobacco, moderate intake of a mixed diet, and half a bottle of wine a day with meals.

lordosis. An abnormally increased concavity in the CURVATURE OF THE SPINE at lumber level; also known as hollow back.

LSD. An abbreviation for lysergic acid diethylamide, a hallucinogenic drug, i.e., one which causes hallucinations. It was originally derived from ergot but was synthesized in 1938. Drug users refer to it as 'acid', 'sugar' or 'zen'. It is one of a class of drugs known as psychotomimetic (simulating mental illness) and such substances have been used by primitive races from time immemorial, being taken during tribal rites to induce frenzy and illusions of supernatural power. Other examples are mescalin, obtained from the

Mexican agave, bufotenin, a skin-secretion of toads, and also marihuana.

LSD has been employed therapeutically in mental illness with the purpose of improving the attitude of psychiatric patients to psychotherapy, but its unauthorized use in 'taking a trip' is both illegal and very dangerous. Devotees claim that the episodes of hallucination and temporary insanity, produced by even minute amounts of the drug, are an enlargement of experience because of the profound alterations which occur in their perceptions and emotions.

There is however substantial risk of causing a prolonged psychotic illness resembling schizophrenia or toxic psychosis, and of inducing delusions and impaired judgement which may lead to fatal results. There have, for instance, been incidents in which individuals have thrown themselves from a height under the delusion that they were able to fly. There is also evidence that the drug can produce genetic damage with effects on subsequent children.

The hallucinogens are not drugs of addiction leading to dependence, but they are more immediately harmful because of their effects on the brain and the transmission of nerve-impulses.

lumbago. Any pain in the small of the back is commonly called lumbago but the causes may be diverse and include specific lesions such as lumbar strain, osteo-arthritis and prolapsed inter-vertebral disc. The term is best reserved for the condition of fibrositis affecting the muscles and their associated fascial structures in the lumbar region of the back, which is immediately below the waist.

The symptoms, which may be acute or chronic, are predominantly pain and muscular spasm. In acute lumbago the pain and disability may be very severe, the patient being quite unable to straighten his back from a semi-stooping position.

Immediate treatment includes measures such as rest, warmth and physiotherapy, coupled with the use of analgesics to relieve the pain. Prevention of recurrence requires the removal or correction of pre-disposing factors and the treatment of any identifiable general disease.

See also BACKACHE; RHEUMATISM, MUSCULAR.

lumbar puncture. The tapping of the space between the spinal cord and its enveloping membranes in the lumbar region for diagnostic or therapeutic purposes in cases of injury or disease of the CENTRAL NERVOUS SYSTEM. The fluid in the space is drawn off through a hollow needle. Also known as 'spinal tap', the procedure is practically painless in skilled hands.

The pressure with which the cerebro-spinal fluid emerges, its appearance, its composition, and its bacteriological state are all of diagnostic significance and provide evidence about the brain and spinal cord, the presence of fresh or old haemorrhage, and the presence and nature of any infection.

In certain infections the lumbar puncture (intrathecal) route is the best for the administration of selected drugs.

lungs. The pair of organs in the RESPIRATORY SYSTEM where the oxygenation of the blood takes place.

lupus. Originally used to describe a chronic degenerative skin condition with swelling and ulceration, the term is now always used with a second term specifying the type. For example: (1) lupus erythematosus is a general illness which may be chronic (with skin lesions alone), subacute, or disseminated, in which there may be involvement of blood vessels or nerves; (2) lupus vulgaris is a form of tuberculosis of the skin.

lymph. A transparent fluid, sometimes slightly yellow and opalescent, collected from the tissues throughout the body. It flows through the LYMPHATIC SYSTEM and comprises a clear liquid portion, varying numbers of white blood cells and a few red blood cells.

lymphadenoma. See HODGKIN'S DISEASE.

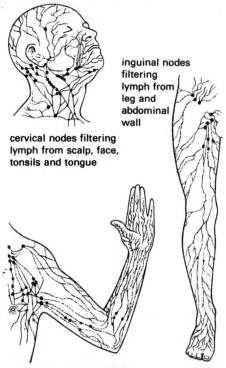

inguinal nodes filtering lymph from leg and abdominal wall

cervical nodes filtering lymph from scalp, face, tonsils and tongue

axillary nodes, filtering lymph from arm and chest wall

The superficial lymphatic system

lymphatic system. The capillaries, collecting channels and trunks that collect LYMPH from the tissues and carry it via the main lymph vessels, the thoracic duct and the right lymphatic duct into veins at the base of the neck.

The lymphatic vessels are absorbent in function, preventing the accumulation of excess fluid in the tissues, and carrying in the lymph a good deal of the fat absorbed during digestion into the blood stream. The lymphatics play an important part in drainage from an infected area, the lymph nodes acting as a filter against the spread of infection. The long-held view that the lymphatics contribute only to the spread of malignant disease is being modified in the light of considerable current research into the nature of body defences against cancer.

Lymph glands. Numerous flattened, oval or rounded structures located along the course of lymphatic vessels. They vary greatly in size, from 1 to 25 mm. in diameter. Several lymph vessels enter on one side of the gland and usually a single vessel leaves on the opposite side, the gland acting as a filter against the spread of infection. Normally, the lymph passes through one or more lymph glands or nodes on its way to the blood stream, and the glands are particularly numerous in the neck, pelvis, and abdomen and around the lungs. They consist of masses of lymphocytes enclosed in a fibrous capsule. The lymph nodes are important in the body's system of defence against disease, both because of their filter action and also because they produce lymphocytes, a form of white blood cell, which help combat infection.

Diseases. These generally take the form of a swelling of the glands, with or without pain.

Acute infection is often associated with painful enlargement of the local lymph glands, while chronic inflammation occurs particularly in tuberculosis and syphilis, in which it is painless. In all cases of infection treatment is by attention to the original cause, with appropriate antibiotic therapy.

Primary cancer of the lymph nodes is not common, while secondary deposits of a malignancy is a frequent cause of lymph node enlargement.

In HODGKIN'S DISEASE and LEUKAEMIA the lymph nodes are one amongst several other tissue groups usually involved.

lymphogranuloma venereum. An infectious disease spread by sexual contact and affecting the lymph-channels and lymph-glands related to the genitalia. It causes enlargement of glands in the groin and this may be followed by the development of pus and ulcers on the overlying skin. Other complications are stricture of the rectum and coarsening of the skin. There may also be general disturbance with fever, chills, headache and loss of appetite.

The condition is due to a minute organism of the genus *Bedsonia;* it occurs chiefly in tropical and sub-tropical regions and may be both protracted and disabling. The incubation period is very variable, from a few days to several months, and the individual is infectious as long as there are active lesions.

Treatment by sulphonamides or the tetracyclines is effective but one attack does not confer immunity.

M

McBurney's point. A rather vaguely defined position low down on the right of the abdomen, first described by the American surgeon, Charles McBurney. It lies about one-third of the way along an imaginary line from the front spine of the right hip bone to the umbilicus. In a typical case of appendicitis, tenderness on pressure is maximum at this point.

macule. A spot or blemish on the same level as the surrounding skin, as contrasted with a papule which is raised above the surface. A rash is commonly described, according to the position of the spots, as being macular or papular.

maladjusted child. A child who shows evidence of emotional instability or psychological disturbance in ways that have a bad effect on himself or his companions and who cannot, without expert assistance, be helped by his parents, teachers or other adults with whom he ordinarily comes into contact.

It has been estimated that between 5 and 10 per cent of children of school age are maladjusted although no simple criteria of diagnosis exist. Maladjustment may show itself through the child's return to more infantile patterns of bowel and bladder control, by timidity or a withdrawal into fantasy, by failure to make progress in class or a sudden deterioration in school work, by playing truant, by temper tantrums, or by dishonest, aggressive or destructive behaviour which may end in delinquency. The variety of symptoms suggests that there is no single cause for the condition.

It is often said that NEUROSIS is responsible for a large proportion of maladjusted children with PSYCHOSIS accounting for some cases and yet others attributed vaguely to personality disorder. Clearly there are many factors involved in the creation of maladjustment: the child's genetic inheritance may make him more able or less able to endure stresses without damage to his personality; long-term psychological and social factors may deprive him of the affection and security needed for personality development; over-forcing by ambitious parents, over-strictness and over-indulgence may play parts; occasionally a sudden event that utterly shocks the child may be a precipitating factor; and perhaps a minor degree of maladjustment is part of the normal process of growing up – with the child increasingly seeking to decide his own actions but lacking an adult's experience of life. Broadly, long-term deprivations seem more important than single shocking events; and study of maladjusted children reveals that many of them come from broken homes or homes in which marital disharmony is marked.

Identification of the maladjusted child depends largely on the awareness and understanding of teachers, school doctors and school nurses, but also on their belief that available treatment facilities are really useful. So the provision of an efficient child guidance clinic in an area may actually appear to increase maladjustment.

Anti-social behaviour among boys tends to come more to notice than among girls, at least until the age of puberty. Hence far more boys than girls receive treatment for maladjustment. Again, teachers and school nurses concerned with secondary education come to expect a little abnormal behaviour among adolescents and to regard it in most cases as not needing prolonged skilled treatment. So there are roughly four times as many referrals of primary as of secondary children to child guidance clinics.

The child guidance clinics of the school health services provide the corner-stone of treatment of maladjusted children. A full investigation of the child by a team consisting of a child psychiatrist or specially qualified medical officer, a psychologist and a psychiatric social worker is normally carried out. When the investigation, which is often long and involved, is completed, the same team institutes treatment. Though a day or residential school for maladjusted children may be recommended it is felt that most children are best helped by being treated in their usual school and home environment. In all cases, the child's psychological disorders require appropriate treatment, and his home circumstances careful assessment and possible adjustment. Treatment is often prolonged and difficult. Reliable estimates of success and failure rates do not exist. In any case, the child often requires support into early adult life.

Although a sizeable slice of the work of health visitors in Britain and public health nurses in the U.S.A. consists in trying to create stable emotional conditions for children and in seeking to educate parents about children's requirements for mental and social development, the general improvement in children's physical health and physical environment does not appear to have been accompanied by a similar reduction in maladjustment. There are at least two possible explanations: (1) that external stresses acting on parents (e.g., wars, unemployment and fear of redundancy) have adversely affected the domestic environment of children; and (2) that standards of diagnosis have altered, so that a child who would have been regarded merely as 'highly strung' twenty years ago is now classed as sufficiently disturbed to need treatment at a child guidance clinic. Probably both explanations contain a considerable element of truth.

malaria. A tropical or sub-tropical disease of man and certain other animals, caused by the presence of the parasite *Plasmodium* in the red blood cells. It is transmitted by the bite of an affected female mosquito of the genus *Anopheles* which has previously sucked the blood of a malaria sufferer. The plasmodia reproduce in the human at frequent intervals, each entry of a new generation of the parasite into the red blood cells giving rise to a further acute malarial attack. Such an attack consists of a chill, accompanied and followed by a fever and general symptoms, and terminates in a sweating stage. Attacks recur at 48-hour, 72-hour or less definite intervals, depending on which of the four species of *Plasmodium* known to affect man is responsible. An attack of malaria may simply end in recovery quite

spontaneously (with or without subsequent relapses months or years later), or it may, in the case of *Plasmodium falciparium* malaria, proceed to involve the brain and also, possibly, the kidneys, leading to severe illness and frequently death.

Those raised in malarious areas develop quite a strong immunity to the more severe forms of the disease, but generally at the cost of being anaemic, emaciated, and depressed as a result of repeated attacks.

Malaria may be prevented by the elimination of anopheles mosquitoes from areas of human habitation by use of insecticides. Hundreds of millions of people have thus been freed, in the last twenty-five years, from the possibility of malarious attack, though permanent watchfulness has to be maintained to prevent the re-establishment of the mosquito. Where the mosquito continues to breed, protection against malaria is obtained by using insect repellents, fitting window screens, etc. to reduce the possibility of being bitten, and above all by the regular use of appropriate anti-malarial drugs. Those visiting a possibly malarious area, however briefly, must take suppressive drugs throughout the visit and for the following four weeks.

Chloroquine has long been the most useful of a number of drugs for the treatment of acute and chronic cases of malaria. It has mostly replaced quinine.

Research into the possibility of immunization against malaria is well advanced.

male climacteric. See CLIMACTERIC.

malignant. From the Latin *malignus*, evil. The term is applied to those tumours (such as cancer and sarcoma) which spread so that the disease appears in other parts of the body. This is in contrast with benign tumours which do not give rise to these 'secondaries' and cause trouble merely by pressure. The term is also applied to abnormally serious forms of disease, e.g., malignant smallpox and malignant hypertension. Malignant pustule is a name sometimes given to the inflamed swelling that is usually the first indication of anthrax.

malingering. Deliberate feigning or exaggeration of illness or injury, usually for one of three reasons – to avoid work, especially unpleasant tasks; to obtain compensation for an injury; or to secure sympathy. Malingering involving physical signs can generally be detected because the person counterfeiting an illness seldom knows or can imitate all its signs and because prolonged maintenance of a sign is difficult: for instance, the person feigning pneumonia may deliberately speed his respiration and may take a drug to quicken his pulse rate, but when he falls asleep the respiratory rate drops immediately. Where the malingerer relies on symptoms, diagnosis is much more difficult: for example, nobody except the victim can be certain whether the suspected case of appendicitis really feels abdominal pain and actually experiences tenderness when a finger is pressed on McBurney's point. In many cases of malingering there is some existing pain or disability which the patient exaggerates, and the diagnosis of malingering and of INCAPACITY TO WORK in such circumstances is one of the most difficult tasks confronting a doctor, especially as people have widely differing degrees of susceptibility and sensitivity to pain.

A doctor who suspects malingering is wise to carry out extensive tests and to seek a second opinion before making an accusation; and even where a person is definitely malingering there may be need for treatment of the psychological condition that causes him to seek to avoid work or to crave for sympathy.

malnutrition. The end result of eating too little of the right kinds of food. Strictly, its use should be restricted to those nutritional disorders, such as rickets and scurvy, which are due to lack of specific nutrients in the diet. However, it is generally taken to include the results of general underfeeding.

The primary causes of most malnutrition occurring in the world are poverty and ignorance. Thus even in affluent, developed countries a comparatively small minority of the population is affected through failure to maintain a good DIET; these include the elderly, migrant workers and their families, the lowest paid, and the chronically unemployed. Severe malnutrition in such countries is uncommon (though it has been estimated that up to 2 per cent of the total population of the U.S.A. suffers from malnutrition, and the percentages in certain groups such as the Eskimos and Indians may be extremely high). In virtually all the underdeveloped countries the overwhelming majority of the population is subject to malnutrition. Uneducated in nutritional requirements, ill-versed in agricultural techniques (or landless and unemployed), and racked by intestinal parasites, hundreds of millions of people are frankly under-nourished or become so with the failure of even one harvest and its attendant food-price inflation.

By far the most important dietary deficiency disease is protein-calorie malnutrition, which affects tens of millions of children in Asia, Africa, the Middle East, the Caribbean, and Latin America. Its effects range from those caused mainly by protein deprivation, i.e., kwashiorkor, to marasmus, caused by severe continuous restriction of calories, protein and other nutrients. Intermediate states are generally found. When protein and energy requirements are most needed to meet the demands of growth, as in infancy, childhood, and at puberty, insufficient protein in the diet, generally accompanied by restricted calorie intake, leads to the development of kwashiorkor. In populations living on minimal protein and calorie intake, kwashiorkor epidemics may be precipitated by outbreaks of feverish illness such as malaria or measles, or by infestation with malarial parasites. The disease may affect people of all ages, but is commonest in children between the ages of 1 and 4 years, occurring after weaning from the breast to an unsuitable diet low in protein and calories, such as maize porridge.   Marasmus, by contrast, principally affects infants under one year of age. It generally follows the early failure or deliberate ending of breast feeding and its replacement by dilute milk, milk products or other diet low in both calories and protein. In addition, unhygienic preparation of such food leads to repeated gastro-intestinal infections, which the mother all too often treats by virtual starvation for long periods.

Protein malnutrition carries a high death rate even amongst those who receive skilled treatment. And though even children with very severe kwashiorkor or marasmus may be 'cured' through careful dietary measures, education of the mother in sound nutritional practice is equally vital if relapses are to be prevented. Treatment should thus include a minimum of modern medical technology, and the maximum opportunity for learning through practice.

Prerequisites for the prevention of protein malnutrition are: general health and nutritional education, the abolition of urban poverty, the introduction of appropriate agricultural technology, malaria and measles prevention programmes, and effective population control. Similarly, the prevention of most nutritional disorders amongst the potentially affected groups in affluent countries requires combined health educational and social measures.

There are a number of medical conditions which cause malnutrition in spite of a good diet. These include steatorrhoea which limits the absorption of calcium and fat-soluble vitamins, cirrhosis of the liver which may interfere with the proper utilization of nutrients, and a kidney disorder in which there is loss of protein in the urine.

In addition, insufficiency of MINERAL SALT causes disease, e.g., anaemia resulting from lack of iron or goitre from lack of iodine; and there are a considerable number of DEFICIENCY DISEASES, caused by insufficiency of one or more of the specific vitamins.

Malta fever. See BRUCELLOSIS.

mammography. An x-ray examination of the breasts, or (more frequently nowadays) examination of the breasts by infra-red rays. This can often reveal the existence of a tumour or cyst at an early stage when treatment is easier and more effective than if diagnosis is not made until the swelling can be seen and felt.

mania. Often used as a loose term, applied to any form of mental disorder or even a strong preoccupation, such as stamp collecting, religion etc.; the medical definition of mania, however, is the manic phase of a MANIC-DEPRESSIVE PSYCHOSIS.

manic-depressive psychosis. A disorder of mood in which excitement and mania alternate with periods of depression; delusions are prominent and suicide is relatively common. A specific cause has not been identified. Inheritance plays some part, about 5 to 10 per cent of sufferers having had a parent similarly affected, but many other factors are also recognized: childbirth, the climacteric, head injury, severe infection (particularly influenza), bereavement, financial problems, and difficulties in personal relationships. These factors may act alone or together; but on the other hand often no cause can be identified. Prevention, except partially by genetic counselling, is not possible.

The depressive phase of the illness usually begins and ends gradually, though abrupt transitions may occur. It is characterized by a general slowing down of all the faculties. Appetite and sexual desire are diminished. Sleep often ends at 3 or 4 am, to be followed by hours of fitful dozing. Confidence and interest are lost, as is the ability to experience pleasure. Slowed down in this fashion, the person's life often becomes filled with preoccupations and worries from which he is unable to escape. Such an attack may last for weeks or months. If more severely affected, the person may become obsessed by past failure and misery, and profoundly pessimistic about the future. Filled with self-reproach and self-depreciation his worries often develop into delusions of, for example, poverty, or his own wickedness, or even that he is dead. Suicidal ideas may be present, and suicidal attempts may occur in any person with more than a mild degree of depression so that some cases do end in suicide. Most, however, gradually recover spontaneously, though a few pass into the manic phase. A substantial number have repeated attacks and a few develop chronic depression. Mild cases may be treated in their own homes with anti-depressant drugs by day, sleeping pills by night, and the pursuance of a regular, undemanding daily routine, including work where possible. The more severely depressed are admitted to hospital and generally receive electro-convulsive and drug therapy.

The manic phase of the illness is uncommon. It is characterized by an increase in activity with lessened self-restraint. Work efficiency is generally unaffected in the mild early stages of an attack, but the person may be indiscreet and extravagant, and unpersuadable, through loss of insight, of the abnormality of his behaviour. If he passes into mania his activity gets out of hand; with incessant speech, shouting and singing, and apparently purposeless activity his state of excitement becomes socially unbearable. Often neglecting his food, he may be unable to sleep, and may have increased sexual desire and decreased sexual restraint. Manic attacks are usually shorter than depressive ones, and most recover spontanously, but relapse is common and a few patients develop chronic mania. Treatment is generally undertaken in hospital and includes the use of tranquillizers.

In all cases of manic-depressive psychosis, consideration of a patient's underlying personality and environment is vital in providing treatment. During the recovery period attention has to be given both to improving the person's adjustment to life and to making changes in his domestic, work and social environment.

Manic-depressive psychosis, including involutional MELANCHOLIA, occurs in about one person in a hundred throughout a lifetime, affecting women about twice as frequently as men.

manipulation. A rather vague term that covers the setting of broken bones, the replacement of dislocated joints, the breaking down of adhesions that have rendered active movement of a joint difficult or impossible and the treatment of various diseases by movement of the spine.

The placing of the broken ends of a fractured bone in the best position for successful healing is a very ancient part of medical treatment – mentioned in the Egyptian *Surgical Papyrus* of about 1600 B.C. and has given rise to the modern speciality of manipulative surgery, while assisted movement of joints stiffened by disease or injury has similarly given rise to physiotherapy.

Outside orthodox medicine lie two systems of manipulation: chiropractic, which is based on the idea that many (or all) diseases are caused by pressure on nerves and can be cured by appropriate manipulation of the spine; and osteopathy (founded by A. T. Still in 1874) which rejects all drugs, serums and vaccines and maintains that all disease is caused by osteopathic lesions that result from pressure of displaced bones or contracted muscles on nerves or arteries.

It is very easy to dismiss both chiropractic and osteopathy as 'quackery' and to argue that any form of treatment given by a person exuding both confidence and sympathy will achieve some successes; but orthodox medicine was perhaps at first over-keen to deny that any diseases might be caused by pressure on nerves. Manipulative methods by persons not medically qualified have had some startling successes (and some often unpublished equally startling failures) and orthodox medicine has learned considerably from them: as a well-known surgeon, Sir James Paget wrote as early as 1867 in a careful description of the work of bone-setters (the precursors of the osteopaths), 'The lessons which you can learn from their practice are plain and useful'. However, in the vast majority of diseases x-ray examination reveals no evidence of displaced bones or of pressure on nerves or blood vessels, and orthodox methods – such as the use of the antibiotics, vaccines, etc., that osteopaths reject – have proved completely successful. The human body and the human mind are too complex to allow of all disorders responding to a single system of treatment.

Mantoux test. See BCG VACCINATION.

marasmus. A disease of MALNUTRITION caused by lack of calories, protein and other nutrients. It is particularly associated with the weaning of infants from breast feeding to an inadequate diet.

marihuana. A form of the drug CANNABIS.

marital disharmony. Discord in marriage which may be overcome or go on to complete marital breakdown. The extent and nature of marital disharmony in our society is unknown. The statistics of such bodies as the Marriage Guidance Council refer only to the minority who seek their help, while divorce statistics refer only to those marriages which end in the divorce courts, which many tens of thousands of very discordant marriages never do. Furthermore, causes of marital breakdown accepted by divorce courts – adultery desertion, cruelty, and so forth – tell little about the underlying causes of disharmony, many of which reflect individual and social expectations of marriage and the extent to which couples are able to fulfil them to their satisfaction. For example, in a society such as our own, which places great emphasis on romantic love and sexual exclusiveness within marriage, a single sexual peccadillo has often been enough to precipitate complete marital breakdown. By contrast, until modern times at least, middle class marriages in France were more often arranged with considerations of birth and fortune in mind, and discreet extra-marital liaisons, albeit only by the husband, were tolerated.

The main causes of contemporary marital disharmony are probably emotional immaturity and sexual dissatisfaction. The younger the age of the couple at marriage the greater is their chance of appearing in the divorce courts. Teenagers are rarely equipped to cope with the demanding relationships of marriage, and seldom have the capacity for sexual relationships mature enough to give their marriage a good start. Husband and wife often develop in conflicting directions as they emerge into emotional adulthood, and the arrival of a baby may mean that the young mother becomes preoccupied with the child while the young father seeks other interests. There is much evidence to suggest that marriage (and, with it, parenthood) should be postponed until the mid-twenties, though not infrequently, unfortunately, emotional immaturity persists through life.

As the expectation of sexual fulfilment in marriage – the giving and receiving of delight which deepens and reinforces the bond between the partners – has increased, so has the disharmony consequent upon sexual dissatisfaction. This dissatisfaction, e.g., when the women has pain on intercourse (usually capable of remedy) or where the man reaches his climax early (again often remediable), is an important cause of breakdown in marriages in which joint conjugal roles operate (see MARRIAGE). Such breakdown generally occurs in the early years of marriage.

Disharmony in segregated-role marriages most often centres around cruelty and financial irresponsibility, particularly by the husband. Here, if breakdown occurs it is usually later, when the children are physically more independent. Though it is generally recognized that harm may be caused to children by the divorce of their parents, many underestimate the potentially harmful effects of continued upbringing by constantly bickering parents.

The appearance of marital disharmony generally calls forth an informal network of advice from relatives and friends, usually to the partners individually. They may usefully seek the help of their family doctor, their minister of religion or a marriage guidance organization. Though most instances of marital harmony are thus resolved some inevitably result in DIVORCE, the number of divorces in a society being more a reflection of the liberality of its divorce laws and the cost of obtaining a divorce than an accurate statement of the number of marriages irretrievably broken down. Something like 20 per cent of British and American marriages end in divorce.

marriage. A union between a man and a woman such that the children borne by the woman are recognized as the legitimate offspring of both spouses.

Forms of marriage. One of the oldest social institutions, marriage in some form is virtually universal in human society. The two basic forms of marriage are monogamy and polygamy. In monogamy a person is allowed only one spouse at a time. The term polygamy covers both polyandry, which is extremely rare, in which a woman is permitted more than one husband at a time, and polygyny, in which a man is permitted more than one wife at a time. In general, monogamy is normal in highly organized modern societies, and polygamy is largely confined to less developed societies. In the latter, monogamous marriage is nevertheless often by far the commonest form, polygyny being practised only by men able to support more than one family. Polygyny is not however confined to less sophisticated cultures: it is upheld as an ideal by Islam, is practised in parts of India and Latin America, and until recently was widespread in China.

Polygamy is not capable of comprehension in a monogamous society, based on sexual exclusiveness. In Muslim society, however, a woman's self-esteem, emotional security, and reputation are fully compatible with being one of several wives since the number of wives a man has is generally a reflection of the social standing of his family, and his wealth and income. However, the tendency even in Muslim societies is for the spread of monogamy to accompany economic development, education, and modern social organization.

Choice of spouse. In all societies pre-marital sexual relationships are strictly coded, choice of spouse is bound by certain rules, and anti-adultery customs are widespread. The taboo against incest appears to be universal nowadays, though brother-sister marriages are known to have occurred amongst the Inca royal family, and the Pharaohs of Ancient Egypt traditionally married their sisters. Strong pressures towards marrying a family member prevailed amongst European royalty until modern times, and cousin marriage is still commonplace in many societies. The desire to limit the spread of power and wealth must be regarded as the main underlying reasons for such practices. Conversely, desire to limit the occurrence of x-linked and autosomal recessive hereditary disease provides contemporary scientific support for the custom (which is widespread in monogamous culture) of marrying out of both the family and, very often, the community.

The choice of spouse may be made by the parents or other close relations of eligible persons, by recognized marriage brokers within the community, or by the couple themselves. The latter is the almost universal practice in modern societies and is, at a greatly varying rate, coming to replace arranged marriages in almost all societies in which these take place. For all its appearance to the contrary, even the arrangement of marriage by the couple themselves operates within strictly defined limits. Because of the basic necessity that the couple have to meet each other, geographical and social limitations operate: thus people tend to marry those of their own district, religion, race, social class, and educational level. Amongst university graduates the last consideration appears to be the most important, whilst the development of greater geographical mobility and the drift towards a single world culture seems gradually to be making the other factors less important.

Conjugal roles within monogamous marriage. These are determined by the social, legal and religious frameworks within which marriage takes place, as well as by the families of origin of the spouses and their own personal attributes. Marriage roles adapt and develop as children are born and the family develops, and particularly as the changes in the social standing and activities of women develop.

In pre-industrial societies the conjugal roles of men and women are separate, distinct and forbidden to one another. The husband provides, takes risks, or performs heavy labouring tasks, and he may indeed, without outraging social conventions, enforce his authority by chastising not only his children but also his wife. Meanwhile the wife keeps house and bears and rears children. In modern industrial society most women engage in wage earning before marriage and after their period of childbearing and pre-school child rearing is over. Decision-making has come to be a shared function, with neither partner dominant, although on any one matter the couple may recognize that one member has greater expertise or experience, e.g., that on failure to reach agreement they will normally accept the husband's view of the best lawnmower or the wife's view of the best cooker to buy.

Yet in spite of their increased economic value to society as a whole, and to their marriages in particular, the ability of women to exercise their rights is limited by their childbearing function, by their exclusion from some traditional male occupations, and by the persistence of traditional attitudes and values. These however are adjusting, though unevenly, where they conflict with new industrial and social developments.

It is sometimes alleged that a common cause of MARITAL DISHARMONY in persons of differing backgrounds or different races is unharmonized ideas of conjugal roles, as when the husband enters matrimony with the idea that he is the dominant partner while the wife starts marriage with the concept of equality. Difficulties of conjugal roles are also liable to arise where one partner is absent for a long period (e.g., the soldier returning from war service) so that, by the time of the return the other partner has become accustomed to making the decisions for the household.

Contemporary patterns of conjugal roles reflect the uneven pace of change in different groups in modern society. The evolution of 'joint' conjugal roles is progressing rapidly throughout the world, with husbands sharing domestic work and child rearing as wives share the role of provider. However, such tendencies are still poorly developed amongst the lower-paid and less educated, where 'segregated' conjugal roles are usual – with wives responsible for housework, child care and budgeting, and husbands for providing basic house-keeping money, doing occasional ardous tasks about the home, and being the ultimate child disciplinarian. Those in joint-role marriages more often take their relaxation in the home, together and with friends of both sexes, and have greater expectations of the sexual satisfactions to be obtained from marriage. Joint- and segregated-role marriages are extreme types; most marriages are intermediate with a bias towards one type or the other.

Trends in marriage. Although marriage generally takes place later amongst the better-off and better educated, for a long time the age at marriage has been dropping amongst people of all social origins, though this trend has shown signs of reversal in recent years. The consequences of early marriage are manifold. Divorce rates are much higher amongst those married in their teens and child management is sometimes poor where the parents are themselves hardly mature. On the other hand the advantages of early completion of families, which accompanies a lower age of marriage, include fewer complications of childbirth and a lower risk of producing a mongol child. Marriage appears to be conducive to better health and, on average, married people who are admitted to hospital are discharged sooner than unmarrieds, marriage providing a valuable social support system. Throughout this century the prevalence of marriage, and the esteem in which the married state is held, have increased steadily. The consequent eagerness of people on the one hand to enter marriage, and on the other to expect to achieve contentment as of right, is reflected in the increasing number of marriages which fail. The considerable liberalization of divorce laws in most industrial societies allows partners in failed marriages to dissolve their marriage contract and become available for re-marriage. In consequence divorce rates are also rising rapidly, and an increasing number of young people reaching marriageable age are the products of marriages which have failed. This cannot but influence the pattern of marriage of the future.

masochism. A sexual PERVERSION or deviation in which the person derives pleasure from being beaten, punished, humiliated or abused, usually by someone of the opposite sex. The term, which is in many ways the opposite of SADISM, is named after an Austrian writer, Leopold von Sacher-Masoch (1836-95), whose books provide copious examples of this abnormality.

Freud called masochism 'The most frequent and significant of all perversions'. In the typical form the individual is controlled by the idea of being completely and unconditionally subject to the will of an attractive person of the opposite sex; he often spends much of his time in fantasies of being whipped or abused, with generally one form of punishment (e.g., beating on the buttocks) and one imagined punisher predominating; he tries to realize these fantasies with the person of his choice or with a substitute; he obtains his sexual pleasure from this experienced (or sometimes imagined) passively endured violence; and he is incapable of finding sexual satisfaction in normal ways. In many cases, however, the desire for punishment never goes beyond the fantasy level, and where the fantasy is realized the whipping is often a preparation for sexual relations rather than a substitute for them.

Early investigators often termed masochism a female characteristic – an exaggeration of the common female desire to run and be captured or to be mastered in a mock-fight; but it has been shown that it is also very common in men. It is difficult to get an assessment of the number of men who let themselves be slapped or caned by their wives, but some writers state that nearly all prostitutes possess a small whip for use on those of their customers who desire it.

Some cases of masochism undoubtedly originate in a child being beaten for masturbating and coming to associate the humiliation and pain of the beating with the pleasure of masturbation. It is sometimes alleged that the deviation may start with the sensuous excitement in childhood when a mother embraces the child and gently pats his buttocks. On the causes of masochism we have a great deal of psychological theorizing and very little proved fact.

While a sadist is potentially dangerous to others, since he enjoys inflicting pain and may do serious damage, a masochist is not dangerous. The pain is inflicted on himself, and there comes a point in which the initial pain-pleasure feeling is destroyed by the intensity of the pain, so that the masochist seeks the cessation of the punishment.

The term is coming to be used in a wider sense that implies enjoying one's own helplessness or suffering, or deliberately denying oneself enjoyment and success, or punishing oneself (e.g., by excessive work) perhaps as a reaction to forbidden desires. It is also increasingly held that sadism and masochism are only the extremes of the spectrum of human attitudes: while few of us would normally enjoy inflicting pain on others and while relatively few of us would enjoy being whipped by an attractive member of the opposite sex, perhaps most of us have a mild streak of sadism (and occasionally enjoy dominating and mastering) and also a mild streak of masochism (so that we at times relish being 'ticked off' by our partners).

massage. Treatment by stroking, rubbing or kneading the superficial parts of the body with the hand or with an instrument, for such purposes as restoring the power of movement, breaking up ADHESIONS, improving the circulation, aiding digestion, or simply in order to produce a sense of relaxation and well-being. Massage is commonly employed in physiotherapy as an important part of an integrated physical rehabilitation programme. It is widely and increasingly available on a commercial basis in many countries.

mastitis. Inflammation of the female breast. It occurs generally in the early weeks of breast feeding as a result of infection developing in stagnant milk which is lying in the broken surface of uncared-for cracked nipples. Part of the breast becomes hard and tender and the overlying skin reddened. Treatment is by antibiotics, prevention of milk accumulation by proper care of CRACKED NIPPLES, and kaolin poultices. Breast feeding need only be interrupted if pus is present, in which case incision and drainage is required. Mastitis rarely occurs when the simple rules of breast care and hygiene are observed.

mastoid disease. A complication of otitis media (middle ear infection), in which infection spreads from the middle ear to involve the mastoid bone behind the ear, leading to pain, increased discharge or its sudden cessation, increasing deafness and general debility. As permanent deafness, meningitis, or even brain abscess may result from neglected mastoid disease, the doctor's advice should be sought if earache is troublesome. Treatment is by antibiotics and sometimes an operation is necessary. Mastoid disease is prevented by prompt recognition and adequate treatment of otitis media. It is now rare in Britain, but still common in underdeveloped countries.

masturbation. Attempted satisfaction of one's sexual urges alone and unaided. Commonly the hands, fingers and thighs are used to stimulate the head of the penis or the clitoris. This generally results in orgasm within a few minutes. It is widely practised from early childhood onwards, and is a harmless substitute for sexual intercourse except when it interferes with the establishment of normal heterosexual relations, or when feelings of guilt resulting from it lead to personality conflicts. Unfortunately, as a result of erroneous opinions expressed by doctors and others in the past, these guilt feelings are quite widespread.

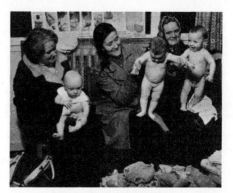

Maternal and child welfare

maternal and child welfare. An omnibus term – nowadays often altered to maternal and child health – for services designed to promote the physical and mental health of both mother and child, and to prevent, recognize and treat departures from health in the expectant and nursing mother, the unborn child, the infant, and the pre-school child. Broadly the term includes antenatal, post-natal and child health clinics, the work of obstetricians and midwives, much of the work of health visitors and part of the work of paediatricians. Essentially the services aim to improve the health of mother and child, so that the mother gives birth to her child with the minimum danger and discomfort and without deleterious effects on her own health, while the child is born healthy and receives adequate care until he starts school.

History of provision for maternal welfare. From the dawn of human history aid has been given to the child-bearing woman. The quality of care it afforded may be considered as a significant index of the civilization of a community. At the height of the ancient Egyptian civilization, and of the Greek and Roman civilizations, the art of caring for child-bearing women was well developed. It later declined and did not regain its former level of development until the sixteenth and seventeenth century. Until the nineteenth century doctors in most developed countries did not attend childbirth. Most deliveries were undertaken by midwives qualified only by experience.

The pattern of development varies from country to country: e.g., in some the profession of midwife remained separate from nursing while in others the intending midwife took a full nursing training followed by a course in midwifery, and in many countries confinement in hospital became almost invariable while in a few home confinement remained common. Development in the U.K. is here outlined as an illustration of progress in a western country.

Following the foundation of the Midwives' Institute in 1881 an Act of 1902 established midwifery training and regulated midwifery practice; and, as the discovery of the causes and means of control of puerperal fever made hospital obstetrics safer, there came a gradual change from private domiciliary practice to hospital confinement. An Act of 1918 made local authorities responsible for providing a full range of services for maternal and child welfare – antenatal care, skilled attendance at confinement whether in hospital or at home (with, in the latter case, midwives entitled to call doctors at need), post-natal care, health visiting services and child welfare clinics.

Apart from the transfer of responsibility for maternity hospital from local authorities to the State in 1948 these services continued and steadily expanded until 1974. Increased provision and uptake of antenatal care and better obstetrics contributed greatly to the reduction of maternal deaths and of stillbirths and early infant deaths. Confinement is nowadays in hospital in over 90 per cent of cases, delivery being mainly by midwives but with obstetric specialists available at need. In recent years increasing stress has been laid on psychological and social preparation for confinement and for the arrival of the baby, on health education classes and on psychoprophylaxis, whether provided by health visitors or by midwives or by both in conjunction.

Achievements of maternal welfare services. The greatest achievement has undoubtedly been to cut maternal mortality from around 10 per cent in mid-Victorian times to 0.2 per cent by the early 1940s with subsequent further reduction in the era of chemotherapy and antibiotics, which completed the virtual eradication of sepsis. The control of haemorrhage and the reduction in mortality from toxaemia (at least partly explained by better antenatal care) have contributed to a continuing decline in the number of deaths. Even so, confidential enquiry reveals that half of all maternal deaths in Britain are still associated with an 'avoidable factor', implying that some aspect of care was inadequate by current standards of practice. The great fall in the perinatal mortality which has accompanied the fall in maternal mortality can be attributed in large part to the provision of good maternal welfare services. Immeasurable is the increase in confidence of expectant mothers which has taken place in the last hundred years.

Two recent developments in the provision for maternal welfare concern the prevention of childbirth. The Abortion Act of 1967 greatly extended the provision of legal abortion in Britain, and has resulted in the substantial reduction of maternal mortality from illegal abortion. The National Health Service (Family Planning) Act of 1967 empowered local authorities to provide contraceptive advice for women on medical and social grounds. In 1974 contraceptives were made available on prescription as a regular part of the Health Service; this it was hoped would help to reduce the growing demand for abortion and discourage its use as a method of birth control.

Development of child welfare services. Child welfare (or health) clinics have developed throughout the world since the last years of the nineteenth century when Infant Consultation and Milk Depots were founded in France. In Britain their introduction by all local authorities was a requirement of the 1918 Act. Prior to that time the voluntary provision for infants consisted of home visiting, depots for the distribution of cheap, safe milk to mothers unable to breast feed, and consultation clinics for medical supervision. The local authorities gradually developed and improved these services. As well as following the progress of pre-school children, under medical and health visitor supervision, many child welfare centres provided cheap or free food; and later, cod-liver oil, dried milk and vitamin supplements became available at the centres. In modern times they have become a focal point for advice and education about all matters affecting the physical and emotional health of young children, as well as for immunization, medical consultation, screening of eyesight, hearing, and general development, and ascertainment of handicap; but, since many mothers seldom attend centres, the home visits of health visitors are perhaps even more important. Since 1948 general practitioners have increasingly undertaken child welfare work, seeing their own patients at their surgery, the local authority clinic, or a health centre. The trend to attachment of health visitors to general practice has therefore been generally welcomed. All local authority Maternal and Child Welfare Services were taken over by Area Health Boards at the reorganization of the National Health Service in 1974.

Welfare services are particularly required by working mothers, unmarried mothers, and their children. Local authority social work departments are required to provide day nurseries and to supervise all other provision of day care of pre-school children. Priority for admission to day nurseries is generally given to children of single parents, including those of unmarried mothers. In addition the social work departments have particular responsibilities in the field of adoption and foster care of children.

Achievements of child welfare services. The development of child welfare services in Britain roughly coincided with other changes likely to improve the health of children – decreased family size, improved living standards and introduction of effective treatment. Nevertheless, many studies have shown beyond a shadow of doubt the enormous value of child welfare services (now more often called child health services), e.g., sharp reduction of infant deaths in areas that had increased their health visiting staffs and their clinics without any similar reduction in deaths in comparable areas that had not achieved increases, and in due course a fall in deaths in the latter areas after they had belatedly extended their staffs. Broadly, these services have been responsible for almost all the education carried out on infant health and well-being – from nutrition to requirements for mental development, and from prevention of burns and scalds to encouragement of immunization. Some visiting of apparently healthy children remains necessary, to maintain rapport with parents, to identify the beginnings of departure from physical or emotional health, and to ensure that a parent to whom such departure is not yet obvious has enough confidence in the health expert to accept advice; but there is likely to be increasing concentration on the underuse of services by the most vulnerable groups, on the early ascertainment of handicap, on the prevention of diseases of affluence such as overnutrition, and on emotional and mental problems.

measles. A very infectious virus disease which few children escaped before widespread vaccination became available. One attack usually leaves the individual immune to further attacks. It is acquired by inhaling infected droplets and, after a ten-day incubation period, produces a chest infection, a rash, and conjunctivitis. It is more serious in children under 3 years who are badly nourished or suffering from other diseases. The most common complication is bronchopneumonia which may be fatal. Otitis media is also common, while measles encephalitis, though rare, is also sometimes fatal. Treatment is essentially directed to relieving symptoms: fourteen days isolation should follow the appearance of the rash, and antibiotics are prescribed for the treatment of complications. Prevention is obtained by a single injection of measles vaccine during the second year of life.

measurement of health. The state of an individual's HEALTH at any particular time can be regarded as a measure of the extent to which he is overcoming the sum of his internal and external stresses. It is not an absolute quality, as can be illustrated by comparing health with disease: for all its frequent appearance to the contrary, disease does not suddenly lay low the healthy (except as a result of sudden trauma). The change is gradual, the affected person passing through intermediate stages between health and disease. These may be very rapid as in the case of certain communicable diseases, prolonged as in the development of tuberculosis, or may even extend over many years as is generally the case in the development of occupational diseases and tumours. In these examples the disease state is often unrecognized until it is fully, or almost fully developed, since the symptoms may appear very late. And yet it has co-existed with apparent health. Consider rheumatoid arthritis, a disease which often develops over many years and, once established, persists throughout life. It generally announces its arrival comparatively early in the disease process and progresses inexorably thereafter, usually with periods of acute painful attacks between which symptoms remit temporarily. Between attacks most sufferers regard themselves as healthy in spite of the acknowledged presence of a chronic disease, whereas the otherwise healthy sufferer from a severe cold is considered ill even though the overwhelming probability is that he will make a full recovery within a very short time.

Individual assessment of health is thus more a reflection of social values, awareness, and personal attitudes than a measure on a health-sickness scale. Nevertheless it is generally accepted that a massive improvement in the health of the citizens of the developed world has occurred in the last two or three hundred years. To understand this point of view it is necessary to consider the means which have been employed to assess the state of a community's health, and how these enable a comparison to be made between past and present, and between those for whom little or no improvement has taken place and the more fortunate.

Though a community's health is as yet impossible to measure it is nevertheless reflected in various measures of sickness. And though sickness resulting in death reflects only the lethal aspect of a community's sickness burden, and not necessarily the major part of that burden, it has nonetheless been the easiest aspect to measure. In Britain the first attempt to register deaths occurred in London in 1532 with the publication of weekly Bills of Mortality. Though these were probably inaccurate and incomplete they laid the foundation for the collection of all vital statistics. The first statistician to analyse them was John Graunt who in 1662 published his findings of the high mortality in childhood, of the rise and fall of death rates in regular sequence, and of the higher mortality of males than females. In addition he was the first to construct a life table – showing per thousand individuals born alive the numbers expected to live to different ages. At the end of the seventeenth century approximately half would survive until they were 10, in the mid-nineteenth century about half could expect to reach their mid-forties (the situation in many developing countries now) whereas about half those born in Britain in 1970 could expect to live to 70 years of age.

In the compilation of health statistics it is necessary that the facts are collected from reliable sources, from large numbers of people observed over sufficiently long periods of time. Even today morbidity (sickness) data are limited, since many non-fatal illnesses never come to medical attention and some which do cause considerable problems of diagnosis and classification. Until recently, knowledge of morbidity was almost restricted to a group of 'notifiable' diseases (smallpox, tuberculosis, diphtheria, etc.) whose diagnosis was comparatively straightforward, and knowledge of whose occurrence was of practical significance to public health authorities.

Assessment of community health continues to rely chiefly on information about death, as it did in Graunt's time. In England and Wales births, deaths, and causes of death have been registered since 1838, and from these data it is evident that mortality has been in rapid decline since about 1870. But another continuing source of data is also available – that of the census started in the U.K. in 1801 and in most developed countries taken every ten years. This showed, for example, that the population of England and Wales doubled in the fifty years up to 1851, a fact which has led most observers to conclude that mortality had in fact already been in steady decline in the hundred years preceding 1870. The steady rise in population continued throughout the next hundred years in spite of a great reduction in the birth rate; this rise is mainly attributable to the continued reduction in mortality which, in turn, has been due almost entirely to a decrease in deaths from the infectious diseases – tuberculosis, typhus and typhoid, scarlet fever, cholera, dysentery and diarrhoea, and smallpox. The decline in deaths from these diseases in the nineteenth century is mainly attributed to a rising standard of living, particularly of improved diet, to sanitary reform which massively reduced the intestinal diseases, and to a decline in the infectiousness of several of the organisms. Only in the case of smallpox is a specifically medical measure (vaccination) regarded as having played the major part. About two-thirds of the continued decline in the mortality rate since 1900 is also attributable to the decline in deaths from infectious desease.

Particularly striking during that period has been the reduction in infant mortality, which had remained at about 150 per thousand live births throughout the latter half of the nineteenth century when overall mortality was in steady decline. The decline in infant mortality in the twentieth century has been attributed to the introduction and great expansion of child health (or child welfare) services, the continued rise in living standards, further control of the physical environment, and, latterly, the introduction of effective prevention and treatment of disease. Hence a community's infant mortality rate has often been held to give a good indication of its general economic health, cultural development, and basic health services. Developed countries now report infant mortality rates of 15 to 25 per thousand live births, while the majority of developing countries have rates comparable to those of Victorian Britain. It is barely appreciated by the Western-oriented health planners in many of these countries that most of the improvement in health in the developed countries is not due to the availability of technologically advanced treatment of sick individuals, but (in order of importance) to a rising standard of living, improved hygiene, specific prevention, and therapeutic measures.

Measures of morbidity are available from a variety of sources in developed countries. Their limitations have been explained. Sources include hospital, general practice, and industrial medical records, special morbidity surveys undertaken for research, notifications of infectious and industrial diseases, National Insurance certification of illness, cancer registration records, army records and school health service records, among many others. It has been strongly argued that if the multiplicity of individual health records is to be put to its fullest use in measuring the health of the community as a basis for rational service planning, then schemes of record linkage utilizing computer facilities should be introduced. A number of pilot record-linkage schemes are now being tested in different countries including Britain.

Identification of pre-morbid states is the function of screening programmes. These have increased in number in recent years and the statistics they provide represent another measurement of health, one that is much nearer 'complete health' and further from lethal illness.

See also INFANT MORTALITY RATE, VITAL STATISTICS, and CHILD HEALTH SERVICES.

median. In anatomy and pathology, midline or central. The median plane divides the body into right and left halves. The median nerve runs down the arm and supplies the muscles that bend the wrist and some muscles of the thumb.

In statistics the median is the middle value which is sometimes a better guide than the average. Thus if the duration of illness in five patients in a ward, all of them undergoing a particular treatment, was two, three, four, five and eleven days, the average (five days) is clearly distorted by the one prolonged illness and the median (four days) gives a more accurate picture.

mediastinum. The collection of tissues and organs separating the two lungs, between the breast bone or sternum in front and the vertebral column behind, and from the base of the neck above to the diaphragm below. It contains the heart and great blood vessels, the trachea, oesophagus, thymus gland, lymph nodes, and other structures and tissues.

medical audit. An objective and systematic attempt to evaluate standards of diagnosis and treatment.

For a number of years some hospitals, especially in the U.S.A., have appointed from their staff a medical audit committee. This committee evolves criteria for particular conditions, e.g., the items in the patient's history, the type of physical examination and the laboratory procedures required for diagnosis, successful methods of treatment, and any procedure or treatment that is unsuitable. In the light of these criteria the committee studies patients' records and brings any manifestly substandard performance to the notice of the doctor concerned. More recently the system has been extended to general medical practice, and in respect of patients whose medical care is paid for by the government it is now a legal requirement in the U.S.A. In Britain systematic assessment occurs in some hospitals but is still rare in general practice.

Some doctors criticize the system on the ground that it creates rigidity, interferes with professional freedom, and inhibits innovation; but on the whole the system is supported by good clinicians as tending to improve the quality of medical care, to help doctors to review the efficiency of their methods and to ensure the best use of available time and resources.

medical officer of health. In countries in which some or all aspects of community health are the responsibility of a local authority or a local health board (as opposed to being a national or state responsibility), the medical officer of health is the doctor in administrative charge of the health services provided by a county, town or district.

The idea of the need for such an official arose largely from the writings of two German physicians deeply interested in the maintenance of good health. Johann Peter Frank (1748-1821) emphasized, in enormous detail in six hefty volumes, that the health of the people is a public responsibility and that officials should be appointed to regulate and supervise matters of health: his concept of health was wide (including for example prevention of accidents, mental hygiene, food hygiene and maternal and child well-being) but he thought of the proposed officer as essentially an advisor of legislators and an enforcer of laws and regulations. Franz Anton Mai (1742-1814) added to that concept the role of educator of doctors and nurses, of adolescents, and of either children or their teachers.

Although designated City Inspector of Health the earliest medical officer of health (MOH) was probably John Pintard, appointed in new York in 1804; but it was primarily in Britain with its strong tradition of local government that medical officers of health first developed. Liverpool in 1847 appointed the first person designated MOH, W.H. Duncan (1805-1863), followed in the next year by the appointment in London of John Simon (1816-1904), and other early appointments were made in Edinburgh (1862), Aberdeen (1862), Glasgow (1863), Leeds (1866) and Manchester (1868). From 1872 in England and Wales and from slightly later in Scotland until 1974 the appointment of MOH was a statutory requirement in the U.K. In 1974 British health services other than certain parts of environmental health were brought under national control and the office of MOH disappeared except, curiously, in the Isle of Man. In many countries, however, the office continues.

There are differences from country to country as to which health and disease services are adminstered nationally, which are run locally, which are entrusted to voluntary agencies and which are left without any formal organization. So no universally applicable description of the MOH is possible. The outline that follows is written with Britain in mind but much of it applies also to other English-speaking countries in which health is a local responsibility, although the post sometimes carries another name, e.g., director of health services.

Until after 1900 the MOH conformed largely to Frank's concept of an advisor of (local) legislators and an enforcer of regulations. He was concerned mainly with control of infectious diseases, establishment of safe water supplies, provision of fit houses, drainage and sewerage, and environmental hygiene generally; and as local authorities began to build fever hospitals and tuberculosis sanatoria he usually also had charge of these. He had no special training in PUBLIC HEALTH but was a clinician, quite often a distinguished clinician, who had an interest in the prevention of disease and was prepared to give up private practice for a salaried appointment. His staff was tiny: in a city with a population of 300,000 he might be aided in the community by one assistant medical officer of health, four or five sanitary inspectors, two or three male clerks and toward the end of the nineteenth century two or three health visitors; and his fever and tuberculosis hospitals might each have a couple of doctors, a handful of nurses and a few domestics. Yet the public health team of that period achieved a great reduction of food-borne infectious diseases and diseases of dirt and poverty, a vast improvement in water supplies, sewerage, street cleaning, and the removal of at least the worst slums of the industrial revolution.

During the first three decades of this century there were extensive new developments. It became a statutory requirement for a doctor appointed as MOH to hold a postgraduate qualification in public health. Concern with the well-being of mothers and babies and of schoolchildren grew rapidly. Health visitors (at first untrained, later qualified nurses with further training and ultimately highly qualified) were appointed in increasing numbers and bit by bit began to replace sanitary inspectors as the right hand of the MOH. There was increasing interest in the health education of the public, although health education was considered rather as didactic instruction than as discussion with a view to the changing of attitudes. Health departments enlarged rapidly and their medical staffs came to include doctors specialized in maternal and child health and (sometimes separately) school health, as well as specialists in infectious diseases. Physicians in private practice, whether general practitioners or consultants, began to see the work of public health doctors,

health visitors and sanitary inspectors as decreasing the amount of illness and, since they depended on patients for their livelihood, became in at least some cases hostile to public health workers.

The twenty years up to 1948 are sometimes termed the finest hour of the MOH In these years the health visitor service was expanding rapidly; the work of health visitors, midwives and medical officers for maternal and child health (supplemented by that of preventive-minded obstetricians and paediatricians not under the direction of the MOH) was producing dramatic results; the physical health both of pre-school and of school children was improving despite the massive unemployment and poverty of the years around 1930; health education was beginning to be understood in at least some areas; the development of immunization and appreciation of methods of inducing the public to accept it were creating enormous potentialities for the reduction of infections; the worst environmental problems were being conquered; and local authorities were establishing general, mental and maternity hospitals, so that before 1948 local authorities controlled more than two-thirds of all the hospital beds in the U.K. With the proposals for a national health service in which consultants would be salaried and general practitioners would receive a fixed annual payment for each person on their lists it looked as though the hostility between curative and preventive workers would die away, as indeed it did, albeit slowly. The MOH was becoming a mixture of administrator, epidemiologist, sociologist and health educator, concerned with all matters pertaining to health in his district.

Yet perhaps his duties had become too diverse, for in the 1940s few medical officers of health, especially in the larger population units, could cope adequately with all their functions. There emerged, at first as mere whispers, ideas that local authority and voluntary hospitals should be linked, with the former divorced from the MOH, that sanitary inspectors (the environmental health officers of today) did not really require to be directed by a doctor, that health visitors were being handicapped by being controlled by a member of a different profession, and that the rising profession of social workers would function better with its own professional head. Perhaps these ideas were merely symptomatic of the advance of social workers, health visitors and sanitary inspectors to full professional status. Perhaps too, in a large city or county, no one person could co-ordinate, without dominating or repressing, large groups of skilled members of different community health professions (e.g., medical officers, dental officers, health visitors, midwives, social workers, physiotherapists, sanitary inspectors and chiropodists) and also administer general and mental hospitals where medical, nursing, technical, auxiliary and domestic staff sometimes together total a couple of thousand for a single hospital.

The creation of the National Health Service in 1948 removed hospitals from the jurisdiction of local authorities and might have led to a renaissance of the MOH as co-ordinator of the swiftly advancing community health service. However there were several difficulties. (1) Salaries in hospital medical posts were considerably higher than those of most local authority doctors, and quite a number of doctors moved from the public health service to become consultants in tuberculosis, infectious diseases or venereal diseases; (2) a doctor aspiring to become a consultant no longer had to face years of penury but was salaried as house officer and registrar, so that good medical entrants to the public health service grew scarcer; (3) at the same time as there emerged a shortage of public health doctors, particularly those of the calibre to fill posts as MOH, the professional preparation of health visitors and social workers was improving rapidly and advanced courses were appearing (e.g., for prospective health visitor administrators and for intending teachers of student health visitors), so that it became increasingly obvious that the work of these professions could no longer be directed by a member of a different profession, with a different background, different attitudes and different priorities; and (4) some of the older medical officers of health, after having spent many years doing good work on hospital administration and control of infectious diseases, had difficulty in appreciating the growing importance of health education and services for the fostering of emotional health.

In the 1950s and 1960s a few local authorities separated sanitary departments from public health departments, and about 1970 separate social work departments were established throughout the U.K. Here and there interesting anticipations of future multiprofessional management appeared (e.g., creation in a health department of an administrative team containing the MOH as chairman, the head of the health visiting and home nursing service, the chief health education officer, and so on) but in general the various community heath professions began to diverge. Simultaneously demands began to grow for integrated planning by hospital and public health services and for collaboration between general practitioners (who were not in public health departments) and health visitors.

Finally in 1974 responsibility for health services, hospital and non-hospital, was transferred to appointed health boards with, as their top managers, an executive group – a medical officer, a nursing officer, an administrator and a finance officer, with others (e.g., dental officer) joining the group when their services were under consideration. So the post of MOH ceased to exist in the U.K.

From 1847 to 1974 the contribution of the MOH to the health of the public was enormous. After all, however outstanding might be a health education officer or health visitor or child health doctor, it was primarily the MOH on whom local authorities relied for advice and it was the MOH who had the difficult task of persuading his authority (always reluctant to spend money) to expand any branch of its health service or to pioneer a new branch; and the MOH was the only person with an over-all view of the health problems and health needs of the district.

In 1974, with the recognition of nursing as a full profession, the portion of his work concerned with co-ordination and deployment of health visitors and home nurses passed to the chief nursing officer of health board, the health education component passed to the chief

health education officer (although he was made responsible to the board's chief medical officer), the sanitary portion went to the director of environmental health of the district local authority, and the strictly medical part passed to the chief administrative medical officer of the board.

The change was perhaps inevitable as the health services grew more complex, but like most changes it had elements of loss as well as gain: chief officers from the various health professions may appreciate more easily the needs and problems of their particular profession, and where time is available a multiprofessional group may take wiser decisions than a single person; and financing from national funds removes the formerly common pattern of an uninterested or penurious local authority depriving its health department of needed funds. But in circumstances of emergency it was useful to have one person who could take an immediate decision (e.g., to detain or release a ship, to close schools and nurseries or leave them open, or to concentrate the whole resources of the public health department or the efforts of one officer on a particular investigation or campaign); and it was useful for members of the public to know – without trying to work out whether their problem was relevant to health visiting, social services, sanitary services or some other portion of a complex department – that they could seek help or guidance from a central source.

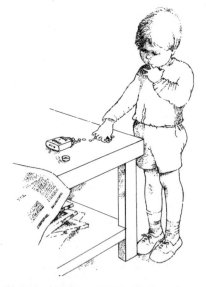

Keep all medicines out of the reach of children

medicines. Substances taken by mouth, or otherwise put into or on the body, specifically for the prevention or treatment of disease.

Their use almost certainly dates from earliest human existence. Preparations of herbs, roots, berries and other substances, from pearls to crocodile dung, known or believed to possess powerful properties, have been employed. Of the huge number of medicines ever used few have had any direct influence on disease, and many have been harmful. Only in the last hundred years or so have scientific principles been applied to the development of medicines, while the introduction of very powerful drugs in the last forty years has necessitated very strict control in their prescription, since almost no medicine with a useful action is without potentially dangerous side-effects.

megaloblastic anaemia. Anaemia in which the blood contains underdeveloped red blood corpuscles termed megaloblasts. By far the commonest of such anaemias is PERNICIOUS ANAEMIA but a similar anaemia occasionally occurs in infants given a diet with insufficient folic acid or in adults unable to absorb that food factor.

megalomania. Preoccupation with ideas of exalted power or wealth, commonly called 'delusions of grandeur'. Minor degrees are common in everyday life and generally represent an over-compensation for a feeling of inferiority. The types of medical interest are essentially those in which ideas of power co-exist with feelings of persecution.

In PARANOIA and the paranoid type of SCHIZOPHRENIA megalomania is often accompanied by delusions of persecution which are systematized, i.e., if a single false belief (for instance that relatives and associates are conspiring to deprive the sufferer of a fortune or are plotting to murder him) is accepted as correct, the delusions appear consistent and logical. It has been suggested that in this form of mental illness the patient, living in an atmosphere of suspicion and hostility and surrounded by imaginary 'enemies', indulges in the delusions of grandeur in an attempt to maintain self-respect. Until the disease becomes advanced it may be difficult to differentiate this dangerous condition from the paranoid reactions discussed later. Yet diagnosis is important because the insane person may seek to kill or injure his 'persecutors' in imagined self-defence.

Commoner are paranoid reactions in which most of the personality remains comparatively intact though rigid and suspicious, but on one particular aspect there are systematized delusions of grandeur or of persecution or often of both. Here the sufferer from megalomania, while perhaps earning his living by normal work, may have delusions of a religious mission, often of a messianic nature, or vast political or social reforms, or of amazing inventions. Religious paranoics, for example, may believe that they have been sent by God on a mission of human salvation and may spend much of their time preaching to attract converts to their cause. Their sermons are frequently filled with dire threats of eternal damnation and similar consequences of non-conversion. Many paranoics become attached to political parties, often to extremist movements, becoming tireless and fanatical and often self-righteous, and frequently do more harm than good to their cause, though they occasionally acquire enormous influence and massive followings. Some paranoics invent remarkable devices which they experience great difficulty in marketing. They then become increasingly convinced that they are the victims of a conspiracy to steal their invention or even the subject of a plot to damage their country by denying it the benefits of their great talents.

Thirdly, there occur paranoid states, usually transient and with spontaneous recovery. Here the individual is perhaps initially suspicious or boastful or both, but temporary delusions of grandeur or of persecution are precipitated by a situation causing acute mental stress.

Whether we think of megalomania or of ideas of persecution, the paranoid state is a temporary, abnormal state, caused in susceptible persons by a stressful situation and with complete recovery highly probable. The paranoid reaction is long-lasting but does not usually necessitate admission to mental hospital, but paranoia or paranoid schizophrenia is a very serious mental disease.

meiosis. See GENETICS.

melaena. The technical term for the passing of black, tarry motions. The condition may be a result of the swallowing of blood, e.g., from bleeding of the nose, or of bleeding from the stomach or intestine. Irrespective of the cause, the blood has remained in the digestive system long enough to be acted on by the digestive juices, and the iron of the haemoglobin has been largely converted into iron sulphide.

By contrast the passing of red blood indicates bleeding near the anus, e.g., from haemorrhoids.

melancholia. A depressed emotional state with abnormal mental sluggishness, apathy, and indifference to one's surroundings. Nowadays it is only usually employed in the term 'involutional melancholia' – a depressive illness occurring for the first time during the period around the menopause, which tends to last longer and be more subject to relapse than manic-depressive psychosis in younger people.

memory. That faculty of mind by which sensations, impressions, and ideas are recalled. Since the brain has to process and co-ordinate information available to it from the external environment, to analyse the best course of action to take on the basis of this information, and to instruct the remainder of the organism to act on the basis of this analysis, it requires to have some way of comparing the information reaching it at any time with that previously encountered describing comparable situations, the responses made to these situations, and the outcome of these responses. It is the mechanism of recording, storing, sifting and comparing information which is referred to as memory.

In evolutionary terms, the more highly developed the animal, the greater the proportion of brain given over to this mechanism (and hence the greater the potential for sophisticated response). The process of fixation of the memory takes place in at least two stages. New information arriving at the brain is placed first in a short-term memory store, probably situated just below the cerebral cortex. It is easily lost from this store. That which remains is transferred after at least a few minutes, probably at about thirty minutes, and possibly up to three hours later, to a permanent long-term store situated in the cortex itself. The natural loss of memory from the short-term store may be increased by shocks to the brain caused, for example, by convulsions or concussion which are known to lead to memory loss for the events immediately preceding them. Memories in the permanent store are not lost in this fashion.

Tests of memory. Psychologists chiefly test span memory, rote memory, and memory of meaningful material. Span memory tests measure how much is retained of unrelated material (such as numbers or letters) after one brief presentation; results are, however, indicative of speed of perception as well as memory fixation and recall ability. Rote memory tests measure how much is retained of unrelated material (such as lists of words or syllables) after they have been seen for some minutes. It is probably a 'purer' measure of the facility of fixation and recall, whereas memory of meaningful material depends to a considerable extent on the patient actually understanding the material. On the other hand, medical investigations are usually concerned with short and long term memory and identifying confabulation (inventions to replace memory gaps). Such tests are useful in the investigation of such cases as head injury, epilepsy, suspected hysteria, and organic psychosis.

Disorders. Memory is referred to as disordered when fixation or recall is disturbed. It often gives the appearance of being disordered when the real problem is one of loss of attention, as in depression or during hallucinations.

Disorders of memory are commonly divided into amnesias, paramnesias and hypermnesias. Amnesia, or absence of memory, may be complete (rarely) or partial: amnesia confined to recent events is characteristic of senile cerebral degeneration, rote memory being better retained than other kinds, while in brain damage there is often persistent amnesia for events immediately preceding and following the accident. Paramnesia, false recollection, may co-exist with amnesia in organic psychoses, such as in the late stages of untreated syphilis. Hypermnesia denotes excessive retention of detailed memories, and is found in some prodigies and in certain mental disorders.

Mendel. Gregor Johann Mendel (1822-1884), a Moravian monk and one of the most curious figures in the history of science.

In his cloister-garden at Brunn he crossed tall and dwarf peas and peas with red and white flowers, and found in eight years of meticulous breeding that the contrasted characters were inherited in numerical ratio according to what we would nowadays call the laws of GENETICS (e.g., that crossing red flowered and white flowered peas gave all apparently red peas, but that interbreeding of these apparent reds gave 25 per cent which bred true, 25 per cent of white which similarly bred true, and 50 per cent of 'reds' which gave rise to off-spring consisting of 25 per cent true reds, 25 per cent whites and 50 per cent of similar 'reds'). Indeed his distributions were so exact that some modern workers have suggested that he may have 'adjusted' his figures: in actual experiments on a few thousand plants 24 or 26 per cent of recessive whites would be a more likely figure than the theoretically correct 25.

Having discovered that contrasted characters (which later generations called characters determined by single opposed genes) did not blend, that the sexual cells remained pure and that the offspring inherited

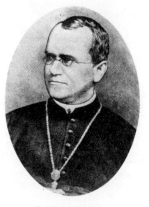

Gregor Mendel

dominant or recessive characters on simple mathematical laws, Mendel published his monograph, *Experiments on Plant Hybrids* (1865) – and it passed absolutely unnoticed. Meantime Mendel was appointed abbot of Brunn and was advised to discontinue his researches, perhaps because the evolution controversy was already alarming religious thinkers; and for his last twenty years the discoverer of the laws of heredity did no scientific work.

In 1900 a group of geneticists chanced to read Mendel's ignored work, and from that time Mendel became one of the great names in biology, so much so that the numerical laws governing the recurrence of inherited characteristics are sometimes known as Mendelism.

Ménière's disease. A condition characterized by fluctuating or progressive deafness, head-noises (tinnitus) and vertigo. For fuller details SEE HEAD NOISES.

meningitis. Inflammation of the membranes (meninges) which cover the brain. Sometimes the inflammation is caused by the spread of infection from a compound fracture of the skull or from chronic middle ear or mastoid disease. More frequently it is caused by micro-organisms that spread in the sub-arachnoid space between the two inner membranes. Meningitis is classified according to the responsible micro-organism, e.g., meningo-coccal or cerebrospinal fever (the commonest), tuberculous (inevitably fatal until after the discovery of the antibiotic, streptomycin) and viral (usually the mildest).

The term meningitis, used without any qualifying word such as 'tuberculous' generally means infection by the meningococcus which causes cerebrospinal fever. The germ can be transmitted by the breathing of infected droplets from cases or more frequently from carriers. The onset of this disease is usually abrupt after a short incubation period of one to three days, with high temperature, rigor, headache, delirium and muscular stiffness particularly of the neck and back muscles which in severe cases may lead to arching of the body. Haemorrhagic rashes also sometimes occur and are the basis for the synonym 'spotted fever'.

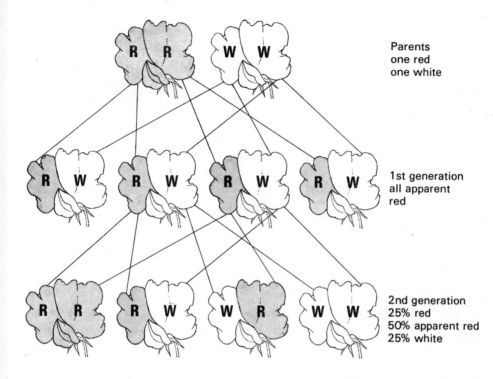

Mendel's inheritance experiment with red and white pea flowers

Precise diagnosis in cases of meningitis depends on examination of the cerebrospinal fluid, samples of which are obtained by lumbar puncture.

Meningitis of all types was formerly a grave condition with a high death rate but the outlook has greatly improved since the introduction of antibiotic drugs. This is even true of tuberculous meningitis, formerly a relatively common and invariably fatal condition in infants and children, but now less often encountered because of the general decline in the sources of tuberculous infection.

menopause. The stage of life in women at which menstruation ceases. It is also known as 'the change of life' or the female climacteric. The menopause usually takes place between the ages of 45 and 50 but there is a considerable range of variation related to race and inheritance. An early onset of menstruation (menarche) is frequently associated with late cessation, and a premature menopause in the fourth decade of life is not very unusual.

The menstrual periods normally cease in one of three ways. They may stop abruptly and never recur; they may continue rhythmically as before with blood loss gradually diminishing to zero; or the regular monthly cycle may progressively lengthen to several months and

finally terminate. Any departure from these typical histories should be regarded as pathological and any form of irregular haemorrhage in women of menopausal age requires careful investigation.

The menopause is due to a decline in activity of the ovaries and this produces various other effects. The sexual organs undergo atrophy and retrogression; e.g., the breasts shrivel and the vagina becomes smaller and its secretion diminishes. This may cause pain on intercourse and diminished resistance to infection. Within the pelvis the tissues become lax and support to the uterus is diminished so that displacement may occur.

In addition there may be general symptoms related to alterations in the balance of the ENDOCRINE GLANDS, such as increased deposition of fat, atrophy of skin, growth of facial hair, and disturbances of the cardio-vascular system. The latter are responsible for the very characteristic menopausal symptoms of 'hot flushes' and excessive tendency to perspire. There may also be headaches, irritability, and depression which occasionally develops into melancholia. In most cases a more normal hormonal balance is gradually re-established and the adminstration of preparations of oestrogen can be reliably expected to relieve the more distressing symptoms of discomfort until this occurs.

In most women the stresses of the menopause are not extreme and they soon subside. Well-being is restored, sexual desire is retained, and there are compensations in the loss of pre-menstrual tension and the recurrent discomforts of menstruation. Occasional cases of continued emotional distress require psychiatric advice.

A parallel but slower and more gradual CLIMACTERIC, with warning of fertility, sexual activity and general vitality, occurs in men, sometimes accompanied by irritability, depression and reduced mental concentration.

menorrhagia. See FLOODING.

menstruation. Througout that part of her life when a woman is capable of bearing children, her sex-organs undergo a regular monthly cycle of events. This is marked by bleeding from the uterus occurring about every twenty-eight days and lasting for four or five days, and is known as menstruation.

The menstrual cycle is controlled by the ovaries, in the REPRODUCTIVE SYSTEM. At the start of the cycle, on about the first day of a menstrual period, a small mass of special cells, known as a Graafian follicle and enclosing an individual egg cell or ovum, begins to enlarge and ripen and project on the surface of the ovary. About the fourteenth day of the cycle the follicle ruptures (ovulation) and the egg cell then enters the Fallopian tube of the uterus and makes its way to the body of the uterus. The Graafian follicle, after it ruptures, undergoes further changes and secretes a hormone called progesterone. This stimulates the lining of the uterus to thicken and develop in readiness for the ovum to become embedded in it, in the event of it being fertilized. The climax of the process is reached on about the twenty-eighth day of the menstrual cycle. If fertilization has not occurred the developed uterus wall breaks down to cause the menstrual flow, carrying the unfertilized ovum with it. The whole cycle then starts again. If the ovum is fertilized the uterus wall is ready to receive it and there the EMBRYO will develop.

It will be noted that ovulation and entry of the ovum into the Fallopian tube occurs about the fourteenth day of the cycle. This is the best time for fertilization, a fact which forms the basis of the 'rhythm method' of BIRTH CONTROL.

During the menstrual period hygiene is important. The flow may be absorbed by sanitary towels or by an internal tampon and a daily bath is important and no longer regarded as unsuitable.

Menstruation may be accompanied by some minor pain and discomfort but this can usually be relieved by rest, warmth and analgesics.

Premenstrual tension. While in many women menstruation starts each month without any previous symptoms, it is not uncommon for the onset of menstruation to be heralded by a few days of irritability, nervousness, feelings of depression, headaches and increased liability to minor accidents. The symptoms are thought to be related in part to retention of fluid. In general a modicum of rest, restriction of salt intake for four or five days and mild analgesics such as aspirin cope with the condition, but in serious cases medical advice should be sought.

Disorders related to menstruation are described under AMENORRHOEA, DYSMENORRHOEA and METRORRHAGIA.

mental deficiency. Variation is a characteristic of all biological activities and this is as true of intelligence as it is of more easily measured physical characteristics such as height or weight.

There are therefore in any population individuals who vary quite widely in their personalities, skills and abilities but who nevertheless can be regarded as normal. Standard INTELLIGENCE TESTS are so constructed that the average intelligence quotient (IQ) is 100 but an actual score which reaches at least 70 to 75 is regarded as still being within the limits of normality.

In addition there are individuals who cannot reach even this level of performance and these are said to be mentally defective or to suffer from mental handicap. It is important to draw a distinction between mental deficiency and mental illness because the latter is a state of abnormal mental function afflicting persons who are usually otherwise of normal mental capacity.

Legally, mental deficiency is defined as a condition of arrested or incomplete development of mind existing before the age of 18 years, whether arising from inherent causes or induced by disease or injury. Four grades were recognized: idiots, imbeciles, feeble-minded persons and moral defectives. A more practical classification however is (1) mildly mentally-handicapped with IQ 50 to 70 and (2) severely mentally handicapped with IQ below 50.

The overall proportion of all types of mental handicap in the community is probably about 25 per thousand. Of these only about 3.7 per thousand can be classified as severely handicapped. The majority of the others although regarded as mildly handicapped within their school environment usually prove to be capable of living independently in the community without the aid of many special services, partly because of their ability to undertake successfully work which does not call for skill and partly because their abilities continue to develop during a substantial part of young adult life.

Those who are severely handicapped present a greater problem. Very many are in special hospitals not only because of their subnormal intelligence but because of social incapacity and deviant behaviour, or very often because there is simply no suitable provision for them elsewhere. A recent survey showed that at least three-quarters were continent, ambulant and had no behavioural problems and that only a few actually required the skilled medical and nursing attention which a hospital provides.

Apart from these facts, there are other considerations such as the effect on personality of the regimentation of hospital life, loss of identity, and under-activity. There is therefore a growing appreciation that large mental subnormality hospitals are 'anti-therapeutic' and that cases of this kind would benefit from being returned to the community and accommodated in small hostels so that they might be enabled to lead as happy and fulfilling a life as possible.

Causes. Many cases are genetically determined. The best known of these are mongolism, due to chromosomal abnormality, and phenylketonuria, a metabolic defect.

Others are related to the mother's health during pregnancy, to obstetric complications, and to the condition of the child at birth, particularly if premature. After birth various cultural and material factors influence development. Amongst these are social practices, education, family size and structure, family stability, housing, and poverty.

Prevention of mental retardation. Causes related to GENETICS can be minimized or avoided by genetic counselling; mongolism can be detected through examination of the amniotic fluid and abortion considered in positive cases; there are also tests for phenylketonuria and similar metabolic conditions. There is still scope for better antenatal and obstetric care and improved post-natal and child health services. Immunization against rubella (German measles) and the detection and treatment of Rhesus incompatability, mycoplasma infections, and placental insufficiency are recent developments which are contributing to a reduction in mental damage. During later development there are opportunities for better child care, with early detection of abnormalities and retardation, backed up by 'preventive education' and organized social care. Measures of this kind can be expected to achieve the identification of children at risk and to provide for their special needs before their behaviour and development deviate too irretrievably from acceptable normality.

mental diseases. The primitive conception of mental illness was that patients were possessed by evil spirits and must be dealt with harshly so that such invaders would be discouraged and depart. This kind of degrading treatment persisted until at least 1793 when Philippe Pinel at the Saltpêtrière in Paris pioneered a more humanitarian approach. Subsequently the study of mental disease and attempts to treat it more rationally became the medical speciality known as psychiatry, still a developing science in which much yet remains to be explained. The early practitioners concerned themselves with descriptive psychiatry – a painstaking attempt to classify mental disease by its symptoms; basically this work is still valid but it is now supported by increasing knowledge of the causes.

Mental disturbances fall into two categories: PSYCHOSIS and NEUROSIS; and there is also a borderland between psychiatry and medicine known as PSYCHOSOMATIC DISEASE.

Of these, the psychoses are much the most serious and only they constitute real mental derangement. Such a mental illness is characterized by marked disruption of personality (or 'affect') and a total loss of touch with reality. A psychotic patient lacks 'insight' and is unable to appreciate abnormalities in his conduct.

The neuroses are essentially different from the psychoses. There is much less personality disorganization and the patient retains his appreciation of environmental realities. His failure to adapt is only partial and he still has an ability to recognize abnormalities in his behaviour and to accept and endeavour to act on the advice of his psychiatrist. The clinical symptoms are those of hysteria, anxiety-neurosis or various types of compulsive

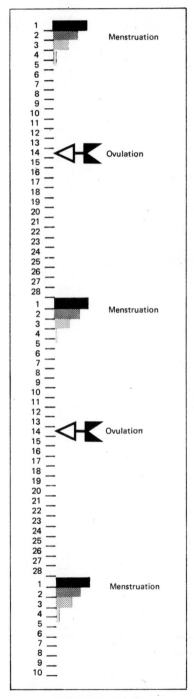

The menstrual cycle

behaviour commonly referred to as 'obsessions'.

Finally, in psychosomatic disease it is increasingly recognized that certain physical illnesses are induced, aggravated or maintained by mental states of tension, stress, or anxiety. Particular examples are peptic ulcer, asthma and certain skin diseases.

mental efficiency. The capacity to cope competently and without excessive strain with ordinary occupational, domestic and social happenings.

Estimation. Although we all have a rough idea of what the term means, exact measurement is extraordinarily difficult. We could start with an intelligence test, on the assumption that it really measures intelligence and not the particular parts of intelligence needed for the test, and could seek to grade mental efficiency simply according to intelligence. Yet some people of very low intelligence appear to manage their affairs well, and conversely some people who have demonstrated high intelligence, e.g., by obtaining degrees and even higher degrees, show a lack of competence in matters of everyday life. Clearly mental efficiency is not just intelligence.

Again it is obviously related not only to the person but to the relevant circumstances or events. A man may display considerable mental efficiency when occupying one post but may show incompetence or excessive strain when promoted to a more difficult post. A woman may appear an efficient housewife and mother in a normal two-parent family but be quite incapable of coping if her husband dies suddenly.

Yet again mental efficiency clearly has different and varying components. One has only to think of the traditional absent-minded professor who shows supreme competence in his teaching or research work but is a simpleton over investing money or can lose himself in a town that he knows well.

In the present state of our knowledge it is probably desirable to limit the estimation of mental efficiency to particular existing or hypothetical circumstances, e.g., to ask, 'is this elderly doctor alert enough to diagnose my illness?' or 'does this women have the common-sense and stability to handle the office during my absence?'

Improvement. Even though we cannot yet measure mental efficiency with any degree of accuracy we know many factors that affect it. Of these a few are mentioned below.

1. Physical health. Body and mind are intimately connected, and mental efficiency presupposes reasonable mental health. A person who has been deprived of adequate sleep for several successive nights, who is undernourished and hungry, who is physically exhausted, who is in a high fever or suffering from considerable pain is not mentally efficient. Clearly the maintenance of good physical health is important for mental efficiency; and obviously it is sensible to try to avoid taking important decisions at a time when our health is below par. Yet, while preservation of good physical health tends to improve mental efficiency, the connection should not be over-rated. On the one hand one can recall a President of the U.S.A. who was a cripple and a British Chancellor of the Exchequer who was alleged to live in almost continuous pain; and on the other hand the person who makes a fetish of physical fitness may have inadequate time to attend to other matters.

2. Drugs, etc. The effect of dangerous drugs in decreasing mental efficiency is obvious, as is the effect of excessive alcohol, although the borderline of excess may be arguable. Clearly avoidance of these drugs and of too much alcohol is conducive to mental efficiency. When we leave the obvious points, however, much is unknown. To give two examples: it is questionable whether the efficiency of a poor sleeper is increased or decreased by a mild sedative at night; and some people would maintain that a pipe of tobacco is conducive to immediate mental efficiency, both by calming the mind and by slightly raising the level of blood sugar, while others hold that tobacco reduces efficiency.

3. Mental exercise. Just as muscles grow weak from lack of use, mental capacities decline if unexercised. Probably most of us have seen the example of an elderly man who showed considerable competence while undertaking a responsible job in which he was keenly interested, but in reaching retirement had few interests and little mental activity, and speedily deteriorated mentally. While excessive mental effort is as harmful as excessive physical effort, it is good for us to have a reasonable amount of cerebral activity.

4. Cultivation of mental poise. Strong emotions and prolonged worry deplete one's stores of mental energy and therefore impair efficiency. None of us would very willingly entrust our lives to an air pilot if we knew that he had on that very day been jilted by a much-loved fiancée, or willingly have an operation performed by a surgeon if we knew that he was about to face a charge of serious professional misconduct. Unfortunately, while it is easy to advise people to avoid excessive anger, fear, worry and jealousy in the interests of both mental and physical health, it is much more difficult to suggest methods of avoiding these things. Certainly a man can strive to face up to the reasonably worst happening that might arise out of his fears and worries, and he will often find that it is much less serious than his vague fears had suggested. Again he can, in the old phrase, 'count his blessings': there are many good and pleasant things in the lives of all of us. Or he can discuss his problems with somebody whom he trusts, not simply to secure the advice of a more emotionally detached person but also to gain relief by bringing his fears and worries to the surface. Not least, he can try to force himself to devote part of his mental attention to the well-being of another person or organization, thus temporarily detaching himself from his own problems.

5. Achieving satisfactions. Probably nothing is more harmful to mental efficiency than continued lack of satisfactions, e.g., the man who feels that he is becoming too old for promotion, that the work he does is really of little value to anybody, that even if he is not made redundant his post will probably be abolished when he retires, that his children have gone their own way, that his wife is much more interested in her job than in him, that he lost his sole recreation when he became too stiff for tennis and that his one attempt to serve

the community failed when he stood for a local council and was not elected. Some experts advocate the pursuit of limited satisfactions, living for the day or the week, e.g., deciding 'I'll complete this particular piece of work today and tomorrow' (and mildly luxuriating in having achieved the goal), or even 'I'll reduce my excess weight by 1 kilo this week'. Others advise the sustained pursuit of larger and more long-term goals. In any case some satisfactions are essential for mental efficiency.

6. Cultivating relationships. The human being is a gregarious animal, and the person who lives entirely for himself and by himself is seldom mentally efficient. For emotional health most of us – though there may be a few exceptions – need the companionship of congenial persons with whom we can discuss joys, sorrows, triumphs and losses. In selecting such congenial persons, initially on grounds of similar views, ideas, tastes or backgrounds, we must of course realize that companionship is a two-way process. People are unlikely to be interested in our ideas or problems unless we can take some interest in theirs.

See also KEEPING FIT.

Legal aspects. The legal aspects pertain almost entirely to the lower end of the wide scale of mental efficiency. Five examples are given here.

1. Dismissal from a post. Where an appointment has any element of security (as opposed, for instance, to week-to-week engagement) the dismissing employer has in most of the developed countries to be prepared to prove – at appeal tribunal or in court – either that the person's work was substantially below what would be expected from a person of similar qualifications and experience or that his conduct was so bizarre as to interfere with the efficiency of other workers. In general this means that dismissal on a single piece of poor work or a single instance of unusual conduct is dangerous and that an employer who suspects mental inefficiency should keep detailed records before taking action. Warnings and rebukes should of course also be recorded.

2. Civil responsibility. Broadly, even if a person's mental efficiency is so impaired that he can be deemed insane, a civil contract holds unless it can be proved that it was of such a nature that it would not have been made but for the abnormal state of mind of the person at the time of the making of the contract. Deterioration of mental efficiency even to insanity does not invalidate a contract made before such deterioration.

3. Criminal responsibility. In the U.K. liability to punishment rests essentially on 'intent' and ability to exercise 'reason'. If a person did not know the nature and quality of his act, or did not know that the act was wrong, or suffered from delusions under which, if they had been factual, the act would have been permissible, he is not subject to punishment but can if necessary be confined for his own protection or that of others.

4. Obligatory transfer to hospital. In most countries this rests on establishing that the person constitutes a danger to himself or to others. In the case of physical danger decision is easy, but very real difficulties arise in other cases, e.g., where an elderly person of allegedly impaired mental efficiency gives away large amounts of his money to the indignation of relatives who expect to inherit.

5. Testamentary capacity. In some respects this presents the greatest problem of impaired mental efficiency, because a will generally becomes known at the time of a person's death but questions about his mental state relate to the time when the will was made. Broadly, a will is likely to stand if it can be established that the person making it understood its nature, understood the approximate extent of his estate, understood which individuals would benefit from the will, was not suffering from serious delusions and was not under undue influence.

mental health. In Great Britain the treatment of mental disorder absorbs about one-eighth of health service expenditure and occupies nearly half the total complement of hospital beds. The suicide rate of the community averages about 10 per 100,000 each year and mental, psycho-neurotic and personality disorders are responsible for fully 10 per cent of the total working days lost through certified incapacity for work. From these facts it will be seen that the health of the population falls far short of reaching the WHO ideal of 'a complete state of physical, mental and social well-being' in its mental component alone.

In developed countries like our own and the U.S.A. the general prevalence of mental disease is about 5 or 6 persons per thousand of population, and mental defectives number as many as 25 per thousand. Although comparable figures for underdeveloped countries are difficult to obtain with any acceptable degree of accuracy they are probably much lower. The reasons suggested for the difference are admittedly somewhat speculative but they illustrate some of the factors contributing to the present massive burden of mental disorder and mental ill-health which constitutes not only a community and individual source of distress, but also a serious drain on economic resources.

Since some psychoses and some types of mental deficiency are genetically determined, the basic prevalence of these should not vary much, though the impact of civilization may activate a latent psychotic tendency. Certainly one effect of better child health services is to ensure the survival of many more children who ultimately prove to be mentally defective. In senile psychosis it is obvious that its prevalence must vary with the age-constitution of the population. If the benefits of civilization ensure more general survival to later ages it is inevitable that more persons will show symptoms of mental disorder resulting from degenerative changes in their brain and blood vessels. However, it is when we leave these clearly recognized conditions and turn to the wide range of other mental illness included in such terms as psycho-neurosis, psychosomatic disease and personality disorder, as well as mere social inadequacy, that we find the greatest difference. It may be that these are more obvious in a civilized environment, but since they are related to stress it is not unreasonable to asume that they will be much more prevalent as a result of the pressures imposed by an increasingly demanding, complex, and changing society.

The factors responsible can be related to culture and social interaction operating in society as a whole, within the family, and at work. Developed countries impose more exacting standards in which the pressures for conformity arouse either rebellion or anxiety and provide innumerable opportunities for conflict not only in personal relationships but in relation to choice of action. There continues to be a decline in religious belief, and faith has been replaced by perplexity, uncertainty, and insecurity. At a more individual level cultural differences between the generations are often irreconcilable. Smaller families weaken the power of kinship. There are not so many aunts and uncles as there once were and the tasks of caring for the aged fall to fewer hands. Housing shortages lead to overcrowding and shared accommodation with all the resulting deterioration in inter-personal relationships. Family ties are loosened by rehousing in distant areas remote from grandparents, relatives and friends. High flats cause social isolation followed by loneliness and depression.

In industry frustration develops from repetitive tasks and lack of creativity; anger is aroused by unsympathetic foremen and uncaring management; anxiety results from considerations of job security.

To these and similar difficulties individuals react in many ways – by rebellion, by 'opting-out', by anxiety, or by developing symptoms of illness. Psycho-neurosis or psychosomatic disease shows as an unconscious escape mechanism, and the possession of a medical certificate of incapacity equates with the former ability of the peasant largely to please himself and not to worry about the problems of maintaining artificial standards and of conforming to a pattern of life with which he was out of sympathy. There is no ready prescription for curing the symptoms of mental distress which stem from the ills of civilization, and perhaps no final solution is even possible. All progress is striving and the less competent members of the community 'resolving hopeless strife, pointing at hindrance and the bare painful escapes of fitful life' tend inevitably to get hurt.

We live however in a period of great secular change during a transition between feudalism and egalitarianism. Ultimately there may emerge a future of greater tranquillity but there is little certainty of this as we contemplate the great problems of over-population and dwindling resources of food and raw materials.

Nevertheless there are still goals to be achieved in the short term: education; improvement of living and working conditions; encouragement of family integrity; adaptation of industry to provide security, satisfaction and a sense of participation; the pleasurable and intelligent use of leisure; and the provision of adequate care services for all kinds of social and medical problems – all these still provide opportunities for great and beneficial advances.

Perhaps the most immediate lines are (1) genetic guidance, coupled where necessary with contraception, to reduce hereditary mental and physical diseases; (2) child health services designed to reduce by timely advice such detrimental factors as over-strictness, forcing, over-indulgence and inconsistency; and (3) education, fitted to the needs and aptitudes of the individual child, and preparing him for leisure as well as for work.

mental hospitals. Until the end of the eighteenth century persons suffering from mental disorder were objects of superstitious abhorrence. When their behaviour was such that they had to be removed from the community they were usually confined under conditions of cruelty and degradation. The authorities had little choice but to consign the dangerously insane to prisons. In London, for example, Bedlam was notorious, and indeed the word has become a synonym for a madhouse or place of uproar.

The more liberal example of Philippe Pinel, who in 1793 struck off the chains of the inmates of the Saltpêtrière in Paris, initiated a dawning recognition that the management of mental disorder required benevolence and humanity. With the growth of towns and cities resulting from the Industrial Revolution a problem which was still being handled casually and unobtrusively in rural communities became concentrated and magnified, and the need for better provision became urgent.

In all developed countries the history of mental hospitals is broadly similar. The U.K. is here taken as an example. Initially there developed 'refuges' usually run as charities or as private retreats and these were supplemented to a small extent by county asylums provided under permissive powers of an Act of 1808. Later during the nineteenth century the efforts of the Earl of Shaftesbury, the recommendations of a Royal Commission, and the enactment of legislation beginning with the Lunacy Act of 1843, gradually led to a general provision of public asylums. The Act also set up, as supervisory authority, the Lunacy Commission which encouraged a new approach to care and treatment and envisaged possibilities for early admission, rehabilitation, and discharge.

This more liberal attitude was frustrated by public concern over improper detention, and the Lunacy (Consolidation) Act 1890, which also replaced the Commission by the Board of Control, introduced new regulations to ensure that asylums could only take certified patients. Since certification was usually deferred until madness was beyond doubt, asylums thus became places of last resort. As they grew into large and isolated institutions dealing only with cases which were largely irremediable, they were increasingly divorced from the mainstream of medical advance and became dedicated only to the custodial care of the seriously deranged.

In an attempt to break down this isolation and segregation, Dr. Henry Maudsley, by his personal generosity, in 1907 pioneered a new type of mental hospital in association with London County Council. This set out to deal with early cases, and to provide for out-patient consultation, teaching, and research. The success of this eventually led to the Mental Treatment Act of 1930 which circumvented the restrictions of the 1890 Act and extended the principle of voluntary admission to all mental hospitals and made possible observation wards and advisory clinics. Meantime medical progress had revolutionized the outlook in mental disorder and the Victorian asylums had to orientate their ideas towards treatment rather than custody. Physical techniques such as electro-convulsive therapy (ECT) and new

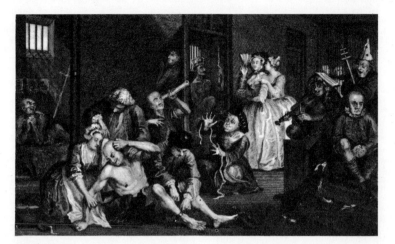

A mental hospital – Bedlam – as depicted by Hogarth in *The Rake's Progress* (1733-35)

drugs reduced durations of stay and opened up new prospects of recovery.

In 1959 (1960 in Scotland) the Mental Health Act repealed all earlier legislation and in effect placed mental hospitals on the same footing as other hospitals so that patients could be freely admitted for treatment and rehabilitation.

The large overcrowded and antiquated institutions of the past have thus become outmoded. Their modernization or reconstruction is a large task but it has begun and future emphasis will be on smaller hospitals, certainly not more than a thousand beds, disposed in smaller units and set in adequate surroundings, with special arrangements for the restless, sick and senile, and for those able to work. They require also to be linked to comprehensive rehabilitation services both inside and outside the hospital.

Although much of this account has been specifically related to hospitals for psychiatric illness similar problems exist in regard to mental deficiency institutions in which the adoption of new ideas and better standards has been even slower. Prolonged incarceration in purely custodial institutions leads to deterioration of the personality, and individuals do not attain their full potential. The aim now is to provide smaller units with the educational, occupational, and recreational facilities to ensure that those who must remain in hospital can participate in a full range of experience and social interaction. Many others with appropriate support from the social care services are capable of being returned to the community to enjoy a more normal pattern of life.

mercury poisoning. Breathing in or swallowing the vapour of metallic mercury is an industrial hazard as most of its compounds are intensely poisonous. In the past most cases of acute poisoning were due to absorption of mercuric chloride (corrosive sublimate) used as an antiseptic douche or lotion, or to its accidental or deliberate swallowing. Symptoms were severe with damage to bowel and kidneys, and death not infrequently followed.

Chronic mercurial poisoning occurs as an industrial disease in such occupations as thermometer, meter, and mirror making, which use metallic mercury; in the fur felt trade which uses mercuric nitrate; and in the manufacture of detonators (fulminate of mercury). The effects are inflammation of the mucous lining of the mouth, increased flow of saliva, loosening of the teeth, and various nervous symptoms such as optic neuritis, minor epilepsy, tremors and mental disturbance. Strict measures of industrial hygiene must be enforced.

Mercury is also becoming an ecological hazard. Outbreaks of acute poisoning (Minamata disease) have occurred in Japan through eating tuna fish caught in waters contaminated by methyl mercury, an industrial waste. Methyl mercury is also used as a fungicide in the treatment of seed-corn and there have been serious incidents causing many deaths where such grain was eaten instead of being sown. One such incident in Iraq in 1971, when near-starving peasants were tempted to consume seed-wheat distributed to small farmers, is reported to have caused at least 100,000 cases of illness with 6,000 deaths.

mesentery. The mesenteries are folds of peritoneum which hang loosely from the back of the abdomen, join the different parts of the intestine and in effect sling them to the back abdominal wall. The mesenteries also contain numerous lymph glands and vessels, and contain the mesenteric blood vessels which supply blood to the intestine. The mesentery of the small intestine is a roughly fan-shaped fold.

metabolism. To sustain its vital processes every living organism requires to extract and use the energy stored in FOOD. By digestion food is broken down into simpler substances which are absorbed into the blood stream and thereafter undergo chemical reactions in the body. These reactions provide for the growth and repair of tissue, the production of heat and energy, the activity of muscle and nerve, the manufacture of essential secretions, and finally the passing of waste-products.

These interdependent activities are collectively called general metabolism. When complex substances are broken down the process is catabolism; their chemical conversion is anabolism. Special metabolism is an account of the changes affecting a particular constituent of the diet.

Chemical reactions may be such as to absorb heat (endothermic) or to give out heat (exothermic). Most of those occurring in the body are exothermic. Even when the body is at rest it has a minimum need for energy to maintain its circulation, muscle-tone, and temperature. This energy, derived from food and food-stores, ultimately appears as heat. Heat so generated by the body can be measured by direct calorimetry with the subject in an insulated chamber, but this is inconvenient and laborious. Since heat is produced by the 'burning' of food, with absorption of oxygen and elimination of carbon dioxide, it is easier to measure the uptake and output of these gases and then calculate how much heat must have been evolved. This procedure is used to determine the basal metabolic rate (BMR), and for purposes of comparison between persons of different sizes this is expressed as Calories per square metre of body-surface per hour. (When considering diets it is the Calorie requirement per day which is quoted.)

Since by far the biggest expenditure of energy during complete rest is on maintenance of bodily warmth, the amount needed varies not only with weight but with the amount of body surface which heat can be lost. The smaller an animal the greater is its proportion of body surface to weight. Thus a man of average height and bulk, weighing about 70 kg. (11 stone) requires approximately 1,100 Calories daily for basic metabolism, or roughly 1,000 Calories per square metre of body surface, while a rabbit, weighing 3 kg. (6 lb.), needs about 150 Calories, or again roughly 1,000 per square metre of body surface.

Basal metabolism varies inversely with fatness, because the stouter the person the greater his total body surface. Thus a fat man whose basic metabolism uses 1,400 Calories daily will at first lose weight rapidly on a 1,800 Calorie diet, because the remaining 400 Calories are clearly insufficient to balance even the mildest of normal activities; but after some weeks of obtaining balancing energy from his own fat and muscular tissues, he becomes appreciably slimmer, has a lessened bodily surface, and perhaps has a basal metabolism of only 1,250 Calories, so that his weight loss on 1,800 Calories daily becomes much slower.

During the first year of life the BMR is about 50, declining to 40 at age 20 for normal adult males and continuing to fall gradually to 36 in old age. Values for women are slightly less at all ages, reflecting their lesser muscularity. Physiologically, BMR is increased by muscular exercise, low environmental temperatures, and by the intake of food, especially protein. The stimulating effect of protein is known as its specific dynamic action. Conversely BMR is reduced by rest, warmth, and starvation, and it falls by about 15 during sleep. Pathologically, BMR is raised by fevers and by hyperthyrodism and lowered by hypothyroidism, under-nutrition, and certain disorders of the adrenal and the pituitary glands, two of the ENDOCRINE GLANDS.

The special metabolism of various foods in the diet is complex and is dealt with under DIGESTION.

Diseases. Metabolic diseases may result from (1) disturbance of the acid-base balance which normally keeps the blood and tissues slightly alkaline; (2) endocrine disorders and defects in metabolizing specific dietary constituents; and (3) excess or deprivation of essential food elements.

1. The acid-base balance may become altered towards acidity or alkalinity. Since blood and tissues are mostly composed of water it is convenient to consider pure water first. Water is composed of hydrogen (acid) and hydroxide (base) ions, in chemical symbols H and OH. If carbon dioxide (CO_2) is added to water it combines with some of the hydroxide to produce a weak acid, carbonic acid, so that the water becomes slightly acid. In blood a change of acid-base balance is a little more complicated because blood contains certain 'buffer' substances such as sodium bicarbonate which tend to neutralize carbonic acid. But if enough carbon dioxide passed into the blood to form more carbonic acid than the buffers could deal with, the blood would become slightly acid. Normally carbon dioxide is breathed out from the lungs, but if respiration is impaired (e.g., by the deliberate holding of the breath or by any respiratory disease) it accumulates in the blood and, when the carbonic acid produced by the action of carbon dioxide on the water of the blood is enough to overcome the buffers, the blood becomes slightly acid (acidaemia). A similar situation can occur when a disturbance of carbohydrate meta-bolism produces excess of aceto-acetic acid, or when inefficient kidneys fail to excrete sufficient of this acid. Conversely, the blood may become too alkaline (alkalaemia) through overdosage of alkalies (antacids) taken for indigestion, or in persistent vomiting with loss of the normal hydrochloric acid from the stomach, or in over-breathing at high altitudes with excessive loss of carbon dioxide.

2. Various endocrine disorders affect the metabolic rate, e.g., insulin deficiency (causing excessive sugar in the blood), and diseases of thyroid secretion (excess raising the metabolic rate, and deficiency lowering it). Examples of defects in the breaking down of specific dietary constituents include gout (in which uric acid accumulates in the tissues), phenylketonuria (in which the body cannot deal with the amino-acid phenyl-alanine), and coeliac disease (in which the body cannot cope with gluten).

3. Excess or deprivation of any food element affects metabolism, e.g., too much carbo-hydrate and fat causes obesity, severe protein deficiency produces kwashiorkor, and carbohydrate insufficiency – whether from low intake or from inability to use it (as in diabetes) – produces acidaemia. See also DEFICIENCY DISEASES, VITAMINS and MINERAL SALTS.

metastasis. The transfer of disease from one part of the body to another by movement of disease particles either in the blood stream or in the lymphatic vessels. In particular in cancer there is a serious danger of a few cells becoming dislodged from the primary growth and giving rise to a secondary cancer elsewhere in the body. Clearly this danger makes it important that cancer is treated early, before any metastasis has occurred.

metazoan parasites. See TROPICAL DISEASES.

metorrhagia. Irregular haemorrhage from the uterus. The condition is sometimes divided into (1) menorrhagia, excessive blood loss during the menstrual period; (2) strict metorrhagia, bleeding between the periods; and (3) bleeding occurring after the menopause. However, the first two often overlap.

Such bleeding is due to some condition of the vulva, vagina or uterus and calls for expert gynaecological investigation. The commonest causes are the presence of uterine polyps (fibroids) or other types of tumour. There should be no delay in seeking advice and appropriate treatment.

metritis. Inflammation of the uterus. Apart from cases due to gonorrhoea, acute metritis is usually the sequel of septic infection occurring after childbirth (puerperal sepsis) or abortion, especially in cases induced without proper aseptic precautions. Chronic metritis may occasionally be due to other pelvic infections but true chronic inflammation of the uterus is not really possible because in menstruation the monthly discharge of its lining ensures that infection drains away with the menstrual flow.

The symptoms of irregular haemorrhage and discharge, with backache and a bulky uterus persisting after childbirth, are considered to be due to dysfunction of the ovaries and are treated accordingly.

microbe. A general name for all micro-organisms too small to be seen by the naked eye. In broadly descending order of size microbes can be classified as protozoa, fungi, bacteria, rickettsia and viruses.

Although hinted at by earlier physicians the idea that infection is similar to putrefaction was first stated by Fracastorius of Verona in 1546, and microbes were seen by Leeuwenhoek using his simple microscope in 1683; but the relationship between microbes and infection was really established only in the late nineteenth century by Pasteur and his German contemporary, Koch.

microbiology. See BACTERIOLOGY.

microscope. An optical instrument with a magnifying lens or combination of lenses for inspecting objects too small to be seen in detail – or at all – by the naked eye.

A simple microscope is merely a single magnifying lens, such as was used by Leeuwenhoek (1632-1723) and Malpighi (1628-94) and is today routinely used by watchmakers. A simple reading glass commonly magnifies about two or three times, but with a very strong lens it is possible to obtain magnification up to about sixteen times without distortion.

The compound microscope, using two lenses, can be traced back to Galileo in 1610, but an effective compound microscope giving a magnification of over two hundred times did not exist until the late eighteenth century. The introduction of an oil immersion lens as part of a compound microscope increased magnification to about a thousand times, but there was still no possibility of seeing objects or structures so tiny that rays of light from them, even in oil which refracted them less than did air, were so bent that they could not come to a focus.

Finally the electron microscope permitted the photographing of objects under vastly higher magnification. To give an illustrative

example, a bacteriologist in the 1920s could see a pneumococcus (a circular bacterium) with magnification and use of oil immersion increasing it to about the appearance of the punctuation mark at the end of this sentence; his successor in the 1970s can not only see a virus of a twentieth of the size of the pneumococcus (by photography, not by direct vision) but can even study its structure.

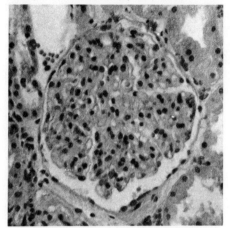

A section of kidney seen under a microscope (magnified 100 times)

micturition. See URINATION.

middle age and health. The life history of any organism follows a pattern in which growth and development rises to a plateau of maximum biological effectiveness followed eventually by gradual decline. In human terms this plateau normally extends from the attainment of adult status to middle age at, say, 45 years. The subsequent decline is due to the progressive ageing of tissues with their increasing susceptibility to adverse environmental conditions and to degenerative changes. This normal progression may be hastened at any stage by harmful circumstances. Of these infection has always been of major importance but many infections can now be controlled and treated much more effectively than ever before, and many other hazards of life have also been greatly reduced.

Conservation of health in middle age and beyond is thus a question of prolonging the plateau of full efficiency and reducing the rate of decline which sooner or later inevitably follows. The main barrier to success is the lack of precise knowledge about many general diseases associated with ageing. Often their causes are complicated and intimately related to life-patterns. In general the wealthier and better educated groups in the population live longer. The death rate, however, is not the only consideration because conditions which do not actually kill also cause much disability and loss of efficiency from recurrent or prolonged ill health. It is necessary to look separately at various diseases:

1. Vascular diseases, i.e., those affecting the blood vessels, are either degenerative or harden the arteries, both of which may be associated with raised blood pressure and tend to cause

damaging disease in the heart, brain and kidney. Coronary thrombosis has shown significant increase in the last thirty years and it seems likely that this has been contributed to by obesity, especially if associated with a high intake of animal fat, by lack of regular exercise, and by excessive cigarette smoking. Cerebral haemorrhage or thrombosis, also related to arterial disease, have not shown increase but nevertheless they continue to be responsible for much residual disability from paralysis.

High blood pressure is at least to some extent a stress-related disease and its ill-effects are capable of being modified by early diagnosis, drugs and suitable adjustment of an individual's way of life, while an enormous role exists for prevention before the blood pressure has begun to rise.

2. Bronchitis and other diseases of the respiratory system are the major cause of illness leading middle-aged patients to consult their general practitioners. The high incidence of bronchitis with its life-shortening effects on the breathing mechanism is perhaps related to our difficult climate (about which little can be done), but there is still scope for progress in the reduction of atmospheric pollution (and of the pollution of the personal atmosphere by smoking), in the provision of better and warmer homes, in the improvement of working conditions, and in the prompt recognition and efficient treatment of the early stages of what could become a chronic disease.

3. Malignant disease is still open to a great deal of research, but although the exact causes of the various types of cancer are still unknown there is much evidence to incriminate sources of chronic irritation: certain occupational hazards, atmospheric pollution, and cigarette smoking are examples. The best hope of reducing the incidence of malignant disease and the risks of a fatal outcome lies in avoiding known hazards and in taking measures to secure early diagnosis (e.g., breast and cervical carcinoma) at a stage when treatment can still be expected to have successful results.

4. Peptic ulceration is in all probability a stress disease aggravated by irregular, hurried, or unsatisfactory meals. These factors again are related to civilization and to the working and living conditions which it imposes.

5. The rheumatic and arthritis group of diseases – such as rheumatoid arthritis, lumbago, sciatica and rheumatism, and the degenerative condition, osteo-arthritis – are not important causes of death but they occasion about 10 per cent of all consultations. Overweight persons are particularly prone to osteo-arthritis. The other diseases probably start with an infection or are related to the body's immunity mechanisms and can be reduced by the finding and possible removal of septic foci, e.g., infected tonsils or bad teeth, and the improvement of tissue resistance by good nutrition and avoidance of harmful environmental conditions such as excessive stress and exposure.

6. Diabetes is in most if not all cases an inherited disease, but reduction of its ill-effects requires early recognition and treatment. If treatment is to be successful, it is necessary to have intelligent and active co-operation from the patient, adequate supervision, and good social conditions.

7. Adequate nutrition is fundamental to good health and the diet of many older persons is deficient in protein, minerals (especially iron), and vitamins.

8. Industrial diseases and industrial, road and home accidents are all essentially preventable.

9. Mental illness, including neurosis and psychosomatic disorders, is in part related to hereditary factors, in part to bad home conditions or poor human relationships in the important early years of life, and in part to current environmental conditions and current human relationships. The scope for prevention is clearly enormous. Early recognition and appropriate help will also reduce the risks of permanently disabling illness.

General. It will be seen that the disabling conditions of middle age and beyond provide vast opportunities both for prevention and for efforts to minimize their ill-effects although many of them cannot be completely prevented. In most instances any worth-while results depend on two essentials: (1) persistent and persuasive health education; and (2) motivation of patients and potential patients to secure active co-operation. Allied to these are schemes for the early detection of disease, as for instance by special surveys, followed by appropriate preventive therapy and advice.

In developed countries and to some extent also in developing countries the last seventy years have witnessed a remarkable improvement in the health of children and young adults, with reduction (and in some cases virtual extinction) of many diseases. It may well be that the next few decades will see similar improvement in the health of the middle-aged.

middle ear disease. See EAR, otitis media.

migraine. True migraine is a paroxysmal nervous disturbance with headache, nausea, vomiting and some sensory disturbance usually related to vision. The name is derived from the Greek word *hemikrania* meaning one side of the head, and indeed, as this indicates, the headache tends to be limited to one side or part of the head the visual phenomena experienced may take various forms such as mistiness of vision, flashes of light, dark or bright spots, and usually precede the onset of headache as an AURA.

Although this is the classical description of migraine any recurrent headache is frequently so-called. Many cases respond quite well to a simple 'headache-powder' containing aspirin, phenacetin and caffeine, especially if given early in an attack. A preparation of ergot (ergotamine tartrate) has some reputation as a remedy either given by injection or in a larger dose by mouth.

milk. A whitish liquid which is the normal secretion of the mammary glands of female mammals and is intended to provide for the nutritional needs of their offspring until weaned.

It consists of a watery solution of protein, lactose (milk sugar) and mineral salts, with small suspended globules of fat forming an emulsion. The relative proportions of these constituents vary in different animals in particular the amount of protein varies roughly in proportion to the rate at which the offspring grows. This can be illustrated thus:

Species	Protein	Lactose	Fat	Minerals	Water
Human	1.7%	7.5%	3.5%	0.2%	87.1%
Cow	3.5%	4.8%	3.7%	0.7%	87.3%
Cat	9.5%	4.9%	3.3%	0.6%	81.7%
Rabbit	15.5%	2.0%	10.4%	2.6%	69.9%

Man has kept domestic animals since prehistoric times and has made use of their milk for his own nutritional needs. Because of its position as a vital natural food it has from time immemorial played a part in religion, legend, and superstition. In *The Odyssey*, Book IX, Homer describes the milking of goats in the cave of Polyphemus, and in the Bible Canaan was the land 'flowing with milk and honey'. Even today a well known wine is still symbolically called *Liebfraumilch*, or Milk of our Beloved Lady.

In the composition of milk as shown above the protein consists mainly of casein and lactalbumen with some enzymes. Milk sugar is lactose, which is easily broken down into glucose and galactose; it is the only source of the latter which is a constituent of brain and nerve tissue. Milk fat is a variable mixture of glycerides – combinations of glycerin with a fatty acid. The principle fatty acid is butyric acid responsible for the characteristic taste of butter and cream. Milk is also a very good source of essential minerals, especially calcium and phosphorus, but it is deficient in iron. Other minor constituents are phospholipids, cholesterol (an alcohol which helps to maintain stability of the fat emulsion), pigments, and vitamins. Usually the latter are all represented to some extent and especially C and D, but it is not a rich or reliable source of these and infants should be given supplementary supplies.

Raw milk is a potential danger as a common vehicle of disease and should always be pasteurized. There are two commercial processes: (1) the Holder method, in which milk is heated to 63 ° to 65.5 °C. (145 ° to 150 °F.) for thirty minutes and then cooled to 13 °C. (55 °F.) or less; (2) the high temperature short time method (HTST), which requires a temperature of 72 °C. (162 °F.) for fifteen seconds with subsequent immediate cooling to 13 °C. (55 °F.) or less. Apart from the risk of disease, raw milk always contains organisms which eventually cause it to sour and curdle. Heat-treated and sterilized milks are available with improved keeping qualities. In homogenized milk the fat globules are broken down and dispersed more finely by forcible spraying against a metal plate.

A wide range of subsidiary products are derived from milk. (1) Cream is produced by centrifuging milk. The fat content is 20 to 40 per cent. (2) Skim milk is the residuum after cream removal. It is used for making cheese and in industry as a source of casein which is used in the manufacture of buttons, paint, bristles etc. (3) Dried milk is milk with water removed by evaporation (spray or roller process). (4) Evaporated milk is concentrated to half volume, sealed in cans and sterilized. (5) Condensed milk is first concentrated to half volume: 40 per cent sugar is then added before it is canned. It is not sterilized and so does not have the brownish appearance and altered taste of evaporated milk. (6) Yoghurt is a sour semi-solid fermented milk, reduced to two-thirds of its original volume. (7) Butter is produced from whole milk by churning, which collects the fat globules together. It must not contain more than 16 per cent water. (8) Cheese is made from the precipitated casein of milk, with varying amounts of milk-fat.

The production and sale of milk in many countries is closely controlled by legislation. Regulations relate to the construction of buildings, the health and care of cows, methods of cleaning and sterilizing equipment, the health and cleanliness of milk workers, and the control of the temperature of milk in storage and transit. The effectiveness of these measures is supervised by periodic inspections and by chemical and bacteriological checks.

Throughout Great Britain the Attested Herds Scheme of 1935 has secured the virtual eradication of bovine tuberculosis in milk herds. Similar measures are now being taken with regard to brucellosis, another bovine and milk-borne disease. The use of antibiotics has also reduced the risks of udder infections transmissible to man by contaminated milk.

milk diet. See DIETS, SPECIAL.

mind. The nature of the mind is something which has engaged the attention of philosophers ever since man began to think about his place and purpose in the universe. It is probable that the distinction between mind and matter had a religious origin and began with the idea that the body came from the earth and the soul from heaven. With advance in knowledge came an increasing tendency to question the origins and relationships of spirit, soul and mind, and to look for explanations based on a fuller understanding of the physical world. Discoveries in physics now make matter seem less material and the study of thought-processes makes mind seem less mental. The differentiation between mind and body thus becomes increasingly dubious as these two areas of study approach each other from opposite directions. These ideas are much debated and it seems unlikely that any amount of discussion will ever lead to general agreement.

It was Aristotle, much before his time, who coined the famous metaphor about a baby's mind being a blank slate, and he received powerful support from Locke in his *Essay Concerning Human Understanding* (1690) who defended the premise that all ideas and all the functions of the mind arise from experience; if this is so, then experience must alter the physical body in some way. By 1870 or so the physiologists were firmly of the view that all human acts could be explained by physico-chemical principles, and that the mind and its actual function were due to electrical and chemical processes initiated by sensory perceptions and further elaborated l association with past perceptions.

Roughly simultaneously with this realization came the knowledge that mental activity takes place in the brain. It is within the brain that we appreciate what the sense organs (e.g., the eyes) have noted, that we associate present information with past experience, that we feel pleasure or anger, that we take decisions, and that we initiate action. The role of the brain was not realized earlier: everyday words like 'sanguine', 'melancholy', 'choleric' and 'phlegmatic' indicate that people used to think of mental attitudes as depending on the 'numours' of the blood and bile. As late as the seventeenth centry Pascal could say, 'The heart has its reasons of which reason is ignorant'.

It gradually became accepted that mind was not a thing but an activity of the brain and on this basis there has been built a scientific discipline which seeks to explore, catalogue, and explain this activity. This is PSYCHOLOGY or the science of mental life.

mind and body. The nervous system of man or any living organism is an instrument of adaptation. Its purpose is to adjust the organism to its environment; and the ultimate object of any sensation, emotion or thought-process is to produce some sort of action appropriate to the circumstances at any given time. Any disturbance received from the environment is technically a stimulus and the action evoked is a response.

Stimuli operate at various levels. Most simply they may produce a reflex action without the mind being involved at all. If for instance a person incautiously touches a hot object the hand is snatched away automatically by a spinal reflex action and closer examination would show that this painful stimulus had also produced physical effects, e.g., in the abdomen. If in addition the person had received a 'fright' from a painful experience of this kind there would be a conscious emotional response, with such symptoms as increased heart beat, sweating, nervous tremor, or by 'shock' with feelings of tiredness, faintness or collapse. Subconsciously the mind might respond by learning as illustrated in the proverbial saying that 'a burned child dreads the fire'.

It is when stimuli produce effects upon consciousness or the subconscious that we can expect adverse reactions between mind and body. In short, emotions profoundly affect the characteristics of bodily adaptation to stress.

The primitive emotions include anger, fear, anxiety (which is a kind of fear), love, and the need to be loved. All of these are accompanied by bodily reactions which prepare the body for action and which may produce either conscious or subconscious effects. Under conditions of civilization the appropriate action cannot always be taken, and so inner tensions develop. These provide the causes for two main groups of diseases. There are first of all those termed psychosomatic which are typically represented by physical conditions such as high blood-pressure, coronary heart disease, asthma, peptic ulcer, colitis and so on, together with less specific symptoms such as fatigue, tenseness, lack of strength, indigestion and insomnia. The second group comprise the neuroses, variously manifested and labelled as neurasthenia, anxiety states, hysteria and obsession.

Conditions of both kinds constitute a very large part of any general medical practice. The treatment which they are accorded is generally only symptomatic and does not influence the root-causes of disability although it may give a measure of psychological support.

Illnesses of these kinds can only be permanently alleviated or relieved by removal of the origins of stress or by psychoanalysis to identify the cause and then to persuade the individual to recognize the causes to appreciate and understand how they have produced his illness, and to induce him to make the calm and resolute efforts necessary to alter his way of life.

Measures for this alleviation or relief are highly important, but clearly removal of the causes of stress (not easy) and successful persuasion of a patient to alter his pattern of living (again not easy) will not reduce blood pressure already dangerously high, nor remove a peptic ulcer that has already eroded the coats of the stomach, nor fully remove a tendency to over-anxiety that has existed for forty years. So, as knowledge of mental factors improves, it becomes more and more important to deal with the causes of psychosomatic and neurotic diseases before the diseases have became established. The fostering of good mental and emotional health is perhaps the biggest task facing health workers today.

mineral salts. A well-balanced DIET must provide not only sufficient FOOD for the energy needs of the body and adequate amounts of fluid and vitamins but it must also supply certain mineral constituents. The basic essentials are salts of SODIUM, POTASSIUM, and magnesium, but these are always present in any reasonable diet and no special measures are required to ensure their adequacy. Next in importance are PHOSPHORUS and sulphur which are mainly derived from protein and which play an essential part in various enzyme reactions. They too are unlikely to be deficient if the diet otherwise contains sufficient protein.

The minerals most commonly lacking are CALCIUM, IRON and IODINE. Calcium is particularly required for the formation of bones and teeth, and infants with calcium deficiency may show symptoms of tetany. Children require at least 1 g. of calcium per day and pregnant and nursing mothers about twice that amount. Milk is by far the best and most readily assimilable source.

Iron is necessary for the synthesis of haemoglobin, the oxygen-carrying pigment of the blood. The daily requirement is from 15 to 20 mg. Deficiency leads to anaemia and the best sources are liver, meat, eggs and some cereals and vegetables including spinach, beans, peas, whole-wheat and oatmeal.

Iodine is an essential constituent of thyroid hormone, and goitre results if intake is insufficient. Sea foods are the chief natural sources but most table salts contain small quantities of sodium iodine (1 in 100,000). The daily requirement is about 15 micrograms. Apart from these well-recognized requirements evidence is accumulating of the importance of 'trace elements' – especially in relation to animal husbandry. Copper in minute quantities has been shown to act as a catalyst in haemoglobin formation and it also prevents a disease called 'swayback' in lambs; sheep become anaemic on pastures deficient in cobalt; chickens develop a bone disease known as perosis when their manganese intake is insufficient.

Although these discoveries may not have direct applications in human metabolism they serve to illustrate a fascinating field of research and to emphasize the importance of minerals in many vital processes not only of the larger animals themselves but of their intestinal bacteria which contribute to the synthesis of special substances which their bodies need.

miscarriage. The accidental or non-deliberate termination of pregnancy before the unborn child has become viable i.e., developed sufficiently to live. The border-line from premature labour is generally taken at twenty-eight weeks after the first day of the last menstrual period, although some children born before that date survive and many born slightly after it die. In contrast to miscarriage the word ABORTION is increasingly associated with deliberate artificial termination of pregnancy.

It is commonly said that about 15 per cent of pregnancies end in miscarriage but reliable figures are hard to maintain because an early miscarriage may be mistaken for a menstrual period. The real figure may well be as high as 20 per cent.

Causes of miscarriage include (1) haemorrhage into the thickened uterine wall or into the foetal membranes, causing separation of the fertilized ovum or death of the foetus; (2) death of the foetus from disease or malformation; and (3) stimulation of the uterine centre (equivalent to the starting of labour), for example through trauma, surgical operation, violent emotion or extreme exhaustion. Among the many predisposing causes may be mentioned endometritis, syphilis, toxaemia of pregnancy, nephritis and uterine malformations.

The main indications of miscarriage are bleeding, usually beginning as a slight staining and becoming more profuse, and sometimes (but not always) pain, radiating round from the back.

In threatened miscarriage, where the bleeding is only slight and the pains are moderate and infrequent, rest and sedatives may permit the pregnancy to continue; and in cases of doubt bleeding in any wanted pregnancy should at first be treated as threatened miscarriage. If miscarriage is inevitable and there is serious bleeding and severe pain the operation of curettage may be needed to complete the process quickly and so end haemorrhage which, if continued, might endanger the mother's life.

Some women are subject to repeated miscarriages, and various measures such as prolonged rest, the administration of hormones, and the treatment of any disease or other conditions which are present may help to secure a more successful outcome. Expert advice should be sought, and good antenatal care is important.

mites. Tiny, eight-legged arthropods, rather similar to ticks, many of which live as parasites on animals or plants, or on decaying organic matter.

Perhaps the best known are the *Sarcoptes scabie* which is responsible for scabies, the *Demodex follicularis* which causes a form of mange in dogs, and the common harvest mite which on occasion causes itching and blisters. A form of typhus – scrub typhus – is caused by a mite.

mitosis. See CELL.

mitral disease. See HEART.

Mittelschmerz. Pain occurring in the middle of the interval between menstrual periods, not yet fully understood but thought to be connected with ovulation. On occasion acute appendicitis has been mistaken for *Mittelschmerz* with tragic results.

mongolism. A common type of permanently retarded growth and mental development in which the face is short and broad, the skull

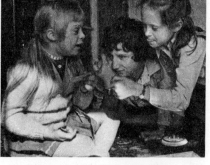

A mongol child with her friends

round and rather small, the eyes slightly slanted and often without eyelashes, the tongue large and often protruding, the hands broad and clumsy, and the fingers short. Sufferers from this congenital condition tend to have, when adult, an intelligence roughly equivalent to that of a child aged 3 to 7 years. They are cheerful, amiable, likeable and more lively than most other types of mentally handicapped person.

Mongols require continuous supervision and protection throughout their life which is sometimes relatively short and they should be provided with interests adapted to their capabilities through occupation centres.

The condition, which occurs in about 1 in six hundred live births, is found most commonly in children born to mothers over the age of 38 or 40 years. It is sometimes due to the possession of an extra chromosome (forty-seven instead of forty-six), and in other cases due to an abnormal arrangement of the chromosomes. The condition, described by the British physician John Down (1828-96), was generally termed mongolism until about 1960 because of the slanting of the eyes, but in recent years 'mongolism' has tended to disappear in scientific usage.

Mongols – now called sufferers from Down's syndrome – constitute about one-quarter of all mentally handicapped children.

monitoring. A term that has recently come into use in Britain for repeated and regular measurement of the concentration of harmful pollutants, to enable us to follow changes over a period and to assess the effectiveness of control measures. Information about increasing levels of pollution in atmosphere, water or soil can provide early warnings before damage to human or animal health occurs. Indication that pollution levels are stationary or decreasing can provide evidence that existing control measures are having satisfactory results.

Airborne pollutants, e.g., factories that emit fumes, can be measured at their source, at various points in the atmosphere and at places where the pollutants tend to fall to the surface. A terrifying example of such pollution occurred in Seveso, Italy, in 1976, necessitating massive evacuation of population. As an example of measurement, for smoke and sulphur dioxide there are some 1,200 sampling points now established in the U.S.A. Similarly pollutant levels in soil are measured, especially in the neighbourhood of industries with emissions of toxic waste that may effect the suitability of the land for agriculture, and certain measurements are made in respect of wild life and foodstuffs. For radioactive substances attempts are made to measure the 'fall-out' from the air and in rain, and to assess the levels of radioactive substances in milk and drinking water.

Possible pollution of fresh water is measured at the points of any discharge of effluent into a river and at various other points, with attention to organic poisons as well as to bacterial contamination. Some internationally co-ordinated work is done on marine pollution, in respect of which it has to be remembered that the sea is the ultimate repository for much of man's waste.

An authoritative account of the present position is contained in an official report, *The Monitoring of the Environment in the United Kingdom*, published in 1974 by Her Majesty's Stationery Office.

monoamine oxidase. An enzyme, commonly abbreviated to MAO, which facilitates the oxidation of adrenalin in the body and thereby reduces the activity – e.g., increased pulse rate and respiration – that would otherwise take place from excess of adrenalin.

One theory of depression is that it is due to deficiency of adrenalin or of a similar substance (a pressor amine). Hence drugs that suppress the production of monoamine oxidase (MAO inhibitors) and so preserve the body's adrenalin are extensively used in the treatment of depression. These inhibitors, should not be used in various diseases of the heart and liver and must be taken only under strict medical supervision; but, so taken, they have a considerable record of at least partial success.

morbidity. The prevalence of disease in a community. Statistics relating to the presence or frequency of disease, or of particular diseases, are of great importance in determining the measures required to improved community health and in deciding how these should be deployed. Figures showing the death rate only refer to events which are past, but morbidity data record current problems of ill-health and may help to identify environmental or social causes.

It is however difficult to collect meaningful information about disease. Death is a clearly defined event and can be certified with reasonable precision, but illness is less easy to define. Symptoms complained of may be vague and not readily assignable to a recognized illness; they may vary from day to day: they may represent a new illness, a recurrence or a relapse. Moreover what one person regards as illness may be tolerated uncomplainingly by another.

The next difficulty concerns the source of information. In virtually all countries deaths are statutorily recorded but except for a few notifiable infections and in some countries industrial diseases there are no legal requirements for the notification of most other conditions. It is necessary to seek other indicators of the prevalence and nature of sickness experience. The most important of these and certainly the greatest in volume are records of incapacity derived in the U.K. from the National Insurance Scheme. Even these suffer from serious defects since they cover only the insured population; illnesses of less than four days' duration are not recorded; occupation is not stated and the diagnosis is often in very general terms either because of uncertainty or because of the doctor's wish not to publicize anything alarming or discreditable. For these and other reasons any calculated morbidity ratios are sometimes too inaccurate to provide pointers to useful action.

In Britain and various other countries national statistics have been supplemented in many ways. Some of these are school and pre-school health records, hospital in-patient and out-patient records, sickness experience in individual firms or industries, general practitioner consultations, cancer registration and special sickness surveys. These fragmented sources help to contribute to the study of illness and its causation.

Of particular interest in Britain is a recent survey of general practitioner consultations which showed that patients consulted their doctors predominantly for conditions relating to disease of the respiratory system, digestive system, locomotory system, heart and circulation, genito-urinary system, nervous system, skin and mental disability in a descending order of frequency. Despite improvements in medical treatment, sickness, absence from work and demands for treatment continue to rise year by year. Such circumstances should not be taken as indicating that the population is less healthy. Rather it means that people, within a different social climate, are less willing to tolerate minor departures from health and more able to seek a remedy now that the costs of advice and treatment, and the expenses of illness, have been shifted from the individual to the community through the availability of a free health service and the provision of social benefits.

morning sickness. Many but by no means all pregnant women experience feelings of nausea on rising in the morning, usually between the second and fourth months of pregnancy. In some cases there is actual vomiting of a small amount of mucus. In the absence of any signs of toxaemia or other abnormality this 'morning sickness' can generally be regarded as of no important significance. Symptomatic treatment by gastric or nerve sedatives is often prescribed or vitamin intake increased by large doses of vitamin C and the vitamin B complex.

Occasionally the condition may progress to the more serious condition of hyperemesis gravidarum but usually in such cases a toxic element is demonstrably present to provide a basis for more rational lines of treatment.

moron. An American term for a mentally defective person corresponding to the British classification 'feeble-minded', with an intelligence quotient between 50 and 75.

morphia. Morphia or morphine (named after Morpheus, the Greek god of sleep) is the chief alkaloid contained in opium. An extremely effective pain-killer, it is one of the most valuable of drugs.

In ordinary dosage it produces a very short period of restlessness and excitement (probably due to removal of the inhibitory effect of the higher nervous centres) and thereafter a dulling of the perceptive faculties, a loss of the sensation of pain and indeed a decreased activity of all sensations, and a state of drowsiness. A characteristic feature – useful for the diagnosis of morphine poisoning – is contraction of the pupils.

The normal dosage for an adult is 16 mg. by injection but children are abnormally sensitive to the drug, so that the dosage has to be far less in proportion to their weight. Many paediatricians consider that morphine should in no circumstances be given to children under 2 years.

The dangers of this extremely useful pain-killer are twofold. (1) It causes depression of the respiratory centre (and therefore shallowness of breathing), of the circulatory system (and therefore lowered blood pressure), and of the alimentary system (and therefore constipation), and in excess the depression of the respiratory centre can lead to death from asphyxia. (2) It is very much a drug of addiction: even three or four doses at intervals of eight or twelve hours can lead to appreciable desire for it, and continuation of dosage for a few days can lead to very definite craving. Hence the use of the drug has to be strictly controlled.

In morphine poisoning – identified by pin-point pupils, shallow breathing and cold skin – the patient should be kept moving and should be given strong coffee if able to drink, and a doctor should be promptly summoned.

mortality. Loss of life. A mortality rate or death rate is the number of deaths in a year per thousand of population. A mortality table shows the average expectation of life at various ages.

mosquito. A general name for gnat-like insects of the family *Culicidae*. There are four principal genera and they are important in medicine as transmitters of certain tropical diseases because of their propensity for biting and blood-sucking. The most important genera are *Anopheles,* many species of which convey malaria, and *Aedes,* whose members transmit yellow fever. *Culex* species are responsible for the spread of filariasis and dengue fever.

Mosquitoes of the *Anopheles* and *Culex* genera occur also in temperate climates but do not spread disease there because of the absence of initial infection. Another non-tropical genus is *Theobaldia. T. annulata* is the large wood-gnat whose bites often cause trouble from subsequent sepsis.

mould. See FUNGUS.

mouth. The uppermost part of the DIGESTIVE SYSTEM. Its function is the ingestion and mastication of food and it also plays a part in speech production.

Inflammation of the mouth is known as STOMATITIS.

Mouth dryness. Dryness of the mouth (xerostomia) is due to deficient secretion of saliva and is a common symptom of any acute feverish illness. It is indicative of loss of body fluid (dehydration), a condition which must be corrected promptly by the administration of additional fluid either by mouth or by injection.

Of less important significance is the dryness of the mouth experienced by mouth-breathers in whom the normal amount of salivary secretion is insufficient to counteract evaporation to the air-flow. Dryness of the mouth may also occur as a result of strong emotion, especially fear. This is the basis of the

traditional witch doctor procedure for identifying from several suspects the actual criminal who is unable to masticate successfully a mouthful of dry food-stuff. Mouth dryness from minor causes may be helped by the use of chewing-gum, acid sweets or by bitter tonics given before meals.

mouth-breathing. Habitual mouth-breathing results from chronic nasal obstruction. In children this tends to produce deformity of the face, naso-pharynx and chest. In most instances it is primarily due to persistent infection and enlargement of the ADENOIDS which are aggregations of lymphoid tissue in the naso-pharynx.

In adults nasal obstruction may result from deflection of the nasal septum (either as a congenital defect or acquired through injury), from chronic infections of the nose leading to swelling of the nasal mucous membrane and sometimes to the formation of bulky growths known as polypi; or from infection and suppuration in the nasal sinuses.

Specialist advice and treatment are generally indicated in order to correct the nasal obstruction by measures appropriate to the individual case.

mouth inflammation. See STOMATITIS.

mouth to mouth breathing. See ARTIFICAL RESPIRATION.

mouth washes. Antiseptic solutions for rinsing the mouth and throat to allay the pain and irritation of septic and inflammatory conditions and to encourage healing. Gargle is a practically synonymous term and gargling is a procedure employed in an attempt to reach the tonsils and posterior pharyngeal wall where infection is common, since the effect of mouth rinsing alone does not extend as far back as that.

Although mouth washes give temporary relief it is doubtful if they have any great effect on infections, which really require specific therapy, and their mechanical cleansing action may be equally well obtained from a simple solution of common salt (one teaspoonful in a tumblerful of warm water). They do, however, have a useful place in dentistry, particularly after extractions, since astringent and antiseptic properties can help to minimize or arrest haemorrhage and combat socket infection.

movable kidney. The kidneys are situated high in the loin on each side of the vertebral column and are kept in position by an envelopment of fatty tissue and by the anchorage afforded by their main blood vessels. Although they move slightly up and down with respiration their lower poles cannot normally be felt through the abdomen. When a kidney has greater mobility than this it can be felt and is said to be movable or floating according to degree. The medical term is nephroptosis which tends to occur in circumstances which cause loss of fat and muscular tone – emaciation for various reasons or repeated pregnancies – and is much more common in women and on the right side because of the longer renal artery.

Symptoms are usually of vague dragging abdominal pain often radiating downwards. Occasionally, more acute colicky attacks occur because of torsion and kinking of the ureter, the duct carrying urine to the bladder. Such an incident may be accompanied by blood in the urine.

Patients are very apt to become neurotic about the presence of a movable kidney. If treatment has to be considered a properly-fitted abdominal support relieves most cases. The operation of nephropexy to sling the kidney from the last rib should only be undertaken in extreme cases and if there is evidence of renal damage. It may not produce much or any improvement if there is a neurotic element in the case.

moxibustion. A method of treatment, employed in CHINESE MEDICINE, in which a moxa (i.e., a heap of dried mugwort) is burned on the skin. The effect, including the raising of a blister, differs from that of ordinary poulticing in that the moxa is not applied over the affected organ but at a point designated by a Chinese physician as likely to influence the disease. Physiology as understood in Europe and America provides no explanation of why the raising of a blister on a particular patch of skin should affect an organ situated far from the patch and supplied by different nerves and different blood vessels.

multipara. a woman who has given birth to more than one child.

multiple sclerosis. A chronic disease of the nervous system in which patches of defective and hardened tissue appear at random in the brain and spinal cord and interfere with the normal function of the affected parts. The condition is also called disseminated sclerosis, insular sclerosis and focal sclerosis. Its cause is unknown.

The onset of the disease is gradual, usually in young adults of either sex, but its course is progressive with increasing disability, although temporary remissions are a feature. The typical symptoms are weakness, uncoordination, rigidity and paralysis of the lower limbs (spastic paraplegia) together with the very characteristic and often associated occurrence of nystagmus, tremor of the arms, and a peculiar scanning or syllabic speech.

There is no effective treatment but it is important to maintain general nutrition and avoid fatigue. Massage and passive movements can help to prevent painful and deforming contractures.

mumps. An acute infectious disease (sometimes known as infectious parotitis) of sudden onset, characterized by fever and by swelling and tenderness of the salivary glands. Usually it is the glands situated in front of the ears which are most affected, so that the resultant swelling produces the typical swollen and distorted facial appearance.

The incubation period is twelve to twenty-six days; the incidence is chiefly in children aged 5 to 15 years; in older persons the testes or ovaries may be affected and symptoms of meningitis or encephalitis occasionally occur. Spontaneous recovery is usually complete within ten days and second attacks are uncommon. Vaccination is available but the immunity is short-lived and it is not generally advised except in special circumstances.

muscle. A type of tissue which has the ability to contract in response to nervous stimuli and which thus provides animals with power for movement of the body and also internal functions, such as digestion.

It occurs in three forms: (1) voluntary

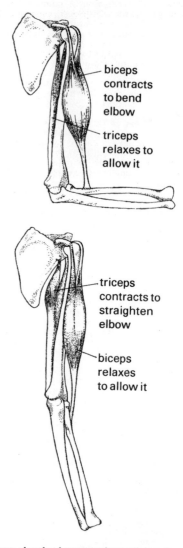

biceps contracts to bend elbow

triceps relaxes to allow it

triceps contracts to straighten elbow

biceps relaxes to allow it

Diagram showing how muscles work in pairs

skeletal or striped muscle; (2) involuntary, visceral or unstriped muscle; and (3) cardiac muscle. The term 'striped' refers to the appearance of voluntary muscle under the microscope when the fibres show alternate light and dark cross-banding. Cardiac muscle has special characteristics of inherent rhythmical contraction and is otherwise intermediate in type since it is both striped and involuntary.

In general, skeletal muscles are either elongated with a roughly cylindrical or spindle shape, or broad and flat. They are connected to the bones, cartilages, ligaments, or skin either directly or by means of tendons. The end of the muscle which is attached to a point relatively more fixed is known as the origin, and its other end is its insertion. When the muscle contracts origin and insertion are necessarily brought closer together and the desired movement results. However, when a muscle is required to contract, its opposing muscle must relax in order to enable it to do so; it may therefore be said that muscles work in pairs.

Visceral muscle forms the walls of hollow organs and ducts including the blood vessels. Cardiac muscle is found only in the walls of the heart.

Voluntary muscles are under the control of the individual and their contraction can be initiated, controlled or inhibited at will. Visceral and cardiac muscle are not subject to such control and react automatically to stimuli from the autonomic nervous system.

Diseases. Paralysis and atrophy of muscle usually result from damage to the nerve caused by infections such as poliomyelitis, by damage to blood vessels affecting the nervous system or by disseminated sclerosis and other diseases of the actual nerves.

Violence may produce rupture of muscle fibres to cause a strain treated by rest and support. CRAMP is a painful spasmodic muscle contraction due to over-exertion or insufficient blood supply. Some cases due to arterial disease may be helped by drugs which dilate the blood vessels. Occupational cramps (writer's, telegraphist's and piano-player's) are caused by constant repetition of small movements. Myalgia is a painful condition in which muscles and their fibrous components and attachments become inflamed by strain and exposure; common varieties are lumbago, pleurodynia (rib muscles) and the stiff neck of acute torticollis. Rest and heat treatment usually relieve symptoms.

Apart from these common conditions there are certain rarer and less well-understood muscular diseases which are often inherited. Myotonia congenita is a disease of childhood characterized by slowness of relaxation after voluntary contraction, and myotonia atrophica is a similar condition of middle age, with wasting of muscle tissues. Familial periodic paralysis is marked by recurrent attacks of extensive paralysis. It occurs mostly in adolescents and tends to improve with age. Myasthenia gravis is characterized by rapid exhaustion of the muscles when movements are rapidly repeated.

Muscular dystrophy (myopathy) affects children and young people as several different clinical types. Most cases are hereditary and x-chromosome linked (see GENETICS) which means that males are mostly affected in the ratio of five to one. Female carriers of the defective gene can be detected by an enzyme test. The condition is one of muscle degeneration. There is no known effective treatment and severe cases may not survive beyond young adult life. Massage, physiotherapy and orthopaedic appliances help to minimize disability.

muscular rheumatism. See FIBROSITIS.

mushroom poisoning. The edible mushroom of commerce is *Agaricus campestris*. It is also found growing under natural conditions, but the gathering and eating of wild mushrooms is fraught with considerable risks unless the collector exercises care and has sufficient botanical knowledge to ensure that poisonous fungi are not included by mistake. There are at least a dozen species which can cause serious illness or death. The most fatal are death cap mushroom (*Amanita phalloides*) and the fly agaric or scarlet fly cap (*Amanita muscaria*).

Eating a poisonous type of mushroom is quickly followed by severe abdominal pain and by vomiting and a cholera-like type of watery diarrhoea which may be blood-stained. The pulse is slowed and there are effects on the nervous system shown by disturbance of vision, dilated pupils, restlessness, and delirium.

Immediate treatment is required by repeated stomach washes and the giving of large doses of atropine which is a specific antidote to the poisonous agent muscarine. There is generally severe and prolonged prostration and in fatal cases the victim gradually sinks into a coma which leads to death within a week.

myasthenia gravis. A disease characterized by rapid exhaustion of the MUSCLES under voluntary control when movements are carried out repeatedly in close succession. With rest, normal power slowly becomes restored although this ability to recover may be lost in later stages. The condition occurs mainly in young adults and the sexes are affected equally. The muscles involved in order of frequency and severity are those in (1) the head and face, especially the ocular muscles, (2) the neck, (3) the respiratory system, (4) the limbs and trunk. In progressive cases death may occur from respiratory paralysis.

Muscular contraction depends on acetyl-choline at the point where the nerve-ending contacts the muscle itself. Its action is limited by the enzyme acetylcholinesterase. By injecting the substance Tensilon (edrophonium chloride) the enzyme is inhibited and the action of acetylcholine is prolonged. This procedure is used as a diagnostic test for myasthenia gravis and temporarily abolishes the tendency to muscle exhaustion.

Various other longer acting anti-cholinesterases are available for treatment, and some cases are also treated by removal of the thymus gland, but the condition is a difficult one to deal with successfully in the long-term.

mydriatic. A drug which causes dilatation of the pupil of the eye. Such medicaments are used in both the diagnosis and treatment of eye diseases. They act by temporarily paralysing the endings of the nerve supplying the muscle which controls the iris. A large dilated pupil facilitates examination of the inside of the eye, and since the power of accommodation or focusing is also rendered inactive, any errors of refraction which could be corrected by spectacles can be more easily and accurately measured.

In treatment the main indication for the use of a mydriatic is IRITIS, in which it is necessary both to rest the iris and to ensure that it neither adheres to the lens in a contracted position nor causes inflammatory deposits on the lens which would damage the sight.

The drugs principally used are solutions of atropine sulphate for treatment or of homatropine hydrobromide for diagnostic purposes because of its shorter duration of action.

myelitis. An inflammatory or degenerative condition of the SPINAL CORD.

myocarditis. Inflammation of the muscle of the heart or myocardium. Acute myocarditis is relatively uncommon and occurs as a sequel to various generalized infections.

myocardium. The specialized muscle which forms the walls of the HEART.

myopia. A defect of EYESIGHT, commonly known as 'short sight', in which, although objects held near the face are seen clearly, distance vision is blurred.

myxoedema. The condition which results from a deficiency of thyroid secretion. In cases which arise spontaneously the gland is small, rather wasted and fibrosed. The incidence is chiefly in women of menopausal age. The signs and symptoms of myxoedema are very characteristic: the features become broadened and bloated with puffy drooping eyelids; there is swelling and thickening of the tissues under the skin (solid oedema); the skin becomes dry and rough with absence of sweating; the hair becomes harsh, sparse and dry; movements and mental activity become slowed; the basal metabolic rate is low and the patient always feels cold. The condition can be effectively treated by the administration of thyroxin.

Myxoedema due to congenital deficiency of the thyroid gland is known as CRETINISM.

N

naevus. The medical term for a BIRTH MARK.

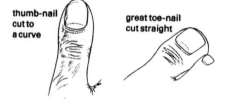

thumb-nail cut to a curve

great toe-nail cut straight

Finger-nails and toe-nails should be cut in different styles

nail. The visible, horny part of the nail consists of hardened and bony epidermic cells, and the nail grows from the nail-bed or matrix which is overlapped by a fold of skin. The half-moons at the base of the nails appear pale because they are not firmly attached to the underlying tissuses.

Excessive paring, especially at the edges, can lead to cracks and bruising with subsequent formation of nail abscesses and whitlow. Painful cracks (hangnails) occurring in the skin at the sides of nails in winter are due partially to insufficient blood supply through the blood vessels being constricted by cold, and partially to insufficiency of natural oil in the skin.

nail-biting. A common compulsive symptom of frustration or repressed aggression. A child, jealous of a younger brother or sister or insecure because of real or apparent lack of parental affection, is unable to vent his aggression on others and gets rid of it by biting his own nails, achieving some satisfaction from his ability to see and feel the results of his actions. In at least a proportion of cases nail-biting, having thus started, persists as a habit after the initial cause has disappeared.

Prevention is essentially the avoidance of insecurity and severe frustration. Nagging and punishment are usually ineffective as treatments. There are essentially two hopeful lines of treatment. (1) Where the initial cause is still operating, careful assessment of parent-child relationships and sometimes of child-school relationships, and thereafter removal of the cause. (2) Where nail-biting has become essentially a habit, an attempt to instil pride in the hands by careful manicuring and nail-cutting.

nail, ingrowing. A condition, mostly of the great toe, in which the nail grows into the flesh on one side or the other, creating considerable pain. The two common causes are badly fitting shoes with pressure on the nail, and cutting the toe nails in a curve (as is normal with finger nails). Prevention consists in careful selection of comfortable, well fitting shoes and in cutting the toe nails straight across, with the sharp points at the side either filed or finely clipped. Where the condition has occurred, treatment usually involves surgical removal of a v-shaped piece from the middle of the top of the nail (so that, instead of growing sideways, it will grow to fill the gap) and the temporary placing of a dressing soaked in collodion between the nail edge and the flesh. If this treatment fails, removal of the nail may have to be considered.

narcissism. Excessive love of oneself. The term derives from Narcissus, a legendary Greek boy who fell in love with his image in a pool of water and was drowned, and subsequently changed into the flower that bears his name. Basically narcissism represents a fixation at (or a regression to) an infantile emotional level, occurring in persons whose intelligence is normal or sometimes above average. Complete narcissism is a form of NEUROSIS and certainly requires psychiatric treatment; but there are many intermediate stages in which a person is self-centred to more than an average extent and is rather childlike in his or her emotional attitudes to life. Whether treatment is necessary depends on the degree of self-centredness. Whether treatment, if needed, is acceptable depends on the extent to which the individual has – or can acquire – insight into the condition.

narcolepsy. A disorder in which a person is subject to uncontrollable drowsiness unrelated to actual fatigue, such as falling asleep while delivering a lecture or immediately after laughing heartily at a joke. In some cases investigation shows that the cause is damage to the hypothalamus of the brain, e.g., from tumour or head injury or following encephalitis; but in quite a proportion of cases clinical and x-ray examinations fail to identify a cause. Apart from treatment of the cause if found (e.g., removal of a tumour) most victims respond well to dosage with amphetamine sulphate, but in general this is a palliative rather than a cure: in other words, the attacks of drowsiness or actual sleep recur if the amphetamine is discontinued.

narcosis. Dulling of consciousness or deep sleep, produced by the action of (1) narcotic drugs such as morphia, and (2) anaesthetics. Continuous narcosis is a method of preliminary or temporary treatment sometimes used in mental disorders associated with excitement or great agitation: the patient is rested in preparation for later treatment by being kept asleep or almost asleep for several days, being awakened only for meals and for the performance of natural functions.

nasal catarrh. see CATARRH.

nasal feeding. A method of feeding a person who cannot swallow. A thin tube is passed through nostril, throat and gullet to the stomach, and liquid is then poured slowly into a funnel attached to the tube.

natural childbirth. Childbirth without anaesthetics or analgesics.

Noticing that childbirth seemed less painful in women in certain underdeveloped countries, Dr. Grantly Dick-Read in the 1930s evolved the theory that the pain was primarily due to fear and could be removed by rational explanation and the teaching of relaxation exercises. For the most part his methods have been replaced by more recent methods of explanation and relaxation generally termed psychoprophylaxis; but the question remains: can psychoprophylaxis or relaxation exercises remove the pain of childbirth?

Some obstetricians deny such removal, but many thousands of women claim to have derived benefit and in many cases to have given birth without requiring any form of anaesthesia. In the present state of knowledge it would seem advisable for expectant mothers to attend health education and psychoprophylaxis classes, to use the exercises in the early stages of labour, but to have anaesthetics available for such women as do not find the measures fully effective.

naturopathy. A superficially attractive system of health care by simple, 'natural' diet, regular exercise, the avoidance of all 'artificial' foods including foods grown with chemical fertilizers, and the rejection of drugs and medicines, although some naturopaths will accept drugs produced from plants but not synthetic drugs. Clearly there are certain advantages in a system that succeeds in avoiding over-eating, under-exercise, cigarette smoking and the over-use of medicines to which many of us are prone. Yet in attributing all disease to artificial foodstuffs and artificial ways of life and in seeking what is essentially a return to nature the naturopaths conveniently forget that primitive tribes suffer from a mass of infectious and nutritional diseases, that their members are quite often stunted or deformed and that in such communities early death is the rule rather than the exception.

Food, however pure, can neither prevent nor cure invasion of the body by a droplet-borne bacterium or virus; a natural way of life cannot stop the carrier of a hereditary defect from passing it to his offspring nor incite a failing pancreas to produce enough insulin for the body's needs; avoidance of artificiality cannot prevent the development of allergy to a particular pollen or remove the pain of a wound or burn. Moreover, if we turn to such naturopaths as accept 'natural' drugs, there seems little difference between treating malaria with the 'natural' bark of the cinchona and treating it with quinine 'artificially' extracted from that bark (except that in the latter case the dose is much more accurate), and little difference between supplementing a winter diet that is deficient in vitamin C with 'natural' lemon juice or supplementing with an equivalent amount of synthetic ascorbic acid.

Every species that has survived has done so by a process of continuous adaptation. Such things as canned foods and artificial heating that enable man to exist under arctic conditions, vaccines and antibiotics that allow him to combat infection, and contraceptives that enable him to cope with the population explosion are all parts of the process of continuous adaptation. The naturopath philosophy, resisting and rejecting adaptation, would, if universally adopted, result in the regression of mankind to its primitive state.

nausea. A feeling of sickness or impending vomiting. This may occur as a result of emotional disturbances (especially fear), unpleasant sights, smells and tastes, indigestion and gastritis, food-poisoning, or severe eyestrain. It may also appear as an early symptom in an attack of migraine, in the early stages of many fevers, in sea-sickness, and in the morning sickness of early pregnancy. In many of these conditions nausea precedes actual vomiting.

navel. The umbilicus or navel is a depressed, button-like scar in the central line of the abdomen. It is the scar resulting from the cutting of the UMBILICAL CORD which originally united the unborn child to the placenta.

near-sight. Short-sightedness or myopia. See EYESIGHT.

neck. The neck is supported by seven cervical vertebrae which are braced by strong muscles that enable the head to be freely moved. The muscles on each side which stand out prominently when the head is turned are the sternomastoids. In the front of the neck from above downwards are the hyoid bone, the larynx and the trachea (windpipe), with the oesophagus (gullet) lying behind the trachea, and the thyroid gland situated in front of the larynx. The main blood vessels in the neck are the carotid arteries and the jugular veins.

Swellings in the neck are most commonly due to enlarged glands, arising from septic tonsils or teeth, from tuberculosis, or from glandular fever. Swelling in the front of the neck is generally due to enlargement of the thyroid gland. See GOITRE. Pain in the neck muscles may result from inflammatory causes, but probably the commonest is rheumatic wry neck or torticollis.

necrosis. Death of a limited portion of the cells or tissues of the body. It may occur from cutting off the blood supply to the affected area, in bacterial poisoning or after severe burns or other injuries. The dead tissue may be discharged to the surface with pus, or may remain and cause prolonged suppuration and so necessitate surgical removal, or may remain and become converted into a harmless lump of bony or fibrous tissue.

negativism. A phase, common around 2½ years, in which requests or commands are bluntly refused. See CHILDHOOD, PSYCHOLOGY OF.

Negativism is also sometimes found in old people who use it as a convenient method of stressing their importance. It usually disappears if the old person is given a little more attention and helped to find interests.

neoplasm. The medical term for a TUMOUR or growth, i.e., an accumulation of cells that serve no useful purpose. The neoplasm may be benign or malignant; in the latter case it is normally referred to as CANCER.

nephritis. Inflammation of the KIDNEY.

nephrosis. A condition in which the filtering mechanism of the KIDNEY is damaged.

nerve. A bundle of conducting fibres through which impulses pass between the brain and spinal cord and other parts of the body. Motor fibres conduct impulses from the brain and cord to the muscles, initiating movement. Sensory fibres carry impulses inwards from the skin, muscles, etc., originating sensations of pain, touch, pressure, heat, cold, etc. See NERVOUS SYSTEM.

nervous breakdown. A common term for any emotional illness which makes it impossible for a person to cope with the stresses and strains of life. The corresponding medical term is NEUROSIS, but the two words tend to differ in breadth of meaning. Neurosis includes also milder forms of emotional disorder in which the person feels tired or depressed or inadequate or persistently anxious or suffers from obsessions, but still manages to carry out his normal work. The non-medical term, nervous breakdown, generally indicates a neurosis that has progressed to a stage at which the victim can no longer carry out the duties for which he has been trained, or can no longer be deemed a responsible member of the community.

nervous child. The terms 'nervous' and 'maladjusted' are both used to indicate children with psychological difficulties, though the second term implies that the instability or disturbance is too severe to be remedied by parents and teachers, while 'nervous' causes no such implication. The difficulties usually manifest themselves in one of four main ways: (1) as behaviour disorders, e.g., temper tantrums, aggressiveness, bullying, stealing and sex difficulties; (2) as habit disorders and physical symptoms, e.g., stammering, thumb-sucking, nail-biting, bed-wetting and sleep-walking; (3) as neurotic disorders, e.g., pathological anxiety, phobias and compulsive acts; (4) as educational and vocational difficulties, e.g., school failure, school phobia, and frequent day-dreaming. Psychotic behaviour (such as extreme withdrawal or manifestations of hallucinations) is not usually classified under the heading of nervous disorders.

In most cases the difficulties originate at home – in parental over-strictness and over-discipline, in over-indulgence, in inconsistency, in lack of demonstrated affection, in quarrels between parents, or in situations creating jealousy of a younger or older brother or sister. Less frequently their origin is in school circumstances.

Prevention is largely a matter of parents becoming aware of a child's need for physical and emotional security, demonstrated love, reasonable parental consistency, freedom to explore and investigate coupled with a kindly, guiding authority, and provision of playthings and playmates appropriate to the stage of development. Most people, however, are occasionally inconsistent or thoughtless, and parents should appreciate that children have considerable resilience. Errors in child management have to be continued or repeated to produce child maladjustment. The advice of the family HEALTH VISITOR can be of great value to parents, e.g., anticipatory guidance about the next stage of development and its problems, current guidance about the handling of existing difficulties, and, not least, reassurance of needlessly worried fathers and mothers.

Where a child's behaviour is for an appreciable time inappropriate to his age and stage of development, detailed investigation and prolonged treatment may be needed. See CHILD GUIDANCE and MALADJUSTED CHILD.

nervous system. The mechanism primarily responsible for the co-ordinated activity of the body as a whole.

A typical nerve cell (or neurone) consists of a small nucleated body, many tiny branching filaments (dendrites), and a long branch (the axon) which in turn ends in branching filaments. Essentially a neurone is a long fibre that collects impulses from the delicate filaments at one end and transmits them to the filaments at the other end; and a nerve is a bundle of such fibres. A single nerve may consist solely of sensory fibres that carry impulses of sensation from the periphery towards the brain, or solely of motor fibres that carry instructions outwards towards the muscles, or of a mixture of motor and sensory fibres.

The transfer of sensory information (e.g., about pain, heat, or cold affecting a toe) to the brain and of instructions back to the relevant muscles is achieved not by a single sensory fibre and a single motor fibre, but by two series of fibres with interlacing endings. The message, whether sensory or motor, can be considered as an electrical impulse which runs along the fibre and then 'sparks the gap' between the ending of one neurone and the beginning of the next.

The cerebrospinal system is said to have two parts: central and peripheral. The central nervous system consists of the BRAIN and the SPINAL CORD. The brain receives information from the cranial nerves (e.g., those serving the eyes and nose) and the spinal nerves (e.g., those receiving impulses from the limbs). The cranial and spinal nerves together constitute what is known as the peripheral nervous system. The brain processes the information and sends out appropriate instructions along the motor nerves (e.g., telling the leg muscles to move the body nearer to an object that the eyes have seen). The spinal cord is the main nerve trunk between the brain and the arms, legs and trunk.

By no means all messages, however, make the full journey to the brain and back. On a level with every pair of nerves leaving the spinal cord there is an alternative system for relaying the impulses within the spinal cord itself without the necessity of involving the brain; this mechanism is known as the reflex arc and is responsible for maintaining the muscle tone as well as for very specific muscle responses known as REFLEX ACTIONS. For instance, if the hand touches a very hot object the sensory impulse (conveying the awareness of pain) results in an instruction at spinal cord level for the muscles of the arm to take appropriate action, so that the hand is actually removed from the hot object before the brain receives the impulse which it interprets as pain.

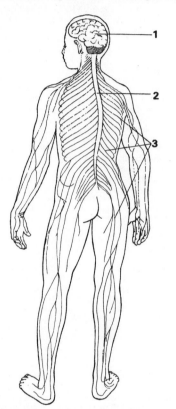

1 brain, which receives information from sensory nerves and transmits instructions via motor nerves

2 spinal cord, protected by the spinal column, which is the nerve pathway to and from the brain

3 spinal nerves, sensory and motor, branching to all parts of the body

The nervous system

The autonomic nervous system conveys messages to involuntary muscles and secreting glands, which is to say that it regulates functions not under the control of the brain, e.g., heart-rate, blushing, sweating and control of digestion. Functionally the autonomic nervous system is divided into two parts. The SYMPATHETIC NERVOUS SYSTEM is connected with the thoracic and upper lumbar spinal nerves, while the PARASYMPATHETIC NERVOUS SYSTEM is connected both with the vagus (tenth cranial nerve) and with the sacral nerve.

Activity of the sympathetic nervous system mobilizes the body to meet physical danger – dilating the pupils and to some extent raising the hair (creating a frightening appearance), widening the coronary and other major arteries (and so increasing the flow of blood to the muscles), constricting skin blood vessels (and so ensuring less blood loss from a superficial wound), increasing the force of the heart beat (thus again making more blood available for the muscles), dilating the bronchi and bronchioles (and so allowing more air into the lungs), and decreasing the activity of digestive organs (for digestion can be postponed until the danger is past). Essentially these nerves act releasing additional amounts of the hormone adrenalin, so that an injection of adrenalin has similar effects.

By contrast the parasympathetic nerves restore peace after the emergency has been tackled, e.g., slowing down the heart, reducing the blood flow, restoring digestive activity, and allowing the sphincters of bladder and anus to relax and permit urination and defaecation. Both these systems are greatly influenced by the ENDOCRINE GLANDS and they both influence and are influenced by the emotions.

nettle-rash. An allergic condition characterized by the rapid appearance of weals and blisters, usually lasting for only a few hours, and accompanied by intense itching.

The rash resulting from actual nettle stings appears to be due to the injection of histamine and acetylcholine; and so-called nettle-rash from other causes (e.g., after the eating of a food to which the individual is sensitive) is thought to be due to release of histamine in the tissues. Antihistamine drugs are generally effective, and calamine lotion will relieve the itching until the drug takes effect.

Where the condition recurs a careful search for the cause is desirable, but the fewer the number of attacks the less the likelihood of identifying the source.

neuralgia. Shooting pain, usually occurring in paroxysms, along the course of any nerve, but most commonly arising in the nerves of the face and head. The condition is often caused or precipitated by a cold draught, or may arise from pressure on a nerve (e.g., from badly fitting dentures) or from irritation of a nerve by disease in its vicinity. In many cases no cause is found.

Hot fomentations usually give some relief, and aspirin and phenacetin are useful, although both merely give temporary relief and allow time for spontaneous cure to occur.

neurasthenia. A vague term denoting an irritable, hypersensitive weakness and depression. A person suffering from the condition feels exhausted and unhappy, cannot concentrate for long, is constantly beset by worries, and is very concerned about symptoms which often include headaches, muscular pains, fullness in the abdomen and tremor of the hands.

Freud regarded neurasthenia as a result of repressed auto-eroticism, or self-love, which finds expression in sexual conflict or sexual difficulty, and so creates exhaustion. Probably that is not the only explanation, but in all cases neurasthenia originates in a disturbance of the mind. Hence, while tranquillizers may play a part in the treatment of mild cases of short duration, for most serious cases some form of psychological treatment is essential, including an attempt to identify and remove the underlying causes.

Traumatic neurasthenia is a similar or identical condition which develops after an injury, e.g., in a traffic accident, with the weakness and proneness to fatigue persisting long after the physical injury has healed. 'Compensation neurosis', as it is sometimes called, does not imply malingering or deliberate deceit. To the victim it is absolutely genuine. Yet in most cases it clears up rapidly after the amount of compensation has been settled.

neuritis. Inflammation of a nerve (localized neuritis) or of several nerves (polyneuritis).

The symptoms vary according to whether the inflammation is of the nerve sheath or of the actual nerve filaments themselves and according to whether the nerve is irritated or incapacitated. Early signs may include numbness (most commonly of the 'glove and stocking' areas) and loss of sensation, or pain and muscle weakness and tenderness. If the condition progresses the skin of the affected area often becomes cold and shiny, while the muscles waste.

Causes of localized neuritis include (1) exposure to cold, found most commonly in Bell's palsy and sciatica; (2) pressure, e.g., from a tumour; (3) poisoning, e.g., lead particularly affects the wrists; and (4) diphtheria, formerly a very common cause of temporary neuritis. Treatment consists largely of identifying and removing the cause, although electrical treatment and counter-irritation may help.

Causes of multiple neuritis include various acute fevers, diabetes, beriberi (the deficiency disease caused by lack of vitamin B₁), and poisoning by alcohol, arsenic and lead. Alcoholic neuritis, commonest in middle-aged women, is probably not so much due to poisoning as to destruction of vitamin B by alcohol (so that it resembles the neuritis of beriberi). It affects the legs mostly, causing foot-drop and poor sensation in the feet, and a compensatory high-stepping gait. Treatment involves identification and removal of the cause, rest, massage and electricity.

neurosis. A very common but rather ill-defined group of psychological abnormalities (also known as psychoneurosis), including excessive anxiety, anger, fear, hate, jealousy, hysterical states and the states associated with phobias and obsessive actions. The distinction from PSYCHOSIS (mental illness) is clear: the psychotic's personality is unbalanced and disorganized, on certain matters he is out of touch with reality and cannot reason properly, and he is usually unaware that he is ill; the neurotic is in full touch with reality, can reason normally and is very worried about his illness. It is more difficult to indicate the border between neurosis and the edge of normality: there is no sharp boundary between the over-anxious person who tends to worry too much and the victim of anxiety neurosis. Broadly, if extreme tidiness, or concern with detail, or anxiety, reaches the stage where it is interfering with work performance and social relationships, it is a neurosis.

While heredity may play a small part, neurosis is in the main due to a combination of unfortunate happenings in childhood and adult stresses. As Freud showed, neuroses originate in unresolved conflicts (e.g., between innate tendencies and parental precepts), and mostly represent a flight from the particular conflict; and the pre-neurotic person (less secure or more apprehensive than others, or described as 'rather a perfectionist' or 'a bit jealous') is precipitated into full neuroticism by the stresses of adolescence, by work strain or by marital problems.

Prevention would seem to lie in the education of parents, and also of teachers and others concerned with children, about the emotional and psychological requirements of children for adequate development of personality, so that a sustained attempt may be made to build personalities capable of standing up to the strains and tribulations of normal life. Some workers claim that, now that most infectious diseases and many physical diseases of children have been brought under control, the teaching of mental hygiene is the main task of the modern health visitor.

The neurotic is unhappy and incapable of good work, and his symptoms are absolutely genuine. He badly needs help, and there is absolutely no point in advising him to 'pull himself together'. If he could do so, he would not be a neurotic.

One form of treatment is to supply tranquillizers and to take such steps as may be practicable to lessen current worries or problems – in other words to seek to restore the patient to his pre-neurotic state in which he managed to cope fairly well with his difficulties. Where the precipitating strains were heavy and can be removed or lessened, and where the underlying conflicts are not too extreme, this may be all that is needed.

Alternatively or additionally, an attempt may be made to discover the underlying factors, to bring the conflicts to the patient's consciousness and to help him to resolve them in a way satisfactory to himself. This may involve a full course of psychoanalysis, but might be achieved much more easily.

Many American experts believe that the first form of treatment alone is inadequate, and that it is essential to help the patient to find his problems and improve his capacity for problem-solving. Many British experts hold that detailed psychological investigation is unwarranted unless simpler methods have failed.

Neurosis is not only very common, but is also particularly common in persons of high intelligence and ability. Hence both prevention and treatment are important, not only for the sake of the unfortunate persons but also in the interests of the community.

neurosurgery. The branch of surgery which deals with operations performed on the brain, spinal cords or nerves, e.g., to remove a tumour of the brain or to treat a prolapsed vertebral disc. Neurosurgery is in the main a development of the twentieth century: only a few simple and relatively speedy operations were practicable before the advent of long-acting anaesthetics. Nevertheless, at least one important neurosurgical operation – that of trepanning the skull, or in other words boring a hole to permit the escape of excess fluid – has been in existence since the dawn of history.

nicotine. An alkaloid in tobacco which stimulates the sympathetic and parasympathetic nervous systems. It is responsible for the nausea, sickness, faintness, etc., sometimes experienced at the initial smoking experiment. In habitual smokers it causes increased pulse rate and raised blood pressure, and it may be the factor in tobacco that contributes to diseases of the arteries.

Nicotine is used as an insecticide, and can penetrate the skin or be inadvertently swallowed. A toxic dose of nicotine produces a burning sensation in the mouth, followed by vomiting and diarrhoea, violent excitement, and presently exhaustion, loss of consciousness and sometimes death. Treatment consists of rapid emptying of the stomach by stomach tube or by emetic, injecting a small dose of atropin, and, if respiration is becoming difficult, using artificial respiration.

night blindness. Inability of the eyes to adapt to partial darkness. While the normal person experiences at dusk a gradual diminution of vision, a person with night blindness passes suddenly from daylight to complete darkness. The common cause is deficiency of vitamin A, but night blindness also occurs as a hereditary condition and in some diseases of the retina and choroid.

nightmare. A dream marked by very acute fear, anxiety or other unpleasant emotion. The second part of the word derives from an Anglo-Saxon term meaning 'demon' and relates to the mediaeval theory of nightmares as caused by evil spirits. In most cases nightmares reflect, often in distorted form, difficulties and emotional disturbances in waking life. See NIGHT TERROR.

night terror. The fundamental difference between a nightmare and a night terror is that in the former the frightening dream is recalled and fear departs when the person reaches full consciousness, whereas in night terror the person wakens suddenly in a state of panic but can give no reason for his fears.

Night terrors sometimes occur in adults but are mostly found in nervous children, especially after unusual excitement or fatigue. For most cases three negative measures prevent recurrences: avoidance of excessive excitement and fatigue, especially in the evenings; adjustment of meal-times or amounts so that no heavy meal is eaten within two or three hours of going to bed; and avoidance of needless or excessive frustration at home and school. Where night terrors persist despite these measures the child should be referred to a child guidance clinic.

nipple. The teat of the female breast; the protuberance from which the milk ducts discharge. During pregnancy the nipple enlarges, simultaneously with the whole breast, and becomes more pronounced and darker in colour. Pigment is also deposited around the nipple during pregnancy and thereafter never entirely disappears.

Cracked nipples are not uncommon during the period of breast feeding, due either to the child being put too much to one breast or to a defect in the shape or size of the nipple. Cracked nipples are painful and can form a channel whereby infection passes to deeper tissues. Careful washing and application of friar's balsam often remedies the condition,

and a metal shield worn between feeds can be useful.

Leaking nipples usually indicate lack of muscle tone, rather than excess of milk. The breasts can be toned up by alternate hot and cold sponging and by gentle massage. Attention to general health and to diet is also necessary.

Paget's disease of the nipple is essentially a cancer of the milk ducts. The affected nipple becomes scaly, thickened and smaller than the other nipple. Treatment is by surgical removal of the breast.

Eczema of the nipple superficially resembles Paget's disease but the nipples remain equal in size. The condition may be caused by scabies or may be allergic in origin. Treatment varies with the cause.

nitrogen. An inert gas which is the largest component of air and also an essential element in all living animals.

Soil bacteria and certain plants utilize nitrogen from the air to synthesize proteins which are the only foodstuffs containing nitrogen. The proteins are broken down in the digestive systems of persons and animals, and in part re-synthesized for replacement of tissue, while waste nitrogen is excreted by the kidneys, mostly as urea.

nitrogen mustards. A group of drugs which delay the multiplication of rapidly dividing cells. In such conditions as Hodgkin's disease and chronic leukaemia they do not constitute a cure but they may appreciably prolong life.

nits. Eggs of LICE. They are coated with a sticky substance and adhere firmly to hairs or clothing. A female louse lays eight to twelve eggs a day during a life span of about three weeks, and the nits hatch in seven to fifteen days.

nocturia. Passage of urine during the night. In a healthy young adult the kidneys are relatively inactive during sleep, so that the bladder does not require to be emptied during the night. Older people often have to rise once nightly, but more frequent need to pass urine constitutes nocturia.

Causes include: (1) various diseases of the kidney resulting in increased secretion of dilute urine; (2) diseases of the bladder, such as cystitis; (3) in men, disorders of the prostate gland; and (4) in pregnant women, pressure on the bladder by an enlarged uterus. Unless the cause is obvious nocturia needs medical investigation.

nocturnal emissions. Involuntary discharge of sperms and fluid from the prostate gland during sleep. The discharge is sometimes, but by no means always, accompanied by erotic dreams, and so the term 'wet dreams' is often used.

During adolescence these discharges often distress boys and sometimes distress their parents. However, they are normal physiological happenings and should be so regarded. They do not harm the person in any way. Where they are frequent (more than about twice monthly) attempts may be made to reduce their frequency by plain living, avoidance of circumstances likely to lead to sexual stimulation and efforts to concentrate the youth's attention on non-sexual matters.

Nocturnal emissions also occur in some celibate men who lead continent lives, and in men subjected to sexual stimulation without gratification.

noise. Sound which is undesired by, or unpleasant to, the recipient. Whether a sound becomes a noise depends on at least five factors:

1. The sound pressure level which is measured in decibels: a quiet bedroom at night (with clock ticking, people breathing and external sound of gentle rain) is often around 25 decibels; a soft whisper at five feet represents around 35; conversation becomes difficult when the level exceeds 55; a heavy diesel vehicle at twenty-five feet produces 90; and in some factories the level exceeds 100.

2. The pitch: if they are at equal pressure levels, a high pitched screech is less tolerable than a sound in the middle of the hearing range.

3. Continuity: although continuous loud noise may be worse for hearing than intermittent noise of equal level, it is easier to become habituated to a continuous noise than to one of the same pitch and pressure level occurring at frequent but irregular intervals.

4. Time: the average person will endure without discomfort 55 decibels in a busy restaurant or 50 in an office but would consider 40 intolerable in his bedroom.

5. Personal idiosyncracy: human reaction and sensitivity to noise varies greatly. One man can go to sleep with the radio blaring; another has sleep prevented by a ticking clock. One woman can make abstruse calculations amid 75 decibels of traffic noise; another has her efficiency impaired by a level of 50.

Excessive noise during work causes slower response to stimuli, more errors in work requiring accuracy or precision, irritability, reduced efficiency and industrial fatigue. While there is considerable individual variation, in general these effects become provable at about 85 decibels and may well exist at lower levels. Continued loud noise in such occupations as riveting and boiler-making ultimately produces impairment of hearing, and the level at which this is provable is again about 85 decibels.

Undesired noise at home constitutes an interference with privacy, and excessive noise at night interferes with sleep. Again, however, individual variation is considerable: of people living near a new airport, about 40 per cent seek to move house (though not all succeed), about 40 per cent grumble but tolerate the noise, and about 20 per cent state that it does not disturb them.

Preventive measures in noisy industries include the wearing of ear-plugs by workers, periodical testing of the hearing of workers and removal from noisy jobs of persons beginning to show loss of hearing, the erection of special walls to screen noisy machines from workers and also from the public, the use of silencers on noisy tools and plant, and the substitution of quieter machines for noisy ones. Similar preventive measures are available in respect of traffic noise, e.g., the building of a 'baffle' wall between a highway and a row of houses.

In Britain noise and vibration can constitute a statutory nuisance under the Noise Abatement Act of 1960, and local authorities are required to take steps to abate noise nuisance on a complaint by three or more occupiers of premises or land. However, the Act does not apply to statutory undertakings (e.g., British Rail, electricity works, and British Airways) and if noise is caused by a trade or business it is a defence to show that the best practicable means of preventing or containing it has been used; and practicability inevitably has regard to financial expenditure. The same Act prohibits the use of loud-speakers on streets between 9 pm and 8 am with certain specified exceptions, such as police and fire service in emergency, and limits some other forms of noise.

To a considerable extent, however, noise nuisance remains one of the untackled problems of urban communities.

normal. Conforming to the standard pattern that exists under reasonably favourable circumstances. Since the primary purpose of the various health professions is to prevent or remedy unfavourable deviations from the normal, the identification of normality is important. In mathematics and physics normal has very nearly the same meaning as average and can for practical purposes be described as the particular range, on each side of the average, within which lie nineteen out of every twenty findings. In measurements subject to biological variation, however, normality is not necessarily indicated by findings evenly distributed on both sides of the average.

Four examples will perhaps illustrate. (1) Patients receiving a particular treatment recover from a disease in 3, 4, 5, 6 and 22 days respectively: clearly neither the average (8 days) nor any strip on each side of the average gives us useful information. (2) Students used to be taught that the normal amount of haemoglobin corpuscles in blood corpuscles, estimated by the Sahli or Haldane method, was 95 to 100 per cent for men and 90 to 95 per cent for women; but when women were given iron to compensate for loss of blood during menstruation their average haemoglobin rose to the same as for men. To accept the average of 90 to 95 as normal would have implied that a slight degree of anaemia should be deemed normal. (3) The average height of American soldiers in World War I was 68 inches, but in World War II it was almost 69 inches. Since human beings do not alter by an inch in a single generation, the obvious conclusion is that a sizeable number of Americans in 1915-18 were stunted, i.e., had not grown to their full potential. A similar finding is obtained by comparison of adults from crowded British cities with adults of the same stock reared in New Zealand. (4) Measurement of thousands of British boys aged 6 years and classification according to height shows that the average 6 year old of 45 inches weighs 45 pounds, and we might unwisely reckon the normal for a 6 year old of that height at 42 to 48 pounds; but the 45 inches tall son, of tall, lean, wiry parents might well be in good health with a weight of only 41 pounds, while the large-framed son of stocky parents might not be over-weight at 49 pounds.

In many biological measurements there is a considerable overlap between the normal and the abnormal. For instance, the normal systolic blood pressure of young adults is generally taken as 115 to 120 mm., and a pressure, of say, 145 mm. would often suggest early hypertension; yet the writer of this article has known a prominent athlete who had a systolic pressure of 145 at the age of 20 years and who forty years later shows no evidence of cardiac or circulatory disease. From this type of overlap it is apparent that successive measurements at different points of time give much more information than single measurements, and also that the health sciences are nearly always dependent on the interrelation of a series of measurements. Medicine would be very much easier and the training for it much less arduous if we could simply take isolated findings and say, for example, 'systolic blood pressure at 35 years – under 150 normal, over 150 – pathological', or 'intelligence quotient – 72 educable, 68 – ineducable.'

In babies and pre-school children developmental screening, records at child health clinics, and health visitors' records have together given us a very good idea of what is normal; and paediatricians and health visitors can generally recognize at an early stage unfavourable deviations from physical or mental normality. For children of school age the differentiation of the normal and the slightly abnormal is not quite so accurate but health workers who examine large numbers of children in schools acquire much skill and make relatively few mistakes. As age advances the range of normality unfortunately widens appreciably and a single set of measurements becomes less and less valuable. A single examination of a person of middle age can identify manifest disease but few clinicians would venture without a repeat examination to categorize a particular non-average finding as 'within the norm for health' or 'indicative of early disease'.

normal saline. A solution of common salt in sterile water made to exactly the same strength as in the cells of the body, i.e., 0.9 per cent. A rough approximation can be made by dissolving a level teaspoonful of salt in two tumblerfuls of recently boiled water. For purposes like bathing an eye or washing a wound this solution is much more soothing than is simple sterile water.

nose. Although normally regarded as the organ of smell because of the olfactory receptors in its upper part, the nose is primarily the organ that warms, moistens and filters air before it passes to the lungs.

Internally the nose is divided into two parts by a cartilaginous septum. Entering each half through a nostril the air passes over a series of folded cartilages lined with mucous membrane and is thus warmed and moistened before travelling on to the nasopharynx. The air is also filtered by minute hairs.

Diseases. Common symptoms of diseases of the nose include discharge ('running nose'), obstructed breathing ('stuffed nose') and impaired or lost sense of smell. Frequent diseases include colds, catarrh, adenoids and polypi.

There are paths of communication between the nose and the hollows (sinuses) in the neighbouring bones of the skull, so that an infection of the nose can pass to the sinuses.

Foreign bodies. Small children quite often insert foreign bodies into their nostrils, and this cause of nasal symptoms should never be ignored in the young. Vigorous blowing of the nose often dislodges the object, or, if it is within sight, it may be removed with small forceps. If it is not in sight and cannot be dislodged by nose-blowing expert attention is required.

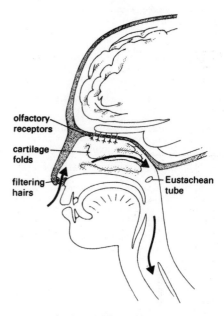

Anatomy of the nose

Fractures. These are not uncommon as a result of direct violence, e.g., a blow, or impact of a cricket ball. There is generally considerable bruising, nose bleeding and displacement of the nose to one side. Immediate treatment includes keeping the patient's head up and applying cold water to the nose. Medical attention is important because without it the fracture will tend to heal with the displacement unconnected.

nose bleeding. Nose bleeding, from rupture of a small blood vessel inside the nose, has many causes. In a child it may follow obstruction by a foreign body, result from a blow on the nose, mark the onset of a severe fever, be due to nose picking, or have no discoverable cause. In an adult most of these causes may operate, but nose bleeding may be a release mechanism in persons with high blood pressure or excess of blood, and it may occur because of exposure to high altitudes.

Immediate treatment is to get the patient sitting with head thrown back and breathing through the mouth, to loosen constricting clothing (e.g., collar) and to pinch the nostrils together for several minutes. If the bleeding continues an ice-bag should be applied to the nape of the neck and another to the bridge of the nose. If the bleeding still continues, medical attention is required.

nose douching. A formerly common method of seeking to get rid of a thick or persisting nasal discharge was by gently douching twice daily with a solution of common salt or sodium bicarbonate, one teaspoonful to a glass of warm water. Douching, however, is not free from danger: the presence of an unpleasant discharge normally implies infection, and douching may push the infection to the air sinuses or to the Eustachian tubes and thence to the middle ear. In general, therefore, douching has been abandoned in favour of more modern methods of treatment.

notifiable diseases. In virtually all countries there are arrangements for notification of specified infections to a person charged with responsibility for their control. British procedure is here given as an illustration.

In Britain certain specified infections must be notified by the general practitioner to the Medical Officer of Health (until 1974) or the Chief Administrative Medical Officer (thereafter) so that he can institute measures for the prevention of an outbreak, the protection of the community, the treatment of persons suffering from the condition and the further study of the causation and prevalence of the disease.

Health education, better hygiene, immunization facilities and improved living standards have made most infections rarities, so that the need for notification is sometimes questioned. Essentially it is required for the following reasons. (1) A general practitioner has no power to deal with contacts who are not even on his list of patients: he cannot, for example, offer them vaccination and keep them under surveillance. (2) Even in respect of his own patients the practitioner has no legal power: he cannot stop the infectious person from attending school, church or cinema. (3) He cannot institute such measures as chlorination of water in a suspected water-borne outbreak or temporary closure and investigation of a suspected bakery in a food-borne outbreak. (4) Where a disease normally occurs sporadically but occasionally becomes epidemic, an outbreak may be quite widespread before any one practitioner is aware that the few patients that he is seeing represent more than normal prevalence of the disease. (5) If thirty practitioners each see anything from one to ten cases in the early stages of an outbreak, no one of them is in a position to estimate requirements, for example in respect of additional hospital beds, extra laboratory facilities, additional nurses or extra supplies of vaccines or antibiotics. (6) As some infections become rare they are easily missed by doctors who seldom encounter them: it is therefore important that there should be one doctor with full knowledge of the infectious situation and able either to alert his colleagues to the presence of a particular disease or to decide that the circumstances do not give rise to such risk as would justify such alerting. (7) Since diseases like cholera and typhoid create much public alarm it is important that there should be a recognized person who can not only tell the public what safety precautions to take but can also allay needless anxiety.

The infections currently notifiable in Britain are: cholera, diphtheria, dysentery, encephalitis, food poisoning, infectious jaundice, malaria, measles, meningitis, ophthalmia neonatorum, paratyphoid, plague, poliomyelitis, relapsing fever, scarlet fever, smallpox, tuberculosis, typhoid fever, typhus fever, whooping cough and yellow fever.

While the general practitioner's responsibility for notification remains clear, the position in respect of investigation is at present a little complicated. Hitherto, especially for food-borne diseases, histories of patients and contacts have been taken mainly by health visitors who have special skill in interviewing; study of food-shops and taking of samples has been mainly the task of public health inspectors; epidemiological considerations have been largely a matter for public health medical officers and laboratory experts in collaboration; and advice on preventive precautions has been a function of health visitors, health education officers, public health medical officers and public health inspectors, according to the nature of the advice and the people advised. The 1974 'integration of health services' split the team that previously controlled infectious diseases, leaving veterinary and meat inspectors and public health inspectors in the employment of local authorities, while the other members of the team passed to Health Boards. Clearly collaboration and gap-bridging are needed.

numbness. A state of altered sensation usually arising from pressure on a nerve, inflammation of a nerve, application of certain drugs to the skin e.g., carbolic acid, or impact of intense cold on the skin. The altered sensation often begins with 'pins and needles' but rapidly progresses to impairment or absence of sensation.

Numbness of the hands and feet may arise in osteoarthritis or may be an indication of impaired circulation, but may also be due to any of the factors mentioned above. Treatment varies with the cause.

nurse. A person professionally qualified in the giving of personal nursing care to persons who are sick or infirm, whether in hospital or at home, and in the teaching of patients, relatives of patients, potential patients and the general public as to the preservation or improvement of health, the prevention of disease and the reduction of relapses and recurrences. For the sick patient the nurse's role is commonly thought of as consisting of doing things for the patient, using technical and ministration skills with, of course, full knowledge of related physical and emotional factors: but it also involves creating an atmosphere of confidence and inducing the patient to try to do things for himself. On the community side, whether engaged in preventive (health visiting) or curative (home nursing) work, the nurse is not merely acting for individuals or families, e.g., intervening between them and the stresses of physical environment and social climate, but also striving to induce them to act and behave in ways that will improve their physical, emotional and social well-being.

The doctor and the nurse were originally undifferentiated from each other and from the priest; but in the Middle Ages medicine came to be increasingly practised by men who were not clergymen, while nursing lay mainly in the hands of monks and nuns, and in northern countries after the Reformation in the hands of untrained persons with a sense of vocation.

Although the unqualified doctor or the doctor qualified only by apprenticeship did not disappear in most developed countries until later in the nineteenth century, medical advances in the eighteenth and early nineteenth centuries reacted temporarily to the disadvantage of nursing, with the separate skills of nursing ignored and the nurse regarded merely as an assistant to the doctor – an attitude which still to a certain extent persists in some European countries.

The first school of nursing in the Western World was established in 1833 in Kaiserswerth by Theodor Fliedner, neither a nurse nor a doctor but a German clergyman; and in 1860 Florence Nightingale, who had herself trained at Kaiserswerth, set up a three year course of training at St. Thomas's Hospital, London.

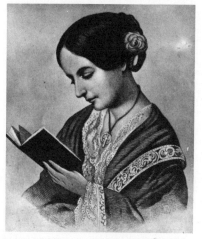

Florence Nightingale, the founder of modern nursing

Amid the enormous technical advances, scientific discoveries, rapid cultural changes and increasing family mobility of the late nineteenth and early twentieth centuries the profession of nursing developed rapidly but unevenly. In Britain, after many hospitals had for years issued their own certificates, there was introduced in 1919 a national examination, taken after three years of training in an approved hospital, leading to the qualification of State Registered Nurse (SRN) in England and Wales and Registered General Nurse (RGN) in Scotland, and in the same year the post-registration certificate for health visitors was established; but for more than sixty years there was intermittent argument about entrance requirements and about the nature of the training. On entrance requirements many nurses maintained that they should be as high as for other professions, and pointed out not only the increasing complexity of technical procedures and the importance of knowledge of psychology and physiology but also the very high wastage rates – higher than in any other profession – among student nurses. On the other hand many doctors, perhaps inheriting the 'handmaiden' idea of the past, claimed that a nurse did not need a full secondary education. So far there is an uneasy compromise: the intending nurse tutor or health visitor tutor, before taking the relevant higher course, needs academic qualifications equivalent to university entrance requirements; the intending HEALTH VISITOR requires considerable but rather lower qualifications; but the academic requirement for entrance to general nursing remains lower than for other professions. With the introduction in the 1960s of courses leading simultaneously to a

university degree (honours or ordinary) and an SRN, and with the introduction in the 1970s of a degree in nursing, it seems likely that the entrance requirement will ultimately rise.

The argument about the nature of the training is essentially on whether it should be (like the medical training) predominantly an academic training in universities or colleges with secondment at appropriate periods for practical experience, or should be pre-dominantly a practical training at the bed-side with release for lectures and tutorials at appropriate periods. With increasing modern stress on health education of the community (in which the health visitor and to a smaller extent other nurses inevitably play a leading role), and with increasing complexity of hospital procedures, it seems likely that professional preparation will move steadily towards the type received by medical students.

In the U.S.A. there has been the same argument but more rapid movement towards university or college courses: by 1973 some 48 per cent of American nurses, including a clear majority of the younger ones, were university or college graduates, with hospital schools of nursing obviously in a phase of decline. The situation in the Scandinavian countries broadly resembles that in Britain, but in France and Italy the nurse's status is lower and her training mostly practical.

Florence Nightingale in her *Notes on Nursing* (1859) declared that nursing 'ought to signify the proper use of fresh air, light, warmth, cleanliness, quiet and the proper selection and administration of diet – all at the least expense of vital power to the patient', and a few years later she stressed the teaching role of the newly created health visitor. To these necessary but rather obvious qualities have to be added a highly developed and accurate observation, technical and ministration skills, capacity to set aside one's own feelings and needs because of the urgent needs of the patient, skill in the use of complicated equipment, insight into cultural and value systems, ability to communicate successfully, and professional ethical standards, together with – for a proportion of nurses – administrative and organizational skills (for the chief nursing officer of an area has to deploy and organize a professional staff numbering thousands), and knowledge of educational psychology and teaching methods (for a tutor has exactly the same functions as has a university or college of education lecturer).

Until 1974 community nurses (health visitors, domiciliary midwives and home nurses) were subject to the over-riding responsibility of the medical officer of health and in some hospitals nurses were under the jurisdiction of the medical superintendent. The 1974 reorganization of British Health Services made nurses unequivocally responsible to their own professional heads and made the chief nursing officer of each area a full member of the Executive Group of chief officers. In other words, the nurse was at last recognized as of full professional status, not an assistant to the doctor but an independent colleague, lacking certain skills which the doctor has but possessing certain skills which he lacks.

Nursing in Britain has been under the jurisdiction of several bodies – separate General Nursing Councils for England and

Wales and for Scotland, separate Central Midwives Boards for these countries, and a United Kingdom Council for the Education and Training of Health Visitors; but proposals have been accepted by the Government for a single U.K. Council for Nurses, Midwives and Health Visitors.

nursing. Since it takes three years of full-time professional education to convert an intelligent young person into a qualified nurse, with further full-time preparation required for entry to various branches (e.g., health visiting, midwifery and home nursing), and since the complexity of a nurse's duties and responsibilities increases with almost every development in the various health sciences, it is no more possible to set down the essentials of nursing in a single article than it would be to specify the fundamental principles of accountancy or personnel management or veterinary surgery. Yet, just as many people have to invest money and prepare tax returns without being accountants or to co-ordinate groups of staff without being qualified personnel managers or to treat the ailments of domestic animals without being veterinary surgeons, so many people have – without specialized nursing education – to care for sick relatives at home.

A few basic points are therefore mentioned here. For simplicity the patient is called 'he' and the unqualified nurse 'she', but of course either could be of either sex.

Attitude. Probably the most important requirements for home nursing of a relative are sympathetic understanding and genuine interest, emotional self-control, alert observation, and respect for the judgment of visiting experts. The patient who is ill and in pain lacks his normal control of himself, he may be very irritable and unkind, he may seek to leave his bed long before it is safe for him to do so, or he may plead for his pain-killer considerably before it is due. It is vital that the person nursing him meets his irritability and difficult behaviour with kindly patience and a judicious mixture of sympathy and firmness. The patient who is beginning to recover is often bored and disgruntled. It is important that the nurse finds means of securing and maintaining his interest. She may be very worried about the serious nature of his illness, distressed about his pain, hurt by his unkind remarks and anxious about her own ability to carry out a particular treatment, but she needs to conceal these feelings. For the time being she is his main contact with the outside world and the person on whom he depends, and she must convey to him an atmosphere of calm confidence.

She sees the patient for hours on end whereas any visiting doctor or nurse sees him for minutes. So it is important that she uses her observation in order to report anything that might have a bearing on the diagnosis or on the treatment.

However skilled she may be in her own professional or commercial field she has to remember that she is an amateur in nursing and that the visiting doctor or visiting nurse is an expert on the treatment, disease and the well-being of the patient, and that the expert's instructions must be carried out completely: the amateur nurse is taking part in a battle for the patient's life or for his health, and a soldier cannot argue with the commander in the middle of a battle. She has to realize, too, that the doctor's expertise and the nurse's expertise are different: a busy doctor or busy nurse can sometimes be induced by a persuasive amateur to concur in an opinion relating to the other person's expertise, but such reinforcement of the amateur's view is seldom benefical to the patient.

Sick-room. To such extent as choice is possible the room should be of adequate size, reasonably warm but well ventilated, though with the bed out of all cross-draughts; and quiet with regard both to outdoor traffic and to indoor noises. The bed should be accessible from both sides. If light disturbs the patient's sleep a screen may shield the window or a partial shade may dim the electric light, while leaving the nurse enough light to see the patient and to read or write. A small table at the bedside for the patient's use and another table for the nurse's use are desirable, and if the bathroom is at some distance a washstand can be very useful. Since the nurse will be present for many hours, it is important that there is a comfortable chair for her use: reasonable comfort is essential for her continued efficiency, but this point is often forgotten by willing amateurs whose initial thoughts, naturally, are concerned with the well-being of the sick relatives. Apart from these items, the less furniture there is in the room the better.

The patient. When removing clothing from an injured patient or putting garments on him it is useful to tackle the uninjured side first, so limiting movement. In most illness the patient should be washed daily all over with warm water, the ordinary bedclothes being removed before the washing and the patient covered with a blanket, and the blanket being raised over individual parts of the body while these are washed and dried. The back should be examined daily for reddening and treated promptly if redness appears, so preventing bed-sores. In some cases various manipulations – such as changing of garments, washing, bed-making, feeding and toileting – cause some discomfort or actual pain, and both gentleness and quiet encouragement are needed.

The bed. Where available a single bed is better, both for the comfort of the patient and for the convenience of the nurse. The bedclothes should be light and changed frequently: as already mentioned the room should be warm and additional heat can be supplied by hot water bottles with, if the patient is too ill to complain of excessive heat, external wrapping. The sheet under the patient should be firmly tucked under the mattress all round, otherwise the patient in bed all day will quickly get it creased, producing discomfort and danger of bed-sores. If there is any likehood of incontinence or indeed if the patient is too ill to move from the bed to the toilet, a draw-sheet and rubber mackintosh are essential.

Bedmaking. To make a bed with the patient lying in it is a skilled art, but bed-making should be done twice daily for the patient's comfort. In general the guidance of a qualified nurse should be sought at first, and when the attendant feels competent for the job the help of a second person should be enlisted if possible. Probably the simplest method is to place a chair at the foot of the bed, to lift each blanket or sheet separately from the top and

If you have been advised to control your weight, avoid the food on these shelves:

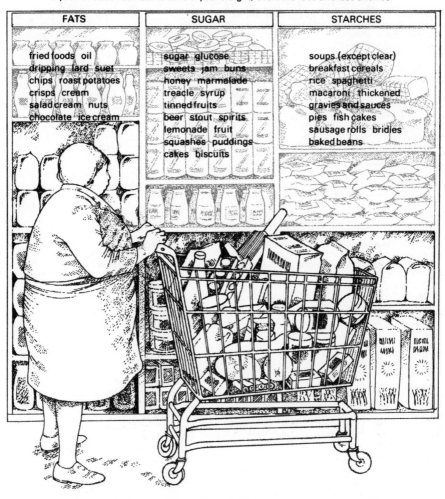

FATS	SUGAR	STARCHES
fried foods oil	sugar glucose	soups (except clear)
dripping lard suet	sweets jam buns	breakfast cereals
chips roast potatoes	honey marmalade	rice spaghetti
crisps cream	treacle syrup	macaroni thickened
salad cream nuts	tinned fruits	gravies and sauces
chocolate ice cream	beer stout spirits	pies fish cakes
	lemonade fruit	sausage rolls bridies
	squashes puddings	baked beans
	cakes biscuits	

Allowances: 3 slices bread daily; 120g. (0.25 lb.) margarine or butter weekly

Nutrition: obesity

fold it over the chair, and when only one sheet remains over the patient for one person to raise him gently while another person straightens the sheet (or draw-sheet) under him. If the patient cannot lie for a minute without pillows he may have to be supported while the pillows are changed.

Temperature and pulse. These are important indications during illness. The person nursing a patient should learn to read a thermometer and record the temperature, always remembering to shake the thermometer down after use, to take the temperature in the same place (the mouth which is slightly higher or the armpit which is slightly lower) and not to record the temperature immediately after a meal or a hot drink or a hot bath. Similarly she should learn to take the pulse at the wrist, placing the tips of her first and second fingers over the artery on the thumb side of the wrist and counting the beats for thirty seconds. In some illnesses counting the rate of respirations can also be useful.

Medicines. Medicines should be kept in a different part of the room from fluids intended for external application, and the nurse should school herself never to pour out a dose without reading the label on the bottle. When one is tired – and for most people home nursing is a fatiguing job and an unusual job – mistakes can occur easily.

Liquid food and solid food. It is important to

appreciate the risk of dehydration and to ensure that the patient has sufficient liquid in a form that he is willing to take. In some illnesses the amount of fluid consumed has to be measured. Solid food is relatively unimportant in a very short illness but is clearly important in any prolonged illness. Attractive serving of food, attention to the patient's likes and dislikes and gentle persuasion may make the difference between food being accepted and refused.

Relief for the attendant. Apart from 'on-call' duties (where they may be relaxing or sleeping but available at need) a qualified doctor or a qualified nurse is usually prepared during a prolonged emergency, such as a major epidemic, to work for about fifty-four hours a week (or nine hours a day for six days a week) or rather longer for an emergency that lasts only ten or fourteen days, but judges that efficiency falls if it proves necessary to exceed these times. The same sort of maximum has been established in industrial work during the pressures of wars or civil calamities. The amateur nurse undertaking the care of a sick relative is tackling an unfamiliar job and is emotionally involved. It is therefore unlikely that, in an illness lasting more than a few days, she can cope efficiently with spells of duty longer than those acceptable to qualified professionals. A common mistake during the illness of a much-loved relative is to be 'on duty' for thirteen or fourteen hours a day for well over a week before seeking help. By that time observation has become less acute (and important signs may be missed), self-control is lessened (so that the patient may become conscious of worries and fears), toleration of unkind remarks or harmful behaviour is reduced, and the possibilities of mistakes over medicines are increased. In other words the amateur nurse's attempt to cope for too long may harm the patient as well as herself. Where a serious illness nursed at home looks like extending substantially over a week it is therefore sound common-sense to start considering what relief can be provided by relatives, friends, paid help or services available from the state.

nutrition. The term is used both for (1) the process whereby FOOD is converted into energy and living tissue, and (2) the state of a person with regard to his absorption and assimilation of appropriate foods.

Each species of animal appears to have its own requirements of food: some, like cattle, are strict vegetarians; carnivorous animals eat only animal flesh; and some – like man – are omnivorous, both meat and vegetables being included in the DIET.

In primitive communities qualitative or even quantitative under-nutrition is common: man has discovered which foods are edible, but depends on successful hunting of animals or successful growth of plants, with winter feeding an annual problem and famine a recurring danger to life. In highly developed communities food production and food preservation have normally removed all dangers of winter shortages, a wide choice of varieties of food is available, over-nutrition is common among the affluent, and people have had leisure to develop many irrational prejudices and taboos, so that under-nutrition can occur either from poverty or as a result of food fads.

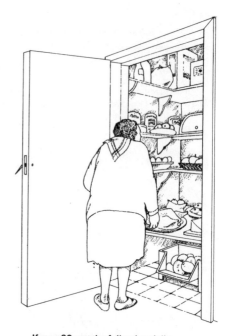

If over 60, eat the following daily:
0.5 litres (1 pint) of milk if possible but not less than half this amount.
1 helping of 55g. (2oz.) of meat, fish, poultry (once a week eat liver and oily fish)
1 egg
28g.(1oz.) cheese
1 tomato or half an orange
1 helping of **root** vegetables or **green** vegetables
1 helping of potatoes
3 to 4 slices of bread (often wholemeal)
1 helping of porridge or breakfast cereal
40g.(1.5oz.) margarine or butter

Nutrition: good food

In the twentieth century, as population growth outstrips increase of food production, under-nutrition becomes commoner, and on a conservative estimate half of the world's population today are appreciably under-nourished.

It can be said that FOOD is needed to supply energy not only for work and movement but also for such purposes as maintaining the bodily temperature and keeping the heart beating: to provide material for growth and for repair of tissue, with the amino-acids of proteins particularly required; and to provide substances – e.g., vitamins and trace minerals – for chemical processes that take place in the body.

While manual work manifestly increases food requirements it used to be said that mental work did not do so, but in recent years it has been established that mental activity does consume some energy.

The nutritional requirements for health are subject to many variations. To take some examples: in cold weather we use more Calories in maintaining our bodily temperature than in hot weather. Alcohol is a good source of Calories and therefore reduces our need for carbohydrate, but conversely it increases our need for vitamins of the B complex. In various infections the metabolic rate is speeded up so that we need more food, but paradoxically many foods are poorly digested, so that – to take one essential substance as an instance – by the time we have recovered from a severe infection our bodily stores of vitamin C are badly depleted.

Good nutrition is essential for health. Particularly vulnerable groups in respect of under-nutrition are: babies; rapidly growing children and adolescents – with the transition from school to work often a point of maximum danger; expectant and nursing mothers; old people – who often have deficiencies of protein, minerals and vitamins; immigrants – who may have difficulty in obtaining foods familiar to them and be reluctant to accept the diets normal in their new country; the very poor – who may have difficulty in affording expensive protein foods; and, commonest of all, the ignorant – whose food purchasing is often faulty and whose food preparation may destroy vitamins and lose minerals. Particularly vulnerable in respect of over-nutrition are persons whose occupations tempt them to over-eat, e.g., cooks and persons travelling on expense accounts.

nymphomania. Abnormally strong and frequent sexual desire in a woman. The parallel desire in a man is termed satyriasis. Nymphomania and satyriasis may become so severe that ethics and will-power lose their controlling influence and the need for relief by the sexual act dominates the imagination, but with actual intercourse providing less satisfaction than in the case of normal people.

The conditions used to be attributed to abnormalities of hormone secretion, but the modern view is that they have a deep-rooted psychological basis and that, while tranquillizers may temporarily subdue the extreme sexual drive, a full course of psychotherapy is usually needed.

nystagmus. Involuntary rapid and jerky movements of the eyeball, from side to side or up and down. Both eyes are usually affected. In children it may arise from diseases of the nervous system, congenital cataract, or inflammatory diseases of the eye. In adults it may appear in multiple sclerosis and cerebellar disease, and it is also found – without other signs of disease – in miners who work underground in semi-darkness. In general its presence suggests the need for immediate expert investigation.

O

obesity. The condition of being over-weight with excessive fat stored in the body.

In addition to being unattractive, appreciable excess of weight is dangerous: it forces the heart to work harder, because a greater volume of tissue has to be supplied with blood; it increases liability to pneumonia and other respiratory infections; it raises the chance of diabetes and arteriosclerosis; and because the stout person is in effect carrying an extra stone or half-stone whenever he moves, obesity increases the likelihood of arthritis, backache and flat feet. Not least, obesity decreases the expectation of life.

The exact borderline of obesity is hard to define. A professional boxer usually knows his best weight – below which he loses strength and above which he loses speed – but most of us can only hazard a guess at our optimum weight. Attempts were formerly made to assess ideal (unclothed) weight by a simple formula.

However, bone structure varies. A man of 172 cm. (5 ft. 8 in.) and heavy frame may be underweight at 68 kg. (150 lb.) while another man of the same height and light frame may be overweight at 63.5 kg. (140 lb.). Modern attempts to divide adults into heavy, medium and light bone structure for each height are more useful, but even these are merely approximations, and rigid application of such tables (see HEIGHT AND WEIGHT) suggests, rightly or wrongly, that about half the adults in Britain and the United States are overweight.

Perhaps more important than any hypothetical ideal weight is whether a person's weight is rising or remaining stationary. Prolonged consumption of rather more food than is needed leads to production of more tissue, but the slightly corpulent person expends more energy in supplying blood to the extra tissue and because he carries additional weight, uses more energy in each physical activity. If his weight becomes stationary he is probably not unduly at risk. If, on the other hand, his weight is continuing to rise, his life and his health are in danger.

Obesity is commoner in some races, for instance, Eskimos, living in icy climates, need a thick layer of adipose tissue. It is occasionally associated with endocrine or glandular abnormalities (e.g., hypothyroidism or hypopituitarism) which reduce the rate of energy expenditure. But in general it represents simply a prolonged disproportion between the quantity of Calories ingested and the quantity utilized by the body. Certainly some people have bodies that use food inefficiently, excreting the excess in faeces, urine, sweat and breath without gaining weight; but in persons whose bodies make efficient use of food weight gain indicates prolonged over-eating.

Over-eating proteins plays little if any part in

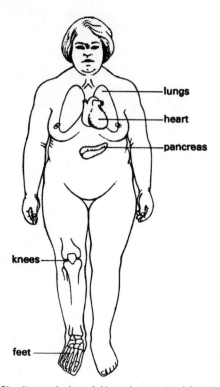

lungs

heart

pancreas

knees

feet

Obesity may be harmful to various parts of the body

obesity: increase of protein foods (e.g., lean meat and white fish) raises the rate of combustion in the body, and excess is excreted rather than stored. Fat plays little part: a disproportionate amount of fat leads to indigestion. The real culprit is excess carbohydrate (starches and sugars) which is stored in the body as fat. Lack of exercise may play a part in persons transferring from heavy manual work (in which many Calories are expended) to sedentary occupations, but it is more often a result than a cause of obesity: to lose one pound by exercise a man would have to walk fifty miles and disregard the increased appetite produced by his exertions.

Causes. The overeating that leads to obesity usually results from specific causes.

1. Over-feeding, especially excess of carbohydrates, in infancy and childhood, with subsequent persistence of the habit of eating too much. Fat babies tend to become fat children and in due course corpulent adults. Parents who systematically over-feed their young children are unknowingly shortening their lives. Obesity is commonly regarded as a problem of middle life, but at least half the cases start in infancy or childhood. In this connection it should be noted that, while obesity is often described as characteristic of affluent societies or of favourably placed groups in mixed societies, it can also occur in the poor because carbohydrate foods are usually cheaper than protein or fatty foods.

2. Psychological disturbances either in childhood or in adult life. The person who is lonely, bereaved, frustrated or otherwise disturbed eats in substitution for some other ungratified emotion. The emotional factors in obesity are only now becoming recognized. To treat a case of excessive weight without attention to emotional factors if they are present means either that the treatment will fail or that, if it succeeds in respect of reducing the amount of eating, it will leave the patient in a worse condition by removing his substitute for the unsatisfied emotion.

3. Nature of work. For instance, it is not unusual for cooks to be stout.

4. Failure to adjust food intake to changing circumstances. A retired athlete often puts on weight, as sometimes do people who move from physical to mental occupations. The elderly are usually less active than they were in their younger days and so require less energy (Calories) from their food.

Prevention. Just as obesity starts in childhood, so should its prevention. Essentially it implies that we should make parents aware of the dangers of over-feeding children, and especially of giving them excessive carbohydrates; that health workers should seek to prevent or alleviate mental disturbances at all stages of the lives of their clients; and that all concerned with health education should point out that even a small additional daily intake – a single extra slice of bread or three extra lumps of sugar – can in time create a considerable burden of overweight.

Treatment. Established obesity inevitably demands a rigorous DIET, with rigid restriction of amounts of bread, cakes, biscuits, milk puddings, sweets, cream and potatoes, limitation of alcohol, avoidance of eating between meals, and weekly weighing. Such a diet by itself almost always fails. To have any hope of success the person who is trying to lose weight also needs much reassurance and encouragement, in addition to attention to any relevant emotional factors. Appetite depressants are sometimes used to help patients to endure restricted diets, but the amphetamines cause excitement and sleeplessness, and undue reliance on drugs often results in reversion to the previous weight after the drug is ultimately discontinued.

objective. Observed by another and not merely felt by the patient. Thus a person's alleged headache is subjective (and may be exaggerated, accurately described, minimized or faked) but the bruise on his forehead noted by an unbiased observer is objective.

obsessional neurosis. An emotional disorder in which the victim's consciousness is dominated by certain ideas or impulses and by resistance to them. The sufferer is aware that his obsession is senseless and undergoes considerable mental anxiety during his fruitless efforts to gain freedom from the particular fear, preoccupation or impulses.

The cause is multiple and not fully understood. There appears to be a considerable amount of parental influence involved: in fully one-third of cases a parent has also been obsessional, and in many other cases a parent has been over-conscientious, excessively orderly, abnormally concerned with cleanliness or a stickler for precision. In such cases the origin of the disorder is probably less a matter of heredity than of the development of personality being impaired by the parental attitudes and behaviour. In other cases the source seems to lie in painful or disturbing experiences. In others, again, the psycho-analysts' explanation of obsessions as symbolic self-reproaches for earlier sexual mis-demeanours is almost certainly true. However, some obsessionals have not had neurotic parents, have not experienced any series of painful happenings and have not indulged in conduct that weighs on their consciences.

The obsessions may consist of ideas; questionings, impulses, phobias or a mixture of these. Ideas vary from tunes 'running in the head' for prolonged periods to obscene associations, such as every hole or cleft reminding the patient of a vulva. Questionings include a persistent and senseless 'Why' about relevant and irrelevant matters, with often a preoccupation with religion or philosophical questions. Impulses may be aggressive or suicidal, or merely a compulsion to count every step walked or to touch every lamp-post passed. Phobias include fear of open spaces, of enclosed spaces, of darkness and of dirt.

Many apparently normal people have persisting ideas, questioning natures, senseless impulses and irrational fears. What differentiates the obsessional from the normal is the domination of the particular fear or idea and the painful effort that he makes to get rid of it.

Treatment involves frank discussion with the patient, avoidance of situations in which the obsession is most marked and where practicable a change of environment. Psychoanalysis, hypnosis and suggestion help in some cases but not in all. Where the obsession is severe, and especially where it is dangerous either to the patient or to others, pre-frontal leucotomy may be considered, though the current tendency in such cases is to try appropriate drugs and to regard leucotomy as a last resort.

obstetrics. The branch of medicine concerned with pregnancy and childbirth. Although a handful of physicians studied obstetrics from the time of Soranus (over two thousand years ago) doctors – all male – were traditionally debarred from attending women in labour, and the midwives of the mediaeval and early modern period were quite untrained except for the passage of information from mother to daughter. William Smellie's classes in 1741 for medical students in afternoons and for prospective midwives in mornings represented a revolutionary breakthrough. He offered twelve lectures, later increased to eighteen. Others followed Smellie's example, but as late as the end of the nineteenth century most doctors had never studied midwifery and most midwives were untrained Sarah Gamps. The specialist obstetrician, the general practitioner with training in midwifery, the qualified health visitor and the qualified midwife all really arrived during the present century.

occiput. The back and lower part of the skull pierced by the foramen magnum through which the spinal cord passes from the brain. Writers of fiction often describe characters as receiving a blow on the occiput. Actually a blow aimed at the head from behind would strike the parietal bones unless the assailant

was shorter than the victim and striking slightly upwards.

occlusion. The term is used in four different ways, all connected with the derivational idea of shutting. (1) Closure of the eyes by drawing the eyelids over them. (2) Blockage of any hollow tube, e.g., in coronary occlusion one of the arteries that supply blood to the heart is blocked by a clot. (3) Temporary closure of the vocal passage in speech, as in formation of the stop consonants. (4) The coming together of the upper and lower teeth in the process of biting. The converse term, malocclusion, is used only in the fourth sense and means inability of the teeth to meet correctly.

occupation and health. Quite apart from certain occupations being associated with the risk of specific OCCUPATIONAL DISEASES, occupation and health profoundly influence each other. This is not surprising in view of the fact that the average employed adult spends about 45 per cent of his time on essential basic activities (e.g., sleeping, eating, dressing and washing) and divides the other 55 per cent fairly equally between work – including travelling to and from work – and all other activities.

The influence of health on work is obvious. A man with poor physical health cannot become a policeman, a colour blind person cannot become a lorry driver, an epileptic cannot take a job that involves climbing ladders, and impaired physical or mental health may make a person incapable of continuing his previous occupation.

Perhaps the first point to be noted about the influence of occupation on health is the need of every person for occupation, not merely for financial reasons but to provide job satisfaction and a sense of being needed. It is common knowledge that a healthy young adult, if unemployed for several years, runs considerable danger of physical and mental deterioration and may become unemployable. However, absence of employment is not really within the scope of this article.

Clearly an over-heated, badly ventilated office or workshop increases the likelihood of spread of air-borne infectious diseases; a cold, draughty building may predispose to rheumatism; an excessively dry atmosphere may lead to catarrh and other diseases of the nose and throat; unguarded equipment of a potentially dangerous nature can cause industrial accidents; working in a very noisy factory may ultimately damage hearing; persistent bad lighting or persistent glare may be harmful to eyesight; an outdoor job with exposure to cold and rain may increase liability to bronchitis; occupations of much mental stress are associated with increased incidence both of the psychoneuroses and of coronary thrombosis; and a job involving much travelling with an expense account increases the chance both of obesity and of alcoholism.

In Britain the Factories Act (1961) specifically covers such matters as cleanliness, overcrowding (prescribing a minimum of 400 cubic feet of air space per person), temperature (requiring not less than 60 °F. after the first hour of work in rooms where most of the work is sedentary), ventilation, lighting and sanitary accommodation. Regulations made under that Act cover such things as lifting of heavy weights, washing facilities, accommodation for clothing, seating, provision of first aid equipment and, if more than fifty persons are employed, provision of an available person trained in first aid. The Offices, Shops and Railway Premises Act (1963) broadly extends the provisions of the Factories Act to these premises.

Inevitably legislation provides only for minimum physical standards. An efficient occupational health service of skilled doctors and nurses, each with specialized knowledge both of occupational health and of the particular industry can go far beyond this minimum standard in ensuring good working conditions. Moreover, since absenteeism can gravely damage productivity, such a service is in the interests of both employers and employees. There is however, the difficulty that industrial doctors and nurses employed by a company and on its pay-roll, are often regarded by the workers as the management's men. On the one hand employees feel that the doctors and nurses will hesitate to make recommendations that might interfere with productivity and profit, and on the other hand workers are sometimes reluctant to implement recommendations, e.g., in relation to protective devices, that might slow down the rate of piecework. To be really effective industrial doctors and nurses must be seen to be impartial and to be fearless in the presentation of their recommendations.

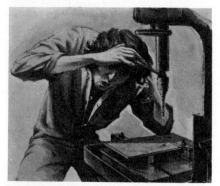

Occupation and health: an easily preventable factory accident

Occupations have enormous psychological effects which are only in the process of becoming recognized. People in cohesive and mutually supporting occupational groups (e.g., coal miners) are less likely to become alcoholics or to suffer from some mental disorders than are persons who work largely in isolation. A sarcastic or unsympathetic senior officer can greatly damage the mental health – and impair the working efficiency – of the more sensitive members of his staff, and this is especially the case in occupations where complete escape from the surroundings during leisure is difficult, as in ships, hospitals and residential schools. Similarly a person who has accepted a job beyond his capacities may ruin his own health and damage that of his juniors. Conversely, a group working together under good physical conditions and with mutual consideration and respect can develop a co-operative spirit and a high morale which enormously benefit the mental health of the individual members as well as improving the standard of work.

Again, sedentary and active occupations influence health. For example, bus drivers have greater liability to coronary heart disease than have bus conductors of the same age, although in large measure an individual worker can counteract adverse influences by adjusting his leisure activities, so that, for example, the desk-bound clerk engages in pastimes that involve abundant physical exercise.

On the sheer evidence of death-rates, clergymen (despite low incomes), senior civil servants (despite heavy responsibilities), school teachers (despite large classes) and farmers (despite exposure to all weathers) are in general long-lived, with doctors reasonably long-lived, while welders, coal-miners, dock labourers and publicans generally have short lives. In thinking of occupational mortality, however, one has to consider the people entering different occupations. A person of dubious physical health is more likely to seek to become a typist than a labourer, a teacher than a nurse, or a tailor than a salesman; a nurse of poor physique or unadventurous disposition is more likely to remain in a hospital post than to enter the more strenuous and climatically hazardous career of a health visitor; and a lawyer of doubtful health is more likely to specialize in conveyancing than in court work.

A useful check of the effects of occupation on married men would be a comparison of a numerically large group with their wives. If, allowing for sex differences, diseases and death-rates are broadly similar in the two groups then – provided the wives do not work in the same occupation – it may be assumed that no specific occupational factor is present. If there is a substantial increase in the morbidity or mortality of the men over their wives, the presumption is that there exists an adverse occupational factor. If, finally, the men on the whole are healthier than their wives or outlive them, there is some presumptive evidence that the circumstances of the particular occupation are conducive to health.

occupational diseases. As early as Roman times there was some awareness of the connection between occupations and diseases: the poet Martial mentions diseases peculiar to sulphur workers and several writers speak of the pallor of miners. Yet Paracelsus in the seventeenth century was probably the first physician to appreciate fully that specific occupations could cause diseases: he identified the miner's liability to lung disorders and the smelter's risk of poisoning by heavy metals. The recognized foundation of occupational medicine, however, is Ramazzini's *De morbis artificum diatribe* (1700). Ramazzini not only identified many occupational diseases but also suggested ways of avoiding or reducing them.

Since then knowledge of illnesses caused by various trades has advanced rapidly. In Britain for instance fourteen industrial diseases are now notifiable to the Chief Inspector of Factories. They are lead poisoning, phosphorus poisoning, arsenical poisoning, mercury poisoning, manganese poisoning, carbon bisulphide poisoning, analine poisoning, benzene poisoning, anthrax, toxic jaundice, compressed air illness, epitheliomatous ulceration, chrome ulceration and toxic anaemia. Following improvement in working conditions all have now become rarities, although chrome ulceration, epitheliomatous ulceration and lead poisoning each amount to about one hundred to two hundred notifications a year in Britain.

The commonest occupational diseases of today are of the skin, lungs and muscles.

Occupational dermatitis - clinically indistinguishable from any other form of DERMATITIS - may occur through the skin becoming sensitive to a particular solvent, oil or dye. Barrier creams carefully applied before work can help to prevent the condition.

Dust diseases of the lungs include pneumoconiosis (in coal miners, graphite workers and boiler scalers), byssinosis (due to inhalation of cotton dust), asbestosis, and silicosis. Preventive measures include substitution of a toxic substance by a harmless one, reduction of exposure to the dust by exhaust ventilation and scrupulous cleanliness, and the use of respirators to prevent inhalation of dust and fumes.

Occupational palsy or *cramp* is a condition of discomfort, pain and fatigue arising from habitual use of one set of muscles in finely coordinated movements; WRITER'S CRAMP and musician's cramp are examples.

occupational pyrexia. A condition, quite common thirty years ago but relatively uncommon today, occurring in workers in textile factories, and characterized by bouts of feverishness, headache, nausea, general weakness and disinclination for food. It is found more in recently appointed workers than in those with long service, and is almost certainly allergic, a hypersensitivity to some of the constituents of the raw materials. Treatment is essentially as for any other ALLERGY with change of work necessary in some cases. An alternative name for the condition is mill fever.

There are at least two explanations of the decrease in occupational pyrexia, both partially correct. Firstly, better ventilation and better hygienic standards generally have made it likely that people with only a mild hypersensitivity to a particular constituent will escape; and secondly, in the past mill fever was a convenient name under which to lump a number of different diseases, such as aspergillosis.

occupational therapy. Treatment of the physically or mentally ill by engaging them constructively in selected activities.

The term was originally used to denote the occupational methods adopted for the relief and treatment of nervous and mental illness, but has come to include similar methods in all forms of prolonged illness. In certain conditions particular forms of occupation are physically desirable to strengthen weakened or unused muscles; and in most illnesses occupational therapy has a considerable psychological effect, restoring the patient's confidence in himself and in his ability to do things.

Properly undertaken, occupational therapy involves attempting to discover the patient's aptitudes, talents or abilities, exploiting these in suitable occupation, and so building up a sense of achievement and satisfaction in the patient's mind. This does not merely relieve the tedium of a long spell in hospital but also actively promotes recovery.

Weaving, raffia and basket work, needlework, toy-making, book-binding and painting are well-established forms of occupational therapy; but in general the occupation has to be geared to the patient, not the patient to the available occupation.

Occupational therapy, which gives the patient something useful and interesting to do, slides imperceptibly into vocational rehabilitation, in which a person who has become permanently unfit for his former occupation learns new skills in preparation for a job suited to his restricted abilities.

oedema. Abnormal accumulation of watery fluid in the body tissues or cavities. Oedema is not a disease but a symptom of disease of the heart, kidney or liver. Perhaps the commonest form of oedema is the slight swelling of the ankles that many people experience after prolonged standing. While this may be an indication of cardiac or renal disorder, it has various other causes, e.g., constriction of veins by tight garters. See DROPSY.

Oedipus complex. During the insecurity of infancy many boys pass through a stage in which they are more attracted to their mother than to their father and are even a little jealous of him. Where this stage persists and becomes exaggerated into a neurosis it is termed the Oedipus complex, named after a legendary Greek who married his own mother without being aware of her identity.

The explanations of Freud undoubtedly cover the fully developed complex and in such cases psychoanalytic treatment can be useful. Much commoner, however, is the almost latent variety in which the young man subconsciously looks for a bride who resembles his mother physically and mentally, compares his wife disadvantageously with his mother, resolutely declines to enter his father's occupation and adopts religious and political views utterly different from those of his father.

The feminine equivalent where a daughter has excessive love for her father and resentment of her mother is called the Electra complex.

oesophagus. The muscular tube, often known as the gullet, which conveys food from the mouth and pharynx to the stomach. It lies in front of the spinal column, behind the windpipe in the neck and behind the upper part of the heart in the chest. Food is propelled down the tube by muscular movements called PERISTALSIS.

It is the narrowest part of the whole digestive tube and swallowed foreign bodies tend to become lodged in it. The oesophagus may also become obstructed for other reasons: the commonest causes of this stricture of the oesophagus are: (1) scarring due to the swallowing of hot or corrosive fluids, (2) malignant disease arising in the oesophagus itself, and (3) external pressure especially from aneurysm of the aorta or malignant disease of lungs, bronchi, or mediastinum.

The gullet can be examined by an oesophagoscope, a tube with a light at the end and working in the same way as a periscope.

oestrogen. The two groups of hormones secreted by the ovary are known by the general names, oestrogen and progesterone. The oestrogens are the substances responsible for the development and maintenance of a woman's sexual organs and breasts, and in preparation for pregnancy they cause a thickening of the inside lining of the uterus.

Several synthetic oestrogens such as STILBOESTROL are available for therapy, e.g., for treatment of painful menstruation and for alleviation of symptoms at the menopause.

Most oral contraceptives contain small amounts of an oestrogen and a progesterone, the relative quantities and the particular synthetic oestrogen varying with the brand of contraceptive.

oliguria. Diminished secretion of urine. It occurs in some diseases of the kidney and in diseases of the heart and liver associated with OEDEMA. It may also occur temporarily in healthy people who have perspired excessively under conditions of abnormal warmth.

omentum. The omenta are double folds of peritoneum which contain fat and blood vessels and which separate abdominal organs from each other. The great omentum is attached to the lower border of the stomach and hangs like an apron in front of the intestines. The lesser omentum separates the liver from the stomach.

one-parent families. Families consisting of one or more children and only one available parent. Common causes of this situation include: (1) the death of one partner, leaving the other a widow or widower; (2) divorce; (3) desertion by one partner; (4) chronic illness or insanity of one partner; (5) not all cases of illegitimacy but such cases as are unaccompanied by any stable union.

The varying causes lead to considerable differences in financial circumstances, mental outlook and attitudes of relations. Thus the widow is in some, though by no means all, cases materially comfortable through inheriting life insurance or obtaining compensation for the accident or injury that killed her husband; the divorced person may have considerable alimony; but the unmarried mother or the woman whose husband has simply disappeared is often in dire financial straits. The widow and her children, if old enough, may look back to years of normal family life; the divorced or separated person may recall unhappy years of discord and bickering and may even have a permanent hostility to the opposite sex; and the unmarried mother has no personal experience of married life. The widower, though he may have to face the cost of employing a housekeeper, will in general receive the sympathy and practical help of his relatives, whereas in some cultures the unmarried mother is the subject of a stigma which may even make it difficult for her to secure employment. Again the widow and the unmarried mother can contemplate marriage but the divorced or deserted person in some cases finds the idea of re-marriage in conflict with long-existing religious tenets.

In most cases the solitary parent has to be the bread-winner for the household involving placing young children in a day nursery or in the daily care of a child-minder (unless there is an available grandmother or aunt of the children) and involving constant worry about children's illnesses. In any such illness there is a conflict between the needs of the children and the requirements of the bread-winner's job. It is easy to say on humanitarian grounds that the children must always take precedence, but the absence of one person in a highly responsible or

highly specialized post may seriously impede the work of sixty other people.

Not least, the one parent has to try to fulfil the role of both father and mother. It might be thought that, with a woman as sole parent, the absence of a father's authority might lead to excessive licence and 'spoiling'; but in many cases the effect is the reverse, the woman over-compensating for the absence of a husband by being over-strict, with harmful effects on the children's later ability to make decisions and exercise initiative.

In most western countries the problems of the one-parent household were largely ignored until recent decades. However, Sweden led the way by providing for such households special flats with adjacent nurseries, several developed countries now offer additional financial allowances in such cases, and helpful associations (such as, in Britain, the Society for the Single Parent and her Dependents) have come into existence. Also the spread of contraceptive measures (reducing the number of unmarried mothers) and improved facilities for the prevention and treatment of illness (reducing the number of deaths of parents) have between them considerably lessened the total number of one-parent families.

Nevertheless the situation of the solitary parent and her (or more rarely his) dependents is difficult; but it is worth remembering that even three generations ago the difficulties could be overcome, e.g., one child brought up in a one-parent family (Ramsay Macdonald) became prime minister of Britain and another (Charlie Chaplin) became perhaps the world's most famous cinema actor. In most African countries, with their tradition of the extended family, the position is much easier. See also DIVORCE.

onychia. Infection of the bed of a nail. Mild cases may clear up spontaneously, moderate cases respond well to antibiotics, and in severe cases removal of the nail may be required. If the nail is removed and the infection cleared, the nail will re-grow; but if the infection remains it may destroy the growing tissue, so that ultimately the nail comes off and does not re-grow. Hence deliberate removal of the nail to facilitate treatment of the infection may well save permanent loss of the nail.

operation, need for. The question of operative treatment arises under two different sets of circumstances.

Firstly, in acute illness the matter may be one of urgency and indeed of life or death. In acute appendicitis, for instance, or in a perforated ulcer of the stomach or duodenum, every hour of delay materially increases the risk to life. A death from an unnecessary operation is extremely rare, but every year hundreds of people die because operation was not performed or was performed too late. In any acute illness where the attending doctor desires a surgeon's opinion and where an experienced surgeon advises operation, neither patient nor relatives should hesitate.

Secondly, operation may be considered for the relief of a long-lasting condition. Examples are infected tonsils and adenoids, prolapse of the uterus, incurable arthritic joint, and ingrowing toe nail. Here there is ample time for consideration of the advantages and disadvantages of operation as opposed to other available methods of treatment. Clearly decision will depend on many factors, including the patient's general health, but it is worth remembering that, with modern anaesthesia and modern surgical techniques, many operations involve little danger and little post-operative pain or discomfort.

ophthalmia. Inflammation of the eye or the membranes lining the eyelid. Conjunctivitis, iritis and trachoma are varieties of ophthalmia. Ophthalmia neonatorum, formerly common in new-born infants, was due to gonococcal infection during the journey through the mother's birth passage. In most developed countries the condition has disappeared, partly because of more efficient diagnosis and treatment of maternal gonorrhoea, but mainly because of routine treatment of the eyes of all newly born infants to prevent it.

Sympathetic ophthalmia is a curious condition in which, after an injury to one eye, the other eye becomes inflamed. Not only does the sympathetic inflammation need treatment, but the inflammation is long-lasting and hard to cure. Indeed, where both eyes were previously normal, it is not unknown for the injured eye to make a greater recovery of sight than the sympathetically inflamed eye. As a preventive measure many eye specialists, when treating an injured eye, use atropin or an antibiotic or both for the uninjured eye.

ophthalmologist. A doctor who specializes in treatment of diseases of the eye. A frequently used alternative name is ophthalmic surgeon, but not all doctors who have specialized on the eye undertake surgical work.

These terms should be differentiated from optician, a qualified, non-medical worker. An optician tests eyesight and prescribes spectacles but, if he discovers evidence of disease of the eye, refers the patient to an ophthalmologist.

ophthalmoscope. An instrument for examining the interior of the eye and especially the retina and its blood vessels. Apart from indicating various diseases of the eye, ophthalmoscopic examination can sometimes provide the first indication of other diseases that affect the retinal blood vessels, e.g., diabetes and nephritis.

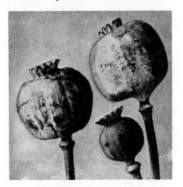

The opium poppy in seed

opium. The dried juice of the seed capsules of the white poppy which is extensively grown in China, Egypt and Iran. Opium contains several alkaloids, the most important being morphine

and codeine. In the past the drug was normally given as a crude powder or as an alcoholic solution, laudenum, but nowadays the purified active ingredients are preferred for greater accuracy of dosage.

Opium has been used to relieve pain since the dawn of history. It reduces or removes pain, slows respiration, constricts the pupils and produces a dreamy state with pleasant imagery or, if the dose is large, a deep sleep. Opium and its main alkaloid, morphine, are of the highest value for relief of pain, but their use has to be carefully controlled because of the danger of addiction. A craving for morphine can begin to appear after as few as three injections, and the drug habit, once established, is very hard to break.

In Britain dilute solutions of opium are readily available, e.g., a mixture of chalk and opium for the treatment of diarrhoea, but morphine and higher concentrations of opium are rigorously controlled under the Dangerous Drugs Act.

opium poisoning. Opium poisoning can occur by accident (especially in children), in attempted suicide or through therapeutic misadventure. After a short initial period of euphoria and mental excitement, the condition manifests itself by increasing drowsiness going on to complete stupor, contracted 'pin-point' pupils which do not alter in size when light is shone on them, blueness and coldness of the skin, and stertorous or irregular breathing. The main danger to be guarded against is respiratory failure.

If the drug has been taken by mouth an emetic to cause vomiting may be useful. Irrespective of how the drug was taken, strong coffee helps if the patient can swallow, and most experts advise rousing the patient by movement. The most essential points in treatment, however, are the application of artificial respiration (aided by oxygen if available) if breathing becomes difficult, and (again if available) injection of 5 to 10 mg. of the specific antagonist, nalorphine. Given prompt treatment recovery from opium poisoning (as distinct from poisoning by its alkaloids) is highly probable, but in morphine poisoning the outcome is not so certain.

opposition. The act of turning the thumb inwards towards the other fingers, thus enabling an object to be grasped. The primates, i.e., man, apes and most monkeys, are unique in having this important capacity to grasp objects.

optic nerve. The bundle of nerve fibres forming the second cranial nerve which carry impulses from the retina to the back of the BRAIN. Inside the skull the nerves join to form a cross, the optic chiasma, so that impulses from the right side of each retina go to the right side of the brain and impulses from the left go to the left side.

optic neuritis and atrophy. Inflammation of the optic nerve is not a disease in itself but a symptom of such diseases as brain tumours, meningitis, chronic nephritis, gout and lead poisoning. It leads to failure of sight with blurring of vision, headache and pain in the back of the eye. Treatment varies with the cause.

Optic atrophy, i.e., degeneration of the nerve resulting in blindness, may follow uncured optic neuritis or may arise as a primary condition in organic nervous diseases, especially in the late stage of untreated syphilis.

orchitis. Inflammation of the testicles, characterized by swelling, pain and tenderness.

Orchitis occurs most frequently as a painful complication of mumps in adolescent boys and young men. Treatment consists of rest in bed with the scrotum supported by a pillow and pain relievers used as required. The inflammation disappears in a week or so but in some cases the disease leaves the victim sterile.

Less common causes of orchitis include gonorrhoea and enteric fever (in both of which antibiotics are useful), and injury.

organ transplant. See TRANSPLANT.

orgasm. The climax of the sexual act. In the male it is produced mainly by stimulation of the penis and results in the ejaculation of semen. In the female it is produced principally by stimulation of the clitoris. In both sexes orgasm is followed by relaxation of sexual tension and departure of blood from the previously engorged genital organs.

oriental sore. Also termed Delhi or Baghdad boil. A lesion, or more usually a number of lesions, of the skin and the tissues immediately below the skin caused by a protozoon (*Leishmania tropica*) normally transmitted by the bite of a sandfly. The sore begins as an itchy papule, enlarges over many weeks and becomes ulcerated, forming a boil which may take months to heal. Preventive measures are as yet almost non-existent in the countries in which the condition is common. There is no particularly effective treatment, although the injection of a 10 per cent solution of mepacrine hydrochloride is said to accelerate healing. If the sore becomes infected, usually as a result of scratching, antibiotics may be needed for the organisms causing the infection, but antibiotics have little if any effect on the protozoon causing the sore.

ornithosis. A feverish illness with symptoms resembling both pneumonia and typhoid fever, and caused by a virus transmitted by birds, especially from their dried excreta. It is sometimes divided into two varieties: (1) psittacosis which is the result of infection by a large virus transmitted mainly by parrots, and (2) ornithosis proper, which is caused by a much smaller virus transmitted by pigeons, hens and other birds. In both varieties the mortality was very high until the advent of the tetracyclines, and even with early treatment with these recovery is by no means certain. Chlorotetracycline, 4 g. daily for two days and thereafter smaller dosage, is probably the drug of choice.

orthodontics. The branch of dentistry concerned with prevention and correction of faulty position of the teeth, usually by gradually moving teeth to better positions by the sustained slight pressure of a brace or a wire.

orthomolecular psychiatry. A school of medical thought, largely founded by Linus Pauling and becoming prominent in the 1970s, which maintains that many mental diseases are caused by a twisting of molecules and which, in particular, emphasizes the importance of large intake of certain vitamins both for prevention and for cure. The adherents of the orthomolecular school point out especially that 94 per cent of schizophrenics excrete abnormally low quantities of ascorbic acid, niacinamide or pyridoxine, and claim that the disease is benefited or cured by massive doses of these vitamins.

As so often happens with pioneers, the founders of this school of thought appear to overstate their case. There exists a good deal of evidence that many psychotic diseases (including at least a goodly number of cases of schizophrenia) are due to genetic abnormalities which, even if identifiable in advance, could hardly be prevented by massive doses of the water-soluble vitamins; and it is a little difficult to understand how much massive doses could remedy a genetic abnormality. Again, such human experiences as prolonged stress, insecurity, rejection and alienation play a large part in the causation of mental disorders (certainly including some cases of schizophrenia) but are disregarded by Pauling and his associates. In other words, the orthomolecular psychiatrists have not established the only cause or even the main cause of mental disorders and have not provided the sole method of treatment.

Nevertheless their published results are impressive, and they have certainly made out a case for trying massive doses of the B and C vitamins on schizophrenics. At the worst the treatment would do no harm and would not be excessively costly, and even if it improved or cured only a relatively small percentage of schizophrenics the benefit to the persons and to the community would be enormous.

orthopaedics. The branch of surgery that deals with the correction of deformities. The deformities in question include both congenital and acquired conditions, and forms of treatment used include massage, electricity, exercises, the breaking and resetting of bones, and a vast number of appliances.

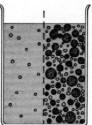

Two solutions of differing concentration separated by a semi-permeable membrane.

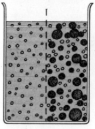

While large molecules cannot pass through the membrane, smaller ones do, thus equalizing their concentration on either side.

Osmosis

osmosis. The diffusion of fluids through a semipermeable membrane into a solution where the concentration of the fluids is lower, thus equalizing the conditions on either side of the membrane. A semipermeable membrane is one of such nature that it acts like a sieve, holding back large molecules but permitting small ones to pass through. The walls of capillary blood vessels, for instance, are such membranes. They permit water, salts, and sugars and aminoacids to pass through but prevent the passage of larger molecules. At the end of a capillary nearer to the heart (and receiving in weakened form the pressure of the cardiac contraction) the concentration in the capillary is greater than in the adjacent cells, so the traffic is from capillary to cell; at the far end of the capillary the concentration is greater in the cell than in the capillary, so the traffic is in the reverse direction.

ossification. Hardening of cartilage into bone, either as part of normal growth or in disease. The term is also used to indicate attitudes or beliefs becoming rigid and unalterable.

osteitis. Inflammation of bone. It may be acute or chronic and is the result of bacterial invasion, either from an external wound or from a local focus of infection e.g., in the mouth, throat or alimentary tract.

Osteitis deformans (Paget's disease) is a disease of later life in which certain bones, especially the long bones, lose some of their calcium and hence their rigidity, and then become deformed through weight-bearing. The first symptom is pain, and diagnosis is facilitated by radiological examination. Corticosteroids and sodium fluoride are currently being used in treatment of the condition and they seem to prevent the advance of the disease.

Osteitis fibrosa is a thinning of bones through over-activity of the parathyroid glands.

osteo-arthritis. Gradual degeneration of one or more joints, with some loss of cartilage (the smooth tissue which lines the joint) and the formation of rough deposits of bone. It is a very common disease from 40 years onwards and is characterized by pain (generally worse at night), increasing stiffness of the affected joints, limitation of movement and in some cases deformed appearance with 'knobbly' joints.

There are three main types which may exist together. The mono-articular type affects the hip or shoulder mostly and is commoner in men; the polyarticular type affects many joints and is more frequent in women; and the spinal type creates a rigid 'poker' back and causes considerable pain.

Faulty posture, injury and excessive weight are predisposing factors, and prevention consists largely of their reduction or avoidance. There is probably also a hereditary factor, and certainly the disease appears to run in families.

In most cases deterioration is very slow and only three forms of treatment are needed: (1) movements and exercises to maintain the mobility of the joint as far as is practicable; (2) mild analgesics to control the pain; and, (3) radiant heat, which not only lessens pain but also appears to have a positive beneficial influence.

In advanced cases surgical treatment may be needed to create a painless, immobile joint: a fixed knee or hip joint is often preferable to one with limited movement and causing considerable pain. A modern advance of striking value is the replacement of a badly damaged joint by an artificial joint. In

successful cases, which are already numerous, the mobility and happiness of the subject are vastly improved.

osteoma. A benign (i.e., non-cancerous) tumour of bone, found most often in the skull or jaw. The tumour grows very slowly indeed. If it presses on a nerve, hinders joint action or causes unpleasant deformity it can be removed by surgery. If it does none of these things it is probably best left in position.

The harmless osteoma should be sharply differentiated from an osteosarcoma, a highly malignant tumour liable to give rise to secondary growths, e.g., in the lungs. Where its situation makes its removal possible, an osteosarcoma should be excised as early as possible.

osteomalacia. A chronic disease, mainly occurring in women, characterized by loss of calcium from the bones so that they become soft and yielding, with consequent bending and deformity.

The main cause is deficiency of vitamin D in pregnancy. The deficiency prevents the adequate absorption of calcium and phosphorus from the intestine, and the foetus gains its quota of these minerals at the expense of the mother. Essentially osteomalacia in an adult corresponds to rickets in a child.

Prevention consists of providing enough supplies of foods containing vitamin D (e.g, milk, butter, cheese and eggs), with artificial supplementation by vitamin pills or cod liver oil if necessary; but it should be remembered that there is also such a thing as over-dosage with vitamin D. Where the condition has occurred, termination of pregnancy is desirable with thereafter a diet rich in calcium, phosphorus and vitamin D.

osteomyelitis. Inflammation of the bone marrow through infection by pus-forming germs. The main symptoms are severe pain, tenderness in the affected part and high temperature. Antibiotic treatment has revolutionized the outlook in this formerly very dangerous disease, but surgical removal of the infected bone may still be required if antibiotic treatment is delayed.

osteopathy. A system of medical practice, founded in 1874 by A. T. Still (1828-1917), an unqualified but experienced doctor who abandoned orthodox medicine in favour of his new methods. As outlined in Still's major book of 1910 and in his earlier writings, osteopathy is based on the self-sufficiency of the human body. It disbelieves in all drugs, vaccines and sera; it places little or no reliance on electricity or radiology; and it accepts surgical treatment in certain cases only as a last resort. Its main tenet is that 'disease is the result of anatomical abnormalities followed by physiological discord', from which it follows that natural healing will occur if the abnormalities are corrected. In other words osteopathy as originally understood holds that most or all diseases are caused by displacements (especially of bones) and are curable by manipulation.

Since on one hand prevention and cure of deficiency diseases by vitamins and of various infections by vaccines and antibiotics respectively are now beyond dispute, and since on the other hand the development of radiology renders virtually all displacements visible, some of the basic tenets of osteopathy are manifestly in doubt. Nowadays most practising osteopaths accept that by no means all diseases respond to manipulation of bones and joints. While most osteopaths have departed from Still's view that osteopathy 'can be applied to all conditions of disease', some orthodox medical practitioners have accepted that osteopathy has had successes not explicable on purely psychological grounds, and that reduction of displacement by manipulation may have a valid place in the treatment of some diseases.

In orthodox medicine manipulative surgeons have undoubtedly learned something from osteopaths, just as osteopaths learned something from the bone-setters of the past. But the medical contention is that to consult an osteopath in the first instance is dangerous because the osteopath, trained only in the manipulative art, may diagnose a condition incorrectly – such as diabetes, anaemia or an acute infection – which will not respond to manipulation and urgently needs appropriate treatment of an entirely different kind.

osteoporosis. A thinning and weakening of bones, common in old people, especially those whose diet is deficient in calcium. The condition is commoner in women than in men, and cessation of ovarian function at the menopause is thought to be a factor in some cases. Excess of adrenal hormones is another possible factor and the condition sometimes occurs after prolonged treatment with corticosteroids. Where the spine is affected the main feature is episodes of backache, with inability to stoop or bend, and sometimes inability to move from the position at the time of onset, but with considerable periods of remission in which there is no pain or only a mild backache. Where a long bone, e.g., the femur, is mainly affected there may be no symptoms until there is a sudden fracture.

Apart from treatment of the fracture in the latter case, treatment involves rest during acute bouts, analgesics for the pain, adequate calcium and vitamin D, and gentle reintroduction of movement as the pain ends. Since, irrespective of the particular cause, loss of calcium from bones plays an important part, an obvious preventive measure is to ensure that elderly people have diets rich in calcium. Milk is an excellent source of calcium and is easily absorbed and digested.

osteosarcoma. See OSTEOMA.

osteosclerosis fragilis. A rare hereditary abnormality of bone growth, in which bones are unusually weak and brittle. The child may be born dead, or the disease may become apparent in the first year of life, or (in a milder type) the condition may not be discovered until adolescence or later. Pathological fractures occur, heal poorly and create deformity. So far no effective treatment is known.

otitis media. See EAR.

otorrhoea. Discharge of pus from the ear. See EAR, otitis media.

otosclerosis. A hereditary condition in which the bones of the middle EAR become thickened and hardened, resulting in increasing difficulty in the transmission of sound impulses from the ear drum to the brain, and sometimes ultimately causing complete deafness. Treatment is either by fenestration, i.e., an operation whereby a new opening is made to the inner ear, or by removal of the affected

bone and its replacement by a synthetic substitute. With either treatment the complete restoration of hearing occurs in most cases.

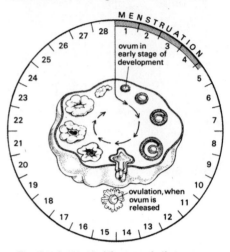

The development of the ovum in the ovary

ovary. The female sex gland, and thus part of the female REPRODUCTIVE SYSTEM. The two ovaries are oval bodies nearly 4 cm. (about 1½ in.) long, situated on each side of the uterus. They contain ova (or egg-cells) and they produce hormones, including oestrogen and progesterone, which give the adult woman her typical physical characteristics and largely regulate the menstrual cycle. During each menstrual cycle one (or occasionally more) of the ova ripens, comes to the surface of the ovary in a little follicle or blister and passes along a uterine tube to the uterus where it may be fertilized by a sperm.

Diseases. 1. Inflammation of an ovary may arise from the passage of infection along the relevant uterine tube. The condition is characterized by abdominal pain and tenderness, with rise in temperature. Treatment is with sulphonamides or antibiotics. Inflammation of the right ovary is liable to be confused with appendicitis.

2. Ovarian cysts are bladder-like growths which sometimes become remarkably large; they are mostly painless but may cause pain if they become twisted. Treatment is by surgical removal of the cyst.

3. Cancer of the ovary is difficult to differentiate from benign solid tumours until after removal, when laboratory tests can be performed on the tissue which has been removed. In most cases it is painless. In view of the diagnostic difficulty and the danger of spread of cancer, all ovarian tumours should be treated by surgical removal or by radiotherapy.

4. Displacement of the ovary can result from stretching or twisting of the ovarian ligaments. There is pain and tenderness, and surgical treatment may be necessary.

5. Insufficient production of ovarian hormones may cause delayed puberty or menstrual irregularity. Hormone treatment is usually effective.

overcrowding. Every person requires adequate air space, good ventilation without draughts and a modicum of privacy. Overcrowding increases the risk of air-borne (droplet) infections and also of contact infections. Hence respiratory infections and most specific fevers reach their peak incidence in winter when people are crowded together indoors and with windows closed for warmth. Overcrowding lowers general standards of health and of resistance to disease; and when a single room has to serve as the living, sleeping, eating and washing accommodation of a family, the resulting irritation, frustration and deterioration of morale is obvious. Tennyson's phrase, 'the crowded haunts of incest in the warrens of the poor', is apt.

Many developed countries prescribe minimum standards for living accommodation. In Britain it is laid down that, disregarding babies under 12 months and counting a child of under 10 years as a half, a house is overcrowded if two rooms contain more than 3 persons or three rooms more than 5 persons; and that to accommodate two adults a room must have a floor-space of at least 110 square feet.

Overcrowding in factories is also prohibited in some countries. In Britain the specified minimum is 40 square feet per person in a room at least 10 feet high, and the same minimum is now required for offices in which people normally work. Standards are also specified for schools and hospitals.

These standards, however, are not easily enforced in declining areas where money for new buildings is scarce or in rapidly growing districts where builders are not simultaneously available for new factories, new houses, new schools, new hospitals and new offices. While the reduction of overcrowding has proceeded apace in the last fifty years, overcrowding still remains one of the major hazards to health.

ovum. The technical term for a human egg-cell. See OVARY.

oxalic acid. Derived originally from sorrel and rhubarb-tops this acid is synthesized for various industrial uses. In appearance it resembles epsom salts and thus may be swallowed accidentally. If so taken, it corrodes the lining of the mouth, throat and stomach. Calcium compounds – such as chalk or whiting mixed with water – are the best antidote, and the patient should be kept warm and treated for shock. Since vomiting would return the corroding acid to the throat and mouth, emetics should never be given.

oxygen. A colourless, odourless, tasteless gas which constitutes one-fifth of our atmosphere and is essential to human and animal life. In respiration oxygen is taken into the lungs and carried in the haemoglobin of the red blood corpuscles to every part of the body.

Oxygen is valuable in any disease in which

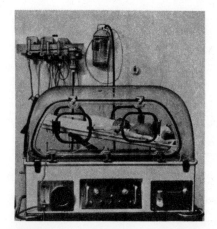

The oxygen for a premature baby is regulated in an incubator

the lungs have difficulty in taking up air and in any condition in which there is insufficiency of oxygen in the arterial blood. For example, it eases breathing in pneumonia and severe bronchitis, and it is useful in congestive heart failure and coronary thrombosis.

Oxygen is normally supplied in compressed form in steel cylinders and is administered to the patient through a mask fitted over the nose and mouth, or through a tube passed through a nostril, or occasionally by a 'tent' covering the patient's head and shoulders.

In major operations the anaesthetist routinely has a cylinder of oxygen available and ready for use in the event of breathing difficulties developing.

Oxyuris vermicularis. The scientific name for the internal parasite commonly known as the THREAD WORM.

ozaena. A chronic inflammation of the nose with crusting and partial wasting of the nasal membrane. It is probably the result of long-continuing untreated infection. Although NOSE DOUCHING (despite its possible dangers), and attention to general health, particularly diet and exercise, may be tried, in many cases surgical treatment is necessary.

ozone. An unusual form of oxygen with three atoms to the molecule instead of two. It has a penetrating odour and is produced by the passage of electrical discharges through the air. In high concentration it is poisonous.

A little ozone is sometimes present in the seaside air, but the odour generally described as ozone comes primarily from seaweed; the health-giving powers of seaside air have never been scientifically demonstrated.

P

pacemaker. The part of the heart, the sino-atrial node, from which starts each wave of contraction of heart muscle. The tiny electrical impulse that originates in the node is conducted to all parts of the heart and causes the muscular contraction, with expulsion of blood down the arteries, that we call the heart beat.

If the natural pacemaker temporarily fails to work, as in certain forms of heart attack, an external artificial pacemaker, if available within a few minutes, can produce similar electrical impulses, thus re-starting the heart and maintaining the beat until the pacemaker recovers.

Where the pacemaker is permanently incapacitated or the conducting mechanism from it is seriously damaged, a battery-driven artificial pacemaker can be inserted under the skin of the chest.

paediatrics. The branch of medical science concerned with the prevention, diagnosis and treatment of diseases of children, and with the physical, emotional and mental growth and development of children.

It is universally recognized today that a child is not simply a miniature adult and that the health care of children, whether preventive or curative, differs from that of adults. To give some random examples: children require to grow and therefore have, in proportion to size, greater nutritional needs than adults; adults can make their wants and symptoms known whereas young children cannot; adults are independent and can even survive periods of solitary confinement without manifest harm while children are dependent, and their emotional development is damaged by deprivation of parental care and by lack of encouragement over attempts at self-expression and use of initiative; children are very susceptible to infections (e.g., whooping cough and measles) and so need to be immunized whereas most adults have developed a considerable immunity to many infections; a raised temperature indicates illness in an adult but in a child a trivial event may throw the temperature-regulating mechanism out of gear for a few hours; and even if an adult and a child one-quarter of his weight have the same illness and can be treated with the same drug the right dose for the child may be greater or less than a quarter of the adult dose.

Some of the early medical writers of Greece and Rome showed faint indications of understanding that children's requirements and children's diseases differed from those of adults, but the idea of the health care of children as a speciality is really a development of the nineteenth century.

Clinical paediatrics, i.e., the specialist treatment of the diseases and disabilities of children, started with the publication of a book on children's diseases by Nils Rosen von Rosenstein of Uppsala in 1765 but it was not until about 1850 that advanced countries began to provide special hospitals for children (e.g., Great Ormond Street in London, 1852) or children's wards in general hospitals; and in the U.K. the first professorship in diseases of children was established as late as 1906.

The timetable for preventive paediatrics, i.e., sustained attempts to improve child health and prevent children's diseases, is very similar. In 1748 William Cadogen of London published a book seeking to offer guidance on the nursing, feeding, clothing and exercise of children, and in 1816 John Davis, also of London, tried to spread such information by engaging a group of home visitors to carry out what we would nowadays call health visiting and health education; but Davis was ahead of his time and the project collapsed after a few years.

The beginnings of more lasting efforts to promote good health in children emanated not from doctors or nurses but from intelligent laymen concerned about the fact that one baby in every six or seven died before the age of 12 months and another within the following four years. Preventive paediatrics can be regarded as starting either when New York City appointed its first female 'sanitary visitor' in 1859 or when HEALTH VISITORS, at first untrained, were appointed in Salford (England) in 1862: and can be deemed to have reached maturity either when New York City Health Department established its Division of Child Hygiene (1908) or when the British health visitor became a qualified nurse with a qualification in public health (in stages from 1919).

During this century the infant death rate in advanced countries has fallen from about 150 deaths per thousand births to around 17 per thousand, with even lower figures recorded in Sweden and Finland; deaths of children above the age of 12 months have declined even more dramatically. These massive improvements have been parallelled by a great reduction in childhood illness and by a general all-round improvement in child health. In terms of lives saved these advances constitute by far the biggest achievement in the whole of medical history, and therefore merit some analysis.

While nobody would deny that better living standards and better housing played a part, the improvements occurred in countries like Finland and Holland that suffered extensive war damage, and study of towns in the U.K. shows that some with a great deal of bad housing and fairly high unemployment were among the leaders in the reduction of child deaths. Clearly services played a larger part than environmental conditions, though the latter can by no means be discounted.

Some credit must go to obstetricians and

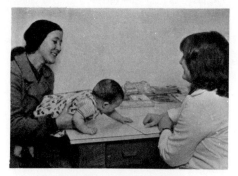

A paediatrician with her patient

midwives for better management of pregnancy and labour, and some to clinical paediatricians for more skilful treatment of children's illnesses, but the largest share of the credit belongs to the preventive services.

It is no coincidence that Sweden, the world leader in improvement of child health, has long had the highest ratio of public health nurses to population, with Finland closely following. In England the health ministry in a formal report as early as 1917 declared that 'the health visitor is the most important element in any scheme for maternal and child welfare'. In Scotland in the 1950s a detailed statistical study of a series of towns over two separate periods of time showed a significant association between generosity of health visitor staffing and infrequency of baby deaths. In the 1960s the few British towns that brought their figures for infant deaths down to something approaching the Swedish level had health visitor staffing appreciably more generous than the average for the country.

In recent decades there have been some interesting developments in preventive and clinical paediatrics.

1. In the first half of this century in all advanced countries such functions as health education and counselling of expectant mothers, assessing of the physical and emotional development of young children, advising of parents about child nutrition and child management, guiding parents about protection against infections, and identifying early departures from normality were in the hands of a team with a doctor specialized in child health as the unquestioned leader. In recent years, while teamwork continues, more and more of these tasks have passed to nurses with subsequent public health training, like British health visitors and Swedish public health nurses. A partial exception to the trend has been France which employs increasing numbers of doctors in child health clinics and tries to make attendance at such clinics virtually compulsory.

2. As children's diseases, especially infections and nutritional disorders, became less common the reduction was partially balanced by more frequent survival of physically and mentally handicapped children. Simultaneously clinical paediatrics became more sophisticated and tended to develop new sub-specialties. So in addition to the general paediatric physician and paediatric surgeon there have begun to appear paediatricians who specialize in heart diseases of children, in nervous diseases of children or in child psychiatry. There has also arisen a new non-medical profession of child psychologist.

3. In some countries there have been attempts to unify preventive and clinical paediatrics. In some cases these have taken the form of providing a post-graduate training that equips the intending specialist for work in both fields. In other cases they have taken the form of seeking to interest selected general practitioners in paediatrics and to provide training for them. On present evidence, however, it seems likely that much of preventive paediatrics will in most countries be undertaken increasingly by nurses with subsequent specialized training. It would be a very costly experiment to train a mass of doctors to do work that public health nurses already perform well; and a very large number of doctors would be required, since much of the best work of the health visitor or public health nurse is undertaken not in clinics or health centres but in the homes of the people. There the visitor can more easily assess cultural, social and environmental factors in addition to advising the parent who is too busy or too lazy to attend a clinic, or who feels readier to discuss problems in the familiar atmosphere of the home than in a consulting room.

There is no fixed age at which paediatrics ends and adult medicine begins. In the clinical field, separate curative facilities for children usually cease at about 12 or 13 years. In the preventive field the age of leaving school is an obvious border.

Paget's disease. Two separate diseases are named after their discoverer, Sir James Paget (1841-99).

(1) Paget's disease of bone, OSTEITIS DEFORMANS, is a softening and later thickening of bones occasionally found in middle-aged or elderly men.

(2) Paget's disease of the NIPPLE is a form of breast cancer, characterized by itching and a rash resembling eczema.

pain. Nature's primary indication that all is not well with the human machine.

The hurt or injury occurs in some part of the body, the message of distress is picked up by specific nerve-endings and carried by two types of sensory nerve fibres, and the brain interprets the message as pain, localizes it to the particular area and initiates necessary action. Biologically pain is very valuable in that it enables us to remove the endangered part from injurious influences, to decide consciously to avoid harmful stimuli and to seek medical aid for an injury or illness that might be disregarded if it were painless. Indeed, one of the unfortunate facts of life is that a few serious diseases (e.g., cancer and tuberculosis) tend to be painless in their early stages.

The sensory nerve-endings called pain receptors are more plentiful in some areas than in others. The cornea is particularly rich in them, so that eye injury causes immediate and severe pain. The teeth have very efficient pain receptors – Burns described toothache as 'the hell of all diseases'. The genitals have abundant pain receptors, so that injury produces intense pain and shock. The finger tips are well supplied, thus the tearing off of nails is an ancient form of torture. The buttocks are quite well supplied, so that, without adjacent vital structures that could be injured, they are a traditional site of chastisement. On the other hand, some internal organs lack pain receptors: for example, diseases of bone which do not affect its outer membrane are painless, as are many diseases of the brain.

Transfer of the message is impossible unless the relevant sensory nerves are intact. Hence in certain diseases of nerves a cut or burn fails to produce any sensation of pain; and in at least one disease – syringomyelia – the sense of pain disappears but that of touch remains, indicating that the nerve fibres for these sensations are different. Once pain has served its purpose in calling attention to the area and helping diagnosis, it can be stopped by blocking the nerves, e.g., by injecting an appropriate drug.

Sensitivity to pain varies. Firstly, it varies with cerebral development: mammals and birds feel pain much more acutely than fishes and reptiles, and it is doubtful whether a worm can experience pain. Secondly, it varies with the degree of injury. Thirdly, it varies with the portion of the body affected, being less in parts poorly supplied with pain receptors. Fourthly, it varies with the individual: some people feel pain very acutely and even faint when subjected to what in others would be only moderate amounts of pain; and at the other end of the scale some people appear to have an unusually high tolerance of pain.

Pain is sometimes differentiated into 'burning', 'stabbing', 'gripping', 'gnawing', 'boring' and 'aching'. In addition there is the psychological anguish that is termed 'mental pain'.

The brain may sometimes ignore the message owing to preoccupation, as when in the excitement of battle a soldier receives a painful injury but remains unaware of it until later. Occasionally, too, the brain can be at fault in localizing pain, e.g., a person whose leg has recently been amputated may 'feel' pain in the absent toes; this is a phenomenon closely resembling referred pain, which is explained below.

Referred pain is that which is felt in a part of the body remote from the site of the actual injury or disease. This happens because the spinal cord is developed in segments, each with its own pair of spinal nerves. In the early embryo these segments are closely related to a similar segmental arrangement of the other developing tissue. Initially, each spinal nerve is thus related to the nearby skin, deep tissues, and viscera.

As growth and development proceed this close relationship is disturbed, with the result that the deeper structures and the skin may become widely separated although they continue to share a common nerve-supply. Pain impulses from the deep structures therefore reach the same point in the spinal cord as pain-impulses from a remote skin-receptor before they ascend the cord to be appreciated in the brain.

Since the brain is much more used to receiving stimuli from end-organs on the skin than from elsewhere, and because the cortex of the brain has a well-developed sensory 'map' of the body-surface and only rudimentary representation of visceral structures, it misinterprets the site of the pain. The actual pain is 'referred' to the segmentally-associated area of skin even although this may be some distance away.

Referred pain also occurs when nerve-trunks are damaged in their course by injury or disease. Pain is then experienced, not at the site of the damage but at the periphery of the nerve-distribution.

Common examples of referred pain are numerous. The heart condition angina pectoris may produce pain radiating down the left arm; abdominal conditions irritating the diaphragm may be felt as pain in either shoulder; the pain of renal colic is felt in the groin and upper thigh; hip-disease may be referred to the knee; spinal caries, according to the level affected, may produce pains in the arms, 'girdle-pains' in the chest, lower abdominal symptoms, and pains in the buttocks and legs; and a blow on the inner side of the elbow may cause a tingling pain in the little finger.

To the physician pain is of great importance as an aid to diagnosis, and he may have to allow pain to continue until he has determined its cause. Thereafter, removal of the cause of pain and relief of the actual pain are the doctor's two primary objectives. Removal of pain is essential – as soon as possible after diagnosis of the cause – not only for reasons of humanity but also because continued severe pain creates shock and can even kill.

palate. The roof of the mouth, consisting of a bony front part, the hard palate, and a fibro-muscular hind part, the soft palate.

In the unborn child the right and left sides of the palate develop separately and normally fuse together. Failure to fuse results in cleft palate, a fairly common congenital defect, often associated with HARE LIP, a failure of the halves of the upper lip to fuse. The voice has a harsh nasal sound and pronunciation of the palatal consonants is indistinct. A repair operation is required and should normally be undertaken during the early months of life.

palliative. A medicine which relieves symptoms rather than curing the underlying disease. The term is often used in a derogatory sense, and certainly simply to relieve pain without ascertaining the cause is bad practice; but many conditions – such as the common cold, shingles and tension headache – are temporary, so that palliation is all that is required. Aspirin (although of specific curative value in certain rheumatic conditions) is the palliative in commonest use, and other palliatives frequently employed are codeine and paracetamol.

pallor. Paleness of the skin, mainly due to constriction of the surface blood vessels. There are many causes, of which the four which follow are probably the most common. (1) Natural or habitual pallor occurs where, although the person is in good health, his skin is a shade thicker or his capillaries lie a shade deeper than in most people. (2) Prolonged pallor is in most cases a result of severe anaemia. It also arises from other causes such as chronic kidney disease and long confinement indoors. (3) Temporary pallor is a common consequence of fatigue. (4) Immediate pallor occurs in shock, fainting and sometimes in severe emotional disturbance.

In immediate and temporary pallor the cause is generally obvious, as is any necessary treatment. Prolonged pallor necessitates investigation unless the explanation is known. Natural pallor needs no treatment but adequate sunshine or a course of ultra-violet rays may improve the appearance.

palpitation. Awareness of the strength, rapidity or irregularity of the heart beat.

Excited action of the heart, creating this awareness, may occur as a result of indigestion, over-smoking, excess of alcohol, excess of tea or coffee, toxic goitre, anaemia or various diseases of the heart. The excited action may continue for a few minutes or for many hours.

Investigation is desirable because palpitation may indicate a condition needing treatment. Even more important, however, is reassurance, because the patient nearly always attributes the symptom to serious disease of the heart.

palsy. Until this century palsy was simply another term for PARALYSIS. In modern usage, however, palsy is generally reserved for conditions characterized not only by loss of power but by quivering of the affected part of the body. Nevertheless, facial neuralgia – a neuritis causing temporary paralysis of the muscles of one side of the face – is still sometimes called Bell's palsy.

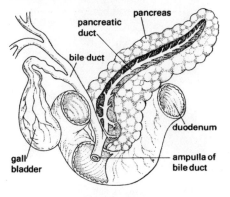

The pancreas

pancreas. An elongated glandular structure lying on the posterior wall of the upper abdomen. Its rounded head is encircled by the curve of the duodenum and its body and tail extend to the left crossing the left kidney and reaching the spleen.

It consists of two distinct types of tissue. The main secretory cells produce digestive ferments which pass by small ducts to the main pancreatic duct and thence into the duodenum to assist in the breakdown and digestion of food. Embedded in the glandular tissue are enclosures of another type of cells, known as the Islets of Langerhans. These produce the hormone insulin required for the metabolism of carbohydrate. They have no collecting ducts and insulin is absorbed directly into the blood stream, so that the Islets of Langerhans can be classed as ENDOCRINE GLANDS.

Animal pancreas is used as a foodstuff under the name 'sweetbread'.

Diseases. Deficiency of the pancreatic hormone insulin produces DIABETES. Absence or insufficiency of pancreatic enzymes which help

digestion in the bowel cause intestinal disturbance and abnormal stools. In the congenital disease cystic fibrosis both lungs and pancreas show fibrosis and cyst formation and the affected child develops poorly and often has respiratory complications.

Apart from these special conditions acute pancreatitis is common, usually in association with inflammation of the gall bladder and gall-stones. Attacks tend to occur suddenly and constitute an abdominal emergency. Sub-acute pancreatitis is sometimes a complication of hypothermia in the aged owing to the effect of cold on the blood vessels and intestines.

The pancreas is a common site for malignant disease. Carcinoma of the head of the pancreas interferes with both pancreatic secretions and that of bile, the latter effect producing jaundice.

pandemic. An outbreak of infectious disease not limited to one community or country but occurring or threatening to occur on a much wider and even world-wide scale. Pandemics are considered to be due to a spontaneous increase in the infective power of the particular organism concerned.

In modern times the best examples are the periodic widespread outbreaks of influenza. Historically, between 1346 and 1351 the Black Death spread through the whole of Europe and Asia as a pandemic of bubonic and pneumonic plague, killing some 60 million persons, or about half of the estimated population at that time.

papilloma. A type of tumour growth which appears as a raised area on the surface of the skin or the mucous membranes lining internal organs, glands and ducts.

Skin papillomata are familiar as warts. Those which arise from mucous membrane are most commonly found in the bladder, larynx, stomach and intestine. Although initially benign, many types of internal papilloma have a considerable tendency to become malignant and should be dealt with promptly.

papule. A pimple or small projection raised above the surface of the surrounding skin.

paracentesis. A minor surgical procedure in which a body cavity is punctured by a hollow needle or a similar tubular instrument of suitable size in order to allow a pathological collection of fluid to escape.

This form of 'tapping' is most commonly employed in the relief of ascites (abdominal dropsy) but other applications are in the treatment of pericarditis, pleurisy, otitis media, and hydrocele.

paracetamol. A mild analgesic generally regarded as a little stronger than aspirin and used to relieve pain, either alone or in combination with aspirin.

paraesthesia. Any unusual sensation (e.g., pain, heat, itching or tingling) experienced without any external cause. Paraesthesia is a common symptom in some diseases in which a nerve is compressed or irritated.

paralysis. Complete loss of the power of movement in any part of the body, produced by some damage to the nervous system or the muscular mechanism. Damage which causes loss of sensory reception is sometimes called sensory paralysis.

Various terms indicate the extent of any paralysis. Thus monoplegia means paralysis of one limb; diplegia: paralysis of both corresponding limbs; quadriplegia: paralysis of all four limbs; paraplegia: paralysis of both legs and the lower part of the body, seen particularly in spinal injury; hemiplegia: paralysis of leg, arm, and face of one side, as seen in the ordinary type of apoplectic stroke; crossed paralysis: affecting leg and arm of one side and the other side of the face, indicative of nerve tract lesions within the brain stem.

Paralysis may be spastic or flaccid. In spasticity there is loss of control of movement, muscle rigidity, exaggerated tendon reflexes, no alteration in electrical excitability, and only minimal wasting of muscle tissue through disuse. In flaccidity there is loss of all muscular power, complete limpness, absent tendon-reflexes, 'reaction of degeneration' to electrical excitation, and ultimately complete wasting away of muscle tissue. Strokes, spinal injuries, spinal tumours and multiple sclerosis are causes of spastic paralysis. An example of a disease that causes flaccid paralysis is poliomyelitis.

paralysis agitans. See PARKINSON'S DISEASE.

paranoia. Emil Kraepelin (1856-1926), a Munich physician who pioneered the systematic study of psychiatry, regarded paranoia as a separate mental illness characterized by a permanent pattern of delusions generally of persecution, but in which there is complete preservation of clear and orderly thought and action, and complete absence of hallucinations. Paranoid delusions also occur in other types of mental illness such as toxic psychosis and schizophrenia, but in these conditions there is also confusion and hallucination. However, many conditions initially regarded as paranoia prove in the fullness of time to be cases of SCHIZOPHRENIA.

It has become increasingly profitless to regard paranoia as a separate disease. Its particular symptoms are relatively rare, and although it may be separately identifiable it has to be assessed and re-assessed in the light of the later trend of the illness.

Bearing in mind the caution that most cases will ultimately prove to be schizophrenia, it is however possible to indicate a condition conveniently described as paranoia. Pronounced mental symptoms do not usually begin until middle life but a careful study of the earlier history will often reveal personality changes from adolescence onwards. In the developed disease the predominant feature is a completely consistent and systematized set of delusions, usually related to persecution, grandeur, personality, or status, which are maintained and supported with such persuasive detail and such unassailable logic as to be extremely convincing and likely to deceive many people. Paranoiacs thus tend to become leaders of religious and political movements, to swell the ranks of regicides and assassins, and to become tireless litigants and general trouble-makers.

It is precisely because they are so plausible. that they are so dangerous. In the present state of knowledge there is no real cure for paranoia and it is often only after many years that increasingly anti-social behaviour or the development of increasing patterns of delusion make the condition recognizable and leave no alternative but to protect society by committing such cases to a mental hospital.

paranoid states. Temporary conditions in which a person of suspicious and boastful

nature develops delusions of grandeur or of persecution as a result of extreme mental stress. See MEGALOMANIA.

paraphrenia. A descriptive term applied to PARANOIA and SCHIZOPHRENIA where the symptoms mainly consist of hallucinations and extravagant delusions.

paraplegia. Paralysis of the legs and lower part of the body due to injury or disease of the spinal cord. Both voluntary movement and sensation are affected. In injury the PARALYSIS is of spastic type, but in other cases progression of disease may lead to a flaccid paralysis. The extent of the paralysis, resulting from injury is determined by the level at which the spinal cord is damaged.

An important aspect of paraplegia is loss of control over bowel and bladder function, with incontinence and liability to ascending infection of the urinary tract.

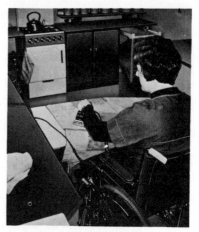

A paraplegic housewife

parasites. Organisms which live on, or in, the body of another animal or plant and derive their sustenance therefrom. Although this definition could logically include the bacteria their presence is conventionally called infection rather than parasitism. If the association between host and invader is of mutual benefit this is recognized by using the term symbiosis.

Parasites of man may conveniently be divided into those living on the skin, ectoparasites, and those existing internally, endoparasites. Ectoparasites include fleas, lice, itch-mites and fungi such as ringworm. Endoparasites range from single-celled protozoans such as those of amoebic dysentery and malaria to the more highly organized flukes (trematodes), flat-worms (cestodes) and round-worms (nematodes) which exist in great variety, especially in tropical countries. Internally fungi also cause conditions like 'farmer's-lung' and actinomycosis.

Parasites vary in their potentialities for producing disease. Ectoparasites are mainly a source of irritation (although lice and fleas spread typhus and plague during epidemics), but biting insects transmit many tropical diseases. Some endoparasites like intestinal tape-worms are relatively harmless at that stage of their life history, but many others produce serious injury particularly in such tropical diseases as schistosomiasis and filariasis.

parasympathetic nervous system. One of the two divisions of the autonomic NERVOUS SYSTEM which is responsible for unconscious regulation of much bodily activity and independent of the brain except for some control by the hypothalamus. The parasympathetic system has two main centres: the cranial, just below the brain, with fibres passing along various cranial nerves, expecially the vagus; and the sacral, at the foot of the spinal cord. While the other division, the sympathetic system, puts the body in a position of readiness for activity, activity of the parasympathetic causes a phase of relaxation, with, for example, slowing of the heart and the breathing, and increase in the activity of the digestive system.

In general the parasympathetic system acts by releasing acetyl choline from its nerve endings. Drugs like atropine and hyoscine suppress or reduce the activity of the parasympathetic, while drugs like physostigmine stimulate it.

parathyroid glands. These ENDOCRINE GLANDS produce parathyroid hormone which controls calcium metabolism. They lie close to the thyroid gland in the neck.

paratyphoid fever. A specific infectious disease due to *Salmonella paratyphi,* which has three varieties, A, B, and C. The symptoms are mainly of gastro-intestinal disturbance with continued fever and sometimes a measles-like rash. It resembles classical TYPHOID FEVER and is difficult to differentiate clinically but the incubation period tends to be shorter, the onset more abrupt, the duration of illness less prolonged, and toxaemia less severe. As in typhoid fever there is a potential risk of the same serious complications – haemorrhage, intestinal perforation, or myocardial toxaemia – but they are relatively rare and generally the fatality rate is low except perhaps in the elderly or debilitated. Often there may be little more than fever, malaise and transient diarrhoea.

While typhoid is spread by water, or occasionally food contaminated by a carrier or a missed case, paratyphoid is spread by food (especially milk and uncooked foods) similarly contaminated. The disease requires isolation and hospital treatment.

General measures of prevention are as for typhoid. Vaccine protection is available, often combined with protection against typhoid, and is a sensible precaution for persons travelling to any country in which the disease is still common.

parent age and child care. The infant death rate is at its lowest among babies born to mothers between the ages of 20 and 30. The rate is slightly greater for mothers under 20 but for those over 30 it begins to rise steadily and increasingly steeply after 40. The same pattern is shown in the incidence of prematurity, and babies born before term are more subject to intercurrent disease (i.e., disease that occurs during the progress of another), and more likely to show developmental problems than the normal full-term infant. Other maternal factors affecting the quality of child life may also be operative. Mongolism, for instance, due

to chromosomal abnormalities, is closely correlated with maternal age.

It follows therefore that maternal age at birth has some influence on the physical aspects of child care and that special attention should be paid to children born to mothers over thirty. To identify departures from normality and to initiate appropriate measures are matters for the appropriate child-care services.

There are, however, other less tangible ways in which parental age can influence child development. On the one hand there is an increasing number of very young mothers aged 16 to 20 or even younger. Apart from the other factor that many such births are illegitimate, there is the problem of ensuring adequate care from a mother who is herself relatively immature and who may have neither the motivation and ability, nor the financial resources to fulfil the demanding tasks of parenthood.

At the other end of the age-scale is the child born to rather elderly parents, and the difficulties there are increased should it be a single late child. In a larger family parental experience with earlier children and the presence and influence of brothers and sisters help to ensure that problems of upbringing are less likely to arise. Any normal child as he grows begins to show qualities of energy, initiative, determination and curiosity, and a desire to explore his environment. These characteristics may conflict with the comfort of elderly parents and their settled way of life. They tend to interpret 'good behaviour' in terms of their own convenience and seek to ensure that their child complies with their wishes quickly, quietly and without argument. To enforce conformity by continual repression, punishment, or threat of punishment, is to curtail initiative and frustrate natural curiosity and the effect in later life is that the child grows up to be either resentful of control or diffident and easily-led. Alternatively parental attitudes may take the form of over-indulgence. A late and only child may be excessively prized and receive more attention than is good for him, both from parents and well-meaning relatives. A steady flow of fussy adulation engenders a subconscious conviction that he can be a centre of attraction without making any personal effort to be endearing and out-going.

Older parents must therefore avoid the two extremes of being too staid and matter-of-fact or of being over-anxious and over-protective. They must strive to know and enjoy their child, and mere training and teaching are not enough. They must learn to play and laugh and enter into the child's world of discovery and make-believe and endeavour to form a companionable relationship in which supervision and care are tempered with fun.

See also INFANCY, PSYCHOLOGY OF and CHILDHOOD, PSYCHOLOGY OF.

paresis. A condition of incomplete paralysis of voluntary muscles. If on testing a muscle or group of muscles feeble contractions can still be elicited the muscles are said to be paretic or in a state of paresis to distinguish their condition from the state of paralysis in which the patient is unable to produce any muscular contraction whatever.

Paresis tends to occur in the early stages of progressive diseases of the nervous system. On the other hand a paretic response after the total paralysis which has resulted from a stroke indicates some recovery of function and is to be regarded as a hopeful sign.

Parkinson's disease. A relatively common chronic nervous disease of later life, chiefly affecting males, characterized by muscular tremors, weakness and rigidity, and by a typical stooped posture, 'shuffling' gait and a mask-like immobile facial appearance. Alternative names for the condition are paralysis agitans or 'shaking palsy'.

The exact cause is unknown but the symptoms suggest that there is a disorder in the cerebral hemispheres of the brain, and within recent years it has been shown that patients have an abnormally low concentration of a substance dopamine in their brain tissue. Dopamine itself does not pass from the blood to the brain but a related substance, levodopa, overcomes this difficulty and cases of Parkinsonism have been substantially improved by the administration of this drug. Levodopa can cause serious side-effects such as nausea, vomiting, and disturbances of blood pressure and heart action, and a search continues for safer preparations. Systematic physiotherapy is also of service.

paronychia. Inflammation of the skin and tissues around a finger-nail or toe-nail, usually arising after an injury of the nail. See WHITLOW.

parotid. The parotid glands, left and right, are the largest of the SALIVARY GLANDS.

parotitis. Inflammation of the parotid salivary gland. Simple acute parotitis is usually due to ascending infection reaching the gland from septic conditions in the mouth and a salivary calculus may dilate or damage the duct making infection easier. Most cases recover spontaneously but local warmth and mouth washes may be prescribed.

Suppurative parotitis can occur as a sequel to simple parotitis, and also by spread from local sepsis in the jaw and adjacent structures or by blood-borne infection in septicaemia and other infective or debilitating diseases. Abscess formation results and may be a serious complication since pus may reach the base of the skull or the deeper structures of neck and thorax. Surgical intervention will be required.

Epidemic or infectious parotitis is a specific infectious disease due to a virus and more usually called MUMPS.

parturition. A term meaning labour in CHILDBIRTH.

passive movement. The movement of a joint by manipulation when, because of paralysis or some other cause, the patient is unable to perform the movement unaided.

Pasteur. Louis Pasteur (1822-95) was the genius who identified the microbe as man's main enemy and devised weapons to fight the foe. His career is fascinating: his ancestry was undistinguished (his father had retired from the army with the rank of sergeant-major and became a tanner) and he showed little childhood promise (his headmaster described him as a good average pupil, hard working and quiet, and at the *école normale* – or training college for teachers – his examiners in chemistry classed him as 'mediocre'). He had no medical and little scientific training (he attended some lectures at the Sorbonne in 1842 while earning his living as a teacher), but was nevertheless offered two separate professorships at the age of 27 (physics at

Dijon and chemistry at Strasbourg). Semi-paralysed from the age of 46 following a hemiplegia and bitterly opposed by the medical profession (as late as 1873 he was elected an Associate of the *Académie de Médecine* by a majority of only one vote) he yet contributed more to medicine than any man of his century, with the possible exception of Freud.

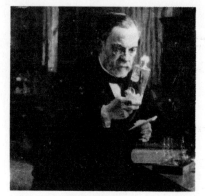

Louis Pasteur

His first researches were in crystallography, where he discovered, initially in relation to tartaric acid, that certain compounds exist in two forms, the molecules of the one being the mirror-image of those of the other. Subsequently, investigating a failure in the manufacture of alcohol from beetroot, he began his major study of fermentation, infection and putrefaction, and demonstrated that all three were due to bacteria. He removed by a heat treatment a disease that had been killing off silk-worms and ruining the silk trade, greatly benefited the wine and beer industries by a similar method, and then turned his attention increasingly to diseases of man and mammals. His most dramatic achievement was the discovery of a vaccine against anthrax: he proved its efficacy publicly by vaccinating twenty-five out of fifty sheep and then inoculating all fifty with anthrax; all the vaccinated sheep survived. His last years were devoted largely to the study of rabies and the production of an anti-rabies vaccine. His work was greatly reinforced by that of his German contemporary, Robert Koch (1843-1910) who identified the actual organisms responsible for various infections. By the time of Pasteur's death the controversy was really over: the bacterial origin of infections was a matter of recognized fact.

pasteurization. A process for ensuring the hygienic safety of milk and for improving its keeping qualities by heating it to a moderate temperature for a prescribed time. Pathogenic bacteria are killed and other bacterial development considerably delayed. There are two approved official methods. (1) Holder method: 65 °C.(150 °F.) for thirty minutes and cool immediately. (2) High temperature short time (HTST) method: 72 °C. (162 °F.) for fifteen seconds and cool immediately.

Efficient pasteurization destroys the enzyme phosphatase in milk and this is used as a basis for the phosphatase test to check that the process is operating satisfactorily.

Pasteurization is also used in treating some other foodstuffs for similar reasons: cream and fruit juices are examples.

patella. The kneecap, an isolated bony structure flattened in profile and roughly triangular in shape, situated in front of the knee joint and incorporated in the tendon of the muscle which brings the thigh forwards. Its back surface, in contact with the lower joint surface of the thigh bone, is covered by articular cartilage. The patella is the largest of the sesamoid bones found embedded in certain tendons and whose function generally is to modify pressure, reduce friction, and change the direction of muscle pull.

Fractured patella is a common injury usually produced by sudden violent muscular action as in attempting to recover balance. Successful repair generally requires open operation to wire the fragments in position.

The patella may also become dislocated, particularly in a leg misaligned through knock-knee deformity. Recurrent cases require operation.

pathogenic. Capable of producing disease.

pathognomonic. Signs or symptoms absolutely characteristic of a particular disease and sufficient to establish the diagnosis. Thus pain in the lower right quarter of the abdomen may be due to a number of causes but the addition of tenderness on pressure over McBurney's point is said to be pathognomonic of acute appendicitis.

pathology. The systematic scientific study of bodily changes produced by disease. Disease is manifested either by visible signs of structural change or by symptoms of disturbed function. Since function depends on structure any disease must basically be due to underlying changes either in structure or in chemical composition.

The methods employed in pathology are those of the anatomist, physiologist, physicist, biochemist and bacteriologist. Changes in physical structure may be recognizable with the naked eye (pathological anatomy) or by the ordinary microscope (pathological histology). Chemical changes may be detectable by ordinary qualitative or quantitative tests or by micro-chemical methods combining some form of chemical reaction with subsequent microscopic examination.

It is important, however, to appreciate that there may be changes which are not detected by any of these methods. The electron microscope now permits further exploration of the details of cell and molecular structure (cytology) while functional responses to infection and tissue interaction require the use of biological reactions classified generally as immunology. Enzyme reactions and the micro-chemistry of the cell also call for increasingly sophisticated chemical procedures.

Pathological investigation is thus two-fold in nature. The first step is to identify a structural difference and trace its evolution and the next is to discover its cause, making use as required of progressively more searching methods of examination until a satisfactory solution is achieved.

With the discovery of the effects of bacteria in many disease processes, pathologists originally fell heir to the new science of bacteriology but this is now generally pursued as the separate discipline of microbiology.

pediculosis. The condition of being infested with LICE.

pellagra. A vitamin deficiency disease found mainly in regions such as the southern states of U.S.A., the Mediterranean shores and the Far East where maize is a staple article of diet. The symptoms are: wasting; inflammation of the mouth (stomatitis) and tongue (glossitis) with other indications of gastro-intestinal disturbance; a symmetrical scaly skin condition often with pigmentation; nervous manifestations such as numbness, tremors or paralysis; and mental deterioration. It is caused by lack of VITAMINS of the B_2 complex particularly nicotinic acid and riboflavin. It is readily cured by an adequate diet and the administration of appropriate vitamin supplements, although the scaly skin condition is slow to resolve.

Pellagra-like symptoms may also occur in patients on anti-biotic drugs which tend to kill off intestinal bacteria that normally assist in the synthesization of vitamin B from foodstuffs.

pelvis. The massive bony ring at the lower end of the trunk which supports the vertebral column above and is itself supported by the legs. The main bone of the pelvic girdle is the ILIUM.

The size and conformation of the female pelvis is of importance in relation to childbirth. *Pelvis* is a Latin word meaning 'basin' and the name is also applied to the hollow interior of the kidney of which the ureter is the outlet.

pemphigus. A name for several diseases of the skin characterized by the formation of blisters.

Three of these types are described here. (1) Pemphigus neonatorum: a form of impetigo seen in new born infants usually due to staphylococcal infection. The delicate, soft skin readily separates to form blisters. There is often quite severe general upset but antibiotic treatment is effective. (2) Acute pemphigus: small skin blisters occurring in association with generalized signs of blood poisoning. It is generally treated by sulphonamides or antibiotics. (3) Chronic pemphigus (pemphigus vulgaris): recurrent crops of watery blisters occurring on both the skin and the mucous membranes with deterioration of the general health. The blisters are usually sterile and the exact cause is unknown. The condition, which is probably one of the collagen diseases, usually heals on treatment with corticosteroids.

penicillin. An antibacterial substance produced by a mould of the genus *Penicillium*. In 1928 Sir Alexander Fleming, Professor of Bacteriology at St. Mary's Hospital, London, noted that a culture plate had become contaminated by a mould and that colonies of staphylococci on the plate showed signs of dissolution. The mould was identified as *P. notatum* and its product which thus inhibited bacterial growth was given the name penicillin. Attempts to obtain this in a concentrated useful form initially failed and the incident at that time was regarded as only of academic interest because of the prevailing view that pus-forming body-invaders once established were beyond the reach of chemicals.

The demonstration that sulphonamides could overcome the pneumococcus changed the outlook and by 1940 Florey and Chain at

Oxford successfully overcame the problem of extracting and concentrating penicillin using low-temperature methods. In 1941 Abraham and his colleagues showed that the extract was therapeutically effective against many serious infections. Because of the difficulties created in Britain by World War II large-scale production of penicillin was started in America and improved strains of mould were sought for and developed. Most commercial production now uses *P. chrysogenum,* first isolated in Peoria, Illinois, from a mouldy cantaloup.

Penicillin is now available in several forms. (1) Benzyl-penicillin or penicillin G, the original form. (2) Acid-resistant phenoxymethyl-penicillin or penicillin V, resistant to gastric juice and effective when taken by mouth. (3) Procaine-benzyl penicillin and benzathine penicillin which are longer acting. (4) Penicillinase-resistant penicillins – some resistant organisms produce penicillinase, an enzyme which destroys penicillin. Synthetic penicillins such as methicillin and cloxacillin have been developed to overcome this difficulty. (5) Broad-spectrum penicillins which are active against a wider range of organisms, e.g., ampicillin. The use of penicillin has been a landmark in the treatment of bacterial diseases. It has proved to be active against pus-forming cocci generally and against the pneumococcus, meningococcus, gonococcus, *B.anthracis,* clostridial types such as *Cl. tetani,* and the treponeme of syphilis. It is essentially non-toxic except that some persons may develop allergic symptoms of asthma, skin eruptions or anaphylaxis.

The importance of its discovery and exploitation was recognized in 1945 by the award of the Nobel Prize for Physiology and Medicine to Fleming, Florey and Chain.

penis. The male organ of copulation and the external organ of the REPRODUCTIVE SYSTEM. It consists of three elongated sections made up of spongy tissue, the spaces of which are occupied by blood sinuses. The middle section is traversed by the urethra, for the passage of urine and semen, and its outer end is expanded to form a bulbous extremity called the glans penis. The skin of the penis is thin and loose and, at the tip, is folded upon itself partially to cover the glans as the foreskin, or prepuce; this is the skin which is removed in the operation of CIRCUMCISION.

Diseases. Congenitally, the penis may be diminutive with the urethra opening on its upper or lower surface instead of at the extremity. These abnormalities are epispadias and hypospadias respectively. When extreme they may give rise to difficulty in deciding the sex of an infant. In phimosis, another congenital condition, the foreskin is lengthened to extend beyond the end of the penis and so narrowed as to obstruct the urinary flow and be non-retractile. A narrow foreskin if forcibly retracted may cause paraphimosis, a partial strangulation of the glans. Both conditions require circumcision.

In the adult venereal infections are the commonest causes of disease. The penis is a common site for syphilitic chancres. Gonorrhoea and other forms of sepsis produce balanitis or inflammation of the glans, and gonorrhoeal infection may extend up the urethra to produce a purulent discharge and later a urethral stricture. Warts are usually a

complication of gonorrhoea. In elderly men the glans may develop papillomatous tumours which have a tendency towards malignant change, and carcinoma also occurs, commonly beginning as an ulcerated area in the groove behind the glans.

All the conditions mentioned require professional advice and treatment but the correction of phimosis, sexual continence, cleanliness and hygiene are important preventive measures.

peptic ulcer. An ulcer occurring in the stomach or duodenum, or occasionally at the lower end of the oesophagus. See DUODENAL ULCER and GASTRIC ULCER.

perforating ulcer. A complication of chronic gastric or duodenal ulcer. The ulcerative process ultimately extends through the whole thickness of the wall of the organ concerned to produce a hole which allows gastric or duodenal contents to enter the peritoneal cavity and cause peritonitis.

Acute perforation produces sudden and intensely violent pain in the whole region accompanied by vomiting and signs of shock. It constitutes an emergency requiring immediate operative treatment.

Sub-acute and chronic perforations occur in similar but less dramatic fashion when there is a small leak which the body defences succeed in temporarily containing. A sub-gastric abscess eventually results which will also require surgical measures for its relief.

pericardium. The membranous sac containing the heart. It comprises two layers, an external one composed of tough and dense fibrous tissue, and an inner serous coat (the parietal pericardium) continuous with a similar layer covering the heart itself as the visceral pericardium. The resultant space between the visceral and parietal serous coats is the pericardial cavity. Serous means 'exuding serum' and the opposed layers are thus kept smoothly lubricated to facilitate the heart movements.

Inflammation of the pericardium is pericarditis. It most commonly occurs in the course of acute and sub-acute attacks of rheumatic fever and also as a complication of septicaemia, pneumonia, empyema, pulmonary tuberculosis, cardiac infarction and penetrating wounds. It may also arise as a terminal incident in chronic diseases such as nephritis and malignant conditions with thoracic spread.

The symptoms are generally pain in the front of the chest, cough and breathlessness, with raised temperature, and rapid pulse rate. Fluids may collect, distending the pericardial sac, which seriously interferes with the heart's action. Acute pericarditis may be followed by chronic adhesive pericarditis where the two layers of the pericardium become adherent to each other and this also reduces efficiency of the heart.

The treatment of pericarditis is that of the underlying disease, and the accumulated fluid may have to be drawn off by tapping (aspiration).

perineum. The area of skin with its underlying structures at the base of the trunk which surround the outlet of the pelvis. It forms a diamond-shaped region between the pubis in front, the buttocks behind and the thighs laterally. Through it pass the urethra and anus and in the female it also contains the external genitalia with the opening of the vagina.

The perineum is liable to be torn during childbirth and unless carefully repaired this may later on lead to incontinence or prolapse. Infected haemorrhoids may give rise to an abscess in the perineum.

period. In precise terms any interval or division of time. In a medical context the following are some common uses of the word.

1. Menstrual period: the monthly uterine discharge during the years of reproductive capacity, otherwise known as menstruation.

2. Safe period: the basis of the rhythm method of BIRTH CONTROL, conception being relatively unlikely except between the tenth and eighteenth days of the menstrual cycle counting from the first day of the menstrual flow.

3. Incubation period: in infectious diseases the interval between infection and symptoms.

4. Quarantine period: in infectious disease the interval which must elapse before an individual who has been exposed to infection can be regarded as no longer liable to acquire or transmit the disease.

periosteum. A fibrous membrane covering and closely adherent to all the surfaces of bones except in areas where there is articular cartilage, which gives a smooth surface at the joints.

In young bones the periosteum is thick and vascular and its deeper layers contain cells known as osteoblasts which form new bone during growth. In adult life its thickness is reduced but is still contains blood vessels which enter and nourish the bone. Hence the tendency of bone to die if the periosteum is stripped off by injury or disease.

Muscles and tendons are attached to bone through their incorporation with the periosteum.

peripheral neuritis. A condition of general inflammation of the peripheral nerves. The early symptoms are numbness, tingling, and tenderness over the nerve-trunks. This is followed by weakness and paralysis, loss of tendon reflexes, and muscle wasting. The condition is caused by a poisoning of the blood by (1) chemical poisons such as alcohol or arsenic, (2) bacterial toxins especially in diphtheria, or (3) metabolic diseases particularly diabetes and beri-beri.

A special feature of diphtheritic polyneuritis is its tendency to affect also the cranial nerves to cause disturbances in focusing the eyes, swallowing, and speech. The conditions which cause polyneuritis also damage the heart-muscle and there is a recognized risk of sudden heart failure particularly in diphtheria and beri-beri.

The treatment in all cases is to remove or treat the cause of the poisoning of the blood, to stimulate the passing of urine and to aid perspiration (in both cases to help get rid of the poisons), to ensure adequate diet and to enforce rest until recovery. Beri-beri requires specific treatment with vitamin B_1.

peristalsis. The rhythmical movements of the small and large intestines by which their contents are gradually impelled downwards during the digestion of food and the subsequent elimination of waste material. Successive ring-like contractions pass slowly along the bowel sweeping forward any intestinal contents.

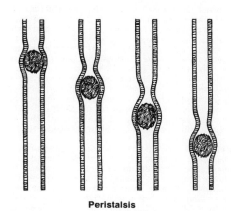

Peristalsis

Similar peristaltic movements occur in the oesophagus and at the pyloric end of the stomach, and they are also seen in the secretory and excretory ducts of other organs.

Anti-peristalsis is peristalsis occurring in reverse of the normal direction of movement and mainly affects the oesophagus during vomiting.

peritonitis. Inflammation of the peritoneum, i.e., the membrane lining the abdominal cavity and covering the abdominal organs. The condition may arise from a ruptured appendix following failure to diagnose appendicitis, from infection of the uterus after childbirth, from a perforated ulcer of the stomach or intestine, or from various less common causes. Symptoms include severe abdominal pain, signs of shock and rigid ('boarded') abdominal muscles. Immediate medical treatment is essential. It includes intravenous feeding and administration of antibiotics, and may include removal of the accumulated fluid by drainage.

pernicious anaemia. A particular form of severe progressive anaemia. Like an earlier synonym, Addison's anaemia, the name is obsolescent and the condition is now better described as megalocytic or megaloblastic anaemia because of the presence of large immature red cells in the blood stream. The disease usually commences in middle life and formerly had a uniformly fatal outcome within a few years; there is also a juvenile form, which is hereditary in origin. Its characteristics were the insidious onset of great weakness and an appearance of typical yellowish pallor very suggestive of the correct diagnosis. Other features were sore tongue (glossitis), dyspepsia from lack of gastric acid, and nervous symptoms from spinal cord degeneration. Death resulted from debility and heart failure.

The blood showed a great reduction in red blood cells to as few as one-fifth of normal with a high proportion of immature forms which correlated with abnormal bone-marrow activity. Haemoglobin was not reduced proportionately so that the red cells remained well-coloured compared with other forms of anaemia (high colour index).

Treatment was to no avail until, in 1926, Minot and Murphy of Boston discovered that the disease could be controlled by giving raw liver. Further work suggested that the liver normally produces substances essential for red-cell formation in the bone marrow and that these result from the interaction of an 'intrinsic factor' derived from the stomach lining and as 'extrinsic factor' from food. These essential substances were ultimately identified as cyanocobalamin (vitamin B_{12}) and folic acid, and their administration now completely restores normal function to the bone-marrow.

Fortnightly or monthly intra-muscular injections of appropriate preparations are usually prescribed with periodic blood tests to check the position. Treatment needs to be continued for life.

personal behaviour.. Since communities began it has been evident that tolerable co-existence depends on general willingness to observe codes of conduct designed to secure harmony, justice and fair treatment between man and man. The alternative is chaos, when only might is right and the devil takes the hindmost. All societies with even a modicum of organization have sets of rules which can be recognized as falling into at least three categories as the laws of state, church, and God. The first two are clearly man-made and developed to meet the circumstances and conventions of their times and they differ from rules with a moral connotation, widely expressed as God's law or accepted more generally as moral law. Moral rules are fundamental to human relationships. Unless they are observed it is virtually impossible to initiate, and continue any organized social activity. To call moral law 'God's law' begs many questions, not least about its origins, but it is significant that many different religions are at one in enjoining honesty, truth, trustworthiness, justice, sympathetic help for the needy, and respect for individual rights.

The universal emergence of basically similar moral codes suggests the influence of some inborn characteristic which for want of a better term is called 'conscience'. Aversion from wrong, and impulses to do good are to some extent outside conscious control and there is evidence of such instinctive behaviour in lower animals. Human adults have a protective and altruistic attitude to their young and males treat females with children sympathetically. Submissive acts of apology and confession disarm aggression and such behaviour has its counterpart in other species. The implication of these behavioural analogues of morality is that conscience has evolved biologically and is represented in the genetic constitution, although like other characteristics it may be over-ridden or reinforced in more advanced organisms by environment or experience. Basic moral behaviour is extended to situations with less direct social consequences, and enlargement of moral concern is represented by religious belief and practice as conformity to the law of God, because people may not be strongly motivated to obey rules unless they feel that they represent the decree of an authority which they respect and fear. Evangelical moralists tacitly accept this view by seeking to awaken a conscience regarded as dormant.

The psychoanalytical school of Freud favoured instead a concept of the super-ego which held up to the ego positive ideals of socially desirable behaviour in order to secure modification or suppression of other impulses.

Human beings constantly face conflicts between duty and inclination. They feel a sense of obligation and when they ignore this or take a contrary course they experience guilt and remorse. The purpose of religious activity is seen as centring on the resolution of such conflicts so that obligation becomes desire.

Finally there is the learning-theory approach which holds that both the foregoing explanations are hypothetical and unproven and that moral behaviour is only learned by example and precept. There is a case, too, for maintaining that moral behaviour is influenced by pressures of society. What people do or say in public may not accord with their inner impulses. Clergymen, for instance are expected to be exemplars of moral rectitude, and other professions and callings impose similar standards of probity. If the factors influencing morality are examined a number of considerations can be identified.

1. Temptation. The Christian religion, and especially its less liberal varieties, sees resistance to temptation as a crucial test of moral strength. At one extreme are persons who are obsessively scrupulous and alert for signs of sin in themselves and others. Conversely, there are those who find any sort of temptation irresistible. Experimental evidence suggests that resistance to temptation is stronger in females and in persons of good intelligence, that it improves with age, and that it is related also to personality, extroverts being more impulsive and less self-controlled.

2. Guilt. A disagreeable emotional condition which follows transgression. Physical punishment is not very effective in upbringing because it provokes feelings of aggression. These submerge the feelings of anxiety produced by guilt. It is anxiety which motivates reformation, producing a desire to secure re-approval and alleviation of guilt by subsequent reward. This approach is also seen in religion which stimulates guilt and offers commitment as a route to peace of mind.

3. Altruism. Actions are altruistic when they are primarily designed to benefit another person. Generous attitudes can be acquired by training. Children are encouraged to share their toys and sweets and rewarded by adult approbation which is gradually reduced in frequency and degree as the child learns instead to reward himself by self-praise and self-satisfaction.

4. Insight and belief. Attitudes to moral rules depend on a person's conception of their status and validity. The adult who is conditioned merely by a unilateral respect for authoritarian decrees is still acting rather like a child. At a more mature stage a sufficiently well-developed conscience will encourage a morality based on self-accepted moral principles. What these principles will be depends on what the individual conceives to be 'right' or 'wrong'. The increasing permissive-ness of society is based on a belief that relationships between responsible adults are not matters for moral judgment provided no third party is hurt.

5. Delinquency and crime. Deliquency rates increase steadily through childhood to a peak in late adolescence and then decline sharply in the mid-twenties. The rising tide of delinquency is seen as indicative of moral decline in society, but in fact most delinquents turn into ordinary

law-abiding adults as they accept the responsibilities of work, marriage and family. Delinquent acts are very often commited with full approval from associates and they occur mainly from excitement, resentment of parental or official control, or from the desire to compensate for feelings of inferiority by 'acting tough'. Repeated convictions often do no more than enhance a delinquent's status amongst his companions. There appears to be no justification for an assumption that delinquency equates with a defective conscience, and membership of a non-delinquent group can prove an effective means of reformation by offering legitimate forms of status and self-expression.

Crime on the other hand tends to be a more or less consciously chosen career or to be evidence of some personality disorder.

personality. It is a matter of everyday observation that people differ individually in their attitudes to life and in their inter-reactions with their fellows. The impression which they make on others and their impact on the community as a whole can be summarized as their personality, which has been defined as 'that quality or assemblage of qualities which makes a person what he is and distinguishes him from other persons'.

To a great extent individual personality represents a summation of past experience and the modifications of behaviour which have resulted therefrom, but underlying this are certain basic attributes derived from inheritance. Many workers have attempted to correlate disposition with physical characteristics. Their observations have sought to identify three types of body build defined as (1) endomorphic: broad muscular and athletic with large body cavities and viscera and an active endocrine system; (2) mesomorphic: soft, rounded and fleshy; (3) ectomorphic: tall, narrow and spindly, poorly-muscled, and with small organs and a relatively stable endocrine system.

At one extreme, endomorphy tends to be associated with a pyknic (from the greek *puknos,* thick) type of personality; ectomorphs on the other hand display a leptic (from the Greek *leptos,* thin) behaviour pattern. Pyknics have an extroverted and out-going attitude to life. They are sociable, active and energetic, 'hail-fellow-well-met', fluent conversationalists with strong, but not lasting, emotional reactions, and they show an ability to take positive decisions, to act on them promptly and generally to get things done.

In contrast, leptics are introverted and unsociable, inactive, ill-at-ease in society, and handicapped by shyness, diffidence, and reserve. Their immediate emotional reactions appear shallow and difficult to arouse but they may sometimes react strongly, and apparently irrationally, to trivial incidents as the result of a sudden release of accumulated resentment. Despite the superficial impression which they make of being misfits in society they may nevertheless be possessed of valuable attributes because their mental vision tends to be of longer range, with abilities to foresee and plan. Introverts have made many valuable contributions to knowledge and to the betterment of humanity.

In the development of personality there is thus a fundamental factor based on *habitus* or physical characteristics (recognized originally by Hippocrates as *habitus apoplecticus* and *habitus phthisicus*), but experience of life superimposes layer upon layer of modifications derived from upbringing (see CHILDHOOD, PSYCHOLOGY OF) and from education and emotional experiences; from the acquisition of enthusiasms, prejudices, intolerances, and bias; from habits and hobbies; and from vocational and non-vocational pursuits. Moreover personality does not remain fixed throughout life. It may alter with age and experience, and through physical, endocrine, and emotional factors. The demure, shy and retiring young girl may become in turn the brisk and competent wife and mother, and later still the frustrated, complaining, nagging spouse. The thrusting ambitious executive may become, through lack of material success, the soured and querulous bane of his colleagues. Physical defects may also profoundly alter personality. Illness, disability, disfigurement, or loss of sight or hearing may completely alter a person's attitude to life.

One of the most interesting features of personality is the difference which exists between the nationals of different countries and there is at least some evidence that this is related to the cultural patterns of the upbringing of children and to the influences of climate. It surely cannot be purely accidental that the residents of cold and temperate regions tend to show passivity and reserve compared with the spontaneity and ebullience found in those who live in a warm or tropical environment. It has been maintained, for example, that the clue to the Russian national character lies in the custom of 'swaddling' their babies. Long periods of immobilization alternating with joyous intervals of play are mirrored in their traditional adult attitudes of stolid, patient self-restraint, interrupted by episodes of explosive emotional release.

Personality tests. An appreciation of the fact that people possess different types of personality has aroused much interest in procedures for assessing their individual attributes, and such tests are now available in great variety. Many are based on structured questionnaires or on situations calling for interpretation by the examinee. One of the latter which has gained a good deal of acceptance is the Rorshach ink-blot test. The difficulty in devising such tests is to ensure that they really measure what they purport to do, that they are properly validated, and that they do not allow of cheating. It is often easy for an examinee to give sociably acceptable answers to a questionnaire in the hope of gaining good marks rather than truthfully record his own attitudes. However, such tests are being increasingly used in research, in vocational counselling, and in personnel selection.

The personal attitudes for success are a good basic intelligence and a well-organized memory but other qualities are less easy to measure. Also required are self-assurance and willingness to listen, a pragmatic cast of mind, a taste for hard work, and the courage to take risks. There is no real substitute for intelligence but it is not enough in itself. Many who are intelligent lack the moral courage to act. On the other hand moral courage insufficiently modified by intelligence produces fanaticism. The task of education in the formation of personality is both to build on native intelligence and to foster desirable moral qualities.

personality, multiple. A disordered state of mind usually occurring in psycho-neurotic illness of hysterical type in which a patient appears to lead several different lives without being aware, at any one time, of the memories and experiences of his or (more commonly) her other identities. Hysterics adopt this type of behaviour in order to fulfil subconscious wishes or to evade difficulties, and multiple personality is only an extension of DOUBLE PERSONALITY caused by a further fragmentation of memory so that different sets of recollection and experience influence immediate behaviour.

personality, psychopathic. A behavioural pattern or relationship between an individual and his environment, characterized by markedly anti-social or asocial tendencies.

The psychopath is egocentric and largely incapable of displaying concern, sympathy or affection for others. His attitude to life is governed by his present needs without reference to the past or future. For him to want something is to take it and he feels neither guilt nor remorse at the consequences of his actions. Psychopaths form an important section of the criminal or delinquent members of society. Their developmental histories may show evidence of severe rejection in childhood and absence of conditions for forming secure personal relationships, but there are often genetic influences as well. As deliquents they are recognized to be most difficult to reform.

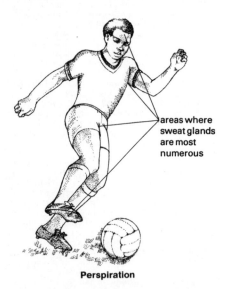

areas where sweat glands are most numerous

Perspiration

perspiration. The term signifies both sweat and the act of sweating. Sweat is secreted by sweat glands present in large numbers in the skin or subcutaneous tissue throughout the body although in some parts, such as armpit and groin, they are particularly numerous. Each gland is a simple tube coiled within the tissues and opening on the skin-surface by a funnel shaped duct. Sweat production contributes to heat regulation since its

evaporation from the body-surface produces a cooling effect. If the surrounding temperature is at, or above, body temperature it is clear that heat cannot be lost by convection or radiation, and sweating compensates for this. If evaporation is poor because of high air humidity, this mechanism will also be ineffective and heat-stroke is threatened.

Sweating is mainly stimulated by the effect of body-heat on the temperature-regulating centre of the mid-brain and resultant impulses conveyed by the parasympathetic nervous system to activate the glands. Warming of the blood stream of a cat will cause its paws to sweat even although these are kept cool. In dogs and cats, sweat-glands are found only on the skin of paw-pads and they compensate by panting which produces increased evaporaton of fluid from the lungs.

'Cold sweats' occur in fear or other emotional stress due to nervous influences disturbing the adrenalin-acetylcholine balance.

Excessive perspiration. Obese persons perspire readily and profusely. This is because the ratio of body bulk to skin surface is greater than in a thin person and so the capacity of the skin to lose heat by radiation and convection is relatively less.

This effect is physiological as it is in the sweating of febrile illness, but excessive sweating also occurs in nervous states, in conditions of toxaemia, anaemia and debility, and in certain diseases of the endocrine system such as diabetes and thyrotoxicosis. The sweat-glands are inhibited by the sympathetic nervous system (adrenergic) and activated by the parasympathetic system (cholinergic) and in these pathological conditions the adrenalin-acetylcholine balance is disturbed.

Excessive perspiration is called hyperidrosis. If it remains on moist skin sites it may become invaded by bacteria to produce odours, a condition known as bromidrosis or offensive sweating.

perspiring feet. Sweat-glands are very numerous on the palms and soles and some individuals perspire excessively from these sites, perhaps because of relative deficiency elsewhere. Just as some persons have a 'clammy' hand-shake, so others have sweaty feet.

It is a personal idiosyncrasy but one which calls for special attention to foot-hygiene because moist skin there predisposes to fungoid infections, 'soft-corns', and offensive odours. The feet should be washed daily and treated with an astringent lotion and dusting powder. Salicylic acid lotion (BPC) followed by zinc, starch and talc dusting powder (BPC) is a suitable régime. Socks should be changed daily and thoroughly washed. In warm weather and under suitable circumstances the wearing of sandals is helpful.

pertussis. See WHOOPING COUGH.

perversion or **sexual deviance.** A condition in which the person obtains sexual gratification otherwise than by ordinary intercourse with a partner of the opposite sex. Since 'perversion' implies obstinacy or wickedness, the older term – sexual perversion – is in the process of being replaced by the modern term, sexual deviance.

As Freud demonstrated, a child goes through stages of interest in the mouth (oral eroticism) through which tastes are felt and food enters the body, the anus (anal eroticism) from which emerge the excreta that appear to give such concern to parents, the genitalia, and later the genitalia of the other sex; and through a phase of great attachment to the parent of the opposite sex with some jealousy of the parent of the same sex, a phase of interest primarily in playmates of the same sex, and a heterosexual phase which gradually develops into adult love which is, of course, partly physical and partly idealistic, tender, romantic and protective. At any stage the emotional development may undergo arrest.

The deviation in which love is reserved for persons of the same sex is known as HOMOSEXUALITY in males or LESBIANISM in females. It may arise in part from strained relations with the parent of the same sex, so that, for instance, the boy with a cold and remote father may feel great need for acceptance by a man; or from over-possessiveness by the parent of the other sex, resulting in too close identification with that parent.

Essentially there are two types of homosexuality or Lesbianism: in one the effeminate man or masculine woman identifies with, and often acts like, a member of the other sex; in the other type the person exhibits the normal characteristics of his or her sex but is strongly attracted to individuals of the same sex. In either case the homosexuality may remain latent and reveal itself only in a difficulty in forming heterosexual relation-ships, or it may lead to actual physical relations – usually anal intercourse in males or mutual masturbation in females.

Most adolescents pass through a stage of latent homosexuality and in adults there are many gradations, e.g., the completely heterosexual "normal' person, the normally heterosexual person who has homosexual desires during prolonged separation from the other sex, the person who oscillates between heterosexuality and homosexuality, the latent homosexual who cannot obtain sexual gratification from either sex, and so on.

Sodomy, common in Ancient Greece and fairly common in Elizabethan England, has for centuries been illegal in many countries and its practice has been a common source of blackmail, but the modern tendency is to regard relations between consenting adults as permissible and that there is no justification for legal intervention and infliction of penalties.

The term SADISM is used where sexual excitement is obtained by inflicting physical or mental suffering on another person, usually, but not always, a member of the opposite sex, while MASOCHISM is the condition in which sexual gratification arises from undergoing actual beating or mental humiliation, again usually by a member of the opposite sex. There is often only a specific portion of the body involved, e.g., a particular sadist may gain satisfaction only from hurting the breast or the genitals, or a particular masochist may be stimulated only by flagellation of the buttocks. Masochistic tendencies may start with early severe punishment for sex play, with excitement and punishment linked; the origin of sadistic tendencies is still somewhat controversial.

In both conditions there are many variations. Examples are the apparently normal teacher or parent who nevertheless gets some pleasure from punishing children, or the apparently normal person who courts humiliation or even (in certain strata of society) blows, the person who beats or is beaten by a willing partner as an exciting prelude to intercourse, and the person for whom the whipping of another or of himself or herself serves as a complete substitute for intercourse.

Clearly a mild sadist and a moderate masochist can form a mutually satisfactory combination. Masochism by itself is not dangerous, since the pain is borne by the person who desires it and will cease when it exceeds the resulting pleasure; but sadism can be dangerous since the infliction of pain is by the sadist and the suffering is by the victim who may be powerless to resist.

There are elements both of sadism and of masochism in all of us. Why, but for sadistic impulses, would we laugh at knock-about comedy or avidly read newspaper reports of murder trials? Why, but for masochistic sensations, would we watch and sympathize with the sufferings of the hero or heroine of a tragedy? Yet in most people the sadistic and masochistic elements are relatively small, with one or other predominating but subordinate to normal sexual desires, and with pain-inflicting or pain-desiring components of the personality restrained by a mass of developmental, cultural and social forces.

Nymphomania, or inordinate sexual desire for a whole series of partners, is another deviation, as is fetishism, where an article of clothing creates erotic impulses, and voyeurism, the 'Peeping Tom' condition.

pessary. Any appliance worn inside the vagina. The term is used mostly for devices that support the uterus when it has been displaced downwards (prolapsed) as a consequence of childbirth. These devices are normally first inserted by a doctor or nurse, but many women quickly learn how to remove a pessary, clean it and re-insert it.

Diaphragms or rubber caps inserted as contraceptive devices, and medicated suppositories inserted into the vagina for the treatment of inflammation are also called pessaries.

Other forms of pessary are those employed to support the rectum.

petit mal. A minor form of EPILEPSY. In this form convulsions do not occur but the patient loses consciousness for a few seconds or even a minute and is subsequently unaware of any gap in his activities.

phagocyte. A cell able to engulf and digest invading bacteria and dead cells. Certain types of white blood corpuscle are phagocytes and can be considered as both the street cleaners and the policemen of the BLOOD: the former because they remove the remains of cells that die in the course of the ordinary wear and tear of the body, and the latter because they constitute the body's first line of defence, surrounding, sealing off, and dealing with invading bacteria.

phalanx. A segment of a finger or the bone of such a segment. The thumb and the great toe each have two phalanges, while all other fingers and toes have three.

phantom limb. The illusion that an amputated limb is still present. In the early days after amputation, sensations of distress in nerve fibres that were cut during the operation are commonly interpreted by the brain as pain in the part that has been removed.

pharmacist. A person qualified in preparing medicines and making up prescriptions. In most countries a person is not entitled to compound and dispense medicines prescribed by a doctor until he has passed necessary examinations. In Britain the appropriate qualification is Member of the Pharmaceutical Society, commonly contracted to MPS. A pharmacist is therefore a professionally qualified person but he is not qualified to practise medicine.

pharmacology. The branch of medicine that deals with the systematic study of medicinal substances, their actions on the body, their chemistry, their appropriate dosage, and the effects of over-dosage. Pharmacology includes both (1) therapeutics, the study of the use of drugs to treat disease, and (2) materia medica, the study of the sources, composition, and preparation of medicinal substances.

Pharmacology should be differentiated from pharmacy which is a narrower but related subject, namely the preparation and storage of drugs.

pharmacopoeia. An official list of approved drugs, their composition, chemical properties, preparation and dosage.

Probably the earliest official publication of this nature was the *London Pharmacopoeia*, first produced in 1618 and continuing until replaced by the *British Pharmacopoeia* in 1864. It is published every few years, lists the drugs approved for medical use in Britain, and is a standard book of reference for pharmacists and manufacturing chemists. The *British Pharmaceutical Codex* contains preparations of probable value that have not yet reached official status. In America the *United States Pharmacopoeia* was first published in 1820 and became official in 1907.

pharynx. The cavity of the throat, lying behind the mouth and separated from it by the soft palate and uvula above and on each side by the pillars of the fauces enclosing the tonsils. It extends upwards to the rear part of the nasal passages, while below it is continuous with the oesophagus. The trachea (windpipe) passes in front of the oesophagus and communicates with the pharynx by way of the larynx, which is protected by an overhanging lid, the epiglottis. The tonsils (commonly quite large in children and shrivelled in adults) are almond-shaped masses of lymphoid tissue which form part of the protective lymphoid tissue in this region.

Diseases. Acute pharyngitis, inflammation of the throat, is among the commonest of infections. It is caused by bacterial invasion and most frequently occurs after exposure to cold or to irritating vapours. Symptoms include dryness of the throat, pain on swallowing, and often aching of the back and limbs. The condition usually clears up within a few days, and severe cases respond well to antibiotics.

Chronic pharyngitis or 'clergyman's throat', results from excessive voice strain, or immoderate use of tobacco or alcohol. The main symptoms are a dry, tickling cough, hoarseness (largely from inflammation of the larynx), and a feeling of dryness in the throat. Avoidance of irritants and rest for the voice are the basis of treatment.

Inflammation of the tonsils, or TONSILLITIS, is

frequent in children in both an acute and a chronic form but is rare in adults.

phenacetin. A synthetic drug used, alone or in combination with aspirin, to reduce fever and to relieve pain.

phenobarbitone. The most commonly used drug of the BARBITURATES. It is prescribed as a mildly sedative drug to reduce nervous tension or anxiety or to relieve insomnia. Like all barbiturates it is mildly addictive; and it should in no circumstances be taken simultaneously with alcohol, since two substances interact and each increases the effect of the other.

phenylketonuria. A hereditary disease in which the body lacks the enzyme necessary for the use of phenylalanine, a normal constituent of protein, so that toxic products from the abnormal breakdown of this amino-acid enter the blood stream and damage the brain and the nervous system.

Detection is by a simple urine test, normally employed for all babies as a matter of routine. Where the condition is ascertained early in infancy a special diet can prevent mental retardation, and sometimes the diet can be discontinued later in life.

The disease is inherited as a recessive, i.e., it appears only if both parents carry the abnormal gene; see GENETICS.

phimosis. A condition, in most cases inherited, in which the foreskin (prepuce) of the PENIS is abnormally tight and cannot be pulled back over the glans. In severe cases phimosis may interfere with urination, and quite often it is a cause of bed-wetting. Mild forms tend to disappear spontaneously, but in severe cases the operation of circumcision may be needed.

phlebitis. Inflammation of a vein. The area around the vein becomes red, painful, and tender, and the swollen vein may be felt as a hard cord.

Phlebitis occurs most commonly in the veins of the leg after childbirth, following a surgical operation, or after a prolonged period in bed. It also occurs in association with varicose veins.

ANTICOAGULANT DRUGS (i.e., those which slow down the clotting of blood) such as heparin are advisable because the condition is often associated with THROMBOSIS of the vein, and a clot, once it has formed, may become detached and cause damage elsewhere. Antibiotics and rest are the essentials for treatment, and warm fomentations (see POULTICES) help to relieve the pain.

phlegmasia alba dolens. White leg. A form of PHLEBITIS or thrombophlebitis occurring as a complication of childbirth and involving painful swelling and pallor of the whole leg. Skilled medical treatment is essential, not only because of the pain and swelling but also because of the THROMBOSIS, with the associated danger from detachment of fragments of the clot.

phobia. Irrational and baseless fear. Examples are AGORAPHOBIA, fear of open spaces; bacteriophobia, terror of germs; CLAUSTROPHOBIA, fear of closed spaces; cynopholia, dread of dogs; and ailurophobia, fear of cats. In a typical case of fear of dirt the victim may feel obliged to wash his or her hands fifty times in the day, is unhappy whenever he does not yield to the compulsion to wash but can give no reason for being more exposed to dirt or more susceptible to its effects than are other people.

These pathological disorders are forms of

NEUROSIS and are usually related to repressed impulses or to submerged guilt feelings. FREUD cast much light on their origin and made the successful treatment of serious cases possible.

In mild cases the victim should be advised to avoid the situations which create or exaggerate the fear: to attempt to 'fight' the fear is useless, and wherever possible the victim should continue his normal daily activities. Where the phobia seriously interferes with work or leisure activities, psychiatric treatment is needed.

phosphorus. A non-metallic element contained along with calcium in bone and also in the sheaths of nerves. Phosphates, i.e., organic compounds of phosphorus, are important MINERAL SALTS ih body chemistry, energy being released by their breakdown and stored by their formation.

The element itself is a dangerous poison. Chronic phosphorus poisoning (phossy jaw) was formerly common in match factories but is now unknown. Acute phosphorus poisoning, e.g., from accidental swallowing of certain pesticides, is characterized by vomiting, abdominal cramp, diarrhoea, intense pallor, and signs of collapse. Atropine sulphate in doses of 1 to 2 mg. sometimes helps but the condition is often fatal. Prevention entails (1) the observation of strict precautions to prevent absorption by persons manufacturing or using phosphorus compounds (e.g., the use of protective clothing and wearing face masks), and (2) care that none of these compounds contaminates any form of food or drink.

photophobia. Intolerance of bright light by the eyes. This is commonly found in inflammatory conditions of the eyes and also occurs in migraine and in meningitis.

phthisis. Wasting of tissues, consumption. The term, now almost obsolete, was formerly used as a synonym for pulmonary TUBERCULOSIS.

physiology. The study of the working or functioning of normal cells, tissues and organs. Physiology can be contrasted with – but shades into – ANATOMY, the study of structure, and PATHOLOGY, the study of changes causing or caused by disease.

Before medicine widened to include mental and emotional disorders (involving study of normal psychology as a basis) and community aspects (involving similar study of social science and environmental hygiene), anatomy and physiology were regarded as the two sciences basic to medicine and they are still essential preliminaries to any understanding of the processes of disease.

Aristotle's grandson, Erasistratus (about 300 B.C.) who identified the main functions of the nerves, muscles and digestive tract, is generally regarded as the founder of physiology; and Galen, some four hundred years later, is considered, despite his many mistakes, as probably the greatest physiologist of the Ancient World. Thereafter physiology languished, because the physicians of the Middle Ages preferred speculation to experiment and investigation. Physiology revived in the seventeenth century, e.g., with Harvey's discovery of the circulation of the blood. Yet it is probably true that knowledge of human physiology, animal physiology, and plant physiology has advanced more in the last sixty years than in all the rest of recorded history.

physiotherapy. Treatment of illness by physical measures, such as massage, heat, electricity, and exercises. Probably its most important contributions are towards restoration of function of joints and muscles after an injury or a stroke. Since 1920 physiotherapy has been a recognized profession in Britain, separate from medicine, nursing, and dentistry, but included in the group of professions supplementary to medicine.

pigeon chest. A deformity in which the breastbone (sternum) juts forward, creating a characteristic appearance, and in severe cases causing some limitation of movement of the heart and lungs. The condition is sometimes congenital but is usually a result of deficiency of calcium or vitamin D in the diet during the early years. See RICKETS.

pigmentation. A pigment is any naturally occurring substance that imparts colour.

The cells of the skin contain a pigment called melanin. The amount varies in different races, and those of fair skin is increased by the action of sunlight. The function of melanin is to protect the skin and underlying tissues against the sun's rays. Absence of pigment occurs in the hereditary condition of ALBINISM. Increased pigmentation is found in Addison's disease and sometimes in diabetes and exophthalmic goitre. In leucoderma there are patches of unpigmented skin surrounded by over-pigmented skin.

The blood pigment, haemoglobin, is responsible for the colour of a bruise or a black eye which follows bleeding below the surface of the skin. In jaundice the yellow pigmentation is due to the circulation of bile pigments in the blood.

piles. A dilated and often inflamed condition of veins at the lower end of the rectum and anal canal alternatively called haemorrhoids. External piles originate in the part of the anal canal that is lined by skin, and in many cases they cause no symptoms except an occasional burning sensation when a constipated motion is passed. Internal piles originate in the part of the bowel and anal canal covered with mucous membrane. They may remain within the anal orifice and only occasion slight and intermittent bleeding, or they may form distinct fleshy masses which are protruded when faeces are passed and cause considerable pain, bleeding and itching.

Most cases are due to constipation and straining at stool, but they are common im pregnancy due to raised intra-abdominal pressure and they may be a symptom of more serious disease causing obstruction to the portal circulation. Extreme pain is usually due to the dilated vein becoming thrombosed and inflamed.

If the bowels are kept open with appropriate diet and bland laxatives, small haemorrhoids often subside with use of suppositories to reduce congestion. For more serious cases injection of an irritant fluid into the haemorrhoid may be required, causing scarring and obstruction of the distended vein. Surgical closure of the veins, first described by Hippocrates 2400 years ago, is seldom necessary.

Avoidance of constipation is an important preventive measure.

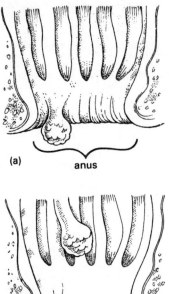

(a)   anus

(b)   anus

Section through the end of the anal canal showing (a) an external pile, and (b) an internal pile.

pimple. A small raised inflammatory spot on the skin, due to infection in a hair follicle or a sweat gland, and in many cases forming pus before healing. A pimple should in no circumstances be squeezed, both because squeezing spreads the infection and because the squeezing of a pimple may result in a permanent scar. Pimples are commonest in adolescence, the common age of victims of ACNE.

pineal gland. A small, red, oval gland, about the size of a pea, situated at the base of the brain. It is probably a vestigial ENDOCRINE GLAND which in our primitive ancestors controlled the darkening of the skin on exposure to bright light. Despite various theories, e.g., that it is associated with sexual development, it has no proved existing function. Descartes regarded it as the place of residence of the soul.

pink eye. See CONJUNCTIVITIS.

pins and needles. The unpleasant sensation which arises in the course of a nerve after irritation, such as is caused by pressure from a limb being kept for a time in an awkward position. If the cause is not obvious and if the symptom recurs, the condition warrants medical attention.

pituitary gland. A small, pea-like body situated in a depression of the sphenoid bone at the base of the skull, the pituitary is the most complex of the ENDOCRINE GLANDS and has been called 'the conductor of the endocrine orchestra'.

pityriasis. A rather vague term used for any bran-like or scaly appearance of the skin.

Pityriasis rosea is a disease characterized by the development of pink spot-like marks which begin to scale in about ten days. The disease ends spontaneously in about six weeks, and the only treatment needed is reassurance and calamine lotion.

Pityriasis alba is a form of impetigo with scaly, whitish discs, mainly on the face.

placebo. A medicine without direct action on a disease, such as water with a harmless colouring agent added or a pill composed entirely of flour. It may be used simply to give the patient the feeling that some treatment is being employed, e.g., to retain his confidence and give. him some comfort during an investigation that takes time but is essential before curative treatment can be started; or to reinforce medical advice where the advice alone would be less likely to be followed; or in alternate members of a series of patients to test the effects of a new drug. In respect of the latter use it should be noted that, if the placebo is given with apparent confidence, more than half of the patients receiving it feel the better for it, a fact which renders difficult the evaluation of a new drug.

The first two uses are of obvious value, but the third raises both practical and ethical problems. Some would argue that it is unjustifiable to give placebos to patients simply to measure their progress against that of other patients. Yet there is sometimes no other way of testing a new drug. For instance, assume that we have a number of patients with a particular illness that normally clears up in four to six weeks with rest and appropriate diet, and that there is a new drug (already established as safe by use on animals and human volunteers) that may well shorten the illness. If we give it to all the patients we learn nothing: even if most of them are restored to health in three to four weeks we may simply have been dealing with a fairly mild variety of the particular disease. If we give the drug to half the patients and nothing to the others, the 'untreated' ones will feel aggrieved, the 'treated' ones will feel better even if the drug is really valueless, and the judgment of doctors and nurses may be affected by knowledge that certain patients had received a drug that the staff hoped would be beneficial. If on the other hand one person gives the drug to some patients and the placebo to others, no patient feels aggrieved and the doctors and nurses who judge progress do not know which patients were given the drug.

Used responsibly placebos are therefore valuable; but in the hands of a lazy, irresponsible or tired doctor they can be an inefficient substitute for careful examination and diagnosis.

placenta. The disc-shaped organ by which an unborn child gains nourishment from its mother. One surface of the placenta is connected to the baby by the umbilical cord, while the other surface is firmly attached to an upper part of the wall of the uterus, so that oxygen and nutrients can pass from the uterine blood vessels to the placenta while carbon dioxide and other waste materials from the baby can travel in the opposite direction.

Shortly after the child is born the placenta separates from the uterus and is expelled as the after-birth.

Placenta praevia. An unusual situation of the placenta where, instead of being attached to the uterine wall high up, it is attached low down and tends to lie across the opening of the uterus. In such a situation, as the birth process starts, there is danger to the mother from bleeding and danger to the child from lack of oxygen because of premature detachment of the placenta. Treatment is usually by CAESARIAN SECTION.

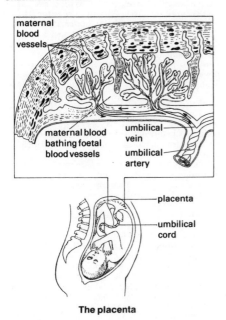

maternal blood vessels

maternal blood bathing foetal blood vessels

umbilical vein

umbilical artery

placenta

umbilical cord

The placenta

plague. A severe and highly fatal infectious disease, caused by a bacterium (*Pasteurella pestis*) and transmitted by rat-fleas. Rats are infected as a result of the bites of the fleas, and as rats die from the disease the fleas seek other hosts, including man, and, by biting, pass the infection to them.

The disease occurs in three main forms. (1) Bubonic plague, transmitted only by bites of fleas and therefore not directly transmissible from person to person, shows itself by painful swellings (buboes) in the armpits, groin and neck, extreme weakness, and high fever, often followed by dark blotches from bleeding into the skin. These blotches account for the mediaeval name, the BLACK DEATH. Until the era of antibiotics more than 50 per cent of sufferers from bubonic plague died and even now the chance of death is high, even in cases with early diagnosis and efficient treatment. (2) Pneumonic plague, transmitted both by bites of fleas and by droplet infection, is a virulent pneumonia which is usually fatal. (3) Septicaemic plague, the rarest form, has no local signs of infection and almost always ends in death within three days.

Treatment of all types involves strict isolation, with attendants wearing gowns, masks, gloves, protective boots, and clothing impregnated with DDT, together with good nursing and high dosage with chloramphenicol (starting with 500 mg. every four hours) or streptomycin, both of which are strong antibiotics.

Preventive measures include periodic surveys in all areas where plague exists to determine the prevalence both of rats and of rat-fleas, measures for the destruction of rats and of fleas, especially those on ships arriving from infected ports, elimination of breeding places, rat-proofing of buildings and ships, periodic examination of rats for evidence of infection, isolation of patients and of contacts of pneumonic cases, and disinfection of the persons and clothing of all immediate contacts. An anti-plague serum, if available in time, confers a passive immunity for about a month, and a vaccine gives at least some immunity for several months.

During the fourteenth and fifteenth centuries successive waves of plague killed approximately half the population of Europe, but the last widespread epidemic was in 1665. Since then there have been only local outbreaks but these have originated in many parts of the world.

plastic surgery. The branch of surgery which deals with the repair of disfigurements and the reconstruction of deformed parts of the body, mostly either by the use of tissue grafts or by the employment of artificial materials. An example of the former is a skin graft, where after an extensive burn of the cheek a flap of skin is partially detached from the arm and placed on the cheek, with the other end of the flap left attached to the arm. It is detached completely from the arm when blood vessels have begun to grow into it from the cheek so that it can live. An example of the use of artificial materials is the insertion of a glass eye.

platelets. Alternately known as thrombocytes, these are small spherical discs present in blood in a density of between 250,000 to 450,000 per ml. They are probably produced in the bone marrow, play an important part in the stopping of bleeding, and are necessary for the clotting of blood. If platelets are insufficient, as in the various types of purpura, multiple haemorrhages occur in the skin and mucous membranes. If platelets are abnormally plentiful, as tends to occur for some days after an operation or childbirth there is a possibility of the occurrence of thrombosis.

plethora. An excess of blood, generally showing itself by a fullness of the blood vessels of the face, and sometimes by nose bleeding and by a sensation of fullness in the head. It occurs mainly in middle-aged persons who over-eat and over-drink, and it is often associated with high blood pressure.

pleura. The double layer of membrane lining the outer surfaces of the lungs.

pleurisy. Inflammation of the pleura, i.e., the double layer of membrane lining the outer surfaces of the lungs. The inflammation is caused by bacterial or virus infection.

Dry pleurisy, where the inflamed membranes rub together, is characterized by sharp, stabbing pain on breathing or coughing, cough and high temperature. The condition occurs alone or may be a result of pneumonia, tuberculosis, or cancer of the lung.

Pleurisy with effusion, where the inflamed

membranes are separated by fluid, commonly follows the dry variety. The pain disappears because the membranes are no longer rubbing, but breathing may be difficult and on inspection the affected side is seen to have reduced movement or to be completely immobile, while sounding the chest produces a note of dullness.

Treatment includes strapping the affected side to reduce lung movement, application of local warmth (e.g., poultices), the giving of analgesics to relieve pain and, if the fluid is present in large quantity, 'tapping' to drain it. The bacterial forms respond well to antibiotics, while virus pleurisy (Bornholm disease) usually subsides spontaneously within a few days. An x-ray examination is desirable after recovery, to eliminate the possibility of the pleurisy having been secondary to tuberculosis or cancer.

pneumoconiosis. A general name for diseases of the lung caused by inhaled DUST.

pneumonia. Inflammation of the lung as a result of infection by bacteria or viruses. The affected air pockets (alveoli), which normally hold oxygen for transmission to the blood and carbon dioxide received from the blood, become water-logged with inflammatory exudate and so incapable of performing their normal function.

Lobar pneumonia. In this condition the whole of a lobe of a lung is affected. The onset is sudden with pain in the side, short distressing cough, rapid shallow breathing, and raised temperature. Without specific treatment the temperature remains high for four to twelve days and then falls abruptly to normal within a few hours, the so-called crisis which is marked by profuse perspiration. Before the era of antibiotics fully 25 per cent of patients died, and pneumonia was particularly fatal in the elderly and was called 'the old man's friend'. Even in the antibiotic era the disease has quite a high death rate. The organisms most commonly responsible for pneumonia are the pneumococcus and the streptococcus. The germ is identified from the sputum and an appropriate antibiotic employed, but good nursing is as important as the right antibiotic.

Bronchopneumonia. Groups of alveoli near larger air-passages are affected in this type of pneumonia, so that there are small patches of inflammation or consolidation throughout the lungs. There are symptoms of severe BRONCHITIS, with increasing shortness of breath, discomfort in breathing, and often pain on both sides of the chest. While bronchopneumonia may occur alone, especially in the elderly, it often arises as a complication of measles, whooping cough, or bronchitis. Antibiotic treatment is important; the room should be kept moist with a steam kettle; and heart stimulants (e.g., brandy or coramine or strychnine) may be needed. As is the case in lobar pneumonia, skilled nursing is essential and for this reason it is generally desirable that the patient be treated in hospital.

Post-operative pneumonia. Formerly common, this third type is becoming a rarity. It arose partly from irritation of the lungs from the older anaesthetics (now replaced by anaesthetics less liable to irritate) and partly from prolonged and complete immobilization in bed (now replaced by minimal bed-rest after most operations).

pneumothorax. Air in the cavity between the two layers of pleura. It may occur from rupture of a tuberculous patch on the surface of the lung or as a result of a penetrating wound of the chest. Artificial pneumothorax is the deliberate introduction through a hollow needle of a measured amount of air into the pleural cavity to make it impossible for a diseased lung to expand and so rest it and facilitate healing.

While the occurrence of a large spontaneous pneumothorax is accompanied by pain, breathing difficulty and often signs of shock, the graded introduction of air into the pleural cavity should produce no symptoms either immediately or later. Patients are often at first afraid of having one lung temporarily put out of action, but most ordinary activities can be carried out perfectly well with only one functioning lung.

poisons. There is no arbitrary division between poisonous and non-poisonous substances. Many drugs which are life-saving in tiny doses (e.g., strychnine) kill in larger quantities; medicines that adults regard as harmless (e.g., aspirin) can poison young children and substances essential to life (e.g., vitamin D, common salt, and even water) can destroy life or impair health if consumed in sufficient quantities.

Excluding the toxins of bacteria and the venom of snakes and insects, harmful substances can be roughly classified into four groups. (1) Corrosive irritants which irritate and inflame the alimentary canal and produce immediate symptoms, e.g., strong acids and alkalis. (2) Non-corrosive irritants which do not produce symptoms for half an hour or longer, e.g., arsenic. (3) Poisons affecting specific tissues, e.g., sodium cyanide, which prevents the transfer of oxygen in living cells. (4) Narcotics which act on the nervous system, e.g., morphia, and prussic acid.

Evidences of poisoning. Symptoms appear suddenly in a previously healthy person. Depending on the type of poison they may appear immediately or some little time after the taking of the affected food, drink, or medicine. If the poison is derived from food several people may be ill simultaneously. Apart from these points the evidences vary with the actual poison.

Treatment of suspected poisoning. Summon medical aid immediately. If the poison is known, give the appropriate antidote, e.g., a solution of baking soda for an acid or of vinegar for an alkali, or if the poison is unknown a drink of milk, which will at least dilute it. Retain all food, drink, and vomited material since these may permit the identification of the poison and of its source. If the patient is conscious ask him what he has swallowed: he may lose consciousness later. If he is unconscious, place him on his stomach with the head turned sideways to prevent suffocation if he vomits. If breathing stops, apply artificial respiration. Combat shock by application of warmth (e.g., hot water bottles) and, if he is conscious stimulants (e.g., brandy or whisky). Emetics, such as a tablespoonful of mustard in a tumbler of warm water, are dangerous if the poison is corrosive – a circumstance often revealed by staining or burning of the mouth – and are again dangerous if the poison can form a vapour, as in poisoning by cleaning fluids. With

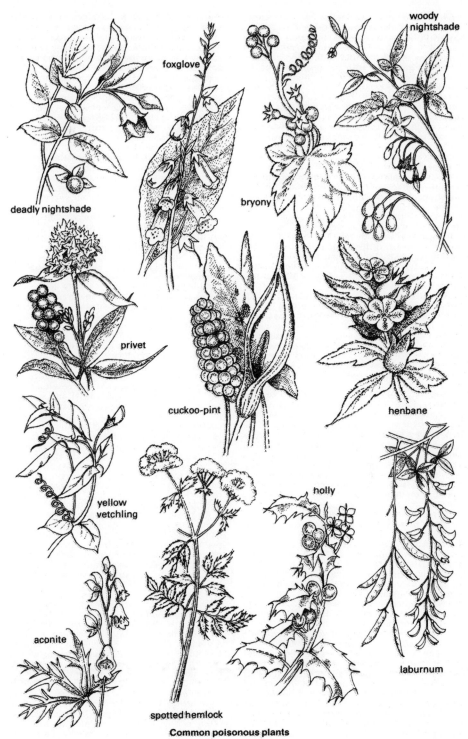

woody nightshade

foxglove

bryony

deadly nightshade

privet

cuckoo-pint

henbane

yellow vetchling

holly

aconite

spotted hemlock

laburnum

Common poisonous plants

these exceptions an emetic may be useful provided that the patient is conscious.

poliomyelitis. An acute infection of the central nervous system, causing no clinical symptoms in the majority of infected persons, fever and headache with some stiffness of the neck or spine in a sizeable minority, and temporary or permanent paralysis in about 2 per cent of cases. The condition was formerly called infantile paralysis, but it affects young adults and the middle-aged as well as children. The condition is caused by a virus which is transmitted mostly by droplet spray from the nose and throat of an infected person, and also to some extent by flies.

Although there are approximately twelve thousand people in Britain suffering from the persisting effects of poliomyelitis in the form of paralysis of one or more of the limbs, paralytic poliomyelitis is essentially a rare complication of a disease that is usually either symptomless or with symptoms resembling those of influenza. Hence both the diagnosis of a non-paralytic case and the tracing of the source of infection are difficult. Using letters to represent people, a typical chain of infection would be: A (with temporary paralysis) infects B, who has influenzal symptoms for a few days; B infects C, who develops no symptoms but infects D, who – also without symptoms – infects E, who dies of paralysis of the respiratory muscles.

Paralytic cases require skilled nursing, preferably in hospital, with special equipment available during the acute phase, e.g., a respirator for use if respiratory paralysis threatens. In some centres specialized care such as KENNY TREATMENT is undertaken. Unless there is spontaneous and full recovery of muscle power within a few weeks, physiotherapy and hydrotherapy will thereafter be required, but in some cases the paralysis becomes permanent.

In Europe and America poliomyelitis was one of the very few infections which increased in prevalence during the middle years of this century, giving rise to a theory, never fully proved, that poliomyelitis was essentially a disease associated with good sanitation, perhaps implying that where sanitation was poor children either died in infancy or else acquired some degree of immunity. The position, however, has been completely altered by vaccination.

Vaccination. In country after country the introduction of poliomyelitis vaccination and the education of the public about its desirability and efficiency have virtually eradicated the disease. To take two years at random and using figures for England and Wales: in 1950 before vaccination had begun there were 5,565 cases of paralytic poliomyelitis; in 1965 there were 55 cases.

There are two types of anti-poliomyelitis vaccine, both originating in the United States.

1. The Salk vaccine consists of killed viruses which retain the capacity to stimulate the body to manufacture antibodies. Two intramuscular injections of 1 ml. are advised at intervals of four to six weeks, followed by a reinforcing injection about a year later and subsequent reinforcing doses at intervals of a few years. The desirable frequency of the reinforcing injections is still a little uncertain, because when vaccination started the poliomyelitis virus was so widespread that persons with immunity conferred by vaccination might have their immunity strengthened by inhaling the virus, thus increasing their production of antibodies; as the virus becomes rare that stimulation of immunity is ceasing, so that we have to rely on reinforcing injections.

A quadruple vaccine – protecting simultaneously against diphtheria, whooping cough, tetanus, and poliomyelitis – is under trial.

2. The Sabin vaccine consists of weakened strains of the virus and is given by mouth: three drops on a lump of sugar. Three doses are advised at intervals of about six weeks, with reinforcing doses later.

Both the injectable Salk vaccine and the oral Sabin vaccine produce a high immunity to the disease. While there is still argument about which is the better – with expert opinion in Britain tending to favour Sabin vaccine – it is highly important that all children and all previously unimmunized young adults should receive one or the other.

pollution. Defiling of the atmosphere, the land, the sea, or rivers by waste materials.

With increasing world population, rising industrialization, aggregation of people in towns, more and more cars and internal combustion engines, and steady increase in waste products and waste materials, pollution is becoming one of mankind's greatest problems, and indeed a problem critical for his survival. On the one hand it is vital that humanity appreciates and tries to counteract the health damage, financial cost, and ultimate results of air pollution by harmful gases, smoke, dust, and grit, the damage done to marine life by pollution of rivers, lakes, and seas, the harm to animal life resulting from widespread use of insecticides, and even the aesthetic damage created by slag-heaps and piles of disused cars, to say nothing of the continuous diminution of arable land by building of houses, factories, schools, and hospitals. On the other hand it has to be realized that urban life depends on a healthy industrial economy, that industry inevitably creates waste materials and waste products, and that to cripple industry by excessive regulations would lead to massive unemployment.

Air pollution. This is caused by smoke, gases, dust, and grit from domestic and industrial chimneys, railway trains, motor vehicles, and pollutants from industrial processes. It is estimated that fully 50 per cent of atmospheric pollution comes from domestic sources, with industry and transport also serious offenders. Some effects of the various pollutants are: (1) Interference with natural light, thereby reducing the manufacture of vitamin D and generally impairing health. (2) Increasing tendency to fog formation, with consequent increase in industrial, traffic, and domestic accidents. (3) Damage to paint work, building structures, etc., and increased rusting of iron. (4) Increased incidence of bronchitis, pneumonia, lung cancer and emphysema. It is notorious that the death-rate in towns is almost everywhere higher than in the country despite rural areas having less variety of available food, more danger from winter storms, and often poorer medical and nursing care. The effects of air pollution on the respiratory system are best seen when a combination of cold, fog, and atmospheric contamination create the condition of smog – as in the 1952 London smog which killed four thousand people.

To some extent the smoke menace is being countered in heavily populated, developed countries by clean air legislation; but petrol-driven engines are beginning to give out more carbon dioxide than can be re-converted to oxygen and carbon by plant life, and are also giving out highly poisonous carbon monoxide – to such an extent that traffic policemen in Tokyo are now supplied with oxygen equipment for their personal use.

Land pollution. An example of land pollution is excessive use of insecticides: various countries, including Britain, have now banned the widespread use of DDT because of its long-term harmful effects on animals and man. Another example is pollution by radioactive materials: for instance strontium-90 passes to the soil, from it to the grass, thence to cows and their milk, and can in due course interfere with blood cell formation in the human bone marrow. Yet another example is the dumping of obsolete cars and other machinery – not only converting beautiful countryside into an eyesore but also using land that could otherwise be agriculturally productive.

Water pollution. The waste materials from factories, such as mercury compounds from paper mills, have enormously damaged fish life and in some areas have rendered the fish that survive dangerous for human consumption. For instance, in Japan people have died from eating tuna fish with high concentrations of mercury, and similar dangers have been identified in the Great Lakes of America and in Britain in the Bristol Channel. Another growing hazard is oil pollution from leaks from tankers and from accidental collisions. Yet another arises from the discharge of untreated sewage into the sea – very common in coastal towns.

Noise pollution. a form of pollution of which society is only in the process of becoming aware is noise – increasing rapidly through accumulation of population, universal use of the internal combustion engine, and increased use of materials that readily transmit sound.

The case for control of all forms of pollution is strong, but industrialists want their profits and their employees want their wage-packets, while householders like to keep their open fires and their cars. In general, therefore, there is a hostility to anti-pollution measures unless they can be achieved cheaply and preferably by the actions of persons other than ourselves. Yet increasingly air, water and land pollution are coming to constitute one of the world's two most fundamental problems, the other being the related problem of steadily rising population. Legislation alone is not the sole answer. The vast problem of pollution will be solved only by a combination of three things: education, to make people aware of the danger and of the need to accept and even demand control; research, to find measures which can reduce pollution with least damage to industrial efficiency and to personal comfort; and legislation, both to bring into line those who are too selfish to comply unless compelled to do so and to provide financial aid for those who could not otherwise afford to take effective steps for the reduction of pollution.

polycythaemia. Presence of red blood corpuscles in abnormally high quantity. The normal figure is about 5 million per cubic millimetre of BLOOD, and anything above 6.5 million is termed polycythaemia,

Apparent polycythaemia occurs in dehydration, where all bodily fluids including blood are reduced, and therefore the red blood corpuscles are more numerous in any measured quantity of blood. Genuine increase in corpuscles occurs in circumstances of any prolonged deficiency of oxygen, such as is occasioned by living at high altitudes or created by various diseases of the heart and circulation: the body manufactures extra corpuscles to cope with the harder work of carrying sufficient oxygen to the tissues.

Polycythaemia vera is an uncommon condition in which an excess of red cells and a thickening of the blood occur from causes as yet unknown. The disease is found mostly in the second half of life, and often creates headaches, dizziness, lack of concentration, purpling of the face, and enlargement of the spleen. True polycythaemia is one of the very few diseases for which bleeding (the blood-letting so extensively used in the seventeenth and eighteenth centuries) is still employed as treatment, although of course the modern method is insertion of a wide-bore needle into a vein, not vein cutting or application of leeches.

polypus. A tumour attached to a mucous membrane by a stalk. Such tumours occur in the nose, bladder, intestine, and uterus. They are benign (non-cancerous) but may cause trouble by obstruction (e.g., of breathing through the nose) and may very occasionally become cancerous if left. In general they are best surgically removed.

Polyposis is a hereditary tendency to form polyps in the bowel.

polyuria. The state in which an excessive amount of urine is passed. The normal quantity in an adult is about 1.5 litres (2.5 pints) daily, but varies with the amount of liquid drunk and the amount of sweat excreted by the skin. Broadly, patients suffering from polyuria may pass anything from 2 litres (4 pints) daily to the 23 to 27 litres (40 to 50 pints) excreted in some cases of diabetes insipidus.

Polyuria with albumin present in the urine suggests disease of the kidneys. Some of the causes of polyuria without presence of albumin are excessive fluid intake (e.g., the person who drinks a great quantity of beer or a large amount of tea or coffee inevitably passes much urine), nervousness, diabetes mellitus (in which the urine contains sugar), and diabetes insipidus. Since polyuria is essentially a symptom, treatment is to remove the underlying cause.

popliteal fossa. A lozenge-shaped hollow at the back of the knee, bounded by the hamstring muscles above and the calf muscles below.

population and health. The complex interactions of population and health are best considered under two headings: national and international aspects, and local aspects.

National and international aspects. For many thousands of years the population of the world increased very slowly, roughly keeping pace with increased availability of food and other necessities. When the number of mouths to be fed in any country began to exceed the food available for these mouths, the balance was adjusted in one of four ways – by increased deaths from gradual malnutrition or acute famine, by lowered resistance to infections such as plague and malaria, by colonization and development of previously undeveloped land, or by invasion of the territory of a less populous neighbour. Governments had no fears about over-population but dreaded under-population as the forerunner of conquest by a land-hungry invader. Such population stimulants as family allowances are really modern evidences of the persistence of old fears of under-population.

In the nineteenth century more and more of the world's 'wide open spaces' were colonized; and in the last 150 years world population has risen dramatically, to the stage where it is doubling every thirty to thirty-five years. This upsurge is largely the result of the life-saving effects of vaccines, vitamins and antibiotics, and improvements in sanitation, hygiene, antenatal care, child health care, and medical treatment. In England and Wales, for instance, now the third most crowded country in the world (the two most densely populated being Holland and Mauritius) the population rose from under 9 million in 1801 to 29 million in 1861 and 46 million in 1961.

Contraceptive education and facilities and the legalized abortion now available in some countries have not yet arrested the growth. World population is now estimated to have reached the startling total of 4,000 million; in Europe the number of people is still increasing in every country except East Germany, while in North America the increase is very considerable, and in some of the countries of Asia and South America the population is doubling every twenty-six years.

Already many hundreds of millions of people suffer from permanent malnutrition and it seems unlikely – with four-fifths of the land surface of the globe uncultivable – that food supplies can be increased sufficiently for the satisfactory feeding of even the present 4,000 million, far less the 8,000 million anticipated by soon after the year 2000. Moreover, as population increases, more and more land is required for houses, shops, factories, schools, and hospitals, leaving less available for food production. Clearly on the population-food balance alone there are only four possibilities: to find rapidly means of vastly increasing food production; to limit population growth, reducing births as we have already reduced deaths; to accept falling nutritional standards until the balance is adjusted by millions of deaths from malnutrition and from infections of persons with lowered restance; or to resort to the mass murder of war, with the victors – if there are any victors – hoping to secure the bulk of the world's food. The densely populated countries, such as Britain, which import most of their food are particularly badly placed in a world of increasing food shortages.

Even if a method is found of enormously increasing food production, the vast upsurge of population is already producing other shortages. The world's raw materials, such as coal, oil and steel, are being used up at an alarming rate. It is no longer merely the dream of a science fiction writer that, given some means of obtaining food and so remaining alive, our grandchildren may have to revert from the motor car to the horse and trap, and from the aeroplane and steam-ship to the wooden sailing-ship. Excluding, however, the

basic and desperate problem of food production, there are certain elements of hope – increased use of electricity and possibly of nuclear or solar power.

From national and international aspects the fundamental problem confronting humanity is the dual one of limiting population growth and increasing food production.

Local aspects. Local changes of population, especially if sudden, have effects on the structure of the community. A steep increase in the birth-rate for a few years produces dependent children in numbers disproportionate to productive workers and to adults in the caring professions. Prolongation of life, e.g., through prevention or successful treatment of some diseases of maturity, produces a parallel disproportion between veterans and productive or caring adults. The simultaneous occurrence of both of these can result not only in a desperate shortage of nurses, health visitors, midwives, teachers, etc., but also in severe scarcity of agricultural and factory workers. Depopulation, such as occurs where young adults move from a country district to towns, can leave the area of dwindling population with a gross excess of old people. Large scale immigration, whether of nationals or of persons from other countries, can produce a mass of social and cultural problems.

Apart from changes in population, the diseases of an agricultural or fishing community differ appreciably from those of persons mainly employed in commerce, finance and technology. The problems and social and cultural patterns also differ. Hence for successful health education the approach has to be different.

It is often said that a change from a rural to semi-urban community tends to raise living standards, increase amenities, render medical and nursing care more readily available, and therefore benefits the physical and mental health of the people. In general that is true, but the benefits may be very uneven. For instance, as South Africa became a 'developed' country the prosperity and health of the White Africans improved greatly, but only one-tenth of cultivable land was reserved for Black Africans, and as their population grew the reservations became increasingly overcrowded and impoverished.

Rapid increase in the population of large towns, as happened in the period of the Industrial Revolution, produces overcrowding and slum conditions – with prevalence of bronchitis, pneumonia and rheumatism, demoralizing strains on parents trying to maintain standards under impossible conditions, and increase of maladjustment, delinquency, aggression and withdrawal in children affected by the tensions, irritability and despair of the parents. Nevertheless, the detrimental effects of rapid population increase in cities like Birmingham, Manchester and Glasgow in the nineteenth century have been over-estimated: living conditions were by modern standards horrifying, but they were only marginally worse than the insanitary rural hovels of the previous century. Every educated person knows something of the horrors of the Industrial Revolution but many of us have an idealized picture of earlier rural Britain – 'Sweet Auburn, loveliest village of the plain.

Where health and plenty cheered the labouring swain'. Actually the labouring swain lived on a bare subsistence income in a damp, poorly lighted hovel and tramped fifty yards to draw his drinking and washing water from a possibly polluted stream.

On balance the extreme rural area lacks cultural amenities and immediately available medical and nursing services, and the enormous city has inevitable problems of congestion, pollution and insufficient access to open spaces. As nuclear power develops and transport becomes easier, it may well be that industry will no longer have to be located close to coal mines, navigable rivers or railway termini, and that the present sharp distinction between large cities and rural areas may disappear. If these developments mean that industry can be situated wherever people like to live, industrial towns of much less than 30,000 population will be unlikely, because we need sufficient population to justify good secondary schools, public libraries and so forth, and cities of much more than 250,000 will be unnecessary, because that population is sufficient to supply hospital services, municipal theatres, etc. We may well see the development of central cities of 150,000 to 250,000 population and associated peripheral towns of 30,000 to 50,000 inhabitants, all sharing to some degree the present advantages of both urban and rural life.

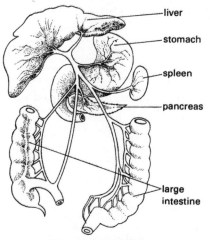

liver

stomach

spleen

pancreas

large intestine

The portal circulation

portal circulation. The passage of blood from the stomach, pancreas, spleen and intestines to the liver by the hepatic portal vein. At the liver gylcogen is extracted for storage before the CIRCULATION OF THE BLOOD continues through the hepatic vein.

port and airport services. Services designed to protect countries from the importation of communicable disease whether conveyed by passengers, crews or cargo. Apart from the general duty of preventing the entrance of infection, port health authorities are responsible for the inspection of imported food, the inspection of ships both for defects of hygiene and for evidence of rat infestation, and the medical inspection of aliens. Authorities responsible for airports have similar duties but also have to be aware of particular risks, such as the arrival of passengers who are incubating an infectious disease but owing to the speed of air travel do not yet show any signs of it, or the inadvertent transport in aircraft of insects harbouring the germs of a particular disease. The modern rarity in developed countries of outbreaks of plague, typhus, yellow fever, cholera and smallpox testifies to the efficiency of port and airport services.

National and international agencies now collaborate effectively on the control of epidemics, the rapid exchange of epidemiological information, the standardization of vital statistics, and in emergencies the provision of medical and nursing aid to countries in danger of being overwhelmed by disease beyond the scope of their normal resources. In particular, 138 countries – almost every nation in the world – are members of the WORLD HEALTH ORGANIZATION.

International regulations, adopted by the World Health Organization in 1951 and periodically revised, seek to give reasonable uniformity and maximum protection against the spread of disease with minimum interference with traffic and trade. An important article of these regulations imposes a duty on the health administration in each country to notify the World Health Organization whenever any part of the country becomes an infected area (and also to indicate when it becomes free from infection). This information is clearly of major significance but it has to be remembered that the information is only as good as the services providing it. Thus if cases of cholera occurring in a particular country are for a week misdiagnosed as dysentery, the port and airport doctors in other countries will for that week be left wholly unaware that persons arriving from the area in question may be in the process of developing cholera.

post-maturity. The condition of an infant whose birth is delayed beyond the normal time for the ending of pregnancy. In such delay there are dangers to the child since the nutriment passing through the placenta may be insufficient, and dangers to the mother especially if the child's bones begin to harden. It is therefore normal practice to induce labour artificially if it does not start within a few days of the expected date.

posture. The position of the body and limbs as a whole. Man's adoption of the erect position has had repercussions which are not wholly to his advantage. While use of the ancestral hind legs for standing and walking has enabled the front legs to be developed for climbing, grasping and throwing, a high incidence of hernia, varicose veins and flat foot is part of the price paid for an upright position.

Correct posture is very important for growth and health but unfortunately bad posture is often initially comfortable, although in due course it does harm by placing stresses and strains on parts of the body that were not intended to bear these burdens.

During the early development of postural defects much can be done by remedial exercises, but a child is apt to be bored by dull repetitive exercises and much better results can be obtained if the exercises are given as a form of interesting recreation and amusement.

Attention should particularly be paid to the posture of the scholarly, unathletic child who ignores the Roman maxim of 'a healthy mind in a healthy body', the abnormally tall boy or girl who so easily develops a stoop, and the short-sighted person whose round shoulders are essentially the result of peering forwards.

potassium. A silvery-white metal, of low density and unusual softness, that oxidizes rapidly in contact with air. The metal does not occur in nature in an uncombined form but potassium compounds are essential MINERAL SALTS for both animal and plant life. One of the things on which the maintenance of human life depends is the correct balance between potassium salts inside cells and sodium salts in the surrounding fluids.

With a normal diet the intake and excretion of potassium are equal at about 2.5 g. per day. Potassium depletion can occur in extensive diarrhoea and vomiting, and potassium excess is found in Addison's disease.

Pott's disease. Tuberculosis of the spine, named after its discoverer, Percival Pott, a London surgeon. The disease was formerly common and was often transmitted by infected milk, with the germ localizing in the spine. Pasteurization of milk and the introduction of tuberculin-tested cattle have made the condition a rarity.

Pott's fracture. See ANKLE.

poultices. Warm, pulpy masses applied to parts of the body to transfer heat in order to reduce inflammation, relieve pain or 'draw' pus from a boil. Nowadays it is customary to use kaolin preparations, such as antiphlogistene, available in tins and ready for application after heating. However, the older bread, mustard and linseed poultices are quite effective.

The mustard poultice is selected here for mention. Take one measure of mustard and five of linseed; mix the mustard into a smooth paste with lukewarm water; pour the linseed, previously kept in a closed tin, into sufficient boiling water to make a smooth paste on stirring; stir the mustard paste smoothly into the linseed paste; spread on linen; apply to the affected part of the body for fifteen minutes; after removing the poultice dry the skin very gently with cotton-wool, dust with powder and cover with wool.

Fomentations. These are applications of cloths which have been heated by being wrung out with hot water (with or without drugs, such as turpentine or laudanum, added to the water). They serve essentially the same purpose as poultices.

prefrontal leucotomy. The operation of cutting nerve fibres in the prefrontal lobes at the front of the brain. The operation, devised by Egas Moniz (1874-1955) of Portugal, had considerable success in relieving some severe mental disturbances. The cutting of the fibres removes certain channels of communication and may end depressive, suicidal or aggressive tendencies. The fibres do not regenerate, so the operation is irreversible; and the person so treated may become rather irresponsible. With the discovery of drugs that act selectively on different portions of the brain, and so produce the effects without the permanency, the operation is now tending to fall into disuse.

pregnancy. The period from conception to labour, lasting for about 39 weeks in the human and for different lengths in animals, up to the 27 months of an elephant. Pregnancy is a natural and physiological state, not a period of invalidism. Despite the occurrence of occasional morning sickness in half the women during the second month, pregnancy is a time when a woman should feel at her best.

Duration of pregnancy. This is usually taken as 273 days, but variations from 240 to 320 days have been recorded, and animal breeders have noted similar proportions of variation. Since the exact date of fertile coitus is seldom known, the expected date of delivery is generally calculated as 280 days from the beginning of the last menstruation. Such calculation itself explains some of the variations in duration, since conception, arbitrarily assumed to occur seven days after the start of menstruation, may actually take place up to ten days earlier (just too late to stop the succeeding menstrual flow) or several days later.

Signs of pregnancy. The commonest presumptive sign is suppression of menstruation, but this is occasionally the result of disease (e.g., tuberculosis) or of fear of pregnancy and very occasionally menstruation continues during the first month of pregnancy. Other presumptive signs include morning sickness (common but far from invariable in the second month); changes in the breast (sensation, fullness, enlargement and pigmentation successively); changes in the abdomen (in particular progressive enlargement); and quickening (the perception by the mother about the fifth month of the movements of the foetus). Absolute diagnosis depends on the feeling and counting of the foetal heart with a special stethoscope, the feeling of the foetal movements or x-ray findings. Since none of these are really practicable before the fourth month, biological tests are much used. The Aschheim-Zondek test, for instance, consists of injecting the patient's urine into an immature female mouse: if the urine contains hormones produced in pregnancy, the ovaries of the mouse become swollen and congested in about four or five days.

Growth of the baby. An ovum fertilized by a spermatozoon is called a zygote. The zygote repeatedly subdivides to form a globular mass of cells which then arrange themselves into an outer layer and an inner cell-mass, separated by fluid. The inner cell-mass develops into the future embryo and the outer wall ultimately becomes the chorion which unites with another sac, to form the amniotic cavity in which the embryo becomes suspended by the body-stalk or future umbilical cord.

Meantime the mucous membrane of the body of the uterus has become thicker and more vascular under hormonal influence and in this the developing ovum becomes embedded. The blood vessels of the chorion are thus brought into relationship with the maternal circulation. At a slightly later stage the blood vessels of the chorion are concentrated at one site opposite the body-stalk to form the placenta, which is supplied with blood from the embryonic circulation. The placenta provides an interchange system between the embryonic and maternal circulation. This stage is reached by about the end of the second month of pregnancy. Simultaneously the inner cell mass has developed into a recognizable embryo, two inches long, and with all its tissues, organs and limbs differentiated. Conventionally it is then referred to as a foetus instead of an embryo.

It should be noted that the placenta also allows infective agents and drugs to cross to the foetal circulation, and so the embryo can be affected by certain diseases such as syphilis or rubella or by toxic agents which can damage its development particularly in the earlier months. X-rays can also have adverse effects.

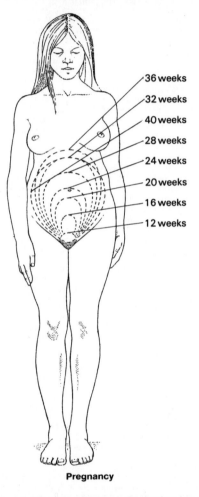

Pregnancy

During the next seven months further intra-uterine growth consists largely of a gradual increase in size and weight. The foetus by its fourth month is about five inches long, ten inches long at five months and about twenty inches long at full-term.

All the materials needed for growth must come from the maternal circulation. A mother therefore needs extra food although quality is more important than quantity. By the end of pregnancy the additional requirement is some 500 Calories per day, and the developing foetus also makes increased demands on her iron and calcium intake which should be supplied by supplements of iron and folic acid and by additional milk.

Health in pregnancy. As already indicated, pregnancy is a physiological state, not a pathological state, and is a time when a woman should be at her best, with every faculty alert and her whole body full of life and energy. Nevertheless it is a very testing time for the woman.

During the nine months of pregnancy her body has to adapt to hormonal changes, to the steady growth of the baby and to an average weight increase (including the weight of the baby) of about 1 kg. (24 lb). In the second and third months of pregnancy she may well have bouts of nausea and sometimes slight actual sickness in the mornings, and may also develop frequency and urgency of urination because of pressure of the enlarging uterus on the bladder: later in pregnancy abdominal pressure may lead to indigestion, constipation, varicose veins, and occasionally piles. Mistaken attempts to 'eat for two' may also lead to indigestion and flatulence. In addition specific diseases of pregnancy may occur, e.g., hyperemesis gravidarum.

While both excessive physical and excessive mental fatigue are undesirable and even dangerous, and while extreme emotional upset in the later months can lead to premature labour, health in pregnancy is best maintained by a continuation of normal activities, coupled with a philosophy of reasonable moderation. Exercise such as walking is useful although the more violent forms of exercise should be avoided. Food should be adequate and nourishing but not excessive: even at the very end of pregnancy a woman needs only about 25 per cent more Calories than before pregnancy. Fresh fruit, green vegetables, milk, butter, cheese and eggs should be plentifully included in the diet; an extra pint of milk daily is a useful source of calcium and provides most of the extra Calories needed. Too much meat is alleged to place a strain on the kidneys. Constipation should be avoided, with mild laxatives used as required. Clothing should not be constricting: belts and garters are not suitable. Adequate rest should be taken and the woman should have plenty of fresh air. Bathing is perfectly permissible but cold baths and very hot baths are undesirable. Sexual intercourse is undesirable during the later months.

Good antenatal care is important and the expectant mother is well advised to attend an antenatal clinic, discussion classes for prospective parents, and classes in psychoprophylaxis (a method of psychological and physical training for childbirth, particularly involving explanation and relaxation); but it cannot be sufficiently emphasized that pregnancy is normally a healthy period, not a time of illness and invalidism.

For false or spurious pregnancy, see PSEUDOCYESIS.

prejudice. An unfavourable opinion formed and maintained without knowledge, justification or adequate reason. Racial, religious and political prejudice is common, e.g., irrational dislike of persons with dark skin, Jews, Roman Catholics or Communists. Sex prejudice is far from rare: in some universities it is almost unknown for a woman to secure a senior post, and in women's professions in the process of being opened to men (e.g., health visiting and nursing) it is sometimes alleged that a good male student tends to receive a lower mark in examinations than a female student of equal merit. Prejudice may even extend to accents and colour of hair.

The term prejudice is also sometimes applied to an unjustified or irrational favourable attitude.

The mildly prejudiced person is usually completely unaware that he is biased, and the strongly prejudiced individual will, if challenged, produce 'justifications' for his attitudes. For instance, he says that his unwillingness to appoint women to senior posts is reasonable because women are usually unfair to their subordinates, but he later casually admits that he has never had close contact with workers responsible to a woman; or he justifies his dislike of Welshmen by saying that they are treacherous, but can produce no examples to justify that belief.

The 'blind spot' normally arises from unconscious factors. In part these originate in childhood and are acquired from parents and early associates, mostly taking the colour of the parental prejudices but occasionally operating in the exactly reverse direction. For the most part however, prejudices derive from the present or recent cultural environment: they are formed through the unconscious influence of friends and work-mates, and are an interesting example of crowd psychology.

A man who becomes aware of his bias, as a prejudice, not as an attitude that he readily justifies, is on the way to overcoming it; but most people remain permanently ignorant either of their deep-rooted dislikes or of the fact that these are irrational.

In health education where the educator is seeking to alter habits and attitudes awareness of the prejudices of the person being taught is vital. Anything that is in danger of running counter to a prejudice has to be tackled subtly and obliquely: it is hopeless to try to alter a person's prejudiced ·attitude by telling him bluntly that he is wrong. It is of course, also important that the educator should try to become aware of his own prejudices. Much health education in the past has been unsuccessful because educators with middle-class attitudes and values have unconsciously sought to impose these on persons with completely different attitudes and values.

premarital conception. While every social group in countries that use the institution of marriage frowns on illegitimacy and imposes penalties that vary from death to social ostracism, the extent of toleration of premarital conception varies enormously. In some rural parts of Scandinavia it was in nineteenth and early twentieth centuries – and to some extent still is – almost a prerequisite for marriage, and in some rural parts of Britain and U.S.A. it is still very common and well tolerated. In many towns it is regarded as quite acceptable in working-class districts so long as marriage follows before the baby is born but is viewed with disapproval in the more affluent or cultured social groups. One British study showed that about 5 per cent of premarital conceptions in first births occurred among professional women, about 25 per cent among wives of manual labourers and about 30 per cent among wives of farm labourers.

Prenuptial conceptions – like illegitimate births – have tended to increase fairly steadily in the period from 1930 to 1970, until around 1970 and 1971 about one-quarter of all first births were allegedly from prenuptial conceptions, as were fully 40 per cent of first births in women under 20 years. These figures may slightly exaggerate the facts, because it is difficult to differentiate a normal birth eight months after marriage (i.e., a premarital conception) and the birth of a slightly premature child the same eight months after marriage (i.e., a post-nuptial conception and premature birth) but the nature of the increase is beyond doubt. There are three possible explanations of the rise over the years: (1) In an increasingly mobile society a girl, away from the influence of parents, deliberately takes the risk of having an illegitimate child to strengthen the likelihood of marriage, believing either that bonds of affection are strengthened by sexual relations or that the man will agree to marriage if a child is on the way. (2) Previous moral and religious conventions are losing their sway and there is less commitment to the old idea of chastity before marriage. (3) With puberty taking place earlier and financial and economic independence arriving later there is a longer period· in which sexual relations may take place, with the possibility either of an illegitimate child or of hasty marriage.

Until recent years there was a broad parallel between prenuptial conceptions and illegitimate births: they were both high or low in the same geographical areas, social classes and age-groups. In the last few years in many districts increasing facilities for contraception, more sex education and reasonably liberal provisions for abortion have combined to cause some fall in the number of illegitimate births – although the fall in numbers is often masked when figures are given as rates per total births, because legitimate births have also decreased – but there has not as yet been a corresponding decline in births following prenuptial conception.

prematurity. Birth occurring appreciably before full term. Since it is generally impossible to ascertain the exact date of conception the convention has been adopted of regarding a baby as premature if its birth weight is less than 2.5 kg. (5.5 lb.). This rough and ready standard is reasonably accurate in cases where the infant at full term would have been expected to weigh between 3 and 3.5 kg. (7 and 8 lb.). Clearly, however, there are many cases in which the arbitrary standard is inaccurate. An infant born to well-built parents from families of above average size might well be premature even though its birth weight was about 3 kg. (7 lb.), whereas if the parents are small by reason of hereditary factors (as opposed to being stunted through poor nutrition or other environmental factors in childhood) the baby might be fully developed although weighing a little less than 2.5 kg. (5.5 lb.).

In some cases the delivery has to be brought on early because of maternal illness, and in other cases premature birth occurs spontaneously. The chance of spontaneous premature birth and the likelihood of early induction of labour becoming necessary are both greatly reduced by good antenatal care.

A premature infant suffers from three main disadvantages. Firstly, a mature infant can do without oxygen for a couple of minutes but the less well equipped premature baby cannot. Hence at the moment of birth, with change from oxygen exchange through the placenta to ordinary respiration, there is increased danger of brain damage. Secondly, protective fat develops only in the last weeks of a normal pregnancy. So a premature baby, lacking this fat, has difficulty in maintaining body heat. The baby should be kept in an incubator at about 24 °C. (75 °F.) or, failing that, in a specially warmed cot protected from all draughts. The baby should not at first be bathed but merely smeared with warm olive oil. Thirdly, since the stomach is small and the infant may be too weak to suck, feeding requires considerable care and patience.

During the first few weeks a premature infant is very vulnerable. Indeed fully one-third of all infant deaths are nowadays ascribed to prematurity. After it has survived the dangerous early weeks, however, it is not at materially greater risk than is a younger mature baby of the same weight or stage of development.

During the first two years or so the prematurity should be remembered in any assessment of the child's intellectual or physical development, e.g., a baby that was a couple of months premature is really only 10 months old at its first birthday. By about three years, however, the fact of prematurity can be forgotten, because the differences between a child of 40 months and another of 38 months (or of 40 months but born two months prematurely) are trivial.

prenatal diagnosis. Ascertainment during pregnancy of whether an unborn child suffers from certain hereditary disorders, with the aim of terminating the pregnancy if the child is abnormal but allowing the pregnancy to continue if the child is healthy. It is alternatively known as amniocentesis.

The method may be used for (1) certain chromosomal disorders (e.g., mongolism, where a mother over the age of 40 years has roughly a one-in-forty chance of giving birth to a handicapped child); (2) certain defects of the spinal cord (e.g., spina bifida, where the mother of a defective child has at least a one-in-ten chance of producing another handicapped child); (3) several diagnosable metabolic disorders; and (4) some severe sex-linked disorders (e.g., haemophilia).

Potential parents at risk may prefer to accept genetic counselling and family avoidance but if anxious to have a healthy child if possible, can be offered analysis of the amniotic fluid at about the sixteenth week of pregnancy on the understanding that they will accept termination of pregnancy if the examination of the fluid shows that the child is defective.

The procedure (called amniocentesis) is to withdraw about 10 ml. of amniotic fluid under a local anaesthetic, and then culture cells from the fluid to study the chromosomes (e.g., for the extra chromosome of mongolism) or examine the fluid for the presence of particular proteins (e.g., the alpha-foetoprotein of spina bifida). Diagnosis is not normally practicable before fifteen weeks, and is not yet possible at all for some genetic conditions, such as cystic fibrosis and phenylketonuria. The withdrawal of the fluid normally causes little discomfort, but very rarely quite serious complications ensue such as maternal haemorrhage, septicaemia and premature labour.

A major advance in 1974 in respect of spina bifida was the finding of alpha-foetoprotein in the maternal blood serum. There are occasional 'false positives', so a mother with the protein in her serum should be offered amniocentesis before the pregnancy is actually terminated.

The procedure is quite expensive in staff time – discussion with a health visitor or general practitioner, discussion with a geneticist, half an hour of the time of an obstetrician and a nurse (for the withdrawal of the fluid), considerable laboratory work, etc.; but the cost in time and money is trivial compared, for instance, with that of caring for many years for a partially paralysed, incontinent, mentally retarded victim of spina bifida.

presbyacusis. Diminution of hearing as age advances. The process starts in adolescence; persons of 17 or 18 years are too old to hear very high-pitched sounds that were perfectly audible to them several years earlier. As age increases more and more high-pitched sounds are unheard and in later life there may be difficulty in distinguishing some consonants, although vowels are still well heard.

In many cases of deafness in the elderly the trouble is simply wax in the ears, and softening with a suitable lubricant followed by gentle syringing will restore reasonably normal hearing. In other cases a hearing aid is needed.

presbyopia. Decreased ability to focus the eyes as age advances. From the age of about 40 or 45 the lens becomes less elastic and it is more and more difficult for the person to obtain a clear view of near objects. Distance vision remains good but spectacles are required for reading and sewing.

preservation of food. Maintenance of the nutritive value and palatability of foods, and prevention of their decomposition by application of heat, extraction of moisture, subjection to cold, or addition of harmless preservatives. Deterioration of food is occasioned essentially by bacteria, yeasts and moulds. In general these thrive in conditions of moisture and warmth, but their growth is inhibited by extreme cold, and they are killed by extreme heat and by various chemicals. Hence the importance of the various methods mentioned above. Whatever method is used the foods to be preserved should be fresh and wholesome at the start of the process.

Sterilization requires a temperature of over 82 °C (180 °F) for only a few seconds for a liquid (e.g., milk) but for quite a number of minutes for solid food (where the heat has to penetrate effectively to the centre of the solid). Drying involves both removal of moisture and slow application of heat. Freezing stops bacterial growth, so that most foods can safely be kept for up to a week in an ordinary domestic refrigerator at about -16 °C. (4 °F). or for many months in a deep-freeze refrigerator at about -18 °C (-1 °F). Common preservatives include sugar (as in jam making), vinegar (as in pickling) and salt (as in the salting of beef or herring). Canning, bottling, refrigeration and so on do not reduce food values except in respect of vitamin c (destroyed both by heat and by oxidation) and to a smaller extent some of the other vitamins.

One of the biggest advances in the history of mankind is the discovery and application of methods of preserving food – so that foods can be stored from years of plenty to cover years of poor crops and perishable foods can be transported to distant markets. Without preservation of food small towns could have developed, with fresh meat, fish and vegetables brought in daily from the adjacent countryside and coast, but the growth of large cities would have been impossible. Similarly, without some means of storing food for the winter and spring mankind would have been restricted to a small tropical strip of the universe and even there would have been liable to destruction by famine in years of poor crops.

preventable diseases. When Lady Mary Wortley Montague (1689-1762), followed more scientifically by Edward Jenner (1749-1823), introduced vaccination against smallpox which had previously killed as many as one tenth of all children, when James Lind (1716-1794) kept an entire ship's company free from scurvy by supplying them with lemon juice, and when explorers of then unknown parts of the world avoided malaria by dosing themselves with quinine or alcohol, a new concept was added to medicine, the concept of preventing diseases. Yet perhaps it was rather the development of an old concept, for Hippocrates in *Airs, Waters and Places* had shown some awareness of the relations between environment and disease, the Romans had drained marshes to prevent malaria, the isolation of lepers had begun as early as 583 A.D., and the Persian-Arab civilization had possessed some slight insight into prevention; but for fully a thousand years prevention was almost forgotten.

Even a hundred years ago the most enlightened of our ancestors thought that a minority of diseases might ultimately be preventable. Today we recognize that the majority of diseases fall into that category. Perhaps by the end of this century there will remain only a handful of diseases not yet preventable.

> Apart from the degenerations of later life, most diseases are preventable, e.g., by genetic guidance, antenatal care, attention to emotional and physical health of child, immunization against infections, good diet but avoidance of obesity, adequate exercise, suitable recreations, avoidance of cigarette smoking and moderation in all things.

Preventable diseases are so numerous that only a few groups can here be selected for mention.

Infections. Until the middle of the twentieth century these were by far the greatest killers of mankind. Plague had several times destroyed a quarter of the population of Europe; malaria was unquestionably the biggest killing disease in the world; typhoid was the commonest fever of the developed countries in the nineteenth century and even in the earliest years of this century; and as late as 1941 Scotland – a relatively small country – had over ten thousand cases of diphtheria and 517 deaths from that disease.

Some of the preventive measures introduced in recent decades have been: (1) eradication of food-borne infections by provision of pure water and uncontaminated food, with the result that typhoid and cholera have virtually disappeared from developed countries; (2) destruction of the breeding grounds of insects carrying infection, the most dramatic example being the removal of yellow fever from Havana and the Panama area, but the world-wide reduction of malaria is perhaps even more significant; (3) production of vaccines and education of the public about their desirability, with subsequent enormous reductions in smallpox, diphtheria, poliomyelitis and many other infections; and (4) virtual eradication of the 'captain of the men of death', tuberculosis, by a combination of better nutrition, better housing, follow-up of contacts BCG vaccination and mass radiography.

To mention two other examples, ophthalmia neonatorum, a formerly common cause of blindness, has responded to routine instillation of drops in the eyes of babies, and rubella (German measles) – which when occurring in expectant mothers caused a high proportion of congenital defects in their offspring – is in the process of being eradicated by vaccination and public education about the need for vaccination. A few infections are not yet preventable. Gonorrhoea (unless we can prevent it by sex education and moral education) and the common cold are examples, but most infections are now deemed preventable in developed countries, although it has to be remembered that health education about immunization and about food hygiene becomes more difficult as the particular preventable diseases become more rare.

Diseases of nutrition. Lind used lemon juice to prevent scurvy some 160 years before Szent-Györgyi isolated vitamin C, and Goldberger established pellagra as a nutritional disease considerably before the existence of a group of B vitamins was known. It is, however, essentially in the last fifty years that improved knowledge of nutritional needs, better available food supplies, identification of vitamins and other trace substances, education of the public about diet and budgeting, and the addition of minerals and vitamins to certain foodstuffs have combined virtually to eliminate from highly developed countries such diseases as rickets, scurvy, iron deficiency anaemia and simple goitre. We still occasionally find nutritional disorders in the very old, especially if living alone, or in immigrants still using a diet suitable only for a climate with greater sunshine and more warmth; and in the underdeveloped countries many deficiency diseases (e.g., kwashiorkor) are still very common. However, given a proper balance between population and food production so that enough food is quantitatively and qualitatively available per head of population, and given adequate health education of the public about dietetic needs at different ages, virtually all nutritional diseases can now be prevented.

Most diseases of pregnancy, labour and the puerperal state. Antenatal care, better

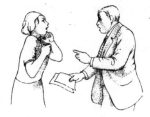

domestic tension

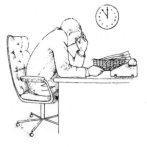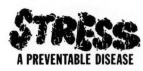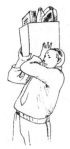

STRESS
A PREVENTABLE DISEASE

overwork   unusual exertion

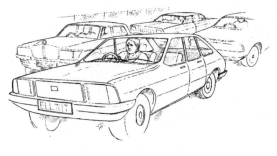

travel strain

nutrition, health visiting and midwifery services, and better obstetrics together reduced maternal mortality (on figures for England and Wales) from about 6 per thousand births a hundred years ago to less than 3 in 1941 (before the advent of antibiotics) and to 0.2 in 1971; and simultaneously infant deaths fell from 158 per thousand births in 1871 to 60 in 1941 and 18 in 1971, with most Scandinavian towns and a few British towns reaching a figure of about 12 per thousand. In other words, deaths of mothers through causes associated with pregnancy or childbirth have fallen from 60 to 2 per ten thousand pregnancies (a fall to one-thirtieth) and infant deaths have fallen from 16 per hundred births to less than 2 (a fall to less than one-eighth). In terms of lives saved these reductions rival the savings from infections and utterly outstrip the saving of lives from any forms of medical or surgical treatment.

Home accidents. These were formerly the commonest cause of death from 1 year to 21 years and a very common cause of death and of disability in the elderly. Recent work in Aberdeen, Stirlingshire, London and Helsinki has demonstrated that by studying the causal factors operating in different social groups and age groups and then educating persons at risk or persons responsible for children or veterans at risk, the incidence of home accidents serious enough to need medical treatment can be reduced by more than one-third. Particular value is placed upon home visits and one-to-one discussions by the health visitor. There is some evidence that the same techniques can be successfully applied to the reduction of traffic accidents and industrial accidents.

Hereditary diseases. It is becoming possible to identify many carriers of serious genetic defects (such as Huntington's chorea, spina bifida, deaf-mutism, the main variety of mongolism, and the main type of schizophrenia) and to reduce their transmission by a combination of genetic counselling, health education and contraceptive facilities.

Of the five groups so far mentioned it should be noted that the first two could be virtually eliminated and the last three very greatly reduced, although some home accidents would still occur and some developmental abnormalities would still take place.

Problems in the process of being solved. The psychoneuroses, aggressive behaviour and crimes of violence are very common today, and their treatment is unsatisfactory. For example Eysenck produced evidence in 1952 and again in 1965 purporting to show that neurotics receiving treatment by psychotherapy responded very little better than neurotics not receiving such treatment, and Brown demonstrated in 1968 that multiproblem families 'helped' by intensive social case-work were only marginally better than parallel families not receiving such aid. However, simultaneously with evidence of the limitations of clinical and social treatment there have appeared strong indications of the value of prevention. There are indications, for example, that aggressive behaviour and violence are often a response to arbitrary frustration and attacks on a child's self-esteem, and can be prevented by a warm, affectionate relationship with parents and associates. Delinquency on the whole appears to be caused by parental rejection, harsh or inconsistent discipline or broken homes, so that it can be reduced by campaigns to make every child a wanted child, by education of parents and prospective parents about child management, and by measures for the prevention of marital breakdown. It begins to seem quite likely that education of children, prospective parents and parents of young children may very substantially reduce the psychoneuroses, aggression, violence, delinquency and maladjustment.

Again, although man is mortal and diseases of old age can be postponed rather than avoided, there are enormous possibilities for the reduction of diseases at present associated with middle-life and the earlier portion of old age. We are beginning to understand, for example, that coronary thrombosis is in large measure caused by excessive stress, over-eating, heavy smoking and lack of exercise, and that all four factors are largely under human control. Again, we are in the process of realizing that chronic bronchitis – the 'English disease' – can in most cases be prevented by a combination of positive and negative factors: good nutrition, avoidance of obesity (both in the middle-aged who might develop bronchitis this year and in the child whose bronchitis may be half a century ahead), clean air, avoidance of cigarette smoking, warm and well-ventilated houses, immunization against diseases liable to produce effects on the respiratory system, and use of clothing that affords adequate protection against the elements.

The limitations of prevention. Although a few conditions so far afford scant possibilities of either prevention or treatment – with the common cold perhaps the disease for which there is least justifiable hope – it seems likely that the next half century will be the era in which disease as a whole, mental and physical, becomes recognized as preventable; that admission to hospital before the age of 75 or 80 will become increasingly infrequent; and that, within the next seventy years the occurrence of death in a person under the age of 75 years may well be so unusual as to warrant a special enquiry when it occurs. If this last suggestion at first seems fantastic, it may be noted that our grandparents would have thought the idea of a special enquiry into all deaths associated with pregnancy and childbirth utterly impracticable, and yet we already have it. It is also worth noting that long-term prevention of disease (e.g., reduction of senile psychosis sixty years later by fostering a child's capacity to form friends and develop fresh interests) is a science only still in its infancy.

Yet perhaps we need some moderation even in the application of measures designed to prevent mental and physical disorders. Perhaps the continued progress of mankind demands that some youngsters with personal unhappiness should challenge the beliefs and standards of their elders; that some adolescents should endanger life and limb, whether by attempting to climb an unscalable cliff or by experimenting with a new drug; and that some middle-aged people should continue to be regarded as eccentrics. PREVENTIVE MEDICINE has enormous potentialities for human health and happiness, but human progress may require that some people should not fully share in that health and happiness but should feel what Shelley called 'divine discontent'. Every health worker rightly aims at decreasing illness and improving well-being, but to some extent it is the unhappy, dissatisfied people – the people on the verge of neuroticism – who make scientific discoveries, produce works of art or change the patterns of human life.

preventive medicine. The science that seeks to reduce disease by identifying, removing or altering the causes or by modifying the response of the person on whom these causes operate. Preventive medicine is gradually evolving its own techniques and methods but was originally a combination of applied physiology, psychology, biology, sociology and medicine, with the persuasive methods on which it has increasingly relied taken at first from education and commerce.

Most people appreciate the general need for health to be improved and for PREVENTABLE DISEASES to be prevented. For instance, the World Health Organization states in the preamble to its constitution that 'The enjoyment of the highest available standard of health is one of the fundamental rights of every human being, without distinction of race, religion, political belief, economic or social condition' and also that 'the health of all peoples is fundamental to the attainment of peace and security and is dependent upon the fullest co-operation of individuals and States'. Again most intelligent people accept the importance of maintaining health and eliminating preventable diseases in individuals and families, because illness produces pain, disability, lowered morale, reduced earning capacity and in some cases untimely death.

Many people also understand our need for better health as a nation, since illness on a large scale hampers industrial production and damages the international balance between imports and exports, lowers the efficiency of the armed forces, and reduces the standard of living both through lessened productive work and through the heavy burden of medical and supporting services. In connection with the last point it is worth noting that in Britain in the early 1970s the loss of productive work through illness was each year about fifty times the loss through strikes and lockouts.

Yet terms like 'cure', 'therapy' and 'surgical operation' have such glamour by comparison with the more prosaic 'improvement of health' or 'prevention of illness' that even the words for well-being and its improvement periodically change their meaning. 'Health' (by derivation and original meaning akin to 'wholesomeness') is nowadays often employed to mean merely 'services for the prevention, diagnosis, treatment relief and support of illness', with the major part of Britain's 'health' expenditure devoted to treatment of illnesses that already exist. 'Sanitary science', although initially embracing all human well-being, has been increasingly narrowed to the environmental aspects of hygiene. 'Hygiene' itself, despite its original meaning of 'a healthy mind in a healthy body' has been reduced, unless clumsily prefixed by an adjective (as in mental hygiene), to mere cleanliness of the person and the surroundings. 'Public health' – which a great Prime Minister, Disraeli, called 'the foundation upon which reposes the happiness of the people and the strength of the nation' – has gradually been narrowed from the combined concern of the clinical doctor, the preventive doctor, the health visitor, the health education officer, the dietitian, the midwife, the nurse and the sanitary inspector to simply the province of the last of these. 'Epidemiology', although strictly concerned with the occurrence, age and occupational distribution, causes and prevention of all mental and physical diseases, is still in the minds of most people associated with 'epidemics' and the infectious diseases. 'Social medicine' carries, quite wrongly, political implications and also conveys the impression that social factors outweigh psychological and physiological factors. And the newest term in Britain, 'Community Medicine' is already beginning to imply mainly the administration of hospitals (for the sick), health centres (largely for the investigation of persons who consider themselves sick) and other services for treatment and support of those who are ill.

'Preventive medicine' is an unsatisfactory term for two reasons. Firstly 'preventive' is far too narrow. Improving, fostering and maintaining emotional, social and physical health are quite as important as the preventive aspects, though strict separation of 'promotion of health' from 'prevention of disease ' is not easy: we provide a good diet for a child to foster its growth and development, but incidentally the adequacy of calcium and vitamin D in the diet prevents rickets; and we give the same child plenty of warm, demonstrated affection, security and reasonable freedom to explore and make decisions in order to improve mental and emotional development, and we incidentally do much to prevent maladjustment, delinquency and sexual deviance. Secondly, 'medicine' seems to imply that the work is mainly that of doctors, whereas perhaps the biggest contributions can be made – and in part have already been made – by workers other than doctors, e.g., health visitors, health education officers, school teachers, personnel officers, and so on. However, until a better term is devised for the systematic improvement of psychosocial and physical health and the reduction of disability and disease, 'preventive medicine' is perhaps the best available phrase.

Preventive medicine can be considered as consisting partly of investigation and partly of application of remedial measures. Firstly, why do certain illnesses occur in particular races, in particular social groups, in particular age groups, in particular occupations, under particular circumstances of stress or grief, in people who are geographically or socially isolated, or in people subjected to certain environmental or climatic hazards? Secondly, what measures can we devise to reduce particular diseases or to improve the mental or physical health of potential victims, and how do we induce the people involved to make use of these measures?

On the investigating side the term includes epidemiology, i.e., the study of disease in the mass and of the factors that may lead to the development of a particular mental, psychosomatic or physical illness or to its avoidance, and to the creation of patterns of good health. To some extent the whole of the behavioural and biological sciences can be considered as being included. To take a single example, the study of tuberculosis from the aspect of preventive medicine would include investigation of the following factors: the causal organism (leading among other things to the production of the vaccine, BCG; the means of destroying the organism (leading for instance to pasteurization of milk); its methods of spread (leading to isolation of cases, contact tracing and the extermination of infected cattle); the conditions favouring spread (leading to improvement of housing and attention to nutrition): the age-groups most affected (leading to the use of BCG for older school children); reservoirs of infection (leading to mass x-ray campaigns to identify mild but infectious cases in elderly persons); psychological factors that lower resistance (leading to careful attention to persons recently bereaved); the social groups most affected (leading, where staff and funds are limited, to concentration on the less affluent portions of society); and the motivational factors and techniques which make one form of health education effective for a particular group of persons but less effective for another group. Clearly the investigating side includes a great deal of evaluation of methods both of prevention and of treatment. For instance, sticking to the same example of tuberculosis, is the success rate of the moderately serious operation of removal of an affected lobe of a lung sufficient to justify the use of that treatment as against artificial collapse of a lung (pneumothorax) until it heals spontaneously; or is a mass radiography campaign to find undetected infectious persons financially justifiable in a town where the incidence of tuberculosis has fallen to one case for every ten thousand inhabitants?

On the application side the old classification into personal and community aspects is unsatisfactory because of enormous overlap. It is probably better to classify simply into measures for promotion of better health and measures for prevention of illness, although even these overlap.

Promotion of good health includes both motivation and HEALTH EDUCATION. Motivation is important because, once we have passed beyond the fairly elementary stage at which improvements can be affected by legislation, co-operation of individuals is essential. In a democratic society even legislation – for clean air, or clean food, or to reduce road accidents by measures relating to speed, alcohol or seat-belts – requires the consent of the public; and legislation can hardly ensure that parents do not over-discipline or over-protect their children or bully or cajole them to excessive mental efforts, or that middle-aged people do not eat too much or smoke excessively or try too hard to 'keep up with the Joneses'. Motivation is vital because successful education for physical or emotional health is impossible unless the person to be educated actually desires improved health; many people, including many who are apparently well-educated in other fields, make the mistake of regarding good or bad health as a matter of luck and as unrelated to their previous actions.

Once a person desires to improve his own health or that of his children, health education becomes possible. It has essentially three broad aspects: individual discussion (as between health visitor and client or doctor and patient), group teaching (as with school classes or discussion groups for prospective parents) and use of mass media (e.g., pamphlets, press articles, TV interviews, posters and exhibitions). Three points should perhaps be noted in connection with education for health. Firstly, in respect of many common causes of illness most adults and older children know the facts (e.g. the relationship between stress and coronary thrombosis or between cigarettes and chronic bronchitis) so that what is needed is not statements of the facts but unobtrusive persuasion to alter attitudes and behaviour. Secondly, the subjects that the public wish to discuss are not necessarily those on which the health educator thinks they need enlightenment, e.g , in a district in which food hygiene is poor, parents may arrive in crowds to discuss prevention of delinquency but ignore a meeting on food handling. Thirdly, in the semi-educated, critical, argumentative community of today people are prepared to discuss subjects and to form their own conclusions but are wholly unwilling to be told dogmatically what to do.

The other large branch of the application side of preventive medicine, namely prevention of physical and mental disease, can be considered under various overlapping headings. Specific prevention (aimed at the actual and fairly certain removal of risk of a particular disease) includes such things as inducing parents to provide a child with enough calcium and vitamin D so as to prevent rickets, or persuading them to have the child immunized against diphtheria. Presumptive prevention (acting on the highly probable) may be exemplified by decreasing the chance of maladjustment by permissive feeding, lack of stress on toilet training and wise handling of a child's early aggression. Relative prevention (arresting of disease in an early stage) includes, for instance, contact-tracing to detect early cases of tuberculosis. Prevention of relapse has an obvious meaning but has social as well as clinical connotations, e.g., a family rescued from threat of eviction for rent arrears may be in danger of relapse unless the causes of the arrears are investigated and removed.

As indicated under PREVENTABLE DISEASES the majority of ailments are now regarded as potentially or actually preventable. Hence preventive medicine (including its health promotion aspects) is undertaken by health workers from many professions and is in process of becoming the biggest branch of the health and disease services.

However, there is still a long way to go before this happens. On recent British figures the country's health and welfare services cost £2,700 million a year, of which approximately £1,400 millions were expended on hospital services (almost wholly curative and palliative, and employing nearly 800,000 persons), with £335 millions spent on social services (mainly supportive), £238 millions on pharmaceutical services, and smaller sums on general practitioner, local health authority and general dental services.

priapism. Persistent and painful erection of the penis unaccompanied by sexual stimulation. The term derives from Priapus, the Greek God of fertility and procreation. The condition is sometimes due to a blood clot in the veins of the erectile tissue of the penis; sometimes it is a symptom accompanying stone in the bladder or urethra; it is occasionally a result of gonorrhoea, and has been known to occur, without other apparent cause, after prolonged sexual activity. Whatever the cause, the organ becomes woodenly hard, painful and extremely sensitive, and there may be difficulty in passing urine. Treatment varies with the cause, ranging from sedative drugs to anticoagulants.

prickly heat. An itchy rash of small watery blisters and red pimples, due to blocking of sweat glands, occurring through excessive perspiration in humid, tropical conditions, and affecting particularly the neck, face, chest, back, armpits and thighs. The rash usually disappears slowly after the body cools, but bathing – without soap – may help, as may the application of a dusting power. In climatic conditions conducive to prickly heat alcohol and heavy meals should be avoided, especially by a newcomer in his first month or so, clothing should be light and porous, and the person at risk should endeavour to keep cool, e.g., by avoiding needless exertion and moving at a slow pace.

primary. There are two uses of this term. (1) The initial defect or disease from which may arise 'secondary' or subsequent trouble, e.g., the primary focus of cancer is in one part of the body but unless promptly treated it may lead to secondaries elsewhere. (2) The main disease from which a person is suffering or the main factor in his treatment, with the implication that other diseases or factors are subsidiary and less important.

primipara. A woman who has given birth to a child for the first time, in contrast to a multipara, the mother of more than one child. In recent years, however, some medical writers have tended to employ the term for a woman who is bearing her first child. Strictly such a woman is a primigravida and does not become a primipara until after the birth.

private practice. Medical, dental or other treatment provided outside any National Health Service and for which the patient pays directly. Some aspects of private practice are almost universally accepted and virtually non-controversial. Others are highly controversial.

The points below apply specifically to Britain but similar problems occur in various countries.

General practitioners and private practice. Discounting a tiny and diminishing number of general practitioners who remain outside the NHS and treat only fee-paying patients, GPs receive fixed payments for all persons on their National Health Service lists, are debarred from charging these persons for any service coming within the terms of the NHS, but are otherwise free to undertake private work. This falls mainly into two groups. (1) A GP may provide and charge for any service – even to a person on his list – that is outside the National Health Service: examples are the supplying of a medical certificate for an insurance company or the giving of a form of vaccination that the patient desires but that is not nationally advised. (2) A GP can provide and charge for any medical advice and treatment for a person not on his list, irrespective of whether the person is or is not on the list of another doctor, although ethical problems may arise if the person is on the panel of somebody else. The provision of services outside the NHS is fairly small, because most needed advice and treatment are included in the NHS, and is fairly non-controversial. The provision of private medical care for a person not on the GP's list occurs mostly in the case of people who seek to avoid the inconvenience of visiting the consulting room and are prepared to pay for the time the doctor spends in visiting them at home: it is analogous with the position of a parent who elects to send his child to a public school rather than to a free local authority school. Such private practice is tending to decrease in an era of inflation, and is rendered more difficult by the creation of primary additional payment for visiting someone for whom the doctor receives private fees.

Consultants and private practice. A very few consultants are wholly outside the NHS, see only private patients and have no access to hospitals; if their patients need institutional treatment it is given in nursing homes with medical, nursing and other staff outside the NHS. Nearly all consultants, however, work within the NHS and are paid for their national work either on a full-time or on a part-time basis. Where a consultant is full-time no question of private practice normally arises. Roughly half of all consultants work on a part-time basis, being remunerated for perhaps eight sessions weekly in the NHS and free to treat patients privately in the rest of their time. Where a patient receiving private care from a consultant is treated in a nursing home outside the NHS little controversy arises; but as medical and surgical procedures, diagnostic and curative, become more complex it grows increasingly difficult for nursing homes to provide bacteriological and biochemical services or highly skilled, specialized nursing services of a standard equal to that of hospitals. Where controversy becomes acute is over the situation that a consultant who sees a patient privately can have him admitted to a pay-bed in a hospital, the patient being responsible not only for the consultant's bill but also for hospital charges which – varying with the type of hospital – average about £100 a week. Approximately five per cent of adults in Britain are members of insurance schemes that wholly or partially cover the cost of such treatment.

Supporters of this form of private practice claim it saves the country money, since the state would otherwise have to pay for the patient's treatment; that a patient who desires to have his operation at a time suitable to himself and to have a private room and a telephone is entitled to spend his money on these things; and that the existence of private practice in hospital gives the consultant more freedom than in a purely salaried service. Opponents of the system argue that it is mainly used for queue-jumping, e.g., that a private patient needing a tonsillectomy or a ·hernia repair will receive it in a fortnight whereas a public patient may remain for months on a waiting list; that nurses, junior doctors and paramedical staff have to treat the private patients – often more clamorous in their demands for attention – without any extra remuneration, simply for the benefit of the consultants; that if a consultant gives better treatment to fee-paying patients than to others, he is not giving of his best to the latter; and that if the consultant's care of private and public patients is equal, there is little reason other than queue-jumping for a person to pay fees.

The crucial long-term factor would appear to be the persisting national shortage of professional staff, especially nursing staff: not only is there a serious and gradually increasing shortage of nurses, but more than one third of Britain's nurses are from underdeveloped countries – people who come to Britain for nursing education and work for a few consolidating years before returning to their own countries – and this source of supply is diminishing as these countries establish their own schools of nursing. Given a continuing shortage such that some hospital beds must remain closed and some patients must wait a long time for necessary treatment, it is difficult to argue for the full retention of the private bed system, since a patient in a private room and with higher expectations of care inevitably occupies a higher proportion of nursing time. Possible solutions appear to be: (1) the gradual phasing out of private treatment in hospital, with part-time consultants able to treat private patients only in nursing homes after a period of transition; (2) extension of the system of fees for private patients to nurses, junior doctors and paramedical staff, so that private practice becomes in effect rationed by price; or (3) an attempt to continue on present lines, possibly with a slight reduction of the number of private beds, but with rigorous safeguards against queue-jumping.

problem children. A rather outmoded term to describe 'difficult' or 'maladjusted' or 'highly strung' children. See BEHAVIOUR DISORDERS, and CHILD GUIDANCE.

problem families. Families whose habits, behaviour, values and ways of life fall appreciably below those of the community in which they live. They have to be differentiated on the one hand from eccentrics who depart appreciably from ordinary families in one or two important respects and on the other hand from families with only one or two serious problems (e.g., illness, or lack of money) which respond easily to treatment.

In a true problem family the problems are so multiple that a worker hardly knows where to begin to help, and there is not so much an unwillingness to respond to treatment as a tendency to relapse as soon as there is a temporary cessation of help. A typical problem family shows most of the following characteristics: the house is very sparsely furnished, with carpets, rugs, table cloths and armchairs unknown luxuries and coats often replacing blankets as covering of beds; the house is filthy and generally smells; there are often unrepaired broken windows and blocked water-closets; uneaten food tends to remain on the table, with children, cats and flies having free access to it; there are no set times for meals; budgeting is non-existent, with protein foods mostly bought and eaten in the two days after the week's income is received and cheaper foods used for the rest of the week; the garden is a wilderness; both adults and children are unclean, poorly clothed and often lice-infested; the adults have a bad work record; the children miss much schooling, partly from many minor ailments and partly from truancy; and yet the children – dirty, unsuitably fed and with no regular bed times – are often both loved and happy. Debts are numerous and rent arrears the rule, not the exception.

Booth called them the 'submerged tenth' (although numerically they are nowadays nearer the submerged hundredth) and Blacker described them as the 'social problem group'.

Causes are multiple, probably the commonest being a sort of emotional and social immaturity: the adults often behave very much as children of 10 or 11 years might behave if left unsupervised for long periods. Other causal factors include low intelligence, over-large and unspaced families, prolonged illness of one or both parents, and housing so inferior that it would tax the ability of a normal family to maintain standards. Carelessness with money plays a bigger part than lack of money: a problem family does not improve when its main bread-winner obtains a well-paid job, and often such a family forgets to collect allowances, such as pensions or unemployment allowance. Alcohol is seldom an important factor: the available money has all 'disappeared' a couple of days after it has been received.

Punishment is rarely effective. For any hope of even partial success treatment has to begin with helping the family to meet its material needs and so gaining their confidence. Thereafter the worker, now accepted as a family friend, can try to induce the family to collaborate, e.g., in cleaning or decorating the house. The Family Service Units, a Quaker organization, have had a measure of success in rehabilitating some problem families. Training homes where mothers can learn cooking and budgeting have also claimed some successes. Family planning advice by health visitors and readily acceptable contraceptive facilities have sometimes broken the vicious circle of ineptitude and procreation; and specialized home helps have been used in some areas. In general, however, these families remain a constant source of work and worry for health visitors, social workers and environmental health officers. A worker who is both enthusiastic and efficient will be lucky to secure an apparent response rate of 20 per cent, and half of these will relapse when the frequency of visiting diminishes.

It is sometimes argued that the work on problem families is so unrewarding that they should simply be left, or perhaps that the children should be taken into care and the adults left, although in that case further children will probably be produced. Unfortunately, however, one problem family can damage a neighbourhood, lowering the value of adjacent houses, spreading weeds to adjacent gardens and causing infection or infestation in work-mates or school-mates. Hence continued treatment of these families is essential.

The most fruitful preventive measures would appear to be sustained education about family planning and oral contraceptives, teaching of children about child care and home economics, and early identification and treatment of incipient problem families.

proctitis. Inflammation of the rectum. It usually occurs along with itching of the anus and may be due to threadworms, fungal infections, louse infestation or allergy. It may also occur in association with diabetes or with inflammation of the colon. Treatment varies with the cause, but the application of a towel soaked in warm water often relieves the symptoms and the avoidance of constipation usually helps.

progesterone. A female sex hormone secreted by the corpus luteum which develops each month in the ovary at the site from which an ovum has been released. The hormone stimulates the development of the uterus and prepares it for the implantation of the fertilized ovum. If pregnancy occurs progesterone prevents further menstruation and the release of more ova. If pregnancy does not occur the secretion of the hormone stops in a few days.

Because of its action in preventing the release of ova, progesterone is one of the basic elements in oral contraceptive pills. The hormone is also useful in the treatment of threatened or habitual miscarriage.

prognosis. A prediction of the probable future course and outcome of a disease. The prediction is based partly on the history of the disease in other people, partly on the previous health and constitution of the patient, partly on the drugs available and partly on the patient's response to these drugs. The antibiotics have enormously improved the prognosis in many diseases formerly highly dangerous to life.

progressive muscular atrophy. A disease characterized by progressive wasting of the muscles, most frequently the muscles of the arms, associated with degenerative changes in the central nervous system. The condition, commonest at 30 to 50 years, often causes paralysis within a few months, but in quite a number of cases there are long stationary periods each followed by a further deterioration. The cause is as yet unknown, no effective treatment or method of prevention has been devised, and so far all that can be done is to maintain the general health of the patient, e.g., by massage and passive movements.

projection. Unconscious reading into the minds of others of feelings, opinions and desires which we ourselves experience, e.g., blaming others for our own guilt or failure, or attributing to others our own stinginess or untidiness. Essentially projection is a defence mechanism which helps us to maintain our conception of our own dignity and merit, but it can lead to considerable bias in our judgment of others.

prolapse. Any protrusion or downward displacement of an organ. The term is most frequently used for downward displacement of the rectum or the uterus.

Prolapse of the rectum, with protrusion of a piece of bowel through the anus, is not uncommon in children and sometimes occurs in adults in association with haemorrhoids. In most cases replacement is possible without surgical operation.

Prolapse of the uterus, common in women who have given birth to several children, is usually a delayed result of injury during childbirth, e.g., stretching or tearing of the supporting muscles or ligaments. Possible lines of treatment include the fitting and wearing of a ring pessary, surgical reconstruction, and removal of the uterus.

Prolapse of an intervertebral disc is usually called SLIPPED DISC.

prontosil. Prontosil was the first drug found to have a specific effect on acute bacterial infections when administered by mouth. The sulphonamides have been developed from it and have taken its place.

prophylaxis. The medical term for prevention of disease. While prophylaxis may be anything from a vitamin tablet to a course of exercises or a complete reorganization of a person's way of life, the term is often used specifically for three types of preventive measures: (1) immunization and vaccination (specific prophylaxis of various infections); (2) the wearing of a condom and subsequent douching (prophylaxis of venereal disease and also of conception); and (3) teeth cleaning (dental prophylaxis).

proprietary medicines. Patent medicines, with undivulged constituents and often claiming remarkable curative or preventive powers, were formerly very common in virtually all countries. They were intensely disliked by doctors because (1) if they were valueless they not only defrauded the patient but delayed his attempt to secure proper treatment; (2) if they had a value they were employed largely as a result of a self-diagnosis by the patient and therefore liable to be used for conditions in which they would not help; (3) if they had value and were selected for disease in which they would help they were in competition with the physician and liable to affect his income; (4) if a patient used a patent medicine and subsequently consulted a doctor, the doctor had no easy means of ascertaining whether the drug that he desired to prescribe was compatible with the drug already in the patient's system; and (5) it was basic to medical ethics that a doctor, having found a particular drug useful in a particular disease, should make the fact known to his colleagues so that patients in general could benefit from his discovery.

The history of proprietary medicines in Britain in recent decades is interesting.

Around the 1920s there were attempts – especially that of Professor A.J. Clark – to analyse patent remedies and to publish their ingredients, their pharmacological action, their approximate manufacturing cost and their retail price. Many of the firms brought unsuccessful legal actions but had greater success by indicating that they would no longer advertise in any newspaper or journal that mentioned the publication. On a short term basis the firms won, but in the longer term Clark and his associates tolled the death knell of proprietary medicines.

The Pharmacy and Medicines Act, 1941, made it an offence to advocate a proprietary medicine for the treatment of certain serious diseases, required disclosure of the ingredients of each patent medicine in precise terms and to some extent restricted the sale of these medicines; and the Food and Drugs Act, 1955, made it an offence to sell any food or drug which is not of the nature, substance or quality demanded by the buyer, and also made it an offence to use false or misleading labels. In addition, a trade association of manufacturers of proprietary medicines – The Proprietary Association of Great Britain – has devised a code of advertising standards, and in recent years the *Monthly Index of Medical Specialities* has provided a fairly complete indication of the composition of all marketed medicines.

Medicines in Britain are divided into those advertised solely to the medical profession and those advertised also to the general public, but the purchaser is fairly adequately protected, although occasionally an unscrupulous manufacturer can find a loophole in the law.

In some other countries matters are very different. One learns, for example, of alleged cures for cancer, with concealment of the actual drugs employed, and with orthodox medical practitioners having no easy means of ascertaining whether the alleged 'cure' is a discovery as important as that of vitamins or antibiotics or is merely a money-making fraud.

proprioception. Sensations coming from the muscles, ligaments, tendons and joints and from the labyrinths of each ear. These impulses – often never reaching the realm of consciousness – give information about the position of various parts of the body, so that posture is adjusted as required.

prostaglandins. Substances, produced in the body, which affect the nervous system and the blood flow in the kidneys, and also stimulate the contraction of uterine muscle. Because of this latter property it is possible that they may be developed as a contraceptive for use after sexual intercourse – a 'morning after' pill. Trials of synthetic prostaglandins are, however, still at only an early stage.

The most hopeful technique so far is instillation of 4 to 8 mg. of a prostaglandin into the uterus, via the cervix. This usually produces bleeding resembling normal menstruation and if a pregnancy test is carried out in a fortnight it is negative. However, in some cases the prostaglandin has side effects such as vomiting and painful uterine cramps.

prostate. A glandular structure, normally about the size of a chestnut, lying at the neck of the bladder in males and surrounding the outlet of the urethra. The prostate secretes a clear, viscous fluid which lubricates the urethra and mixes with the sperm cells to form semen.

Diseases. By far the commonest disease of the prostate is enlargement, characterized at first by frequency of desire to pass urine, and later by partial obstruction of the flow of urine and sometimes by incontinence as a result of the bladder never being completely emptied. In most cases surgical removal of the gland is required, although a course of antibiotics should first be tried, because there may well be some inflammation which makes a relatively slight enlargement appear worse than it really is. As yet little is known about the cause of enlargement, so prevention is not practicable.

Acute prostatitis, inflammation of the gland, is an occasional complication of infection elsewhere in the urinary system. The condition is characterized by high temperature, pain in the lower part of the back and frequency of urination. Treatment is that of the original infection.

Chronic prostatitis, with similar symptoms but less fever, is often associated with cystitis. Both acute and chronic inflammation of the gland respond well to antibiotics.

Cancer of the gland occurs most frequently at 50 to 70 years. It is characterized by symptoms of enlargement (see above) but often exhibits more pain and leads to traces of blood in the urine. Rectal examination reveals a hard, irregular swelling. Until a few years ago surgical removal was recommended as the only effective treatment, but in recent years it has been found that treatment with stilboestrol in many cases results in complete cure. In addition to being important for the actual condition, the success of hormonal therapy in this form of cancer gives reason to hope that in due course drugs – possibly synthetic hormones – will be found that are effective for cancer in other parts of the body.

prosthesis. The replacement of an absent or amputated part by an artificial one. Dentures, glass eyes and artificial limbs are examples of prosthetic devices.

In general artificial limbs are moved by the muscles of the remaining stump, but nowadays some are powered by electric batteries.

prostration. Complete physical or mental exhaustion.

protein. The complex FOOD substances containing nitrogen, and essential constituents of protoplasm of which all animal cells are composed.

On average the human body consists of approximately 70 per cent water, about 15 per cent fat and 12 per cent protein, with the muscles composed almost entirely of water and protein. Hence protein is constantly required for the building and maintenance of the body tissues.

Each protein molecule in the body is itself composed of a chain of amino-acids of which some twenty-two have been identified, including eight which the body cannot manufacture and which are therefore essential requirements in diet.

Food containing protein can be divided into two types: those containing first class protein (i.e., protein with all the essential amino-acids) such as meat, fish, cheese, eggs and milk; and those containing second class protein (i.e., protein which is useful but lacks some of the essential amino-acids) such as peas, beans and lentils. During digestion the complex proteins of the foods eaten are broken down to their constituent amino-acids and then rebuilt to constitute the proteins of the bodily tissues. Surplus of protein can be used as bodily fuel and in conditions of starvation, protein will be used for fuel to the detriment of maintenance of tissues.

In communities where there is no shortage of food it should be remembered that excess protein in the diet is simply used as fuel which could just as well be supplied by the far more plentiful (and, incidentally, much cheaper) carbohydrate. Under these circumstances the nitrogenous portion is converted to urea and excreted in the urine. Indeed for energy purposes protein is an uneconomical food because considerable energy is used in its digestion, which is the basis of its employment in 'slimming' diets.

In developed countries many affluent people eat more protein than necessary, whereas in underdeveloped countries where MALNUTRITION is common, insufficient protein is usual. Severe protein deficiency leads to general weakness, swelling of the abdomen and lowered resistance to disease.

protozoa. Single-celled organisms, the smallest creatures that can be called animals. An example is the amoeba, found in most ponds, the largest of which are just visible to the naked eye and slightly smaller than the dot at the end of this sentence; the smallest may measure only 0.005 mm. They are usually regarded as the lowest form of animal life, just as fungi are regarded as the lowest form of plant life, with bacteria and viruses regarded neither as animals nor as plants. In general they do not reproduce sexually (most protozoa do not have male and female members of the species) but merely swell and then split into two, a process technically called multiplication by simple fission. Thus the amoeba that we see today is immortal in the sense that it has never lost an ancestor by death.

The vast majority of protozoa are harmless, but malaria, sleeping sickness and a form of dysentery are carried by parasitic protozoa.

The study of protozoa is known as protozoology.

prurigo. A vague term for a group of intensely itchy conditions in which the main physical signs are pimples with the tops scratched off and thickening of the skin. While the precipitating cause may be a trivial local irritant, the condition is in most cases fundamentally emotional in origin – a sort of direction of anger, thwarted elsewhere, against the self. Anti-itching ointments, steroid hormones and tranquillizers may all help, but the essential treatment, and equally the essential means of prevention, is relief of the underlying emotional tension and therefore investigation of its causes.

pruritis. The medical term for ITCHING.

prussic acid. An intense and rapidly acting poison of the narcotic group occurring naturally in the oil of bitter almonds and identifiable from its characteristic almond-like smell. It is alternatively called hydrocyanic acid.

When taken internally the acid and certain of its salts (cyanides and isocyanides) cause a momentary sensation of burning in the mouth and are absorbed with extraordinary rapidity. Breathing becomes spasmodic, there are a few convulsive movements, unconsciousness supervenes and – usually within a couple of minutes – death results from paralysis of the respiratory and central nervous systems. On post mortem examination the blood is a curiously bright red.

The poison, in addition to being very rapidly absorbed, is quickly destroyed by the tissues, so that, if the patient is still alive, artificial respiration should be tried, and continued until he has recovered or definitely died. If an oxidizing agent, such as hydrogen permanganate or potassium permanganate, is available it can be given in the hope of converting the prussic acid to a harmless oxamide. Intravenous injection of methylene blue (50 cc. of a one per cent solution) has proved effective in some cases.

Although factual information is hard to obtain, it is commonly said that spies, who might, if captured, be tortured to force them to release information, carry capsules containing prussic acid, place them in their mouths if capture seems likely, and at need secure a quick death by crunching them.

pseudocyesis. Spurious or false pregnancy. This curious condition occurs in neurotic women, in women near the menopause who are very anxious to have a child, and in some eastern countries in women whose husbands could divorce them for barrenness. It is primarily emotional but the emotion affects the formation of hormones by the pituitary and other glands.

All the symptoms of pregnancy appear and many of the physical signs, e.g., the breasts and abdomen enlarge and menstruation may cease. Often the condition is so like a genuine pregnancy that examination under a general anaesthetic is necessary to establish the diagnosis. Under anaesthesia the hysterical fixation of the abdominal muscles collapses and vaginal examination reveals that the uterus is of only normal size. Treatment is essentially psychological and is far from easy.

The condition is not confined to human beings, but is sometimes seen, for instance, in female dogs.

psittacosis. A severe infectious disease with the general symptoms of pneumonia, but also with extreme weakness, slow pulse and often delirium, so that it may be mistaken for typhoid. The disease is caused by a virus, transmitted by parrots, parakeets, canaries and some other birds, and infection occurs through close contact with the birds or with their recent excreta. In most cases infection arises from sick birds, but occasionally an apparently healthy bird can act as a carrier.

Treatment consists of isolation of the patient and prompt and adequate administration of tetracyclines or other appropriate antibiotics. Although patient to patient transmission is rare, nurses handling a patient should wear thick gauze masks and all discharges from the patient should be disinfected. Infected birds and their carcases and cages should be destroyed.

There is as yet no method of immunization, but the condition is preventable by strict regulation of the import of, and traffic in, birds of the parrot family, with both a period of quarantine and a laboratory examination before any such bird is offered for sale.

psoriasis. A fairly common skin disease characterized by the formation of red patches which are covered by fine silvery scales. The disease often runs in families and is not infectious, but its cause is still uncertain. The most widely accepted theory is that the condition is due to an inherited defect in the formation of the cells of the skin.

The guttate variety, which occurs in children, often follows an infectious disease which seems to trigger off the condition. Application of oily calamine lotion and administration of vitamin supplements often effect a cure within a few months.

Psoriasis of extensor surfaces (e.g., knees or elbows) may occur at any period of life. There is usually no itching and the patient should be encouraged to accept the patches as harmless and non-infectious. Many treatments have been advocated without much success, e.g., ointments containing coal tar and local application of steroid drugs. Exposure to sunlight is probably as useful as any other treatment.

Psoriasis of the flexures (e.g., armpits, genital area and below the breasts) is commonest in the obese, and treatment of the obesity may help.

The disease also occurs in the nails, palms and soles.

psyche. The human spirit or mind, including all its emotions, perceptions and activities. The term is derived from the name of a beautiful nymph in Greek mythology who was beloved by Cupid and subsequently granted immortality. The term is used by psychologists and psychiatrists mainly because 'soul' has become restricted to spiritual or religious connotations and 'mind' is overwhelmingly associated with reasoning and remembering.

psychedelic drugs. Drugs which produce abnormal states of consciousness or hallucinations.

While opium and drugs derived from it tend to produce sleep and pleasant dreams, the hallucinogenic or psychedelic drugs achieve their effects while the person who has taken them is awake.

Some, like marihuana (better known as hashish or cannabis), have been used for many centuries in certain religious cults to produce ecstatic states. In general cannabis and similar drugs do not produce immediate harmful effects and do not lead to true addiction although they may produce some degree of psychological dependence.

A very different hallucinogen is lysergic acid diethylamide, usually known as LSD. It causes swirls of bright colours and of sounds, and it profoundly alters judgment, so that a person under the influence of the drug may attempt to 'fly' from the window of a high building or may believe that he can cross a busy street without bothering about the traffic. Moreover, use of LSD on a number of occasions can permanently damage the entire personality.

psychiatry. The branch of medicine concerned with the diagnosis and treatment (and in some cases the prevention) of emotional and mental disorders. Broadly it includes the study of five main groups of illness:

1. The psychoses, in which the loss of touch with reality is so severe that even untrained persons describe the patient as 'insane'.

2. The psychoneuroses, in which the person suffers from compulsions, obsessions, morbid fears or chronic invalidism without a physical basis. In general the distinction between psychotics and neurotics is clear enough: the psychotic is unaware of his derangement, whereas the neurotic is very unhappy about his illness. Differentiation of the mild neurotic from the extreme end of the spectrum of 'normality' is more difficult, e.g., it is hard to determine the point at which perfectionism and attention to detail become so marked as to constitute mental illness.

3. A rather vaguely bounded group of illnesses characterized by social inadequacy, emotional instability and abnormalities of behaviour. Many alcoholics, many drug addicts, most delinquents, some criminals and many multi-problem families fall into this category. As with the previous group it is hard to specify a border line, e.g., to decide whether the friendless woman who shuns her neighbours or the man who dresses or behaves eccentrically is mildly mentally ill or is still at the limit of 'normal'.

4. Mental handicap or deficiency, varying from complete idiocy to a condition in which the person can cope with a simple, repetitive job but needs help in every situation of difficulty. Although the intelligence quotient is a convenient yardstick in the case of persons whose life experience has been fairly normal, there is clearly not a very wide difference between the mentally handicapped person with IQ of 69 and the very dull 'normal' person with IQ of 76.

5. Such disorders of children as severe temper tantrums, persistent bed-wetting, maladjustment, school phobia and juvenile delinquency. Here again it is very difficult to differentiate from the limit of 'normality'.

Psychiatry is essentially a science of the twentieth century. Until the nineteenth century mental illness was usually regarded as evidence either of favour by the Deity (so that the afflicted person should be respected) or of possession by an evil spirit (so that flogging and starvation were advocated to drive away the spirit). Treatments, such as bleeding and purging, were usually ineffective, and in most cases the mentally sick were either left to fend for themselves or, if deemed dangerous, rigorously confined, often with manacles. Pinel (1792) in France, Fricke in Germany and Tuke in Britain initiated humane reforms, introducing air, light and the beginnings of occupational therapy; and a few decades later an American, Dorothea Dix, had great success in abolishing needless restraint and humanizing the care of mental patients. Yet it was not until 1854 in Britain (at the Crichton Royal Hospital, Dumfries) and 1877 in America (at the McLean Hospital, Boston) that any training for mental nurses was introduced. Certainly some patients recovered in an atmosphere of kindness and security but the nineteenth century was essentially the era of merely custodial care.

Charcot (1825-1883) really formulated the idea that certain disorders arose in the mind. Janet advanced this view by showing that consciousness can be split into a number of separate currents and that action of these currents in different direction can produce various mental disturbances. The dominant figure in modern psychiatry, Sigmund FREUD (1856-1939), focused attention on the unconscious and on repressed impulses. He showed the effects of conflict between the conscious and the subconscious on behaviour and health, demonstrated how repressed impulses could reappear in distorted form, and indicated the enormous influence of childhood experiences (especially those in the very early years) on later life. He was really the founder of psychoanalysis, and produced for the first time methods of curing many cases of psycho-neurotic illness. Jung and Adler in some

respects widened Freud's work. Kraepelin in 1913 and Bleuler in 1920 evolved reasonably satisfactory classifications of mental illnesses. During the 1920s Anna Freud, and others began to study child psychiatry, and Myerson's work on inherited mental disease was another landmark. By 1930 psychiatry had become a well recognized medical speciality and by 1960 it was on the way to becoming the largest of the specialities.

Of the five main groups mentioned at the beginning of this article, the psychoneuroses became treatable after Freud's work was accepted (although some psychologists have claimed recently that other methods are as effective as psychoanalysis), and it soon became evident that the emotional and behaviour disorders of childhood could in large measure be corrected by detailed investigation and treatment. Such investigation and treatment were (and are) inevitably slow and costly. An enormous advance was the application of prevention, with which the name of John Bowlby is greatly associated, but reaching a peak in Gerald Caplan's work in the 1960s. Essentially the approach of Caplan and his co-workers is based on the assumption that many mental disorders result from maladaptation and maladjustment, and that by early alteration of the balance of forces – including of course education of parents and teachers on child management – healthy adaptation and adjustment is possible. On the whole not only children's disorders but also the psychoneuroses and the vague group of inadequacies and abnormalities of behaviour are now regarded as preventable at long range; and indeed, now that most infections and nutritional diseases have been conquered, such prevention is perhaps the main task of health visitors and other health educators.

While some forms of mental handicap are occasioned by happenings to the unborn child (e.g., maternal rubella – German measles), by birth injuries and by events after birth, for the most part mental handicap is hereditary, so that its diminution is very much dependent on GENETIC GUIDANCE. Mongolism is a typical example, due to a chromosomal defect. However, not all feeble-minded parents give birth to mentally handicapped children and in some cases apparently normal parents have handicapped offspring. Hence on present knowledge preventive methods can reduce, but by no means eliminate, mental handicap. Some cases of mental handicap fully respond to early diagnosis and treatment, e.g., cases of cretinism and of phenylketonuria; but in the majority of cases of unprevented handicap all that can be done is to bring up the child in a suitable environment and develop his limited capacities to their fullest extent.

By far the most difficult problem is both the prevention and the treatment of the psychoses. Some of the organic types can be prevented: the psychosis of late syphilis is now virtually unknown, mental disease due to brain injury can be made less common by measures for reduction of home accidents and traffic accidents, and the incidence of senile psychosis can perhaps be reduced by ensuring that elderly people have good nutrition and adequate social contact. The really common types, however, are manic-depressive psychosis (with alternations of excess mental activity and melancholy), schizophrenia (split personality and withdrawal from life) and paranoia (systematized delusions) although the last two slide into each other.

Manic-depressive psychosis has in many cases a hereditary background, although Kraepelin's finding that this existed in 60 to 80 per cent of cases is nowadays regarded as exaggerated. Manic phases can usually be controlled with tranquillizers and depressive phases with isoniazid and similar drugs, but recurrences are common. Neither prevention nor cure can as yet be regarded as very successful.

Paranoia may be, as Freud thought, a result of repressed homosexual longings, or simply the result of downward progression of a suspicious, distrustful personality, or indeed the name may really cover a number of different conditions. Until more is known about causes neither prevention nor treatment is likely to yield much in the way of effects.

The commonest of the major psychotic diseases, schizophrenia, is also the source of most argument among psychiatrists. Most workers agree that there is a large hereditary factor – e.g., in identical twins if one has schizophrenia the odds are more than three to one that the other also suffers from it – so that genetic counselling would seem to offer great hope for reduction of the condition. Others, from Anna Freud onwards, have stressed the role of unfortunate childhood experiences as causal or precipitating factors, so that mental hygiene in the formative years may be important. Many treatments have been tried, with some degree of success.

Perhaps a fair summary of the present position is this: emotional and behavioural disorders of children are preventable and also treatable; similar disorders in adults are in large measure preventable at long range but very hard to treat when fully developed; psychoneurotic diseases are in the main preventable at long range and are also in most cases curable; the reduction of mental handicap is fundamentally a matter of genetic counselling and in most cases existing mental handicap is incurable; the organic psychoses can be prevented; and there are some hopeful signs for the future prevention or cure of the other psychotic diseases.

psychoanalysis. A special method of exploring the unconscious mind, originated by Freud. It aims at bringing to the surface forgotten memories and hidden fears and conflicts. By so doing it often precipitates an emotional crisis, after which the patient is in a position to understand and cope with his problems.

After the analyst has taken a careful history and carefully noted any gaps in the patient's narrative, the usual method is 'free association'. Here the analyst may occasionally direct the patient's thoughts by a word or a phrase, but in general the analyst merely listens while the patient says anything that comes into his mind, however foolish or objectionable it may seem. Gradually his words begin to reveal the repressed matter lying in his unconscious, and so help to indicate the origins of his psychoneurotic or psychosomatic illness. The process is inevitably slow, perhaps taking two hours a week for a year.

Under hypnosis the procedure can be quickened, but the success rate is reduced, because in this case it is really the analyst who does the uncovering, whereas part of the value of the free association method lies in the patient uncovering hidden memories for himself.

A psychoanalyst is a doctor (or occasionally a non-medical psychologist) who has undertaken special training and has himself been analysed, so as to become aware, for instance, of his own prejudices.

Although disliked by some non-analytical psychiatrists and although very slow and therefore costly, psychoanalysis is of proved value in the treatment of the psychoneuroses (e.g., hysterias and obsessions), and some of its practitioners have claimed a measure of success in paranoia. It has limitations, however: firstly, it is useless unless the patient is willing; secondly, it tends to fail if the patient is too uneducated or too unintelligent to communicate well; and thirdly, it becomes difficult after the age of 45 to 50 years because of the patient's increasing mass of experiences.

psychology. The study of mental life, of behaviour and of all the activities of the individual, not only at one point in time but throughout his life span. Probably the science, which has developed enormously in the last sixty years, is best indicated by enumeration of a few of the problems with which it is concerned. Some examples are: how a child becomes 'socialized', acquiring the language, values and culture of the group in which it is brought up; how and why a child plays; how a child or an adult learns, and what things facilitate or impede the learning process; how and why we remember or forget; how people are influenced by instincts or innate drives; how we are motivated, both consciously and unconsciously; how we can measure intelligence (or measure something that we call intelligence; how we think; what factors stimulate our imaginations; what kinds of sensation contribute to feeling; what circumstances or factors create personality disorders in which the individual in effect turns against himself; and what circumstances or factors create behaviour disorders in which the individual turns against society.

Psychology is investigated both subjectively (by reasoned analysis, the usual method last century) and objectively (by observation and planned experiment).

An appreciation of psychological principles is essential to the understanding of all human relationships, from salesmanship to marital relations, and from personnel management to the education of children. Just as a knowledge of physiology is necessary to understand the functioning or malfunctioning of the body in physical disease, so a knowledge of normal psychology is essential to understand mental diseases and the many diseases in which body and mind interact.

Psychology is a vast subject, perhaps indeed the widest of all the sciences. There is certainly such a science as general psychology – just as there is such a thing as general medicine – but, like medicine, psychology is becoming increasingly divided into specialties.

Thus educational psychology is particularly concerned with teaching and learning. A practical example of its interests might be to investigate whether the traditional forty-five 'minute teaching periods in secondary schools and the traditional fifty to fifty-five minute lectures in universities and polytechnics are best, or whether more shorter periods or fewer but longer periods would facilitate learning and the retention of learning material.

Child psychology includes some of the matter of educational psychology but is also concerned with assessing children's personalities (as well as their intelligence) and helping children with emotional or behaviour problems.

Abnormal psychology deals, as the name implies, with the actions and behaviour of persons who are mentally ill or sexual deviants or otherwise removed from the average behaviour and values that we all call 'normal'.

Social psychology is concerned with the interaction of groups, the influence of the group on the individual and the influence of the individual on the group. It clearly comes near to sociology, just as clinical psychology (including the work of non-medical psychologists in mental hospitals and clinics) approaches psychiatry, and just as industrial psychology impinges on personnel management.

psychoneurosis. A general term covering anxiety states, obsessions, compulsions and causeless fears. See NEUROSIS.

psychopath. A rather vague term describing a person whose behaviour is habitually or repeatedly antisocial. In Britain the Mental Health Act of 1959 defines the term as a persistent disability of mind which results in abnormally aggressive or seriously irresponsible conduct, and needs medical treatment. Violent criminals and moral delinquents are examples.

Despite evidence that a few criminals have an abnormality of the sex chromosomes and that some others show anomalies on an electroencephalogram, it is beyond dispute that most psychopaths are made, rather than born. Rejection in childhood and lack of affection from parents or substitute parents play important parts.

psychoprophylaxis. Strictly the term simply means prevention or reduction of illness or pain by affecting the mind, but usually it is reserved for the psychological measures employed to prevent or diminish the pains of childbirth.

The pregnant woman loses much of her fear through being taught that childbirth is a natural and not particularly unpleasant process. Also she is encouraged to perform certain exercises again and again until she does them as routinely as a soldier stands to attention or shoulders arms. When the uterine contractions start she begins to perform these exercises and, apart from any actual help that they give, has her attention directed more to the exercises than to the 'labour pains'.

With adequate psychoprophylaxis some women voluntarily undertake childbirth without any analgesic or anaesthetic, while many others find that the anaesthetic can be given later and in smaller dosage than would otherwise be the case.

psychosis. Mental disorder involving sufficient loss of touch with reality to render a person 'insane', i.e., incapable of functioning independently in society. In descriptive terms the main types of psychosis are: (1) Manic-depression, in which the patient is either excited or depressed or alternates between these two states of mind. In this group there can also be included involutional melancholia where there are marked symptoms of depression associated with ageing. (2) Schizophrenia, in which there is a retreat from reality, an emotional nihilism, and often bizarre and incongruous behaviour combined with silliness, mannerisms, mental inertia, personality deterioration and often purposeless activity. (3) Paranoia which is characterized by suspicion and delusions of persecution, often well-constructed and systematized, maintained with apparent intelligence, and giving rise to appropriate emotional responses. (4) Dementia, in which there is a general decline of mental capacity and memory.

These purely clinical types of mental illness can develop in a variety of ways and a classification based on the cause may be described as follows: (1) organic psychosis, in which there is some demonstrable structural pathology of brain tissue or its vessels; (2) toxic psychosis, in which there is some exogenous or endogenous intoxication (i.e., intoxication originating from outside or from within); and (3) functional psychosis, in which no sufficient toxic or organic cause can yet be demonstrated in the present state of knowledge.

To these can usefully be added the 'defect reactions' in which there are constitutional absences or deficits rather than an acquired disease. These include patients with mental deficiency or with constitutional psychopathic inferiority as manifested by various types of unstable personality, the alcoholics and drug addicts, the kleptomaniacs and pyromaniacs, and those who exhibit other forms of antisocial behaviour.

Because of the growing appreciation that much mental illness arises from demonstrable causes it is absolutely necessary that practising psychiatrists must also be good general physicians, competent to track down the bodily conditions which are affecting the mind. Conversely, the general physician must be equally aware of the psychiatric effects of organic brain disease.

A clear distinction has to be drawn between psychosis and mental handicap. In the latter conditions the brain has been defective from birth or early childhood and the person can at no time think or reason like an ordinary individual. In the case of the psychotic the intelligence is normal and may indeed be véry high. See PSYCHIATRY.

psychosomatic diseases. Diseases in which mental events or disturbances cause physical effects.

No definition is wholly satisfactory because in all diseases and injuries there is an interaction of mind and body, e.g., the soldier in the excitement of battle may not even realize that he has received a serious wound, the person with toothache often finds the pain decreasing as he enters the dentist's surgery, and the recovery of a seriously ill person depends considerably on whether he actually desires to recover. Broadly, however, a disease is termed psychosomatic when its main causal factors are in the mind.

In any normal person conscious emotion produces physical results, such as blushing from embarrassment, feeling a sinking sensation in the pit of the stomach from dismay, or having a quickened pulse rate during anger. These physical results are caused partly by action of the nervous system (including the sympathetic and para-sympathetic nerves) and partly by release of hormones from the endocrine system.

Perhaps the easiest disease in which to indicate a ·mental element is gastric ulcer. Prolonged emotional stress causes increased acidity of the gastric juice, with gradual erosion of the mucous membrane of the stomach wall by the highly acid juice, so producing an ulcer. Moreover, a study of patients suffering from gastric ulcer shows that they are on average more conscientious, more prone to worry, more rigid in attitude and keener to strive for success than are most people. In other words, although there are some physical factors predisposing to gastric ulcer (e.g., faulty diet) the disease occurs mainly in persons of a particular type of personality and the mechanism is known.

In most organic diseases of mental origin the connection is not quite so clear-cut. Much emotion occurs at an unconscious level. This hidden and unfelt emotion nevertheless stimulates the sympathetic nervous system (altering, for instance, the rate of the flow of blood) and changes the rate of production of hormones (e.g., by the pituitary). Many – but perhaps not all – cases of asthma are produced by unconscious emotional factors. Thus a patient who has no conscious dislike of cats develops asthmatic attacks whenever he is in the presence of a cat and is thought to be allergic to the animal; but on being asked to study a picture of a cat he develops an attack, demonstrating that the condition in his case is psychosomatic, not allergic.

Apart from gastric ulcer and asthma, diseases in which emotion can play a large part include migraine, duodenal ulcer, colitis, hypertension, many skin diseases, and perhaps coronary thrombosis.

There is considerable argument about the number and prevalence of psychosomatic diseases. Some doctors maintain that about one-half of all physical illnesses fall into that category, while others would restrict the figure to nearer one-tenth. In a sense both are right. For perhaps 10 to 15 per cent of all persons consulting doctors because of physical symptoms, stress, fear or anxiety (conscious or unconscious) is the dominant causal factor; in perhaps another 10 to 15 per cent the mind plays an important part; and in yet another 10 to 15 per cent it contributes appreciably to the disease. Even a disease as physical and as clearly bacteriologically caused as tuberculosis has its mental causal factors: in any particular age-group living under similar social and environmental circumstances there are relatively more cases of tuberculosis in persons who have recently been bereaved or jilted or lost their jobs than in persons in whom these factors have not operated.

It should be clearly understood that there is no question, in a psychosomatic disease, of the condition being imaginary. The man with a gastric ulcer has a definite ulceration of the membrane of his stomach: the woman with asthma has a definite constriction of the smaller bronchioles and consequent difficulty in breathing out; the individual suffering from a psychosomatic disorder may die from it, in which case the pathological findings are demonstrable on post mortem examination.

If a disease is wholly or largely psycho-somatic it may well need physical methods of treatment (e.g., drugs) to reduce or remove the symptoms; but for complete cure and avoidance of recurrence it will manifestly also need investigation and treatment of the underlying emotional problems, which – as already mentioned are sometimes below the level of consciousness.

The best hope for the prevention of diseases of emotional origin would appear to lie in the fostering of strong and stable personalities in the early formative years, always remembering in such fostering the need for demonstrated affection (without 'smothering with love'), consistency, security, freedom to explore and investigate, and sufficient kindly authority to enable the child to learn without too much trauma that the needs and wishes of others have to be considered in addition to his own needs and demands.

psychotherapy. Treatment of emotional and mental disorders by verbal means, as opposed to drugs and physical measures. Essentially psychotherapy began with Freud's techniques of psychoanalysis but it nowadays also includes many less elaborate measures, such as simple counselling (by psychiatrist, doctor, health visitor or even social worker), group therapy (where a number of patients discuss their problems under the chairmanship of psychiatrist or psychologist, who in most cases keeps the discussion going but deliberately makes little personal contribution), and play therapy (in which children indicate, and sometimes solve, their conflicts in play).

ptomaine poisoning. An outmoded and inaccurate name for food poisoning. Decomposing proteins such as game hung for an unduly prolonged period produce alkaloid substances called ptomaines, and it used to be thought that these were the main cause of food poisoning. Certainly ptomaines are mildly poisonous (and one rather rare variety of shellfish poisoning is caused by a ptomaine), but they are produced when the food is in such a state of decomposition that it would be rejected by the palate. The real cause of food poisoning is specific bacterial contamination of food.

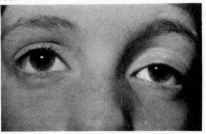

Ptosis

ptosis. Sagging or drooping of the upper eyelid in consequence either of weakness of the muscle which raises the eyelid or of damage to the nerve supplying that muscle. Some cases are congenital; some follow shingles or certain other infectious diseases; some occur as a result of damage to the nerve, e.g., from tuberculosis, syphilis or tumour; a few cases are of hysterical origin; sometimes the condition is observed only on awakening from sleep and disappears within a few minutes. Treatment varies with the cause. In some cases where the defect is very disfiguring a small operation may be advised.

ptyalin. An enzyme present in saliva which converts starch into sugar and thus plays an essential part in DIGESTION.

ptyalism. Abnormal secretion of saliva. Common causes include oral sepsis, decaying teeth and trigeminal neuralgia. The condition also occurs in overacidity of the stomach, is sometimes caused simply by excessive smoking, and frequently occurs in the early months of pregnancy. Since saliva when swallowed carries air with it, there are usually symptoms of flatulence as well as excessive salivation. Treatment depends on discovery and removal of the primary cause, but 0.3 ml. of tincture of belladonna thrice daily, half an hour before meals, is often helpful in reducing the inconvenience of the symptoms, although it does not affect the cause.

puberty. The period of onset of sexual maturity. The time at which sperms and ova are first produced and adult sexual characteristics appear, such as the deepening of the male voice and the enlargement of the female breasts. In girls it is usually reckoned as being established by the first menstrual period, whereas in boys its onset is less definite. For consideration of the mental and physical changes in more detail see ADOLESCENCE.

pubis. The front portion of the innominate or pelvic bone. It consists of a roughly square body and two branches, one passing backwards and upwards towards the acetabulum, and the other backwards and downwards to join a similar branch of the ischium. In the middle line of the body the two pubic bones join together to form the symphysis pubis.

public health. The science that studies individuals and families in their domestic, social and occupational groupings and in their working and living conditions, and seeks to promote mental and physical health, to reduce disease and to create the conditions for healthy living.

The beginnings of public health services in the past are interesting. Conduits and aqueducts were built during the Cretan-Mycaenean civilization. The Greeks studied the epidemiology of what we now call infectious diseases. Both the Old Testament and the Koran stress the importance of personal cleanliness and hygiene. The Romans built reservoirs, aqueducts, water pipes and drainage systems, and also appointed public physicians – ten to each large city and five or seven for smaller cities. Under the Persian-Arab civilization there were paved and lighted streets and well-designed hospitals, where different types of disease were separated. In some ways the Romans in the second century A.D. and certainly the Arabs in the eleventh century (e.g., Avicenna's interest in prevention as well as cure and his stress on forming and moulding the character of a child) were ahead of developments in Western Europe and America until the latter part of the nineteenth century.

Isolation of lepers existed in the Middle Ages, and quarantine measures for plague suspects developed in the fourteenth century or possibly earlier; from about that time some large towns made sporadic efforts to improve street cleaning and environmental hygiene, and occasional writers attempted to instruct the public – or those of them who could read – on health, sometimes with a surprisingly modern slant. For instance, an Elizabethan book advises:

'From care his head to keep, from wrath his heart,
Drink not much wine, sup light and soon arise....
When moved you find yourself to Nature's needs,
Forbear them not, for that much danger breeds,
Use three physicians still: first Doctor Quiet,
Next Doctor Merry-man, and Doctor Diet.'

Yet concern with public health in the modern sense can be considered as having its vague beginnings in the writings of eighteenth century French thinkers (and not least in Rousseau's educational novel, *Emile*, 1762) and more specifically in the very detailed publications of two German physicians, Johann P. Frank (1748-1821) and Franz A. Mai (1742-1814). In practice real attention to the health of the people began after – and in consequence of – the industrial revolution.

In some ways public health can be regarded as still in its infancy. Apart from the degenerative conditions of old age most diseases are in large measure preventable – coronary thrombosis, chronic bronchitis, mongolism, schizophrenia, spina bifida, most infections and the psychoneuroses are examples, yet even in the most advanced countries the average worker loses twelve to fifteen days of productive work every year through illness, with the total work loss through illness about fifty times the average loss through industrial disputes: and, with an optimum life span of over a century fully a quarter of us die before the age of 65 years. Yet in other respects the advances in public health in the last hundred years have been dramatic beyond the imagination of persons living in previous centuries. The conversion of most infections (except influenza, the common cold and gonorrhoea) into rarities in advanced countries, the conquest of diseases of dirt and destitution, the doubling of the average duration of life and the reduction of infant deaths from one in six to one in sixty are striking examples of these advances.

In the outline that follows, the history of public health is considered in four overlapping stages with the stages described mainly as they occurred in the U.K., but, with a few alterations of dates and names, the stages – or certainly the first three of them – apply on the whole to the English-speaking countries generally.

The legislative stage. To secure safe, adequate and wholesome water supplies, proper systems of sewage disposal, clean and uncontaminated food, fit houses, reduction of overcrowding to tolerable limits and diminution of water-borne and food-borne infections, it was necessary to persuade people that public money should be spent (e.g., on water supplies and sewerage systems) and that legislation should be passed (e.g., on adulteration of food), and thereafter enforced by appropriate inspectors, with penalties for infringement. The later nineteenth and early twentieth century was essentially the era of the sanitary legislator, the medical officer of health (working on his own without sizeable numbers of either medical or nursing colleagues) and the sanitary inspector (later renamed in the U.K. the environmental officer). To these officers is largely due the elimination of such diseases as cholera and typhoid.

The legislative phase is not yet ended. For instance we still have problems of air pollution and noise pollution; but in the main the diseases preventable by legislation have been prevented, and in some countries – such as Sweden – the sanitary inspector is now almost a rarity.

The stage of interest in the physical health of mother and child. Services to identify and treat, and later to prevent, deviations from health in expectant mothers, infants, pre-school children and school pupils developed rather irregularly in the latter years of the nineteenth century and very steadily in the first third of this century. The health visitor arrived on the scene in the 1860s (but was not a registered nurse with a further professional qualification until after 1919), and the district nurse arrived at about the same time. Child health clinics began to appear around the turn of the century and the first rudiments of a school health service were established about 1905-1910, while qualified midwives appeared in England in 1902 and in Scotland in 1915. By 1940 there were vast reductions in the maternal death rate and the infant mortality rate, and corresponding improvements in the general physical health of mothers and children. The phase of interest in the physical health of mothers and babies – the era of the public health medical officer and of the earlier type of health visitor reached its peak in the 1930s but is not yet ended. For example, education on family planning and genetic counselling are very much things of the present.

The stage of interest in the emotional and physical well-being of the family. Advances in the sciences of psychology and sociology, as well as improved knowledge of motivation and health teaching techniques, revolutionized public health in the middle third of the century. The post-registration preparation of the nurse aspiring to become a health visitor widened and deepened beyond recognition, and she became no less concerned with the prevention of maladjustment and the psychoneuroses than with the prevention of nutritional diseases and infections, and as involved with the health of the elderly as with the young. Health education departments were established within many public health departments, with courses gradually evolving whereby selected health visitors or selected graduates in the behavioural sciences could qualify as health education officers. New workers also began to appear in public health departments, e.g., dieticians, speech therapists, physiotherapists and chiropodists.

While development was irregular, by the early 1970s the emotional and social – as well as the physical – health of citizens of the most progressive towns had improved enormously; and experts in finance were beginning to point out that increases in health education and health visiting services paid dividends in the shape of a reduced burden of disease.

The splitting of public health in Britain. Almost inevitably health visitors (concerned primarily with promotion of good health and prevention of physical and mental illness) and general medical practitioners (largely concerned with the curing of illness in the same people) began to work together, although each retained his or her separate aims and kinds of priorities. Both workers began to see the hospital not as a separate institution but as an extension, implying a continued need for two-way communication. The 1974 integration placed all doctors, nurses and paramedical workers under the same management, although of course community physicians (essentially the public health medical officers with a different name), health visitors, health education officers, and so on retained their specialist trainings and their particular functions.

Slightly before the integration, however, the social work services, including old people's homes, day nurseries and the home help service – had been separated off to form social work departments. Hence the new integrated health services were concerned with promotion of health, prevention of illness, treatment of disease and medical and nursing supportive services, but supportive services not requiring medical or nursing skill were the concern of social work services.

In 1974, too, sanitary inspectors (public health inspectors) did not pass into the integrated health services but remained in environmental health departments of local authorities. Most of the sanitary inspector's sampling, inspectorial and enforcement functions are clearly separable from those of other health workers, but problems may arise in the case of outbreaks of food-borne disease in which previously medical officers, health education officers, health visitors and sanitary inspectors worked as a united team.

Some alternative names. There is a tendency for meanings of terms to become narrowed to the most widely known portion of their original significance, e.g., for 'mental health' to become associated with services for the mentally sick and mentally handicapped (as opposed to the improvement or maintenance of mental health), and for 'hygiene' to lose its old meaning of the complete science of health and to become synonymous with personal cleanliness and environmental aspects. Similarly 'public health' is sometimes used for simply its large-scale and impersonal aspects, such as purity of water and food and adequacy of drainage and sewerage: an example is the renaming of sanitary inspectors or environmental health officers in the U.K. as public health inspectors during the 1960s although their training and duties were unconcerned with emotional health, mental health, social well-being or personal aspects of physical health.

Because of these partial changes alternative names are appearing, such as community health, community medicine, social medicine and preventive medicine. However, none of these is completely satisfactory. 'Community health' is a term of doubtful meaning, as indicated in COMMUNITY HEALTH SERVICES, and neither 'community health' nor 'community medicine' is a really suitable term to cover such individual and personal aspects of health as genetic counselling, contraceptive advice and antenatal care; names including the word 'medicine' seem to put undue stress on medical aspects, as opposed to psychological, sociological and health educational aspects; 'social medicine' appears in some countries to carry political implications, as if it were 'socialized medicine'; and 'preventive medicine' puts the whole emphasis on the stopping of illnesses as contrasted with the fostering of good emotional and physical health. So perhaps the old term 'public health' should continue to be used.

puerperal fever. Any condition producing after childbirth a rise of temperature to 38 °C. (100.4 °F.) maintained for twenty-four hours or recorded on two consecutive occasions. The term is generally applied to the septicaemia that was formerly common after labour. A synonym in the Victorian era was childbed fever.

In the process of childbirth the linings of the uterus and vagina are bruised by the passage of the child's head, and the separation of the placenta leaves a raw area. So the whole area is eminently suitable for the reception and multiplication of germs if they enter, e.g., from the hands or throat of the doctor or midwife.

During most of the nineteenth century hospital confinement was extremely dangerous because infection passed from patient to patient. In some hospitals as many as one mother in every four died from childbed fever. The arrival of antiseptics, with routine disinfection of the hands of doctors and midwives and of all instruments, brought the death rate from the condition down from one in four to nearer one in a hundred; and by 1900 the maternal death rate from all causes had fallen to about five per thousand total births. Antiseptic techniques, aseptic methods, better understanding of how bacteria spread, better maternal care and better obstetrics together made puerperal fever an extreme rarity, and with the advent of the sulphonamides and the antibiotics that rarity, when it does occur, is usually curable.

The reduction of hospital deaths from childbed fever from about one in every four births to about one in every hundred thousand births is one of the great triumphs of preventive medicine.

puerperium. The period immediately following labour during which the uterus and other organs return to approximately their previous sizes and positions. In normal circumstances the period lasts for six to eight weeks.

The uterus is about 15 cm. (6 in.) long at the close of labour and can be felt quite distinctly in the abdomen; it dwindles by about a finger's breadth a day during the first seven or eight days and thereafter decreases more slowly. The bloodstained discharge from the uterus, the lochia, becomes paler and less copious after the first week. Bit by bit the organs return to normal, although lines remain on the abdomen and the vulva stays a little stretched.

Although childbirth is a normal process it is a .strenuous one, and the puerperium is essentially a period of rest and recovery of strength. Apart from the husband and the patient's mother, visitors should normally be

excluded for the first three days, and during the next few days the nurse should use her discretion, limiting visitors to such persons and numbers as will not tire the woman. Adequate rest, preferably including an afternoon nap, is an important feature of the puerperium. The resumption of household tasks should be gradual.

After the stress of pregnancy and childbirth transient mild depression is not uncommon in the puerperium, and in a very small number of cases there develops a form of manic-depressive psychosis known as puerperal insanity. This requires skilled treatment on the same lines as for other affective diseases, but the outlook is hopeful.

pulsation. The throbbing caused by the beating of the heart. Pulsation of the apex of the heart can usually be seen – as well as felt – between the fourth and fifth ribs. Abnormal pulsation of an artery may be due to an ANEURYSM, and capillary pulsation may occur in some cases of heart disease.

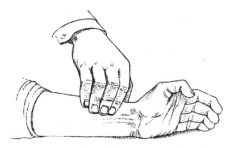

Taking the pulse

pulse. The pressure wave in an artery corresponding with each contraction of the heart. As these contractions push blood onwards into the arteries the increased pressure (systolic pressure) can easily be felt in any artery that can be compressed against a bone. Between each contraction less blood is pushed along the arteries and the considerably lower pressure (diastolic pressure) can again be felt.

The pulse is generally most conveniently felt on the thumb side of the wrist in the radial artery. Each pressure wave reaches the wrist about one-tenth of a second after the particular beat of the heart. A doctor or nurse feeling the pulse seeks to ascertain several things: the rate, the regularity or irregularity, the force of the systolic contraction, the strength of the diastolic relaxation or rebound, and the condition of the arterial wall.

The normal pulse rate in people who have been at rest for some minutes varies between sixty and eighty per minute. The pulse accelerates with exercise (but in a healthy person rapidly returns to normal after the exertion is over), fear and excitement, and most fevers, with typhoid and diphtheria notorious exceptions. Irregularity of the pulse may be due to various diseases of the heart, some digestive disorders, overindulgence in alcohol, excessive smoking or excessive consumption of coffee. While the systolic and diastolic blood pressure can be more accurately measured by a sphygmomanometer, an experienced person can obtain a good approximate estimate from the pulse. In normal persons the arterial wall cannot be felt unless the patient is very thin, but in disease thickening, hardening and twisting may be noted.

pupil. The rounded aperture in the centre of the iris of the eye. Through this aperture light reaches the back of the eye. In dim light the pupil dilates to allow more light to impinge on the retina, and dilatation is also caused by action of the sympathetic nerves on the iris, by secretion of adrenalin (as in fear and excitement) and by drugs which temporarily block off the sympathetic nerves (e.g., belladonna and atropin). In bright light the pupil contracts to protect the sensitive retina, the contraction being initiated by action of the parasympathetic nerves. The pupil also contracts as the eyes are brought to focus on an object near to the face, and certain drugs, such as morphine, constrict the pupil.

In health the pupils are regular in shape and equal in size, and should contract briskly when exposed to bright light. The size, regularity and contracting power of the pupils are altered in certain diseases of the nervous system.

purgatives. See LAXATIVES.

purpura. A general name for a group of diseases in which blood leaks from capillary blood vessels causing purple spots under the skin or in mucous membranes.

Idiopathic thrombocytopenic purpura, occurring mostly in children and old people, is caused by an inadequate number of blood platelets. Salient features are multiple haemorrhages in the skin, and on blood examination a reduced platelet count and an abnormal fragility of red blood corpuscles. For the acute form of the disease transfusions of fresh blood or of suspensions of platelets are useful and ACTH often helps. For the more chronic form surgical removal of the spleen is usually necessary.

Purpura simplex, sometimes called 'rheumatic purpura' but really unrelated to rheumatism, occurs mostly in pre-school children and appears to be due to a deficiency of the capillary walls, not to a shortage of platelets. Corticosteroids and ACTH sometimes help, but there is really no specific treatment and relapses are common.

Heavy dosage of aspirin occasionally causes another form of purpura; and the small haemorrhages found in association with scurvy were originally thought to be due to deficiency of vitamin C but are now sometimes attributed to inadequacy of an alleged vitamin P with lack of C causing the scurvy but lack of P responsible for the purpuric spots.

purulent. Containing or discharging pus.

pus. A thick, yellowish fluid consisting of blood serum, broken-down blood cells and tissue cells, and killed bacteria. When bacteria invade any part of the body a process of inflammation begins: additional blood is rushed to the part bringing large numbers of white blood corpuscles whose function is to engulf and destroy the bacteria. The pus that is formed essentially consists of the 'corpses' from the battle.

The process of pus formation is called suppuration. When pus has formed and is under pressure it tends to track to the exterior of the body or to a hollow organ, and there form an abscess. The introduction of antibiotics has greatly decreased suppuration, because in many cases the antibiotic successfully kills the invading bacteria; but the old maxim, 'Where there is pus let it out' still holds, i.e., where there is any substantial amount of pus, incision, free evacuation and drainage are needed.

pustule. A tiny blister containing pus. Typical pustules are seen in acne vulgaris and in smallpox. The characteristic blister of anthrax is termed a malignant pustule.

pyaemia. A form of blood poisoning with formation of multiple abscesses throughout the body, and due to septic emboli – usually containing either staphylococci or streptococci – travelling from one point of infection. Symptoms include shivering, high temperature, rapid pulse, exhaustion and sometimes delirium, together with symptoms from the local abscesses. Treatment involves identification and usually surgical removal of the original infection, the use of an appropriate antibiotic and the provision of ample fluids both to dilute toxins and to prevent dehydration.

pyelitis. Inflammation of the central part (the pelvis) of the kidney. It results from infection which can progress upwards from the urinary tract or downwards from any part of the body. Stone in the kidney and inflammation of the bladder are common causes, and the condition is not infrequent in pregnancy.

Characteristics include raised temperature, pain and tenderness in the loins, and frequency of passing urine; but in many cases there is merely a vague malaise, so that the condition is identified only by examination of the urine for bacteria.

The sulphonamide drugs are generally effective.

pyelography. An x-ray examination of the kidneys after they have been temporarily rendered opaque by injection of an iodine compound which concentrates in the kidneys. If the kidney that is to be examined is functioning well the compound may be injected into a vein and reaches the kidney via the bloodstream. If the kidney is not adequately filtering material from the blood, the compound has to be introduced into the bladder using a cystoscope.

pyloric stenosis. Obstruction of the outlet of the stomach, the pylorus, through which food normally passes to the duodenum on its way through the DIGESTIVE SYSTEM. The common form occurs in young babies in the first few weeks of life, with cases in boy babies thrice as numerous as in girl babies. The affected infants suffer from projectile vomiting (i.e., true vomiting rather than the customary dribbling of feeds), steadily lose weight, and die if untreated. Some cases respond to atropin and similar antispasmodic drugs which relax the muscle of the pylorus. Other cases require a surgical operation which, while quite serious, is life saving. The condition is known to be of genetic origin.

A rather similar condition arises occasionally in adults as a result of scarring after a duodenal ulcer.

pylorus. The opening at the lower end of the stomach through which the stomach contents pass to the duodenum. The opening is controlled by a band of circular muscle fibres known as the pyloric sphincter. In PYLORIC STENOSIS the pylorus is narrowed and the passage of stomach contents becomes obstructed.

pyogenic. Pus-forming.

pyorrhoea. The term means simply a discharge of pus but as commonly used it usually refers to pyorrhea of the sockets of teeth. In this condition there is chronic infection and ulceration of the gum margins which may extend into the tooth-sockets, destroying the lining of the teeth, invading the bone, and loosening the teeth.

In its earliest stages it commences as inflammation of the gums usually caused by poor dental hygiene but sometimes aggravated by other local factors such as mouth breathing and irregularity of the teeth, or by general diseases which lower tissue resistance. Once

pyorrhoea has become established its ill-effects are irreversible because destroyed tissue cannot be replaced, but its further progress can be retarded by measures taken by a dental surgeon such as removing tartar and cutting away redundant gum-margin which forms pus-retaining pockets. The co-operation of the patient in carrying out gum-massage and maintaining satisfactory care of the teeth is also very important.

pyrexia. A synonym for FEVER or any febrile condition in which there is elevation of the normal body temperature.

pyrosis. See HEARTBURN.

pyuria. The presence of pus in the urine. This always indicates some inflammatory condition in the urinary tract: nephritis, pyelitis or cystitis. Pus is detected in the urine by laboratory tests and the treatment is that of the underlying condition.

Q

Q fever. A specific infectious disease caused by a rickettsia-like organism, now called *Coxiella burneti,* with an incubation period of two or three weeks and characterized by fever, headache, and usually chest pain, cough and scanty expectoration, indicating some lung involvement. The name 'Q' stands for Queensland, where the condition was first identified.

Ticks, wild animals, cattle, sheep and goats are natural reservoirs of infection, and the condition mostly occurs in persons working with animals or animal products; it is caught from air-borne spread of infected discharges or from direct contact with infected material. Patients suffering from Q fever are therefore mainly found among veterinary surgeons, farmers, and employees of dairies, stock-yards, meat-packing plants and wool-processing factories.

Exact diagnosis depends on blood-tests. The duration of the disease is variable and relapses are frequent, but it very seldom kills and treatment by antibiotics is effective. Pasteurization of milk destroys the organism. A satisfactory protective vaccine is available and should be used for persons at risk; where the disease occurs there is a need for investigation and hygienic control of sources of infection.

quarantine. The period during which persons who have been in contact with an infectious disease require to be isolated in order to make sure that they themselves are not going to develop the disease and so become a fresh source of infection to others. The duration of quarantine periods varies with different diseases but for any one disease must cover its longest incubation period.

There is ancient authority for the idea of quarantine: since the fifteenth century the sanitary laws of Venice, conforming to the Mosaic Code, enforced a period of forty days

isolation on all foreign shipping – hence the derivation of the word from the Italian *quaranta,* meaning 'forty'.

Nowadays quarantine is increasingly being replaced by SURVEILLANCE.

quickening. The stage of pregnancy at which the mother first becomes conscious of the movements of the developing child within her womb. Usually this awareness begins about the sixteenth to eighteenth week, which is approximately mid-term. By this time the uterus has enlarged and risen sufficiently to be in contact with the abdominal wall, and it is the transmission of impulses to the latter which enables the mother to sense them. The movements are initially quite feeble and have been picturesquely likened to 'the fluttering of a bird in the closed hand'.

quinine. A bitter-tasting alkaloid derived from the bark of the cinchona tree, originally from South America but subsequently grown in many warm countries. From 1638 it was used in Western Europe for both the prevention and the treatment of malaria. Essentially it renders the blood unsuitable for the multiplication of malarial parasites, so regular dosage in a mosquito-infested district will usually prevent malaria and larger dosage will generally cure the disease. In recent years, however, quinine has been largely replaced for prevention and treatment of malaria by synthetic substitutes which are even more effective and have fewer toxic effects. Nevertheless quinine is a drug that has saved millions of lives.

Apart from its specific effect on malaria, quinine helps to reduce any high temperature and is a favourite preparation in colds and other febrile illnesses, e.g., as the liquid ammoniated tincture of quinine or as quinine sulphate tablets. Large doses may produce ringing in the ears, temporary deafness, headache and giddiness; and extremely large doses may cause death by paralysing the brain and the respiratory centre.

quinsy. A complication of severe tonsillitis resulting when infection causes pus to form within the tonsillar capsule, creating an abscess. Inflammation and accumulation of pus leads to severe pain and difficulty in swallowing. The fauces are swollen and discoloured and the affected tonsil is displaced towards the mid-line.

Early cases may sometimes be treated successfully by prompt administration of antibiotic drugs but a developed case will usually require the opening of the abscess and evacuation of pus followed by antiseptic gargling. Immediate treatment should be followed later by removal of the tonsils since otherwise recurrence is common.

The word itself is interesting since it is a corruption of the French *esquinancie.* It is also related to the rather old-fashioned medical equivalent 'cyanche' which comes from two Greek words *kyon* and *angchein* meaning 'to throttle a dog' which emphasizes the great difficulty in swallowing caused by a well-developed quinsy.

quotidian fever. A form of MALARIA with bouts of fever almost every day.

R

rabies. A virus disease mainly affecting carnivorous animals (dog, cat, fox, wolf, jackal, skunk, opossum, mongoose, stoat, weasel, etc.) and also common in bats. It is widely prevalent throughout the world except in Australia. In Europe only Britain, Scandinavia, Iceland, Spain, Portugal and Cyprus are free from it, because of quarantine regulations and constant surveillance. Elsewhere the disease is a real or potential hazard of serious importance.

Affected animals show restlessness, snapping, difficulty in swallowing (hence the alternative name 'hydrophobia' – fear of water), excessive salivation, fury, or lethargy, followed by paralysis, coma and death. In man infection results from being bitten by a rabid animal and causes severe inflammatory reaction in the central nervous system (encephalomyelitis).

The incubation period is very variable (three weeks to six months or more) depending on the site or severity of the bite. Symptoms in man are similar to those in animals with sudden onset of fever, headache, restlessness, muscular spasm (specially of the muscles used in swallowing and breathing), and in due course paralysis of these muscles, coma, and death, usually within a week. Once the condition has developed far enough for the symptoms to appear, the outcome is invariably fatal. Early treatment of suspected cases by anti-rabies vaccine provides, therefore, the only hope.

Precautions. If there are special risks of contact with animals vaccination to develop immunity should be advised. Otherwise the ordinary traveller abroad should regard any animal with circumspection and seek immediate competent advice if bitten. If this happens the animal should if possible be caught and kept under observation to see if it develops rabies. In many countries vaccination of dogs is compulsory so it is also helpful to identify the owner and find out if the dog has been recently vaccinated, since such a dog is unlikely to be developing rabies.

If there is any doubt whatever a course of anti-rabies inoculation should be started immediately. The success of treatment depends entirely on its initiation as soon as possible.

If rabies is imported to a country previously free it can easily become endemic. Its eradication would involve massive destruction of wild creatures and vaccination of domestic animals. So rigorous control of the importation of dogs and cats is very important.

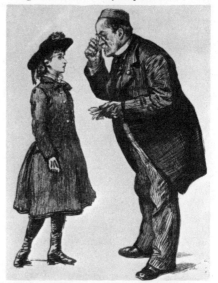

Rabies: Louis Pasteur examining a young English girl bitten by a mad dog. Rabies remains a killer disease

radiant heat. When light rays at the red end of the visible spectrum or the slightly longer infra-red rays beyond are absorbed by the skin their energy is transformed into local heat.

Infra-red radiation is given off by any hot body, but for therapeutic purposes heat cages or special lamps with a curved reflector are used for convenience and accuracy of local application. The heating elements of such appliances usually consist of ordinary electric bulbs blackened or reddened, or of porcelain cores wound with resistance wire which heat up on passage of an electric current exactly as does an ordinary electric radiator.

The action of infra-red radiation is to warm the skin and superficial tissues, producing redness from swelling of small blood vessels and increased circulation of blood. The rays also act as a sedative to sensory nerve-endings and induce perspiration. Because of these effects radiant heat is used to relieve pain and relax muscle spasm. The improved circulation helps to reduce inflammation, and increased perspiration aids the excretion of toxins and waste products through the skin.

Conditions in which such treatment is prescribed are neuritis, neuralgia, arthritis, fibrositis, inflammation caused by injury, cellulitis and superficial sepsis; it is also used as a preliminary to massage and movement in injuries and paralysis, and occasionally in nephritis.

radioactive drugs. Medicines which exercise their effect through the RADIOACTIVITY of their constituents. Radiotherapy, mainly employed for treating malignant disease, has until recently utilized radiation given by x-rays from outside or applied internally by implanted radium needles. These methods are rather imprecise and also tend to damage skin or other tissue within the field of radiation.

Various elements that are needed by particular cells or organs pass directly to them, e.g., iodine passes to the thyroid gland. So, if artificial radioactive isotopes of these elements are given as drugs they can convey radiation exactly to the diseased organ. Moreover, because they are later eliminated or have known short periods of decay, their effects can be predicted or controlled.

The most successful example of this technique is in the treatment of persons suffering from hyperthyroidism or from cancer in the thyroid. A carefully calculated dose is given of a draught containing radioactive iodine (iodine 131) and the thyroid gland, performing its normal function, concentrates this radioactive substance within itself and so destroys its over-active or abnormal cells. Similarly radioactive phosphorus can be used for the treatment of certain blood diseases such as chronic leukaemia and polycythaemia. Other radioactive drugs are also used in diagnosis as 'tracers' to study how certain elements are being absorbed or altered and to localize tumours.

Patients undergoing such treatment need careful supervision because their waste-products may be radioactive and require special measures for disposal. Incontinence raises additional problems.

radioactivity. All matter consists of atoms of various elements. Each atom has a central nucleus, providing almost all its mass, and made up of positively-charged protons and uncharged neutrons. Around it are negatively charged electrons and, since the atom is held together by electrical forces, the electrons are equal in number to the protons. The atomic weight of an element depends on the total of protons plus neutrons (M) but its atomic number (z), which determines its chemical identity, depends only on the number of protons. Some identical chemical elements exist as isotopes always with the same z number but with different numbers of neutrons and hence a different atomic weight or M number. Most of the common elements are stable isotopes and undergo no change because any unstable variants in their geological past have long since broken down to stable residues with protons and neutrons bound together by nuclear forces so strong that no particle ever escapes.

In general, nuclei are stable if the total number of particles is not too great and if the proportions of protons and neutrons are about the same. In certain naturally occurring elements, such as uranium, with unstable isotopes, these requirements are not met, and the atom breaks down liberating particles and energy. This is radioactive disintegration and it results in radioactivity characterized by the emission of alpha, beta, or gamma 'rays', although it is now known that the first two consist of particles, being helium nuclei (two protons plus two neutrons) and electrons respectively. Radioactive decay decreases with time, and each radioactive isotope remains active for a period which varies enormously, from centuries to a fraction of a second.

Many new radioactive isotopes can now be made artificially by bombarding stable nuclei with atomic particles in an atomic reactor. This alters the z or M numbers, or both, to values incompatible with stability. These isotopes are important in medicine both for diagnosis and for treatment because radioactivity affects cell function. They also have research uses as 'labelled atoms' which facilitate studies in physiology, chemistry, genetics and many other subjects since the behaviour of an otherwise indistinguishable sample of a particular chemical element can be traced by its radioactivity.

radiotherapy. Treatment by means of x-rays or by the use of RADIOACTIVE substances. Radiation has the effect of damaging any tissue by ionization but cells are particularly susceptible at times when they are undergoing rapid growth and multiplication. Radiotherapy therefore has particular application in the treatment of malignant disease. The dose of radiation is adjusted so as to destroy the active cancerous cells without permanently harming the less active normal tissue.

The methods employed rely on conventional x-rays or on radium or the release of radium (radon). Deep x-ray therapy is applied by placing the patient under a beam of x-rays directed, usually from several different directions, to the site of tumour growth. With radium or radon, hollow needles containing the radioactive material are imbedded in the tumour. Now that it is possible to make radioactive isotopes, variants of this basic treatment have become possible. For general irradiation radioactive cobalt (cobalt 60) may be employed in a positioning device like a large x-ray machine (cobalt bomb).

Sometimes x-rays are also employed for the treatment of superficial skin diseases, especially those like ringworm which are due to fungi, but safer methods using new effective drugs are now more generally preferred. A complication of deep x-ray therapy is radiation sickness which usually manifests itself as a feeling of intense lassitude, sometimes accompanied by vomiting and diarrhoea, and by fever, a burning sensation in the mouth, and loss of hair. It may be necessary to stop the treatment temporarily or to reduce the frequency and intensity of applications. Radio-isotopes are also now used in the form of RADIOACTIVE DRUGS, to be taken internally for certain specific purposes.

radium. In 1896 Antoine Becquerel (1852-1908), a French physicist, showed that uranium salts could act upon a photographic plate. This work was followed up by Marie Curie and her husband Pierre, and they eventually succeeded in isolating a new element from pitchblende, a black mineral containing uranium oxide. This element proved to be radioactive and was given the name radium. Radium gives off alpha and beta particles and gamma rays all of which have produced effects on living cells. Because of this, radium and one of the substances produced by radium (radium emanation or niton) are used in medicine for the treatment of malignant disease in RADIOTHERAPY.

radius. One of the two long bones of the forearm, situated on the outer side of the limb. Its upper end is small and forms a small part of the elbow joint but the lower end is enlarged to articulate with the wrist bones and forms most of the wrist joint. When indirect violence is applied to the forearm it is usually the radius which suffers damage so that a fracture of its lower end just above the wrist joint (Colles' fracture) is a very common type of injury in falls upon the hand.

rash. Any temporary eruption on the skin is known as a rash or exanthem. Similar effects on mucous membranes are called an enanthem. Rashes are produced by the action of toxins on the elements of the skin and particularly on its small blood vessels. They may be produced by external causes such as bacterial and viral infections, parasitic or chemical irritation and drugs, or internally by metabolic abnormalities and allergies.

They vary very much in type, and their appearance and distribution are often highly characteristic of a particular disease or condition. The following terms are used in describing the features of a rash:

Erythema: a uniform redness of the skin.

Urticaria: irregular firm raised patches or weals.

Macules: discoloured spots not elevated above the surface.

Papules: small, solid, round, pimple-like elevations.

Vesicles: small fluid-containing blisters.

Bullae: large irregular fluid-containing blisters.

Pustules: papules, vesicles, or bullae which have become infected and filled with pus.

Petechiae: small pin point haemorrhages into the skin.

Purpuric spots: discoloured areas due to haemorrhages into the skin.

Ecchymosis: a large isolated patch of haemorrhage beneath the skin, usually due to external violence.

A prodromal rash is one which occurs in the early stages of an infectious disease and does not have the full-blown characteristics of the typical exanthem.

Any rash is only a symptom, and treatment must be directed towards identifying and removing the precise cause. Where a rash causes itching calamine lotion or talcum powder sometimes relieves the symptom.

rat-bite fever. This general term includes two very similar diseases which can only be differentiated bacteriologically. Each disease results from being bitten by an infected rat and the organisms responsible are *Streptobacillus moniliformis* and *Spirillum minus*. Most cases occur in India and the Far East, and in these countries are predominantly due to *Sp. minus*. In Europe and America the disease is relatively rare and is generally caused by *Str. moniliformis*. The Japanese name for the condition is *sodoku*.

The disease has an incubation period of three to ten days. Characteristic features are an unhealed, septic and swollen rat-bite, enlargement of the related lymph-glands, a high, swinging temperature, a measly or haemorrhagic rash, and severe joint pains. The death rate in untreated cases is about 10 per cent, but antibiotic treatment (especially with the tetracyclines) is usually effective. Apart from rat-bites local outbreaks have occurred through consumption of contaminated milk. Preventive measures should include rat-control and pasteurization of milk.

rats. Rats are by far the most injurious domestic and commercial pests. They persist as an ever-present menace always ready to increase their depredations when defensive and offensive measures against them are relaxed. They destroy great quantities of stored food and spoil even more; they damage property by burrowing and gnawing; and they are carriers of several important diseases.

Two species are found in Britain: the black rat (*Rattus rattus*) and the brown rat (*Rattus norvegicus*), but colour alone is not a good guide to identification. *R. rattus* is smaller and slimmer with a sharp muzzle, large naked ears and a long slender tail. It rarely weighs over 0.25 kg. (8 oz.). *R. norvegicus* is larger and stouter with a blunt muzzle, small hairy ears and a shorter thicker tail. Adults usually weigh about 0.5 kg. (1 lb.).

Rats are very prolific and breeding starts at about the age of 4 months. It is estimated that an unchecked rat population with access to adequate food supplies will increase by 10 per cent per week, and this increase is of course compound. In other words the population can double every two months.

Diseases. Bubonic plague is a disease carried by rats and transmitted to man by fleas. Although it is rare in developed countries there is always a risk of plague reaching a country by ship-borne rats. The worm disease trichinosis is transmitted by rats to pigs and may then infect man. Rats also transmit tape worms (especially the dwarf tape-worm, *Hymenolepis nana*), spirochaetal jaundice (leptospirosis) and rat-bite fever. Apart from these specific diseases rats contaminate food by their excreta which may contain the organisms of food-poisoning (salmonellosis).

Control. In Britain the Rats and Mice (Destruction) Act 1919 requires the 'occupier' of land to take all necessary steps to destroy rats and mice thereon and to prevent infestation. However, eradication of rats requires expert knowledge and help is best obtained from local authority pest officers or from a commercial specialist. The measures required are the rat-proofing of buildings and systematic extermination by poison-baiting, gassing or trapping. There are also other legal powers to enforce the 'de-ratization' of ships.

Raynaud's disease. An unpleasant condition characterized by spasm of the arteries supplying the fingers and toes, usually affecting both hands and both feet and occurring particularly in cold weather. Young females are the principal sufferers and there is often a considerable psychological element involved. Three stages in the condition of the fingers and toes are described: (1) contraction of blood vessels – the affected parts are pale and numb; (2) asphyxia, i.e., lack of oxygen in the tissues so that they are blue, congested, and painful; (3) gangrene, so that parts become black and may separate, although not many cases proceed to this extreme.

Preventive measures should aim at avoidance of cold and the use of warm clothing even if the dictates of fashion make this difficult to accept. Drugs that dilate blood vessels are also helpful. Severe cases may require surgical measures to divide the sympathetic nerve fibres accompanying the limb arteries.

recessive. The study of GENETICS has shown that particular hereditary characteristics are each determined by a pair of genes one of which is inherited from each parent. If the two genes are different the individual is said to be heterozygous for that characteristic which is then determined by the more powerful or DOMINANT gene. The other gene is unable to exercise its effect and is said to be recessive. Recessive inheritance can thus occur only when the individual is homozygous, having inherited two recessive genes – one from each parent.

A number of common conditions are determined by recessive inheritance including haemophilia, cystic fibrosis, amaurotic family idiocy (Tay-Sachs disease) phenylketonuria and sickle-cell anaemia.

Two persons may appear quite normal but each may carry a recessive gene for, as an example, albinism, and so albinos may appear amongst their offspring in a ratio of one to four. The risks of producing a homozygote are of course increased in marriages between related persons.

Some tests are now available for detection of carriers of recessive genes, notably in phenylketonuria and amaurotic family idiocy. There is as yet no satisfactory method of detecting carriers of cystic fibrosis; this would be a desirable advance since the incidence is about one in two thousand.

rectal douche. A douche is a stream of fluid directed against a part of the body or into any cavity for the relief or treatment of disease.

Instillation into the rectum of liquid intended to be retained and absorbed – such as a solution of glucose and salt where feeding by mouth is impracticable – is normally called injection; and a substance inserted to relieve constipation is termed an enema. Both are douches, but the term is more commonly applied to instillations for the treatment of worms (e.g., threadworms) and to the use of astringent, antiseptic or sedative lotions in inflammatory or ulcerative conditions, such as may arise from haemorrhoids, severe dysentery or malignant disease. The choice of a particular lotion depends on the exact condition and the effect sought.

rectal feeding. The rectal route may be used to supply liquid food when for any reason the normal route is not available or it is desired to afford the stomach complete rest. Rectal feeding is not very effective. It used to be common practice to instil peptonized fluids containing milk or beef extract but it is doubtful if these were absorbed. Rectal infusions for this purpose now utilize only salt and glucose – 5 or 10 per cent of the latter in normal saline. They are given either at intervals by catheter, rubber-tube, and funnel, or continuously by a drip apparatus.

rectum. The terminal part of the large intestine of the DIGESTIVE SYSTEM, it is continuous above with the descending colon and below with the anal canal. It lies entirely within the lower pelvis. Faecal matter entering the rectum from above collects there until distension produces a desire to defaecate. Contraction of the rectum then expels the motion through the anal canal and the anal opening.

Diseases. Imperfect development of the lower opening of the rectum (imperforate anus) is a relatively common congenital defect noted at birth and requiring immediate surgical treatment.

Chronic inflammation ('proctitis') may be a downward extension of mucous colitis or due to dysentery, threadworms, or in tropical countries hookworms (bilharziasis). Less common causes are gonorrhoea, tuberculosis and syphilis. Ulceration may follow, and when it involves the anal canal is known as fissure-in-ano which gives rise to severe pain on defaecation. Sepsis tracking from ulcerated areas causes abscesses around the anus (peri-anal abscess or ischio-rectal abscess). This may ultimately produce a false passage to the exterior (fistula-in-ano).

Carcinoma is the commonest tumour, usually occurring after the age of 60.

Piles or haemorrhoids are varicose veins lying in the wall of the lower rectum and anal canal. Although very common and usually only the result of chronic constipation, their sudden late appearance in a person over 40 rises suspicion of more serious disease and calls for investigation.

reduce. To restore to the natural position, often referring to dislocated joints or factured bones.

referred pain. Pain that is felt in a part of the body remote from the actual injury or disease. This happens because many of the organs of the body first develop in one part of the embryo, but in subsequent development they move to their final positions, taking their nerves with them. Hence pain signals from these nerves are misinterpreted by the brain as coming from their original position. See also PAIN.

reflex action. A rapid involuntary muscular response to some sensory stimulus. It is the result of what might be described as an 'emergency short cut' through the NERVOUS SYSTEM in order to achieve an immediate response to a crisis before transmitting the signal to the brain. This is achieved by using the 'reflex arc' in the spinal cord. Reflex actions are classified as (1) superficial, (2) deep or tendon, (3) visceral. In superficial reflexes muscular action results from skin stimulation. An example is the plantar reflex in which stroking

pain in right
shoulder possibly
due to inflamed
gall bladder

pain in left
shoulder possibly
due to heart
disease

pain in groin
possibly due
to kidney
stone

pain at
side of
leg
possibly
due to
slipped
disc

Referred pain

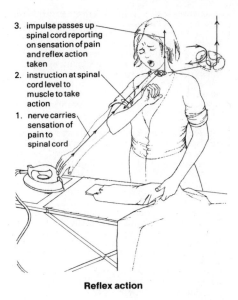

3. impulse passes up
   spinal cord reporting
   on sensation of pain
   and reflex action
   taken
2. instruction at spinal
   cord level to
   muscle to take
   action
1. nerve carries
   sensation of
   pain to
   spinal cord

Reflex action

the sole of the foot causes bending of the toes.
The knee-jerk is a deep or tendon reflex, a tap
on the knee-cap ligament causing straightening
of the leg. Most involuntary physiological
actions depend on visceral reflexes: food
stimulating the pharynx is automatically
swallowed and the need to pass urine or faeces
is a response to distension of the bladder or
rectum.

Investigation of reflex activity is an
important part of clinical examination in
disease of the nervous system and provides
clues to the nature and site of any injury.

refraction. Deflection of a ray of light from its
path when it passes through a transparent
substance, e.g., glass or water. It is this
phenomenon which enables the eye to focus
light onto the retina, and if the eye is so formed
that the focus is not perfect, there is said to be a
refractive error; see EYESIGHT.

registrar. A term with two specific meanings:
1. An official charged with keeping certain
records. Examples are the local authority
registrar who maintains formal records of
births, marriages and deaths in his district, and
the university registrar responsible for
information relating to students, staff and
courses.
2. In the U.K. a doctor who has passed
through the junior post-registration grades of
house officer (house physician or house
surgeon) and senior house officer and is

aspiring to become a consultant in a particular
specialty. A senior registrar in his third or
fourth year normally holds all relevant higher
qualifications and is of consultant calibre, but
has not yet secured an appointment as a full
consultant.

regression. There are three definitions of this
particular term.
1. In psychoanalytical theory regression is a
defence mechanism: in anxiety a person may
retreat to an earlier developmental stage of
greater security. This is particularly seen in
orphaned or neglected infants who regress into
stupor and require stimulation before they will
suck or otherwise respond. This suggests that
there is a return to a pre-natal pattern of life
when breathing and circulation were maternal
responsibilities. Poor breathing and circulation
impair nervous development and this leads to
profound and persisting physiological and
psychological consequences. Nowadays the
usual prescription is a daily dose of TLC - tender
loving care – combined with massage and
sensory stimulation.

Adults may show similar regression
especially in chronic alcoholism and
involutional psychosis, and in schizophrenia
where stupor and a curled-up position are seen
as symbolic of an unconscious attempt to re-
attain the secure and undemanding protection
of the womb.
2. Another meaning of regression is the
subsidence of a disease process.
3. Regression has yet another meaning in the
field of statistics. Here it is employed to
describe the relationship between two variable
quantities.

rehabilitation. The term is applied to
systematic measures that aim at restoring a
person's physical, mental, social and
occupational fitness after illness, injury or
prolonged strain. Clearly there is a certain
overlap with treatment, but essentially
treatment is the curing of the particular
condition or its improvement as far as is

practicable, while rehabilitation seeks to cope with the weakness produced by the condition or by its treatment. The following examples illustrate the difference.

1. A coal-miner sustained a serious injury to an arm and a leg. Treatment involved many weeks in plaster. The fractures have now healed and from the aspect of treatment he is cured; but the unused muscles have become weak, so that he needs a course of exercises – rehabilitation – before being fit to resume work as a miner.

2. A man whose tuberculosis was diagnosed late has spent eighteen months in hospital but is now regarded as cured. No further treatment is required (though as a safeguard he may be asked to attend occasionally for examination). During these eighteen months all his personal needs have been catered for, his decisions have been taken for him, and he has gradually become more and more dependent. He is in no condition to re-enter a community in which personal effort and initiative are demanded. He needs considerable re-education towards energetic independence and the acceptance of full social responsibility. For rehabilitation he may need a period of organized and graded occupational therapy, or intellectual stimulation through prescribed reading, lectures and group discussion, or planned social activites.

3. A bus driver of 21 years whose recreation was football had a serious accident; a leg had to be amputated and he has been fitted with an artificial limb. Treatment is completed and he can walk well with the artificial leg. As part of his rehabilitation he needs to be fitted for a different type of employment, convinced that he can enjoy recreations other than football, and helped to realize that his former associates will not regard him as a cripple.

4. Through shortage of jobs a man has been unemployed for three years but jobs suitable for him are now likely to become available. There was no illness and therefore no treatment; but in these three years of increasing discouragement about posts he has become physically weaker and mentally demoralized. Manifestly he needs a period of mental and physical 'toning up' before becoming fit to undertake the particular form of work for which he is qualified.

In the past the term 'rehabilitation' was mainly understood as the application of physical measures such as physiotherapy, e.g., to improve the muscular action of a person whose leg or arm had been temporarily paralysed as the result of a stroke. These physical measures remain highly important but nowadays recognized as constituting only one part of rehabilitation. As will be apparent from the examples given above, various educational, social, psychological and vocational factors may also be involved.

In most, indeed perhaps all, countries rehabilitation is still very inadequately and patchily developed. There are various reasons for this. In the first place, doctors, especially doctors working wholly or mainly in hospital, are primarily interested in diagnosis and treatment; and in most cases they know little about the requirements of the post to which the patient hopes to return or the social climate in which he will live after the discharge from hospital. Clearly a team approach is needed

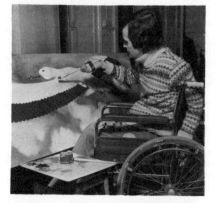

Rehabilitation: this man, severely disabled following an accident, has learnt to overcome some of the resulting handicaps

involving various combinations of the following specialists: the hospital nurse, the health visitor, the social worker, the physiotherapist, the occupational therapist, the speech therapist, the orthoptist (a specialist in the training of the eye-muscles), the remedial gymnast, the chiropodist, and in some cases the psychologist and the personnel manager.

In the second place, several advanced countries already have a considerable shortage of qualified nurses, and such workers as health visitors, physiotherapists and occupational therapists are often in very short supply.

Thirdly, there is a tendency in many countries for physiotherapists, remedial gymnasts, occupational therapists and so on to be based in hospitals; but doctors, faced with a shortage of beds often dependent on a shortage of nurses, naturally seek to discharge patients as soon as clinical cure is complete or has advanced as far as is reasonably practicable; and many of the most important portions of rehabilitation are related to the stage after treatment has ended.

Nevertheless, there are advances in progress, such as the provision of day hospitals where the recovering patient spends the evenings and nights at home but has any necessary treatment and occupational therapy during the day. As a further example of advance the setting up in the U.K. of industrial rehabilitation units and government training centres may be mentioned. Additionally, progressive psychiatric hospitals are developing units for industrial therapy where work can be organized to resemble an industrial situation but can also be carefully regulated to the capacity of the individual patient.

Apart from shortages of skilled personnel, there are many difficulties. For instance, if a financially supported unit begins to produce and sell goods in a time of considerable unemployment, the ordinary (undisabled) producers of these goods begin to question whether it is beneficial or harmful to restore a disabled person to something like full capacity at the cost of making another person unemployed.

A very practical aspect of rehabilitation is the development and use of aids for the disabled. These range from obvious items like artificial limbs and purpose-built cars which can be driven by a person with the use of only one leg or one arm to many ingenious gadgets to deal with the recurrent difficulties of everyday domestic life. Many such devices have been produced by voluntary organizations (e.g., in the U.K. the British Red Cross Society and the National Fund for Crippling Diseases), but in general advice is available from the health visitor, public health nurse or social worker.

rejuvenation. Ageing appears to be an inescapable outcome of the activities of any biological organism, and rejuvenation in the sense of any real renewal of youth remains a mere dream. In extreme old age there is an inevitable deterioration in the efficiency of physical and mental functions.

The main theories advanced to explain this are that ageing is caused by loss of (or injury to) cells that the body has lost the capacity to replace; that cells produced late in life are not as good as the same type of cells developed during youth; and that the changes are not so much in the cells as in structureless components of the body, for instance the walls of blood vessels. These theories may all be true.

Since cell-function in a complex organism is influenced by chemical messengers or hormones, and since ageing of reproductive cells precedes ageing of other tissues, it was only a short step to the hypothesis that if production of sex-hormones could be maintained the ageing of other tissues could be delayed or reversed. This led a Russian surgeon, Serge Voronoff of Moscow, to develop an operation for transplanting to man the testes of anthropoid apes. At that time (1930) this 'monkey gland' form of rejuvenation gained some notoriety and it still retains some status as a humorous metaphor, but the claims of its originator were not fulfilled and his work is now only of historical interest. From what we now know of tissue-matching and tissue-rejection (see TRANSPLANT) it is clear that the procedure was foredoomed to failure. It may be that there are still unexploited possibilities using human tissue but there would be enormous practical difficulties. Experience in the use of sex hormones such as testosterone in the treatment of testicular inadequacy or of the male climacteric has not produced any convincing results.

The most effective practical hopes of delaying the ill-effects of old age lie in the extension of two fields of medical work: (1) efforts to maintain and improve the physical and emotional health of persons around the age of RETIREMENT, e.g., attention to diet, exercise, eyesight and hearing, and the fostering of leisure interests; and (2) identification and treatment of diseases of later life at an early stage, where they can be cured or at least ameliorated.

relapsing fever. A specific infectious disease due to generalized infection by a spirochaete, *Borrelia recurrentis*. Man acquires the disease from infected lice or various species of ticks. Louse-borne relapsing fever may become epidemic and is mainly found in Africa, Asia, and South America. The tick-borne variety is more usually endemic and occurs principally in tropical Africa, but wild rodents such as ground squirrels and prairie dogs harbour ticks which have caused cases in the U.S.A.

The incubation period of the disease is three to twelve days (usually eight) and it shows itself as an intermittent fever in which feverish episodes of two or three days alternate with non-feverish periods of two to four days in up to ten or more 'relapses'. In untreated cases, especially in the epidemic form, as many as half may die, but the infection responds well to antibiotic treatment.

Prevention depends on the control of lice and ticks by insecticides and repellents, and on precautions against tick-infestation by clearing land, reducing small mammal populations, controlling stray dogs, and dipping livestock.

relaxation therapy. Treatment by resting the activity of both body and mind has long been employed in both mental and physical diseases.

1. Anxiety and emotional tension are symptomatic of life in advanced societies. Noise, the pressures of modern life, increasing materialism, and disregard for the individual and of his emotional needs and capacities have all led to an increasing prevalence of psychosomatic disease, depressive, obsessional or anxiety states, phobias, hysteria and hypochondriasis.

A once-fashionable method of treating such 'neurasthenic' conditions was associated with the name of Weir-Mitchell and was based on prolonged bed-rest, a generous diet, massage, and removal of external stimulation. However, this was before the almost explosive development of drugs active on the brain beginning about 1950. Relaxation therapy as now understood and practised in the treatment of mental and psychoneurotic disorders depends on the use of new psycho-active drugs which are used simultaneously with psychotherapy. The drugs employed vary in strength. Powerful ones are used in acute mental illness and have revolutionized the work of mental hospitals. Minor tranquillizers or anti-anxiety agents are nowadays prescribed and taken on an ever-increasing scale.

2. On the physical side muscle spasm is a feature of injuries and various acute and chronic inflammatory conditions. Although it is a protective response it can be a major cause of pain and discomfort; and relaxation by rest, correct posture, massage and infra-red radiation can do much to help. Return to mobility is encouraged by passive movements controlled by the masseur or by active movements performed in a relaxed fashion with the weight of limbs or body supported by slings or by floating in the physiotherapy pool.

3. Systematic training in relaxation is also the basis of the regime pioneered by Dr Grantly Dick Read to encourage painless and NATURAL CHILDBIRTH.

renal. Of the kidneys.

renal colic. Stones may form in any part of the urinary tract through the deposition of urinary salts. The presence of a stone (or CALCULUS) in the kidney causes pain in the loin and blood in the urine. At intervals there may be attacks of more agonizing spasmodic pain starting in the loin, and radiating downwards to the groin. There may be frequency of passing urine and evidence of fresh haemorrhage with vomiting, abdominal rigidity, and all the symptoms of shock and general collapse.

Such an attack of renal colic is due to intermittent contractions of the pelvis, of the kidney and of the ureter in attempting to drive the stone downwards along the ureter. Similar pain may be produced by the passing of a blood clot or of urinary crystals (gravel). Immediate treatment employs sedatives, rest, and local application of heat, but the condition requires full genito-urinary investigation to determine what further measures are needed. Operation may be called for if the stone has not been passed.

renal dialysis. See KIDNEY MACHINE.

reproduction. The fundamental difference between living and non-living things is that only the former possess the ability to grow by assimilation of food and to multiply by reproducing new organisms like themselves.

Reproduction may be either asexual or sexual. The asexual pattern is seen in simple single-celled organisms where the cell and its nucleus become elongated and shaped like dumb-bells and then split into two new individuals, a process known as binary fission. A further development of this is a splitting into several new individuals simultaneously; this is multiple fission. The multiplication in the blood stream of the parasite which causes malaria is an example.

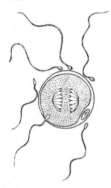

Fertilization: the head of the sperm enters the ovum, creating a single cell

Sexual reproduction on the other hand is preceded by a linking of male and female sex-cells – spermatozoon and ovum respectively. These sex-cells or gametes unite to form a zygote by the process of fertilization. The zygote then undergoes repeated sub-division and gradually grows into a new individual.

Some simple animals and many plants possess both male and female reproductive organs in one individual and are capable of self-fertilization. They are said to be hermaphrodites. In other instances the ovum is capable of development without fertilization and this type of reproduction is known as parthenogenesis. See REPRODUCTIVE SYSTEM, HEREDITY and GENETICS.

reproductive system. Reproduction in the vertebrates, including man, is sexual, that is to say that fertilization requires union between an ovum from the female and a spermatozoon from the male. The result is a zygote or embryo which is then protected and nourished within the female for a period of gestation, varying with the species, until growth by cell-division and differentiation produces a miniature replica sufficiently developed to be born and to survive. The reproductive system therefore provides for the production of ova by the female and spermatozoa by the male, for arrangements to secure their union, and for the accommodation of the embryo until it reaches a required stage of development.

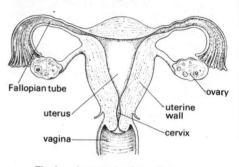

The female reproductive system

The female pelvis contains the uterus or womb, a pear-shaped, hollow, muscular organ designed to accommodate and nourish a growing embryo and to expel it when mature. From its upper border arise two narrow ducts (one on each side) known as the Fallopian tubes; these terminate as trumpet-shaped, fringed extremities close to the ovaries.

An ovum is liberated each month from an ovary and conveyed by the Fallopian tube to the uterus. If it encounters a spermatozoon it may become fertilized and the resultant zygote embeds itself in the lining of the uterus and develops as an embryo. The lining undergoes a regular monthly cycle of change designed to make sure that it is suitable for implantation; this is known as MENSTRUATION.

The lower end of the uterus is the cervix which links these internal organs to the vagina, a muscular tube opening externally at the vulva. This is a cleft bounded in front by the mons veneris, a fatty pad, overlying the pubic bone and carrying the pubic hair; at the sides by two thick folds of skin, the labia; and behind by the perineum. The forward ends of the labia are joined to enclose the clitoris, a small, sensitive organ corresponding to the male penis. In the virgin state the lower vaginal opening is partially closed by the membranous hymen ruptured at first intercourse (defloration).

The male organs basically consist of the sex-glands or testes for the production of spermatozoa and, in addition, other structures to ensure that the spermatozoa can subsequently be deposited within the female genital tract. The spermatozoa are conveyed from the seminal tubules of the testes inside the scrotum towards the base of the bladder by the vas deferens of the spermatic cord. Also at the base of the bladder are the prostate gland and two sack-like pouches, the seminal vesicles. The gland and vesicles produce a fluid which mixes with spermatozoa from the vas to become the seminal fluid or semen.

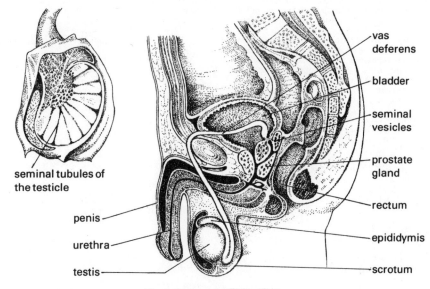

seminal tubules of
the testicle

penis

urethra

testis

vas
deferens

bladder

seminal
vesicles

prostate
gland

rectum

epididymis

scrotum

The male reproductive system

From here the liquid passes along the urethra, a duct extending down the centre of the penis, the external male organ of copulation. The end of the penis has a sheath called the prepuce or foreskin. (This is removed in the operation of circumcision; where it is not so removed it should be pulled back during bathing and the underlying part, in which debris can accumulate, kept clean.)   Part of the structure of the penis is a spongy layer, the spaces of which are occupied by blood vessels. Under sexual stimulation the spongy tissue becomes distended with blood so that the whole organ becomes enlarged, stiffened, and erect, preparatory to copulation. During sexual intercourse the erect penis enters the female vagina and contractions of the vas deferens and seminal vesicles force seminal fluid into the penis from which it is forcibly and rhythmically expelled into the vagina as an ejaculation.

It should be noted that in the female the urinary tract is quite separate from the genital tract, but that in the male the urethra carries both urine and semen.

resolution. A term describing the successful repair of tissue damage by inflammation without the formation of pus, ulcers or gangrene.

respiration. Apart from some insignificant exceptions, like some types of bacteria, all living organisms require oxygen to maintain life. In the chemical changes undergone by living cells oxygen is combined with carbon and hydrogen derived from food materials. This process, known as oxidation, produces carbon dioxide (CO_2) and water (H_2O), and at the same time liberates the energy required for heat production and muscular activity. Oxidation of hydrogen is an important source of body water, but the carbon dioxide is simply waste matter. The whole process in which an organism exchanges oxygen and carbon dioxide between itself and its environment is known as respiration.

In general, single-celled organisms and simple multi-cellular plants and animals live in a fluid, so that this respiration takes place directly between the cells and their surroundings. In larger and more complex organisms that is no longer possible because the area of external surface becomes relatively smaller as bulk increases and the surface itself changes on account of the need for support and protection so that a more complex arrangement needs to be developed. This is provided in all the higher animals by the circulation of the blood. The essentials of such a system are a network of capillary vessels carrying blood to all the cells; lungs or gills to allow the blood to take up oxygen from the environment and get rid of carbon dioxide; and a blood-pump or heart to move the blood from the lungs to the cells and back again.

The process of respiration can be divided into internal respiration, which is the exchange of gases between cells and blood, and external respiration which is the gaseous interchange in the lungs between the blood and the air. Respiration has another important function because the level of CO_2 in the blood helps to determine the pH or acid-alkali balance of the bloodstream, and this is delicately adjusted by the rate and depth of breathing. See METABOLISM and RESPIRATORY SYSTEM.

respiratory system. The elements of the respiratory system are the lungs and the respiratory tract, which comprises the nose, pharynx, larynx, trachea, bronchi and bronchioles and provides a route for air to enter and leave the lungs. Within the nose are the two nasal passages. They open externally at the nostrils and are separated internally by the midline nasal septum. They are designed to humidify and warm air which is breathed in by contact with moist mucous membrane; the area of the mucous membrane is increased by the turbinate bones which are three thin, curved, shelf-like projections into each nasal passage.

Behind the nose is the pharynx, a tubular cavity communicating above with the mouth and nasal passages and below with the larynx. At the upper end of the larynx is a flap of cartilage, the epiglottis, which folds over during swallowing to close the upper opening of the larynx and so prevents the entry of food or fluid.

The larynx, voicebox, or Adam's apple is a hollow piece of cartilage containing the vocal cords which can be drawn together so as to vibrate in the air-stream and produce sounds for the purpose of VOICE AND SPEECH. The channel through the larynx is continued downwards in the neck and chest as the trachea or wind-pipe. In mid-chest it divides into smaller tubes called bronchi. These branch to the right and left lungs and then by further subdivision to the main lobes of each lung – three on the right and two on the left. These main branches again divide and redivide as the bronchial tree or bronchioles and so reach every part of both lungs. They end as very fine tubes less than 1 mm. in diameter, each lying close to a small segment or lobule of the lung consisting of a group of alveoli or air-sacs. The trachea, bronchi and bronchioles are lined by cells with fine hair-like projections, called cilia, the purpose of which is to move secretions outwards with a whip-like action. The alveoli are lined by flattened cells so that air within them is separated from the capillary blood vessels of the lungs by a microscopically thin layer in order to facilitate the movement of oxygen from the air to the blood in the capillaries and of carbon dioxide in the opposite direction.

The lungs themselves appear spongy and are inherently elastic, so that they shrink and contract when not distended by air. In life they completely fill the chest cavity. During the act of breathing in, the size of the CHEST is increased by the muscles of respiration; the diaphragm moves down and the ribs are lifted upwards and forwards. This produces a partial vacuum and air enters the lungs along the respiratory tract; this process is known as inspiration. On expiration the muscles of respiration relax and air is expelled by the natural elasticity of the lungs and by return of the chest wall and diaphragm to the resting position.

Control of respiration is effected by nerve impulses from the respiratory centre in the mid brain. When the centre is stimulated the rate and depth of breathing are increased to meet the demands for greater respiratory inter-change of oxygen and carbon dioxide. The most important stimulus is a rising concentration of carbon dioxide in the blood stream. This normally occurs after exercise or in asphyxia. Other factors also may either inhibit or stimulate the centre: examples are gasping from sudden immersion in cold water, 'winding' by abdominal blows, coughing induced by partial obstruction, sneezing produced by irritation of the mucous membrane, and the rapid respiration which may accompany fear or anger. These are involuntary reactions but the brain also exercises voluntary control to meet the need

for a controlled air-flow during speech and singing.

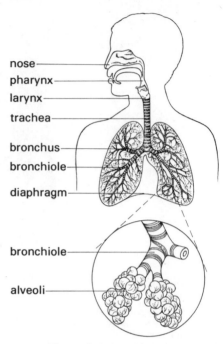

nose
pharynx
larynx
trachea
bronchus
bronchiole
diaphragm
bronchiole
alveoli

The respiratory system

Diseases. Diseases of the lungs and respiratory tract are very common, ranging in severity from the relative triviality of the common cold to conditions of the utmost gravity. In a survey in Britain, National Health Insurance statistics show that they are responsible for more than one-quarter of the total days of work-absence.

The main causes are infection, allergy, tumour and damage by dust, the first-named being by far the most frequent. They may be classified as follows:

1. Infections: these may occur in the upper respiratory tract or the bronchial tree and lungs. Examples of the former include the common cold, sinusitis, pharyngitis, tonsillitis, laryngitis and tracheitis. The infecting organisms are either viruses, as in colds and influenza, or various harmful bacteria, most frequently streptococci. Bronchial tree and lung infections include acute and chronic bronchitis, bronchopneumonia, lobar pneu-monia, pulmonary tuberculosis, pleurisy and fungus infections. These are due respectively to the pneumococcus, *M. tuberculosis,* and various types of moulds. Bronchiectasis, emphysema, and abscess of the lung may occur as later complications.

2. Allergy: responsible for hay-fever and for many cases of asthma.

3. Tumours: these may be simple or malignant. Nasal polypi are common and papillomata occur on the vocal cords, the so-called 'singers' nodes'. Except for these, simple tumours are rare, but the larynx, trachea and

bronchi are frequent sites for carcinoma, particularly in smokers. Although the lungs themselves and their related lymph-nodes may occasionally give rise to primary malignant tumours (endothelioma and lympho-sarcoma) tumours of the lungs are more usually secondary to malignant disease elsewhere.

4. Dust-diseases: these are occupational in origin due mainly to the inhalation of particles of silica or of other kinds of inorganic or organic dust. They produce chronic fibrosis of lung tissue.

rest. Cessation from motion or disturbance. A fundamental need of all living organisms is that their activity should be interrupted or reduced at appropriate intervals in order to allow recovery of strength by the elimination of waste products and the replenishment of energy resources. In addition, more prolonged periods of freedom from disturbance may be required for repair of tissue.

All this is a matter of common knowledge and experience. The whole body needs a nightly period of repose which we recognize as sleep. Muscles become fatigued by excessive exercise, and recover when rested; the mind becomes tired by long-continued mental effort; the special senses become blunted by over-use. If the objection is raised that this principle does not apply to the heart, which beats uninterruptedly from birth to death, the answer is that it secures its necessary respite not only from diminished activity during sleep but also in small amounts between each heart-beat, as it relaxes completely during the phase of diastole.

The above are examples of the need for rest as a normal physiological provision, but in disease rest becomes an essential aid to any form of treatment in order to secure reduced activity, either of a particular tissue or organ, or of the body as a whole. In many conditions, particularly those associated with fever and toxaemia, there is wasting and tissue destruction. These impose strain on the circulatory and excretory systems and this strain must be reduced as far as possible. Healing of diseased organs depends on tissue repair; unnecessary movement extends the area of infection, increases damage, and discourages or delays attempts at restoration.

In certain circumstances rest can be secured by mechanical or therapeutic means. Fractured limbs can be splinted; a lung can be immobilized by temporarily collapsing it; iritis can be treated by paralysing the ciliary muscle with appropriate drugs; and rest of the mind, important in many illnesses, can be secured by psychotherapy or by the use of tranquillizing drugs. The degree of rest which should be imposed depends on the particular condition under treatment. It may range from the absolute bed-rest necessary for the patient with a heart-attack to the holiday which is recommended to complete a period of convalescence. Professional advice must be the guide.

A person seeking to organize his own rest should note various points. Physical rest should include adequate time in bed each night and at least an hour of complete relaxation at some time during each day. Mental rest is often the most difficult to achieve: it involves the deliberate fostering of a determination not to think at night about the worries of today or the problems of tomorrow; it also involves a certain reorientation of attitudes – a conscious creation of degrees of priority and a firm decision to omit or postpone tasks or engagements for which there is not adequate time available.

The subject of rest is inseparable from that of sleep, which if inadequate will not only delay the cure of disease but will also undermine previously good health. The causes and treatment of sleeplessness are more fully discussed under INSOMNIA.

restlessness. Excessive or relentless activity occurs most often at night and in association with sleeplessness (INSOMNIA), which is itself a feature of many illnesses and largely a problem of good nursing. Over-activity by day, with or without sleeplessness at night, is an important feature of certain diseases, e.g., hyperthyroidism, the manic phase of manic-depressive psychosis, and a form of brain damage that leads to constant jerky movements. It may also occur in adults and children who are physically uncomfortable, over-tired or over-anxious.

It is sensible to look for simple causes first. For instance the person who is restless in bed – especially if he is a young child or an invalid unable to remove causes of discomfort – may be hungry or thirsty, his feet may be cold, or he may be too hot or too cold generally. His bed may have an uncomfortably hard mattress, wrinkled sheets, unremoved crumbs or badly placed pillows. He may need to pass urine or empty his bowels. If he is a patient his bandages or splints may be too tight. If such causes are eliminated, the restlessness may be a result of fears, persisting anxiety, or over-fatigue.

Restlessness may be more specifically related to his disease. The patient may be fevered, with a hot dry skin or, conversely, excessive perspiration. He may have pain, headache, breathlessness, palpitation, flatulence or abominal discomfort. If he has had an operation restlessness is an important warning of internal haemorrhage.

It is essential to identify the cause of the distress and take steps to afford relief. Drugs should be a last resort. By depressing vital functions they delay the elimination of toxins and are no substitute for the beneficial effects of normal sleep and rest if they can be secured by simpler methods.

resuscitation. Emergency restorative measures applied to a person who is unconscious or apparently dead as a result of respiratory or cardiac failure.

The need for resuscitation as a first-aid procedure usually arises from some accidental or unexpected cause as in drowning, choking, gas or narcotic poisoning, electrocution, or a heart attack. In these circumstances ARTIFICIAL RESPIRATION should be started immediately; mouth-to-mouth breathing is effective and simpler to carry out than the older standard methods. Where the heart has stopped external cardiac massage may be of use but requires care and experience. The heart is compressed by rapid rhythmical pressure on the breast bone (see FIRST AID). Most ambulances now carry oxygen and resuscitatory appliances as standard equipment.

Resuscitation may also be needed for newborn infants, and in the course of anaesthesia for surgical operations, but in these circumstances specialized equipment and resources are provided as a precaution.

retention. In retention of urine there is a stoppage of voiding of urine through a defect in the urinary apparatus. As urine accumulates, the bladder becomes distended and painful. If hot hip baths or hot fomentations applied to the abdomen do not give relief, it may be necessary to pass a catheter into the bladder.

retina. The light-sensitive inner lining of the EYE.

retirement. It is now a generally accepted pattern of British life that men should give up work at 65 and women at 60. This is a development quite uncharacteristic of less advanced societies and even of our own recent past. By adjusting pace to age and physical capacity, men used to work for as long as they were reasonably effective. Although their output might diminish they retained respect as sources of knowledge and skill, as local oracles, and as peacemakers in disputes. In the domestic field much the same was true of the older woman who often maintained or increased her sway.

Various factors have operated to change all this. Social legislation has introduced retirement pensions at a fixed chronological age and technological advances have also had their effect. The older worker may be steadier, more accurate, and more conscientious, but he is also slower, less strong, and less adaptable. His skills and knowledge soon become outmoded by progress. We live in a world where machines rapidly become obsolete or disposable and there is perhaps a tendency to view men in a similar light – 'superfluous lags the veteran on the stage'.

The position of women has also changed radically with their increasing employment outside the home, not only before marriage, but in later life after their main family responsibilities have been fulfilled. They too find themselves with problems of retirement unknown to their mothers and grandmothers. Changes in society have undermined the status of the older woman as a respected figure in home or village. The younger generation tends to move away to new housing areas and grandparents are left alone in a world with which they are out of sympathy and which they cannot influence.

In the past an elderly person was more of a rarity and to that extent more likely to be accorded respect. In 1900 only 6 per cent of the population was over pensionable age. In 1970 the figure was 16 per cent and still increasing: the average man who reaches the age of 65 can look forward, on British statistics, to thirteen years of rich, zestful life, and the average woman to sixteen such years. This change has been due not to any spectacular increase in longevity but simply to there being fewer deaths in infancy, childhood and young adult life.

The average expectation of life at birth is now 68 years for men and 75 years for women. This is a remarkable difference between the sexes and in large measure appears to be accounted for by the fact that attainment of retiral age generally forces on men a much more dramatic change than on women who have to remain active and interested in domestic tasks which to some extent they have done all their lives whether or not they also had paid employment. For men, however, retirement means that their feelings of usefulness and importance are suddenly taken away. This may be a shattering and demoralizing experience with rapid onset of boredom and loss of interest in life. Lack of mental stimulus soon has its repercussions on physical well-being; it was Nelson who said that it was better to wear out than to rust. Most parents try to prepare children for the first big change in life, from home to school; and the bulk of formal education should be a preparation for the change from dependent child to self-supporting adult, spouse and parent. Yet curiously little attention is paid to preparation for the equally big change from worker to pensioner. Full discussion of preparation for a healthy old age is beyond the scope of this article but six very important points are here selected for mention.

1. Attention to physical health. In particular the person around retirement age may find his hobbies and interests becoming limited by deteriorating vision, often easily corrected by suitable spectacles and good lighting. His communication with others may be lessened by poorer hearing, sometimes improved by removal of wax from the ears and in other cases helped by an appropriate hearing aid. He may begin to suffer from corns or bunions, requiring the attention of a chiropodist.

2. Decisions about food, drink and exercise. The overweight person and the person who is retiring from a physically strenuous job should cut down their intake of starches and sugars. The person who is facing a serious reduction of income should become aware of the need for adequate protein (with milk, eggs and fish often cheaper than meat) and for sufficient vitamins (with the possibility of much of the fruit and vegetables being supplied from his own garden). He may have a tendency to constipation through insufficient roughage in the diet or inadequate exercise. As he ages his dentures may cease to fit his shrinking gums and need renewal, since chewing difficulties can discourage him from maintaining a healthy diet. An occasional drink does no harm but alcohol may have to be reduced because of its cost to a retired person. Regular but moderate exercise is important: non-strenuous activities like walking and bowls are best.

3. Need for creative activity. Considerably before retirement he should begin to consider how he is going to occupy his vastly increased leisure time. Interests that appeal to different types include studying a subject for which time was not available earlier, painting, gardening, piano playing and sewing. Bowling is an excellent recreation and helps to create social contacts. Walking is good exercise but is more solitary.

4. Maintenance of social contacts. If he contemplates moving house, e.g., to be near his children, he should do so while still active enough to make new friends, and he should in any case consider how he is going to find substitutes for the many contacts that he had in the course of his work. Whether he moves house or not he should try to join some form of congenial social organization. One way in which he can very usefully make new contacts is by joining one of the many organizations that seek to help persons who are older or more handicapped than himself.

5. Financial matters. Monetary preparation

for retirement should begin at least five – preferably ten – years earlier, since some savings can make the difference between physical comfort and bare existence. It may also be possible to work out other economies for the future period of lessened income. For instance, the house may be too large, and transfer to a smaller house may reduce housework and save money. The heating system may be wasteful of fuel, and the cost of installing a more economical system could perhaps be met during full employment but not after retirement. Not least, skilled advice should be sought regarding the best way of investing any savings.

6. Finding people and organizations that can help. Before retirement a person is wise to familiarize himself with agencies that can help him. In the U.K. the family HEALTH VISITOR can do much to suggest methods of maintaining physical and mental health, preventing accidents and injuries, and rearranging the domestic budget; the local office of the Department of Health and Social Security can give information about pension and possible supplementary allowances; and the local education department may organize pre-retirement courses.

In retirement the person should continue to follow the lines indicated in the six points above, to lead a reasonably active life, and to realize that he is entitled to call on the services available – whether on his general practitioner (who in Britain receives a larger annual payment for an old person than for an ordinary member of his list), or on his health visitor, or on the social work department. In looking ahead he has to face the fact that all men are mortal, but he should also appreciate that advances in modern medicine should make the suffering of severe pain unnecessary.

Two further points may be noted. Firstly, age tends to accentuate the traits of earlier life. Hence the person of advancing years may need a self-assessment. If, for example, he tended earlier to give vent to rages, raising his blood pressure, he may now have to cultivate self-discipline lest he creates the circumstances for a stroke. If he over-smoked, he may now grossly over-smoke and create a danger of chronic bronchitis; or if he was careless over his clothing and appearance, he may have to take pains lest he become an unshaven, unwashed, disreputable looking old man.

Secondly, if he lives with a younger relative, he should remember that the relative needs a private life and adequate time to enjoy it. At least some old people change their image from that of beloved parents to that of hated tyrants by seeking to have a younger relative available for twenty-four hours in each day.

Measures are therefore necessary to ensure that retiral from work is not followed by the tragedy of physical and mental deterioration. Industry should seek to make retirement more flexible and abandon the rigidity of a set chronological age. Re-training for non-manual jobs, the provision of sheltered or part-time work and the organization of outwork for the house-bound are possibilities which might be studied so that pensioners could be meaningfully employed. Training for leisure is as important as training for work and can diminish many of the problems and ill-effects of enforced idleness.

There is immense scope too for organized effort by social agencies. Adequate retiral allowances linked to cost of living indices are of course a first essential but equally important are all the measures now being developed, all too slowly, to ensure that elderly people are integrated with the community and do not become prey to loneliness and isolation. The significance of the whole question of retirement becomes very clear when it is remembered that about half the people who reach pensionable age can expect to have more than a quarter of their lives ahead of them.

retrolental fibroplasia. The death-rate among newly born infants, which had been almost stationary for many years, suddenly started to decline substantially about 1940. This was due in part to improvements in the resuscitation and care of premature infants with the use of incubators which provided an oxygen-rich atmosphere.

Unfortunately, some surviving infants were found to be blind or to have severe visual defect because of increase in fibrous tissue behind the lens of the eye. Most surprisingly, it was discovered that this effect was caused by high concentrations of oxygen which nobody had even suspected might be harmful.

Since then the practice has been to limit oxygen-concentration, or to give it intermittently, and the condition of retrolental fibroplasia has virtually disappeared as suddenly as it came.

retroversion. A particular variety of displacement of the UTERUS out of its normal position.

rhesus factor. A substance present by inheritance in the blood of most people but not of all.

In 1900 Karl Landsteiner (1868-1943), a New York pathologist, and other workers elsewhere showed the existence of four BLOOD GROUPS. These were known as A, B, AB and O according to the factors (agglutinogens) which could cause red blood corpuscles to clump together.

However, a subsequent and equally significant development was the discovery (by Landsteiner and Weiner in 1940) that red cells from rhesus monkeys when injected into laboratory animals produced agglutinins which in turn would react with red cells from 83 per cent of human blood samples. Persons with such cells were designated rhesus-positive (Rh + ve); the other 17 per cent were rhesus-negative (Rh–ve). These proportions vary with race.

Demonstration of this rhesus factor next led to an appreciation of the cause of haemolytic disease of the new-born (erythroblastosis foetalis). If a Rh–ve woman is bearing the child of a Rh + ve man, the unborn child may inherit the Rh factor from the father. Normally foetal and maternal bloodstreams remain quite separate so that no difficulty need arise if their Rh grouping is different. However, if the placenta is damaged even minimally (e.g., by toxaemia, accidental haemorrhage, or obstetrical operations or manipulations), Rh + ve foetal red cells gain access to the Rh–ve maternal circulation and cause an antibody to form. This antibody then diffuses back into the foetal circulation and destroys foetal red cells so that the infant is either still-born or shows signs of severe anaemia at birth, with jaundice and other symptoms which may cause death or disability.

This does not happen in the first pregnancy. Several stimuli are required to produce significant amounts of antibody, so it is the second and succeeding infants who are most likely to be affected. For good antenatal care it is very important to identify the Rh–ve mother and assess the formation of antibodies so that steps may be taken in good time to treat the infant by exchange transfusion, replacing its damaged blood. This can now be done even before birth. Another procedure that aims to prevent the development is active Rh immunization in Rh–ve mothers by giving injections of appropriate immunoglobulin shortly after delivery. The object of this is to neutralize the antigenic effects of any Rh+ve foetal red cells which may have crossed the placenta.

rheumatic fever. An alternative name is acute articular rheumatism. Streptococci cause various diseases: upper respiratory tract infections, tonsillitis, scarlet fever, erysipelas, and puerperal fever are specific examples but the germs are also a common cause of impetigo, wound infections, cellulitis, osteo-myelitis, otitis and septicaemia.

Rheumatic fever may occur as a sequel to streptococcal infection, usually of the upper respiratory tract. Although the actual infection may be insignificant or may have gone unrecognized, the fact that it did occur can almost always be demonstrated by laboratory blood-tests.

So rheumatic fever differs from conventional infection by being a reaction brought about by toxin from previous or present streptococcal conditions. Its main clinical features are fever and arthritis of many joints, very often heart involvement shown by rapid pulse, chest pain and breathlessness, usually anaemia and loss of weight, and sometimes twitching movements, nodules below the surface of the skin, and rashes. Mild and unrecognized attacks may occur and definite and even severe heart disease may develop even in the absence of obvious rheumatic fever.

The acute stage is usually treated with salicylates and sometimes with cortisone to reduce inflammation in the joints, but prevention is all-important. Any initial or predisposing infections should be promptly and adequately treated by antibiotics. Since acute rheumatism is particularly prone to recur, the long-term use of prophylactic penicillin is now standard practice with the object of removing or minimizing the risk of heart complications.

rheumatism. A general term for a group of disorders that cause pain in the joints, muscles and bones. RHEUMATIC FEVER, which is a specific infection though sometimes called rheumatism, is considered elsewhere, as is RHEUMATOID ARTHRITIS. The present note deals essentially with muscular rheumatism and so-called chronic rheumatism in adults, and with rheumatism in children.

Muscular rheumatism. An ill-defined term which may be regarded as synonymous with fibrositis, a condition of acute or chronic inflammatory change affecting the fibrous tissues of the body, and in particular those which form the muscular sheaths and tendons, and the joint capsules and ligaments. The symptoms are predominantly pain and muscle spasm. Lumbago is perhaps the most familiar example of the condition but any group of muscles may be affected.

An exact cause is often difficult to identify, but sepsis, diet, metabolic defects, trauma, occupation, fatigue and climate may all play a part. The condition is common in cold countries and especially in persons whose occupations involve exposure to damp, cold, and excessive strain. Damp and cold act by depressing the circulation, so encouraging the accumulation in the tissues of the end-products of metabolism.

Many patients claim that they can forecast the weather by the exacerbation of their pains and stiffness.

Treatment depends on accurate assessment of the causes but principles to be observed are: removal or correction of any predisposing factors, treatment of any identifiable general disease, local treatment relying mainly on rest, warmth and physiotherapy, and analgesics.

Chronic rheumatism. To such extent as it can be differentiated from muscular rheumatism, chronic rheumatism is usually taken to mean subcutaneous fibrositis or panniculitis. This is characterized by painful and tender hard nodules under the skin at various sites, but commonly over the inner aspects of knees, the back of the neck, and the outer aspects of arms and thighs. These are particularly frequent in over-weight persons and may also be associated with menopausal changes and hypothyroidism.

To secure relief the nodules should be dealt with locally by massage. This must be as vigorous as the patient will tolerate and may be assisted by the application of local heat. Treatment must be persistent and prolonged in order to break up and disperse the condensations of fibrous tissue.

Rheumatism in children. When children are alleged to be suffering from 'rheumatism' (with swollen, painful joints and a raised tem-perature) the condition is generally RHEUMATIC FEVER, a disease caused by streptococcal infection and liable to damage the heart unless promptly and efficiently treated. There is, however, a less acute condition in children characterized by recurrent pains in limbs and joints, fatigue, pallor and loss of weight. In general this should be regarded – and treated – as a mild form of rheumatic fever, and not dismissed as 'merely growing pains'. In a picturesque phrase a French physician, E.C. Lasegue (1816-83) said of childhood rheumatism that it 'licks the joints but bites the heart'.

Predisposing heredity or environment? Many workers have suggested that adult rheumatism and for rheumatism in children that certain people have an inherited tendency to develop the disease. In particular it has been claimed that where rheumatism – whether true rheumatism or rheumatic fever – occurs in childhood one or other parent often has rheumatism, and that two types of children are particularly susceptible – the red or sandy-haired youngster with freckled complexion, and the child with lank dark hair, long eyelashes, a pale complexion, bluish sclera of the eyes, massive teeth, and a nervous disposition.

Rheumatism, however, is a disease with a well-defined 'social pathology'. Statistics related to social class show a greatly increased incidence in the lower socio-economic groups. Poverty is associated with bad housing, dampness, inadequate heating, deficient light and ventilation, over-crowding and poor nutritional standards.

Much research has been done on the relative importance of these factors and it is clear that over-crowding is the most potent. The fact that outbreaks of 'acute rheumatism' occur in residential schools, barracks, and training-ships where general hygiene, nutrition, and medical supervision are usually good, supports this view. Limitation of cubic space is not perhaps the sole factor because infrequent air-changes, lack of daylight, and dust accumulation all help to maintain a harmful concentration of bacteria. Disturbed sleep, and lack of opportunity for open-air exercise may also impair resistance to infection. In short, contact is probably more important than constitution in the bacterial form; and in the common muscular rheumatism or chronic rheumatism of adults climate, occupation and environment undoubtedly play the main part.

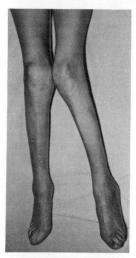

Rheumatoid arthritis

rheumatoid arthritis. A particular form of arthritis of many joints affecting chiefly the smaller joints of the hands and feet and generally showing a symmetrical distribution. All the structures within the joints may be involved. Women are chief sufferers (five to one) and the age-incidence is mainly from 20 to 50 years, although there is a variety which affects children known as Still's disease.

In the acute stage painful joint symptoms may be accompanied by a low or variable fever and by fatigue, loss of weight and anaemia. Later on there is severe muscle-wasting with deformity and loss of movement resulting from contractures, fusing together of joint cartilages, or partial dislocations.

The exact cause is still unknown but indications point to the influence of infection or toxaemia, possibly streptococcal. In many cases there is some obvious point of infection such as decayed teeth or diseased tonsils which can be dealt with. A large proportion of patients have absence of gastric hydrochloric acid which would favour chronic intestinal infection.

It is a formidable disease because of its serious crippling potentialities. The acute stage requires treatment by rest, analgesics to relieve pain, and immobilization of affected joints, with daily passive movement. A wide range of more specific therapy has been employed at various times with varying degrees of success and failure. Salicylates, vaccines, and injections of gold salts have all had their advocates. Gold salts are to some extent back in favour but most current treatment largely relies on the new anti-inflammatory drugs based on phenylbutazone, with or without the help of steroid compounds.

rhythm method. A non-contraceptive method of birth control in which intercourse is restricted to the time of physiological sterility ('safe period') in each menstrual cycle. Generally, the ovary expels only one ovum per cycle, approximately fourteen days before the start of the next menstrual period, and the ovum is only available for fertilization for twenty-four to forty-eight hours. Spermatozoa only remain viable in the female genital tract for three to five days. There is thus a maximum period of seven days during which conception is theoretically possible, but in practice this may be longer because of menstrual irregularity.

In applying the rhythm principle by the calendar method a woman must first keep a prior record of her menstrual history for six to twelve months. From this she determines her shortest and longest cycles. In a regular twenty-eight day cycle the period from the tenth to the eighteenth days, counting from the first day of the period, is unsafe. With irregular cycles the following example will show how to calculate the unsafe period. Shortest cycle, say 25 days: subtract $18=7$; longest cycle, say 31 days: subtract $10=21$; unsafe period between seventh and twenty-first day from the start of last period.

The alternative temperature method depends on the fact that the body temperature rises slightly immediately after ovulation and remains up for three days until the ovum starts to disintegrate. A record of morning temperatures is kept and the safe period can then be determined as extending from the fourth day after the initial temperature rise until the next cycle commences. An obvious weakness is that many factors other than ovulation can cause a slight rise in temperature.

The rhythm method has the approval of the Roman Catholic Church but is troublesome to apply and mistakes occur more often than with any other form of contraception. It should not be relied on if menstruation is very irregular, after childbirth, near the menopause, or during illness, dieting or medication.

riboflavin. One of the VITAMINS of the B-complex, also known as vitamin B_2.

ribonucleic acid. See RNA.

ribs. The twelve pairs of curved bones which enclose the chest-cavity. The upper seven pairs are the true ribs which articulate behind with vertebrae of the spinal column and join the sternum or breast-bone in front. In addition to forming the thoracic cage of the chest, the ribs move upwards and forwards ('bucket-handle action') by muscular action when breathing in,

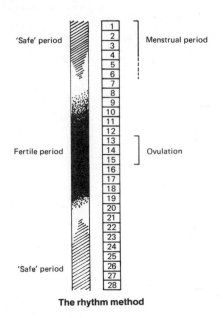

The rhythm method

'Safe' period — Menstrual period

Fertile period — Ovulation

'Safe' period

Rickety infants are prone to develop complications due to other infections, but otherwise early cases, adequately treated, make complete recovery. If neglected, any bony deformities are likely to persist.

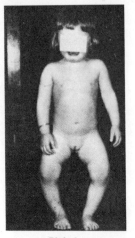

Rickets

so increasing the size of the chest and sucking in air from the exterior. The reverse takes place when breathing out.

The lower five pairs are the false ribs and three of these, instead of reaching the sternum, have their front ends attached by cartilage to the rib immediately above. The last two pairs have no attachment in front and are therefore known as floating ribs.

A fractured rib is a common type of injury, and ribs may also be malformed or deformed by disease, especially in rickets, pulmonary diseases of the lung or spine, and in some kinds of paralysis. In the so-called 'rickety rosary' the front ends of the ribs become enlarged and bulbous to form a bead-like row of projections along each margin of the sternum. This also occurs in infantile scurvy and is known as 'scurvy-beading'.

rickets. A deficiency disease in which lack of vitamin D upsets calcium and phosphorus metabolism. This vitamin may be obtained from a suitable diet or it may be produced by the body itself through the action of sunlight on precursors in the skin (photosynthesis).

Rickets occurs in infancy and early childhood. In the initial stages there is mainly retarded physical development and failure to thrive. The infant tends to be either lethargic or fretful, his muscle development is weak and he is reluctant to sit, crawl, or walk, the appearance of teeth is delayed, the abdomen may appear distended, and there is often excessive sweating. Later on, bony changes appear: bulging of the forehead; delayed closure of the skull fontanelles, enlargement of ends of long bones; curvature or deformity of limbs; and deformity of chest or spine.

Both breast-milk and cow's-milk tend to be deficient in vitamin D, especially in the winter months. Artificial milk powders are usually fortified to some extent but all infants should be given a vitamin concentrate in addition.

rickettsia. A specific group of micro-organisms, intermediate between the bacteria and the viruses, named after their discoverer, Howard T. Ricketts (1871-1910), an American pathologist. Many different species have since been identified and incriminated as the causal agents of such diseases as Rocky Mountain spotted fever (*R. rickettsi*), boutonneuse fever (*R. conorii*), Siberian tick typhus (*R. sibericus*), rickettsiapox (*R. akari*), marine typhus (*R. mooseri*), Tsutsugamushi disease (*R. orientalis*), louse-borne typhus fever (*R. prowazeki*), and trench fever (*R. quintana*). Brill's disease is typhus recrudescent after an earlier infection. *R. australis*, the cause of Q fever or Queensland tick typhus, has now been reclassified as *Coxiella burneti.*

Rickettsia organisms are widespread in wild and domestic animals and then become parasitic in various arthropods, such as ticks, lice, fleas, and mites. Infection spreads to man through bites by these insects, by contamination of his skin from their crushed bodies or their faeces, and by inhalation of infective dust. The various diseases are broadly similar, with a short incubation period, followed by an intermittent or remittent fever of some weeks duration, and the appearance of some form of rash. Exact diagnosis often depends on blood tests.

Most of the infections clear up even without special treatment with only a small or negligible mortality, but epidemic typhus may have a fatality rate of 40 per cent, and untreated cases of Rocky Mountain fever also produce a substantial number of deaths.

The use of antibiotics (chloramphenicol group) is, however, now very effective in cutting short the course of these diseases and has significantly reduced the former risks of mortality.

For some observations on prevention see also Q FEVER.

rigor. An ague, or severe shivering attack, produced by the effect which toxins in the blood-stream have on the temperature-regulating centre in the mid-brain. Rigors may occur during the early stage of any infection, or during the course of a disease associated with organisms circulating in the blood, as in septicaemia or malaria.

In the first or 'cold' stage of a rigor the patient appears pinched and blue, he shivers uncontrollably, and his teeth chatter. His temperature rises to perhaps 40 °C. (140 °F.) and he passes into the 'hot' stage, with restlessness, thirst, a hot dry skin, and further rise of temperature. There then follows the 'sweating' stage with profuse perspiration and gradual decline of temperature.

A rigor may also sometimes be produced by shock (e.g. following an accident involving breaking a limb) and is quite common after some surgical operations.

rigor mortis. A Latin phrase meaning 'rigidity of death'. It usually develops about six hours after death and gradually passes off within a day or so. It is due to chemical and enzyme reactions which cause the muscles to become fixed in a state of general contraction so that the corpse is absolutely stiff and inflexible.

ringworm. A general term applied to fungus infection of the keratinized areas of the body – the hair, skin and nails. Various genera and species of fungi are responsible and collectively they are called dermatophytes. The scientific name for ringworm is tinea.

Tinea capitis (ringworm of the scalp) is due to various species of *Microsporon* and *Trichophyton*. It begins as a small papule and spreads concentrically leaving scaly bald patches. Initial infection is usually from animals – cattle, cats, dogs – but person-to-person spread may follow.

Tinea corporis (ringworm of the body) is due to a species of *Epidermophyton*, *Microsporon* or *Trichophyton*, and appears as flat, scaly, spreading, ring-like lesions. Infection is by indirect or direct contact, especially in gymnasia and swimming-baths.

Tinea pedis (athlete's foot) is mainly due to *Epidermophyton floccosum*, and is characterized by scaling and cracking of the skin between the toes. Spread is by contact with contaminated floors in shower-stalls and swimming-baths.

Tinea unguium (ringworm of the nails) is usually seen as a spread from toes in which the nails thicken, become brittle, and disintegrate.

In the past ringworm was notoriously difficult to treat and potentially hazardous forms of therapy, using x-rays or thallium acetate were sometimes employed. However, standard treatment now uses a new antibiotic drug, griseofulvin. Prolonged courses may be required for more resistant types of the disease.

Prevention depends on hygienic measures of disinfection in swimming-baths and similar places, the avoidance of contact with affected animals, and the regular changing, disinfection, and washing of clothes and footwear.

Areas of fungal infection show fluorescence under ultra-violet light, and this can provide useful diagnostic help.

RNA. These initials stand for ribonucleic acid which forms part of the chromatin in every cell and is concerned with the process by which the inherited genes in the cell-nucleus control cellular growth, development, reproduction, and behaviour.

The cell nucleus holds information about how the cell should behave, and this information is derived from its predecessors and passed on to its successors when the cell divides. Each item of information is a gene and collectively these genes form the chromosomes. The effect of a particular gene is to instruct the cell to manufacture a particular kind of protein.

Genes are composed of short lengths of deoxyribonucleic acid (DNA) which is a long chain-like molecule. The characteristics of each gene are determined by the arrangement of four chemical groups attached to the DNA chain. Taking these three at a time sixty-four different arrangements are possible and this number of 'triplets' is sufficient to specify and determine the particular arrangement of some twenty amino-acids of which every different protein is composed.

Within the cell, and separate from the nucleus, are other aggregations of chromatin material called ribosomes. They contain RNA and are the site of protein synthesis as the cell grows and develops.

The problem is to transfer instructions from the genes in the cell nucleus to the ribosomes in its cytoplasm. This function is carried out by RNA 'messengers' which are molecules of ribonucleic acid carrying the pattern determined by the genes. Messenger RNA leaves the cell-nucleus and attaches itself to the ribosomes.

Amino-acids then find their appropriate 'triplets' and arrange themselves in a chain as specified by the RNA to form the particular protein required.

The basic details of this process were worked out by the M.R.C. Unit for Molecular Biology at the Cavendish Laboratory in Cambridge about 1961. Other workers have also discovered how to make synthetic pieces of RNA and these have proved capable of controlling the assembly of a predetermined protein. It is possible that in the future further developments will provide a direct means of controlling heredity, at least to some extent. This opens up the prospect of being able to breed individuals to pattern who might be monsters or geniuses or immune to disease. Even although this may never be practicable it is no longer mere science fiction.

Rocky Mountain spotted fever. A communicable disease caused by *Rickettsia rickettsii*, and transmitted by species of hard TICKS (*Ixodidae*). It occurs during spring and summer in most of the United States and also in Canada, Mexico, Colombia and Brazil. It is the prototype of several similar conditions known generally as tick typhus, due to other species of RICKETTSIA, and occurring in Southern Europe, the Levant, Africa, India, Siberia and Queensland.

Onset is sudden with fever and headache, followed on the third day by a rash of elevated and non-elevated spots, appearing first on the extremities and then spreading to the whole body and forming tiny haemorrhages.

In untreated cases, 20 per cent of cases died, but the disease now responds well to appropriate antibiotics. Blood tests are helpful in the diagnosis.

Preventive measures aim at reduction of tick populations, avoidance of tick-infested areas, and the use of protective clothing to prevent tick-bites. A vaccine against infection is available but annual reinforcement is required and it is less used than it was, now that treatment is more effective.

rodent ulcer. A relatively common type of malignant ulcer arising from proliferation of cells in the deeper layers of dermis or true skin. Since these are epithelial cells the condition is technically a carcinoma but it differs from other tumours of similar origin in being only locally malignant and it never spreads by metastasis to related lymph-glands.

It chiefly affects the skin of the upper face in elderly persons and starts as a flattened hard nodule which breaks down and ulcerates on the surface. Over a period of years, if untreated, it gradually invades and destroys the tissue beneath and may produce great disfigurement.

Early treatment by wide excision and subsequent skin-grafting affords good prospects of complete cure, while x-rays or radium are also successfully employed.

Romberg's sign. See ATAXIA.

Rorschach test. A specialized form of intelligence test for the assessment of emotional elements of personality. It was devised by a Swiss psychiatrist, Hermann Rorschach (1884-1922) and is now extensively employed in psychological investigation. The patient is shown a series of ten 'ink-blot' designs and asked to describe what the irregular patterns suggest to his mind. The responses elicited are then studied and interpreted as clues to significant aspects of his personality. It is an example of a projective test, so-called because the patient is unconsciously forced to reveal his own personal attitudes.

rosacea. A condition of chronic congestion of the blood capillaries affecting particularly the skin of the nose and the surrounding central area of the face. It is usually related to persistent indigestion, and it is aggravated by alcohol, strong tea, and too hot or spicy foods.

Eventually it leads to thickening of the skin, giving a lumpy red appearance to the face, and to over-action of the sweat-glands whose follicles become distended with secretion and may become infected (acne rosacea). In late stages the overgrowth of skin and the tissue beneath it converts the nose into a bulbous swelling known as rhinophyma or, popularly, 'brandy-nose'.

Treatment requires investigation of gastric function and the correction of excess or deficient acidity, the avoidance of unsuitable food or drink, and applications to the nose of such preparations as calamine lotion. Rhinophyma can be treated surgically with expectations of a good appearance after the operation.

roughage. In addition to nutrients any normal diet also contains material which is not disgested and not absorbed from the human intestine. Such material, derived mainly from cereals, fruit, and vegetables, is variously described as dietary fibre, residue, or roughage. Although everyone knows that 'an apple a day keeps the doctor away', professional opinion has varied about the value and importance of roughage, and distinguished gastro-enterologists have been prepared to maintain that the human gut is designed for a meat and not a vegetable diet.

However, at the moment, fibre-containing diets are in favour. Studies of primitive races have suggested that diverticulitis, appendicitis, and cancer of the colon are less frequent when there is a high intake of vegetable fibre. It is also known that fibre influences fat digestion, so that persons on high-fibre diets have lower levels of blood cholesterol and therefore might be expected to be at less risk of developing arteriosclerosis of their blood-vessels and subsequent heart disease. There are effects also on water retention and on the metabolism of bile.

Much research remains to be done, but evidence is accumulating that roughage is a valuable protective constituent, and that a good diet should include suitable sources such as whole-meal bread, vegetables, and fruit.

roundworms. A general name for worms of the class Nematoda which are characterized by being cylindrical in shape, without segmentation or appendages and by having separate male and female forms, the latter being larger. Some smaller species are also called thread-worms or whipworms.

Roundworms reproduce from fertilized ova which develop into adult worms either directly or through intermediate larval stages. Many are parasitic in man and cause symptoms either from the presence of mature forms in the gut or tissues or by movement of larvae about the body.

In temperate countries, the genera of importance are: (1) *Trichinella* which causes TRICHINOSIS, generally acquired by eating infected pork. (2) *Ascaris* which usually develops in the intestine and may produce effects from pressure or blockage or cause pneumonia or nephritis as larvae move around. (3) *Enterobius,* the common THREADWORM is a common intestinal parasite of children especially in institutions.

In tropical countries the range is much wider and the effects are frequently disabling not only to individuals but to whole populations. *Ankylostoma* and *Necator* (HOOK-WORM), *Filaria* (elephantiasis and 'Calabar swelling'), *Oncocerca* (lesion of deeper surface of skin and blindness), *Trichuris* (whipworm) and *Dracunculus* (Guinea-worm) are some examples.

Different species of round worms are spread in various ways: by direct eating of their eggs, by larval penetration of the skin, and by bites from insect-carriers. Control requires expert knowledge of some complicated life-cycles, but many effective drugs are now available. The vermicidal drugs actually kill the worms and the vermifugal ones expel them from the body.

rubella. See GERMAN MEASLES.

rupture. A popular term more or less synonymous with HERNIA, which is any protrusion of an organ from within the cavity in which it is normally contained, usually occurring through an abnormal opening or weak place in the walls of the cavity. A hernia is further described according to its position. Rupture usually means some form of abdominal hernia, but hernia can mean a protrusion of any organ from any cavity, as for example hernia of the brain after accidental or surgical opening of the skull.

S

Sabin vaccine. A vaccine against polio-myelitis, prepared by cultivating successive generations of the three main types of poliomyelitis virus under artificial conditions until they lose their virulence. An appropriate dose of the resultant harmless, inactivated virus (usually three drops of the vaccine on a lump of sugar with two further repetitions at intervals of four to six weeks) is given by mouth and confers a high immunity for several years. The immunity can be supplemented by a single reinforcing dose three or four years later.

The Sabin vaccine has the advantage of being given by mouth. It has been criticized on the ground that it is a live vaccine, that the harmless virus is excreted by vaccinated persons and that, just as it lost its virulence by growth under artificial conditions, it might conceivably regain its virulence by passage through a series of people; but no such evidence of regained virulence has been found. The alternative is the Salk vaccine, for the manufacture of which the three main types of poliomyelitis vaccine are killed by formaldehyde. Two intramuscular injections of 1 ml. some four to six weeks apart create a high immunity, but a reinforcing dose is desirable three or four years later.

The use of one or other of these vaccines has almost eradicated poliomyelitis in several countries.

sacrum. A large wedge-shaped bone at the lower end of the spinal column formed by the fusion of five sacral vertebrae.

As viewed from behind it is situated between the two hip-bones, and its concave front aspect forms part of the cavity of the lesser pelvis. It articulates above with the fifth lumber vertebra and below with the coccyx or rudimentary tail. Its lateral articulations with the hip-bone are the sacro-iliac joints, frequently the site of pain and disability arising from sacro-iliac strain. See BACKACHE.

sadism. A manifestation of abnormal personality in which pleasure, and especially sexual pleasure, is derived from the infliction of cruelty upon another. As a sexual PERVERSION or deviation, sadism may involve the whipping, beating, or maltreatment of a sexual partner in order to achieve arousal, but the term is also used to describe an attitude of mind which derives satisfaction from contemplating or securing the discomfiture of others.

The name derives from descriptions of the condition which may be found in the writings of the Marquis de Sade (1740-1814).

Treatment requires the employment of psychotherapeutic methods.

safe period. See RHYTHM METHOD.

St. Anthony's fire. A name formerly applied both to erysipelas and to ergot poisoning. In the twentieth century erysipelas, a diffuse inflammation of the skin and cellular tissue caused by haemolytic streptococci, is still quite common, but ergot poisoning is almost unknown. The serious epidemics of St. Anthony's fire in the Middle Ages were, however, almost certainly due to poisoning with ergot, a fungus disease of rye.

St. Vitus's dance. An old-fashioned name for SYDENHAM'S or rheumatic CHOREA.

salicylates. Salts of salicylic acid which in general reduce temperature in fevered conditions, lessen pain and promote sweating. Sodium salicylate, a white crystalline substance soluble in water, is employed in the treatment of rheumatic fever, but in large doses may cause dizziness and head noises. Methyl salicylate or oil of wintergreen is sometimes used externally as a liniment for inflammation and sprains. Acetylsalicylic acid, better known as aspirin, is one of the most widely used of all medicines.

saline. See NORMAL SALINE.

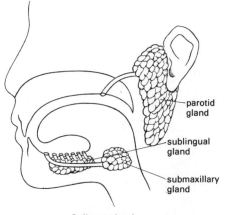

parotid gland

sublingual gland

submaxillary gland

Salivary glands

salivary glands. Saliva is secreted by three pairs of glands and passed to the mouth by ducts. The submaxillary glands are situated beneath the floor of the mouth, and close to the inner surface of the angle of the lower jaw. Each has a duct known as Wharton's duct, opening beneath the tongue. The sublingual glands lie beneath the tongue on each side of the mid-line and have a number of small ducts. The parotid glands lie below and in front of the ear, overlapping the vertical part of the lower jaw; each has a duct known as Stenson's duct, which reaches the mouth at a point on the inner surface of the cheek opposite the second upper molar tooth.

Secretion of saliva is a reflex phenomenon

caused mainly by stimulation of taste-buds in the tongue and mouth, but also by the anticipation or smell of food.

The functions of saliva are to keep the mouth moist, to assist in the swallowing of food and to start the process of digestion.

The chief disorders of the salivary glands are inflammation (PAROTITIS) produced by ascending duct-infection or by MUMPS, and the occurrence of calculi in the ducts.

Salk vaccine. See SABIN VACCINE.

salpingitis. Inflammation of a tube. Although sometimes referring to the Eustachian tubes, which pass from behind the eardrum to the back of the nose, without qualification the term normally relates to the Fallopian tubes which extend between the ovaries and the upper part of the uterus.

Most cases of Fallopian salpingitis are due to infection ascending from the uterus, and caused either by gonococci or by pus-forming organisms associated with septic conditions of the uterus. Abortion and childbirth may be complicated by this condition. Tuberculous salpingitis is also not uncommon, either blood-borne from elsewhere in the body, or spreading from the membranes surrounding the abdominal contents.

The symptoms are deep-seated pelvic pain, vaginal discharge and menstrual irregularity, with tenderness on either side of the abdomen and hardness detectable on vaginal examination.

Treatment can be aimed at preservation or may eventually require surgery, but the availability of suitable antibiotics has revolutionized the management and outcome of the condition. In salpingitis the ovaries are usually involved as well and there is always a substantial risk of subsequent sterility either from ovarian damage or because the Fallopian tubes have become blocked.

salt. In chemical terms, a salt is any compound of a base or inorganic radicle with an acid, but ordinarily 'salt' is taken to mean common salt or sodium chloride (NaCl). Sodium chloride is an essential constituent of the blood plasma and tissue-fluids because of its role in maintaining these at the correct osmotic tension to ensure that the water-content of cells remains stable. See OSMOSIS.

Normal saline is a solution of salt, having the same osmotic pressure as blood plasma, and containing 0.9 gm. of common salt per 100 ml. of water. It is used to raise the blood-volume, and hence the blood-pressure, in conditions of shock and collapse. It may be given by various routes, but is usually given rectally, or by injection into the skin or into a vein.

In ordinary circumstances any normal diet provides adequate amounts of sodium chloride, but bacon, milk, and milk-products are especially good sources.

Salt is excreted in the perspiration, and excessive sweating (as in hot climates or occupations) may so reduce the osmotic tension of the blood that muscular cramps result. Additional salt must be taken to restore the depletion.

A salt-free or salt-poor diet is sometimes ordered in kidney disease where the inability of the kidney to excrete salt leads to water-retention and oedema.

salts, mineral. See MINERAL SALTS.

sand-fly fever. A disease, resembling influenza, with fever lasting three or four days, headache, malaise, nausea, and limb pains. The virus which causes it is transmitted to man by the common sand-fly, *Phlebotomus papatassi,* a small, hairy, blood-sucking midge, which bites at night, and is found on the Mediterranean coast and also widely in sub-tropical and tropical parts of Africa, Asia, Central and South America.

The incubation period is three to four days; one attack confers a lasting immunity; there are no specific measures of immunization or treatment; the disease simply runs its course, causing no danger to life.

Preventive measures include insecticidal spraying of, and around, human habitations, with personal use of insect-repellents and mosquito-proof bed-nets.

sarcoma. A type of malignant tumour or CANCER resulting from the unregulated proliferation of connective-tissue cells such as those of ordinary fibrous tissue, bone, cartilage, muscle, and pigmented tissue. It is to be distinguished from carcinoma, which always arises from epithelial cells.

Sarcomata, as a rule, are very malignant, fast-growing, and vascular. They are apt to spread rapidly, either directly, or by blood-borne and lymph-borne metastases.

Various terms are used to describe special types according to their origins. Osteosarcoma, chondrosarcoma, myosarcoma, and melanotic sarcoma arise from bone, cartilage, muscle, and pigmented tissue respectively.

satyriasis. A psychological abnormality in which a man has an abnormal desire for sexual relations. It is very similar in cause, effect and symptoms to the condition of NYMPHOMANIA in woman.

scabies. A skin infestation caused by a small spider-like parasite, the itch-mite or acarus (*Sarcoptes scabiei*). The female acarus is about 0.4 mm. in length and the male rather smaller; they are just visible to the naked eye as glistening white dots. The female burrows into the horny layer of the skin to lay her eggs and she prefers the thin parts such as the finger-webs, the fronts of the wrists, the armpits, and the breasts. At the affected sites small vesicles form and the burrows tend to fill up with dirt and so may be seen as fine twisting lines.

The main symptom is itching and as the patient scratches he inflicts further skin-damage which usually becomes infected. The disease is very contagious and newly-hatched mites readily migrate from person to person and also contaminate bedding.

Treatment is relatively easy and effective, using lotions based usually on benzyl benzoate, but it must be thorough, and it is advisable to treat a whole family simultaneously. Clothing and bedding should be washed and disinfected to prevent recurrence.

scalds. Tissue damage or destruction caused by moist heat through contact with hot liquids or hot vapours such as steam. Scalds do not differ essentially from burns and their effects are classified in six degrees of severity (Dupuytren) in exactly the same way, although carbonization does not occur. See BURNS.

Most scalds are of first, second, or third degree, with reddening, blistering, and skin destruction respectively, they produce local symptoms of pain and inflammatory reaction, together with the general effects indicative of shock, and these may be severe since large areas of skin are often involved.

Minor scalds can be satisfactorily treated by the application of medicated tulle with a protective dressing and bandage. Extensive injuries require admission to hospital and first-aid treatment should be limited to the provision of a sterile dressing covering the whole area, either dry or moistened with normal saline or sodium bicarbonate, together with measures to relieve pain and combat shock. See FIRST AID.

Severe scalds of third degree or worse cause serious skin damage and lead to subsequent scarring and contraction. Skin-grafting may be required to achieve a satisfactory functional result and to restore an acceptable appearance.

scapula. The shoulder-blade, a flat, triangular bone situated on the upper rear aspect of the thorax between the levels of the second and seventh ribs. It forms part of the shoulder-girdle, articulating at the point of the shoulder with the collar-bone. The upper end of its outer border is expanded to form the shallow glenoid cavity into which fits the head of the humerus, the long bone of the upper arm.

Fractures of the scapula are rare because it is mobile and well-surrounded by muscle layers. A congenital elevation of one or both scapulae is sometimes seen and is known as Sprengel's shoulder. In 'winged scapula' or scapula alata, which may occur in persons of feeble muscular development, or as a result of damage to nerves, the lower angle of the scapula projects unduly.

scar. A mark left on the skin or on other tissue after a wound or sore has healed. Cicatrix is an alternative name. If tissue has been destroyed the defect is made good by ingrowth of fibrous tissue instead, and it is characteristic of the latter that it contracts, thus producing the puckered and depressed appearance which scars usually have.

Extensive scarring, especially near joints, may cause disabling contractures. Occasionally there may be some overgrowth of scar tissue to produce an unsightly raised appearance known as keloid scar.

Troublesome or disfiguring scars can be treated by excision and skin-grafting.

scarlet fever. Haemolytic streptococci cause various infections differentiated by the method of infection, the tissue affected, and the presence or absence of a rash. Development of a rash depends on the balance between toxin-formation by the organism, and antitoxin immunity in the patient. Although bacteriological tests show the same infection as other cases of streptococcal sore throat, scarlet fever or scarlatins has very clearly recognizable characteristics so that it can be distinguished among the variety of streptococcal infections.

Usually of sudden onset, its features are fever, constitutional disturbance, inflamed throat with exudate on tonsils and pharynx, tender, swollen neck-glands, a generalized rash (a general blush with fine darker points) which avoids the face (circumoral pallor), and the so-called 'strawberry tongue' – initially with white fur and red papillae and gradually peeling to appear generally reddened.

The incubation period is one to three days and it is mostly likely to occur in young children, although infants under one year are seldom affected. Severe cases are less often seen nowadays, and treatment with antibiotics cuts short the disease and lessens the risk of serious heart and kidney complications. Cases should be isolated for at least seven days from onset, or until symptoms disappear. Peeling of skin begins during the second week and may take some weeks to be complete, especially on the soles and palms. The dead fragments of skin flaked off do not convey infection.

In epidemic outbreaks search should be made for some common source of infection. It is often possible to trace it to contaminated milk or food, or a chronic CARRIER.

Schick test. A test of susceptibility to diphtheria, devised by Bela Schick. A tiny dose of diphtheria toxin is injected into the skin of one forearm and a similar dose of inactive toxin is injected into the other forearm. The arms are inspected in forty-eight to ninety-six hours. A positive result, i.e., a red spot on the arm, indicates susceptibility to the disease, while a negative result (i.e., no spot) indicates immunity. Very occasionally a red spot appears on both forearms, indicating sensitivity to the protein injected and making the test valueless for the particular person.

For diphtheria contacts the test is often combined with attempts to grow diphtheria germs from nose and throat swabs. A Schick negative person with no diphtheria germs in his throat is neither a case nor a carrier but a healthy, immune person who need have no restrictions placed on his movements. A Schick positive person without germs has so far escaped but needs immunization. A Schick positive person with germs is probably incubating the disease and should be admitted to hospital. A Schick negative person with germs is probably the carrier responsible for the outbreak.

schistomiasis. See BILHARZIASIS.

schizoid personality. Since sufferers from schizophrenia tend to be incapable of feeling or expressing emotion and to live in a dream world of their own, the term schizoid personality is sometimes used for persons mildly approximating to that condition, i.e., for persons who, although within the bounds of normality, are cold, unemotional, self-sufficient, aloof and withdrawn. In a small minority of cases the adolescent of this shy, retiring, introspective disposition develops into a schizophrenic, but in the great majority of cases he simply develops into a rather solitary, self-sufficient and unemotional adult.

schizophrenia. A type of mental illness or psychosis. From derivation the term means a splitting of the personality. Schizophrenia is perhaps the commonest of the serious mental illnesses since it accounts for about one-quarter of all admissions to mental hospitals. Its significance for society, and for the individual, is even more important because it principally affects young people on the threshold of their lives and careers. For this reason it is sometimes referred to as dementia praecox.

Most cases begin between the ages of 15 and 25 and onset after 40 is very rare (except in the paranoid type). It is slightly more common in males than in females.

Its exact cause is still unknown but there is undoubtedly a considerable hereditary factor. The inherited defect appears to be some inborn metabolic abnormality, and this hypothesis is strengthened by the similarity which exists between the disease and the effects of certain hallucinatory drugs such as mescaline and lysergic acid.

Although mental stress, in the form of overwork, a broken love-affair, or other tragic experience, may sometimes be regarded as a starting-point of breakdown, it is usually possible to show from a detailed clinical history that this was only the latest of a series of disturbing events which fostered or accelerated a latent disposition. In retrospect, the schizoid personality may be indentifiable from an early age: the quiet, shy, solitary, model child, who is introspective, submissive, or sentimental, and the adolescent who is unusually touchy, suspicious, obstinate or resentful of advice are both suspect, though not all of these will later show signs of the disease.

The essential feature of schizophrenia is a retirement from reality into a world of fantasy. To the outside observer this change appears as a disorder of thought, emotion or lack of emotion unrelated to actual circumstances, and domination by hallucinations which lead to abnormal impulses and conduct. It is usual to describe four main types of the disease according to its principal manifestations. These are:

1. Simple schizophrenia: deterioration of emotional reaction with apathy and withdrawal.

2. Hebephrenia: 'silly' behaviour, inappropriate smiling and laughter, coining of words, and hallucinations.

3. Catatonia: stupor, negativism, suggestibility and impulsive conduct.

4. PARANOIA: preservation of thought and emotion to a late stage, but with delusions of persecution or grandeur.

The treatment of schizophrenia is rather unsatisfactory. Many methods have been tried. Shock therapy by insulin or electrical devices has enjoyed a vogue which is now being replaced by the use of new drugs and more intensive psychotherapy.

Although some cases do recover, at least to some extent, there is great likelihood of permanent damage to personality. Acute cases and those which commence at later ages are rather more hopeful. There may however be some scope for prevention of the condition. If the schizoid type of child is identified, the child guidance service and child health services can help to foster his social integration and to safeguard him from situations of mental stress.

school health services. Since children of school age constitute about one-fifth of the population in countries of stationary population and more than that fraction in countries of rising population, and since the child is proverbially father of the man in health matters as in other aspects of life, it is clearly important that effective steps should be taken to foster the physical and mental health of pupils. Indeed for long-term benefit to the community provisions for school health services must rank second in importance only to antenatal and pre-school health services.

Moreover, school children are an organized and accessible group and therefore an obvious target for sympathetic efforts to improve their present health and future attitudes to health maintenance.

Yet these services developed late. In France, school medical examinations were required by the republican Convention in 1793 and again by a law of 1833, but they only began in some – not all – Paris schools in 1842 and elsewhere in France started in 1879 or later. The first nation to establish school medical inspection throughout the country was Sweden in 1878. In the U.K. development was very sporadic until after 1907 (England and Wales) and 1908 (Scotland), although an association of medical officers of schools was formed as early as 1884. In the U.S.A. development was – and to some extent still is – even more haphazard: the first school medical officer was appointed in New York in 1871 but his post was abolished in 1873 and there were no subsequent school medical inspections until 1894.

All these inspections were primarily to detect disease, especially infectious disease, and to New York belongs the credit of appreciating the importance of educating children and their parents on health: in 1902 a nurse, Lina Rogers, was appointed to New York schools, and similar appointments rapidly followed in the U.S.A. and the U.K.

There was and is considerable variation in the services provided. In the U.S.A. for instance the services in most areas have been the responsibility of boards of education, but in some areas the services have been supplied by the county or city health department; in some cities (e.g., New York) there was a functioning service before 1910, while in others there was little half a century later (e.g., Chicago appointed its first school medical officer 1950).

The following paragraphs are based on the services of the U.K. but in large measure also apply to the services of the Scandinavian countries and of Australia and New Zealand.

Broadly the services seek to provide preventive care designed to ensure that the welfare of children is supervised throughout their school career and that any necessary action is taken to safeguard their health, to secure early and adequate treatment of remediable defects, to minimize the physical and educational handicaps imposed by disability, to concern themselves with the creation in the children of attitudes and habits conducive to maintenance of health, and to keep a watchful eye on the hygiene of buildings, meals and equipment.

Commonly all children receive full routine medical examination soon after school entry and shortly before they leave school, and special medical examinations are undertaken at the request of the school nurse, school teacher or parent. At the routine examinations all systems of the body are studied by the school doctor and particular attention is paid to posture, nutrition and orthopaedic defects. Sight and hearing are also examined, usually by technical personnel using appropriate equipment. Following examination, steps are taken to arrange for the correction of any defect or for modification of the educational programme to minimize the foreseeable effects of any limitations likely to result from irremediable handicap. Where doubt arises about a child's mental ability he can be referred to an educational psychologist for special assessment.

A very important member of the school health team is the school nurse. There are essentially three patterns. (1) The health visitor for the district may act for part of her time as school nurse: this arrangement preserves continuity of care and uses her knowledge of individual families and her specialized training in health teaching and counselling. (2) A health visitor works full-time in the school and is virtually a member of the school staff, being heavily involved in health education and health counselling, and communicating with her district colleagues about problems involving family and home circumstances. (3) The school nurse is a qualified nurse without subsequent training in health teaching and psychology: she carries out routine checks of cleanliness and infestation, investigates outbreaks of infection, maintains unobtrusive watch on the health of children and brings forward children for special medical examination, but in general has to rely on a visiting health visitor for either actual participation in health education or acting as resource health education expert advising teachers.

The school health team is also responsible for routine immunization procedures against diphtheria, tetanus, poliomyelitis, tuberculosis and, in girls, rubella.

The child with a specific handicap requires special attention, and decisions on educational requirements necessitate consultation between the school health team and the teachers. In the U.K. handicapping conditions are classified as: blind; partially-sighted; deaf; partially-hearing; delicate; educationally sub-normal (ESN); maladjusted; physically-handicapped; epileptic; speech defective.

Although a school health service is primarily preventive and diagnostic in concept, most authorities provide minor ailments clinics, and usually additional special clinics for sight-testing, hearing testing, speech-training, orthopaedics and chiropody.

Every authority also makes arrangements for preventive dentistry. Ideally, every child should be inspected dentally every six months so that any necessary treatment, including orthodontic work (i.e., prevention and correction of faulty position of the teeth), can be promptly provided. The efforts of the dental surgeon are frequently supplemented by the employment of dental hygienists who are qualified to carry out simple routine procedures such as scaling and small fillings.

With a comprehensive and free national health service it might be thought that children should perhaps look to their family practitioners for their medical and dental treatment, but the philosophy of still providing for this treatment within the school service in a systematic way is that abnormalities and defects are most rewardingly dealt with as early as possible and by specially experienced personnel. Moreover, the ready availability of suitable facilities directed exclusively to the school-child helps to ensure that school-attendance and educational progress suffer least interruption, and avoids the delays of waiting-lists and parent procrastination.

In addition to all these activities, which are primarily related to personal health, the school doctor and nurse are also concerned with the influence of the school environment, the suitability and adequacy of buildings and class-rooms, their heating, lighting, cleaning and maintenance, ablutionary and sanitary pro-

vision, the conduct of school-kitchens and dining facilities, and indeed every aspect of general hygiene.

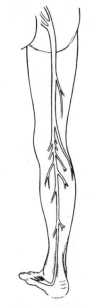

The sciatic nerve

sciatica. Neuralgic pain occurring in relation to the sciatic nerve. The roots of the nerve arise from the lower part of the spinal cord and emerge between the lumbar vertebrae and through openings on the inner surface of the sacrum, the wedge-shaped bone at the base of the spine. The composite nerve-trunk which they form then passes through the lesser pelvis and, including its main branches, follows a course down the back of thigh and leg.

Sciatica is due either to inflammation of the fibrous tissue enclosing the nerve-fibres (neurofibrositis) or to pressure on the nerve-roots and nerve trunk from various causes including 'slipped' intervertebral disc, osteo-arthritis, or disease within the pelvis.

Investigation is required to determine the exact cause. Cases due simply to neuro-fibrositis may respond to rest, warmth, counter-irritation, analgesics, and physiotherapy, but the condition is apt to respond poorly to treatment. Stretching of the nerve is sometimes advocated. A SLIPPED DISC and other physical causes of pressure may require an operation to relieve the pressure.

sclerosis. A hardening (induration) of any tissue. It arises as a sequel to tissue damage caused by inflammation, toxaemia, or restriction of blood-supply, and is characterized microscopically by proliferation and condensation of the supporting or interstitial tissue. Common examples are arteriosclerosis, in which blood-vessels become hardened and inelastic; cerebral sclerosis in which diminished blood-supply leads to nerve damage and overgrowth of neuroglia, the connective tissue of the central nervous system; and multiple (or disseminated) sclerosis, a disease of unknown cause in which sclerotic patches occur in the brain and spinal cord and produce serious functional disturbances.

scoliosis. A sideways or lateral CURVATURE OF THE SPINE.

scrofula. An old-fashioned and obsolete name for TUBERCULOSIS of the lymph-glands, usually in the neck (tuberculous adenitis), which become enlarged and then break down to cause chronic suppuration, with thickened, unhealthy overlying skin and discharging sinuses. The condition is rarely seen nowadays because it was due to bovine tuberculous infection derived from milk and has now been largely eradicated by control of herds and pasteurization of milk.

Another name for scrofula was 'king's evil' because of the irrational belief that it could be cured by the touch of a king.

scrotum. A pouch of skin, situated in the male crotch, and providing two separate compartments for the right and left testicles and the lower end of the corresponding spermatic cords. Its external appearance varies with circumstances. Under the influence of warmth, and with age and debility, it is roomy and flaccid; with cold, and in the young and robust, it is contracted, corrugated, and closely applied to the testes. This is due to the contraction of muscle-fibres in its wall. Apart from its normal contents the scrotum may be enlarged by the presence of the lower part of an inguinal HERNIA, by the fluid accumulation of a HYDROCELE, by a VARICOCELE due to varicose veins of the spermatic cord, or by disease of the testes and their appendages.

scurvy. A deficiency disease due to insufficiency or lack of vitamin c (ascorbic acid). The early symptoms resemble those of a severe anaemia with weakness, lassitude, dizziness, and a tendency to bruising from slight injuries. The most striking subsequent changes are in the mouth where the gums swell, bleed and ulcerate, with eventual loosening and loss of teeth. The effects are primarily due to interference with blood-formation in the bone-marrow, and to increased fragility of capillary blood-vessels.

Adult cases mostly occur in elderly persons on an inadequate diet. Vitamin c is chiefly obtained from fresh fruit and vegetables, and it is easily destroyed by over-cooking.

Treatment is simple and rewarding: administration of ascorbic acid effects a dramatic cure within a few days. After that it should be ensured that the diet includes enough fresh fruit and green vegetables.

Infantile scurvy (Barlow's disease). Like adult scurvy, this is essentially due to lack of vitamin c in the diet and it is particularly apt to occur in artificially-fed infants unless steps are taken to ensure an adequate supplementary intake. It is seldom seen in breast-fed infants unless the mother herself suffers from vitamin c deprivation.

The symptoms are those of anaemia with a tendency to bleeding. Haemorrhages into the skin occur, and sometimes also from the digestive and urinary tracts. In the absence of teeth, the mouth effects are less noticeable, but the ends of long-bones are usually painful and become swollen because of haemorrhage into them and derangement of bone-formation.

The condition responds rapidly to the administration of vitamin c. To prevent it occurring, all infants should receive 20 to 50 mg. ascorbic acid per day, and this applies to breast-fed infants too, since the vitamin content of breast-milk is quite variable. Fresh orange-juice contains nearly 1 mg. per ml. and commercial concentrates usually supply 2 mg. per ml.

sea-bathing. Cold baths have a tonic effect and induce a general feeling of well-being and exhilaration. In sea-bathing the salt makes little difference and the benefits are essentially those of a cold bath, although sun, wind, wave-movement and the usual presence of other participants all contribute to the degree of pleasure and mental stimulation which results.

Sea-temperature commonly varies from 4.5 ° to 21 °C. (40 ° to 70 °F.) and the first effects on entering the water are a contraction of skin blood-vessels, a feeling of chilliness, and a tendency to gasp from reflex disturbance of respiration when water reaches chest-level. Reaction sets in on leaving the water. The skin 'glows' as its vessels dilate, pulse and respiration increase, and the individual feels active and stimulated. If immersion is over-prolonged, chilliness may persist, with shivering and a 'blue' skin, and activity may be depressed even to the stage of collapse.

Moderate bathing is thus bracing and beneficial to those who are healthy and robust, but it should be indulged in cautiously by the young, the old and the debilitated, and children in particular should be supervised to ensure that their enthusiasm does not lead them to stay in too long. It is also inadvisable to bathe soon after meals. The risk of cramp or collapse are increased because of blood being already diverted to internal organs for the purposes of digestion.

sea-sickness. See TRAVEL SICKNESS.

sebaceous glands. The sweat glands of the body, which are present all over the body surface but are most numerous on the palms and soles. They consist of coiled tubes in the deep layers of skin with corkscrew-like ducts running through the outer layer and ending in tiny cup-shaped depressions on the surface. These glands are one of the main excreting channels getting rid of body waste as SWEAT, normally to the extent of about 0.85 litres (1.5 pints) of 'invisible perspiration' daily, a process which is also important for regulating body temperature.

seborrhoea. Excessive secretion of sebum, the oil produced by sebaceous glands. The condition, commonest at and soon after puberty and often decreasing with advancing age, is partly hereditary, partly due to hormonal upset and partly the result of faulty diet. The skin becomes greasy, thickened, coarse and muddy-coloured, and acne vulgaris is a common complication. The most effective treatment is to decrease the fats and carbohydrates in the diet, with corresponding increase in proteins, vitamins and minerals, and to wash frequently with soap and water.

secondary. Arising as a result of some other ('primary') defect or circumstance.

secretion. A term used both for a substance formed and released by a gland or organ and for the process by which the substance is formed and released. To mention some examples, endocrine glands secrete hormones, the liver secretes bile and the tear glands secrete tears, and each of these products of an internal manufacturing process is a secretion.

sedative. A drug, or less often another agency such as a warm bath, which reduces over-activity of the nervous system and therefore diminishes mental excitement and irritability. Moderate doses are often useful in periods of emotional stress, while larger doses are prescribed to induce sleep or to reduce sensitivity to pain.

The borderlines between sedatives and HYPNOTICS and TRANQUILLIZERS are not very clear. Essentially a hypnotic aims to produce sleep (as does a large dose of a sedative) and a tranquillizer aims to calm excitement (as does a smaller dose of a sedative).

Sedatives, such as the various barbiturates and the bromides, are extremely useful drugs but are perhaps employed too frequently nowadays. In conditions of serious distress or excitement they are invaluable, but they are sometimes used in situations in which ten minutes of calm discussion between patient and doctor would be equally effective.

semen. A thick, whitish fluid containing spermatozoa (produced in the testicles) and also containing secretions from the seminal vesicles (situated beside the prostate). During the process of ejaculation semen is discharged from the penis.

semicircular canal. Part of the balancing mechanism of the inner EAR. There are three such canals at right angles to each other. When the body moves backwards and forwards, or upwards and downwards, or sideways, hairlike cells in the appropriate canal detect movement of the contained fluid and information about the movement is transmitted inwards to the brain.

senescence. The process of AGEING.

sensation. Perception of stimuli, irrespective of whether these are of light, sound, smell, touch, pressure, pain, heat or cold. The mechanism of sensation starts in the relevant receptors, e.g., the rods and cones of the retina of the eye or the nerve-endings in the skin. From the receptors electrical currents pass along nerve fibres to the brain, and the experiencing of the sensation actually occurs in the brain.

sentiment. In colloquial usage a sentiment is a thought, feeling or mental attitude influenced by emotion. In psychological writings the term is used rather more precisely for any complex emotional attitude towards a person, object or situation which has been built up in the course of experience. Thus a normal parent's sentiment towards his child usually combines tenderness, affection and at times sternness; and hatred of persons of different colour or different religion is a complex and often permanent attitude largely created by personal experience and by social surroundings. Many feelings and actions that we deem logical and rational are really inspired by our sentiments.

septicaemia. Blood poisoning caused by the entry of disease germs into the blood stream and their survival and multiplication there. The original infection may be in a wound of the skin (sometimes apparently trivial) or inflammation of a bone, joint, vein or heart-valve. The symptoms include high fever, shivering, sweating and pains in joints and muscles. The condition was very serious indeed before the era of sulphonamides and antibiotics and is still

serious, but timely and adequate treatment with an antibiotic or sulphonamide to which the germ is sensitive usually effects a cure.

serum. The clear, yellowish fluid which separates from the blood corpuscles when a blood clot is formed. Serum contains several proteins, including gamma globulin which may contain antibodies against a particular infection.

Serum may be obtained from a person or animal convalescing from – or highly immunized against – a particular infectious disease (e.g., measles or diphtheria). It may be used for injection to prevent the disease in contacts or to reduce its severity in those who are actually suffering from the disease. In a small minority of cases there may be a SERUM REACTION to injection.

serum reactions. Allergic reactions to the injection of SERUM occur in a proportion of people. With the unconcentrated serum of the past, where large quantities had to be injected to provide the necessary amount of antibodies, the proportion was as high as one person in six, but with modern concentrated serum it is much lower. Reactions are of two main types.

1. *Serum sickness* occurs mainly in patients sensitized by a previous injection of the same protein. After a latent period of six to fourteen days following the injection, a rash appears, sometimes localized to the site of the injection but more often generalized or patchy. There is itching, rise of temperature, sometimes joint pains and occasionally nausea and vomiting. The condition, if untreated, seldom lasts for more than twenty-four hours; application of calamine lotion relieves the itching and a hypodermic injection of adrenalin usually relieves the condition completely.

2. *Serum shock* occurs within two hours of the injection of serum and is characterized by shivering, chilliness and signs of collapse. An extreme form of this reaction is called anaphylaxis with breathing difficulty and sudden collapse, usually within minutes of the injection. Adrenalin can be life-saving here, and the general treatment is that of SHOCK. The best preventive measure is attempted desensitization before injection of persons known to be sensitized or known to suffer from allergic conditions. For desensitization a small injection of the particular serum is given under the skin about half an hour before the main injection.

sex education. Sex is an inescapable part of life and a happy and well-balanced sex life is essential for the health of both body and mind.

The Victorians tried to conceal sex under a mass of dogma, convention and secrecy, so that some men and many women embarked on matrimony with little awareness of sexual matters. Frigidity, marital unhappiness, extra-marital relations, high illegitimacy rates and high incidence of venereal diseases were one result, while over-large, unspaced and often unwanted families with exhausted mothers were another.

Today sex is freely discussed, and books and films on sexual matters are freely available, but every study of adolescents reveals gaps and misconceptions in their knowledge even of the physical aspects. Clearly, therefore, we need substantially more sex education. In particular, we can no more rely solely on parents – some of them ignorant even of anatomical terms and ignorant also of aesthetic and moral aspects – to teach children about sex than to teach them about geometry or physics.

It seems essential for a start that every child should be taught the anatomy and physiology of sex with full realization of how the male and female organs complement each other for the achievement of nature's primary purpose, the perpetuation of the species. It seems desirable that such instruction should be given in some detail before hormonal changes arouse sexual desire. Such instruction should obviously include consideration of menstruation and its hygiene, explanation of nocturnal emissions and their harmlessness and full discussion of masturbation.

This physiological approach is, however, only a beginning. On sexual relations are built marital love, home and family, and many of the finest things of life. The aesthetic aspects have to be taught and fully discussed. The world is already over-populated and over-large families are common: the importance of family postponement, family spacing and family limitation has to be considered, with due discussion of contraceptive techniques and their advantages and limitations. Heavy petting has to be considered from the aspect that it is normally a prelude to sexual intercourse and that arousal of passions without their normal release may be physically and emotionally harmful and may also lead to exaggeration of the physical responses in sexual relations and under-valuing of the intellectual, emotional, temperamental and aesthetic sides of relationships between the sexes.

Promiscuity has to be discussed with due attention both to the religious and moral arguments in favour of chastity, and to the claims by advocates of 'freedom', i.e., that the sexual instincts should not be unnaturally dammed up by continence and that repression and inhibition may produce neurosis and maladjustment. The dangers of venereal diseases, abortion and emotional disorders have to be considered in respect of pre-marital and extra-marital relations.

Marriage has to be considered as the general foundation of society, with discussion not only of sexual adjustment in marriage but of wider aspects of mutual consideration.

Perhaps not least, sex education should include an introduction to parentcraft and a consideration of the emotional and physical needs of young children.

Parents can do a great deal in children's early years by answering questions honestly and with brevity of detail appropriate to the child's age and mental development, and by realizing that – since sexual matters do not appear important to the child – he may well forget the information and later ask the same questions. As the child grows older, parents who have devoted some thought to the points mentioned earlier in this article can clearly regard their continuing sex education of the child as part of the general process of helping him to progress to physical, emotional and intellectual maturity, and indeed as part of good family relationships.

It is a common mistake, however, to assume that a thoughtful and well informed parent can undertake the whole of the child's sex education and that sex education outside the home is needed only for children whose parents are ignorant or embarrassed. There are times when discussion between the child and an emotionally detached adult can be more fruitful than discussion with a parent, and times when an adolescent is more prepared to accept the statements of an 'outsider' with some claim to expertise than to accept those of mother or father. Also, since full sex education extends into many different fields (physiology, ethics, population problems, marital adjustment and child psychology are examples) very few parents would feel competent to do justice to all aspects.

Ideally sex education in the home and outside the home should supplement and reinforce each other; but in some homes sex education is virtually non-existent; and some parents who would never assume that they alone and unaided should give their child his total knowledge of religion or music or citizenship, resent the participation of professional workers in the sex education of the child.

Not every secondary school teacher, perhaps not every health visitor and certainly not every school doctor is competent to tackle the vast subject of sex education, including for example the elements of counselling for children with suspected genetic defects, discussion of the relative merits of oral and other contraceptives, and dispassionate consideration of the arguments for and against pre-marital intercourse. Yet these three individuals – teacher, health visitor and doctor – reinforced by the health education staff of the local health board and themselves reinforcing and supplementing intelligent parents can vastly improve future marital happiness, can reduce premarital conceptions, can decrease the births both of unwanted and of illegitimate children and can curtail the incidence of venereal disease.

sex hormones. A person's sex is determined by the sex chromosome from the father at conception (see GENETICS). The mother's sex chromosomes, normally designated X and X, are both female, while the father's are an X chromosome and a rather smaller Y chromosome. If the child gains an X from both parents it becomes a female with ovaries. If it gains a Y from the father it becomes a male with testes.

All the other sex characteristics are determined by hormones which are chemical secretions from the glands of the ENDOCRINE SYSTEM; the sex hormones are formed in the ovaries or testes but influenced by hormones of the pituitary. Both males and females produce two groups of sex hormones, androgens and oestrogens, but in different proportions. If androgens predominate, male characteristics appear, such as deepening of the voice at puberty and the appearance of facial hair; and these may appear in women in whom the hormones are out of balance. If oestrogens predominate, female characteristics appear, such as development of the breasts.

sex instinct. The inborn urge which impels animals of the opposite sex to approach each other at certain times and, by sexual intercourse, to effect the union of the male germ cell (sperm) and the female germ cell (ovum) so that the species may be reproduced and continue.

In human beings the operation of the instinct is modified by sentiments, ideals of conduct, social conventions and acquired codes of behaviour; and the instinct is generally regarded as including not merely 'lust' (as in the mating of some lower animals) but also certain protective impulses and tender emotions. The sex instinct, in short, falls into at least three separate categories – physical or sensual attraction between the sexes, mental or intellectual attraction, and the domestic complex concerning family and home. Any one of these three may be dominant and the three may be in conflict.

It was formerly thought that the sex instinct was non-existent or dormant until puberty, but the investigations of Freud and his followers have shown that in some measure sexual life begins in infancy. It is at first concerned with gaining pleasure from the stimulation of the oral and then the anal regions of the body, the 'auto-erotic stage'. Next the child's interests are temporarily directed towards himself, the stage of narcissism. This is followed by a period of interest in persons of the same sex, the homosexual phase. From about 7 years until puberty there is a latent period under favourable conditions of environment and training, and at puberty there is a marked increase in strength of the sex interest with, in most cases, a change of interest from the same sex to the opposite sex. An over-development or exaggeration of one of the natural stages in sexual development tends to lead to sexual peculiarities in adult life.

The picture of childhood sexuality given above is, however, complicated by the fact that the child has two parents and tends to develop an affection for the parent of the opposite sex and a resentment, sometimes below the level of consciousness, of the parent of the same sex. In most cases this over-concentration on one parent and resentment of the other disappears without trace, but in some instances an excessive fixation of the son on the mother (or the daughter on the father) makes it difficult for the youngster to fall in love or makes the youngster seek an exact counterpart of the qualities of the loved parent. This is the cause of much marital unhappiness and lies at the root of many neurotic illnesses.

In puberty and the years of economic dependence that follow it there is often a conflict between the powerful sex instinct and the forces of tradition and social convention that oppose its gratification. ADOLESCENCE is a time of stress and conflict, and many adults, forgetting their own teenage difficulties, are unsympathetic in their attitudes and reactions.

In most societies gratification of the sexual instinct is secured by marriage, with subsequent procreation and protection of offspring, increasing bodily and mental harmony between man and woman and mutual expansion of personalities. Mutual adjustment of the sexual instinct in marriage is a primary factor in the creation of long years of trust and happiness. Failure of such adjustment may lead to prolonged unhappiness, psychoneurotic illnesses, infidelity and disease.

In women the sexual appetite tends to wane after the menopause although there is considerable individual variation. In men there is no definite period of decline of sexual desire and sexual potency but decrease between 50 and 60 years is fairly common, although some men of over 70 retain full sexual vigour.

sex-linked characteristics. See GENETICS.
sex perversion. See PERVERSION, SEXUAL.
sexual development. See DEVELOPMENT.
sexual deviance. See PERVERSION, SEXUAL.
sexual relations. Sexual reproduction is the means whereby two individuals of opposite sex combine their genetic material to form new individuals who are not genetically identical with either parent. In complex animals, including man, the sexual act is influenced by hormonal cycles, instinctive drives, affection, the pleasure of touch and the relief of tension through orgasm. Reproduction is a natural process, essential for the preservation and perpetuation of the species, but it may quite often be detrimental to the immediate well-being of its practitioners – from the male mantis that is eaten by the female after he fertilizes her to the human couple faced with a young child's needs, implying less available money, less leisure and temporary inability of one of the couple to engage in remunerative employment.

In primitive communities the change from polygamy and polyandry to something approaching monogamy probably followed the establishment of settled homes, and was in part a recognition of woman in the role of home-maker and in part a response to the need to restrict the rate of growth of the population. In the earliest civilizations there was certainly nothing shameful about sexual relations, and woman was not devalued: goddesses were worshipped no less than gods, illegitimacy carried no stigma, female queens and priestesses were common enough and indeed matriarchy may have been the commonest form of rule.

Somewhere around the fourth century B.C. there began to develop new attitudes: politically, that the warrior was the only person fit to rule, with woman being bit by bit demoted to a chattel, without rights and even without a soul; and aesthetically and morally, a prudishness and guilt about matters of sex and a concept of virginity as the ideal state.

The early Christian church, while following both the Greeks and the Jews in supporting monogamy against polygamy for those who must marry, greatly devalued women, glorified virginity and continence, and deemed all pleasure in sexual intercourse wrong. Extra-marital relationships became associated with guilt and the fear of hell-fire, and even marital intercourse was considered something that should not be enjoyed and that should be undertaken only with a view to the procreation of children.

The rehabilitation of woman came very slowly: the right to vote and the right to own property came within living memory, equal pay does not yet fully exist, traditionally female professions (such as nursing) are still paid less than comparable traditionally male professions, and it is only very recently that a woman's passport has ceased to indicate her marital status. Throughout this very slow process of rehabilitation enormous efforts were made to protect the 'innocence' of girls, to limit male company to well chaperoned occasions, to teach self-denial and self-discipline, and to ensure that girls came to matrimony knowing little or nothing about sex and with a vague idea that sexual relations should be reluctantly tolerated rather than enjoyed – and inevitably a large amount of frigidity, marital unhappiness and psychosexual disorders resulted.

The Second World War probably did more than anything else to change attitudes: there were jobs for all, and the woman who became an unmarried mother no longer feared poverty; with death quite likely for the civilian as well as for the soldier there was a freer 'live for the present' atmosphere; and the preachers and moralists who had failed to prevent two wars lost status in the eyes of the young.

The allegedly permissive society of the last thirty years or so, the spread of sex education and the availability of contraceptives have combined to produce a new attitude to sex – an enjoyment of a natural function, a reduction in prudery and a separation of sexual relationships from reproduction of the species. These changes occurring gradually over a century might have been purely healthy, a reversion in fact to the attitudes of ancient Greece and Egypt before the subjugation of women; but, occurring in a single generation, they have sometimes produced confusion and conflict.

sheath. A contraceptive or prophylactic condom or sheath worn over the penis during sexual intercourse.

Since explorers in the eighteenth and nineteenth centuries found that condoms were worn as a protection against diseases, for contraceptive purposes or even as badges of rank by members of many primitive tribes in various continents, it seems remarkable that they were apparently unknown in ancient Greece and Rome and in the emerging civilizations of the Middle Ages. Perhaps indeed they were known and used but not described in writing.

Fallopius (1523-62), the discoverer of the female oviducts or Fallopian tubes, claimed to have invented a linen condom, not to prevent conception but to reduce the likelihood of the transmission of syphilis; and historians still argue about whether he originated the condom or merely applied an already common device to the reduction of a disease that had become widespread in Europe. At any rate, Saxonia in 1597 suggested impregnating the linen sheath in a suitable chemical and then allowing it to dry. Although linen gave place to sheep gut and sheep gut to fine rubber, the sheath was essentially in its modern form from 1597.

It was widely used in many countries in the seventeenth and eighteenth centuries, and curiously became called in Britain a 'French letter' and in France 'le chapeau anglais'. Even today it is probably the most widely used contraceptive device in virtually all countries.

If filled with air (like a balloon) to check for leaks before being placed on the penis prior to intercourse it is a reasonably good contraceptive and also lessens the chance of transmission of syphilis or gonorrhoea. If additionally it is coated with a spermicidal cream its efficiency as a contraceptive rises to about 99 per cent, a figure outstripped only by the modern contraceptive pill. The use of a spermicidal cream also prevents vaginal discomfort from friction.

The best patterns have a teat-shaped end to collect the ejaculate and minimize risk of backward seepage to the free margin of the sheath. Sheaths must be of reliable quality, and since rubber perishes with age, they should also bear a date beyond which they should not be used.

The advantages of the sheath include the very small effort required, as contrasted for instance with the physical effort needed for insertion of an intra-uterine device or the mental effort needed to remember to take an oral contraceptive every day. A second advantage is the fact that no doctor is required, the sheaths being purchasable without prescription (a matter of some importance in Britain and America because some persons who contemplate sexual intercourse may be reluctant to approach doctors, and of enormous importance in Asian and African countries where the number of doctors in proportion to population is very small). A third advantage is that a sheath considerably lessens the likelihood of transmission of venereal disease.

Although a few men and women maintain that even a very fine sheath on the man's penis reduces the pleasure of intercourse, the main disadvantage is of course that it is worn by – and normally purchased by – the man, whereas it is usually the woman who is the more anxious to avoid bearing a child. A further disadvantage is that, as with all contraceptive devices, the unsolved difficulty remains of the highly moral youngsters who have no intention of indulging in premarital sex and therefore use no contraceptives but who subsequently succumb to the temptations created by a combination of soft music, alcohol, proximity and opportunity.

shellfish poisoning. Essentially there are three types of shellfish poisoning.

1. *Bacterial.* Shellfish that grow near sewage outlets are liable to harbour infecting organisms from the sewage, e.g., the organisms of typhoid, dysentery and food poisoning. In Britain, local authorities have power to declare contaminated areas unsafe and to forbid the sale of shellfish from these sources. Where contamination is possible but less severe, authorities also have power to provide tanks in which shellfish may be cleansed by immersion for several days in water sterilized by chlorine. Where bacterial poisoning from shellfish occurs treatment is that of the particular disease.

2. *Toxic.* Mussel poisoning is sometimes caused by a ptomaine, mytilotoxin, produced by bacterial activity and not destroyed by cooking. Symptoms are those of collapse, with giddiness, coldness, lividity and often an itching nettle-rash. The stomach should be washed out with large quantities of water, the patient needs to be kept warm, and stimulants should be given freely.

3. *Allergic.* Some individuals have an idiosyncratic reaction to crabs, lobsters, mussels and oysters, developing within a few hours of eating them an irregular raised rash, diarrhoea and vomiting, and sometimes signs of collapse. The patient should be kept warm, anti-histamine drugs may be tried, and subsequently the person should avoid shellfish.

shell shock. An acute anxiety neurosis following exposure to extreme danger. There are usually underlying or contributing emotional factors but a traumatic experience is the final trigger in the production of the disorder. Common symptoms include headache, anxiety, depression, nightmares and fatigue.

The term was frequently used in the the First World War but has subsequently been replaced by broader terms such as anxiety neurosis, traumatic neurosis and effort syndrome.

shingles. The colloquial name for herpes zoster, an acute infection of a nerve root causing very severe, stinging pain in the skin served by the particular nerve, and in due course a crop of blisters appears over the same area. Pain and raised temperature occur for three or four days before the appearance of the blisters and the latter tend to dry off and shrink during the next week or ten days, although in frail or elderly people the pain may persist for months.

A dusting powder of starch or zinc oxide is helpful, and pain may be relieved by aspirin or phenacetin, or if necessary by pethidine. Claims have been made that costosteroids are helpful. When it affects the nerve supplying the upper face and eye, there may be danger of damage to vision and special care must be taken to reduce this risk.

The virus which causes shingles is identical with that of chickenpox. A person with shingles may infect children with chickenpox, but it is very rare for a child with chickenpox to cause shingles in an adult.

shivering. Uncontrollable trembling or quivering. It is a normal reaction to sudden intense cold and is beneficial in that it generates heat in the muscles. Shivering, or rigor, also occurs in the early stages of many feverish diseases, such as influenza and pneumonia, and bouts of shivering are particularly associated with malaria and glandular fever.

shock. A condition associated with failure or collapse of the circulatory system. Common causes include injuries (especially in the neighbourhood of the heart, lungs, intestines and genitalia), burns, failure of the pumping mechanism of the heart, severe haemorrhage and occasionally serious emotional upset. The symptoms vary with the degree of shock but typically include prostration and exhaustion; nausea and abdominal discomfort; headache and giddiness; and coldness and shivering. The patient is pale, his pulse is rapid and feeble, his breathing is shallow and his pupils are dilated.

Essential features of treatment are to lay the patient flat, preferably with the head a shade lower than the feet so as to increase the supply of blood to the brain, and to keep him comfortably warm; this is most easily done by placing warm (but not uncomfortably hot) water bottles at the feet, armpits and the inside of the thighs. Provided that he is able to swallow and provided also that the digestive organs are undamaged he should be given hot tea or coffee, and reassurance is even more useful. If the breathing becomes enfeebled, artificial respiration may be needed (see FIRST AID), and in serious cases blood transfusion could be required.

The term 'shock' is used colloquially in Scotland to mean apoplexy or STROKE.

shock therapy. Treatment of certain mental disorders by inducing convulsions, either by drugs or (more often) by electrical stimulation of the brain. The treatment – generally known as ECT (i.e., electrical convulsive therapy) – was originally introduced for schizophrenia in which it had little success, but it has proved very effective in ending obstinate melancholias and prolonged attacks of depression. In a number of cases, however, the therapy is only temporarily beneficial and has to be repeated in one or two years.

short sight. The common name for the defect of EYESIGHT known medically as myopia.

shoulder. The part of the body surrounding the ball-and-socket joint between the head of the humerus and the glenoid fossa of the scapula or shoulder-blade. Movement of the shoulder joint is usually good in all directions but mobility is paid for by lack of stability: dislocations of the head of the humerus, usually downwards and forwards, are commoner than dislocations of any other joint. Fractures are also not uncommon. Inflammation of the tendons of the joint leads to the painful condition known as frozen shoulder.

Siamese twins. See TWINS.

sickle-cell anaemia. See ANAEMIA.

side-effect. A secondary and usually undesirable result of a particular drug or other treatment, e.g., a sulphonamide may cure a particular infection but in a small number of patients produces a rash as a side-effect.

silicosis. A disease of the lungs caused by breathing dust from rocks containing silica for prolonged periods. The condition occurs in rock miners, quarriers and sand-blasters. It develops gradually, with the sufferer becoming progressively shorter of breath and having a persistent dry cough.

The silica dust particles form silicic acid in the tissues of the lung and this results in scarring and thickening, with ultimately the signs and symptoms of chronic bronchitis and emphysema.

Treatment is essentially that of chronic bronchitis and emphysema. Prevention is largely a matter of providing special ventilation; where that is not practicable, breathing masks should be worn.

sinew. A synonym for the tendon of a muscle, i.e., the fibrous tissue between the meaty part of the muscle and the bone into which the muscle is inserted. For example, the fleshy soleus and gastrocnemius muscles in the back of the calf combine to end in a bundle of tough fibres, called the tendon of Achilles, running down to the heel bone. This tendon, although it is occasionally torn, is probably the strongest sinew in the body.

Colloquially the term has lost its technical meaning and is often employed to describe muscular strength or vigour.

sinus. This term has two meanings.

1. In anatomy, a hollow space or cavity, usually in bone. The term is applied mainly to the cavities in the skull – the frontal sinuses in the forehead, the maxillary sinuses in the cheeks, the sphenoidal sinuses at the back of the nose and the ethmoidal sinuses behind and below the frontal sinuses. Inflammation of the mucous membrane lining a sinus, whether because of infection or because of allergic reaction, is termed SINUSITIS.

2. In pathology, a burrowing, elongated ulcer, which starts at a blind end (e.g., in bone) and opens on the skin or on a mucous membrane. A sinus differs from a fistula in having one blind end.

sinusitis. Inflammation of the mucous membrane lining one of the SINUSES which connect with the nose, i.e., the frontal, ethmoidal, sphenoidal or maxillary sinuses. Such inflammation often occurs during a cold in the head or other upper respiratory tract infection but may also be caused by allergic reaction or by prolonged irritation by dry air. The nose feels stopped up and has a copious thick discharge, the face and head have a sensation of heaviness, and there may be headache or pain behind the eyes if the frontal or ethmoidal sinuses are involved and pain in the cheek if a maxillary sinus is affected. Treatment consists of rest in a reasonably even temperature, a nasal decongestant spray, and in severe cases an antibiotic. If the symptoms fail to clear after a week's treatment, it may be necessary to consider inserting a needle into the affected sinus (working under local anaesthesia) in order to wash and drain it.

skeleton. The rigid scaffolding to which the body owes its shape.

In the process of evolution two types of skeleton have developed. (1) The exoskeleton or hard outer shell, as in crustaceans: this provides an excellent passive defence but limits movement and has to be cast off at times as the animal grows, leaving it temporarily defenceless. (2) The endoskeleton or inner scaffolding of vertebrates: the endoskeleton of man and other vertebrates, while essentially a central framework, nevertheless provides very complete protection for the brain and considerable protection for the thoracic and pelvic organs.

The human skeleton can be considered as consisting of an 'axial' and an 'appendicular' part.

The axial portion includes: (1) the SKULL, i.e., the eight bones of the cranium and the fourteen bones of the face; (2) the thirty-three bones of the vertebral or SPINAL COLUMN; (3) twelve pairs of RIBS, each joined behind to the vertebral column and the upper ten joined in front to the sternum; and (4) the STERNUM, or breast bone.

The appendicular portion consists of (1) the pectoral girdle, consisting of SCAPULA (shoulder blade) and clavicle or COLLAR BONE, with the bones of two upper limbs attached; and (2) the PELVIS, or pelvic girdle of ilium, ischium and pubis, with the bones of two lower limbs attached. Each upper limb has one HUMERUS (arm-bone), two forearm bones the RADIUS and ULNA, eight WRIST bones, five bones of the palm and fourteen finger bones (three for each finger but only two for the thumb). Each lower limb has one FEMUR (thigh bone), one small PATELLA (knee-cap), two leg bones the TIBIA and FIBULA, seven ankle bones, five bones of the sole and fourteen bones of the toes.

Every movement of the body is brought about by contraction of muscles anchored to particular bones.

Perhaps the most significant features of the human skeleton, as compared with that of most vertebrates, are firstly the relatively enormous size of the skull, and secondly the position of the metacarpal bone at the base of the thumb, allowing the thumb to be opposed to the fingers, as in climbing or gripping an object.

skin. The outer covering of the body consists of two main layers, the dermis or true skin and the outer layer of epidermis or cuticle. The dermis has a framework of tough fibrous and elastic tissue and contains loops of blood capillaries and nerve fibres with endings specialized for sensations of pain, touch, pressure and temperature. It also contains the sebaceous glands which excrete sweat. The epidermis is a protective outer layer without blood vessels. The deeper part of the epidermis contains growing cells but the surface consists of dead cells which are constantly shed and replaced from the growing cells. Hairs are epidermal growths which emerge from little pits called hair follicles. Nails of the fingers and toes are hardened and horny modifications of epidermis.

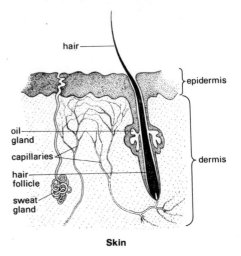

hair — epidermis

oil gland

capillaries — dermis

hair follicle

sweat gland

Skin

The skin is a tough, waterproof, elastic outer covering which protects the soft structures beneath from dehydration, soaking, minor injuries and bacterial invasion. It is an important sense organ, making us aware of such things as pain, heat, cold and touch. The sweat glands play an important part in the excretion of waste products. Both by dilating or contracting its blood vessels (so that more or less heat is given off by radiation), and by adjusting the amount of perspiration, the skin helps to regulate body temperature. In sunny climates it is the main source of manufacture of the body's vitamin D. Not least, it is the organ that is seen – the organ that attracts or repels other people by its beauty or ugliness, the organ that reveals emotions, and the organ that often provides indications of bodily health or disease.

An index of health. In many respects the skin is a useful guide to the body's well-being, constitutional changes being quickly reflected in the appearance and functioning of the organ that is most easily seen. Thus pallor occurs in the anaemias (although some people who are not anaemic have a natural pallor) with a curious lemon-yellow tint in severe cases of pernicious anaemia; yellowing of the skin and mucous membranes characterizes the various types of jaundice; bronzing is seen in Addison's disease; in cancer and advanced syphilis there is a characteristic earthy hue; and in chronic heart disease and chronic bronchitis there is a dusky, bluish tinge. Many acute infections are diagnosed mainly by their skin eruptions, e.g., the blotchy rash of measles, the rather finer rash of rubella, the fine reddening (except around the mouth) of scarlet fever, and the

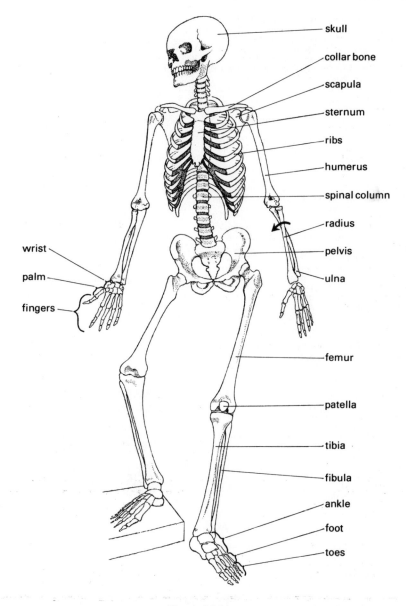

skull
collar bone
scapula
sternum
ribs
humerus
spinal column
radius
pelvis
ulna
wrist
palm
fingers
femur
patella
tibia
fibula
ankle
foot
toes

The skeleton

crops of papules and pustules of chickenpox. Again, the skin of a diabetic is often dry and inelastic; the perspiring forehead of rickets is almost proof of the diagnosis; and a thick, harsh skin suggests deficiency of the thyroid gland.

Diseases. As the most exposed organ of the body the skin is subject to so many disorders that classification is almost impossible. A few out of several hundreds are mentioned here:

1. Skin infections: bacterial, e.g., impetigo, boils, erysipelas; virus, e.g., warts; fungal, e.g., ringworm; and parasitic, e.g., scabies.

2. Rashes arising from acute infections, such as those of measles, German measles, chickenpox and scarlet fever, and the rose-spots sometimes seen in typhoid.

3. Increased sensitivity or pruritus (itching), sometimes occurring by itself in the elderly, and often appearing as a symptom of diabetes, gout, renal failure or cirrhosis of the liver.

4. Decreased sensitivity, as in syringomyelia, leprosy and peripheral neuritis.

5. Changes of pigmentation, either an increase, as in pigmented moles (melanomata),

which are birth marks, and freckles (ephelides) or a decrease, as in albinism.

6. Disorders of secretion: increased perspiration (hyperidrosis) in conditions of abnormal heat, exertion or fear, and also in association with hyperthyroidism and acromegaly; increased oiliness (seborrhoea), often due to hormonal influences; and abnormal dryness (xeroderma), often hereditary.

7. Disorders of skin circulation, e.g., chilblains and rosacea.

8. Dermatitis of various types, including contact dermatitis, the commonest of all occupational diseases.

9. Eruptions of large blisters, as in pemphigus.

10. Cancer of the skin, e.g., rodent ulcer.

11. Miscellaneous other conditions among which are psoriasis, acne vulgaris.

skin grafting. See GRAFTING.

skin writing. A curious condition, otherwise known as dermographia, in which the slightest scratching of the skin produces a red weal, so that it is possible to write on the skin with a finger, with the marks remaining visible for some minutes. The condition is allergic and is akin to urticaria or nettle-rash. Stimulation or injury of cells liberates histamine which causes a dilatation of skin blood vessels and localized reddening and swelling, and often occurs in persons with other allergic symptoms such as asthma.

skull. A general name for the eight domed bones of the cranium that protect the brain and the fourteen bones of the face; the upper jaw is part of the skull while the lower jaw is hinged to it. In most animals the cranium is placed in the back part of the head and the face looks upwards as well as forwards. In man, because of the enormous development of the cerebral hemispheres of the brain, the cranium is above the face as well as behind it, and consequently the face looks straight forward.

The ratio of length to breadth of the skull varies in different races. For instance, the Australian Aborigines are long-headed (dolichocephalic), American Indians are broad-headed (brachycephalic) and most Europeans are round-headed (mesaticephalic).

In any one race a woman's skull tends to be on average rather lighter and with less marked prominences than that of a man, and with a capacity of about 90 per cent of that of the male skull.

Disorders. The commonest disorders of the skull are congenital malformations and fractures.

Since the bones of the skull develop round the brain and gaps for growth are present in the early years, congenital malformations are not caused by defects of the skull but result from disorders of the brain which in turn cause alterations of the skull. In microcephaly the brain is of abnormally small size and therefore a small skull develops to house it. In hydrocephaly there is excess fluid round the brain and so the skull enlarges to make room for it.

Fractures of the cranium are common, although slightly reduced by the wearing of crash helmets by motor-cyclists; such fractures are very important because of their complications. Since there is no available space between the brain and the skull relatively

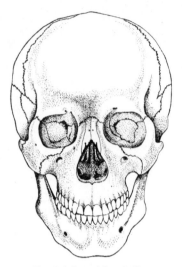

Frontal view of the skull

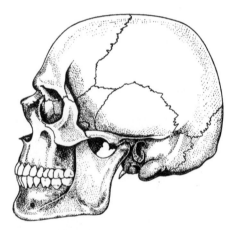

Side view of the skull

minor bleeding can create enough pressure to cause death. Hence operation may be essential to stop the bleeding or to allow excess fluid to escape.

Fractures of the bones of the face are also quite common, as is dislocation of the jaw.

sleep. The partial suspension of the activities of the nervous system which normally occurs at regular intervals and leads to restoration of the body's energy.

Although the transition from waking to sleeping may be abrupt, sleep is usually preceded by a feeling of langour, a heaviness of the eyelids, a relaxation of the muscles and a decreasing acuteness of the senses, with sight fading first and touch being the last to go.

An infant in the early weeks of life sleeps for over twenty hours out of each twenty-four; a child of 1 year sleeps for around fourteen hours daily; a child of 8 years needs at least ten hours a child of 12 on average requires nine hours although individual differences are beginning to appear by this age; and most adults need about eight hours, although a few adults require substantially more or less and there are two or three cases on record of adults who appear able to exist without sleep. As a rule continued deprivation of sleep causes symptoms resembling those of drunkenness and is injurious to physical health as well as to mental health.

During sleep all the chemical processes of the body are slowed, but brain activity – as demonstrated by the electroencephalogram – undergoes a change but does not cease. Whereas electrical waves from the waking brain are rapid and irregular, in deep sleep they are slow and regular but with occasional periods of increased electrical activity associated with rapid movements of the eyes. Some workers suggest that these active periods are associated with dreaming but evidence is hard to obtain since most people do not remember their dreams or even whether they have been dreaming.

Slumber is encouraged by conditions of comfort, darkness and silence, in other words by an absence of strong sensations, but paradoxically it is sometimes aided by monotonous repetitive sensation, such as a sound occurring every thirty seconds. Most of all, sleep is influenced by physical and mental tiredness and by habit.

Inability to sleep or INSOMNIA, is often a result of pain or other physical sensation, or of anxiety, or in some cases of over-intense cerebral activity immediately before going to bed.

sleep walking. The occurrence during sleep of certain muscular actions which imply activity of the portion of the brain controlling the relevant muscles. In the most marked form the person may rise from bed and perform a complicated series of actions (like Shakespeare's Lady Macbeth walking and washing her hands in imaginary water). If the eyes participate in the activity the person may see and avoid objects in his path.

Minor forms of sleep walking – or somnambulism, to use the medical term – include talking during sleep and such actions as sitting up in bed while still asleep. As a rule there is on wakening no recollection of the nocturnal activities.

Sleep walking is sometimes regarded as allied to hysteria but in most cases it is probably an expression of deep emotional conflict. Where it occurs as a single episode it is worthwhile to try the effect of reducing cerebral activity for the last couple of hours before the time of going to bed and avoiding heavy meals in that period. Where somnambulism continues or recurs medical advice is desirable.

sleeping sickness. An infectious disease of tropical Africa, caused by a minute parasite called a trypanosome and transmitted by the bite of an infected tsetse fly. The incubation period varies from one to three weeks. The early stages of the disease are characterized by irregular fever and rigors, intense frontal headache, areas of puffiness on the legs and face and enlargement of the lymph glands. After some months further symptoms appear: mental and physical inertia, shuffling gait and a

tendency to fall asleep. Untreated cases usually die within a year. Various arsenical drugs are useful in treatment but the doses required for therapeutic effect come dangerously near to the poisonous level. The tsetse fly that carries the parasites usually acquires them by biting antelopes or other wild animals, or by biting infected persons.

Preventive measures include mass injections of the local population with one of the appropriate drugs (to prevent the tsetse fly from becoming infected when it bites); clearing of bush around villages and beside roads (to remove flies); and fly control by suitable insecticides. Tsetse flies mainly bite by day, so journeys across infested country should be made by night.

A rather similar disease – American trypanosomiasis or Chagas' disease – occurs in Central and South America. Here the organism is transmitted in the excreta of various bugs and the disease, although often fatal in children, is less deadly in adults.

The disease should not be confused with 'sleepy sickness' a colloquial name for ENCEPHALITIS LETHARGICA.

sleeplessness. See INSOMNIA.

sleepy sickness. A colloquial name for ENCEPHALITIS LETHARGICA, a serious infectious disease caused by a virus, which in recent years has apparently become extinct. The disease should not be confused with SLEEPING SICKNESS.

slimming. A deliberate and sustained attempt to lose weight. In underdeveloped communities where malnutrition is common and plumpness is a sign of affluence and power, slimming is virtually unknown. In the affluent societies of Western Europe and North America, and especially in the middle and upper classes in these countries, people are becoming increasingly aware of the dangers of obesity. Excessive weight puts a strain on the heart (which has to pump blood to a gradually enlarging territory), the kidneys (which have to remove waste products produced in that enlarging territory) and the joints and muscles (which have to bear more weight). Obesity raises the chance of such diseases as chronic bronchitis and diabetes, and it increases the severity of conditions like pneumonia. Furthermore, it diminishes prowess in sport and looks unsightly. Hence attempts to reduce weight are very common.

Persons seeking to lose weight should remember certain basic points.

1. Excessive eating is often employed to camouflage life's problems. If a person eats as a form of compensation for bereavement or loneliness or sexual frustration or lack of work satisfaction, a reduction of food, however achieved, merely removes the compensation without tackling the basic cause. Attention to underlying factors may be far more important than attention to the diet, and slimming in the presence of sympathetic and encouraging associates is far easier than slimming without support and help.

2. Our weight depends essentially on our intake of Calories. If for our particular body size and amount of exercise we need 2,600 Calories daily and eat 2,300 we shall lose weight; if we need 2,600 and normally eat 2,800 we can expect to gain weight, unless we are the kind of person – lucky in an affluent society conscious of avoirdupois but in dire straits in

famine conditions – who makes inefficient use of our food.

To lose weight the fundamental need is to consume fewer Calories. Certainly we can seek to increase our calorific needs by more exercise, but violent exercise can be dangerous for those not accustomed to it and even mild exercise, while increasing Calorie expenditure, also increases appetite. Again, we can temporarily remove some weight by getting rid of excess fluid, as by saunas or Turkish baths, but the fluid – being the amount that is normally needed for our bodily size – will in due course be replaced. For sustained weight reduction we need a Calorie intake less than our Calorie expenditure, with gradual increase to balance expenditure after the weight loss has been achieved.

For weight maintenance an average-sized, middle-aged man of fairly sedentary occupation needs about 2,600 Calories daily, and a similar woman, being rather smaller, needs about 2,300 Calories. Tables giving the Calorie values of different foods and drinks are available in many textbooks on nutrition and dietetics. In general a slow reduction of weight (through eating perhaps 200 Calories a day less than are expended) is desirable over a number of weeks, with ultimate return to a Calorie intake that will simply maintain the reduced weight without either increase or further reduction. Sudden dramatic reduction of food intake may cause illness or exhaustion and is in any case likely to be followed by increased eating and restoration of the overweight condition after the period of extreme dietetic effort. Broadly, an overweight person can seek unaided to cut his Calorie intake by about one-tenth, but for more drastic reduction he would be wise to enlist the help of a doctor, health visitor or dietitian.

3. In attempting to reduce food intake we cannot afford to reduce all food components equally. The adult DIET should contain about 75 g. (2.5 oz.) daily of protein, or – since no food is pure protein – about three times that weight in lean meat, white fish, cheese, eggs and legumes (i.e., peas, beans, etc.). Unless our intake of protein has been grossly excessive its reduction would be dangerous to health. Again, sharp curtailing of our intake of animal fat (e.g., butter and cheese) could create a deficiency of the fat-soluble vitamins A and D; reduction of bread consumption may lead to a shortage of the vitamin B complex; most of us get 40 per cent of our needed vitamin C from potatoes, so that omission of potatoes from the diet may lead to deficiency of vitamin C unless we are eating plenty of lemons, oranges, tomatoes and green vegetables; and cutting down on milk and milk products may create a deficiency of calcium. Yet again, to prevent constipation we need a reasonable amount of ROUGHAGE - foods of low dietic value but appreciable residue.

Having ensured that we have adequate protein, adequate vitamins (possibly by addition of vitamin supplements to the diet), adequate calcium from milk and milk products, and adequate roughage, we can reduce our Calorie intake by particular attention to the reduction of carbohydrates (e.g., sugar, sweets, cakes, scones, white bread, to a lesser extent brown bread and potatoes), secondarily to the reasonable reduction of fats (e.g., butter and fried foods), and thirdly to the reduction of proteins to such extent as they were previously excessive. In arranging such reduction we can very much please ourselves so long as the total reduction is adequate: for instance, we may need to curtail our combined Calorie intake from whisky, potatoes, bread and cakes, but there is no particular virtue in cutting out the two that we happen to enjoy and leaving the two that we could happily do without. What we should aim at is a palatable, personally satisfying diet that will gradually reduce our weight over a number of weeks and that thereafter, with slight additions, can be maintained permanently.

The many 'slimming diets' in current vogue are mostly based on maintenance of adequate protein supplies and adequate vitamins, and reduction of total Calories by diminution of carbohydrates and, to a lesser extent, of fats.

Appetite depressants can help at the beginning of a period of weight reduction but some are addictive and some produce side effects. If needed, they should be taken under medical supervision. Usually, however, psychological help is more important than the use of drugs. Such help includes attention to the underlying causes of the obesity, encouragement to persevere with the diet, sympathy with occasional dietetic indescretions and relapses, and even pleasant conversation at meals to make a relatively small meal take longer to consume.

slipped disc. The vertebrae of the SPINAL COLUMN are separated by cartilaginous discs, and slipped disc is the painful condition that occurs when a disc cracks or becomes slightly displaced and so presses on a nerve. The dominant symptom is pain, occasionally felt near the site of the injury, as in lumbago, but more often experienced in the muscles which are supplied by the nerve concerned, e.g., displacement of the fourth or fifth lumbar disc is felt as sciatica, i.e., pain in the back of the thigh and the calf. Common causes include sudden, abrupt movement, for instance lifting a heavy case to the rack of a railway compartment may injure a lumbar disc, and the 'whiplash' injury when a stationary car is run into from behind, causing the head to jerk backwards and then quickly forwards with possible cracking of a cervical disc. Often, however, no cause is found and there is only a vague attribution to prolonged bad posture.

While heat, massage and analgesics all help the pain, they affect the site where the pain is felt and not the site of injury, so they afford only temporary relief. These temporary measures are usually necessary, and most cases respond to rest, sometimes including the wearing of a supporting collar for a neck injury, and often including the use of a board under the mattress for a back injury and occasionally the wearing of a spinal brace. Where these measures are not followed by return of the disc to its normal position and shape, manipulation by an orthopaedic surgeon (or by an osteopath) sometimes helps.

Young or early middle-aged adults with long backs, the commonest victims of slipped disc, can to some extent console themselves with the knowledge that the ageing process renders recurrence of the injury less likely. On the other hand, where the condition occurs after the age of sixty and fails to respond to rest and

measures to relieve pain, a surgical operation
may be required.

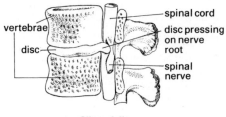

Slipped disc

slough. A portion of dead tissue (e.g., the core
of a boil) that is cast off from the living tissue.
Sloughing is the falling away of such dead
tissue.

smallpox. The most infectious of all diseases,
caused by a virus and characterized by a rash
of pimples which become filled with pus and
finally dry with crusting and often leave
permanent pitting of the skin. From the time
when it was first identified by Rhases (in the
tenth century) it has been one of the major
killing diseases.

Spread is by droplet infection from persons
sick with the disease or incubating it, by
articles recently contaminated by discharges
from such persons, and possibly by aerial
transmission for very short distances. The
incubation period is eight to sixteen days with
twelve days normal.

The rash tends to be most prominent on the
face and limbs, and takes the form of papules
(solid pimples) for two to four days and then
vesicles (watery blebs) for two to four days.
These points used to be emphasized as
differentiating smallpox from severe
chickenpox, but nowadays laboratory facilities
for diagnosis make them less important.

There are two main varieties of the disease.
The minor type (variola minor or alastrim) is
quite serious, with a death rate of around 1 per
cent. The more severe type (variola major) has
a death rate of up to 30 per cent. Persons
vaccinated within the previous three years
practically never develop the disease, and
persons vaccinated even many years earlier
tend to have only mild attacks.

Treatment includes rest (in very strict
isolation), good nursing (by far the most
important ingredient in successful treatment),
analgesics for pain, sometimes stimulants for
prostration, attention to the eyes because
ulceration leading to blindness is one of the
possible complications, and use of appropriate
antibiotics to prevent or treat complications
such as pneumonia. Against the disease itself
there is as yet no useful antibiotic.

Subject to what is said below, prevention is
essentially by vaccination of as many of the
child population as possible (aiming at the
production of an insusceptible community) and
by re-vaccination of such adults as are exposed
to special risk. Where a case occurs, there
should be strict isolation of the case in a
hospital exclusively for smallpox, with
medical, nursing and other staff debarred from
contact with the general public until the period
of infectivity is over. Prompt detection and
vaccination of all contacts and their
surveillance for sixteen days is essential. The
fears of the public must be allayed and there
should be provision of mass vaccination in the
district if some of the contacts cannot be
identified.

Vaccination has been available since
Jenner's publication of his discovery in 1798,
and vaccines of guaranteed purity and potency
have been available for at least 120 years. In the
last 30 years, however, it has been appreciated
that, since smallpox is solely a disease of man
and not transmitted by any animal, education
of people in all countries in which the disease
exists to accept vaccination could eliminate the
disease from the world. The eradication of this
grave disease in country after country has been
one of the greatest triumphs of health
education and preventive medicine, and has
succeeded to such an extent that smallpox is
now normally present in only two countries in
the world. Consequently, in many countries –
including Britain – vaccination of children is no
longer deemed necessary. Instead, vaccination
is reserved for the relatively small number of
people who are travelling to the countries in
which smallpox still exists, and for such
doctors and nurses as are likely to be in contact
with any case that occurs in the district. Until
smallpox is eradicated from the entire world
the latter precaution is essential, because a
person incubating smallpox may travel from a
country in which the disease still exists to a
country free from smallpox but with
inadequate airport health services, and may
infect someone who – still within the
incubation period of the first case – travels
from an apparently free country to another free
country before showing signs of the disease.

smegma. A soapy-like mixture of dead skin
cells and oil from the sweat glands that collects
in folds of the skin, and especially around the
clitoris and the foreskin of the penis. It is
important that the genitals should be kept
clean, because there would appear to be an
association between the presence of smegma in
a man and the occurrence of cancer of the
cervix in a woman with whom he has frequent
sexual relations.

smell, sense of. Smells are identified by
delicate, hair-like endings of the olfactory
nerves in the mucous membrane of the upper
and back part of the nose. From these smell
receptors impulses pass inwards to the
olfactory tract, which is an outgrowth of the
brain. In many animals the olfactory tract is
hollow and of considerable size; but in man it is
much smaller and more solid, so that man has a
relatively poor sense of smell, summed up in
Kipling's phrase, 'the noselessness of man'.

Nevertheless our perception of smell, weak
as it is, accounts not only for our perception of
odours but also for much of our taste. Certainly
the taste receptors on the tongue identify the
four basic taste sensations (sweet, sour, salt
and bitter) but most of what we normally
regard as taste is actually smell. Hence if the
upper part of the nose is blocked with excessive
mucus, as in a severe head cold, we have
difficulty in differentiating by taste foods of the
same consistency. Loss of the sense of smell is
known as ANOSMIA.

Many attempts to classify smell have been
made, the most recent being into burned,
fragrant, rancid, sour and blends of these.

Sensitivity to scents and odours increases when the atmosphere is moist (explaining why flowers smell more perceptibly after the dew has fallen) and when the temperature rises. For some smells there is differing sensitivity between the sexes, e.g., men can in general detect the odour of coffee more quickly than women. There are, however, considerable individual differences, and even in any one person there may well be some day to day variations of sensitivity to odours.

smoking. While many dried plants can be smoked (e.g., opium) the term normally means the drawing into the mouth of the smoke created by burning tobacco.

The smoking of tobacco is essentially an American contribution to civilized life. Practised by American Indians it was imported to England about 1600, allegedly by Sir Walter Raleigh, and to Portugal by Johannes I. Nicotius whose name is perpetuated in 'nicotine'. In the seventeenth and eighteenth centuries smoking was mostly by pipe although cigarettes were made in Spain as early as the middle of the seventeenth century. During the nineteenth century there was a fairly steady increase in smoking by men, with the cigarette becoming more popular than the pipe towards the end of that period. Smoking by women was rare until after the First World War but in the last fifty years or so there has been an almost year by year increase in smoking by both men and women.

Attitudes to smoking have varied over the centuries. King James I with his *Counterblast to Tobacco* heralded the first of many condemnations, and the Puritans in general disliked smoking. Interest in smoking revived about the time of the Restoration (1660) and a few decades later the idea evolved that smoking was beneficial to health. Some doctors claimed that it could cure many diseases and, more specifically, that it helped to prevent fevers.. Boys at Eton school were actually beaten if they did not smoke. Gradually a converse view began to spread – that over-indulgence in tobacco could lead to chronic inflammation of the throat, hoarseness, excessive secretion of mucus and an irritating cough; that it could impair the appetite and make the complexion 'muddy'; that smoking a clay pipe (the stem of which grew very hot) could lead to cancer of the lip and tongue; that very heavy smoking could cause tremors, palpitations, faintness and giddiness; and – a statement often made but never adequately proved – that smoking by children could stunt growth. With the exception of clay pipes, however, tobacco smoking was not significantly associated with the occurrence of serious diseases until after the middle of the present century.

Smoking is an expensive pastime but its devotees claim that the expenditure is well worth while. Oscar Wilde called a cigarette 'the perfect type of the perfect pleasure', and Charles Darwin said 'nothing soothes me more after a hard day's work than a cigarette'. Smoking certainly facilitates social intercourse, and indeed one of its dangers is perhaps that all smokers tend to smoke more when in company. A pipe, and perhaps a cigarette or a cigar, is alleged to be emotionally calming, and smoking certainly gives a nervous person something with which to occupy his hands.

Undisputed physiological effects of smoking are that it raises the blood sugar (so that it is satisfying to a hungry person who is temporarily unable to obtain food), that it tends slightly to quicken the heart rate and to increase the blood pressure, and that it after a time raises the level of blood platelets and appears to increase their adhesiveness (a point which may explain the relation of heavy smoking to coronary thrombosis).

Over the last twenty-five years or so evidence has been accumulating about the relationship between smoking and various diseases, but widespread publication of the facts has produced singularly little change in smoking habits – perhaps because virulent anti-smokers have damaged their cause by exaggerating the dangers. It is probably fair to say that smoking is not the sole cause or even the main cause of any disease, but that smoking, especially heavy smoking and in particular heavy cigarette smoking, increases the likelihood of various diseases. Here are a few points.

1. Influence on duration of life. Heavy cigarette smokers have an appreciably greater chance of early death. Fletcher in *Common Sense about Smoking* summarized the British evidence by expressing the percentage of men aged 35 who may expect to die before the age of 65 as – non-smokers, 15; smokers of 1 to 14 cigarettes per day, 22; smokers of 15 to 24 per day, 25; smokers of over 25 per day, 33. The American Framington study which followed up a cohort of men for eighteen years showed little difference in the life expectation of non-smokers, ex-smokers, pipe smokers and smokers of under 10 cigarettes per day but confirmed the reduced life expectation of heavy cigarette smokers.

2. Influence on coronary thrombosis, a very common disease of middle and later life. Various studies, including a massive study of British doctors by Doll and Hill, have shown that the ratio of coronary attacks in heavy cigarette smokers to that in non-smokers is approximately 14 to 10. Coronary thrombosis is common enough in non-smokers, so smoking is certainly not the main cause, but the ratio should certainly cause the heavy smoker to think.

3. Influence on lung cancer, still a relatively uncommon disease. Here the evidence is much more definite. Lung cancer is about thirty times as common in heavy cigarette smokers as in non-smokers, and tobacco has been proved to contain several substances liable to cause cancer (carcinogens).

4. Influence on other respiratory diseases. A smoker's cough (commoner in cigarette smokers than in pipe smokers) is indicative of irritation of the respiratory system, and chronic bronchitis is much more frequent in smokers than in non-smokers. Other respiratory diseases, such as asthma, appear to be no more common in smokers than in non-smokers.

In general it appears that cigarette smoking is much more associated with harmful effects than pipe or cigar smoking, possibly because a cigarette burns at a higher temperature, or because different portions of the tobacco leaf are used.

Some advocates of smoking have pointed out that comparison of smokers and non-smokers is not necessarily of like with like. Psychological studies have suggested that heavy smokers are more energetic, restless and extroverted than non-smokers, so that (irrespective of smoking) they might be more liable to coronary disease. That, however, hardly holds true for lung cancer which has been produced experimentally in animals by measures equivalent to heavy smoking.

Again, advocates of smoking have indicated that smoking depresses the appetite, that most people who stop smoking gain weight and that obesity may be more dangerous than continuation of smoking. Anti-smokers maintain that the death rate in ex-smokers (despite possibility of obesity) is less than in continuing smokers, but the question once more arises of whether we are comparing like with like.

Everything written about smoking is controversial. It has some proved and some probable associations with diseases, it is expensive, it gives personal pleasure and is an easily acquired mild addiction, and while about 80 per cent of people can discontinue it easily if they so desire, the other 20 per cent find discontinuation extremely difficult. Many doctors and other health workers have reached the position of saying: (1) that they unhesitatingly advise children not to start and adolescents and young adults who are light smokers to discontinue; (2) that they do not advise long-continuing smokers in older age-groups (say from 60 years upwards) to seek to discontinue unless they have diseases actually harmed by smoking; and (3) that they are in some doubt about how to advise persons between 30 and 60 years.

If the undesirability of smoking is accepted various measures need to be considered:

1. Fiscal measures that increase the tax until people hesitate to pay the amount demanded. Duty on tobacco, already very heavy in countries like Norway, Sweden and Britain, now amounts in Britain to about one-fifth of the Government's revenue. Against this, the cost in Britain of diseases directly attributable to smoking was officially assessed in 1974 at the very small sum of £30 million a year. It would be a very bold Chancellor of the Exchequer who would so vastly raise the tax as to deprive himself of a large slice of national income, and a very fervent anti-smoker who would advocate such action with a balancing steep increase in income tax. Moreover, sudden cessation of purchases of tobacco would have serious effects on the economy of tobacco-growing countries.

2. Restriction of advertising. This has been tried in Britain in respect of television advertising with very doubtful results. There was no marked drop in the sale of cigarettes. Also a study by a health visitor of children's smoking habits just before the ban of television advertising showed no relationship between the brands bought and the brands advertised. Equally, a formal warning on cigarette packets that smoking may damage health has proved ineffective. Just as a child will climb a particular tree if told that it is dangerous, so perhaps many of us respond to the challenge of taking a risk.

3. Health education of adults. The value of campaigns is a little questionable. (1) It is possible that the adult who increases weight by stopping may be at greater risk than before. (2) The person who gains real or imaginary consolation from tobacco may substitute more dangerous consolations, e.g., drugs. (3) Anti-smoking campaigns concentrating on mass media have in general failed. (4) Anti-smoking clinics have not really proved their value. Since smoking by expectant mothers has detrimental effects on babies and since most expectant mothers are still fairly young, an approach to them might be useful. Again a campaign to influence selected groups that in turn influence the community – e.g., doctors, nurses and teachers – might be worth trying.

4. Health education of those who are not yet confirmed addicts. Campaigns directed to school children and adolescents are probably the most useful line of approach. In such campaigns two things should be avoided: (1) health arguments – about disease thirty years later – make little impression on the young or merely worry them about the risks that their parents are taking; and (2) it is fatal to associate health education with a kill-joy attitude consisting of a series of negatives – a condemnation of cigarettes, alcohol, sweets, cannabis, promiscuous sex and so on. Perhaps the best hope lies in an appeal to the boy's athletic strength ('wind' for football and racing) and to the girl's beauty (stained teeth and tobacco-laden breath).

5. Production of a carcinogen-free cigarette. This would seem obviously desirable, but in countries like Britain every time that a firm announces the manufacture of a cigarette free of cancer-producing substances, it fails to appear on the open market and the Treasury intimates that it will be subjected to exactly the same taxation as ordinary tobacco.

6. Encouragement of changing from cigarettes to a pipe or small cigars. This would seem clearly desirable but most of the exponents of the dangers of smoking appear to have an 'all or nothing' approach.

7. Encouragement of moderation in smoking. Some of the many published investigations show little if any differences between light smokers and non-smokers, and all published studies highlight the danger of heavy smoking. There might well be a far better response to appeals to keep cigarette consumption to under ten per day and not to inhale than to appeals to stop smoking altogether.

snake bite. Poisonous snakes occur in all tropical and sub-tropical countries and to some extent in more northern climates. Not all snakes are poisonous, but identification of the biting snake is important because a specific antidote, if available, is more effective than a general one for all snake bites. In general the poison is injected from hollow fangs which connect with poison glands, and identification involves study of the fangs.

The highly poisonous cobras and mambas have fangs fixed in the upper jaw with few or no other teeth in that jaw, and these snakes usually have heads covered with large scales. Vipers and pit vipers (such as the rattlesnake of North America) have erectile fangs which when relaxed lie in a sheath of mucous membrane, and most of them have heads covered with small scales; some are very poisonous but the adder of Europe is seldom fatal to adults. There are also several varieties of highly poisonous sea snakes.

In general snake bites are indicated by two clean puncture wounds, often about an inch apart. Immediate treatment consists of the application of a tourniquet between the bite and the body (to reduce circulation of venom) with subsequent loosening of the tourniquet for a few minutes every quarter of an hour. If practicable, the patient should be immediately transferred to hospital, with reassurance given meantime, together with any available measures for relief of pain. The affected part should be put at rest and the patient's breathing safeguarded during removal to hospital. Incision of the wound and sucking away of the venom is no longer considered useful, although it has a long history.

The symptoms vary according to the type of snake but after initial shock and pain usually include the development within twenty minutes of swelling and paralysis of the bitten part. Generalized effects include colic, pallor, vomiting and sometimes collapse with both respiratory and circulatory distress. Specific antivenom (or failing that, polyvalent antivenom) can be life-saving; stimulants can help the flagging respiratory and circulatory systems; as much rest as is practicable is essential, and corticosteroids can also be of help. Antivenom, so useful for the bites of many tropical snakes, is of doubtful value for adder bites: in almost all cases the victim recovers without serum treatment about as rapidly as with it, and in a few cases serum produces a violent allergic reaction.

In the absence of prompt skilled treatment the outlook varies from a 50 per cent chance of death from the bite of a black mamba to a 1 per cent chance from that of a European adder.

sneezing. Sudden expulsion of air through the nose, occurring as an involuntary reflex action to remove irritation. Sneezing may be caused by the presence of irritating particles (e.g., pepper, snuff, and the pollen of some flowers) or may be an early symptom of cold in the head, influenza, hay fever or certain infections (e.g., measles). When a person with an infection, such as a head cold, sneezes otherwise than into a handkerchief he is liable to spray infectious droplets around for as much as a couple of yards.

Repeated sneezing may imply that control of the relevant muscles has been lost and has to be regained, as in the case of continued hiccough. A cold sponge pressed against the face sometimes helps.

snoring. Noise due to vibration of the soft palate, generally occurring from sleeping with the mouth open, especially when lying on the back. Occasional snoring can often be stopped if the sleeper can be induced to turn on to his side. In children snoring is usually due to the presence of enlarged adenoids.

The term is normally reserved for noisy breathing during sleep. Similar noisy breathing, also due to flapping of the soft palate, occurring when a person is not asleep is called stertor and arises in apoplexy, drunkenness and morphine poisoning.

snuffles. Noisy breathing through the nose (in contrast to snoring where the breathing is through the mouth). The condition is associated with nasal catarrh. In the past snuffles was often described as one of the manifestations of congenital syphilis, but by no means all children with that now very rare affliction had snuffles and many non-syphilitic children suffer from snuffles.

social aspects of health. An awareness of the relationships between social conditions and disease is not new. For instance, in the U.K. in the middle of the nineteenth century there was frequent conflict between Local Boards of Guardians and Poor Law Medical Officers because the latter again and again tried to prescribe decent food and drink as medical necessities.

However, advances in the scientific aspects of medicine, (e.g., the introduction of antiseptic and aseptic techniques, the discovery and acceptance of anaesthetics, the identification of bacteria and then of viruses, the development of vaccines for prevention of infections and the introduction of sulphonamides and antibiotics for treatment) deflected emphasis for many decades from social factors. In all the developed countries treatment became increasingly concentrated in hospitals and in the hands of consultants with expert knowledge of the particular disease but little knowledge of the individual patient or of the underlying social conditions and pressures affecting him. The general practitioner, trained in hospital by hospital consultants and continuing to regard them as his professional leaders, was in most cases much more interested in clinical advances than in social pathology.

Even in the preventive field many of the nineteenth-century administrative and socio-economic reforms owed relatively little to doctors: medical officers of health, aided by sanitary inspectors and engineers, implemented programmes for pure water supplies, sewage disposal and slum clearance, but only a few of them actually initiated programmes. Certainly the early public health workers contributed enormously to the reduction of water-borne and food-borne diseases, but even for a condition as common as tuberculosis then was, they were more interested in decreasing the risk of infection (e.g., by identification and isolation of cases) than in studying the factors that made large sections of the community very prone to infection. Again, it was not until the second half of this century that any health worker was sufficiently interested in the causes of home accidents to work out that they were commonest in the least affluent section of the community.

Interest in the relationships between health and disease on the one hand and social factors and circumstances on the other spread gradually. In part it was due to the social awareness of some forward-looking public health medical officers and of a smaller number of general practitioners, in part to the rising professional status of health visitors (e.g., in the U.K.) and public health nurses (e.g., in Sweden) who from the nature of their work could not avoid becoming aware of the social circumstances and attitudes of their clients, and in part to the emergence of sociology as an independent science and to the slightly earlier emergence of modern psychology. By the middle 1950s the medical officer of health had been described as 'a sociologist with clinical insight' and the post-nursing training of student health visitors was beginning to include some sociology.

Interested health workers began to realize that some diseases (e.g., coronary thrombosis) were associated with affluence and others with poverty, and that many less obvious factors played a part, e.g., susceptibility to tuberculosis is increased in persons suffering from serious bereavement. Health workers and social scientists in collaboration also established many points. To give two completely different examples, they showed that upbringing and life style from birth onwards had as strong an effect on an expectant mother as had the nine months of pregnancy, and they demonstrated that in industries handling asbetos safety precautions to reduce the intake of asbestos particles were not enough by themselves since workers often regarded masks and other devices as uncomfortable and as hindering productivity and so reducing income.

Physical and environmental factors affecting health are nowadays well recognized, e.g., the adverse effects of over-nutrition, under-nutrition, faulty diet in respect of individual constituents, overcrowding, excessive noise and inadequate exercise. Mental and social factors are in the process of becoming recognized, e.g., it is now appreciated that during the comradeship and collaborative effort of the Second World War various mental and psychosomatic diseases became less common, and that these diseases are more frequent in conditions of obvious loneliness (such as a lighthouse keeper) or partially disguised loneliness (like a clergyman in a remote district with no other persons of good education near him) than in close-knit communities (such as a miner in a mining town).

Many difficulties still interfere with the full application of social knowledge to the improvement of health and the reduction of disease. A few may be mentioned here. Firstly, skilled medical treatment is inevitably given mainly in hospitals, where neither doctors nor nurses can know much about the social circumstances, values and cultural pressures affecting a short-stay patient, never having seen his home or place of work. Secondly, health workers, especially doctors, often unknowingly seek to force middle or upper class ideas and values on their patients: an example is the almost hysterical medical attitudes in the nineteenth century towards masturbation, contraception and sex as pleasure; and another is the reluctance of some doctors today to prescribe contraceptives to single people. Again, health workers may not be consulted in illness: a woman with severe backache may decide against investigation and treatment because of the anticipated costs (in a country without a national health service) or because of the feared impact on her family if she is temporarily transferred to hospital. Yet again, some people – especially some social scientists – question whether the doctor should be the sole arbiter of what is or is not perceived as illness, e.g., deciding whether a person whose behaviour is at variance with that of the surrounding neighbourhood should be diagnosed as insane and removed to a closed institution, or deciding which of two equally ill patients should be admitted to the only available hospital bed; and these criticisms gain strength in countries in which some

patients pay their doctors while others are publicly financed patients of the same doctors.

Even in health education, the branch of the health and disease services to which sociology has made the largest contribution, there are still some educators who fail to change attitudes and habits because they unconsciously attribute their own beliefs and values to the people whom they are trying to teach.

Moreover, in the U.K. the rigid separation of health services and social services has certainly not contributed to increased awareness of the interaction of health factors and social factors.

Nevertheless it is becoming generally appreciated that nearly all illnesses involve social factors (just as nearly all social conditions and social problems involve health factors) and that their impact may be of crucial importance for the prevention, identification and treatment of actual or potential ill-health.

societies, peasant and urban. By derivation a peasant is one who lives upon the land and who supports himself and his family by rural labour. Before the Industrial Revolution this was the common lot of the majority of mankind since towns were small and scattered and mechanical transport had still to come. The peasant had a sense of security derived from attachment to his land and family, and from age-old customs which determined his pattern of life; his society was held together by established practice and belief. Life depended on home-grown produce and home-made goods from village crafts practised by individuals in their own homes. Any surpluses were marketed or bartered at local fairs or through contact with pedlars or travelling dealers. The sense of community was strong because adversity and prosperity affected all. Pestilence, famine or climatic difficulties were no respecters of persons, but when harvests were good the benefits were general.

Industry in itself was not incompatible with a peasant society. The pottery and textile industries flourished in England long before the Industrial Revolution and the fabrics made by Indian peasants clothed all Southern Asia from early times. It was industrialization rather than industry which changed the scene because the advent of industrial power made it essential to concentrate work into factories. Cottage industries could be practised at home in accordance with inclination and opportunity, but factories forced migration to the towns and accelerated the growth of urban societies. Impersonal discipline replaced the personal freedom and easy-going pace of village life and rigid time tables imposed unaccustomed strains.

With industrialization during the eighteenth and nineteenth centuries, towns became overcrowded and squalid. Unhygienic living conditions led to spreading diseases and high death rates, family ties were loosened and moral standards became abased, workers were exploited under conditions little better than slavery and child-labour was a deplorable commonplace.

In the present day, much of this is still happening in the emergent nations but in more advanced countries the glaring abuses have been, or are being, eradicated. The afflictions of modern urban society now take different forms. The aged, and those who are physically or mentally handicapped, become social problems instead of being inconspicuously accepted in a simpler and more sympathetic setting. The worker experiences frustration from repetitive tasks lacking any creative satisfaction, and develops a sense of insecurity knowing that loss of employment may mean destitution or poverty without any of the support which the peasant derives from the extended family and his heritage in the land.

These conflicts are the roots of anxiety now well-recognized as the underlying cause of psychosomatic disease and neurotic illness. But even prosperity is not without its ill-effects. Surplus income and the temptations of the town lead to unwise expenditure in ways which are socially or physically harmful: gambling, promiscuity, alcoholism and smoking, to name only a few. Increase of population, a rising standard of living, and universal demand for goods and services all require mass-production and ever more industrialization.

Urban societies therefore need to be planned so that industry is adapted to the needs of the community and the aspirations of its members. The mutual support and social relationships afforded by a peasant society can be replaced by adequate measures of social security and by the development of cultural and recreational facilities for the profitable and companionable use of leisure.

These are the lines of current thought and practice in advanced countries but to ensure 'the good life' for countless millions now being introduced all too rapidly to the pressures of a wage economy is a task of mammoth proportions.

sodium. A metallic element of remarkably low density and great softness and one of the essential MINERAL SALTS in the diet. The element does not exist in pure form in nature, and is best known in the form of some of its salts, e.g., sodium chloride (common salt), sodium bicarbonate (baking soda), sodium carbonate (washing soda), sodium hydroxide (caustic soda), sodium citrate and sodium salicylate.

Sodium chloride is present in all bodily fluids and the maintenance of its level is essential to life. Where excessive salt is eaten in the diet the surplus is largely excreted in the urine, although in part the level may be maintained by retention of fluid, so that too much salt may contribute to weight-gain and oedema. Where salt intake is low the urinary excretion of salt diminishes rapidly to maintain the balance. In hot countries, however, and especially in persons unacclimatized to these countries, considerable salt loss occurs through perspiration, which makes it necessary to increase the salt intake.

sodomy. A sexual PERVERSION or deviation in which love is reserved for persons of the same sex. It is known as HOMOSEXUALITY in males and LESBIANISM in females.

soft sore. See CHANCROID.

softening of the brain. A colloquial rather than a medical term, often used as a synonym for cerebral syphilis. Actual softening of patches in the brain may arise from a burst blood-vessel (apoplexy) and from certain types of brain tumour.

somatic. Pertaining to the body as opposed to the mind. In medicine the term is used when differentiating physical or corporeal ailments from mental or psychological illnesses, and psychosomatic is the word employed when mental or emotional causes produce physical effects. In biology the term somatic is used to describe all the cells of the body except the reproductive cells (which are in one sense immortal).

somatotype. A term sometimes employed in attempts to classify physique. A big-boned, well-muscled person is described as being of mesomorphic somatotype and a small-boned, poorly-muscled person is of ectomorphic somatotype, while a third type is called endomorphic. Determination of somatotype involves a complicated series of measurements – width of head, shoulder to shoulder distance, hip distance from iliac spine to iliac spine, circumferences of neck, arm, midthigh, calf and ankle, and thickness of fat at various parts of the body.

Undoubtedly we need some classification of physique: for instance the old idea of saying that a man of a particular height had a particular optimum weight was clearly faulty, since large-boned and small-boned persons of equal height would have appreciably different ideal weights. Nevertheless, many workers consider that the twenty separate measurements required for determination of somatotype are too elaborate for general use.

somnambulism. See SLEEP-WALKING.

sore throat. Inflammation of the tonsils, pharynx, oesophagus or larynx, with pain and usually reddening. Common causes include excessive talking and shouting, excessive smoking, and bacterial and virus infection. Serious throat conditions include quinsy, Vincent's angina and cancer of the oesophagus.

The value of gargling and of various types of slowly dissolving lozenges is in some doubt, but they can be tried, along with avoidance of the causal factor, if known. In general the continuation of a sore throat for more than three days justifies the seeking of medical advice, and if there is any breathing difficulty associated with the sore throat the doctor should be consulted at once.

spa. An institution specializing in the regulated drinking of (and bathing in) natural water, usually with a high content of mineral salts. The aim of the treatment is the removal of the waste products of faulty metabolism through the kidneys, the bowels and the skin.

Spa treatment, e.g., for rheumatism, is a very old method of attempting to combat disease. In so far as any benefit accrues from spa treatment it is probably due not to the drinking of the water but to the ordered discipline of spa life, the complete change of diet and the mental peace resulting from the removal of ordinary daily cares and worries.

space medicine. The conquest of space, to the extent that a manned space-ship can circle the earth not in Jules Verne's eighty days but in a couple of hours and that already men have walked on the Moon, raises a mass of completely new medical problems. To mention a few examples: what are the food requirements of a man spending weeks in a condition of weightlessness? Does the change from earth gravity to very much reduced gravity and later the return to earth gravity impose any strain on the heart and cardiovascular system? Are there radiation hazards once a space-ship has gone beyond the protecting envelope of the earth's atmosphere?

Does complete isolation, including the knowledge of being thousands of miles from other human beings, produce any long-term or immediate psychological effects? Remembering that bacteria in the Arctic are alleged to have shown signs of life and capacity to multiply after having been frozen for an estimated period of 10,000 years, are there any pathogenic bacteria, viruses or fungi on the Moon? Not least, what physical and mental qualities render a potential recruit suitable or unsuitable for selection for space-travel?

Knowledge of the physiological and psychological effects of space-travel is still in its infancy, but the return of every man or animal from a flight in space produces additional information, and some space conditions can be simulated on earth. Already space medicine is becoming a recognized medical speciality.

Spanish fly. A popular name for cantharides, a powder made from the body and wings of a dried bettle, *Cantharis vesicatoria*. It is an irritant, sometimes used as a paste for blistering the skin surface, and sometimes given orally in a mistaken belief that it acts as an aphrodisiac.

spare-part surgery. A term sometimes used for the replacement of damaged parts of the body by parts made of stainless steel alloys, silicones, plastics or other inert materials. False teeth are the oldest and best known example. Steel alloy replacements are already quite common for the hip joint and are occasionally used for the elbow joint and the knee. Plastic tubes are sometimes employed to replace diseased portions of blood-vessels. Silicones are used to repair damage to the ear, the chin bone and the testicle, and battery-run cardiac pacemakers coated with silicone can replace a defective natural pacemaker in the heart.

In many cases replacement of a damaged joint or organ by inert material is easier and simpler than TRANSPLANT surgery from a very recently deceased person, because transplant surgery (involving living tissue) often produces a rejection reaction, whereas inert materials do not produce such reactions and do not irritate neighbouring tissues.

spasm. A sudden involuntary contraction of a muscle or group of muscles. If contraction persists it is called tonic spasm; repeated alternate contraction and relaxation is clonic spasm. The muscle fibres in the walls of blood vessels and other tubes may also develop spasm to obstruct blood-flow or otherwise affect function; arterial claudication produced in this way occurs particularly in the heart and brain and in the limbs. Bronchial spasm produces asthma.

Spasm is also seen in a variety of more specific illnesses. It occurs in epilepsy and other diseases of the central nervous system; it is a feature of such conditions as chorea, meningitis, tetanus and rabies; it is characteristic of strychnine poisoning; and spasm of the hands and feet is a symptom of infantile tetany. Various occupational cramps such as writer's or telegraphist's cramp are similarly the result of muscular spasm.

Spasms of psychogenic origin are described under TIC.

spastic. A form of paralysis in which the affected muscles are kept taut or in spasm.

While a spastic paralysis can occur at any age (e.g., as a result of brain injury or of stroke) the term spastic is usually applied to a form originating before birth though not always recognizable in the first few months of life. In a typical spastic the legs are usually more seriously affected than the arms and the person walks with a curious stiff gait. Mental development is sometimes also retarded.

The causes of the condition include shortage of oxygen to the brain in the interval between the baby getting his oxygen from the mother's blood and starting to breathe for himself, jaundice of the new born, and birth injury, all in large measure preventable. Yet the condition is not uncommon, although the emphasis on it in developed countries nowadays implies not that it is increasing but that other forms of handicap in children (e.g., those due to rickets, tuberculosis and poliomyelitis) have decreased sharply. In general a severely affected child is best educated in a special school for spastics.

specialization. In the study and treatment of disease, disability and injury, there has been a basic distinction between medicine and surgery since the earliest times. From the evidence of archaeology and from ancient writings we know that surgery was a well-developed craft when the practice of medicine still rested largely on superstition. From the time of Hippocrates, and later on with the influence of the mediaeval schools, medicine gradually acquired a more commanding status and surgery was relegated to humbler and less-esteemed practitioners who as barber-surgeons plied their rather despised and separate trade. It was not until the eighteenth century that their particular expertise gained full recognition as a comparable professional discipline.

In the context of disease and its treatment, specialization means that particular knowledge and skills have come to be differentiated into increasingly narrow fields recognized as specialities and practised by individuals who concentrate on 'knowing more and more about less and less' and who follow careers as specialists.

The original distinction between medicine and surgery is no longer adequate in the modern context. The growing scientific complexity of medicine is leading to ever greater specialization and this is absolutely necessary if a practitioner is to keep in touch with the latest developments and be able to utilize them for his patients in terms of medical care.

The range of recognized specialities is now immense. In broad terms the nine 'families' within the whole range of the medical profession are: general medicine; general surgery; obstetrics and gynaecology; general practice; psychiatry; community medicine; pathology; anaesthetics; radiology and radiotherapy. Many are still further subdivided. General medicine for instance includes sub-specialities in: internal medicine; cardiovascular disease; clinical pharmacology; communicable diseases; dermatology; endocrinology; gastro-enterology; geriatrics; clinical haematology; neurology; renal disease; respiratory disease; rheumatology; and venereology. Medical paediatrics under the same general classification is rapidly developing a similar range of paediatric sub-specialties. Much the same can be said of the other main divisions as well.

Specialities must not be regarded as rigid concepts. Some which were formerly regarded as disciplines in their own right have returned to the fold of other major groups as their work contracted or changed. New specialities arise when new developments replace purely clinical art by the need for specialized hospital facilities and laboratory resources.

Even the general practitioner is not immune from the advancing march of specialization and he now has opportunities in health-centre and group practice to develop special skills and to practise these through joint appointments in the hospital service and in general practice, to the benefit not only of his own patients but to the general staffing needs of the hospitals.

Specialization now occurs also in other health professions. For instance the health visitor and the midwife are specialized nurses with extensive post-qualification trainings, and in each of these professions there is further specialization, e.g., the specialist health visitor concentrating on health education of groups or on the well-being of old people, or the midwife with specialized experience of premature babies.

On the whole, specialization, as indicated above, improves and increases skills and is therefore beneficial to the patient; but a stage may be reached at which many people have expert knowledge of the various diseases from which members of a family suffer but nobody really understands the particular family and its problems and interactions.

species. A group of animals or plants possessing common characteristics and capable of reproducing others with these characteristics. A species is often divided into races or breeds, the two terms being identical in meaning. Interbreeding of races within a species will produce fertile offspring of mixed race, whereas interbreeding of two species will either fail, or produce offspring that are not fertile.

Related species are grouped together as a genus. Thus rabbits and hares are of the genus *Lepus,* the ordinary rabbit is of the species *cuniculus* and is therefore scientifically called *Lepus cuniculus,* while the common hare is called *Lepus timidus* and the mountain hare *Lepus variabilis,* with the genus name often shortened in writing to its initial letter, e.g., *L. variabilis.*

However arbitrary (and sometimes misleading) the Latin names adopted, they at least give a useful international classification for multicellular organisms and even for protozoa; but for bacteria and viruses exact classification is difficult, unsatisfactory and from time to time altered by bacteriologists.

spectacles. A set of two glass or plastic lenses in a frame, worn in front of the eyes to improve the clarity of the EYESIGHT.

A short-sighted (myopic) person who cannot see distant objects clearly, because the light rays from them come to a focus in front of the retina, needs concave or diverging lenses. A long-sighted (hypermetropic) person who cannot clearly see near objects, because the rays from them would come to a focus beyond the retina, needs convex or converging lenses. As the lens within the eye begins to harden with advancing years (presbyopia) most people

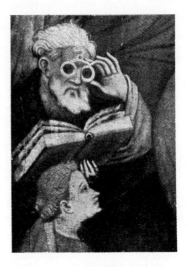

St Luke holding spectacles to his face, painted in 1404 by Konrad von Soest; this is believed to be the earliest painting of the use of spectacles

of middle age require convex lenses for such functions as reading or sewing, and some require bifocal lenses, with the upper part concave for distant vision and the lower part convex for near vision. Where one eye needs help but the other is normal, the glass for the normal eye may be plain, like window glass.

Additionally, an eye – whether normal, myopic or hypermetropic – may be astigmatic, i.e., unable to focus vertically and horizontally at the same time, because of lack of symmetrical curvature of the cornea. Hence the glass – in addition to being convex, concave, plain, or convex below and plain or concave above – may have to be differently curved in different directions, so as to bring vertical and horizontal rays together to a focus on the retina.

Again, the glasses may be tinted to afford some protection from strong light, or may be made of non-splinterable material to reduce risk of eye injury.

Archaeologists have found a crystal considered to have been used as a magnifying glass three thousand years ago in the ancient Assyrian city of Nimrud, and Nero is reputed to have used an emerald as a lens to improve his sight. However, a pair of lenses which were actually inserted in frames for reading were probably used by the Chinese in the tenth century; they first appeared in Europe in the late thirteenth century when they were introduced in Florence, becoming popular among the high ranking clergy as well as the aristocracy. At first only convex lenses for hypermetropia or presbyopia were used, but a portrait of Pope Leo X painted by Raphael in 1517 shows His Holiness wearing concave lenses for myopia; bifocals were not invented until the eighteenth century, when the first mention of sun-glasses is also found.

Probably the commonest error of spectacle users is to forget to clean them frequently. Dust from the atmosphere easily settles on the lenses, as does grease. Yet people who would never dream of facing the day's activities without washing their faces will frequently put on spectacles that have lost half their effectiveness through being uncleaned.

speech. The power of articulating words intelligibly. Many animals possess some power of vocal communication. Most people who keep dogs or cats can identify the different sounds that express need to go out, desire for food and so on; and it is likely that canine or feline ears can differentiate quite a number of sounds that we deem identical. Yet the ability for exact and detailed communication in words – the ability to say 'A tall, white-haired man wearing spectacles is coming up the garden path' – is specifically human.

Words are formulated in the speech centre of the cerebral cortex, a centre which lies on the left-hand side of the brain in right-handed persons and on the right-hand side in left-handed persons. The sounds themselves, i.e., the VOICE, are produced by vibration of the vocal cords of the larynx; and essentially the vowel sounds are formed by the larynx but produced by the shape of the mouth, while the consonants depend mainly on the position of the palate, tongue, lips and teeth.

Some of the many causes of speech disorders are as follows.

1. Deafness. A person deaf from infancy will not learn to speak unless taught by special methods. A person who becomes deaf later in life may gradually undergo changes in speech because he no longer hears himself pronouncing words.

2. Mental handicap. In extreme cases the person does not have the intelligence to understand what is said or to formulate answers. In less exteme cases his vocabulary will be small and his articulation poor.

3. Emotional disorders. These may produce stammering or stuttering, or sometimes complete absence of speech.

4. Damage to the speech centre, e.g., from a stroke, a brain tumour or multiple sclerosis. Depending on the nature of the damage speech may be totally absent, or slurred, or unrecognizable gibberish.

5. Abnormalities of the larynx. Examples are the hoarseness or even temporary speechlessness of laryngitis, and the loss of voice following surgical removal of the larynx.

6. Abnormalities of the mouth, palate, tongue or teeth. Examples are the defective speech associated with hare lip and cleft palate, and the milder articulation difficulties associated with badly fitting dentures.

Treatment manifestly varies with the cause; but except in cases of serious brain damage it is likely that speech therapy, or psychological treatment, or any necessary dental or surgical attention will at least materially improve the speech.

spermatic cord. A bundle of fibrous tissue and rudimentary muscle fibres containing the duct of the testis and the blood vessels of the testis and epididymus and thus forming part of the male REPRODUCTIVE SYSTEM. The passage of the cord from the abdomen to the groin, through the subcutaneous inguinal ring, creates a weak spot at which a hernia sometimes develops.

spermatorrhoea. Involuntary discharge of seminal fluid occurring at times other than during copulation. Seminal emission is common during adolescence and young adult life and has no sinister significance. At these ages the testes are very active in sperm-production and the distended seminal vesicles periodically discharge excess secretion.

Spermatorrhoea is also sometimes a symptom in neurasthenia and becomes a matter of further needless anxiety to the patient.

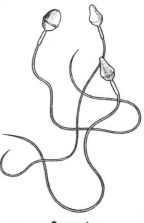

Spermatozoa

spermatozoon. A mature male germ-cell. Spermatozoa develop in the testes and are the essential germinal or fertilizing element of male seminal fluid where they are present in great numbers. Each is a single modified cell with a flattened oval head, an elongated cylindrical neck and body, and a long filamentous tail. Their overall length is about six-hundredths of a millimetre.

Spermatozoa are actively mobile by using their tails and so are capable of ascending from vagina to uterus and Fallopian tubes of the female REPRODUCTIVE SYSTEM. Fertilization of a mature ovum generally occurs in the Fallopian tube; a single spermatozoon pierces the capsule of the ovum, achieves fusion with the female nucleus and so starts the development of a new individual.

sphincter. A ring-like band of muscle-fibres found at the entrances or exits of hollow organs and ducts. Muscle contraction reduces the diameter of the ring, narrows or closes the opening or passage and thus controls the flow of any contained material.

The best known examples of sphincter muscles are the cardiac sphincter at the junction of oesophagus and stomach; the pyloric sphincter at the lower end of the stomach; the anal sphincter at the lower end of the anal canal; and the urethral sphincter at the outlet from the bladder. Sphincter oculi is a term sometimes used to describe the circular muscle fibres in the iris which constrict the pupil and so control the amount of light passing through to the retina.

sphygmomanometer. A clinical appliance for measuring arterial BLOOD-PRESSURE. An inflatable cuff is wrapped around the patient's arm and air pumped into it until it constricts myelocele the unprotected and malformed nervous structures lie exposed in a central cleft.

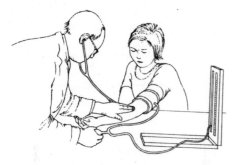

Sphygmomanometer

the arm sufficiently for the pulse-beat to be stopped. This air pressure is meantime also raising a column of mercury against a scale and the blood pressure is recorded according to the height of the column of mercury.

spider. A name applied to eight-legged, wingless, predacious arachnids, most of which spin webs in which to trap their prey. In general the first pair of legs are poison-claws, the second pair are organs sensitive to touch and the remaining legs are the real organs of locomotion. The spinnerets, from which are secreted silken threads to form webs, are situated near the hind end of the abdomen.

Although most varieties, like the ordinary garden spider, are harmless to man, fear of spiders is remarkably common.

Dangerous varieties whose bite can sometimes kill include the American black widow, also found in some European countries; the Russian karakut spider; and the Australian night stinger. After initial local pain, swelling and reddening, bites from these insects are followed by a general reaction of muscle pains and spasms, sweating, fever and rapid pulse, and danger of circulatory collapse. If available, an injection of calcium gluconate into a vein helps the muscle pains and spasm; and antivenines have been prepared and are available in some countries.

The notorious tarantula, much utilized by writers of fiction, gives a very painful bite but is unlikely to prove fatal to any animal as large as man.

spina bifida. A congenital abnormality affecting the spinal cord and spinal column. During the early life of the embryo the outer layer of cells running down the back of the body curls over to form the neural groove and this closes right over, becoming a tube lying just below the surface skin. As development continues, this tube forms the spinal cord with the vertebrae of the SPINAL COLUMN protecting it. The cord lies within the vertebral canal, formed by the neural arches of the vertebrae. In spina bifida the primitive neural groove fails to close and the vertebral canal becomes deficient at the back because of the faulty development of the vertebral arches. These defects lead to anatomical and functional abnormalities of varying degree. In spina bifida occulta involvement of the cord and its membranes containing cerebrospinal fluid; in meningomyelocele the protrusion also involves part of the spinal cord and associated nerves; in

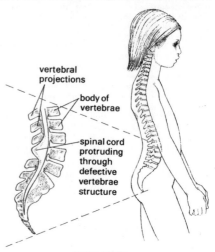

Spina bifida

About 2,000 new cases of spina bifida occur in Great Britain each year. The incidence varies from 1 in 500 to 1 in 250 births and it is a major handicapping condition of childhood. Its cause is largely genetic but partly due to other factors, since social class, birth order, nutritional state, maternal age, and infections during early pregnancy have also been shown to have significant effects.

Before the introduction of early surgical treatment in the 1950s most cases died in early life but many children are now reaching school age and adolescence and a long-term survival rate of 50 per cent may be expected.

Survival, however, raises great problems not only of clinical management but of educational, social, and emotional adjustment. Some 60 per cent of the survivors require special education because of physical and mental handicap since the effects of spina bifida include defects of movement due to paraplegia, urinary and faecal incontinence, sensory defects, skin ulceration and brain damage resulting from hydrocephalus, often an associated condition. The care of a child with spina bifida is a team effort involving medical and nursing skills, together with guidance in relation to educational, social and employment difficulties. The parents also require help and social support. In view of the substantial hereditary element in the condition there is need for GENETIC GUIDANCE and family planning advice.

spinal column. The vertebral column or main axis of the body consists of a series of bones called vertebrae, united to one another by intervertebral fibro-cartilaginous discs and by ligaments. The vertebrae number thirty-three and, although conforming to a standard pattern, they have individual characteristics as the cervical (seven), thoracic (twelve), lumbar (five), sacral (five), and coccygeal (four) vertebrae. In the first three groups the twenty-four vertebrae are each separately mobile so that the column is flexible. It can bend in all directions and rotate to a limited extent, but the sacral and coccygeal vertebrae are fused to form the sacrum and coccyx respectively.

Each of the vertebrae has four projections, two upper and two lower, which form the joints with the corresponding parts of the adjoining vertebrae and, in the case of the lowest of the lumber vertebrae, with the sacrum below. Between these joints there are firmly attached pads of fibro-cartilaginous tissue known as the intervertebral discs.

The vertebrae each have an arch towards the back and these, lying as they do one above the other, form the vertebral canal in which lies the spinal cord, which ends at the level of the first of the lumbar vertebrae. The spinal nerves leave the cord and emerge pair by pair, from between the vertebrae and from openings on the inner surface of the sacrum.

The bones of the spinal column are supported and laced together by fibrous ligaments and attached to this composite structure are the muscles which provide the power for voluntary movement – bending forwards (flexion), backwards (extension), and sideways (lateral bending), and also some rotation.

Viewed from the side the column has certain natural curves, concave backwards in the cervical (i.e., neck) and lumbar (small of the back) regions and concave forwards in relation to the thorax (chest) and sacrum (low back). The size and massiveness of the vertebrae increase progressively from above downwards and the upper two cervical vertebrae – the atlas and axis – are particularly specialized in form to support the skull and to permit rotation of the head.

Injuries. The spinal column is very strong but indirect violence may produce fracture-dislocations with risk of injury to the spinal cord, which runs within the vertebral canal, but in lesser injuries the continuity of the column is preserved.

Such comparatively lesser injuries consist of sprains, twists, partial and complete dislocations of the joints between vertebrae, and fractures of the vertebral bodies, neural arches (the parts of the vertebrae which enclose the spinal canal), or of the articular, spinous or transverse processes (the projections from the neural arch which provide anchorage for the muscles of the back). Sprains are commonest in the more mobile cervical and lumbar regions and are produced by sudden and excessive stretching of ligaments as in 'whiplash' car accidents or over-lifting. There is pain and muscular spasm but no x-ray evidence of injury. Fractures result from direct blows, sudden excessive bending, or abnormal stresses. An x-ray will confirm bony injury and such cases require rest and orthopaedic measures to secure repair, followed by physiotherapy.

In complete lesions the column is broken and displaced (fracture-dislocation), a common result of falls or of riding and traffic accidents. The chief risk is to the spinal cord itself which gets crushed between the arch and body of the adjacent vertebrae, so that PARAPLEGIA results. Skilled and prolonged treatment is needed but prospects are poor. The cord ends at the level of the first lumbar vertebra and lesions below this involve only the leash of nerve-roots known as the cauda equina and some subsequent restoration of function is more possible.

Deformities and diseases. Deformities of the spinal column may result from congenital defects, from diseases of the bone, or from the effects of soft-tissue changes. Apart from SPINA BIFIDA congenital conditions are rare. There may be absence of a part or whole of one or more vertebral bodies, fusion of adjacent vertebrae, or other defects. In disease there may be defective ossification, bony softening (rickets, etc.) or bone destruction (tuberculous osteitis, etc.).

However, most of the postural defects are due to muscular or ligamentous changes, and CURVATURE OF THE SPINE, arising from any cause, is classified according to appearance. In kyphosis the spine arches or angulates with convexity to the rear; in lordosis the convexity is to the front; in scoliosis the column is bent laterally to one side or the other and the vertebral bodies are rotated.

The small joints of the spine are also prone to develop arthritic changes, especially in later life, producing spondylitis (inflammatory changes) or spondylosis (joint fixation); and damage to an intervertebral disc is a frequent cause of disability known as slipped disc.

spinal column, tuberculosis of. Tuberculous infection of the vertebrae is sometimes called Pott's disease after Percival Pott (1713-88), a surgeon of great repute in his day. Bacilli reach the affected site through the blood stream from a pre-existing focus, usually in the lungs or in the lymphatic glands of the neck or abdomen. Such primary lesions are now rare in most developed countries because of better control of sources of bovine and human infection. Consequently the incidence of any type of bone or joint tuberculosis has dramatically declined.

In the past most cases occurred in children below the age of puberty. The disease usually affects the vertebral bodies, especially in the thoracic and lumbar regions, and these become eroded, with symptoms of pain and rigidity, and then collapse to reduce the deformity of kyphosis. In the thoracic region this appears as the typical angulation commonly called 'hunch-back'. Lumbar involvement causes less obvious deformity but pus produced may track down within the sheath of the psoas muscle (the muscle attached to the front of the lumbar vertebrae and passing in front of the hip-joint to the femur) to appear at the pelvic brim as a psoas abscess.

The treatment of spinal tuberculosis requires prolonged rest, orthopaedic appliances to immobilize the affected area, and anti-tuberculous drugs. With an adequate regime most cases eventually make a good recovery.

spinal cord and nerves. The spinal cord is an elongated cylindrical part of the central nervous system occupying the canal in the spinal column from the base of the skull to the level of the first lumbar vertebra. In an average adult it is about 45 cm. long and 1.25 cm. in diameter, tapering towards its lower end, and is enclosed within three layers of membranes corresponding to the meninges of the BRAIN. It is composed almost entirely of nerve-tissue with a core of grey matter or nerve cells surrounded by white matter consisting of nerve fibres which are disposed as 'tracts' conveying impulses up or down its length.

At regular intervals there arise thirty-one pairs of spinal nerves each having an anterior and posterior root, the latter distinguished by an oval swelling or spinal ganglion containing nerve cells. These spinal nerves are bundles of both motor and sensory nerve fibres which respectively relay outward impulses to related muscles and carry incoming sensory stimuli. The motor fibres leave the cord by the anterior root and fibres carrying sensory impressions enter by the posterior root.

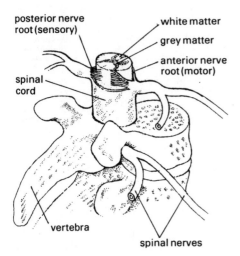

posterior nerve root (sensory)

white matter

grey matter

anterior nerve root (motor)

spinal cord

vertebra

spinal nerves

Anatomy of the spinal cord

Within its membranes the cord, like the brain, is also surrounded by cerebrospinal fluid acting as a water-cushion for support and protection. Since cerebrospinal fluid may show changes in certain diseases, a sample may be helpful for diagnosis. This is obtained by lumbar puncture, a hollow needle being inserted between the lumbar vertebrae. Similarly drugs may be injected for treatment or for the induction of spinal anaesthesia.

Diseases. The brain and spinal cord are continuous, lined by the same membranes and subject to the same diseases but with great differences in frequency. This article deals only with diseases of the cord, but see also BRAIN, DISEASES OF.

Haemorrhages and tumours (both common in the brain) are very rare. Such tumours as occur are seldom tumours of the cord itself but either meningiomas (growths in the lining membranes) or bony tumours which press on the cord. However, nerves which run from the spinal cord to the various parts of the body are often involved in certain general diseases, some of which (like poliomyelitis, locomotor ataxia and shingles) are due to specific infections.

For most of the other diseases of the spinal cord the causes are less clear.

Some, like Friedrich's ataxia, are familial or hereditary, some, such as syringomyelia, are due to congenital defect, and a particular type of hardening of the nerves at the side of the cord is associated with pernicious anaemia. Other common conditions include multiple (or disseminated) sclerosis and progressive muscular atrophy, the causes of which are still uncertain.

Special mention must be made of spina bifida, since improved surgical techniques are now saving a proportion of children born with this congenital condition in which the spinal canal fails to close during development so that the child suffers from a degree of paralysis.

Injuries. Fracture dislocations of the vertebral column are very likely to injure the spinal cord and because of its small size the damage usually severs the cord with complete paralysis below the site of injury. The spinal cord does not heal and the results are a permanent loss of movement and sensation (paraplegia).

spirochaete. A general name applied to any long, filamentous, spirally-coiled bacterium. Organisms of this kind are members of the Spirochaetales and require to be distinguished from the Spirillaceae, another family of curved and sinuous shape but which have other characteristics, and cause quite different diseases.

Of the spirochaetes the clinically important genera related to infections of man are:

1. *Borrelia. B. recurrentis* (relapsing fever); *B. vincenti* (Vincent's angina or stomatitis).

2. *Leptospira. L. icterohaemorrhagiae* (Weil's disease or spirochaetal jaundice); *L. canicola* (canicola fever – infection mainly from dogs).

3. *Treponema. T. pallidum* (syphilus); *T. carateum* ('pinta', a South American skin disease); *T. pertenue* (yaws); other species such as *T. refringens, T. gracilus,* and *T. balanitidis* are found in association with venereal disease and *T. microdentium* is often found in ill-cared-for mouths.

spleen. A large organ situated in the left upper part of the abdomen and of an elongated flattened oblong shape. Its size and weight are very variable but in the adult it is about the size of two hands placed palm to palm and weighs some 200 g. (7 oz.). It is soft, friable and very well supplied with blood vessels.

Although not essential to life it has several important functions. It acts as a blood-reservoir to augment the blood-volume when the need arises; it breaks down and disposes of damaged or worn out red cells and sets free their haemoglobin which passes to the liver for conversion to bilirubin; it produces new white cells especially in intra-uterine life and in infancy, and it protects against infection by removing micro-organisms from circulation.

The spleen is well protected by its situation high up under the ribs but it is sometimes ruptured by direct or indirect violence. Because of its friable and vascular nature haemorrhage is usually severe. The damage is difficult to repair surgically and it is often necessary to remove the whole organ.

Diseases. The spleen may undergo atrophy in old age or from debility and arterial degeneration, and it may suffer damage to its blood vessels from embolisms in endocarditis and septicaemia, but the usual sign of splenic disease is enlargement of the organ, often to a gross extent – it may reach a weight of 4.5 kg. (10 lbs.). Enlargement (splenomegaly) is easily detected clinically and always calls for further investigation. Its cause is complex because the spleen has several distinct functions.

Its role in bodily defence mechanisms

involves the filtering out and destruction of bacteria, protozoan parasites and worn out blood corpuscles. This explains the enlargement seen in acute and chronic infective conditions such as typhoid fever, miliary tuberculosis, malaria, kala-agar, hookworm disease, haemolytic anaemias and polycythaemia.

In post-natal life, its foetal function in blood formation is normally assumed by the bone-marrow but there may be renewal of its primitive activities in diseases such as leukaemia and lymphadenoma. Other splenic cells play a part in the metabolism and storage of fat, haemoglobin and iron. Derangement of this mechanism is seen in Gaucher's splenomegaly and other similar diseases. There is also a condition known as splenic anaemia or Banti's disease characterized by splenomegaly, anaemia, fibrosis of liver and spleen, and jaundice, sometimes controlled completely by removal of the spleen.

Apart from these more individual diseases, the spleen may be affected by amyloid disease, a form of waxy degeneration occurring in chronic toxaemia, as from long-standing suppuration, chronic tuberculosis or tertiary syphilis. It may also be enlarged from the effects of cirrhosis of the liver.

spondylitis. Inflammation of one or more of the vertebrae, often leading to permanent stiffness of the spine (spondylosis) and deformity (kyphosis), and characterized by recurrent severe episodes of backache or, less commonly, of referred pain in the leg. Spondylitis may be due to some infections, e.g., tuberculosis, but the majority of cases are of anchylosing spondylitis, a condition possibly allied to rheumatoid arthritis, thought to be genetic in origin, and affecting mostly young men of athletic habits.

The old treatment of immobilization and use of back supports and braces is now seldom advocated, and deep x-ray therapy is also largely discontinued, partly because of the high relapse rate and partly because of the danger of producing leukaemia. Aspirin and other analgesics are useful; a hard mattress is desirable; and the modern drugs phenylbutazone and oxyphenbutazone are valuable. In general, if the patient endeavours to maintain mobility in the long periods between spasms, the disease appears to burn itself out by about the age of 45 years.

sporadic. A term derived from the Greek word for 'scattered' and used mainly in relation to infectious disease to differentiate the isolated case or small local outbreak from the presence or occurrence of disease in endemic or epidemic prevalence.

spotted fever. A colloquial name applied to several different specific infectious diseases whose common feature is the occurrence of a rash showing spots which are the result of small localized haemorrhages into the skin (petechiae).

The term is most commonly employed as a synonym for cerebrospinal fever (meningococcal meningitis or meningococcal septicaemia) but Rocky Mountain fever and typhus may also be so described.

sprains. If excessive force or violent movement forces a joint beyond its normal range of action in any direction the supporting ligaments may be over-stretched or torn and the result is a sprain. In a sprain-fracture fragments of bone may be simultaneously torn from the point at which the ligaments are attached. In most cases the synovial membrane surrounding the joint is also damaged with the effusion of blood and synovial fluid into the joint cavity. Muscles and tendons may also be torn. There is usually severe pain and some degree of shock shown by feelings of faintness and nausea.

Sprains should be x-rayed to see if there has been injury to the bone. Otherwise the principles of treatment are to put the affected joint in a position of ease and to limit effusion and provide support by a firm, well-padded bandage. Sometimes a splint will be required to ensure adequate fixation. Once effusion subsides (four to five days) passive movements are commenced, followed by gradual active use, avoiding the production of pain or muscular spasm. Other measures may also be required to protect injured structures until they are soundly healed. In general, sprains require to be treated efficiently to avoid persistent or recurrent disability.

sprue. A disease or group of similar diseases characterized by chronic diarrhoea due to unabsorbed fat, loss of weight (both from failure to absorb fats and from voluntary restriction of intake of food because of the diarrhoea), anaemia (from failure to absorb folic acid, vitamin B_{12} and iron), inflammation and soreness of the tongue, and sometimes bone pains and mental apathy.

1. Non-tropical sprue. Best treated initially with a gluten-free diet, i.e., exclusion from the diet of ordinary wheat flour and of all articles made from it. In about 60 per cent of cases the dietetic treatment effects a complete cure but the gluten-free diet has to be continued. In the 40 per cent that do not respond, a high protein, low fat diet is useful and a course of such antibiotics as tetracycline or neomycin should be tried.

2. Tropical sprue. Has similar manifestations but appears to respond better to adequate dosage of folic acid, although a diet containing high protein and low fat is also useful.

squint. For accurate binocular vision (i.e., using both eyes together) the visual axis of both eyes must be correctly aligned so as to converge and meet at the point on which vision is directed. If this does not occur one eye must be in a faulty position. This condition is strabismus; the eye is said to 'squint' and its deviation is either obvious to the observer or, when slight, may be demonstrated by optical tests.

Strabismus produces double vision and because this is confusing the brain tends to suppress the image produced by the squinting eye, which gradually loses its visual acuteness. Squints may arise from actual paralysis of muscles controlling the eye movements but in the common squint of childhood there is no paralysis and the squinting eye moves with the sound one but maintains its deviation. Hypermetropia, or long sight, is often associated with the condition.

Squints require supervision by an ophthalmologist, and any persistent deviations observed should be attended to immediately. Various lines of treatment are employed according to circumstances. These include the wearing of spectacles, measures to enforce use of the squinting eye such as a patch or certain drugs that temporarily diminish the vision of the sound eye, exercises, and surgical procedures on the eye muscles.

stammering. Halting or hesitant speech due to spasm or incoordination of the muscles involved. Frequently the first consonant or syllable is repeated several times and this is STUTTERING. Speech is composed of words, and words are formed from vowels and consonants. Vowels are produced in the larynx by the vocal cords vibrating in a flow of air and their sounds are modified by changes in the shape of the mouth. Consonants are formed by interruptions of the air-flow at various 'stop' positions by the lips, teeth, tongue and soft palate. Speech thus depends on an air-flow provided by the respiratory muscles and muscularly controlled by other movements of the mouth, tongue, and adjacent structures. Consonants are interpolations in vocalized sounds; the stammerer adopts the correct 'stop' position for the one he intends to say but he maintains this too long and fails to allow the vowel to follow without delay.

Stammering affects about 1 per cent of children and is more frequent in boys. It is often associated with left-handedness, particularly if the child has been forced to use his right hand for schoolwork. It may appear either at speech-learning stage or later after some stressful experience. Occasionally it may be familial or imitative. Stammerers can usually sing or whisper without difficulty. In verse or song the metre demands orderly management of breath and attention is diverted from articulation to respiration. Other neurotic disorders may be associated indicating that it is a symptom of anxiety or repressed aggression.

Treatment requires much patience. The dominant hand should be determined and the child allowed to use it. Otherwise the emphasis is upon speech training and on child guidance methods. The speech therapist determines which of the 'stop' positions particularly give trouble and then concentrates on exercises and practice for breath-control, voice production, and correct 'stopping' until speech becomes automatic and not a conscious and laboured effort. Child guidance seeks to uncover hidden conflicts. These two activities complement each other. Conquest of speech difficulties gives confidence in other directions and vice versa.

standardized death rates. Death-rates are lowest at young adult ages and highest at the extremes of life. Males on the whole die younger than females and therefore have higher death rates. Hence a population with a high proportion of young adults or a preponderance of females has a low death-rate which is not strictly comparable with other communities having a different age and sex constitution.

To overcome this difficulty the local death rates for various age and sex groups are applied to a standard or national population and the mortality figures are recalculated to arrive at totals which represent the expected deaths if the local population had been of the same age and sex constitution. From the number of 'expected deaths' it is then possible to determine an adjusted or standardized death rate, and to make meaningful comparisons.

staphylococci. Cocci are minute spherical micro-organisms about one-thousandth of a millimetre in diameter. *Staphylos* is a Greek word meaning a bunch of grapes, and staphylococci are so called because microscopically they can be seen to occur as little compact groups, in contrast with the long chains formed by streptococci.

The two principal species of staphylococci are *Staph. albus* and *Staph. aureus* which develop in culture as white and golden-yellow colonies respectively. *Staph. albus* is ubiquitous and relatively harmless, and can almost always be found on the skin. Both types may however be found in superficial skin infections such as pustular acne, boils, carbuncles, styes, ear infections and so on. *Staph. aureus* is more invasive and is common in such conditions as osteomyelitis. It may subsequently reach the blood stream and cause septicaemia. Contamination of food stuffs with these organisms and their toxins can also cause staphylococcal food poisoning.

starvation. The result of denying to the body nutriments adequate to provide its requirements for food and energy. Deprivation may be absolute as in voluntary fasting, hunger-strikes or severe famine; partial when food is scarce; or it may result from disease processes interfering with the intake, digestion, or assimilation of food.

In starvation the body initially secures its needs by drawing upon its own reserves of glycogen and fat. Metabolism of fat in the absence of carbohydrate causes acidosis. When these stores are exhausted tissue protein is then used and extreme wasting develops. Starvation associated with disease is known as cachexia.

Three weeks may be regarded as the average length of survival from starvation if water is available, but the Irish hunger-strikers (Cork Prison, 1920) recovered after 94 days. Deprivation of water cannot be withstood more than a few days. A case is recorded of a patient who fasted for 382 days receiving only fluids and vitamins, but as his weight fell from 210 kg. to 64 kg. (33 stones to 10 stones) he was obviously subsisting on his exceptionally large reserves.

statistics and health services. The use of statistics to measure the efficiency of health services is discussed in the articles on MEASUREMENT OF HEALTH and VITAL STATISTICS. This article considers some implications for the health services of changing population figures. Statistics for Scotland are used below, but the data for England and Wales and for the Scandinavian countries are very similar, and although the U.S.A. and Australia have a rather younger age structure, they are moving in the same direction. On the other hand, available data for many developing countries are greatly different.

Scotland's main population increase occurred in the nineteenth century (from 1,600,000 in 1801 to 4,470,000 in 1901) but there has been a further 16 per cent rise of population this century, with numbers tending to rise sharply in and around towns and with the population of rural areas declining or remaining fairly level. Apart from this over-all and unevenly spread increase the five salient population changes of this century have been as follows:

1. A very marked and fairly steady drop in the birth-rate throughout the first forty years

(from 30 per thousand population to 17 per thousand) followed by a very slight rise (to a peak of 20 per thousand in 1963) and thereafter – in the era of family planning – a steady fall to about 13 per thousand. These changes imply a steady fall in the pre-school population until about 1944 and a second fall from the middle 1960s, a fall in school population (unless modified by other factors) until the 1950s and a further fall in the 1970s, and a year by year decrease in the numbers entering employable age-groups until about 1960 with a second year by year decrease beginning about 1980.

2. With better antenatal, maternity and child heath services, vitamins, vaccines, antibiotics, social improvements and health education, there has been a dramatic fall in the deaths of babies and children and to a lesser extent of adolescents and young adults – from about a quarter of all persons dying before the age of school entry (in 1900) and another quarter dying before the age of 25 years, to the situation in the middle 1970s where under 5 per cent die before school entry and only about 25 per cent (including the 5 per cent) die before the age of 64. This change, while slightly modifying the effects of the decreases in the birth-rate, implies the continued survival of many physically and mentally handicapped persons who would have died in an earlier decade.

3. Increased survival in late middle-age and early old age, so that by the 1970s a person who attained the age of 65 years had an average expectation of living for another 12 years if male or 16 years if female. This change implies a quite remarkable rise in the numbers of old people requiring care and attention.

4. An increase in the proportion of non-earning dependents, despite the decreases in the birth rate. This has arisen both from the raising of the school leaving age to 15 and then to 16 and from a vast rise in numbers of students attending universities, central institutions, colleges of education and further education centres – with consequent reduction in the proportion entering employment.

5. A change in the ratio of the sexes: about 104 boys are born per 100 girls, but in the era of high child mortality substantially more boys (the weaker sex) died and women were more numerous than men from about the age of 16 (so that 'surplus' women staffed such professions as teaching and nursing and provided the upper and middle classes with an abundance of maid servants) whereas today women are fewer than men up to about the age of 34 years.

The effects of these changes on the population structure include: (1) over the last seventy years considerably more than a doubling of the proportion of the population of pensionable age (over 65 male and over 60 female), a rise from about 7 per cent at the end of last century to over 16 per cent today and with 17 per cent anticipated in a few years – with consequent need for increased hospital staff, staff of old people's homes, general practitioners, health visitors, home nurses, chiropodists, home helps, etc.; (2) a rise in the proportion of non-earning young to almost 34 per cent, despite reductions in the numbers of children aged 0 to 4 years and 5 to 9 years – with consequent need not only for more university, college and school teachers but also for other people catering for the needs of the

young, from school nurses to authors and sellers of children's books; and (3) a reduction of the proportion undertaking the productive work of the country and providing services for the young and the old to between 50 and 51 per cent of the population – but with that percentage including mothers with young children, adults in mental and general hospitals, and persons in prison.

In respect of manual workers this apparently desperate situation is fully countered by automation, so that, although there are fewer available persons of working age, there are actually more available workers than jobs. However, the health professions, the teaching profession, the civil service, many numerically smaller professions and the higher posts in commerce and industry all have to be staffed from the more intelligent 10 to 15 per cent of the gradually dwindling group of 'earners'.

Until about 1960 the numerical deficiency was in large measure made good by increased educational opportunity, because in the past a considerable number of children of ability had left school at the minimum age on account of adverse home circumstances. The 'slack' so provided has now been pretty fully taken up, and there is an increasing shortage in many professions. The shortage is probably greatest in nursing, where, without any increase in establishments to cope with greater numbers of old people and greater survival of handicapped persons, the shortfall in existing establishments is around 20 to 24 per cent in 1975, even though one-third of Britain's nurses are from overseas, a source of recruitment that will gradually dry up as the developing countries open their own schools of nursing. Similar but lesser shortages exist in other health professions and indeed in most other professions, although a few (such as midwifery and school teaching) are beginning to be affected by the fall in the birth-rate.

Some of the many implications are as follows. (1) We can no longer hope to staff professions like nursing with 'surplus' women but are forced to ensure that salaries and conditions become such that shortages will be equitably spread among all professions. (2) In all professions (and not merely in the health professions) we must recognize the need to conserve the skills acquired by long training and must face the problem of dilution of staff and delegation of functions not demanding full professional skill. (3) In all professions we have to consider whether reorganization and reallocation of functions can save professional time without damaging the people served: to take two examples out of many, in an era when general practitioners, health visitors and home nurses work in association we have to determine whether complete freedom of patient choice is practicable or whether there is excessive waste of skilled time if eight doctors, six health visitors and five home nurses visit the same short street on a single day; and (to take an instance outside the health field) we have to determine whether every secondary school and every university requires staff to teach Greek to about three pupils or students, or whether one school in each region and one university in Scotland should be the centre for a subject that attracts few students.

Questions of salary alterations, reallocation of functions, private beds and dilution of staff are often deemed political, but in reality there lies behind each of them as the inescapable factor the slowly diminishing proportion of persons in the working group.

status lymphaticus. The thymus gland, consisting of lymphoid tissue, is situated in the lower neck and behind the upper part of the breast-bone. It is one of the ENDOCRINE GLANDS and is concerned with antibody formation and defence against infection. It increases in size until puberty and then gradually atrophies.

Some children who are fat, anaemic and lethargic have enlargement of the thymus with overgrowth of lymphoid tissue elsewhere and sometimes die unexpectedly, especially under anaesthesia. Such 'thymic deaths' were once ascribed to status lymphaticus (the lymphoid state) but this is no longer regarded as a satisfactory diagnosis. However, an enlarged thymus can cause respiratory difficulty by pressure on the air-passages, producing respiratory stridor or thymic asthma. Death may thus result in a mechanical way from acute respiratory failure, the likelihood of which is obviously enhanced by anaesthesia.

Thymus enlargement if demonstrably causing symptoms is treated by x-ray irradiation.

stenosis. A narrowing or restriction of any vessel, duct, tube, or canal in the body. The term is most commonly used in relation to disease of the valves in the heart which may result in aortic, pulmonary, mitral or tricuspid stenosis. Arteries may also be narrowed by degenerative disease of their walls and this is of particular importance for the blood supply to heart and brain.

Another frequent site for stenosis is the pylorus or lower outlet of the stomach. Pyloric stenosis occurs as a congenital functional defect in infants, and in older persons as a result of other disease of the stomach, particularly peptic ulcer and tumour growth.

sterility. Although also used medically to indicate a condition of being free from germs (e.g., in phrases like 'the sterility of the operating theatre') the word normally means inability to have children. In males sterility is essentially a failure to produce living spermatozoa, and should not be confused with impotence, i.e., the inability to achieve successful intercourse; and in females it is inability to give birth to a viable child.

In an infertile marriage both husband and wife need investigation since the cause of sterility may lie in either.

Female sterility. In primary sterility conception has never taken place; secondary sterility is infertility after one or more previous pregnancies, often as a result of infection following labour or damage to the uterus.

The general causes are complex because a woman has not simply to provide an ovum ripe for fertilization. Before conception her other organs must be able to receive spermatozoa from the male and facilitate their ascent in the genital tract; and after conception they have to provide for the nourishment and protection of the developing embryo during pregnancy.

The basic essential is ovulation or the production of mature ova by the ovaries. Normal menstruation is an indication that this is occurring and confirmation can be obtained by a laboratory test on a tiny portion of the womb-lining which shows the monthly series of changes related to hormone output by the ovary. Hormone disorders and chronic ill-health may affect ovulation.

A comprehensive gynaecological examination of the reproductive system should uncover causes likely to prevent access of spermatozoa. These may be malformed or underdeveloped states of the vulva, vagina, cervix or uterus and the nature of the vaginal secretion is also important.

Fertilization usually takes place in the Fallopian tubes and any factor which prevents descent of the ovum or ascent of the spermatozoa will prevent a union of these germ-cells. Salpingitis (inflammation of the Fallopian tubes) is much the commonest cause. Evidence of blockage or obstruction can be obtained by air-insufflation or by x-ray examination.

Finally, there is the problem of the uterus inadequate to the demands of a full-time pregnancy: conception occurs but pregnancies repeatedly abort. The uterus may be small and poorly developed, malformed or malpositioned or the seat of some pathological process such as fibroids. Many such cases can be rectified by appropriate surgical treatment.

It will be clear that female sterility is a condition of very diverse causation and that decisions about possible treatment must rest primarily on a painstaking investigation of each individual case.

Male sterility. This not uncommon problem is usually due to some organic disease of the sexual organs. A primary cause is non-production of living spermatozoa by the testes. Testicular atrophy results from certain genetic conditions; from developmental faults as in undescended testes; and from fibrosis of the testes with destruction of the germinal tissue. The latter may occur as a sequel to mumps and other generalized infective conditions, or as a result of x-ray exposure, or in other local diseases affecting both testes.

Secondary causes are those which prevent spermatozoa reaching the exterior. These are practically always due to past inflammatory disease, usually gonococcal in origin, which causes blockage or obstruction. The sites of this may be in the vas deferens, the urethra, or the tubules between testis and epididymis.

Diagnosis of male sterility depends on microscopical examination of seminal fluid for actively mobile spermatozoa. Although some of the obstructive causes may prove to be temporary or intermittent and resolve with treatment or by spontaneous recanalization, there is little hope of any improvement in the cases of non-production of living spermatozoa.

sterilization. There are two definitions of this term.

1. In relation to reproduction. Any procedure whereby an individual is rendered sterile or incapable of fathering or bearing children. See BIRTH CONTROL, permanent methods.

2. In relation to surgery. The elimination of micro-organisms from instruments and dressings in contact with wounds and, in special circumstances, even from the air of operating theatres. See ASEPSIS.

sternum. The breast-bone, a long flat bone extending from the neck to the abdomen and forming the centre of the front wall of the chest. It is in three parts and, although 'sternum' is derived from the Greek word for 'chest', its fancied resemblance in shape to the short Roman stabbing-sword (gladius) has inspired the names given to these sections as the manubrium (handle), the body or gladiolus (little sword) and the pointed lower extremity or xiphoid (sword-like) process.

It articulates at its upper end with the clavicles and its margins unite successively with the cartilaginous ends of the seven upper pairs of ribs.

Fracture of the sternum is uncommon but it is often distorted or displaced by disease, as in rickets, abnormalities of the spinal column, or disease of the respiratory tract. The junctions of ribs and sternum become enlarged in rickets and infantile scurvy to produce the characteristic 'rickety rosary' or 'scurvy-beading'.

stethoscope. An instrument employed to convey sounds, especially of the heart and lungs, to the ear of the examiner. A modern stethoscope consists of two ear pieces attached to flexible rubber tubes which in turn lead to a conical mouthpiece. The mouthpiece is placed against the appropriate part of the body and the sound is transmitted along the tubes to the ears. The stethoscope was invented by LAENNEC.

stiff neck. The common variety of this condition is acute rheumatic torticollis. It is generally caused by exposure to damp, cold or draughts which precipitate or aggravate an attack of fibrositis involving the neck muscles and their fibrous sheaths. The onset is usually sudden with considerable pain on head-movement and the affected muscles can be felt to be rigid and tender. In chronic torticollis or wry-neck the head assumes an abnormal attitude usually tilted to one side and slightly rotates to the other side, but cases of stiff-neck generally show this deviation as well since it represents an attempt to relax and ease inflamed structures.

Minor injuries to the neck muscles and intervertebral ligaments produce similar signs and symptoms. 'Whip-lash' strains arising in traffic accidents are a common cause.

Another variety is reflex torticollis induced by inflammation of adjacent structures such as inflamed glands, cervical abscess, decaying teeth, or disease of the spine.

Rheumatic torticollis usually responds well to rest, local heat and analgesics. Injuries should be investigated to exclude fracture. Other causes require appropriate treatment based on the exact diagnosis.

stilboestrol. Oestrogens are female sex-hormones produced by the ovaries. They are responsible for maturation of female sex-organs and development of secondary sex-characteristics and they also control ovulation.

Three oestrogens (oestrone, oestradiol and oestriol) were originally isolated from the urine of pregnant mares and found to have valuable therapeutic uses. Subsequently (1938) a much simpler and chemically unrelated substance, stilbene (di-phenyl-ethyl), was found to have similar properties and from it were made three derivatives, stilboestrol (di-ethyl-parahydroxy-stilbene), hexoestrol and dienoestrol. In 1948 synthetic oestradiol derivatives were achieved starting with ethinyl oestradiol. Although still available, stilboestrol is now less used. It tends to cause loss of appetite, nausea, vomiting, diarrhoea and skin-rashes. The newer preparations are better and are active in smaller doses.

Oestrogens are used for contraceptive purposes, for the suppression of lactation, for the treatment of menstrual disorders, in certain skin diseases, in senile degeneration of the vulvar and vaginal mucous membrane and in cancer of the breast and prostate.

still-birth. A child born after the twenty-eighth week of pregnancy and showing no signs of life. Twenty-eight weeks has been generally assumed to be the shortest period of gestation which can produce a viable child, defined as 'one capable of leading a separate existence'. However, there is a growing body of opinion that even younger foetuses can now be regarded as viable because of improved methods of resuscitation and post-natal care. In Britain the Lane Committee on Abortion (1974) has suggested that twenty-four weeks should now be the criterion.

Since a still-born child has developed successfully until at least its twenty-eighth week, its death must have occurred either from pathological conditions within itself or from extrinsic factors affecting it during subsequent intra-uterine life or at birth. The possible causes within itself are comparatively rare and chiefly due to developmental abnormality.

In intra-uterine life and during labour the child's safety depends on the health of the mother; on the proper functioning and adequacy of the placental circulation; and on the absence of complications during labour which lead to insufficient oxygen reaching the baby or to birth injury. The causes of foetal death or of premature birth with its attendant risks can be summarized thus:

1. In the mother: malnutrition, pre-eclamptic or eclamptic toxaemia (an infection of the blood), high blood pressure, heart disease, diabetes, thyrotoxicosis (resulting from disorders of the thyroid gland), syphilis and sometimes other infections.

2. Affecting the efficiency of the placenta: several previous pregnancies, multiple pregnancy, haemorrhage before labour, and umbilical cord abnormalities.

3. During labour: prolonged and difficult labour; abnormal position of the foetus; some sedatives; injury to the brain either through the size of the head being disproportionate to that of the birth canal or through over-vigorous use of forceps to assist delivery.

The prevention of still-birth depends on several factors: (1) supervision of the mother's physical and emotional health and education about diet, exercise, and so forth - all aspects in which the health visitor can play an important role; (2) adequate and skilled antenatal care to anticipate, uncover, and treat threatened departures from normal; (3) hospital resources to provide at need in-patient antenatal care and planned delivery; and (4) skilled help to ensure effective resuscitation of the baby if needed.

The reduction in the numbers of still-births in the third quarter of this century is in large measure an indication of the success of heal services in such countries as Sweden, Norwa and Britain; but in these countries th proportion of still-births remains higher among the poor than among the wealthy, higher in women over 35 years than in younger mothers and higher in women who have already had four or more children than in those having their first or second.

Still's disease. A type of rheumatoid arthritis occurring in children and first described by the

English physician Sir George Frederic Still (1868-1941). It usually commences between the ages of 2 and 4 years; onset may be abrupt with high fever and painful swelling of many joints, or more insidious with gradually increasing stiffness and swelling of the small joints of fingers, hands and wrists. Other special characteristics are enlargement of lymph-glands and spleen and often heart complications, particularly pericarditis (inflammation of the membranous sac containing the heart).

Wasting, anaemia, muscle contractures and deformities usually follow. Although remissions or arrest do occur the course of the disease tends to be progressive and may lead to complete invalidism. Rest is essential and other treatment is usually by salicylates, steroids and physiotherapy. Surgery may be required to deal with contractures. A proportion of cases die from intercurrent infection or cardiac complications.

stimulant. Any substance that temporarily quickens the rate of a mental or physical activity. If a stimulant is to be effective there clearly must be a certain amount of reserve power in the organ that is to be stimulated. To use a stimulant where there is no such reserve power is simply the equivalent of whipping an exhausted horse.

In a sense, any substance that is not simply a food (which remedies wear and tear and provides energy-producing material) is likely to have either a stimulating effect or reduce mental or physical activity; therefore a vast number of drugs could be called stimulants. Thus digitalis stimulates heart muscle, producing stronger and slower contractions; oxytocin stimulates contraction of the uterus in childbirth; purgatives, cholagogues and diuretics stimulate the action of the intestine, the liver and the kidneys respectively. Since such stimulants act in a variety of different ways the word is seldom used in medicine.

In common parlance the term is generally employed for two types of substance. (1) It is used (correctly) for drugs which temporarily increase mental alertness, such as the amphetamines and to a smaller extent the caffeine contained in coffee and tea. They have after-effects of course, because the central nervous system cannot be overworked for some hours without cost, but are genuine stimulants. (2) The term is very commonly used for alcohol. Alcohol has many uses: it provides a very rapid source of energy in exhaustion, it creates bodily warmth after exposure to cold (although it should not be given while the person is still exposed to cold), and it removes inhibitions and decreases shyness; but it actually lowers reaction time and mental and physical activity, and is therefore really the reverse of a stimulant.

stings. See BITES AND STINGS.

stitch. A severe pain, usually experienced on one side of the abdomen just below the ribs, and commonly brought on by unaccustomed running or other excessive exertion. It is due to cramp of the abdominal muscles which are maintaining firm contraction in order to protect the abdominal organs from being jolted about. It rapidly recovers with rest and no special treatment is required.

The word 'stitch' is also synonymous with a surgical SUTURE, used in sewing up wounds.

stomach. A capacious musculo-membranous pouch forming part of the DIGESTIVE SYSTEM below the lower end of the gullet, or oesophagus, and the duodenum, or beginning of the small intestine. Situated in the upper abdomen, it is J-shaped with the vertical part expanded to form the fundus and the hook of the J narrowing to the pyloric antrum and sphincter. Food enters through the cardiac orifice just below the diaphragm and is retained for digestion for about four hours. Ferments and hydrochloric acid for this purpose are secreted by multiple glands in the mucous lining of the organ. Muscular movements of the stomach churn and mix its contents with the digestive secretions.

When gastric digestion is complete, the pyloric sphincter, or lower opening, relaxes to allow the prepared contents to pass to the small intestine for further treatment and subsequent absorption.

Diseases. Minor disorders of the stomach are very common.

Indigestion or dyspepsia may be due to acute or chronic gastritis caused primarily by stomach irritants which include dietary indiscretions, alcohol, and chemical and bacterial toxins. It is a symptom also of other diseases accompanied by infection, fever, or metabolic upset. Actual erosion of gastric mucous membrane occurs in gastric ulcer producing both pain and dyspepsia.

Disorders of secretion may produce either an excess or deficiency of hydrochloric acid. Excess (hyperchlorhydria) is usual in gastric ulcer; deficiency (hypochlorhydria) is common in anaemia, debility and malignant disease.

Gastric ulcers may bleed, causing either frank haematemesis (vomiting of blood), or detectable traces in the stools.

Pyloric stenosis is obstruction to the outlet from the stomach. A congenital form occurs in infants but in adults it results from chronic ulceration or malignant disease.

A malignant tumour or carcinoma may arise from the cells lining the inner surface of the stomach. It is a common disease, with an incidence which is higher in males. Indeed it is the most frequent malignant disease in men. No adult age is exempt but it tends to occur in older persons, and while many cases are a sequel of chronic gastric ulceration, others arise without any history or evidence of previous gastric disease.

Early symptoms are often vague with indigestion, loss of appetite, anaemia, weakness and wasting. Such a history in a previously healthy person over 40 should arouse suspicion and suggest a need for x-ray investigation. Further effects depend greatly on the actual site of tumour growth. At the pyloric end of the stomach early obstruction produces vomiting. The vomit is often characteristic ('coffee-grounds' from altered blood). Other late features are absence of gastric hydrochloric acid and development of enlarged lymphatic glands at the root of the neck on the left side from direct spread along the thoracic lymph duct.

Treatment is surgical removal of the organ (gastrectomy), but success depends on early diagnosis.

stomatitis. See TONGUE.

stone. A stone-like mass, technically called a calculus, formed within the body, usually in hollow organs or secretory ducts.

Calculi commonly occur in the gall-bladder, the kidney and urinary bladder, and the ducts of the salivary glands.

Gall-stones are composed either of cholesterol or bile-salts; stones in the urinary tract are derived from the precipation of salts normally held in solution in the urine and vary in composition – calcium oxalate, uric acid and urates, phosphates of calcium, magnesium and ammonia are the most usual constituents. Salivary calculi are generally composed of calcium carbonate or phosphate or a mixture of these.

Gall-stones and urinary caculi often give rise to much pain and ill-health, and appropriate surgical treatment is required.

stools. The faeces, or material evacuated from the bowel. The characteristics of stools may provide important diagnostic clues. Normally a single stool of about 100 g. (3.5 oz.) is passed each day. It should be of semi-solid consistence, neither fluid nor hard, and roughly cylindrical; ribbon-shaped stools may indicate some constriction higher up; there should be no excess of mucus nor any other abnormal constituent; the colour, which tends to be darker on a predominantly meat diet, should range from light to dark brown. Inspection of the stools may show obvious blood, pus, bile, mucus, or parasites such as tape-worm segments. In addition attention should be paid to:

1. Colour: clay-coloured in obstructive jaundice; green in digestive disorders, especially of young children; black and tarry (melaena) from altered blood.

2. Consistency: resembling pea-soup in typhoid fever and intestinal infections; like rice-water in cholera; hard, rounded and separate (scybala) in chronic constipation.

3. Appearance: slimy with mucus in colitis; purulent in chronic dysentery; pale, bulky and oily from excess of fat which may be present as neutral fat in pancreatic insufficiency or as fatty acids and soaps if there is defective absorption, as in sprue or coeliac disease; frothy in carbohydrate fermentation which may follow intestinal infection.

Infant's stools present special features. For the first few days they are dark green and fluid from bile and mucus from the intestine, known as meconium. They then become soft and yellow and only gradually faeculent as a mixed diet is introduced. By two years they should be formed and definitely faecal. During digestive upsets they are often green and may contain curds from undigested milk or froth from fermentation of excess dietary sugar.

Laboratory examination by microscopical, bacteriological or chemical methods will provide still more information, and a specimen of faeces is frequently requested for these purposes. It is usually collected in a special sterile glass container equipped with a scoop or spatula attached to the cap and should be transmitted to the laboratory with the minimum of delay.

strabismus. See SQUINT.

strain. The result of tearing or over-stretching muscle fibres, usually by a sudden or unusual movement. A strain manifests itself by sudden pain which increases on movement of the muscle, swelling, and sometimes bruising. Treatment includes rest of the part, cold compresses to reduce swelling, a firm bandage for a few days, and analgesics if the pain is severe: aspirin or paracetamol usually suffices. The essential difference from a SPRAIN is that the latter involves tearing of ligaments and is in general more severe.

strangury. Painful and ineffectual effort to pass urine. By derivation the word means 'to squeeze out urine' and this describes the difficulties of the patient who makes frequent paroxysmal, painful and spasmodic attempts to urinate but each time only succeeds in voiding small quantities which are often mixed with blood or pus.

Strangury (or dysuria) is a common symptom of such conditions as renal colic, acute cystitis, urinary retention from prostatic obstruction, and especially of acute urethritis, usually of gonorrhoeal origin.

streptococci. BACTERIA are tiny; single-celled organisms which multiply by simply dividing into two. Cocci are varieties of bacteria roughly spherical in shape. Streptococci are cocci in which division occurs always on one axis, so that a single streptococcus after three successive divisions appears as a chain of eight.

Streptococci cause many diseases, from scarlet fever to septicaemia.

streptomycin. An antibiotic derived from the soil-fungus *Streptomyces griseus* and prepared for clinical use as the crystalline sulphate or chloride. It requires to be given by injection into a muscle as it is absorbed from the digestive system.

Streptomycin has a wide range of antibacterial activity but its main use is for the treatment of tuberculosis in which it is very effective. Its chief drawback is a liability to induce severe deafness. Both it and its derivative, di-hydro-streptomycin, have a specific action on the auditory and vestibular nerves. Signs of toxicity such as a ringing in the ears, vertigo, nausea and nystagmus (involuntary rapid and jerky movements of the eyeball) may appear within a few days on high dosage (3 to 4 g.), but they are mostly seen in tuberculous patients under prolonged treatment if the daily dose exceeds 1 g. A decision to continue treatment despite such symptoms means acceptance of a risk of severe deafness but may be justified by the severity of the actual disease.

Another important feature is its tendency to encourage the emergence of strains of the infecting organism which are resistant to the drug, thus leading to the failure of the treatment. For this reason it is usual to give streptomycin in association with other anti-tuberculous drugs such as para-amino-salicyclic acid.

These considerations make it essential that any course of streptomycin treatment should be expertly controlled; the drug is nevertheless an important advance in the treatment of tuberculosis.

stress. Anything which disturbs the natural balance of the body and its tissues. While the term usually means mental stress, it is perhaps useful first to consider physical stress.

Bodily health depends on the health of individual cells and they in turn need a constant internal environment ('le milieu intérieur' of Claude Bernard) provided by the tissue fluids in which they are continuously immersed. When the body is functionally over-taxed it is said to be under stress and the symptoms of such stress can be related to adverse changes in the internal environment induced by untoward or excessive physical or mental activity.

Physical over-exertion causes stress because muscular function requires adequate supplies of fuel and oxygen and rapid elimination of the resulting metabolic waste-products, e.g., carbon dioxide and water. If the elimination is insufficient for the needs of a particular situation the result is fatigue which persists until relieved by rest. To give a simple example, in running we consume more oxygen and build up carbon dioxide in the tissues faster than we can breathe it out; so immediately after running we still breathe fast to get rid of the carbon dioxide and our muscles feel tired because of the excess carbon dioxide. Within physiological limits no harm results.

Repeated physical stress tends to produce HYPERTROPHY so that a particular tissue becomes more capable of dealing with the loads imposed upon it: for instance, long distance runners tend to develop enlarged hearts by the end of their athletic careers. In some cases of prolonged and repeated physical stress there may also be trends towards accelerated degeneration and these can be compared to physiological ageing. There may also be other man-made and external factors which reinforce the effects of this accelerated degeneration. Amongst these are environmental pollution, the physical contacts which encourage infection, and sometimes new habits and new ways of life.

The influence of mental stress is more subtle. Society too has its 'milieu intérieur' which influences individuals as the tissue-fluids influence individual cells. It provides a regulating mechanism to preserve its harmonious functioning, and each individual is subject to these regulatory pressures. It prescribes codes of acceptable behaviour and it tends to discipline, persecute, or ostracize those who will not or cannot conform; alternatively it grades its members by systems of value and prestige, based on race, religion, language, occupation, or wealth, from which escape is difficult. Those who conform avoid pressures and conflict; those who rebel and those who prove inadequate are equally liable to suffer unpleasant consequences.

External social or cultural pressures, e.g., attempts by parents and teachers to induce a non-academic boy to fit himself for entry to a profession, or intolerance of the person whose religious or political views differ strongly from those of his associates, or hostility to the incomer from a different background and with different traditions and customs, all evoke primitive responses and fundamentally these represent preparation either for flight or fight.

Under these emotional drives the body liberates hormones which stimulate its capacity either to escape or conquer. These hormones come chiefly from the pituitary and adrenal glands but also include other secretions with specific 'target organs' such as the skin, stomach, colon and cardio-vascular system. Unfortunately the problems which beset the individual in an organized community can seldom be satisfactorily resolved by direct action, and the hormonal stimuli, if repeated,

eventually lead to a state of peristent reaction or over-reaction shown by symptoms of anxiety, fear, frustration, hate, anger, or rage.

Anxiety is perhaps the commonest manifestation of stress. It stems from conflict and conflict may arise from various causes: from the need to exercise a difficult choice; from unsatisfying personal relationships; from competitive standards of living which bring financial worries and may force husbands to accept promotion posts for which they are unfit or wives to undertake full-time work in addition to looking after children and house; from insecurity and dissatisfaction at work; from the isolation of young families and the loss of kinship networks in a mobile society; and from the many other complexities and perplexities of modern life.

Emotional upset of this kind may lead on to obvious disease. The end result of chronic anxiety may eventually be a neurosis, but more commonly it produces physical symptoms affecting various bodily systems. This is psychosomatic disease and a wide range of modern complaints are so determined. Headaches, insomnia, twitches, tics, skin-rashes, digestive upsets, peptic ulcers, colitis (inflammation of the colon), palpitation, high blood pressure, coronary thrombosis, dysmennorhoea (menstrual pains) and infertility are common examples, but there are many other less well-defined conditions. Repeated absence from work for apparently trivial causes may itself be a sign of such illness and may represent an appeal for help in escaping from some intolerable work situation.

Skin diseases are of particular interest in a psychosomatic context because the effects of emotions on the skin are easily observed, as in blushing in shame, pallor in fright, sweating in fear, and hair-erection and goose-flesh in apprehension and horror. Exteriorization of such emotions when experienced in excess is reflected in such conditions as pruritus (itching), urticaria (nettle-rash) and rosacea (chronic congestion of the blood capillaries leading to a lumpy red appearance of the face).

It is sometimes said that stress is largely a result of modern civilization; that in the simpler cultures of the past the peasant or artisan could work at his own pace, seldom moved away from his relatives and early associates, and had his major decisions taken for him by a possibly benevolent feudal superior, landlord or priest; in short, that stress is in large measure a consequence of emancipation, education, greater opportunity and 'progress'. This is probably an over-simplification, since the peasant of the past was subject to the stresses occasioned by the sheer difficulty of survival in years of poor harvests, together with the strains caused by living in an overcrowded, insanitary dwelling, the physical stresses created by unremitting toil and the mental stresses of constantly trying to please an overlord of often uncertain temper and little benevolence. The stresses today are different, but not necessarily greater. Anyway, even if a return to nature could remove some of the stresses of a mobile, competitive, highly mechanized and highly specialized culture, very few people would be willing to abandon such 'luxuries' as modern heating, lighting, transport and methods of communication, and fewer still would be prepared to have major decisions taken for them by a military or ecclesiastical superior.

Yet, instead of merely treating stress diseases, and often treating them very ineffectively, perhaps we should as a society be directing our attention to the reduction of needless stress. It may be, for instance, that academic education has concentrated too much on fitting children for a career, and has produced on the one hand the 'drop-out' and on the other hand the over-ambitious, over-concentrated career worker without leisure interests or healthy recreation. Perhaps, since most people work for only one third of their waking life up to the age of retirement, education should be for leisure as well as for work. Perhaps again, as machinery increasingly takes over repetitive tasks, work can be made more enjoyable and more meaningful to the persons engaged in it. Yet again, having in large measure conquered death except in extreme old age, perhaps we can use family planning facilities to prevent the continued growth of population and to give the individual (even in cities) a modicum of privacy and reasonable access to green fields and woods. Not least, perhaps we can re-establish compassion, tolerance and unselfishness as desirable qualities to some extent lost in an era of material progress.

We have to realize, however, that some stress (and its accompanying diseases) is the penalty for human advance. Without some stress we would have fewer reformers, inventors or poets.

stricture. An abnormal narrowing of any duct or passage in the body occurring as the result of disease. The usual causes are spasm, inflammation, scarring and tumour, and the commonest sites are in the oesophagus, ureters, urethra, and rectum.

Urethral stricture leads to retention of urine and is perhaps the condition most likely to occur suddenly with urgent symptoms. Cases due to spasm or inflammatory congestion can be treated by inserting a catheter to release urine from the bladder; partial stricture due to scar tissue after urethral infections such as gonorrhoea may be relieved by gradual dilation with appropriate instruments; other conditions may require surgical measures to relieve or remove obstruction.

Strictures elsewhere will generally need operative treatment eventually.

stroke. Damage to the brain, mostly occasioned by (1) bleeding from a weakened artery (cerebral haemorrhage), (2) clotting of blood in a diseased artery (cerebral thrombosis), (3) blockage of an artery by a plug of fat or mass of bacteria or bubble of air (cerebral embolism), or (4) pressure on the vessel by a tumour. Associated underlying conditions include arteriosclerosis and high blood pressure.

The onset is usually sudden in embolism and gradual in thrombosis, while in haemorrhage it may be gradual or, if the bleeding is sudden and profuse, very rapid indeed. Manifestations vary according to the amount and situation of damage but often include unconsciousness and heavy breathing.

A stroke causing only minimal brain damage may cause a few minutes of haziness and confusion, with no later symptoms, but a massive stroke may result in immediate death.

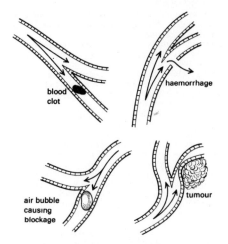

Some causes of stroke

Where the damage is serious but not fatal within the first week – the danger period in respect of death – some paralysis of the arm or leg is common; this is known as HEMIPLEGIA.

In any case of suspected stroke the patient should have restrictive clothing, such as the collar, loosened and should be placed on his side to remove the danger of his choking on his own saliva. Medical help should be summoned immediately. In serious stroke both skilled medical treatment and skilled nursing care are required and it is not possible in the early weeks to forecast how much paralysis of limbs and possible speech impairment will remain.

Prevention of stroke is largely the prevention of arteriosclerosis and high blood pressure, and essentially the same measures are desirable as are mentioned in the article on CORONARY THROMBOSIS. Additionally, since stroke often occurs during or just after violent exertion or strong emotion, persons with high blood pressure should seek to avoid these factors.

Alternative names for the condition are apoplexy and cerebrovascular incident.

stupor. A condition of extreme mental apathy in which the person does not respond at all to his surroundings. It may arise in such diseases as melancholia, schizophrenia and epilepsy, and also occasionally in hysteria. The stuporous patient makes no effort to take food or to attend to the calls of nature, so that measures like spoon-feeding may be necessary. The condition is usually transient, but where it persists for more than a few days, electro-convulsive treatment is worth considering.

stuttering. A condition, allied to STAMMERING, in which a person has difficulty with the initial word of a sentence or phrase and tends to repeat the word or the first syllable of it. The condition is sometimes caused by sudden fright or other emotional shock, and it occasionally occurs after debilitating diseases.

Stuttering in childhood is commoner in boys than girls, and in left-handed rather than right-handed people, and it is sometimes associated with homes with such disturbing factors as parental discord, jealousy or over-strictness. Probably the most important factor in treatment is the fostering of self-reliance and confidence, but in addition a good speech therapist can often help.

stye. Essentially a boil in one of the skin glands of the eyelid. It begins as a hard, painful swelling, the pain (which may appear before the swelling is visible) being caused by the formation of pus under pressure. As the stye develops a cyst filled with pus begins to protrude above the surface, and finally the cyst ruptures, releasing the pus and relieving the pain.

In some cases an early stye may be aborted by pulling out the associated eyelash. Alternatively the stye may be brought speedily to a head by application of warm, antiseptic compresses, e.g., for ten minutes every two hours. Rubbing of the eyelid is undesirable as it may cause the infection to spread.

Repeated styes within days or weeks of each other are an indication of poor general health and lowered resistance to infection.

styptics. Preparations for applying to a wound to check bleeding from a skin surface either by constricting the capillary blood vessels or by inducing clotting of blood. Alum, perchloride of iron, tannin, copper sulphate and silver nitrate are common styptics. In the absence of an available styptic, applications of cold or very hot water will often check an oozing of blood.

subacute. A term used to describe a condition intermediate between acute (which describes an incident of a sudden and severe nature) and chronic (which indicates a longstanding condition).

subarachnoid. The fluid-filled space between the middle of the three membranes lining the brain (the arachnoid) and the innermost membrane (the pia mater).

Subarachnoid haemorrhage. Bleeding into the subarachnoid space with consequent pressure on the brain; it may occur through rupture of an aneurism on one of the small cerebral arteries or through collapse of the weakened wall of one of these arteries. There are two sharply demarcated types. The apoplectic type is characterized by intense headache followed by unconsciousness, and can in some cases be differentiated from stroke only by lumbar puncture (the taking of a sample of cerebrospinal fluid, in which blood is found if the condition is a subarachnoid haemorrhage). In this type about one-third of the patients die, mostly within forty-eight hours, and most of the others make a full although often slow recovery. Where the haemorrhage is less in quantity the meningitic type occurs, with symptoms and signs rather like those of meningitis. In both types surgery may be necessary to deal with the cause of the bleeding.

subconscious. The totality of mental experience and activity operating beneath or beyond consciousness and therefore without the awareness of the person. The term is sometimes employed to include activity under the control of the autonomic nervous system and of hormonal activity, (e.g., involuntary acceleration or slowing of the heart rate or the respiratory rate) but it is generally used to cover deep-seated drives (especially sexual and aggressive) and ideas and memories that have been repressed because they are incompatible with the standards or beliefs in the conscious mind.

The deep-rooted tendencies in the subconscious often come into conflict with the standards of morality, ethics or aesthetics that an individual has acquired from his parents, teachers and associates. The repressed ideas and impulses are prevented by a psychological mechanism called the censor from reaching the conscious mind in direct form, but frequently reach it in distorted forms or by roundabout methods. Many (but not all) dreams and many mistakes in speech are explicable in terms of the emergence of items from the subconscious.

Behaviour, far from being completely rational, is to a considerable extent a compromise between acquired standards and values and impulses from the subconscious.

See also UNCONSCIOUS MIND.

subcutaneous. Under the skin. A subcutaneous injection is one given just under the skin as opposed to the more superficial intradermal injection, which raises a bleb in the skin, and the deeper intramuscular injection.

subjective. Noticed only by the person concerned, in contrast with 'objective'. In general a symptom is subjective while a sign is observed by others.

sublimation. The process whereby prohibited or repressed tendencies, especially sexual and other biological energies, are diverted into channels that are permissible, realizable and socially constructive or creative. For instance, the unmarried woman who has a strong maternal instinct may sublimate by diverting her desire to care for a child of her own into the acceptable channel of working in a children's nursery, or may lavish on a pet animal the affection really intended for a non-existent child. Similarly a man who has a very strong power-drive but cannot gain a top-ranking post in his profession or business may sublimate by becoming the dominant figure in a particular social, political or religious organization.

Sublimation is an important psychological mechanism and its successful employment prevents much misery. Like any other mechanism, however, it can be misused. The man who would badly like to hit his boss but instead beats his children for trivial misdemeanours is sublimating in an unfortunate way, as is the man who compensates for a feeling of inferiority by heavy consumption of alcohol. Conversely, the man with similar feelings of aggression who names a golf ball after his employer and then drives it round the golf course is getting rid of his impulse without harming anybody; and some Japanese firms even make effigies of the manager available, so that an employee who feels aggrieved can strike the effigy.

subliminal. A sensation too slight or transient to be consciously perceived. Such a sensation may enter the subconscious and so may subsequently affect behaviour.

subluxation. Partial dislocation of the bones of a joint without separation being complete. Probably the commonest example is subluxation of the head of the radius (one of the two long bones of the forearm), following a sudden wrench to the elbow, especially of a child; the head of the radius is pulled forward, and the elbow is very painful and the forearm useless until the bone has been restored to its natural position.

subphrenic. Below the diaphragm. A subphrenic abscess is an abscess in the space between the diaphragm and the upper part of the liver. It occurs most commonly as a complication of gastric ulcer or other disease of the stomach; it is characterized by pain and high temperature, and is both hard to diagnose and difficult to treat.

suckling. The term used for BREAST-FEEDING a baby.

sudden death. Death, sudden or otherwise, is signified by cessation both of breathing and of blood circulation, with consequent total cessation of the activity of the brain. Breathing alone can stop for a number of minutes and be restored by artificial respiration, and the heart can stop for several minutes and be restarted by cardiac massage or electrical stimulation.

The commonest causes of sudden death are coronary thrombosis, strokes and accidents. In the last of these the cause of death is, of course, very obvious.

Where a person dies in Britain without having been treated by a doctor within the previous fourteen days, or where the doctor involved is not satisfied as to the cause of death, certain legal formalities are required and in circumstances of suspicion or uncertainty a post mortem may be demanded.

suffocation. Unconsciousness or death resulting from lack of air to breathe or blockage of the respiratory passages. See ASPHYXIA.

suicide. The intentional taking of a person's own life. The recorded incidence of suicide, the methods used and the occupational and age groups mainly involved vary considerably from country to country and from year to year. Broadly, recorded suicides are commoner in highly developed countries (with Sweden particularly high) than in developing countries; in some advanced countries they account for something like one in every fifty deaths of adult males and one in every hundred deaths of adult females. They tend to be commonest at around 55 to 60 years of age, although not uncommon around the ages of 18 to 30. In general, recorded suicide is most frequent in people whose occupations involve strain, responsibility or overwork, or whose occupations make the persons accustomed to violence, or whose occupations provide ready access to easy means of suicide. In at least some countries chemists, doctors, publicans, lawyers, butchers and soldiers have in proportion to their total numbers considerably more cases of recorded suicide than have clergymen, teachers, civil servants and gardeners. Methods vary greatly, e.g., coal gas poisoning is popular in countries in which the gas contains poisonous carbon monoxide; doctors, nurses and chemists who contemplate suicide usually think of drugs; soldiers tend to think of shooting themselves; and persons living near the sea consider drowning.

Figures for recorded suicides are probably not particularly accurate. In the first place, an unknown but perhaps considerable number of suicides, especially at the upper end of life, are certified as having died from natural causes: if a person has been suffering from an incurable and painful disease, and if the attending doctor finds that he had died earlier than had been expected and mildly wonders whether the patient has contrived to take an overdose of pain-killing drugs, there is clearly a likelihood that the doctor will simply certify the death as due to the disease, rather than distress the bereaved relatives by refusing to certify and demanding a post mortem examination. Secondly, an intelligent person can sometimes make a suicide appear like an accident: for instance, his gun appears to have gone off while he was cleaning it. Thirdly, there occur quite a number of unintentional suicides; e.g., in order to call attention to his distress and need for help in a dramatic way a person jumps into the sea with every intention of being rescued or, failing a rescuer, of regaining the shore by his own efforts, but no rescuer appears, the current is stronger than he had realized, and he drowns.

Some psychologists have attempted to link suicide with the extreme end of the spectrum of masochistic inclinations, and to talk of the turning of sadistic aggression upon the self.

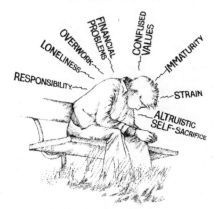

Some causes of suicide

While there may be some truth in these statements, it is perhaps wiser for the present to stick to the long-standing classification of Durkheim. As early as 1897 he divided deliberate self-destruction into three forms which he designated altruistic, egotistic and anomic.

Altruistic suicide, where the person places a higher value on the maintenance of society than on the preservation of his own life, is rare in Europe and North America. Examples are the suicide of Japanese officers after defeat or capture, and the formerly common custom of suttee in which Hindu widows threw themselves on their husbands' funeral pyres.

Egotistical suicide, generally to punish relatives or associates for some real or imaginary injury, is probably commoner than is often appreciated. It clearly implies immaturity or defect of personality and is probably the form of self-destruction that has led to suicide being associated with the phrase 'being of unsound mind'.

Undoubtedly, however, the common variety of suicide is the anomic type, with anomie defined as a state of confusion of values and lack of social cohesion. It is because this type vastly outnumbers the other types that the proportion of suicides to the total population of a community is to some extent an indication of the degree of stress and the amount of social breakdown. To give two examples: despite the worries, fears and dangers of a war the number of suicides often fall during a war, when people tend to collaborate and experience a sense of common purpose; conversely, there are more suicides in periods of heavy unemployment and financial stringency.

Suicides of anomic type are proportionately commoner in single, divorced and widowed persons than in the married, in persons in solitary occupations than in those working closely with others, and in immigrants (whether from overseas or from distant parts of the same country) than in persons with firm roots in a neighbourhood.

The general pattern of anomic suicide is fairly clear – a decision to end things, fostered by loneliness, unwantedness and confused values, with often the moral and social standards of the suicide's upbringing clashing with those of the community in which he has been living. Many statements about suicides are, however, largely unproved. For instance, it is often alleged that there are more suicides among Protestants than among Catholics, but for Catholics certification of death as suicide raises problems of sanctified burial and these problems may well influence certifying doctors in cases that are not absolutely clear-cut. Similarly, statements about social class differences in suicide rates disregard the greater opportunities of the intelligent, the educated and the affluent of making a self-destruction appear a natural death.

Prevention of altruistic and egotistic suicide is clearly very difficult and involves long-term alteration of the whole attitudes and system of values of the person. Prevention of anomic suicide is not easy, although companionship and acceptance reduce its likelihood.

Unsuccessful attempts at suicide are many times commoner than successful attempts and are probabably in many cases never intended to succeed but are essentially a desperate cry for help. Obviously any unsuccessful attempt at self-destruction warrants full investigation of the person's background and problems to ascertain whether there is any acceptable way of giving him the help that he needs.

While on general principles dangerous drugs should be kept under strict control, a great deal that is said about their use in suicidal attempts is of highly doubtful value. In the few cases where the attempt is sudden and unpremeditated it may be facilitated by the availability of a particular drug, but in most cases the attempt is not the result of sudden impulse. In general to lock away hypnotics and sedatives without tackling the basic problem leading to suicidal impulses is merely to compel the intending suicide to substitute drowning or cutting of his wrists for what might have been an easier form of death.

sulphonamides. A group of drugs that prevent the multiplication of bacteria and so enable the defence mechanisms of the body to destroy the invading organisms.

In 1932 Domagk showed that a red dye, prontosil rubrum, controlled certain infections. By 1936 there was considerable experimental use of the active constituent of prontosil, sulphanilamide. Various modifications followed, and these rendered curable many infections of former high fatality, and until the advent of penicillin and other antibiotics they dominated the treatment of infections caused by bacteria. Since some bacteria have now acquired a resistance to several antibiotics, the sulphonamides are still of the highest importance.

With sulphonamides as with antibiotics correct dosage is important. Excessive dosage is liable to produce toxic side-effects. Insufficient dosage or too early cessation may create organisms that have acquired a resistance or immunity to the particular medicament.

Sulphanilamide. Now used mainly as a dusting powder for wounds or burns, often in combination with penicillin powder.

Sulphapyridine. The original M&B 693 which, for example, reduced the mortality of cerebrospinal meningitis from 30 per cent to under 3 per cent; it is now little used because of its tendency to cause rashes and gastric disorders.

Sulphathiazole. At present usually deemed the drug of choice for most serious bacterial infections in which sulphonamides are for any reason considered preferable to antibiotics.

Sulphamezathine. An alternative with remarkably few toxic or side effects.

For most infections soluble sulphonamides are needed, as above, but for bacterial infections of the gastro-intestinal tract (such as bacterial dysentery) what is needed is a sulphonamide that is not easily absorbed. Here sulphaguanidine and sulphasuxidine are the sulphonamides of choice.

The sulphonamides are not effective in diseases caused by viruses.

sunbathing. Attempts to improve health or acquire bronzing by exposure to the sun's rays.

In any such efforts gradualness is the key to success, with initial exposures of only five or six minutes, with the eyes protected by dark glasses, and preferably with the exposures in the morning or evening when the rays are not at full intensity. Injudicious exposure can cause painful SUNBURN and even sunstroke. The danger is particularly acute where a person goes on holiday to a warmer and sunnier climate and, ignoring the change from his normal surroundings, exposes himself to the direct rays of the sun.

sunburn. The painful reddening and ultimate peeling of the skin that results from excessive exposure to bright sunshine. Very fair persons are abnormally sensitive to sunshine, as are victims of some diseases (e.g., porphyria) and persons taking some of the sulphonamide drugs.

Prevention of sunburn is essentially by avoidance of exposure, and this may include skin protection by long sleeves and a broad hat, as well as the use of various creams and lotions as well as caution in SUNBATHING. Where the skin is red and sore, cooling lotions such as calamine and witch hazel are useful. Where there is in addition weakness and giddiness, with feeble and rapid pulse and hot, dry skin, the patient requires treatment for HEAT STROKE.

In tropical climates repeated sunburn with peeling of the skin often leads to wrinkling and sometimes leads to skin cancer.

sunlight treatment. Since vitamin D is produced by activation of ergosterol in the skin by the ultra-violet rays of the sun, sunlight is obviously of value in preventing rickets in children whose diets are low in that vitamin. In general, a moderate amount of sunshine is certainly invigorating, has some general tonic effects and produces psychological benefits, although a graduated increase of exposure to sunshine is essential to avoid sunburn.

Many experts, however, are now a little sceptical about the value of sending a patient with such a condition as tuberculosis of the bones or joints to a sunny and dust-free atmosphere (such as the High Alps) and even more sceptical about the merits of sunlight lamps which produce ULTRA-VIOLET RADIATION in the privacy of the patient's home. Certainly both natural and artificial sunlight treatment (or heliotherapy) have their place in the prevention and treatment of some diseases, but their role was grossly exaggerated in the early decades of this century, and there is a salutory lesson in the saying, 'Mad dogs and Englishmen walk out in the midday sun'.

sunstroke. See HEAT STROKE.

superego. The portion of the unconscious mind which acts as a censor, preventing repressed ideas and impulses from rising from the unconscious (the id) into consciousness (the ego). There are clearly very close connections between what the psychoanalysts term the superego and what religious persons call conscience.

superinfection. A second infection by a different germ arising during the course of an initial infection. For example, smallpox is caused by a virus but most of its complications are caused by bacterial superinfection.

In any severe infection the bodily resistance is weakened so that 'the soil is ripe' for invasion by another organism; and, while the particular antibiotic or sulphonamide employed for the first infection is presumably of known effectiveness against the initial germ, the second invader may well be resistant to it.

Where fever and other symptoms recur, after having begun to respond to treatment, it is often useful to check – by sending appropriate specimens for laboratory investigation – that there has not been a secondary infection requiring a different treatment.

suppository. A cone-shaped mass, usually made of cocoa-butter or gelatin or glycerine, which is used for the introduction of drugs into the rectum. A suppository is solid at room temperature but melts at body temperature, liberating the contained drug. A suppository may be used (1) to initiate action of the bowels in constipation, (2) to allay the inflammation and congestion of internal piles, (3) to reduce pain in any disease of the rectum, or (4) to get a drug into the circulation.

To introduce the suppository it is placed with the pointed end nearest the anus and gently propelled forwards with a screwing movement of the finger. It must be pushed inwards beyond the sphincter muscle, because otherwise it will not be retained.

suppuration. The formation of PUS.

suprarenal glands. Otherwise known as adrenal glands, and lying on the top of each kidney, these are very important members of the system of ENDOCRINE GLANDS.

surgery. The treatment of injuries, diseases or deformities by manual operation or instrumental appliances.

While surgery is essentially the last medical resort, and an admission that both prevention and medical treatment have failed, it has an ancient and honourable history. A papyrus of around 1600 B.C. describes the splinting of fractures, the replacement of dislocated joints, the drainage of abscesses and the need to stitch clean wounds and leave contaminated wounds to drain. Hippocrates (400 B.C.) discusses in detail many aspects of surgery from the treatment of head wounds to that of piles. Surgery made some progress in Roman times but – unlike medicine – developed little in the Persian-Arab civilization.

In the Middle Ages most of the physicians (generally priests) declined to soil their hands, and surgery passed more and more into the hands of barbers – hence the red-and-white pole, suggesting blood-letting and bandaging, found outside hairdresser's shops; hence, too, the tradition that a surgeon in Britain, although always a qualified doctor, is addressed as 'Mister'.

In the eighteenth and nineteenth centuries surgery came back within the fold of medicine, and the successive discoveries of anaesthetics, antisepsis and asepsis rendered the period 1850-1940 the supreme age of surgery. Before the introduction of anaesthetics any operation lasting for more than a few minutes was impossible because of the amount of pain, and before the era of antisepsis and then asepsis any surgical operation was highly dangerous.

During the last half century advances in prevention, exemplified by vitamins and vaccines, and advances in medical treatment, exemplified by sulphonamides and antibiotics, have perhaps gradually removed the pre-eminence of surgery; but brain operations that would have been unthinkable thirty years ago, kidney transplants and even heart transplants are among the many indications that surgery is still advancing.

surveillance. A watch kept over a person regarded as liable to develop a particular infection.

Under the formerly common system of quarantine, persons who had been in contact with a case of serious infection were required to remain isolated in their homes for slightly longer than the incubation period of the disease. That measure checked the spread of diseases transmitted from person to person, but where the contacts were numerous it could damage the entire life and productive work of a community. Furthermore, in the cases of diseases of long incubation periods it served little purpose in the earlier part of these periods since the contacts – whether in the process of developing the disease or not – would not yet be infective.

Quarantine is increasingly being replaced by surveillance. Under this system the persons regarded as contacts remain at work, or in the case of children remain at school, but are inspected daily by doctors or health visitors and are excluded from work or school if any symptoms or signs of the disease appear. Essentially surveillance depends for its success on the idea that a particular infection can be identified just before the person becomes infectious. There are inevitably some diseases for which surveillance is not applicable, and where applicable the system depends entirely on the expertise of the inspecting doctor or health visitor. The saving to the community is, however, enormous: under the quarantine system a hundred contacts might be kept off

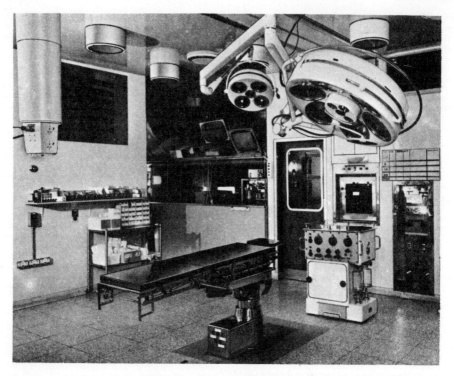

Surgery: a modern operating theatre

work for a fortnight (losing the community the equivalent of four years of a man's work) and then one might develop the disease; under the surveillance system the hundred remain at work and about the thirteenth day perhaps two are excluded – the man who is developing the disease and another who has symptoms warranting momentary suspicion.

suture. The drawing together of two sides of a wound by stitches or clamps. The term is also used for the stitches so employed. Cotton and linen stitches, used for centuries, have nowadays been largely replaced by silk thread, nylon thread, catgut and metal clamps. Catgut has the advantage that it is ultimately broken down in the tissues and absorbed, whereas other stitches have to be removed after the wound has healed sufficiently, in most cases after about a week.

Suturing promotes rapid healing and helps to prevent the formation of unsightly or disfiguring scars. In general it is needed whenever a wound is too large to heal readily by itself.

swab. Essentially a solid stick with cotton wool, gauze or cloth wrapped round one end. Swabs are employed (1) to clean out natural cavities, such as the ear or nostril; (2) to clean wounds, e.g., to mop away blood or pus during an operation; and (3) to obtain samples for bacteriological examination, as in swabbing the throat of a person suspected of early diphtheria or tonsillitis. In major operations, especially on the abdomen, it is standard procedure that all swabs used are counted so as to ensure, before the wound is closed, that they have all been removed.

swallowing. The passage of food from the mouth to the stomach.

One cannot simultaneously breathe and swallow, because in the act of swallowing the epiglottis blocks off the respiratory channel to prevent food from entering the trachea. Thereafter involuntary contractions of the pharynx and oesophagus force the food downwards towards the stomach.

If the epiglottis fails to perform properly its function of sealing off the trachea, as can happen when a person tries to talk or breathe with food in his throat, there is danger of a particle of food passing into the respiratory tract and causing choking.

swallowing difficulty. Difficulty in swallowing may arise (1) in a baby as a result of congenital defects such as a cleft palate; (2) from any painful or inflammatory condition of the throat such as quinsy; (3) from paralysis of the muscles concerned in swallowing, as in certain organic nervous diseases; (4) from pressure of a tumour in the vicinity of the throat; and (5) in hysteria. Where the difficulty persists for more than a few hours medical investigation is desirable. Treatment varies with the cause.

sweat. The salty liquid secreted by the sebaceous glands in the skin. The evaporation of sweat from the surface of the body takes up a great deal of heat and is therefore an important factor in regulating the body temperature. In a reasonably dry atmosphere sweating and evaporation of sweat occur easily after exercise or if the surrounding air is warm, although there is great individual difference in the amount of exercise or degree of warmth that produces any specific quantity of sweat. In a humid atmosphere where the air is already almost saturated with water vapour, the evaporation of sweat is virtually impossible; hence exercise to a degree that is endurable and even pleasant in a hot dry climate is intolerable and even dangerous in an equally warm but humid atmosphere.

Apart from its role in regulating temperature sweat is also an important source of excretion of waste matter from the body.

Sweating and perspiration had originally the same meaning, but some modern writers try to use 'sweating' for the visible process in which beads of moisture appear on the skin, and to restrict 'perspiration' to the invisible secretion and evaporation of much smaller quantities of liquid.

sycosis. See BARBER'S RASH.

Sydenham's chorea. See CHOREA.

sympathectomy. The operation of cutting over-active nerves of the sympathetic nervous system to prevent the effects of their activity, e.g., to avoid constriction of a particular artery.

In most cases it is possible to block the nerve temporarily with a local anaesthetic, and so to verify before the operation that surgery will be likely to have the anticipated effects.

sympathetic nervous system. One of the two branches of the autonomic or involuntary NERVOUS SYSTEM (the other being the para-sympathetic) which operate below the level of consciousness and control many bodily activities. The sympathetic nervous system consists of a right and a left trunk which extend from below the base of the skull to the inner surface of the coccyx; many small branches including branches which communicate with all of the spinal nerves; and several plexuses of many communicating branches, of which the most important are the coeliac or solar plexus in the abdomen, the superficial and deep cardiac plexuses and the hypogastric plexus on the sacrum.

Sympatholytic drugs, such as tolazoline or propanolol, inhibit some or all of the activities of the sympathetic nervous system.

symptom. A manifestation of disease or disorder noticed by the patient or prospective patient, e.g., pain, swelling, cough, abnormal sweating, itching, backache, fatigue or irritability. Although the difference is a very fine one, the symptoms reported by the patient are normally differentiated from signs, i.e., things noted by the doctor or other health worker. The distinction is made because the patient according to his temperament may exaggerate or minimize his symptoms, or even fake them to secure an excuse for being off work or to gain compensation for a non-existent injury, whereas the signs are noted by an impartial and skilled observer. Yet many manifestations of illness can be both symptoms and signs. Nose bleeding, high colour, pallor and breathlessness on exertion are examples.

A symptom, especially pain, is what usually induces a person to seek medical help. However, one of the tragedies of existence is that symptoms develop after – and in consequence of – pathological changes which may be irreversible. Thus the person in the

early stage of pulmonary tuberculosis may look and feel heathy: the characteristic cough, night sweats and loss of weight do not appear until the disease is well-developed in the lung. The first symptons of duodenal ulcer appear after the mucous membrane has been so eroded as to produce a definite patch of ulceration. Cancer in almost any part of the body may be symptomless until the tumour has not only grown to an appreciable size but has started to cause secondary growths elsewhere. The first evidence of disorder of the coronary arteries may be sudden death from coronary thrombosis.

There are hundreds of different symptoms. To mention a few examples, symptoms probably related to the head include the various types of headache, dizziness, fainting, sleep disturbances, skin disease of the scalp, various types of baldness, changes in the colour and texture of the hair, and so on. There is no simple classification, and a single symptom may be produced by any one of several disorders. Even the organ affected may not be directly indicated by the symptom, e.g., pain over the heart in a young person is more often than not caused by a disorder of the stomach, coughing may be evidence of wax in the ear, and pain in the leg may be a manifestation of a damaged intervertebral disc. So a doctor before attempting to make a diagnosis has usually to consider not merely the particular symptom of which the patient is complaining but also all the other symptoms and signs that are present.

Until the twentieth century the whole system of medical care was normally based on the appearance of symptoms which induced the sufferer to make a layman's diagnosis of illness and consult a doctor. Nowadays opinion in the health professions increasingly recognizes that intervention merely in a crisis is unsatisfactory, and favours paying substantially more attention to preventive measures. (1) Health education, in an effort to maintain and improve physical and emotional health, seeks to create habits and attitudes compatible with good health. (2) Prevention of disease may be achieved by several means, either specific prevention such as immunization against various infections or presumptive prevention such as avoiding the main causes of child mal-adjustment or of postural defects. (3) Health screening in advance of any symptoms, as in the periodical medical examination of pre-school and school children, is most rewarding. Attention to health education, disease prevention and health screening has already greatly improved the physical and mental health of persons in the first two decades of life, but most adults still have no contact with the health services until they themselves initiate that contact after symptoms have appeared.

syncope. Temporary loss of consciousness through deficient blood supply to the brain. The term is synonymous with FAINTING.

syndrome. A group of signs and symptoms which are together characteristic of a particular disease and have been given a specific name, generally that of the person who first described them. For instance, the Stokes-Adams syndrome of unusually slow pulse (10 to 20 per minute) and sudden loss of consciousness for a few seconds, followed by a period of stertorous breathing, is characteristic of a particular form of degenerative heart disease.

The recognition of a syndrome can be of great value for accurate early disgnosis. Thus in the example just given, consideration of any of the symptoms by itself would ultimately lead to examination of the heart, probably by an electrocardiograph, and in due course the making of the correct diagnosis, but the existence of the syndrome enables the doctor to make that diagnosis immediately.

synergy. Co-operative or reinforcing action, as when two or more nerves or muscles work together. An example is the movements of forefinger and thumb to grasp an object. The term is also used for two drugs that reinforce each other.

synovitis. Inflammation of the lining membrane of a joint cavity. Causes include infection following wounds or injuries and also transmission of germs from other parts of the body. Symptoms include pain, reddening and swelling, and the joint is usually kept bent. Rest and hot fomentations help, but sulphonamides or antibiotics are often required.

syphilis. A dangerous venereal disease of slow development, caused by a spirochaete, the thread-like *Treponema pallidum.*

A disease confined to human beings, it was unknown in the Old World until 1493 when it was introduced into Spain by Columbus's crew who had been infected in Haiti. Thereafter the disease – the 'pox' of the Elizabethans – spread rapidly throughout the world, causing enormous amount of illness and suffering. The condition was first fully described not by a doctor but by a poet, Fracastorius, in 1536. The causal organism was identified in 1905 and the first effective treatment was introduced in 1910.

Transmission occurs in four ways: (1) during sexual intercourse with an infected person, not only the commonest way, but the way in about 99 per cent of cases; (2) from mother to unborn child via the placenta (see congenital syphilis below); (3) very rarely from kissing a person with a syphilitic lesion on the mouth or by contact with very recent and still moist discharges from an infected person, as in the communal use of drinking cups; and (4) even more rarely from infection of an unnoticed scratch on the hand when treating a patient – an occupational hazard of doctors and nurses.

The incubation period is one to six weeks. Thereafter the disease may be conveniently divided into three stages.

The primary stage is characterized by the appearance of a hard, painless, red papule at the site of infection - usually the foreskin or glans penis in the male and the labia in the female. The papule enlarges to the size of a pea and then breaks down to form an ulcer with sharply cut edges and a hard base, while the adjacent lymph glands become enlarged and 'shotty'. At this stage diagnosis can usually be confirmed by the Wassermann test of blood, and the disease is fairly easily cured, but because of the absence of pain the victim may not seek treatment and may not even know that he has the disease.

The second stage, in six to twelve weeks, is characterized by general symptoms indicating the presence of spirochaetes in the bloodstream – mild feverishness, lassitude, headache and a non-itchy rash which can be mistaken for various skin diseases. Where the skin is moist,

raised patches, called condylomata, may appear with a highly infective discharge. The Wassermann test, if made, is always positive and the disease is still easily curable, but the condition may be missed and the stage subsides without treatment although infection still lurks.

In untreated or inadequately treated cases the third stage may appear between five and twenty years later. It may take various forms – the appearance of a gumma, a chronic abscess which causes symptoms by compressing healthy tissue; an attack on the blood-vessels, causing, for instance, aortic aneurysm (a bulge in the wall of the main artery of the body) which may be fatal; and in particular two different diseases of the central nervous system. Of these, tabes dorsalis (or locomotor ataxia) is characterized by loss of the reflexes that co-ordinate voluntary movement, curious stamping gait, sudden intense stabbing pains in the legs, and impairment of bladder control. Antisyphilitic treatment, analgesics and special exercises all help but the outlook is not very good. The other syphilitic disease of the nervous system, general paralysis of the insane, shows itself successively in gradual deterioration of the personality with increasing loss of emotional control and increasing lack of concentration, delusions of grandeur, and finally paralysis and complete absence of mental activity. Heavy dosage of penicillin can arrest the disease but little or nothing can be done to remove such mental deterioration as has already occurred.

Until 1910, when Ehrlich discovered arsphenamine, syphilis was incurable. Arsenical treatment (arsphenamine and neoarsphenamine) helped as did mercurial treatment, but these have now been replaced by treatment with penicillin and other antibiotics. With adequate dosage of penicillin syphilis is definitely curable in the first and second stages; and in consequence of early diagnosis and efficient treatment tertiary syphilis has now become an extreme rarity.

Prevention of syphilis is inevitably linked with reduction of promiscuity. The non-promiscuous couple, whether married or unmarried, clearly run no risk of the disease; if one of that couple acquires the disease through an act of promiscuity – perhaps during a prolonged absence of the normal partner – only two people are likely to become infected, and if the disease is identified in one the treatment of both is a virtual certainty; but in casual promiscuity or prostitution one infected person may infect many partners. Preventive measures include health education (including sex education and education both about the avoidance of syphilis and about recognition of the primary sore); moral education (to reduce casual sexual relationships); advice about the use of condoms, which afford a partial protection, and about chemicals for use after intercourse; provision of facilities for healthy recreation (to reduce the likehood of casual sexual encounters); efficient contact tracing (very difficult where the couple have met on the street or in a public house and do not even know each other's names); and registration and periodical medical examination of prostitutes.

It should be recognized, however, that promiscuity – of which syphilis and other venereal diseases are a consequence – is fostered by several features of modern life,

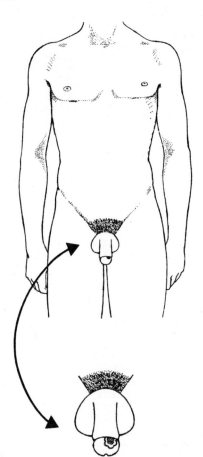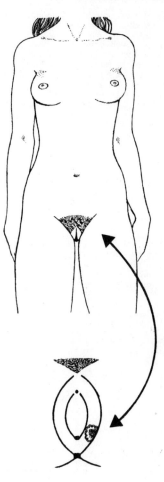

The primary stage of syphilis

such as longer financial dependence so that physical maturity is reached long before matrimony is economically possible, separation of young men from their homes and families (e.g., soldiers in a foreign country), and surplus wealth in any susceptible group (e.g., sailors receiving pay after a long voyage).

Congenital syphilis. Where the mother has uncured secondary syphilis, transmission of infection to unborn children through the placenta is highly probable. In congenital syphilis the disease is found in many internal organs, and in many cases the child dies in the uterus. Indeed the classical picture in a syphilitic mother is a series of pregnancies resulting successively in early miscarriage, later miscarriage, still birth, a living child with syphilis and a healthy living child. Although that is an average picture the variation is great: there are even cases on record of one twin being born with typical syphilis and the other being born healthy.

In a surviving syphilitic child common manifestations include emaciation and sallow complexion, 'snuffles' (a syphilitic inflammation of the lining of the nose), 'saddle-nose' (from destruction of the nasal bones) and 'bossing' (a heaping up of spongy bone on parts of the skull), while affections of the eyes and ears are not uncommmon.

Apart from prevention of infection of the mother by measures to reduce syphilis, prevention is by adequate and timely treatment of the mother. Where a child is found to have congenital syphilis, penicillin treatment is usually effective if given early.

syringe. An instrument, consisting of a hollow barrel, a plunger and a hollow needle, which is used for injecting fluid into a muscle, vein or body cavity, or for drawing off a sample of blood or cerebrospinal fluid. Formerly syringes were made of glass and required very careful sterilization, but nowadays disposable syringes are normally employed; these are used once and then discarded.

syringomyelia. A chronic disease in which irregular cavities develop in the spinal cord and brain stem. The condition is almost certainly congenital but symptoms do not appear until late childhood or early adult life. The characteristic early feature is a loss of sensation, so that the hands often have several painless cuts or burns, and on examination portions of the body are found unable to detect pain or heat, although they can still appreciate touch and vibration. Later there is some atrophy of muscles, especially of the arms, and sometimes a thickening and brittleness of the bones.

Progress of the disease is very slow, with sometimes long periods in which the condition becomes no worse; but as yet no useful treatment or means of prevention has been discovered.

systole. The rhythmic contraction of the muscle of the heart which normally occurs about sixty to eighty times per minute and has the effect of pumping blood into the arteries. The converse phase of relaxation in which blood flows into the heart from the veins is termed diastole.

T

TAB. A combined vaccine used against typhoid and the two common types of paratyphoid, A and B. If given several weeks before the person is at risk, i.e., early enough to permit of the development of immunity, it gives a reasonable protection for at least a year. If given to persons at immediate risk, e.g., in an outbreak where they have consumed the same food or drink as the early cases and are therefore in the position either of incubating the disease or of having escaped, it is useless and indeed, by invalidating the Widal test, makes the diagnosis of cases appreciably more difficult.

In a highly developed country with good standards of hygiene TAB is rarely necessary, but in unhygienic conditions and particularly in the potential disruption caused by war it can be of enormous value. Few experts in Britain, Scandinavia or the U.S.A. would deem the introduction of TAB comparable with that of smallpox vaccination or diphtheria immunization or sulphonamide or antibiotic treatment. Yet a South American physician in a book on *The British Contribution to Medicine* gives the place of honour to Sir Almroth Wright who developed a typhoid vaccine in 1896 and was largely responsible for the introduction of TAB in 1916.

tabes. Any disease involving wasting of tissue. The term, however, is nowadays virtually restricted to tabes dorsalis, a degenerative condition of the spinal cord that occurs in advanced stages of untreated or inadequately treated syphilis.

tachycardia. Unduly rapid beating of the heart. It occurs as a normal event after considerable exertion and in emotional excitement, but may also be a sign of hyperthyroidism or of disease of the heart. To set a borderline is difficult because the normal heart rate at rest varies from about sixty to about eighty beats per minute, but broadly a rate in excess of eighty-eight, occurring more than five minutes after the end of exercise or the occurrence of emotional excitement, can be termed tachycardia.

Paroxysmal tachycardia, in which the heart suddenly starts to beat at perhaps twice its normal rate and equally suddenly reverts to its normal speed, is usually indicative either of hyperthyroidism or of heart disease (especially mitral stenosis). The state may, however, be precipitated by excessive exertion, strong emotion, heavy smoking or heavy consumption of tea, coffee or alcohol. Reassurance is essential because the patient, especially in a first attack, tends to be very anxious, but attacks nearly always end spontaneously without doing much harm. Drinking iced water sometimes ends an attack as does massage of the heart. If the attack continues, quinidine (300 mg.) and a sedative are useful.

taenia. Certain species of TAPEWORM. Care should be taken to distinguish *Taenia* from *Tinea,* which is the scientific name for RINGWORM.

talipes. See CLUB FOOT.

talus. Formerly called the astralagus. One of the seven bones of the foot. With the lower ends of the tibia and fibula it forms the ankle joint.

tapeworms. Intestinal parasitic worms, each consisting of a head, neck and many segments.

Less frequently encountered are the *Bothriocephalus latus* of Central Europe, which enters man through the eating of infested fish, and the *Echinococcus granulosis* or dog tapeworm, which causes hydatid cysts in man.

The common tapeworms are *Taenia saginata,* (the beef tapeworm) and *Taenia solium* (the tapeworm of pork). In the former case the patient usually becomes aware of the infestation only by seeing segments of the worm in his faeces, although in time he begins to lose weight and to have vague ill health. The eggs are normally discharged in the faeces and form cysts in the tissues of animals that swallow the larvae but not as a rule in man. In the case of *Taenia solium* the larvae are liberated within the human body and cysts – cysterci – may form in any muscle or organ, causing symptoms which depend on the site.

Prevention is by adequate inspection of meat and pork and by proper cooking of these foods.

tarsus. The base of the foot. It consists of seven bones with a covering of compact tissue. Nearest the leg are the talus and the calcaneus; intermediate is the navicular; and nearest the toes are the three cuneiform bones and the cuboid. These seven bones support the weight of the body in standing and walking.

taste. The sensation of taste depends on tiny elevations of skin in the tongue, palate and epiglottis, each containing a taste-bud; this is a

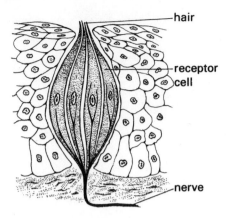

A taste-bud

cluster of spindle-shaped cells from which nerve fibres pass to the facial and glossopharyngeal nerves. The taste-buds detect only four tastes: sweet, perceived best by buds at the tip of the tongue; sour, appreciated best by buds at the sides of the tongue; bitter, identified by buds at the back of the tongue; and salt, for which the buds are more widespread but are largely near the tip and sides of the tongue. Solids are not tasted until at least partially dissolved by saliva.

The finer distinctions of taste are really dependent on the sense of smell. Hence the apparent blunting of taste when the sense of smell is impaired, as by a cold in the head.

tattooing. Pricking indelible pigments into the skin to form words or pictures. Tattooing is much favoured by older adolescents and young adult males, who are sometimes embarrassed later by, for example, an arm branded with the name of a girl who is now only vaguely recalled as the subject of a long past and only temporary infatuation. Removal of tattoo marks is difficult and usually requires minor surgery.

While not illegal in Britain, although prohibited in some countries, it is frowned on by doctors and other health workers because an inadequately sterilized needle can transmit serum hepatitis or occasionally syphilis. In this connection it should be remembered that qualified doctors found the sterilization of syringes and needles both difficult and time-consuming, and gladly began to use disposable ones when these became available. Moreover, the virus of serum hepatitis can be transmitted to the tattooing pigment from an infected person undergoing tattooing, so that, even if a fresh needle is used, the next person tattooed may be at risk.

Tay-Sachs disease. See AMAUROTIC FAMILY IDIOCY.

teenager. A person whose age is over 12 and under 20 years. The term is seldom used for persons of 18 or 19 years but commonly employed for youngsters of 13 to 17 – the difficult phase in which they are in some respects regarded as responsible young adults

and in other respects treated as dependent children. See ADOLESCENCE.

teeth. Every person develops two sets of teeth during life.

The twenty temporary, deciduous or milk teeth consist in each jaw of four central, chizel-shaped incisors for biting food, two conical canines on each side of the incisors for tearing food, and, further back, four cuspid-shaped molars for grinding. The temporary teeth begin to erupt at 6 to 9 months, a lower central incisor being usually the first to appear, and dentition is complete by about 2½ years.

The thirty-two permanent teeth consist of four incisors, two canines, four premolars and six molars. The first molars begin to emerge, further back than the temporary teeth, at about six years and thereafter the temporary teeth are gradually – and usually painlessly – pushed out by their successors. Dentition is usually completed by 14 to 15 years, except for the third molars (wisdom teeth) which appear around 17 to 25 years.

A tooth consists primarily of the hollow interior or pulp, soft connective tissue containing a mass of blood vessels and nerves, and a thick outer shell of dentine (or ivory), a hard cellular substance. On the outside the dentine is lined with enamel, an even harder non-cellular material on the exposed surface or crown, and with bony cement at the root.

Tooth development is impaired by deficiency of any of the following: calcium, vitamin C, vitamin D, fluorine, and manganese and other trace elements. Since teeth begin to develop before birth, although not erupting till long afterwards, these deficiencies are also important in the expectant mother.

Disorders of the teeth. Dental decay (caries) is the commonest cause of toothache. The bacteria normally present in the mouth produce enzymes which act on starches and sugars, both creating acid and forming a 'plaque' of debris on the surface of the tooth. The acid, kept in contact with the tooth by the plaque, gradually destroys the enamel and dentine of the tooth.

For the most part it can be prevented by

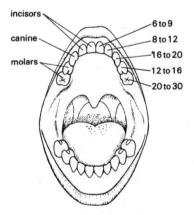

Milk teeth, showing the age, in months, when they usually appear

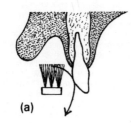

(a)

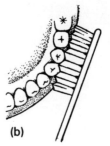

(b)

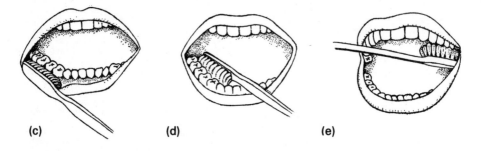

(c)   (d)   (e)

When cleaning the teeth the brush should be swept down from the gums (a) so that the bristle-heads clean between the teeth (b). There are three movements required: on the outside (c), the inside (d), and the tops (e) of the teeth

careful dental hygiene. Where unprevented it leads to the formation of a cavity which provides access for the food products to the pulp. A small cavity may be closed by a filling but a large cavity may well necessitate extraction of the tooth.

Gingivitis and peridontitis (inflammation of the gum) are usually painless until an abscess begins to form, generally necessitating removal of the tooth after the abscess has passed the acute stage, although in a reasonably early

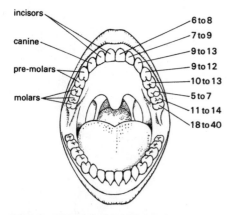

incisors

canine

pre-molars

molars

6 to 8
7 to 9
9 to 13
9 to 12
10 to 13
5 to 7
11 to 14
18 to 40

Permanent teeth, showing the age, in years, when they usually appear

stage the abscess may respond to treatment with antibiotics.

Malocclusion occurs when the teeth grow unevenly, largely through over-crowding; this happens because the human jaw has receded in the course of evolution. In a case of malocclusion the teeth are unsightly and also useless because they do not meet their opposite numbers. Orthodontic treatment at the age of 9 or 10 years can often remedy the defect.

Dental hygiene. Care of the teeth includes at least seven points:

1. Vigorous and thorough gum brushing, preferably morning and evening, but particularly in the evening, with the entire front and back surfaces of the teeth vigorously brushed with a reasonably hard toothbrush containing many bristles – about fifteen forwards and backwards horizontal strokes, i.e., sixty double strokes in all. In this brushing tooth-pastes are quite useful, especially those that contain added fluoride, but the brushing is far more important than the paste.

2. Eating foods that require adequate chewing to clean the teeth. Examples of such foods are rye bread, Scandinavian flat bread, toast, and such raw vegetables as cucumber and carrots.

3. ·Eating plenty of fruits and green vegetables to ensure sufficiency of the water-soluble vitamins, especially vitamin c.

4. Taking a diet containing adequate amounts of calcium and vitamin D.

5. Normally drinking water in which any deficiency of fluoride has been corrected, to bring the fluoride content to approximately one part per million.

6. Limiting the consumption of sweets, cakes, sweet biscuits and sweet puddings, and ensuring that they are eaten before – and not after – tooth brushing.

7. Having a dental inspection, with scaling of the teeth if necessary, twice every year.

In general the standard of dental hygiene in Britain is not high. As a nation we tend to eat far too much sugar and white flour, many of our water supplies are deficient in fluoride, too often tooth brushing is forgotten or undertaken in a very perfunctory manner, and visits to the dentist are postponed until pain indicates the presence of unprevented dental caries. As a whole, therefore, British adults and children have bad teeth. By the age of 2 years, half the children in Britain show signs of tooth decay, and by the age of 12, less than 4 per cent of children are free from decayed, filled, or missing teeth.

On the other hand, it is possible to carry insistence on dental hygiene to excess. Our teeth will not suddenly decay because we were so tired last night that we did not brush them properly, or because we succumbed to temptation and ate a couple of sticky sweet cakes. It is the general and habitual attention to dental hygiene that matters, not the occasional deviation from it.

teeth, artificial. See DENTURES.

teething. The stage of eruption of the teeth, starting at about 6 to 9 months in the case of the milk teeth and continuing until about 15 years for the permanent teeth, with the last of the permanent teeth (the wisdom teeth) erupting at between 17 and 25 years.

Many young children are fractious and irritable during teething, but it is a mistake to attribute all illnesses in such children to teething. The teething process can sometimes be hastened by giving the child a rusk or hard crust to try to chew, and the diet during teething should contain adequate quantities of vitamins A and D (e.g., from appropriate dosage of cod liver oil or halibut oil drops) and adequate calcium (e.g., from a pint of milk and an egg daily).

teleology. The doctrine that all things in nature are created for special purposes and that things happen because it is necessary that they should happen. This is fundamentally the same as saying that it is God's will that a child should die of diphtheria, irrespective of the availability of immunization which would prevent the disease and of diagnostic facilities and serum treatment which could cure the unprevented disease.

In medicine, as in other sciences, teleology conflicts with the study of causes, and so with the means of prevention of disease: teleologically the maladjusted child is inevitable and unpreventable; scientifically the behaviour and attitudes of that child are largely due to one or more factors, such as lack of demonstrated parental affection, over-domination by parents or teachers, over-indulgence, insecurity, and jealousy of brothers and sisters, and attention to these factors can in considerable measure prevent malad-justment.

Yet we all use the language of teleology at times: the doctor hurrying to catch a train says unthinkingly that he breathes faster to bring more oxygen to his muscles, whereas actually increased muscular activity as a result of his decision to hurry creates more lactic acid in the muscles and this stimulates the nerve centre controlling the respiratory rate, with that centre utterly unaware of the train, the railway station or the need to hurry.

television and health. Many criticisms, mostly casual and unproved, are made of the effects of watching 'the box'. In excess it reduces access to fresh air, limits the taking of healthy exercise, converts people from active providers of their own entertainment to passive viewers, limits discussion and family conversation, damages the creative imagination by imposing pictures and scenes as visualized by someone else, and may harm the eyesight, although probably no more so than does intensive reading. On the other hand its supporters say that it brings to the viewer a much wider view of life, that it raises for consideration aspects of problems that a person in a narrow cultural atmosphere may never have encountered or imagined, and that it is a profound educational influence.

There is a modicum of sense in both attitudes. Clearly extreme viewing – like other extremes – can be harmful; but there is little if any concrete evidence that a moderate amount of viewing does any damage either to parents or to their children. The wise parent will, however, try to exercise unobtrusive censorship not only over quantity but also quality, ensuring, for example, that an excitable child does not see an alarming play shortly before going to bed.

temperament. Natural disposition. The tendency of a person – partially inherited and partially created by relationships with others in the formative years – to be easily angered or slow to anger, optimistic or pessimistic, extroverted or introverted, and cautious with strangers or 'hail-fellow-well-met'.

Hippocrates regarded the body as being composed of four elements, air, water, fire and earth, with these corresponding respectively with blood, phlegm, yellow bile and 'black bile', the last being the dark viscous blood of the spleen. Later Galen classified temperament according to the alleged predominance of one element – sanguine or optimistic (with predominance of blood), phlegmatic or slow and inactive (with much phlegm), choleric or peppery (with excess of yellow bile) and melancholic or gloomy (with much 'black bile').

These classifications, though still sometimes used by non-medical writers, are long out-dated, and William James's division into tough-minded and tender-minded takes only one aspect into consideration, as does Jung's division into extroverts and introverts. In seeking to assess a person's temperament we have to consider the frequency and strength of emotional swings (e.g., between depression and elation), the extent of ability to maintain control in periods of crisis, the general sensitivity or insensitivity of the person, the intensity of his feelings and various other points.

While careful study of temperaments helps to predict behaviour, few people are always tough-minded or tender-minded, or complete extroverts or introverts, and ability to maintain control varies with the nature of the crisis. In other words, temperament is only a rough guide to behaviour.

It is often said that natural temperaments

become exaggerated in old age: the extrovert becomes even more sociable and garrulous, the easily frightened person becomes more readily scared, the peppery individual becomes even more prone to anger, and the generous person even more generous.

temperature. The normal temperature of the body varies with time of day (lowest in the early morning) and with the part of the body (lower in the armpit than in the mouth and higher in the rectum). The average mouth temperature of the human is 36 ° to 37.2 °C. (97 ° to 99 °F.). Some warm-blooded creatures, especially birds, have higher temperatures, although all mammals, including humans, fall into the warm-blooded class; and cold-blooded creatures, e.g., reptiles and fishes, have much lower temperatures.

Temperature is kept fairly even by maintenance of a balance between heat production (e.g., by muscular exercise) and heat loss (e.g., by sweating), with the amount of heat loss regulated by a centre in the brain.

In some diseases, such as most fevers, the mechanism for regulating heat loss is thrown out of control, so that the temperature rises. It may rise as high as 43 °C. (110 °F.) but there is risk to life after it reaches 41.6 °C. (107 °F.).

In extreme cold, starvation, severe loss of blood and some diseases the heat regulating mechanism cannot cope with the heat loss, and so the temperature falls. It may sink to 32 °C. (90 °F.) but there is danger when it passes below 35 °C. (95 °F.).

Old people are peculiarly liable to suffer from a cold environment with which their heat regulating centre cannot cope. Their temperature falls gradually, often without them becoming aware that they are cold. The condition is called HYPOTHERMIA.

temper tantrums. Episodes of uncontrolled rage, usually in small children, but occasionally also occurring in old people. A tantrum may be sheer blackmail, or it may be an attempt to express a very genuine and clamant need, as in emotional starvation, or again it may be a reaction to a terrifying situation. In the last case the situation, which may not appear in any way alarming to an adult, calls for prompt separation of the child from the situation. That being excluded, neither immediate demonstrated affection nor punishment is particularly useful: to kiss and cuddle the child may be to yield to emotional blackmail and ensure repetition; to smack or scold him is unfair, since his emotions are temporarily out of his control, and it is a cruel response to what may be an expression of desperate need. It is generally best to ensure that the child is so placed that he cannot seriously hurt himself, to show neither resentment nor concern but to leave him to howl for a few minutes, and then to seek to divert him with a new toy or a favourite game. Where tantrums are frequent psychological investigation may be needed.

Much of our understanding of child behaviour stems from the pioneer work of Dr. Arnold Gesell and his collaborators in the U.S.A. between 1930 and 1940. Another careful enquiry showed that some form of ostensibly angry behaviour occurred at all ages up to 18 but that it was most common in the pre-school years.

In general, temper-tantrums are a reaction to frustration, and most parents experience some

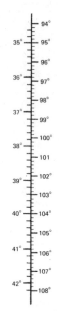

Temperature conversions

such worry when their children disregard prohibitions and make a scene when they are not allowed to do as they wish. This sort of behaviour is very common in the toddler and is characteristic of his stage of development. It must be handled intelligently and not allowed to become an invariable pattern of reaction because this leads to the eventual emergence of the petulant, childish and resentful adult.

The child of this age taxes his parents' forbearance because he has become able to understand what is said to him and his offence is greater when he ignores it. His temper-tantrums must be dealt with by insistence on a sensible regular routine maintained with firmness and patience. Restrictions should be as few as possible and must not reflect parental whim, impulse or inconsistency. They should also be explained by simple reason and logic capable of being appreciated by the child, and they must be adhered to and enforced. Children are also influenced by simple cause-and-effect punishments such as taking away their crayons if they refuse to stop scribbling on the wallpaper.

Conformity may be secured by compromise such as the imaginative substitution of some pleasurable alternative activity instead of adopting coercion which only aggravates anger and obstinacy. When a full-blown tantrum develops it is best dealt with by standing aside and letting the child expend his wrath without interference. To give in is fatal, but after the emotional outburst has subsided of its own accord the parents ought not to scold or show disapproval – comforting and pleasurable distraction are required instead. It is important to try to avoid making issues and having direct clashes. Imagination and ingenuity will suggest alternatives to divert a child from his immediate frustration. Many prohibitions result from fears for a child's safety. It is better to arrange the environment so that safety is inherent and the prohibitions unnecessary.

At a somewhat later age (3 to 7) tantrums sometimes result from what is known as the Oedipus (or Electra) complex: boys try to replace their father in their mother's affections and vice versa for girls.

Demonstrations of affection between the parents arouse envy and anxiety and may result in unexplained bouts of temper or nightmares. Usually these anxieties can be resolved if the child is treated particularly affectionately by the parent who is envied and whose removal is secretly desired.

Reactions of anger occur at other ages too. Even in the infant, too many caresses and too much emotional involvement may so condition it to being fondled that subsequent relationships seem cold and unsatisfactory by comparison. Thus the 1-year-old, suddenly deprived of intimate nursing contacts, feels neglected and strives for attention by inordinate demands which turn to sulkiness and temper when not fulfilled. Over-indulgence is particularly likely when a mother's own emotional life is unsatisfactory. Although adequate nursing intimacies are important for proper psychological development they should not be excessive and should be withdrawn gradually and replaced by other satisfactions if trouble is to be avoided.

Older childhood and adolescence are periods of growing independence. The school child increasingly desires to make his own decisions and do things for himself. Inevitably he is much slower and less accomplished than an adult, but if he is laughed at, or ignored, or prevented, or given no encouragement, he again becomes bewildered and angry. Nevertheless, to be allowed to decide for himself is the only way to develop beyond the stage of impulse. If he is prevented from carrying out his own ideas he reverts to the childish practice of temper tantrums or other aberrations of behaviour.

Similarly, adolescence is a period in which there is still further rebellion against established ways of life and this may be reflected in vandalism and delinquency unless constructive outlets are provided for the impatience and enthusiasms of youth.

tendinitis. Inflammation of a tendon, often caused by unusual and excessive use. The tendon becomes both painful and tender and may creak on movement. Rest is the main treatment, but severe cases may be helped by injections of hydrocortisone, and in some cases physiotherapy is needed after the inflammation has subsided – but not before – to restore normal functioning.

tendon. A tough band of dense connective tissue which attaches a muscle to a bone. Typical tendons are the short, thick ones attaching the biceps muscle to the shoulder, and the long, thin ones that run from the forearm across the back of the wrist and hand to the fingers.

tenesmus. A constant sensation of weight and discomfort in the lower bowel, with desire to visit the lavatory, accompanied by straining in attempts – often unsuccessful – to empty the rectum. Tenesmus may be caused by the bowel being loaded with hard masses of faeces or by various diseases of the rectum, e.g., fissure or polypus; and it is also common in dysentery and other forms of diarrhoea. Warm hip baths or hot fomentations often help, but if the symptom continues it requires investigation.

tennis elbow. See ELBOW.

tenosynovitis. Inflammation of the sheath surrounding a tendon and also of the tendon itself. Causes include a focus of sepsis (bacterial infection) elsewhere, damp, draughts and over-use of the muscle. The main symptom is pain, which is worse on movement, and in later stages worse in cold or damp weather and also worse on going to bed at night. Treatment involves looking for and removing the focus of sepsis, providing local heat and massage, supplying analgesics for the pain, and sometimes giving injections of hydrocortisone.

tension. Mental or emotional strain or strained personal relations. Tension arises mainly from the non-satisfaction of various needs (e.g., for affection, work success or social status). It sometimes expresses itself in outbursts of temper or in prolonged irritability, in which case the person is getting rid of his tension, however unpleasant the process may be for others. In other cases the tension is repressed into silent brooding or worrying, and in this eventuality it may lead to headaches, backache, cramps and various psychosomatic diseases.

Physical activity is often a good way of providing relief from a domestic or work situation that is creating tension. So is discussion of the particular problem with a trusted friend or relative.

terminal. At the end; when used describing an illness it indicates the approach of death.

tertian fever. See MALARIA.

testicle. One of a pair of glands in the male reproductive system, also known as the testis. The right and left testes are suspended in the scrotum by the spermatic cords which contain blood vessels and a secretory duct, the vas deferens. Each testis is an egg-shaped glandular body about 2.5 cm. by 3.8 cm. (1 in. by 1.5 in.) in size, made up of germinal tissue which produces spermatozoa or male germ cells and other tissue which supplies the internal secretion or male hormone testosterone.

Attached to the rear border of the testis is the epididymis which is a twisted tube receiving spermatozoa from the seminal tubules and continuing into the vas deferens.

Diseases. Inflammation of the testicle (orchitis) may occur in gonorrhoea, in almost any infection spreading from the urethra or prostate gland, or – quite often – in mumps. The main symptoms are swelling, pain and tenderness. Orchitis of bacterial origin responds well to antibiotics. Orchitis as a complication of mumps subsides in a few days without treatment other than rest and warm applications but may cause permanent sterility.

Cysts are of two types, dermoid cysts, which are essentially foetal remnants, and spermatoceles, which are swellings due to obstruction of the central tubes of the testis and are usually found in elderly men. Solid tumours occur rarely and are more often benign than malignant.

Varicocele is essentially a varicose condition of the veins of the spermatic cord, and hydrocele is an accumulation of fluid in the capsule of the testis.

Treatment of cysts, tumours, variocele and hydrocele varies with the cause and the size of the swelling, but in some cases surgical treatment is needed

testicle, undescended. Retarded or absent descent of the testicles (medically known as cryptorchism). The testicles are formed in the abdomen of the developing male child and remain there in fish and birds. In man and other mammals they normally pass downwards into the scrotum before or soon after birth. In about 7 per cent of boys one testicle or both fail to descend by the age of one year. Causes of failure include anatomical abnormalities, endocrine deficiencies, and possibly abnormalities of the sex chromosome. In most of these cases the descent occurs spontaneously before the age of 8 years but in cases where descent does not occur by that age (about 1 boy in every 500) hormone treatment or surgical operation may be needed, because the internal temperature of the abdomen is too high to allow the testicles to function normally, so that the person with undescended testicles may be unable to manufacture live sperms.

test meal. A procedure for investigating the chemical function of the stomach by the analysis of small fractions of its contents at intervals during the process of digestion.

In the morning the patient swallows a thin rubber tube (Ryle's tube). The fasting gastric juice is withdrawn and measured, its content of bile and mucus is noted, its acidity is determined and it is also tested for starch (because presence of starch suggests some degree of obstruction at the ring of muscle that separates stomach from duodenum). A measured quantity of gruel is then given and further samples of gastric juice withdrawn at intervals for the next three hours. The acidity of each sample is measured and the sample is tested for starch, bile and blood.

Consideration of the results is of help in diagnosis because characteristic findings are obtained in such conditions as gastritis, gastric ulcer, duodenal ulcer, cancer and pernicious anaemia.

A test-feed for infants suspected of suffering from UNDERFEEDING involves assessing only the quantity of milk taken.

testosterone. Male hormone, an internal secretion produced by certain cells (cells of Leydig) in the testis and responsible for the development and function of male sexual characteristics. Originally extracted from bull's testes (by McGee in 1929) it can now be prepared synthetically from cholesterol. A range of similar substances (androgens) has been developed and of these the one mainly used therapeutically is either testosterone propionate or methyl testosterone. Androgens are employed as replacement therapy in castrated males and in those with similar symptoms from other causes. In the male climacteric they are of doubtful value. In the female they are used for the treatment of inoperable breast cancer, some cases of uterine bleeding, and dysmenorrhoea (pain during menstruation) because they counteract excess of the female hormone oestrogen, but they may cause signs and symptoms of masculinization. They are given by intramuscular injection, but more prolonged effects can be secured by using androgens in oily solution, or by implanting pellets below the skin.

tetanus. An acute specific disease caused by toxin of the tetanus bacillus (*Clostridium tetani*) which multiplies in infected wounds after contamination from soil and dust. Punctured or deep wounds are particularly suspect but it is also common after burns and sometimes may follow mere grazes or trivial disregarded injuries. A special type, tetanus neonatorum, occurs in infants through infection of the umbilical stump.

The incubation period is variable with an average of ten days and the initial symptoms are stiffness of the neck and jaw (lockjaw) followed by generalized rigidity and spasmodic contractions of the whole body which eventually lead to death from respiratory and cardiac failure.

Treatment of the established disease is by anti-tetanic serum, penicillin and sedation, but cases should rarely arise if adequate attention is paid to prevention. Children should be actively immunized by tetanus toxoid from infancy and anti-tetanus injection should form an essential part of the routine treatment of injuries involving breaches of the skin.

tetany. A rare disease of the nervous system produced by a deficiency of calcium in the blood.

Infantile tetany or spasmophilia occurs in young children usually as a complication of rickets or of diseases which lower the absorption of calcium, such as coeliac disease and severe diarrhoeal conditions. The condition may begin with a convulsion or series of convulsions. Spasm of the larynx may cause 'crowing' sounds (laryngismus stridulus) and result in breathing difficulty which may prove fatal. The hands and feet tend to adopt a characteristic posture (carpopedal spasm). Once recognized the symptoms yield readily to intravenous calcium and vitamin D.

Tetany in adults is usually due to injury or disease of the parathyroid glands or to gastrointestinal diseases interfering with calcium absorption. Long-term treatment with calcium and vitamin D is required. The apparently logical use of parathyroid hormone has not been very successful in practice.

thalamus. A part of the brain which acts as a relay station for sensory impressions, since it has extensive nervous connections with the cortex above and the spinal cord below, as well as with the cerebellum, optic tracts, and auditory nerves. Its functional level can be regarded as intermediate between the voluntary activity of the cortex and the reflex activity of the cord.

thalassaemia. A chronic progressive anaemia caused by a hereditary inability to use iron to manufacture haemoglobin. The disease is common in the Middle East, India and China, and is quite often found in immigrants from these parts.

There are two forms. In thalassaemia major there is very severe anaemia, enlarged abdomen through swelling of the spleen and liver, and often prominence of the forehead and sunken appearance of the bridge of the nose. This form of the condition is usually fatal during infancy, and there is no specific treatment although surgical removal of the spleen appears to help in some cases.

In thalassaemia minor the anaemia is only

mild, the spleen and liver are only slightly enlarged, and the expectation of life may be normal.

thalidomide. Extremely favourable reports about this drug (alpha-phthalimido-glutarimide) were first made public at a symposium in Germany in 1955. It was claimed to be an entirely new form of sedative and hypnotic free from the disadvantages of barbiturates, bromides and alkaloids. As a derivative of glutamic acid, a substance naturally involved in brain metabolism, it was regarded as particularly safe. In animal toxicity tests it had proved impossible to determine a lethal dose, and in clinical trials it was well tolerated even in severe liver insufficiency.

It was subsequently widely marketed under various trade-names, in Germany and elsewhere, either alone or in compound formulations for the treatment of anxiety, insomnia, migraine, asthma, and so on. It soon became well-established as a sedative producing calmness without confusion, and as a hypnotic restoring normal sleep-patterns.

Unfortunately, no one had done preliminary tests to determine if it was a drug affecting the foetus. The first note of alarm was sounded about 1960 when it was noticed that many mothers who had taken it during pregnancy were producing babies with serious deformities, particularly the absence or faulty development of limbs, the condition called phocomelia (meaning 'seal-limb' because of the flipper-like result).

As soon as it was appreciated that this was due to thalidomide the drug was, of course, withdrawn (1961). Since then there have been prolonged legal battles to apportion blame and secure compensation for the victims (about four hundred in Great Britain alone).

It is easy to be wise after the event but perhaps it should have been foreseen that a drug which depressed adult nerve-cell activity so efficiently might also interfere with the function of embryonic nerve tissue on which other development depended.

therapeutics. The science and art of alleviating or curing disease. The term includes not only the giving of medicines and drugs but the use of other methods of treatment.

Therapeutics may therefore be (1) rational when the expected result of a remedy is based on accepted scientific knowledge of pathology and pharmacology; (2) empirical when a remedy is known to be effective although its action may not be fully understood; or (3) general when remedies are employed which are not medicines or drugs. This last includes measures like diet, climate, spa and bath treatment, massage, medical gymnastics and the use of physical agencies such as heat, light, electricity and radiation.

Therapy is the application of the principles of therapeutics. Usually a prefix indicates its precise nature, as for example physiotherapy, hydrotherapy, electrotherapy, deep x-ray therapy and so on.

thermometer. An instrument for measuring temperature. In principle, a simple conventional thermometer consists of a glass bulb containing a liquid (usually mercury or alcohol) which on heating expands along a very fine graduated and calibrated tube to give a reading indicative of the bulb's temperature.

Various thermometers are used in medical and nursing practice. Clinical thermometers measure body-temperature and are graduated from 35 °C. to 44 °C. or from 95 °F. to 110 °F. The ordinary oral type is used in mouth or armpit, and a stouter rectal type records temperature in the rectum. In clinical thermometers, the capillary-tube has a constriction so that the mercury-column separates when the bulb cools and remains in position until a reading can be taken. The column must then be shaken down before re-use. Low-reading clinical thermometers are graduated from 21 °C. or 70 °F. and are required for the detection of hypothermia, usually in infants or the aged. Normal body TEMPERATURE is 36.9 °C. (98.4 °F.).

Other instruments are lotion, food, and bath thermometers, and room-thermometers. On the Fahrenheit scale water freezes at 32 °F. and boils at 212 °F. Comparable points on the Centigrade scale are 0 °C. and 100 °C.

Conversion rules. To convert Fahrenheit to Centigrade first subtract thirty-two from the Fahrenheit reading, multiply the answer by five and then divide by nine; to convert Centigrade to Fahrenheit first multiply the Centigrade reading by nine, divide the answer by five and then add thirty-two.

thiamine. A complex organic compound more familiarly known as vitamin B_1 or aneurin. Deficiency causes the disease beri-beri.

Good sources of the vitamin are yeast, wheat and wheat-germ, brown rice (but not polished rice), egg-yolk, liver, chocolate, bacon and ham. Beri-beri does not occur in Britain, but the intake of vitamin B_1 may be marginally insufficient under poor dietary conditions or in alcoholics. Signs of deficiency may include heart weakness and neuritis.

The daily requirements are 200 to 300 International Units for adults and proportionally less for children (1 IU = 3 micrograms). For prevention of deficiency one 3 mg. tablet daily is a usual prescription.

thigh. The upper part of the leg extending from the trunk to the knee. Its central support is a single bone, the largest in the body, known as the FEMUR.

thinking. Purposeful activity of the mind. It used to be common to divide conscious mental experience (i.e., ignoring the UNCONSCIOUS MIND) into feeling, willing and thinking, or in psychological jargon the affective, conative and cognitive aspects; but these tend to be very intermixed. Broadly, however, thinking presupposes two preliminary steps: first, perception, the stimulation of our sense-organs by external sights, sounds and so on, the transmission of impulses from the sense organs to the brain, and their meaningful interpretation (e.g., as a distressed cry or as the appearance of a person); and second, the relation of perception to past experiences or to ideas (e.g., deciding that the distressed cry means that our child is hurt or in danger or that the person is the neighbour whom we desire to avoid). Real thinking begins when our perceptions and recollections of parallel experiences, ideas or imaginings alert us to a problem. The solution to the problem may be simple (e.g., that we should pick up and comfort the crying child or cross the street to avoid the neighbour) or it may be extremely complex and even beyond our abilities, but the attempt to solve it is the essence of thinking.

The thinking may be misdirected if the perception is false (as in optical illusions) or if the relation to past experience is incorrect (as when we mistake the child's cry of joy for one of distress), but it is still thinking.

The purpose of thought is to solve problems by using and manipulating knowledge derived from immediate and stored perceptions. Many situations demand immediate action, and previous experience ensures that there is an answer ready. Thus a car-driver regulates his responses in accordance with traffic conditions and may appear to act almost reflexly, but actually these responses are being thought out on the basis of current stimuli and earlier perceptions. If no answer is immediately forthcoming the second stage of thought is to examine the problem more closely – we 'stop and think'. The next stage is to attempt to resurrect from the mind the facts and principles necessary for a solution. This may take time – recognized by the traditional advice to 'sleep on it'. The recovery of latent ideas depends largely on association. If two ideas occurred together in the past, the calling up of one will tend to recall the other also but what emerges may be affected unexpectedly by the immediate trend of thought. The crossword addict knows only too well how his thinking can be misdirected by such clues as 'European flower' which turns out to be a river and not a blossom.

Like other biological activities, thought can be influenced in many ways. It is for instance adversely affected by disease or by emotion which narrows the span of consciousness. When afraid or anxious we are unable to turn our thoughts from the object of our fear or anxiety. Mental disease in particular is essentially a disordered way of thought. On the other hand increased efficiency of thought can be developed with practice by building up our store of associations and by exercising our minds with problems so that we acquire an increased facility for the recovery of these associations from our subconscious. As Aristotle put it, 'For the things we have to learn before we can do them, we learn by doing them'.

thinness. Body-build is determined largely by constitutional and genetic factors. Many people in perfect health remain consistently thin despite an adequate or even generous dietary intake. This need cause no concern because the tall slender child and the 'skinny' adult with little or no subcutaneous fat are both within the limits of normality. Tabulated weights for height and age usually show only average values and a normal range can be 10 per cent above or below. There are some advantages in being thin; on the whole, thin people have fewer illnesses and live longer, because there is less strain on important systems, notably those of the heart, circulation, and joints.

Sudden or gradual loss of weight is, however, another matter. Thinness which develops as a result of this may be due to a variety of causes including disturbances of the endocrine glands, disorders of the digestive system, diabetes, tuberculosis, anaemia, malignant disease, alcoholism and depression. It calls for investigation.

Excessive thinness is known as emaciation when there is no suspected internal cause (e.g., the thinness that occurs in famine conditions), or cachexia when it is accompanied by signs of disease (e.g., the thinness found in cancer of the stomach). The emaciation which results from a neurotic refusal to eat is known as anorexia nervosa.

thirst. The sensation of thirst arises from nerve-endings in the pharynx. It may be caused by drying of the mucous membrane in that area due to hot atmospheres, by over-breathing, or by drugs such as atropine which inhibit secretion; or it may indicate a real need of the body for water replacement. The latter is of course the plight of travellers stranded in the desert, but this kind of true thirst also arises in a variety of diseases and in various ways.

In feverish conditions there is generally excessive fluid loss because of high temperature and perspiration; and increased metabolic rate with sweating is also a feature of hyperthyroidism. Diarrhoea and vomiting occur in many diseases such as gastritis, enteritis, pyloric stenosis and cholera, and fluid loss in such cases is obvious.

Two specific diseases particularly characterized by thirst are diabetes mellitus and diabetes insipidus. In the former additional water is needed for urine which excretes some of the excess sugar, and in the latter a defect of the pituitary gland leads to massive passing of urine.

Infants often suffer from thirst more often than is realized if kept too warm and given over-concentrated feeds. Crying and restlessness should not be interpreted indiscriminately as a demand for extra food if the requisite Calories for weight are already being provided. A bottle of sterilized water instead will often relieve the situation.

thoracic duct. The main channel by which lymph and chyle are conveyed to the bloodstream. Chyle is the milky fluid taken up by the lymphatic vessels of the intestine and is a mixture of lymph and emulsified fat. The thoracic duct drains the greater part of the body and discharges its contents into the veins in the root of the neck. A smaller right lymphatic duct drains the right upper half of the body and similarly joins the same veins on the right side.

thoracoplasty. An operation on the chest-wall to reduce the size of the underlying thoracic cavity.

Since lung-tissue is spongy, disease of various kinds may result in the formation of cavities. The sides of these cavities. must be brought together so that they may heal over and this is achieved by compressing the affected lung tissue in a chest which has been made smaller by thoracoplasty. The scope of the operation required depends on the site and extent of the lung disease and may be done in stages. In complete thoracoplasty the upper nine or ten ribs are removed so that the chest-wall can move inwards and compress the lung.

The procedure was formerly much used in the later stages of recovery from pulmonary tuberculosis but is now less necessary because of the introduction of effective drugs capable of arresting the disease before the occurrence of extensive tissue-destruction.

The operation is also employed in other conditions such as lung-abscess and bronchiectasis.

thorax. See CHEST.

drained by right lymphatic duct

drained by thoracic duct

The action of the thoracic duct

threadworms. The thread or pin-worm, *Enterobius* (*Oxyuris*) *vermicularis* is a very common intestinal parasite especially in children. The male is about 0.5 cm. and the female 1.0 cm. in length and they may often be seen in the faeces resembling short pieces of whitish thread. They inhabit the lower bowel and at night, with the patient warm in bed, may cause great discomfort and itching by emerging on to the skin around the anus where the female deposits her eggs. The skin becomes damaged and eczematous from scratching. Bladder irritability, frequency of passing urine, vaginitis and mucoid discharge from the anus may also occur. General health may be impaired by restlessness and sleeplessness. Persistent infection is maintained and spread to others by swallowing eggs transmitted on the hands contaminated during scratching. Diagnosis may be confirmed by microscopical identification of eggs in anal smears.

Effective treatment is available by appropriate drugs but complete eradication of the worms requires scrupulous attention to hand-washing, disinfection of night attire and bed-clothing, and simultaneous attention to other members of the household.

thrombocytes. See PLATELETS.

thrombosis. The clotting or coagulation of blood within living blood vessels. This may occur in the heart, arteries or veins, but it is commonest in veins where the blood is relatively slow-moving. If the clot remains attached it is a thrombus; if it floats away to lodge elsewhere it is called an embolus. Thrombosis results from altered blood conditions as in anaemia or infection; from venous stagnation as in varicose veins or in prolonged bed-rest enforced by operation or illness; and from inflammation and degeneration of vessel walls.

Common sites of arterial clotting are the blood vessels of the heart (leading to CORONARY THROMBOSIS) and of the brain (leading to STROKE). Elderly persons with deteriorating blood vessels may also develop thrombosis of the retinal artery with loss of vision or of leg arteries leading to gangrene.

Venous thrombosis is most common in leg or pelvic veins and carries a risk of subsequent pulmonary embolism. It may occur after childbirth or abdominal operations and is one reason for the policy of encouraging early mobility in such patients.

The treatment of established thrombosis is by anticoagulant drugs and rest.

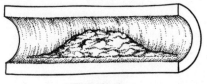

Thrombosis

thrush. Infection of mucous membrane by yeast-like fungi of the genus *Monilia* (sometimes known as *Candida* or *Oidium*). The common species is *M. albicans*.

Thrush occurs mainly in young bottle-fed infants and appears as white patches of the fungus firmly attached to tongue, palate, or cheek. In premature or debilitated infants the patches may spread extensively to the pharynx, oesophagus or even the intestine. However, in most cases the extent of infection is limited to the mouth and its principal effect is to make the infant reluctant to feed and suck properly.

Treatment is relatively easy and effective. The traditional remedy was to paint the affected areas with a 1 per cent solution of gentian violet, but the fungicide nystatin as Nystatin Mixture applied locally by dropper is now generally preferred. Scrupulous attention must be paid to the cleaning and sterilization of equipment used in feeding infants.

thymus gland. A two-lobed ENDOCRINE GLAND lying at the base of the neck concerned with combating infection and possibly also with growth and development.

thyroid gland. An important ENDOCRINE GLAND lying in the neck and concerned with regulating the body's metabolic rate. Enlargement of the gland produces the condition known as GOITRE, and excessive secretion of thyroid hormone results in the condition known as THYROTOXICOSIS.

thyrotoxicosis. The condition which results from hyperthyroidism or excessive secretion of thyroid hormone by the thyroid gland.

Primary thyrotoxicosis occurs in exophthalmic goitre (Graves' disease) which is characterized by enlargement of the glands, increased pulse-rate, prominent eyeballs, loss of weight, nervousness and tremors and an increased metabolic rate, which in turn causes sweating, thirst, increased appetite and sometimes other evidence of disordered metabolism – such as the excretion in the urine of sugar and the reduction of the level of cholesterol in the blood.

Secondary thyrotoxicosis is not essentially different. It results not from general over-functioning of the gland but from thyroid tumour, the so-called toxic adenoma. Signs of hyperthyroidism are less obvious and effects fall mainly on the cardio-vascular system. Auricular fibrillation (a type of disordered heart action) and signs of heart failure may develop before it is appreciated that these have a thyroid basis. In older patients this is a possibility to which cardiologists are alert.

The treatment of thyrotoxicosis is now a very advanced speciality involving the use of drugs like thiouracil which stop or reduce the manufacture of thyroxine, and radio-active iodine which destroys over-active thyroid tissue; and sometimes surgery is necessary to excise part of the gland or to remove a tumour. Each case requires individual expert assessment.

tibia. The inner and larger of the two bones in the lower part of the leg. At its upper end it is enlarged to articulate with the thigh bone or femur as the knee-joint, and its lower end forms part of the ankle-joint. Its front edge or crest lies just beneath the skin and is prominent at the shin and rather exposed to casual injury in such activities as football and cricket. It is also the bone most liable to show deformity as a result of rickets.

tic. Any sudden, rapid, twitching, involuntary movement that occurs repeatedly. Essentially tics are a group of nervous diseases in which there occur: (1) repetitions of sudden twitch-like movements, (2) sudden involuntary utterances, or (3) deliberate repetitive co-ordinated actions related to an imperative idea. Combinations of these types occur.

Simple tic usually shows in 'nervous' children by repeated blinking, grimacing, head-jerking, shoulder-shrugging and similar actions. Most cases recover spontaneously.

In convulsive tic (Tourette's disease) spasmodic movements are more extensive and often accompanied by grotesque attitudes or apparent miming.

In psychic or verbal tic there is an uncontrollable impulse to repeat irrelevant words.

These two types affect older persons and often progress to mental deterioration.

The co-ordinated tic, sometimes seen in highly competent persons under stress, takes the form of purposeless repetition of complicated co-ordinated movements such as twiddling a pencil, jingling change in a trouser-pocket or fidgeting with a tie.

tic douloureux. See TRIGEMINAL NEURALGIA.

ticks. Arthropods of the class Arachnida which also includes scorpions, spiders and mites. Ticks and mites are similar and are grouped together as acarids. Most are very small, many are parasitic on a wide range of wild and domestic animals and some, in tropical and sub-tropical countries, are carriers of disease.

Ticks are usually oval or circular because their neck and abdomen are fused. Adult forms have eight legs and beak-like mouth parts adapted for sucking blood Hard ticks

(*Ixodidae*) have a shell while soft ticks (*Argasidae*) have no shell.

Hard ticks transmit tularaemia and rickettsial infections and soft ticks spread African relapsing fever, and some animal diseases are also tick-borne. In countries where ticks are prevalent, preventive measures include the destruction of animals likely to infect sheep and cattle, and the dipping of flocks and herds. Workers in infested areas should wear a one-piece suit with tight fitting wristlets and anklets.

tinea. The scientific name for RINGWORM, derived from the Latin word for a moth in recognition of the moth-eaten appearance of the affected hairy parts of the body. Care should be taken to distinguish the term *Tinea* from *Taenia*, the latter being a generic name of TAPEWORMS.

tinnitus. The subjective impression of persistent or recurring HEAD NOISES – 'a ringing in the ears'.

tobacco and health. In 1964 an Advisory Committee appointed by the Surgeon-General of the American Public Health Service published an exhaustive report on the adverse health effects of smoking tobacco. It showed that cigarette smoking was associated with a 70 per cent increase in the death-rate of males and to a lesser extent with increased death-rates in females. The diseases associated with smoking were lung cancer, laryngeal cancer, chronic bronchitis and emphysema, coronary thrombosis, high blood pressure and arteriosclerosis. It was also suggested that there might be some relationship with cancer of the oesophagus and bladder and perhaps of the stomach.

The best known British investigations are those of Doll and Hill. Broadly they showed that deaths from lung cancer were about ten times commoner in moderate cigarette smokers and about twenty times commoner in heavy smokers than in non-smokers; that for other respiratory diseases the ratio of deaths was roughly fourteen in heavy cigarette smokers to eleven in moderate smokers and eight in non-smokers; and that in coronary thrombosis (which causes about twice as many deaths as lung cancer and other respiratory diseases added together) the ratio of deaths was about six in heavy smokers to five in moderate smokers and four in non-smokers.

These studies form the basis for the banning of cigarette advertising on television, the printing of Government warnings on cigarette packets and intensive health education efforts to persuade young people not to start smoking, or – less hopefully – to induce smokers to stop. Prohibition of cigarette smoking, advocated by some, is probably undesirable – because many smokers live to a ripe old age without any obvious damage to their health, and because the drop in revenue would be enormous and cessation of tobacco-growing and cigarette manufacture would create massive unemployment in some countries. Yet efforts to achieve voluntary reduction in the number of smokers have so far had relatively little success. See SMOKING.

toe. One of the five terminal members of the foot, corresponding to the fingers, and consisting essentially of two bones in the big toe and three in each of the other toes, with surrounding muscles, nerves and blood vessels.

The toes play an important part in enabling us to maintain balance, e.g., when leaning forwards, and, where not stiffened by the habitual wearing of shoes, can bend considerably and so be of help in such activities as climbing trees. In communities habitually using footwear much of the mobility of the toes has been lost, but some people who have in early life lost the use of hands through illness or accident have learned to paint pictures and to operate typewriters with their toes.

Diseases. Congenital defects of the toes may take the form of extra toes (polydactylism), webbing or fusion of adjacent toes (syndactylism), contracted little toes, or enlargement of one or more toes. If any of these cause troublesome symptoms, they should be treated surgically.

Other conditions are related to the use of unsuitable footwear and symptoms are aggravated by the consequent development of corns, bursae, or arthritis. Gangrene of toes is quite frequently seen as a complication of diabetes and of diseases of small blood vessels. Acute arthritis, especially of the great toe, is common in gout, and ringworm may affect the nails and the skin between the toes (athlete's foot).

Onychogryphosis is a condition in which the toe-nails become enlarged and distorted, usually in elderly persons as a result of neglect.

Hallux valgus or bunion. Outward deflection of the great toe so that it may come to lie either above or below the second toe. The joint at the base of the toe is distorted and the head of the metacarpal bone projects on the inner side of the foot. Pressure on this causes arthritic changes and the overlying skin becomes thickened. A BUNION may develop and may subsequently become inflamed and infected. The condition can cause a good deal of pain and disability and is largely caused and aggravated by tight, pointed, or ill-fitting footwear.

Early cases can be relieved by wearing properly-shaped shoes and stockings with a separate compartment for the great toe, and by the use of a 'toe-post' between first and second toes to restore normal position. More severe cases require an operation.

Hammer toe. A common deformity, usually affecting the second toe, in which the toe is bent in different directions at its various joints so that it takes the shape of an inverted 'v' with the apex projecting above the line of the other toes. The condition usually appears in adolescence and may be caused or aggravated by unsuitable footwear – too short, too pointed, or with excessively high heels. The subsequent development of corns, caliosities or bursae over pressure-points will produce pain and disability.

In mild cases strapping down the toe or wearing a night-splint may secure improvement.

The surgical treatment of more severe cases is to remove the first joint (the apex of the 'v') and allow the bones to unite in a straight position. Amputation of the toe is not a good procedure since it allows the great toe to diverge sideways as in hallux valgus.

Ingrowing toe-nail. This condition mostly affects the great toe and is misnamed because it is produced by the skin and soft tissues overgrowing the edge of a normal nail. Unsuitable footwear compresses the toes and causes the tissues to overlap and in time the pressure against the nail causes a painful ulcer.

Early cases can generally be arrested by correcting the footwear and by cutting the nail square across instead of rounding the troublesome embedded corner which is instead raised and under-packed daily with a small piece of cotton wool.

In more resistant cases it may be necessary to cut out the overlapping tissue, split the nail longitudinally and remove a small strip of it with the corresponding part of the nail bed.

toilet training. See INFANCY, PSYCHOLOGY OF.

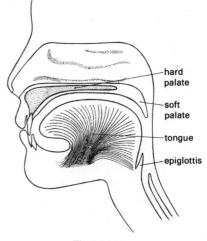

hard palate

soft palate

tongue

epiglottis

The tongue

tongue. A muscular organ lying in the floor of the mouth. Its rear or pharyngeal part (the base) is relatively fixed but the front and oral part is freely mobile. It is covered by mucous membrane which is somewhat rough owing to the presence of projections called papillae. These are of various types, being small and velvety in front and much larger and more obvious behind. The tongue is concerned with SPEECH, SWALLOWING and TASTE.

Diseases. Superficial inflammation of the tongue is glossitis, usually associated with STOMATITIS, which is inflammation of the mucous membranes of the mouth. It may result from local sepsis as in dental caries and pyorrhoea; from gastric disorder and excessive smoking and drinking; or, in children, from infections by viruses and fungi (see THRUSH). A chronic variety is leukoplakia, where there are raised white hardened patches which may ulcerate and may become malignant.

Treatment varies with the cause, but usually the most important part of the treatment is the allaying of the fear of cancer, either by reassurance or, if necessary, by taking for laboratory examination a small scraping of the cells lining the tongue.

Deep inflammatory conditions of the tongue (parenchymatous glossitis), which may lead to abscesses, occur when infection spreads to the substance of the tongue from superficial injuries or ulcers; they are also seen in mercurial poisoning, syphilis and actinomycosis.

Ulcers are usually the result of injury from teeth or of dyspepsia, but may be tuberculous, syphilitic or malignant.

Of tumours the commonest varieties are dermoid cysts, maevi and papillomata; cancer of the tongue is most often seen in men over 40 who are heavy smokers.

Black hairy tongue (melanoglossia) is a striking but unimportant condition due to overgrowth and staining of the papillae. An enlarged tongue is often seen in mongols and other mental defectives and is a congenital abnormality. TONGUE-TIE is described separately.

tongue-tie. On the under surface of the tongue the mucous membrane in the mid-line is raised up to form a crescentic fold known as the fraenum ('bridle') or frenulum. If this is so formed as to restrict the movements of the tongue the condition is termed 'tongue-tie' and the front margin of the fold is sometimes snipped with scissors to free the tongue. However, a degree of tongue-tie sufficiently severe to interfere with sucking, or later with speech, is very rare. Usually the operation is carried out in ignorance of the normal appearance of the tongue and fraenum of the young infant. The operation is generally unnecessary and carries some risk of haemorrhage or infection.

tonsillitis. Inflammation of the tonsils from bacterial infection. Tonsillitis is a specific feature of diphtheria and measles but its occurrence in scarlet fever and rheumatic fever is due to infection by haemolytic streptococci, and the same organisms can nearly always be incriminated in less specific conditions such as outbreaks of pharyngitis and sporadic attacks of severe sore throat. Most cases occur in childhood and adolescence and are rare in infancy.

The symptoms are pain in the throat, especially on swallowing, general upset with malaise, fever and raised pulse-rate, and often enlarged neck-glands. The tonsils appear swollen and red with spots of watery exudate. Pus may then develop producing an abscess or quinsy which will generally require surgical treatment.

Tonsillitis responds well to antibiotic drugs and should always be treated efficiently because of the risk of cardiac and rheumatic complications resulting from infection of the blood. Analgesics and antiseptic gargles also help to relieve the pain. Repeated attacks result in chronic tonsillitis and are usually an indication for removal of the tonsils and the associated adenoidal tissue in the pharynx, popularly termed the adenoids.

tonsils and adenoids. The tonsils are two bean-shaped masses of lymphoid tissue lying on the side walls of the soft palate on each side of the back of the tongue. They are easily visible when the mouth is widely opened. They are relatively large in children and usually shrink about the time of adolescence. Adenoids, possessed by all children, are pads of lymphoid tissue in the upper part of the throat behind the nasal passages. The pads tend to shrink about the age of 11 years. Tonsils and adenoids are part of the defence mechanism of the body. They help to waylay and destroy invading bacteria and also help to create immunity.

By a common misuse of words, 'tonsils and

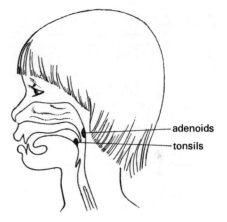

The tonsils and adenoids

adenoids' is frequently employed to mean 'enlarged tonsils and adenoids'.

During pre-school and early school years both tonsils and adenoids often become enlarged as a result of repeated minor infections. Many children develop large smooth tonsils which cause no symptoms and later shrink. On the other hand, enlarged, rough-looking tonsils can be a focus of infection, causing enlargement of neck glands and general deterioration in health; over-growth of adenoids can cause nasal obstruction and mouth breathing, snoring, a stupid or vacant appearance, hoarse nasal speech and sometimes deafness.

In the past enlarged tonsils and adenoids were removed almost routinely, but, while the operation is simple, removal of merely enlarged tonsils and adenoids deprives the body of organs that could perform useful functions. So the modern tendency is to remove them only if they are causing appreciable symptoms or if they are so chronically infected that they are harbouring germs instead of destroying them.

toothache. Sensations related to the teeth are transmitted by branches of the fifth cranial nerve, and dentists distinguish between odontalgia, or pain arising from effects on individual teeth, and neuralgia, in which pain may seem to arise in the teeth but is really from other conditions within the area of the face supplied by the same nerve, such as the nose and sinuses.

In odontalgia, disease of (or injury to) TEETH may expose the dental pulp, which is very sensitive to heat or cold and to the sweet, salt or acid constituents of food. Initially the pain is of a transitory twinge-like character, becoming more persistent and unbearable when the pulp becomes infected, inflamed, and begins to die. The usual cause is dental caries.

Gingivitis or inflammation of the gums leads to gum recession exposing the dentine below the necks of the teeth. This is particularly sensitive to stimulation by food substances which may produce severe pain and prolonged aching thereafter. The onset of toothache in any form is an indication to seek early dental treatment.

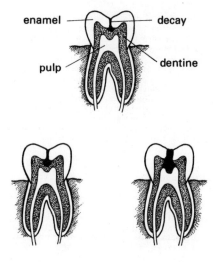

enamel — decay

pulp — dentine

Toothache

torticollis. See WRY NECK.

touch. The skin can feel and differentiate touch, pressure, pain, heat, and cold. Of these, touch is the sensation elicited by, for example, brushing the skin with a wisp of cotton wool or applying a stiff hair, and as a further refinement, sensitivity is tested by using hairs of graded thickness and determining which one is just felt when applied with just sufficient force to bend it.

Touch is appreciated by special skin receptors (Meissner's corpuscles) and these 'touch spots' are not evenly distributed over the body. They are most numerous over the tips of the fingers, palms, soles and lips, and less so over areas such as the back and shoulders. On their closeness depends discrimination or the ability to recognize whether any contact is single or multiple. This is tested by a device like a pair of mathematical dividers or compasses in which the distance between two points can be adjusted. The finger-tips can feel two separate contacts when the points are 1 mm. apart; over the back a separation of 5 cm. may be required.

The very sensitive areas of the skin are characterized by hairlessness, but elsewhere the skin surface bears hairs which are either obvious or rudimentary. Hairs always slant in a definite direction and touch-spots are found in the skin on their 'windward' side. Light contact with hair tips causes a sensation of touch since the hair acts like a tiny lever transmitting movement to its base and stimulating the touch receptor.

Sensations of touch travel from the receptors by nerves from the skin back to the spinal cord and thence upwards to the brain and its sensory centres.

Musicians attach importance to 'touch' as a refinement of technique, but physiologically this is dependent on the quite different sensory impressions conveyed by receptors in muscles and joints. These provide consciousness of position, timing, effort, and the relative position of different parts of the body.

Diseases. Alterations in skin sensitivity, of which touch is only one component, provides the neurologist with important diagnostic clues. Departures from normal may be (1) anaesthesia: loss of sensation, (2) hyperaesthesia: increased sensitivity or (3) paraesthesia: abnormal sensations such as burning, prickling or itching.

Each of these may be produced in many ways. Anaesthesia, for instance, may be caused by conditions as diverse as disease of the blood vessels of the brain or leprosy of cutaneous nerves; hyperaesthesia occurs in hysteria, the early stage of poliomyelitis, shingles, tabes, and often over inflamed underlying organs; paraesthesia is experienced in many skin diseases, in sciatica, and in degenerative conditions of the spinal cord. These are only given as examples; unexplained disorders of skin sensation require investigation.

tourniquet. Any appliance used to control haemorrhage from an injured limb by encircling it and applying pressure to its arterial blood-supply. There have been many different designs, usually named after their inventors, but most are now obsolete or becoming obsolete. Basically they provided a broad canvas band, tightened round the limb, and a pad which could be screwed down upon the main artery.

For first aid use a tourniquet can be improvised from a narrow-fold triangular bandage tied round the limb and tightened by passing a short rod through the knot and twisting. In surgical practice the principal devices now employed are (1) Samway's tubular rubber tourniquet, which is wound twice round the limb on the stretch and secured by the clip provided, and (2) Esmarch's elastic bandage, which is a rubber roller bandage applied under tension.

Tourniquets are dangerous pieces of equipment in unskilled hands. Left on for more than half-an-hour they will cause gangrene of the limb. They must be loosened at least once every thirty minutes to flush the limb with fresh blood, and only re-tightened if absolutely necessary. In most cases it will be found that clotting and retraction of injured vessels have either arrested the haemorrhage naturally, or have so reduced its force and volume that the slight pressure of a pad and bandage will be effective.

toxaemia. The presence or effects of poisonous substances in the blood-stream.

In bacterial toxaemia the multiplication of micro-organisms at some site of infection produces toxins which are then absorbed into the tissues and blood-stream with harmful results. These may be general, with fever, rigor, headache and vomiting, or related to individual tissues such as the heart or nervous system because of the special affinities of the particular toxin.

Non-bacterial toxaemia arises in a variety of ways from deficiency or failure either in the body's breakdown of food substances or in its excretion of waste products. Toxic substances are absorbed into or accumulate in the blood stream and exercise harmful effects either by their abnormal presence or by their abnormally high concentration. Examples are uraemia in kidney disease; hyperglycaemia and acetonaemia in diabetes; thyrotoxicosis in toxic goitre; and cholaemia in obstructive jaundice.

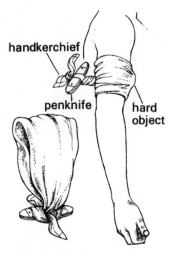

handkerchief

penknife

hard
object

An improvised tourniquet

toxic goitre. See GOITRE.

toxicology. The scientific study of POISONS, including their classification, action and identification, and the treatment of their effects. Medical or clinical toxicologists concentrate on the treatment of poisoning usually in special poisons units associated with a general hospital. The forensic toxicologist is concerned with the legal aspects of poisoning; it is he who determines whether the poisoning is essentially accidental, self-inflicted or felonious. Both depend greatly on help from chemists and pharmacologists.

toxin. Although the term is often used in a general way to include various harmful substances, toxins in the strict sense are poisons of complex protein nature produced by micro-organisms. Essentially they also act as antigens, i.e., they have the ability to induce the body to form specific antitoxins.

Toxins may be either exotoxins or endo-toxins. The former are external products of bacterial growth which diffuse into the medium in which the organism is growing. When absorbed into the circulation they cause specific effects as in diphtheria, tetanus, and botulism. Endotoxins are poisonous con-stituents of the actual organism, liberated when it dies or disintegrates as the result of its destruction by body-defences. Their effects are less specific and shown by fever and tissue-degeneration.

The distinction is a fundamental one in treatment because exotoxins can be neutral-ized by appropriate antitoxin but endotoxins can be removed only by eradication of the germ itself.

toxoid. Some pathogenic bacteria produce soluble TOXINS or exotoxins which diffuse into the surrounding tissues and enter the circulation to cause harmful effects throughout the body. When such organisms are grown artificially their exotoxins can also be detected in the laboratory tests.

Toxins also act as antigens. Their presence in the body brings about an immunity response and this normal defence mechanism results in the production of neutralizing antitoxin.

If toxins are mixed with formalin and incubated their toxicity is destroyed but their antigenic or immunizing properties are retained. Filtrates of bacterial cultures de-toxicated in this way are known as toxoids, formol toxoids, or anatoxines and can be injected to induce active immunity against various diseases, particularly diphtheria, tetanus, and gas-gangrene.

Toxoid can be further modified in order to lessen the risk of possible reactions, and to improve its immunizing properties. In the case of diphtheria, ordinary formol toxoid (FT) is also available as alum-precipitated toxoid (APT) and toxin-antitoxin floccules (TAF).

toxoplasmosis. Infection by *Toxoplasma gondi*, a protozoon, first discovered in paddy-birds in 1900 and now known to be a common parasite of many animals and birds. Human infection is perhaps mainly from cysts in meat but the parasite is easily destroyed by heating to 60 °C. (141 °F.) so cooking should protect. However, it has been shown that a large proportion of domestic cats harbour the organism in their intestinal tracts.

In the adult severe symptoms are not common, as resistance develops rapidly, and diagnosis depends on laboratory tests. There have, however, been cases with fever and swelling of glands, and a few of these cases have been fatal.

Congenital cases are common and more important. Here an infected and often symptomless mother passes infection to her unborn child. In early pregnancy the parasite invades the developing nervous system and may cause brain damage or even death. Later in pregnancy it may cause enlargement of the liver and spleen. After birth the affected child may have swollen lymph glands for a few weeks, or in more severe cases may have permanent damage to brain and eyes.

Preventive measures are as yet uncertain. It is generally assumed that expectant mothers and very young children should avoid intimate contact with sick animals and birds and should probably also avoid close contact with cats and kittens.

trachea. The trachea or windpipe is a tube of cartilage and membrane which provides a channel for the passage of air to and from the lungs. It is about 2 cm. in diameter and 10 cm. long and extends from the larynx in the neck downwards into the upper part of the chest where it divides into the right and left bronchi. Its cartilaginous elements are a series of some twenty rings, incomplete behind. Their purpose is to stiffen the wall of the tube and prevent its collapse, especially while breathing in.

The emergency operation known as tracheotomy may be required when there is obstruction of the air-passage in or above the level of the larynx. Tracheotomy is carried out by cutting into the trachea in the neck and inserting a tracheotomy tube.

tracheotomy. A surgical operation to provide an alternative airway directly into the trachea or wind-pipe in the lower neck. Tracheotomy (or tracheostomy) is required if there is dangerous difficulty in breathing due to obstruction of the upper air-passages. This may arise from foreign bodies, laryngeal oedema, diphtheria or tuberculous laryngitis, tumours of larynx or neck, and from some forms of laryngeal paralysis.

Surgical procedures on the mouth, tongue, pharynx or larynx sometimes require preliminary tracheotomy so that the airway may be packed off to prevent blood or septic matter from reaching the lungs.

In tracheotomy the skin and soft tissues are divided in the mid-line of the neck, the trachea incised and a special tube inserted (intubation). This has an inner sleeve that can be removed for cleaning.

A tracheotomy tube should be removed as soon as possible but some cases may require a permanent artificial opening. After a tube has been worn for some weeks the wound will heal with an established and well-defined track and patients soon learn to carry out routine management themselves and experience little inconvenience except from loss of voice, as air no longer traverses the larynx. Care must also be taken to avoid obstruction of the external opening by clothing.

trachoma. Severe, contagious inflammation of the membrane lining the eyelids, caused by a virus.

Trachoma is a disease of hot dry climates and therefore very rare in the U.K. The incubation period varies from four to seven days, and the inflammation, usually of both eyes, is generally mild at first and sometimes heals of its own accord without treatment. For some reason this spontaneous healing is commoner in children than in adults. More often the inflammation if untreated goes on to scarring of the eyelids, inability to close the eyes, and distortion of vision as a result of inflammatory tissue encroaching on the cornea.

Infection results from direct contact with eye discharges and is sometimes also spread by flies. High prevalence is associated with poor hygiene and crowded living conditions, and the disease is an immense problem in many under-developed countries. In other countries imported cases are occasionally seen, especially in sea-ports and amongst immigrants.

One attack confers no immunity to subsequent re-infection.

Unlike most virus diseases, trachoma responds well to treatment with either antibiotics or sulphonamides. The treatment most favoured nowadays is a combination of two antibiotics: one, e.g., sulphadiazine, by mouth for a fortnight in decreasing dosage, and the other, e.g., tetracycline, given as eyedrops or eye ointment. With early treatment the outlook is good.

In warm developing countries where the disease is common it may be desirable to apply an antibiotic ointment to the eyes of contacts for five days a month for several months. Such preventive treatment is costly, however, and contacts can be very numerous.

traction. In fractures of the long bones of the limbs and of the fingers or toes, the muscles are put out of balance and often move the broken ends of the bone out of alignment. Healing in this faulty position will produce serious shortening or misalignment, and so in treatment the limb must be supported in a suitable splint or cradle and the muscle-pull overcome by extension in order to secure correct reposition.

Application of longitudinal counter-force to extend the limb and reduce the displacement is known as traction, generally provided by means of a cord, pulley and weights, or by elastic. The main problem is how to attach the extension force to the limb.

In skeletal traction this is done by the use of pointed calipers, wires, or pins of various design, which grasp or penetrate the actual bone of the lower fragment, and so provide a secure anchorage for the extension. This method is particularly required to oppose powerful muscle-groups as in thigh fractures. In skin traction the extension apparatus is attached to the skin of the limb by means of adhesive strapping.

The principle of traction also has other applications in the treatment of various bone and joint conditions when it is desired to rest the parts in a good position, to relieve pain, and to promote healing. Spinal fractures, 'slipped disc' and tuberculous hip-disease are examples.

traffic accidents. See ACCIDENTS.

traffic medicine. Casualties from traffic ACCIDENTS constitute a major part of the work of the emergency admission department of any general hospital. They are an enormous source of individual distress and a formidable social evil, but they also pose great problems for hospital administrators in terms of finance, physical resources, and suitably trained staff. In dealing with an ordinary admission a surgeon is normally faced with a single problem, but the traffic accident case may show a multiplicity of typical effects such as head-injury, damage to the face and jaw, crushed chest, ruptured abdominal organs, limb-fractures and other relatively straight-forward orthopaedic conditions, any or all of which may demand separate treatment of a highly specialized kind, if the patient is to be assured of survival or of a good recovery.

To minimize such difficulties public co-operation is essential and much can be done to relieve the present situation by a safety-first attitude of mind on the part of drivers and pedestrians alike, by sensible behaviour (e.g., having one's drink after driving and not before driving, stopping for a rest when tired, and trying to avoid driving when emotionally upset) and by the observance of sensible precautions such as the wearing of crash-helmets and the use of seat-belts.

trance. A state of profound or abnormal sleep, from which an affected individual cannot easily be roused, and not due to any organic disease or drugs. There is loss of voluntary movement, but consciousness and sensibility may be unaffected. Such a condition is particularly associated with hysteria, a psychoneurotic disease, in which symptoms of illness are assumed (albeit unconsciously) in order to secure some advantage. A trance represents therefore an extreme attempt to escape from some awkward real-life situation.

Stuporous conditions are common in mental disease and the problem in relation to diagnosis and treatment is to differentiate a trance which is a symptom of hysteria from similar manifestations in true psychosis like schizophrenia. This is a matter for expert assessment based on careful study of the patient's past and detailed observation. Hysterical and psychotic trance states have very different outlooks. Hysteria is likely to yield to effective psychotherapy, but in psychotic illness there are basic disorders much less easy to overcome.

tranquillizers. Ideally, a tranquillizer is a drug capable of allaying feelings of tension, worry, anxiety, restlessness and panic without impairing normal alertness and intellectual capacity. It is therefore expected to have a selective action on brain-function and this was largely lacking in the hypnotic or sleep-inducing drugs available before 1950, although a start had been made in developing barbiturates and other sedatives. Since then there has been a veritable explosion of synthetic psychotropic ('mind-altering') drugs each with its particular properties and place in therapeutics.

There is now a wide choice and the sedative range of such drugs has been classified by the World Health Organization as follows: (1) Hypno-sedatives: barbiturates; carbromol BP; glutethimide BP; methyprylone BP. (2) Tranquillo-sedatives: benzodiazepine type; propanediol type; diphenylmethane type. (3) Minor tranquillizers: phenothiazine derivatives such as promazine and promethazine. (4) Major tranquillizers: phenothiazine derivatives such as chlorpromazine and chlorprothixene; reserpine; butyrophenones.

Barbiturates are widely used for mild symptoms but often an adequate dose causes sleepiness or incoordination. The benzodiazepines induce tranquillity without much sedation. Chloropromazine is particularly used in the treatment of mental illness, especially schizophrenia and depressive states, but is probably not as effective as drugs of the benzodiazepine type in anxiety states.

The scientific names of all these drugs are very confusing. The following are some trade equivalents in the various groups now so widely prescribed and known that they have practically become household words: (1) Hypno-sedatives: Luminal, Gardenal, Medinal, Nembutal, Carbrital, Doriden, Noludar. (2) Tranquillo-sedatives: Librium, Valium, Mogadon, Miltown, Atarax. (3) Minor tranquillizers: Sparine, Phenergan. (4) Major tranquillizers: Largactil, Taractan, Serpasil, Harmomyl, Serenace.

transfusion, blood. See BLOOD TRANSFUSION.

transplant. Any tissue or organ transferred from one individual to another. The rectification of disabilities by the replacement of diseased parts is an attractive and logical idea. Transplant surgery has therefore developed considerably in recent years, but the difficulties are formidable and of three kinds: (1) limitations of surgical technique; (2) the tendency of the body to reject tissue which its immune-system regards as 'foreign'; and (3) the supply of sufficient healthy tissue or organs to ensure that reasonably well-matched material, in fresh condition, can be provided promptly when required. Blood-transfusion is a form of transplantation and its early success came about because these difficulties were minimal. It was easy to carry out; blood-types could be matched very exactly; and donors were readily available because they did not suffer and were able to regenerate what they donated.

Popular interest in transplantation has centred on more spectacular examples, such as heart and lung replacement, but some simpler procedures are becoming routine. The grafting of non-cellular tissues is relatively easy because they do not cause rejection reactions, and they are readily accepted by the living tissues of the recipient and become incorporated in their new position. Included in this category of transplant surgery (using healthy tissue from someone who has recently died) are the grafting of blood-vessels, heart-valves and bone, and also corneal replacement.

The other large field with a considerable unsatisfied need is in kidney transplantation, still limited by problems of matching, rejection, and the supply of suitable organs. The matching problem is being tackled by a computer-system, Eurotransplant, which retains a record of the tissue-characteristics of patients awaiting a transplant, and selects for operation the one who most closely matches an available kidney. The use of immuno-suppressive drugs and sera depress rejection responses, but an accurate match is of prime consideration because immuno-suppressive measures have the undesirable effect of simultaneously lessening body-defences against other infection. In the U.K. the problem of supply of kidneys has given rise to the Kidney Donor Scheme, which seeks to improve the supply of kidneys, usually taken from young healthy subjects who have died suddenly in accidents.

Heart transplantation gives rise to argument in respect of two of its aspects. Firstly, determination of the exact point of death: it is important that the heart be removed from the body of the donor immediately after death, and this being so, some people claim that, if a national celebrity is in urgent need of a transplant, there may be a temptation to expedite the death of the fatally injured victim of a traffic accident. Secondly, the expenditure of professional time: apart from follow-up, a heart transplant occupies a team of about seven doctors and nine nurses for the best part of a fortnight; some thinkers hold that, when most hospitals have long lists of patients awaiting less complicated treatment and in some cases dying for lack of such treatment, the heavy expenditure of staff time on one patient is unjustifiable.

The replacement of damaged parts of the body by structures made of metal silicone or plastic is known as SPARE-PART SURGERY.

transvestism. A form of PERVERSION or sexual deviation characterized by the wearing of clothes appropriate to the opposite sex, and by the adoption of social and sexual behaviour conforming to the outward appearance so achieved. See HOMOSEXUALITY.

trauma. A Greek word which means 'wound' and hence used in medicine to designate the effect on the body of any harmful external agency including violence, chemical substances, and physical phenomena such as heat, cold and radiation. By analogy the term has also become extended and qualified as 'emotional trauma', a term which embraces the ill-effects resulting from disturbing mental experiences which may be the root cause of psychoneurotic disorders.

travel sickness. Sensations of nausea, sometimes accompanied by actual vomiting, produced in susceptible persons by the irregular or rhythmical movements to which the body is subjected during travel in vehicles,

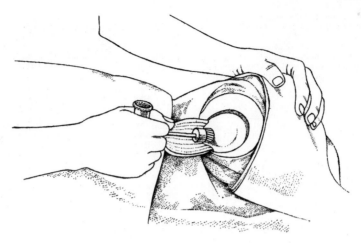

A flap of skin is folded back to reveal the skull before a disc of bone is removed by the trephine

ships or aircraft. It is due to the effect on the central nervous system of excessive stimuli received from the semi-circular canals (a balancing mechanism forming the labyrinth of the inner ear) especially if these conflict with impressions received from the eyes or other sense organs.

The well-known symptoms consist of a feeling of insecurity and visual disorientation, with dizziness, headache, loss of appetite, nausea, vomiting, double vision, and ultimately signs of shock, such as pallor, sweating, and prostration. The importance of visual stimulation is shown by the fact that very susceptible persons can become sea-sick on dry land merely from the sight of wave-movements. An attack closely resembles migraine, and migraine sufferers are generally bad travellers. Apprehension, anticipation, cold, travel smells and the sight of other victims all help to induce an attack.

Fresh air, or good ventilation, is very important, while for sea-sickness to lie down near the centre of the ship in a darkened cabin may help delay onset or minimize effects. Many effective sedatives are now available but travellers who have taken such drugs should be cautious about driving a car within four hours.

tremor. Involuntary muscular trembling or quivering, usually most obvious in the limbs, where alternate contractions of muscle-groups and their anatomical antagonists produce oscillations either general or limited in extent. Tremor may be physiological: shivering, for instance, is a normal reaction to cold or infection since muscular activity generates heat and warms the body; it also occurs when the body is tensed by nervous anticipation as in athletes and racehorses.

Otherwise, tremor is pathological; it may be caused by disease, such as multiple sclerosis, paralysis agitans, dementia paralytica, encephalitis, poliomyelitis, and certain brain diseases. Toxic effects on the nervous system cause tremor, as in alcoholism, metallic poisoning, hyperthyroidism, pernicious anaemia, vitamin B deficiency, many infections, and often in conditions of debility.

The type of tremor may provide diagnostic help. It may be either 'fine' or 'coarse', the former more easily felt than seen. It may be induced by voluntary effort ('intention tremor'), as in multiple sclerosis, or inhibited when purposeful movements are made, as in chorea.

Treatment depends on the cause. Toxaemic tremors improve when toxaemia is removed or corrected but tremors caused by nervous disease present more difficulty. Advances have been made by the development of new drugs of which levodopa has achieved notable success in the management of PARKINSON'S DISEASE

trephine. A special type of bone-saw used for opening the skull by removal of a circular disc of bone. Basically it is a hollow steel cylinder one end of which is formed as a ring of saw-teeth extending upwards on the outside of the cylinder. At the other end is a cross-handle by which the cutting-edge can be rotated against the bone.

This rather old-fashioned instrument is laborious and difficult to use and has largely been superseded by electrically driven burrs and osteotomes (bone cutting tools). Larger areas of bone can be removed by drilling a succession of burr-holes and dividing the intervening bridges of bone by a flexible thread-saw.

trichinosis. A disease produced by the nematode worm *Trichinella spiralis,* a parasite of swine and many wild animals including rats. Human infection is mainly from undercooked pork or pork products containing living worm-cysts. In the intestine, encysted larvae mature to adult worms. These produce new larvae which migrate and encyst in muscles and organs of the human host.

Symptoms are mainly gastro-intestinal, but these are followed by oedema and nettle rash, and the affected muscles become painful, tender, and hard; swallowing, speech and respiration are also affected. In severe cases, fever, toxaemia and cardio-respiratory paralysis may lead to coma and death. Unless the disease is suspected, the diagnosis is easily missed, but it is confirmed by blood tests and laboratory investigation of muscle tissue.

Treatment is largely a matter of dealing with symptoms but vermicidal drugs should be given to destroy worms still in the intestine. Prevention is all important. Although natural distribution of the disease is world-wide it is now rare in most developed countries through control of pig raising (boiling swill; rat eradication, etc.), meat inspection and adequate cooking. However, in the U.S.A., with its rural population, it is said that 1 in 20 post mortem examinations still show evidence of past infection.

trigeminal neuralgia. The trigeminal (fifth cranial) nerve provides sensory fibres to face and scalp and motor fibres to the muscles of the jaw. Neuralgia is paroxysmal pain radiating in the area supplied by a sensory nerve and it frequently affects the trigeminal nerve to produce the condition sometimes known as tic douloureux.

This occurs mainly in older people and causes recurrent pain, which may be distressing and incapacitating, together with tenderness of face and scalp, often concentrated on eyebrow, nose and chin over the sites of the nerve branches. The condition is not fully explained, but it tends to be related to cold, damp, debility and overwork, and may be connected with the blood supply.

In treatment, potential causes such as decaying teeth or sinus infection should first be checked. If pain persists regular use of suitable analgesics is required. More radical surgical procedures are also available. These include injection of the nerve with alcohol or local anaesthetic, and severing the sensory nerve root.

tropical diseases. Conditions particularly prevalent in tropical countries or only found in such countries. A few of these diseases are wholly tropical infections, e.g., the tsetse fly that carries the organism of sleeping sickness does not breed in temperatures below 25 °C. (77 °F.). Many are infections which can occur anywhere but have been wholly or largely stamped out by preventive measures in temperate countries with adequate resources: malaria, cholera and leprosy are examples. Some are not infectious at all but diseases of malnutrition, e.g., pellagra, kwashiorkor and beri-beri. In other words the diseases commonly termed 'tropical' are in part due to climatic conditions under which various organisms (and the mosquitoes, flies, ticks, mites, fleas and lice that carry them) can breed easily; in part due to ignorance, poor hygiene and absence of preventive measures, in part due to poverty; and in large measure due to a combination of these factors.

For the visitor to a tropical country, some precautions are obvious. Where the particular infections are still prevalent, vaccination is advisable against cholera, yellow fever, the typhoid group of fevers, poliomyelitis and tetanus. Appropriate antimalarial drugs should be taken when visiting malaria-infested areas (and for some weeks afterwards) and mosquito-nets should be used. Unless the water supply is known to be safe, as it now is in most large centres of population, water should be boiled or otherwise sterilized before being drunk or being used to wash food utensils. Care should be exercised in respect of all food that is not going to be thoroughly cooked. The danger of bites from snakes and poisonous spiders can be reduced by keeping feet and legs adequately protected. It is inadvisable to bathe in inland waters without assurance of their safety.

To prevent or treat tropical diseases occurring in the indigenous population is an enormous problem. Essentially it involves three things: (1) money, because schools, clinics, sewerage systems, agricultural machinery, etc. are all costly; (2) general education, e.g., with a view to improving agriculture and horticulture; and (3) health education to combat ignorance and harmful tradition.

Tropical diseases form a vast speciality and it is only possible to mention some illustrative examples, some of which are separately described elsewhere under their own headings.

1. Nutritional: beri-beri; kwashiorkor; pellagra.

2. Bacterial and viral: smallpox; cholera; plague (fleas); yellow fever (mosquitoes); leprosy; yaws; tularaemia (deer fly); relapsing fever (ticks); typhus (lice and ticks); typhoid fever; bacillary dysentery.

3. Protozoan: malaria (mosquitoes); kala-azar (flies); sleeping sickness (tsetse flies); amoebic dysentery.

4. Metazoan. Important metazoan parasites are mainly worms of three classes: (1) trematodes (with adhesive suckers): fluke infestation; schistosomiasis or bilharziasis (blood fluke disease); (2) cestodes (ribbon-like): many species of tapeworm; (3) nematodes (thread-like): ankylostomiasis (hook-worm disease); filariasis (elephantiasis from mosquito-borne worms in lymph-channels); dracontiasis (guinea-worm under the skin – spread by cyclops, a small crustacean, in water supplies); Calabar swelling (subcutaneous infestation by mangrove flies); oncocerciasis (subcutaneous nodules caused by flies).

In the conquest of tropical diseases it has to be remembered that the introduction of methods and attitudes from advanced countries is not wholly a gain. There is some loss as well as much profit: for instance, as yaws declines syphilis increases, as leprosy becomes rare tuberculosis becomes commoner, and as malnutrition recedes the diseases of obesity begin to appear.

truss. A surgical appliance designed to give support to the site of a HERNIA (rupture), and to prevent its contents from protruding again after they have been replaced.

Design varies according to the site and size of the hernia, but the device is commonly used for the retention of inguinal, femoral, or umbilical hernias.

In adults, such treatment is merely for comfort, and an operation to cure the condition is generally preferable unless indicated inadvisable by age, ill-health, or the technical difficulties of securing a satisfactory result. In infants with inguinal or umbilical hernias the continuous use of truss for some time may eventually lead to a permanent cure.

trypanosome. A protozoan parasite conveyed to man and animals by bites from infected tsetse flies. Trypanosomes are found in the blood-stream (haemoflagellates) and appear as elongated organisms (30 to 50 microns), which can move by means of a 'keel-like' undulatory

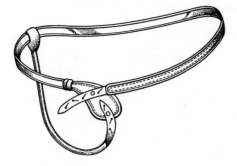

Truss for inguinal hernia of the right side

membrane and a flagellum or tail. They cause trypanosomiasis or SLEEPING SICKNESS of which there are three types, each with a well-defined geographical distribution: (1) Gambian or West African sleeping sickness, due to *Trypanosoma gambiense;* (2) Rhodesian, due to *T. rhodesiense;* (3) South American or Chaga's disease, due to *T. cruzi.*

trypanosomiasis. See SLEEPING SICKNESS.

tsetse fly. A biting and blood-sucking fly of Central Africa. The name includes various species of the genus *Glossina* which are of great importance because of their role in the spread of TRYPANOSOMES (which cause SLEEPING SICKNESS) to man and domestic animals from the many kinds of wild animals which harbour the parasites.

West African sleeping-sickness is spread by *Gl. palpalis* and *Gl. tachinoides* and the Rhodesian variety by *Gl. morsitans* and *Gl. swynnertoni.*

The prevention of sleeping sickness (trypanosomiasis) depends on tsetse fly control and on measures to avoid being bitten, such as fly-proofing and protective clothing. The tsetse fly mainly bites by day, so journeys across fly-infested country should be undertaken at night.

tuberculin. Robert Koch (1843-1910), a German bacteriologist and discoverer of the tubercle bacillus, found that the fluid in which the bacilli grew contained their toxins in solution. He gave the name tuberculin to the thick yellowish fluid (Koch's lymph) which he obtained after filtering off the organisms. This old tuberculin is now prepared as a sterilized liquid containing the standardized growth products of the tubercle bacillus, but some modifications have since been developed. The various products containing tuberculin are used in the diagnosis of tuberculosis both in man and animals and also to a diminishing extent in treatment.

For a tuberculin test a standard quantity of tuberculin is injected into the skin. In non-tuberculous subjects no effect is produced (tuberculin-negative), but with pre-existing infection an inflammatory reaction results (tuberculin-positive).

tuberculosis. A communicable disease resulting from infection by the tubercle bacillus, *Mycobacterium tuberculosis,* of which there are four types – human, bovine, avian and piscine; only the first two usually affect man. As phthisis or pulmonary tuberculosis it is particularly likely to affect the lungs, but may

affect any part of the body. Lymph-glands (scrofula), bones and joints, skin (lupus vulgaris), nervous system (tuberculous meningitis) and larynx are all common sites, as are the intestinal, urinary and reproductive systems.

The disease is contracted by inhaling bacilli from an existing case, or by mouth from contaminated food, especially untreated milk. The bacillus was discovered by Robert Koch (1843-1910), a German bacteriologist, and from among many other distinguished workers special mention must also be made of Karl Ranke (1870-1926) of Munich, whose classification of the evolutionary stages of tuberculosis contributed significantly both to our understanding of the disease and to its clinical management.

As a first stage, a small inflammatory patch forms (the primary focus), usually in a lung but sometimes in the intestine or in a tonsil. The neighbouring lymph glands may become swollen but there are no other symptoms, and in course of time the primary focus becomes surrounded by fibrous tissue and shrinks to a small scar, When the disease was widespread (as it still is in many countries) most people developed the primary foci. The scar could be seen on x-ray examination and the TUBERCULIN test would indicate that the persons had been infected and had developed a defensive reaction. The person was not ill and was not infectious to others.

In the minority of cases the primary focus does not become walled off. Instead organisms spread through the lungs ('galloping consumption') or spread by the blood stream to various parts of the body (causing generalized or miliary tuberculosis, or tuberculosis of bones or joints, or occasionally tuberculous meningitis).

In yet other cases the walling off process starts but a sort of drawn battle ensues. The body develops sufficient resistance to prevent galloping consumption or miliary tuberculosis, but in the lung the pockets of infection (from the initial primary focus or from further infection) enlarge, forming cavities in the lung, with the development of such symptoms as fever, sweating at night, cough and loss of weight. In the absence of effective treatment the person, especially if young, may go downhill fairly quickly or, especially if elderly, may for years have practically no symptoms except a cough. In either case he is infectious to others.

Which of these three results will happen in a particular case depends on various factors. Some of these are: (1) the quantity of invading bacilli: most people have the bodily defence to ward off a few bacilli, but close and repeated contact with a highly infectious person may convert the invaders from a squad to an army, especially if the contact occurs in conditions of overcrowding and bad ventilation; (2) the body's health and capacity to resist: malnutrition greatly lowers this capacity, as do simultaneous illness and deep-seated grief; (3) age: in general susceptibility is greatest at 18 to 35 years (as Hippocrates pointed out 2400 years ago) and lowest in the middle-aged; (4) racial or family resistance or susceptibility: the disease was long deemed hereditary but it probably occurs in families mainly because one member infects another, and even the alleged

Reduction in tuberculosis before antibiotics in England and Wales
(deaths in thousands)

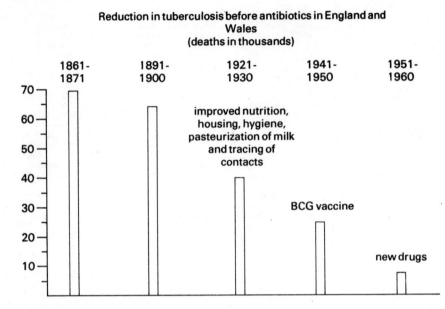

susceptibility of some races may be explicable mainly on grounds of malnutrition.

In most infectious diseases invading bacteria either win rapidly or lose, but tuberculosis is different. Despite its activity in galloping consumption and tuberculous meningitis the bacillus is usually fairly inactive, but it has a waxy coat which in part protects it from the body's defences. So it often causes little in the way of symptoms unless the patient's health declines from some other cause such as malnutrition or another respiratory disease; but though quiescent it nevertheless remains alive. Before the era of effective drug treatment it was rightly said that 'tuberculosis is never cured but only halted'.

Bones and glands. While the usual focus of infection is in the lung, so that 'tuberculosis' in ordinary speech generally means 'pulmonary tuberculosis', the disease can also affect bones, usually at or near joints: the spine (Pott's disease), hips, knees, ankles, shoulders and elbows are most commonly affected. Where joints are involved, the term used is tuberculous arthritis; bone disease alone is tuberculous osteomyelitis, and infection of lymph glands is tuberculous adenitis.

Either the human or the bovine organism can cause any form of tuberculosis, but it used to be held that the human type, mostly breathed in, usually selected the lungs, and that the bovine type, mostly drunk in infected milk or eaten in infected uncooked meat, affected bones and joints more often. Certainly, in countries with pasteurization and similar measures for the partial sterilization of milk, and policies for eradication of tuberculosis from cattle, tuberculosis of bones and joints has become a rarity.

Prevalence. Rightly called the 'captain of the men of death' tuberculosis in the nineteenth century caused one fifth of all deaths in developed countries like the U.K., and its dramatic reduction in such countries is due to a combination of social amelioration, health education and preventive measures, rather than to treatment. In less highly developed countries it is still common, and increasing, and is beginning to replace malaria as the biggest killing disease. It still infects at least fifty million people a year in the world, mostly in countries with a combination of poverty, overcrowding, malnutrition and rapidly growing population, and it causes about three million deaths annually.

Treatment. Until the middle of this century there was no specific treatment for pulmonary tuberculosis. Sanatorium treatment relied mainly on physical rest (complete bed rest at first, followed by carefully graded amounts of exercise), on absence of emotional and mental stress, on provision of a good and attractive diet, on ample fresh air (though its value was exaggerated) and, where appropriate, on artificial pneumothorax to collapse all or part of an affected lung and so facilitate its rest. Similarly the treatment of tuberculosis of bones and joints relied chiefly on immobilization of the affected parts in plaster to limit further damage and to promote healing. These treatments, continued for about a couple of years, resulted in a fair proportion of recoveries. As for acute miliary tuberculosis it was regarded as almost always fatal, while tuberculous meningitis was always fatal.

The development of sulphonamides (1935) and penicillin (1941) gave physicians drugs which were active against many infections. It was a disappointment that they did not influence tuberculosis, still a widespread and dreaded disease. However, by 1944 intensified research produced streptomycin which proved active against the tubercle bacillus. Unfortunately there were some difficulties in its use because the bacilli tended to develop drug resistance and some patients showed toxic effects. By 1946 para-amino-salicylic acid (PAS) was discovered and the effectiveness of this was first reported to the Scandinavian Congress on Tuberculosis at Copenhagen in June, 1948. A further development shortly afterwards was isoniazid, not only very potent but readily diffusible, and so able to reach infective sites.

It was found that the use of one drug alone rapidly leads to the emergence of resistant bacilli so treatment schedules now depend on suitable combinations. Still more new drugs continue to be produced. The selection of a suitable regimen is a matter for the chest-physician; he must consider the patient's progress, any evidence of drug intolerance, and the result of sensitivity tests on the particular organism harboured. In a relapse or with multiple drug resistance it may become necessary to prescibe 'second-line' or 'reserve' drugs, and many are available. In developed countries tuberculosis now seldom kills. For instance, as late as 1946, in England and Wales, 900 girls aged 15 to 25 years died from tuberculosis, as compared with 9 in 1961. Yet drugs, while reducing deaths, have not reduced cases. The reduction of tuberculosis is primarily due to prevention.

Prevention. Although appropriate drugs for treatment are available in many hospitals in India and Pakistan, over 2 per cent of the population develop tuberculosis each year; and although no specific treatment was available until after 1945 there was a remarkable decrease in tuberculosis in Scandinavian countries and to some extent in the U.K. before that time. In other words, the reduction of tuberculosis in developed countries has depended primarily on prevention, rather than on treatment, and this will also be the case in countries where tuberculosis is still widespread.

Reduction of malnutrition has played the biggest part in combating tuberculosis. In the U.K., for instance, the submerged tenth (below subsistence level) of the nineteenth century rose to nearer a submerged fifth in Glasgow, Tyneside and South Wales in the massive unemployment of the early 1930s, and tuberculosis increased steadily, until Glasgow and adjacent counties had the highest tuberculosis rates in Europe with the possible exception of Spain; this was followed by a dramatic fall over the next twenty-five years as undernutrition decreased. Again, reduction of overcrowding has contributed enormously: in towns that vigorously replaced slums with corporation housing (like Barnsley in England and Aberdeen in Scotland) the disease dwindled. Not least, health education has made its contribution both by the primitive but accurate line of emphasizing that 'Spitting spreads disease' and through the advice of health visitors on budgeting and nutritional requirements and on matters like the importance of fresh air. In industry, attention to occupational hazards has helped. Pasteurization of milk and persuasion of the public to use it has greatly reduced tuberculosis of bones and joints. By 1951, when BCG was not yet available and when the new drugs for treatment were still in their infancy, the number of deaths from tuberculosis in England and Wales was 13,000, as compared with thrice that number even seventeen years earlier, and the number of notifications had fallen to 45,000 in the year.

As the prevalence of tuberculosis declined in developed countries two further measures became available: (1) mass radiography, i.e., efforts to persuade entire communities to accept x-ray examination in the hope of identifying the relatively few undetected carriers of the disease, with, in some areas, as much as three-quarters of the entire adult population being persuaded to accept the examination; and (2) the offer of BCG vaccination to children aged 13 years and also to such new born infants as were deemed at special risk. By 1971 in England and Wales the number of deaths had fallen from the 13,000 mentioned above to just over 1300, and notifications in the year were down to 11,000. A problem, however, has arisen among immigrants in Britain and other developed countries: frequently undernourished in their strange new country, sometimes having a higher susceptibility to tuberculosis, and often living in overcrowded conditions, they suffer from about twelve times the proportion of tuberculosis found in indigenous citizens.

tularaemia. A specific infectious disease, primarily of wild animals, but also affecting man in North America, the U.S.S.R., parts of Europe, and Japan. It is transmitted by biting arthropods, particularly the deer-fly (*Chrysops discalis*), by ticks, and in Sweden by the mosquito *Aedes cinereus*. Infection may result also from handling infected carcases, and from eating imperfectly cooked rabbit-meat or contaminated water.

It is due to a bacterium, *Pasteurella tularensis*. The incubation period is one to ten days and the onset is sudden, with chills, fever and prostration. Bites usually ulcerate and there may be enlargement or suppuration of lymph-glands. Untreated cases run a long-continued varying fever with a 5 per cent death rate, but antibiotic treatment is effective and one attack protects. Both live and killed vaccines are available.

Apart from direct infection during hunting and other open-air activities, cases occur in rabbit-handlers since infection persists even after refrigeration. Precautions should be taken against bites, and against casual infection from wild meat and water. An alternative name is deer-fly fever.

tumours. The term tumour is often used to mean any localized swelling, but strictly it should be applied only to growths of new tissue (neoplasms) and not to cysts, inflammatory swellings or simple hypertrophy.

Development of new cells is a normal occurrence, as when tissues grow to repair an injury, or a muscle enlarges to cope with repeated extra strain. Tumours, however, consist of cells that on microscopic examination often display abnormal or primitive characteristics (and are sometimes described as 'normal cells gone wrong'); in general they multiply much faster than do normal cells and are in no way an advantage to the body.

Benign or innocent tumours. These develop singly or, very rarely, in small groups; they displace adjacent tissues by size and pressure but do not infiltrate them, and they do not give rise to secondary growths (metastases). Examples are uterine fibroids and nasal polypi. Benign tumours usually have definite walls, so that their removal is relatively easy. Depending on their situation these neoplasms may cause no symptoms or cause symptoms only by pressure, e.g., a tumour situated on the root of a spinal nerve will gradually compress the soft spinal cord and so lead to paralysis.

As long as they do not produce symptoms through pressure and do not become unbearably unsightly, these tumours can be left in reasonable safety, although in a small proportion of cases an initially benign tumour later becomes malignant. If removal is desired, because of symptoms or appearance or fear of future malignancy, the surgical operation is normally straightforward, and there is no danger of secondaries and little chance of recurrence.

Malignant tumours. On the other hand this type of neoplasm infiltrates adjacent tissues, for example producing ulcers by breaking down subcutaneous tissues and skin, and the cells tend to travel by the lymphatic vessels or the blood vessels to create secondary tumours in other parts of the body. For fuller details, see CANCER.

twilight sleep. A popular name for a regime of sedation and analgesia once much used to allay anxiety and diminish pain during the first stage of labour. The drugs used were scopolamine and morphine given by injection under the skin and repeated at intervals according to the progress of labour and the condition of the patient. Although this form of treatment helped the mother it suffered from the great disadvantage that it also depressed the child's respiratory centre making it difficult to ensure resuscitation and natural breathing.

It has now largely been abandoned in favour of safer methods of analgesia.

twins. A pair of individuals whose birth results from the same pregnancy. The average frequency of twins in the general population is about once in ninety confinements but a tendency to bear twins is inherited and in some races and in some individual families the incidence may be considerably greater.

Twins are of two types. Normally the ovaries release only one ovum during each menstrual cycle but when two or more are released each may be fertilized separately and a corresponding number of embryos will develop. Double or multiple ovulation may occur naturally but it is also particularly likely to happen if pituitary hormones or other 'fertility drugs' are being employed to stimulate ovarian activity for the treatment of infertility. If two separate ova are thus fertilized the result is fraternal, binovular or dizygotic twins. The ova are often released a month apart, so that one twin is really a month younger than the other, although they are born the same day. Whether really of the same age or not, fraternal twins are not necessarily of the same sex and are no more alike than are children of the same parents born at different times.

If, however, a single ovum is fertilized and during subsequent development it divides into two, this will produce identical, monovular, or monozygotic twins, with an identical genetic inheritance and resembling each other so closely in bodily and mental characteristics that they are difficult to distinguish. They do, however, have individual finger print patterns. The study of identical twins, especially where they have chanced to experience different environment in their early years, can do much

to differentiate the influence of nature and nurture, since all differences in their personalities, careers and even diseases are clearly the result of factors affecting them after birth.

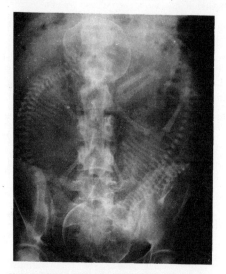

X-ray of twins in the womb: their heads can be seen at the top and bottom of the picture, and their spinal columns on either side.

If this division into two separate embryos should not be complete, the result is undifferentiated or Siamese twins which are joined together to a variable extent. In many examples of this abnormality the degree to which organs are shared may mean that either one or both twins cannot survive, but many examples of surgical separation have been recorded. In some instances survival of one twin can only be achieved by sacrifice of the other.

The most famous examples of Siamese twins (and hence the name) were Chang and Eng Bunker born in Thailand in 1811, who lived to the age of 62. They were however, only joined superficially at the chest by a cartilaginous band and their separation would have been a simple procedure for modern surgical technique although it would have ruined an outstanding career as circus freaks.

Twins may present some problems of upbringing. Initially they may be small and difficult to rear because of their tendency to be born prematurely. If they are breast-fed a mother will seldom have sufficient milk for both and complementary feeds will generally be required. In most instances the exigencies of the situation with its large demands on maternal time and energy will make it desirable to resort entirely to artificial feeding with careful supervision of the intake of food, vitamins and iron.

There is also a great tendency to treat twins as a unit rather than as two individuals and to enhance their appeal and emphasize their similarity by dressing and treating them exactly alike. This is psychologically unwise. Each should be given a chance to acquire an individual personality with individual interests, accomplishments and friends. They should not be ostentatiously compared with each other to the disadvantage of one because this will inevitably engender feelings of inferiority.

tympanites. Distension of the abdomen from the presence of gas in the intestines (from the Greek word *tympanon,* meaning a drum). This may be either trivial or grave. Transient and insignificant cases are due to flatulence (commonly experienced with dyspepsia, gastritis and enteritis) and are also produced by over-consumption of fizzy drinks and fermentable foodstuffs, and by the nervous habit of air-swallowing. Appropriate dietary measures and carminative drugs usually bring relief.

More serious cases are the result of impaired intestinal function, resulting from obstruction, surgical shock after abdominal operations, local toxaemia as in typhoid fever, or general toxaemia caused by pneumonia or other infections. Cessation or reduction of intestinal movements from such causes is known as paralytic ileus and distension is aggravated by the proliferation of gas-forming organisms in the bowel. Treatment depends upon the exact cause. Obstruction requires operation but other measures available include enemas to encourage intestinal activity and the injection of muscle stimulants.

typhoid. The enteric fevers include both typhoid and PARATYPHOID fevers, which are specific infections caused by swallowing bacteria of the *Salmonella* group. Similar organisms are associated with certain types of food poisoning, but both *S. typhi* and *S. paratyphi* (A, B, and C) cause disease which has well-defined clinical characteristics. Paratyphoid fever differs from typhoid in being a less severe illness of different incubation period.

Both diseases are frequently seen in epidemic form. Infection is derived from patients or CARRIERS and is spread by contaminated water or food. Shellfish, raw vegetables and unwashed fruit, and milk and milk products are often involved and flies may act as carriers between infected excreta and food awaiting consumption. Even tinned foods have been incriminated as a result of faulty processing. Carriers are a particular danger as food-handlers, and are also a risk to water-supplies. Enteric fevers have a world-wide distribution and are common in undeveloped countries with primitive sanitary arrangements.

In typhoid fever an incubation period of about two weeks (the range is from five days to over three weeks) is followed by an insidious onset with general discomfort, lassitude, abdominal uneasiness and increasing tempera-ture with relatively slow pulse. Organisms within the bowel invade the lymphoid tissue (Peyer's patches) of the intestine and soon spread to the blood stream as a bacteraemia. This wide-spread infection is shown in the second week by continued temperature, the occasional appearance of a few pink spots, enlargement of the spleen, increased intestinal disorder (pea-soup stools) and prostration, wasting, delirium, heart weakness, and other signs of severe blood poisoning. Intestinal haemorrhage or perforation may also occur and these contribute substantially to the death-rate, which may reach 20 per cent. In the third

week temperature declines and symptoms abate, but convalescence is prolonged and relapses frequent. Bacteria may persist in faeces or urine for months and 2 to 5 per cent of cases may become permanent carriers.

Clinical diagnosis is often difficult: the disease can resemble various other conditions. However, if typhoid is suspected, the organism can be grown in a bacteriological laboratory and after the first few days blood tests become practicable.

Treatment in the past consisted mainly of skilled nursing and attention to symptoms, but in recent years the development of appropriate antibiotics has both reduced the number of deaths and shortened the course of the disease. The disease is notifiable in virtually all countries and patients are normally isolated in hospitals for infectious diseases.

Preventive measures include purification of water supplies; sanitation, fly-control; super-vision of the processing, preparation and serving of food in public eating-places; control of shellfish; washing of food eaten raw; discovery and supervision of carriers; and health education of the public in general and food handlers in particular. These measures between them have virtually eradicated typhoid in many of the developed countries, although a century ago it was the commonest of all fevers.

Specific vaccine protection is available by TAB vaccine. Travellers to countries in which the disease is still endemic should ensure that they observe this precaution with a primary course reinforced at not less than three-year intervals by subsequent injections.

typhoid carrier. A 'carrier' is a person who continues to harbour organisms of an infectious disease but displays no signs or symptoms of the disease.

The carrier state is particularly common after typhoid fever: between 2 and 5 per cent of cases after clinical recovery continue to discharge bacilli often for months or years. The organisms persist in the biliary or urinary system and are excreted in faeces or urine. Some 80 per cent of chronic carriers are women because of their greater liability to gall-bladder disease. The most famous carrier, 'Typhoid Mary', who was responsible for a large outbreak in New York (1903) finally had to be permanently isolated from 1915 until her death in 1938.

Prolonged courses of antibiotic therapy may ultimately cure the carrier state but for faecal carriers the most effective procedure is surgical removal of the gall-bladder.

Carriers need to be kept under regular supervision, precluded from acting as food-handlers, and specially instructed in personal hygiene. In Britain there are statutory powers for their control, and health departments maintain a register of former cases of typhoid to ensure supervision and suggest lines of enquiry in subsequent outbreaks.

typhus fever. The term now includes a variety of similar diseases caused by various species of *Rickettsia* and these are discussed under that heading. However, classical typhus fever, sometimes known as gaol fever, camp fever, or epidemic house-borne typhus fever, is caused by *R. prowazeki* and is one of the great epidemic diseases of history, always ready to appear under conditions of famine, war, and refugee movement, when deprivation, crowding and lack of hygiene, especially in cold or temperate climates, provide opportunities for lice to disseminate infection from man to man.

The onset is usually sudden with headache, shivering fever, general pain and a macular rash (i.e. a rash of discoloured spots not raised above the surface) on the fifth day. Toxaemia and prostration are pronounced. Untreated cases run a course of about two weeks and may recover spontaneously, but the death rate is high and may reach 40 per cent. Modern antibiotic treatment is very effective and there is a protective vaccine, but prevention by hygiene and louse-eradication is still essential.

Murine typhus or endemic flea-borne typhus has a world-wide distribution. It is less severe than classical typhus fever. It is caused by *R. mooseri*, and spreads from rats to man by fleas.

U

ulcer. An open sore on the surface of skin or mucous membrane where infection, inflammation and bacterial toxins cause gradual destruction of epithelium (surface cells) and underlying tissues, often with larger areas of dead tissue which fall away.

Ulcers are of many types. The common causes are: (1) superficial wound infections especially in tissues damaged by trauma, pressure, impaired circulation, disease or conditions affecting the spinal cord and nerves. Examples are slow-healing burns; mouth ulcers from jagged teeth or dental plates; bed-sores; varicose ulcers of the leg; and ulcers in various nervous diseases. (2) Specific infections such as tuberculosis or syphilis and, in the intestine, typhoid fever, cholera or amoebic dysentery. (3) Malignant disease. (4) DUODENAL ULCER, GASTRIC ULCER and ulcerative colitis in which psychosomatic factors may be involved.

Treatment necessarily depends on diagnosis but the principles of dealing with an accessible chronic pus-forming ulcer are to determine and remove the cause and secure rest, to improve circulation by posture, and to treat the accompanying disease. Locally mild antiseptics are usually followed by stimulating applications, and skin-grafting may be of help in the final stages of healing.

Ulcers of more specific causation require therapy appropriate to the exact diagnosis.

ulna. The larger of the two long bones in the forearm. It extends from elbow to wrist on the inner (or little finger) side of the limb. The relatively massive upper end articulates with the lower end of the humerus or upper arm bone and forms the greater part of the elbow joint. This is a hinge-type joint and its stability is maintained by two bony projections of the ulna, the coronoid process in front and the olecranon process behind. The ulnar shaft runs parallel to the radius and diminishes in cross-section from above downwards to terminate at the wrist-joint. The prominent knob on the back of the wrist is the ulnar styloid process.

The olecranon process forms the 'point of the elbow', often fractured by direct violence in falls on the elbow. The shaft is subcutaneous and also liable to fracture by direct violence. Indirect violence, as from falls upon the outstretched hand, more commonly fractures the radius, but either the ulnar shaft or coronoid process may be involved if displacement is severe.

ultrasonics. Sound-waves whose frequency exceeds about twelve thousand cycles per second are inaudible to the human ear but may still be heard by other animals. Such waves are utilized in the so-called 'silent dog-whistle' and are also employed by bats as a sort of 'radar' helping them to navigate in the dark. It is however possible to produce high-energy sound waves of much higher frequencies by means of the electrical excitation of a quartz-crystal (piezo-electric effect). These waves and their practical applications are called ultrasonics.

They are used in navigational echo-sounding and for such purposes as detecting flaws in castings, but they also have a use in medicine. Since depth of penetration and strength of return echo depends on the type of underlying tissue it is possible to scan parts of the body and by suitable recording equipment to map out underlying structures in a similar way to marine echo-sounding. By this method suspected tumours or abnormal situations of the placenta may be identified, and the technique is also proving useful for identification of conditions such as spina bifida in the early stages of pregnancy (with a view to termination of the pregnancy if necessary). The record produced is not unlike an x-ray plate, but the procedure is free from radiation hazard and is superior in soft-tissue examination.

Surgical applications of ultrasonics have also been pioneered by Professor Arslan of Padua and are now in use at other centres. With suitable generating and localizing equipment waves are focused to a point, and small but accurately delineated portions of tissue can thus be destroyed without harming overlying structures. This technique has been employed for the treatment of Ménière's disease and is being developed in neuro-surgery, particularly in connection with Parkinson's disease.

ultra-violet radiation. A form of radiation occupying a position in the electromagnetic spectrum just beyond the violet end of the visible light band and with shorter waves in the range of 3900 to 136 Angstrom units (one AU is one ten-millionth of a millimetre).

Ultra-violet rays are present in sunlight and are produced artificially by electric arc-lamps. Early types used open arcs between carbon or

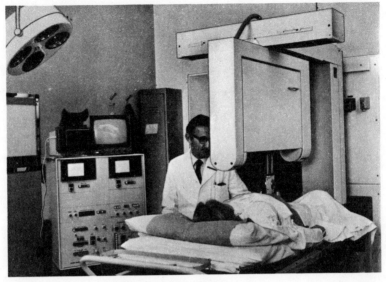

Ultrasound examination

tungsten electrodes. Modern appliances have mercury-vapour arcs in quartz tubes.

The rays are absorbed by the skin, and as in sunburn, according to length of exposure, produce reddening or blistering followed by desquamation (the shedding of superficial layers of the skin) and tanning. They kill superficial germs, stimulate blood-supply to the skin, produce vitamin D by action on skin ergosterol, relieve pain by counter-irritation, and exercise some general tonic effect.

Therapeutically they are used locally or generally. Local applications are used for slow-healing ulcers, impetigo, acne, lupus and psoriasis and for the relief of fibrositic or neuritic pain. General irradiation is employed in rickets, malnutrition, anaemia, debility, recurrent respiratory infections and neurasthenia; but while it has its place both in prevention and treatment, the value of ultra-violet radiation was exaggerated in the past.

Proper supervision is required because of the risk of skin-burns and conjunctivitis (goggles are essential), and also because of potentially harmful effects in certain conditions such as pulmonary tuberculosis, eczema, and some systemic diseases.

umbilical cord. The cord connecting the embryo to the placenta of the mother and containing the vessels – two arteries and one vein – through which nourishment reaches the child and waste products are removed from the child. The cord is normally tied with two ligatures immediately after birth and then cut between the ligatures.

Occasional abnormalities include knots, caused by the foetus slipping through loops in the cord and sometimes drawn so tight as to impede the circulation, thus damaging or even killing the unborn child; twisting may also occur, including twisting round the neck or round a limb.

umbilical hernia. The umbilicus or navel is a potentially weak area of the abdominal wall

through which part of the intestine, enclosed in the peritoneum (the membrane lining the abdominal cavity), may protrude as an umbilical HERNIA.

Umbilical hernia is very common in infancy. The projecting umbilicus is well covered by skin and lined by peritoneum to form a small sac which quite often is not strictly a hernia since it may have no contents. The smallest sacs disappear spontaneously and the traditional treatment is to try to encourage this by the application of adhesive plaster strips either to retain a small pad or to invert the mid-line of the abdominal wall and so compress the sac between the opposed skin folds. These measures usually prove quite effective, but if the hernia persists, or is markedly unsightly, or poses a risk of damage to the protruding intestine, a repair operation will be required. This is best delayed until the age of 2 or 3, since abdominal operations in small infants are frequently followed by respiratory complications.

Occasionally infants are born with a large protruding sac of the peritoneum containing intestine or other organs. This congenital umbilical hernia (or exomphthalos) is a developmental defect. It requires immediate and difficult surgery.

umbilicus. The navel or depressed scar in the centre of the abdomen which results after birth from the severance of the UMBILICAL CORD.

unconscious mind. There is an apocryphal tale of a centipede which became immobilized when it began to think about how it actually walked. Fanciful though this is, it serves to illustrate the unconscious nature of many activities. The impulse producing a movement or action may originate consciously but the detailed execution is controlled unconsciously at a lower level. Similarly, incoming impressions are unconsciously monitored before they reach consciousness as perceptions. Both activities are influenced and modified by the stored-up results of earlier experience. To take a simple example, my eyes see seven people on the pavement; six do not really impinge on my consciousness, but the seventh is brought to my conscious mind as a friend whom I want to see, and I start walking without consciously telling my legs the order in which to move.

The existence of mental activity of which we are not conscious was only grudgingly admitted by the experimental physiologists of the nineteenth century, and even by the early schools of experimental psychology which followed them. These workers studied living systems from the outside and the operations of the conscious mind by introspection. In their views, physiology and psychology dealt with the same phenomena from different angles. The physiologists sought to explain how the brain and nervous system functioned, entirely in terms of reflex acts integrated and conditioned by experience, and the psychologists dealt only with what appeared in consciousness.

However, psychology soon altered out of all recognition and the concept that we take action only when our ideas are fully formed was turned round, so that it became accepted that we only have ideas when our unconscious mind has reached a state of readiness to act. Gradually it was realized that we are unaware of many of the factors which make us act in a particular way. Investigation, description, analysis, and measurement of consciousness had quite failed to explain important aspects of behaviour. It came to be recognized that since all experience was highly personal, sub-conscious abilities and attitudes were built up by the selection and classification of information continuously collected from the outside world. This background of experience is the basis of 'feeling' generated in the unconscious mind and the mainspring of its influence on action. The mental processes involved in desires and emotions are never conscious. It is only the end-products of motivational drives which ever become known directly, and the nature of underlying impulses can only be inferred from their conscious and behavioural consequences. That they do exist can be shown by their emergence in dreams and in states of consciousness modified by hypnosis or drugs.

Psychologists differ slightly about the levels of mental activity that occur without us being conscious of them, but the various terms – pre-conscious, fore-conscious, subconscious and unconscious mind – all mean nearly the same thing. They have been developed to fit explanations that are not widely different. Some see the unconscious as a seething cauldron of passion and desire; others regard it rather as a passive repository of instincts, habits and silent mental functions. At any rate, unconscious mental activity exists at various levels, some of which can be brought to consciousness. However, a distinction may profitably be made between the contents of the subconscious mind – symbols and feelings which can arise in consciousness but which at the moment are absent – and unconscious operations which are never appreciated consciously. Forgotten information, for example, may be dredged up by an effort of will; and names are recalled to consciousness with perhaps a transient feeling of strain, but with no exact awareness of how they are actually recovered.

From this it follows that behaviour is not simply conscious response to a stimulus or reasoning from that stimulus, but is in part based on feelings and ideas derived from past experience, with some of these never coming to consciousness.

Later workers were quick to realize that this provided a means of explaining the difference between logical thinking and the emotional thinking of complexes, so elucidating much that was mysterious in human behaviour. The fruition of this was psychoanalysis, dominated perhaps a little unfairly by Sigmund FREUD (1856-1939) since valuable but less sensational contributions were also made by many others.

Freud's theories were based on a distinction between the id, or unconscious mind, and the ego, or conscious mind. To this he later added the superego, which controlled the moral and judicious aspects of personality, and he also elaborated his definition of the id by recognizing two further principles. Emotional tensions resulting from sexual and other basic instincts he ascribed to an inner force which he called the libido. The conscious impact of this force was painful and unpleasant and its relief gave pleasure. The second principle concerned destructive instincts which stimulated aggression and produced irrational hatreds and violence. Functionally he conceived that both the id and the superego operated by what he called cathexis or anti-cathexis to stimulate or restrain the ego. Anti-cathexis for example operates in connection with memory. If a person fails to recall something or makes a verbal slip it is because this unconscious censor is protecting the ego against some painful or disturbing association and so from the anxiety which recall would otherwise arouse. This is known as repression.

Anxiety is a crucial concept in the explanation of neurosis. Freud distinguished between objective, neurotic and moral anxiety. Objective anxiety is aroused by the recognition of a real danger, and moral anxiety results from shame induced by an active conscience, but neurotic anxiety is an expression of ill-formed fears resident in the id – so-called phobias. In the face of such stresses the ego develops various defence mechanisms designed to suppress or redirect the unpleasant, painful or anxiety-inducing cathexes – these impulses of sub-conscious origin. Such defence mechanisms include identification (adoption of discordant images as one's own), sublimation (the projection of an unworthy impulse on a more acceptable object), reaction formation (doing the exact opposite), fixation (persistence of a primitive mode of gratification) and regression (reversion to a more primitive personality).

However one now regards Freud, it was he who was largely responsible for first exploring the recesses of the unconscious mind. Others have built upon and adapted his fundamental ideas. Since man first emerged from his caves a cardinal tenet of human faith has been the belief that upward progress is inevitable through constant growth of knowledge and an increasingly rational approach to the problems of daily life. The developing theories of psychology do little to sustain this view. Rather they enforce the reflection that human conduct, to a great extent, still appears to be motivated by blind instinctual forces.

underfeeding. A common cause of failure to thrive in both breast-fed and bottle-fed infants. The underfed child fails to gain weight and is either fretful or apathetic; the skin is thin, inelastic, and wrinkled from loss of subcutaneous fat; the eyes appear sunken; muscular development and activity is poor; the abdomen appears relatively large; and the stools ('hunger stools') are often small and green.

In breast feeding, the mother's lactation may be insufficient, the nipples may be retracted or otherwise unsatisfactory, or there may be errors in nursing technique. The baby itself may be unable to suck properly because of a defective airway, congenital defects such as hare-lip or cleft palate, mouth infections, mental defect or intracranial injury. In artificial feeding, undernourishment results from giving insufficient or too dilute feeds, or from the infant failing to take in correct feeds through sucking difficulties, caused either by the disabilities already mentioned or by unsatisfactory equipment, particularly in relation to the design and patency (openness of the passages) of teats.

A breast-fed baby should be weighed before and after a feed to determine how much milk it is actually getting; this is known as a test-feed. If underfeeding is confirmed a complementary artificial feed should be given after each breast feed. In artificially-fed infants the whole procedure should be carefully reviewed in detail and steps taken to ensure that the appropriate Calorie intake for the expected weight is both provided and taken.

Extreme degrees of underfeeding result in marasmus (extreme emaciation) and consideration should be given to the possibility of other diseases being present, such as congenital syphilis, chronic infection (especially tuberculosis or chronic enteritis), coeliac disease, parasitic infection or nervous and mental defect.

In primitive communities underfeeding may be particularly related to the protein component of the diet. This results, for example, in kwashiorkor, a condition characterized by malnutrition, anaemia, oedema and abnormalities of skin and pigmentation.

undeveloped countries, health in. Countries with a high standard of living expect to have ready access to medical advice and to hospital and nursing services, and they have adopted elaborate practical and legislative measures to safeguard their environment. In the emergent countries the situation is still very different. Undeveloped societies are characterized by high infant and child mortality, chronic nutritional disease, widespread parasitic and infectious disease, complete lack of sanitary provision, and no community action against adverse influences. Many such societies still exist but they are becoming increasingly anxious to discard their undeveloped state, to build up their own health services, and to emulate their more advanced neighbours by achieving comparable standards of health. This demand has become explosive since unprecedented population growth and rapidity of communications have together ensured that knowledge of their shortcomings has developed much faster than their ability to provide what is needed in terms of finance, physical resources and skilled personnel.

The health problems of underdeveloped countries stem from: (1) defective nutrition in respect of protein, minerals, vitamins and water; (2) parasitic disease such as hookworm infestation; (3) insect-borne or rat-borne infections like malaria, yellow fever and plague; (4) other epidemic and endemic diseases such as tuberculosis, smallpox, diphtheria and poliomyelitis; and (5) degenerative diseases. Urbanization and industrialization are indications of development – most of Europe has 50 to 80 per cent of its population in towns compared with 10 per cent or less in places like Ghana – but development of this kind is only tolerable if health services keep pace with the new hazards which result.

The basic essentials are thus food, sanitation and disease-prevention. Persons responsible for planning and allocation of community resources must be health-minded rather than disease-minded. The spectacular appeal of curative medicine may otherwise lead to exaggerated and disproportionate hospital provision. In terms of value for money, resources are much better spent in the less glamorous activities of water supply, proper sewerage, dietetic education and other health education.

Scattered populations, large distances, poor transport and little or no organization all create great difficulties in providing either preventive or curative services. Nevertheless there are some advantages in being able to start from scratch: it is possible to build up a uniform administration able to integrate prevention and cure and to develop medicine as a social service with community participation. In developing areas there is no immediate prospect of supplying a family doctor and universal hospital service of the type familiar in more advanced countries. The essential is to provide for each community an organization utilizing less highly trained workers, preferably drawn from the people themselves, who can give basic instruction in hygiene and healthy living and deal with minor complaints and immunization programmes. This has been called 'barefoot doctoring' which can then be backed by progressively more advanced facilities for trained advice and treatment in relatively local 'health centres', reinforced in centres of population by simple but adequate hospitals served by sufficient transport. Prototypes of such an organization now exist in many countries largely through the efforts of the World Health Organization which has provided advice and practical assistance to the responsible governments and also helped to coordinate the efforts of voluntary organizations.

Consideration must also be given to population control. Primitive populations tend to remain stationary because a high death-rate cancels a high birth-rate. When deaths are controlled a rapid expansion of population takes place and the problems imposed by poverty and scarce resources become multiplied rather than relieved. In many parts of the world this is already the situation and the future difficulties loom large.

undulant fever. 'Undulant' means 'wave-like', descriptive of a temperature chart showing successive periods of fever and remission, but as a diagnosis undulant fever usually means the condition normally called BRUCELLOSIS.

uraemia. A condition of toxaemia due to retention in the blood stream of toxic waste-products normally eliminated by the kidneys. The symptoms generally include headache, nausea, vomiting, diarrhoea, diminished urinary output, itching, cramps, panting respiration with urinous smelling breath, restlessness, mental confusion, and eventually convulsions, coma and death.

Uraemia is not always due to kidney disease but may also be caused by metabolic disorders, poisons, or circulatory failure. In treatment the primary need is to identify the cause of the condition and give appropriate treatment, but the actual toxaemia may be relieved at least temporarily by the procedure of renal dialysis using an artificial KIDNEY MACHINE. Blood tests are employed to assess the gravity and progress of the condition.

urea. The breakdown of the protein in the diet produces urea, which enters the blood stream. Chemically, urea is carbamide [$CO(NH_2)_2$], an organic compound of nitrogen; nitrogen is an essential constituent of protein. The normal level of urea in the blood is 20 to 40 mg. per 100 ml. and any in excess of this amount is excreted in the urine by the kidneys. This means that a diet rich in protein increases the urea in the urine, but a proportion of the daily output is also derived from the normal continuous disintegration of tissue-protein.

On an adequate diet, the healthy body maintains a nitrogen balance. Lost tissue-nitrogen is replaced from food and excess is excreted as urea. In starvation, nitrogen is lost by tissue-wastage without replacement and the result is a negative nitrogen balance. Conversely, with an adequate diet, growth, pregnancy, physical training and convalescence all lead to a positive nitrogen balance.

In kidney disease urea excretion may be reduced. The estimation of blood-urea levels and the use of urea-clearance tests provide convenient methods of assessing renal efficiency, but urea retention alone is not wholly responsible for the toxic condition known as URAEMIA.

ureter. A tube which conveys urine from each kidney to the urinary bladder. Each ureter is about 25 to 30 cm. (10 to 12 in.) in length and is a relatively thick-walled narrow canal continuous with the lower end of the collecting funnel (or renal pelvis) of the kidney; it opens into the upper part of the bladder. See URINARY SYSTEM.

Calculi or 'gravel' produced by the precipitation of urinary salts may pass through the ureter or may become impacted or stuck at some point. The thick wall is composed of smooth muscle fibres and this muscular tissue makes spasmodic efforts to force the material downwards to the bladder or to overcome the impaction, so producing the painful symptoms usually called renal colic or more accurately ureteric colic.

urethra. The passage through which urine from the urinary bladder is voided to the exterior.

In the female the urethra is short – only 4 cm. (1.5 in.) – and leads directly to an external opening situated immediately in front of the vagina. Its wall contains circular muscle fibres,

particularly concentrated near the neck of the bladder to form the urethral sphincter.

The male urethra is much longer – 18 to 20 cm. (7 to 8 in.) – since it extents from the bladder to the end of the penis. Its first section, the prostatic urethra, is surrounded by the prostate gland and is there joined by ducts from that gland and from the seminal vesicles. The penile or cavernous part traverses the length of the penis. Between the prostatic and penile urethras is a short narrow and compressible section, the membranous urethra, encircled by the muscle fibres of the urethral sphincter. In the male the urethra serves not only for the voiding of urine but also for the transmission of seminal fluid. In both sexes the outflow of urine is controlled by the sphincter muscle.

Urethritis. This is a condition in which there is inflammation of the urethra due to invasion of its mucous membrane by pus-forming organisms; there is a discharge with pain and difficulty in passing urine. In men, if the infection passes inwards to the posterior urethra, it may lead to further serious effects involving the prostate gland, seminal ducts, epididymis, and peri-urethral tissue, with possibilities of urethral stricture and deep abscess formation.

Most cases arise by infection from the exterior and the commonest cause is gonorrhoea transmitted by sexual contact. Infections due to intestinal organisms are not infrequent in women and also occur occasionally in elderly men. The condition may also follow use of a catheter or be a complication of cystitis.

In treatment the initial need is to identify the infecting organism, to give appropriate antibiotics, and to maintain a copious urinary flow by a large fluid-intake and diuretics. Before the advent of effective antibiotics intensive antiseptic washes were used but these are now seldom required.

uric acid. A nitrogenous compound ($C_5H_4N_4O_3$) normally present in blood and urine. It is formed both by the wear and tear of body cells (endogenous or tissue-wastage production) and by the breaking-down of the nucleoprotein in certain foods (exogenous production). Fish, liver, kidney and sweetbreads are foods particularly rich in nucleoprotein, and tissue-wastage is increased in various acute fevers and in leukaemia.

In gout the excretion of uric acid in the urine is reduced and deposits of sodium urate occur in and around joints, causing the characteristic painful arthritis.

Pure uric acid is colourless, but in acid-urine deposits of it may sometimes be seen as small reddish crystals ('cayenne pepper' deposits). Larger aggregations occasionally form stones (calculi) in the urinary tract.

urinary system. Excess water and soluble waste products are eliminated from the body as urine, a pale yellow and usually slightly acid fluid. About 1200 to 1800 ml. (2 to 3 pts.) of urine are excreted per day. Urine is produced by the two kidneys and flows by the two ureters to the urinary bladder, where it is held until it is convenient to void it. Bladder emptying (technically termed micturition) is normally under voluntary control, urine being passed to the exterior through the urethra, which is short and direct in females but in males traverses the penis.

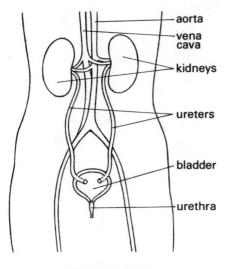

The urinary system

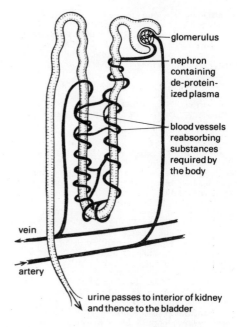

Urinary system: structure of a nephron in the kidney

The complex part of this process is urine formation by the kidney, which consists of very many separate, microscopically small filtration units called uriniferous tubules or nephrons. Each nephron is associated with a tuft of blood vessels called a glomerulus (see diagram). Surrounding this tuft is the blind expanded upper end of the tubule, indented to enclose the glomerulus. The rest of the tubule is long and convoluted and finally opens into the interior of the kidney (known as the 'pelvis'). The glomerulus and surrounding tubule together act as a filter, removing from the blood stream water and all soluble constituents except protein. The upper end of the tubule thus contains, in effect, de-proteinized plasma. As this fluid passes along the convoluted part of the tubule, selective reabsorption takes place. Substances still required are recovered in accordance with body needs, while the excess water and unwanted waste products that remain pass on as urine, first to the hollow interior of the kidney, and thence to the bladder.

The main diseases of the urinary system are those involving the secretory organs, or KIDNEYS. Other structures have simpler functions related purely to collection, storage, and evacuation of urine. Congenital kidney defects are not uncommon and often prove rapidly fatal in infancy, but some may persist unsuspected to later life until symptoms make investigation necessary.

Other kidney disease occurs as acute, sub-acute, or chronic NEPHRITIS and may result from inflammatory, degenerative, or circulatory changes. Symptoms, results, and outlook depend on which elements of kidney structure are involved. Thus, acute glomerulo-nephritis is a common inflammatory complication of acute fevers and streptococcal infections; toxaemias tend to produce changes which are degenerative (nephrosis) rather than inflammatory (nephritis) and generally have a more favourable outcome; and some types of chronic nephritis result from arteriosclerosis associated with high blood pressure.

Bacterial infection can occur anywhere in the urinary tract. The resulting conditions are pyelo-nephritis (kidney and kidney-pelvis), cystitis (bladder), and urethritis (urethra), the last-named very often of gonococcal origin.

Obstructions are common. They cause pain, frequency of passing urine, urinary retention, and local injury. They are usually due to stone (calculus), enlargement of the prostate, or stricture, and tend to lead to secondary infection. Chronic obstruction of urinary outflow from the bladder is practically confined to men with enlarged prostate or urethral stricture. Obstruction at any level eventually gives further trouble as back-pressure dilates ureters and kidney (hydronephrosis), thinning out and destroying kidney tissue.

Primary tumours affect mainly the kidney and bladder. Simple kidney tumours are rare, although occasionally cysts of congenital origin create symptoms in adult life. Hypernephroma is the commonest malignant tumour, usually occurring in older men, and often reaching a large size. Sarcoma and carcinoma are both rare except for one form of sarcoma (Wilm's tumour) found in young children.

The common bladder tumour is a papilloma, which has a strong tendency to undergo malignant change. Bladder carcinoma also occurs in some special circumstances as a sequel of hookworm disease (bilharziasis), and in industries which use carcinogenic solvents. Prostatic enlargement is frequent in older men. It is usually benign but may progress to malignancy.

urination. The act of passing urine. Urine, produced by the kidneys, flows to the bladder through the ureter. As the bladder distends the pressure rises and this invokes reflex contraction of its muscular wall and the accumulated urine is voided through the urethra. In the normal person the reflex mechanism can be voluntarily restrained or initiated in accordance with circumstances.

Disorders of urination are obstruction, frequency (with or without pain) and incontinence. Obstruction may be due to urethral stricture, enlarged prostate or an impacted calculus (stone). Frequency is usually a symptom of cystitis. Incontinence occurs in the young child before control has been learned, in the aged because of failing control and lack of mental awareness, in spinal cord disease or injury, and often in women because of damage resulting from pregnancy.

urine. Normal urine is a fluid secreted by the kidneys and containing urea, uric acid, creatinine, phosphates, chlorides, and sulphates. It is straw-coloured (due to the presence of urochrome derived from the bile-pigment bilirubin), usually faintly acid, and possesses a characteristic odour; its specific gravity varies from 1.015 to 1.025. The average daily adult output is 1200 to 1800 ml. (2 to 3 pts.).

Abnormal constituents indicate disease, and urine-testing should be a diagnostic routine. Alterations in colour may be due to blood or bile, but black urine occurs with certain tumours and various drugs may colour it blue, yellow, green, or red. Bacterial infections split urea to give the smell of ammonia; and alcohol and some drugs also produce characteristic aromas. The specific gravity rises in diabetes mellitus and is reduced in diabetes insipidus and cirrhosis of the kidney. Urine of normal colour and smell may on examination be found to contain albumin, bile, sugars, or ketone bodies.

When allowed to stand a sediment collects in most normal urines; this is mainly phosphates, carbonates or urates, and occasionally uric acid. In diseased conditions the sediment may include blood-cells, pus-cells, bacteria, tumour cells, fragments of tissue resulting from ulceration, and tube-casts, i.e., plugs formed in the kidney tubules as a result of inflammatory or degenerative kidney disease.

Incontinence. Loss of voluntary control over the passage of urine. This is common with the debility and muscular weakness of old age, but it can also occur in prostrating diseases and in surgical shock; in disease of the urinary tract; in pelvic injuries which damage bladder, urethra, or associated muscles; in mental stress from excitement or fear; in disease of the central nervous system; and in injuries to the spinal cord.

In true incontinence the bladder is empty and urine dribbles away as it is produced. In overflow incontinence the bladder is distended and small quantities of urine are passed involuntarily at intervals as pressure overcomes the obstruction. Overflow incontinence is often found in cases of enlargement of the prostate.

Stress incontinence usually occurs in women with pelvic muscles damaged by childbirth. Lifting weights or coughing tightens the abdominal muscles and raises the pressure within the abdomen, so compressing the bladder; and the extra strain overcomes the resistance of the spincter muscle of the urethra.

In stress incontinence a small operation to repair the damaged muscle may be needed. Nocturnal incontinence in old people can sometimes be helped by avoiding all drinks for three hours before bed-time (but taking care not to reduce the total daily intake of liquid). Where the condition persists incontinence pads are useful.

Suppression. Suppression of urine (anuria) is cessation of urinary secretion by the kidneys. It is a very serious condition, rapidly fatal if not relieved, since it leads quickly to uraemia. Anuria may occur in acute nephritis, whether caused by infection or by toxic substances; in the terminal stages of chronic nephritis; in severe fluid loss by other routes (e.g., with the diarrhoea of cholera or the vomiting of hyperemesis); in obstruction of both ureters (e.g., by stones); and occasionally after operations on the urinary tract, following severe surgical shock or in association with circulatory failure in a disease of the heart. Treatment varies with the cause, but may include treatment with a KIDNEY MACHINE.

Retention. In urinary retention, urine cannot be passed although it continues to accumulate in the bladder. Lower abdominal pain results from distention of the bladder which can usually be seen and felt as a rounded swelling above the pubis, and there may be strangury, or painful attempts to pass urine.

Retention may be caused by the following: (1) mechanical factors such as calculus (stone), enlargement of the prostate, or stricture due to spasm, inflammation or such infections as gonorrhoea; (2) the effect of drugs, alcohol, shock, nervousness or hysteria on the centre of the brain controlling the bladder; (3) damage to the spinal cord which impairs the nerve supply to the bladder; (4) over-action of the sympathetic nervous system, especially after surgical operations; (5) pain inhibiting the passing of urine – this may be the result of such conditions as inflammation of the urethra; (6) muscular weakness in the aged and debilitated, or after childbirth, affecting the bladder itself or the muscles of the abdomen.

The condition may require relief by inserting a CATHETER, but if possible this should be a last resort because of the attendant risks of infection.

In cases due to temporary causes difficulty can often be overcome by simple nursing measures to encourage relaxation (hot applications, a hot bath, or an enema).

urticaria. See NETTLERASH.

uterus. The uterus or womb is a hollow, thick-walled muscular organ of the female pelvis, lying between the bladder in front and the rectum behind. During pregnancy it accommodates, protects, and nourishes the growing foetus. In the non-pregnant state it resembles a flattened pear (stalk end down), 7.5 cm. long, 5 cm. wide, and 2.5 cm. thick (3 in. by 2 in. by 1 in.) and weighing 25 to 55 g. (1 to 2 oz.). At its upper end on each side arise the uterine or Fallopian tubes through which ova, discharged from the ovaries, are conveyed to its hollow interior. Its lower third is named the cervix, a conical structure with a central canal, projecting into the upper end of the vagina.

The uterine cavity is lined by cellular tissue

which is influenced by ovarian hormones and undergoes a regular cycle of changes, being shed each month during menstruation; however, if conception occurs it provides a lodging for the developing ovum. The lower part of the cervix has a different, more flattened type of cellular tissue, prone to degenerative or malignant change, and it is this which is sampled in the preventive procedure of cervical cytology.

During pregnancy the uterus enlarges enormously. After childbirth it rapidly returns almost to its original size.

Diseases. Congenitally, the uterus may be duplicated, malformed developmentally, or undersized (hypoplasia). Sterility or difficulties with pregnancy or labour may result.

Normally the cervix and uterine body are directed upwards and forwards (anteversion), and the body is bent slightly forwards in relation to the cervical canal (anteflexion). Backward displacement (retroversion and retroflexion) is not uncommon after childbirth, following stretching of ligaments and weakening of muscles. It is in part preventable by good obstetric practice (avoiding injury), avoidance of over-long inactivity after the birth, prevention of bladder distention, and restoration of muscle-tone by appropriate exercises. Where the displacement occurs it may cause backache or menstrual pain and irregularity. Downward uterine displacement is partial or complete prolapse, usually following pelvic floor damage during childbirth. Pessaries or operative treatment may be advised.

Actual disease affects the cells of the wall of the cervix, the lining (endometrium) of the uterus, or its substance (myometrium). Erosion of the cervix is generally due to chronic inflammation (cervicitis) and produces vaginal discharge. Treatment may involve local

applications, cauterization, or operation. Acute endometritis usually results from infection following childbirth, but may be gonorrhoeal or tuberculous in origin. Persistent chronic endometritis may be indicative of some other uterine condition. The appropriate treatment of endometritis varies with its cause.

Uterine tumours may be benign or malignant. Of the former, polyps grow from the cervical canal or from the endometrium, and fibroids, which may be multiple or of large size, develop from the myometrium. Malignant tumours are mainly carcinomata, arising either in the cervix or uterine body. Cervical carcinoma is commoner, most often seen after several pregnancies, and tends to spread rapidly to adjacent tissues. Conversely, carcinoma of the uterine body more often affects older women who have had no pregnancies and is slower to develop. The treatment of all these conditions is surgical and radiotherapy may also be employed.

The general symptoms of tumours are initially haemorrhage and discharge. Irregular bleeding or its post-menopausal recurrence indicates a need for full investigation.

Cervical cytology is a very simple procedure intended to detect pre-cancerous changes in the cervical epithelium so that treatment can be undertaken in good time. It should be a routine three-yearly precaution in all women over 35 years of age.

uvula. A flattened, conical projection, hanging downwards from the middle of the free border of the soft palate at the back of the mouth. It consists of muscle-fibres covered by mucous membrane. The function of the soft palate is to cut off the nasal passage from the mouth and throat, particularly during the act of swallowing; the uvula ensures that a more efficient seal is achieved.

V

vaccination. The term is derived from the Latin word *vacca,* meaning 'cow', and its original meaning was the development of IMMUNITY to smallpox by inoculation with cowpox, a procedure which proved to be the first great triumph of preventive medicine in relation to infectious disease.

From earliest times smallpox has been an endemic disease of the Middle and Far East. It is said that returning Crusaders imported it to the West, and from the sixteenth century onwards it displayed a rising prevalence throughout Europe and produced many widespread outbreaks. Since as many as 50 per cent of cases died it was a matter for serious concern.

Cows were commonly subject to cowpox, a disease affecting the udder, and milkers often became infected and suffered a similar condition on their hands. Edward Jenner (1749-1823), a Gloucestershire physician (and grad-

uate of St. Andrew's University), noticed that dairymaids often escaped smallpox and he correctly deduced that this was because they had become immune through an earlier attack of cowpox. In 1796 he successfully demonstrated that inoculation with material from cowpox blisters did protect against smallpox.

It may, however, be interesting to note that a less efficient and more dangerous method of vaccination – namely inoculation with matter taken directly from a smallpox vesicle or crust – had previously been used for many centuries in China and other eastern countries and had been introduced to Britain by Lady Mary Wortley Montague in 1718. That fact should not, of course, detract from the credit due to Jenner who produced an effective method of preventing smallpox a century before the existence of viruses was known.

Many European countries promptly accepted

Jenner's findings although at home his work had a mixed reception and aroused scepticism, distrust, and even outright opposition, which to some extent persists today. However, the value of the procedure has been convincingly demonstrated by the complete eradication of smallpox from country after country, until it is allegedly extinct in all countries except Bangladesh and Ethiopia, and may be an absolutely extinct disease in a year or two. If vaccination can be universally applied in these areas, total elimination of the disease will be assured.

In the U.K. the National Vaccine Establishment was set up in 1807 and produced calf-lymph from calves artificially infected with cowpox, but modern lymph is now prepared from variola, or actual smallpox virus, modified by sub-culture; sheep and rabbits are also used in production.

It was not until 1853 that vaccination was made compulsory in England and Wales (1863 in Scotland), but later enactments introduced exemption on the grounds of conscience. When a Royal Commission on Vaccination reported in 1896 it showed that in various years 25 to 50 per cent of infants were actually not being vaccinated. However, the marked decline in smallpox clearly demonstrated that vaccination had achieved results. Compulsion was finally repealed in 1948 and in Britain routine infant vaccination is no longer advised. It is considered that the extremely slight risks of smallpox importation can now be contained by surveillance and local action, and that the very occasional adverse effects of vaccination outweigh in importance any slight chance of contracting the actual disease.

Although, strictly speaking, vaccination means anti-smallpox inoculation using smallpox vaccine administered intradermally (i.e., into the skin) by scratch or multiple-puncture technique, the term is now widely used to include any procedure for inducing active immunity which relies on preparations of killed or treated bacterial or viral cultures. These are usually given by injection under the skin, or even by mouth, as in active immunization against poliomyelitis.

vaccine. A bacterium or virus so modified as to be no longer dangerous but capable of conferring immunity to the disease that it would normally cause. A dead or killed vaccine is one prepared by cultivating the organisms in an artificial medium and then killing them, e.g., by heat or by an appropriate chemical; there is no possibility of the vaccine producing the disease but it stimulates the defence mechanisms of the body to produce antibodies capable of dealing with invading organisms of the particular type. A live or attenuated vaccine is one prepared by cultivating the organism for many generations in an unnatural environment so that it completely loses its virulence but can still stimulate the defence mechanisms of the body. An autogenous vaccine is one prepared from organisms found in the patient's sputum, urine or other secretions; autogenous vaccines had a considerable vogue after their introduction by Wright in 1903, but as knowledge of the typing of organisms increases the need to prepare a vaccine specially for a particular patient clearly diminishes.

The earliest vaccine used was for smallpox: see VACCINATION. Early examples of successful vaccines are: anthrax vaccine introduced by Pasteur in 1882 to protect sheep and cattle against the disease; rabies vaccine also introduced by Pasteur in 1885; cholera vaccine introduced by Haffkine in India in 1894; plague vaccine also intoduced by Haffkine; and typhoid vaccine introduced by Wright and Semple and nowadays used in the form of TAB (i.e., a combined vaccine against typhoid and the two commonest varieties of paratyphoid). More recent examples are the vaccines used against diphtheria, tetanus and whooping cough (these three being usually tackled by a combined vaccine nowadays), poliomyelitis, tuberculosis, measles, rubella, mumps and influenza.

Some vaccines produce an almost perfect immunity: for instance it is virtually unknown for a person successfully vaccinated against smallpox to develop the disease during the next seven years, and the occurrence of diphtheria in a person immunized within the previous three years is an extreme rarity. Some, like rabies vaccine, are useful but by no means a hundred per cent effective. A few, like influenza vaccine, have to be altered frequently: there are many strains of influenza virus, and the vaccine prepared against a strain prevalent in one year may give only a partial protection against the strain prevalent a couple of years later.

Vaccines have played an enormous part in the conquest of infectious diseases. Examples are the eradiction of smallpox from all countries in the world with (at the time of writing) only two exceptions; the reduction of typhoid and paratyphoid by TAB - for, although in highly developed countries pure water, pure food, good sewerage systems and good hygiene render the use of TAB seldom necessary, some experts in tropical medicine deem it the greatest of all medical discoveries; and the reduction of diphtheria in Britain from over fifty thousand cases and nearly five thousand deaths a year to around twenty cases and one death. There are however, some infections – from LASSA FEVER to the common cold – against which no vaccine is yet available.

vaccinia. See COWPOX.

vagina. The word means 'sheath', and the vagina, or female copulatory passage, is a musculo-membranous tube 10 to 12.5 cm. long (4 to 5 in.) extending upwards and backwards from its opening at the vulva to the uterus, the cervix of which projects into it at its upper end. It lies between the bladder and urethra in front and the rectum behind. In virgins the lower orifice is partially closed by the hymen. Besides its function during intercourse it serves as a channel for the menstrual discharge, and, much distended, as the birth-canal during childbirth.

Diseases. Inflammation of the vagina is known as vaginitis. The main symptom is vaginal discharge, but the vulva is usually involved as well (vulvo-vaginitis), giving rise to pain, irritation, itching, swelling, tenderness, and pain on intercourse. Long-standing cases sometimes develop mental depression. An abnormal discharge of white fluid from the vagina is known as leucorrhoea. The discharge of a little milky or watery exudate a day or so before the beginning of the menstrual flow is not abnormal and simply indicates pelvic congestion, but persistent and copious discharge indicates infection or inflammation of the genital organs. Causes include chronic inflammation of the uterus or of its cervix, chronic infection of a cervical tear, gonorrhoea, and – if the discharge is purulent – either cancer of the cervix or presence of a sloughing fibroid. Since leucorrhoea is not a disease but a symptom, treatment clearly varies with the cause; but any persisting discharge demands medical investigation.

Smears should be examined to ensure a correct diagnosis. Treatment may require antiseptic douching, but many cases can be adequately dealt with by appropriate medicated pessaries and the use of systemic antibiotics and hormones. Tights, impermeable pants, and the imperfect rinsing of underwear washed in biological detergents have been blamed for a rising prevalence of vulvo-vaginitis.

vaginismus. A condition in which attempts at sexual intercourse produce spasms of the muscles of vulva, vagina, and surrounding tissues, frustrating penetration or causing painful intercourse (dyspareunia).

Minor degrees of vaginismus may result from painful conditions such as lacerations of the hymen, caruncles (small fleshy excrescences), vulvitis, or vaginitis, and appropiate treatment should effect a cure. However, typical cases more often have a psychological basis due to a subconscious dread of intercourse. Psychotherapy may be required, combined with the use of vaginal dilators which the patient herself, after preliminary demonstration and instruction, can insert regularly, to implant in her mind a conviction that there is no physical basis for her difficulties.

vaginitis. Inflammation of the VAGINA.

vagotomy. Surgical severance of the VAGUS NERVE, certain fibres of which stimulate the stomach glands to produce gastric juice (pepsin and hydrocholoric acid). In peptic ulceration of stomach or duodenum a basic factor is excess acid secretion and the operation of vagotomy is designed to diminish or inhibit this. It has to a large extent replaced partial gastrectomy, an operation to remove the part of the stomach in which secretory cells are most abundant.

vagus nerve. The vagus or tenth cranial nerve contains both afferent and efferent fibres, i.e., fibres bringing sensations to the brain and fibres conveying instructions to organs. It also contains fibres of the parasympathetic system. While other cranial nerves are concerned with the special senses and with the skin and muscles of the head and neck, the vagus – the name means 'wanderer' – travels downwards to the chest and abdomen, and supplies the pharynx, larynx, oesophagus, stomach, intestines, heart and lungs. Activity of the vagus slows the heart, narrows the bronchi and stimulates the process of digestion.

Valium. A kind of TRANQUILLIZER.

valve. Any flap-like fold of the lining of a blood vessel or duct acting as a one-way traffic director. When the pressure becomes higher on one side of the valve it forces the valve open so that fluid flows through to the other side. When the pressure rises on the other side it forces the valve shut, so that the fluid cannot flow backwards.

Perhaps the best-known valves are those of the HEART, but veins and lymphatic vessels also contain valves.

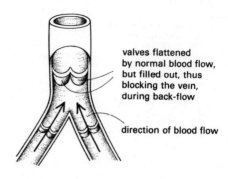

valves flattened by normal blood flow, but filled out, thus blocking the vein, during back-flow

direction of blood flow

Valves in the veins of the leg

valvular heart disease. See HEART.

varicella. A specific generalized infection, commonly called CHICKENPOX, due to the same virus that causes herpes zoster or SHINGLES.

varicocele. A varicose condition of some of the numerous, inter-communicating veins in the spermatic cord. They drain ultimately to the renal veins, and simple varicocele is almost invariably found on the left side because of anatomical differences between the venous junctions on the two sides.

There is usually no other particular cause for varicocele but it does occur as a complication of renal tumour and the possibility of this should be investigated if it appears suddenly, or on the right side.

Although the condition causes swelling of the scrotum and can be easily felt, giving an impression described as like a 'bag of worms', it generally gives little trouble and operation is rarely required. Any feeling of uncomfortable weight or strain can be relieved by wearing a net suspensory to support the scrotum. This is most often needed by young adults participating in athletic activities, or in older men, as ageing tissues provide diminishing support.

varicose veins. See VEINS, diseases of.

variola minor See SMALLPOX.

vascular. Containing or made up of blood vessels.

vasectomy See BIRTH CONTROL.

vector. Derived from the Latin word for a carrier or conveyor, vector really means any living carrier of infection, but the term is usually limited to insects and animals that transmit infection to human beings. Thus mosquitoes are vectors of malaria and yellow fever, lice are vectors of typhus, and flies can be vectors of typhoid and other food-borne infection. Some animals are themselves victims of the disease that they transmit, e.g., rabies reaches man through the bite of an infected dog, cat or wolf. In many cases the eradication of an infection transmitted by a vector depends more on control of the vector than on the much more difficult task of controlling the causal agent.

vegetables. Dietetically, a vegetable is a plant, or part of a plant, used for food, but excluding the parts surrounding its seeds, which are called fruits. This definition sometimes conflicts with ordinary usage. For instance, a marrow, although called a vegetable-marrow, is really a fruit; a tomato is also a fruit although some would regard it as a vegetable; and rhubarb, which is used as a fruit, is a leaf-stem and certainly a vegetable. Cereals are also a problem: they are usually described with the vegetables, but they are the fruits of grasses.

If cereals are included, vegetables may be classified as follows:

Cereals. The seed-grains of a variety of cultivated grasses – wheat, rye, barley, oats, maize, and rice. They consist mainly of carbohydrate (in the form of starch), with variable amounts of protein, fat, minerals and vitamins. The protein is 'second class', in that it does not contain all the essential amino-acids. Wheat and rye contain the protein, gluten, which causes coeliac disease in susceptible persons. The minerals and vitamins are chiefly present in the husk and are largely lost in milling – hence the superiority of wholemeal bread, and also oatmeal, for which whole grains are ground or rolled. Cornflour is made from maize starch.

Pulses or legumes. Peas, beans, and lentils. These contain considerable amounts of carbohydrate and protein but are generally low in fat, with the exception of soya beans which have about 15 per cent fat. When fresh, the pulses are good sources of vitamin C.

Tubers and roots. Potatoes, carrots, parsnips and beetroot are all good sources of carbohydrate; carrots supply vitamin A; turnips provide little nutriment. The roots of certain tropical plants supply arrowroot and tapioca. Sago, also largely carbohydrate, is prepared from the pith of sago-palm stems.

Green vegetables. The commonest are cabbage, cauliflower and Brussels sprouts. They provide few Calories but are good sources of minerals and vitamin C. Lettuce and watercress are eaten without cooking and are particularly good since they do not suffer the losses caused in the others by over-boiling. Spinach contains about 3 per cent iron.

Vegetables thus form an important part of a normal DIET, and by their carbohydrate content contribute significantly to the total Calorie requirement. They have another important function in providing roughage or residue – the plant material which is not digested and not absorbed from the human intestine. In the past the importance of this has been largely unappreciated and disregarded: since it provided no nourishment and was not metabolized, it was ignored by the nutritionists. The influence of Burkitt and other workers has enforced a revision of this attitude, and it is now recognized that dietary fibre reduces constipation, prevents various colonic diseases, and plays a part in the burning up of fats.

vegetarian diet. A diet that excludes the flesh of animals, birds and fishes. There are two main types.

A lacto-vegetarian diet. This type rejects all forms of meat, fish, etc., but accepts milk, butter, cheese and eggs. Such a diet can easily provide a sufficiency of first class protein, vitamins and mineral salts. Although some people would find it a little monotonous to obtain all their first class protein from milk products and eggs, a lacto-vegetarian diet can be as adequate as any other diet. As an example, a day's ration containing 680 g. (24 oz.) of bread, 170 g. (6 oz.) of cheese, 280 g. (10 oz.) of milk, 56 g. (2 oz.) of butter and 85 g.

(3 oz.) of watercress would provide approximately 3,000 Calories, about 100 g. of protein (half of it first class), adequate water-soluble and fat-soluble vitamins and reasonable amounts of most minerals.

A strictly vegetarian diet. Such a diet rejects all foods other than those of plant origin. Such a diet is subject to at least four main defects.

1. Since no vegetable food, however rich in second class protein, contains all the required amino-acids, the strict vegetarian cannot obtain all his protein from one or two sources (e.g., peas and beans or nuts and lentils) but requires to consume a judicious mixture of those vegetables that are rich in protein.

2. Much of the body's mineral requirements is normally supplied from animal sources, e.g., calcium and phosphorus from milk and cheese, iron from meat and eggs, and iodine from fish. The strict vegetarian requires rather a lot of green vegetables and nuts to supply his calcium, a quantity of peas or oatmeal to provide his iron, sufficient wheat germ to supply his phosphorus and water plants such as watercress to provide his iodine.

3. Much of the body's requirement of fat-soluble vitamins is normally obtained from animal fat. Hence the strict vegetarian may be in difficulties unless vitamins A and D are added to foods of vegetable origin, such as margarine.

4. A purely vegetarian diet tends to be very bulky: our nearest animal relations, monkeys, are essentially vegetarians but they devote their waking lives to finding food and eating it.

Nevertheless many people seem to exist in good health on a carefully balanced vegetarian diet.

veins. The vessels which carry blood from the tissues of the body back to the heart. Veins have much thinner walls than arteries but the walls consist of the same three coats, i.e., an outer fibrous coat, a middle layer of muscular and elastic fibres, and an inner coat of elastic membrane. Most veins have VALVES which control the direction of the flow of blood.

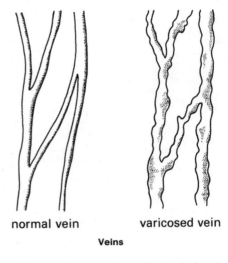

normal vein   varicosed vein

Veins

Diseases. Veins are thin-walled and often lie near the surface, so that they lack support and are exposed to injury.

Varicose veins are very common. Increased internal pressure produces dilation and lengthening. Lengthening causes twisting; and dilation, by further weakening the vein-wall and making internal valves incompetent, encourages further varicosity. Most frequently affected are the long veins of the legs, especially in persons whose occupation involves prolonged standing. Other common sites for varicose veins are around the anus (haemorrhoids or piles), the spermatic cord (varicocele) and at the junction between the oesophagus and the stomach, where they may rupture to cause gastric haemorrhage.

Severe varicose veins require surgical treatment either by removal or tying, or the injection of sclerosing (hardening) solutions. Elastic stockings help minor cases.

Inflammation of veins is called phlebitis; it may be either simple, from local injury or in prolonged exhaustion, or infective. Infective phlebitis of leg-veins is common after childbirth, and is known as phlegmasia. Phlebitis causes clot-formation (thrombus) within the vein, and detached clots may be carried elsewhere by the circulation as an embolus.

Phlebitis calls for rest and local symptomatic measures, with antibiotic cover for any infection.

venereal disease. Disease which is spread predominantly by sexual contact. The specific conditions named in the Venereal Disease Act (1917) of the U.K. are syphilis, gonorrhoea, and soft chancre (chancroid), but some other conditions are spread in a similar manner. Lymphogranuloma venereum and granuloma inguinale (due to virus-like organisms) are diseases of sexual intercourse, and venereal clinics are also called on to treat non-specific urethritis and trichomonas infections.

Venereal diseases are a social problem with implications of morality and guilt. There are possible references to gonorrhea in Leviticus and Proverbs, and it appears in European literature from at least 1378 as 'the burning' or 'the clap'. The crews of Columbus are sometimes blamed for importing syphilis from America in 1493, and it certainly spread rapidly in Europe thereafter; it was sometimes known as the 'French disease'. By the sixteenth century even the Town Council of Aberdeen was attempting to arrest it by branding and segregating those affected. Syphilis and gonorrhea were often confused, even by the eminent John Hunter (1728-93), whose attempts to prove by self-inoculation that they were one and the same probably hastened his death. However, in 1879 Albert Neisser discovered the gonococcus, and in 1905 Fritz Schaudinn isolated the spirochaete of syphilis.

Treatment has great influence on venereal epidemiology. The old remedy for syphilis was mercury, uncertain and toxic but used until 1909, when Ehrlich discovered 'Salvarsan 606', followed by the development of further arsenical compounds. These in turn were superseded in the mid 1940s by the safe and effective penicillin. Up to 1937 the treatment of gonorrhoea largely relied on many weeks of washing out the genital tract, but it often failed to achieve complete cure. Subsequently, sulphonamides and penicillin provided therapy which is effective in a few days.

By the end of World War II it therefore seemed that venereal disease would be steadily reduced and perhaps ultimately eradicated, but this has not happened. Indeed, after a considerable decline for a number of years, the tide seemed to turn. Syphilis remained fairly rare in the U.K. (around 1700 new cases in a typical year) but increased by about 300 per cent in the U.S.A., and in the early 1970s experts estimated that there were about 50 million cases of infectious syphilis in the world (as compared with an estimate of about 20 million at the close of World War II). Gonorrhoea rose even more, to around 70,000 cases in the U.K., about one and a half million cases in the U.S.A. and an estimated 150 million cases in the world, making gonorrhoea the commonest infectious disease after the ordinary cold and influenza. Other venereal diseases also showed a rise. Most alarming of all is the increase – especially of gonorrhoea – in teenage youngsters.

Many factors are involved in attempts to control and reduce the venereal diseases, though clearly spread depends on the extent of promiscuity and on the size of the infector pool, i.e., the number of persons already infectious. Both moral and religious education and sex education should contribute to the reduction of promiscuity, but a trend operating in the reverse direction is prolonged separation of workers in our mobile society from their partners: venereal disease is notoriously common in merchant seamen, servicemen, air pilots and air hostesses, persons working on oil rigs and long-distance lorry drivers. Again to some extent the professional prostitute, who could in many countries be legally subjected to periodical medical examination and who in any case would want to avoid infection or have it promptly treated, is being replaced by the 'good time' promiscuous girl, and this promiscuity is in large measure a part of the antisocial behaviour of adolescent rebellion. So anything that helps to reduce juvenile delinquency should be useful here. Although the increase in venereal disease started considerably before the contraceptive pill was in common use, removal of fear of pregnancy may contribute to the increase in promiscuity; however, experience in various contraceptive clinics suggests that they are used by socially responsible people who are married or 'going steady' and virtually ignored by promiscuous girls.

As for reduction of the infector pool, clearly it is essential to provide adequate, accessible, confidential and free treatment centres; to ensure that these centres are open at hours suitable to the potential users; to spread information about the centres and about the dangers of untreated disease; and, in so far as is possible, to trace contacts and persuade them to undergo treatment.

In the U.K. the current stress is on contact tracing and contact persuasion. The former involves something of the interviewing skill of a detective and is difficult since the infected person may have met the contact casually, may not know the surname and may be poor at description; and contact persuasion involves much of the motivating skill of a health visitor and is even more difficult since the contact generally does not feel ill and in the majority of cases is found on examination to be uninfected. Perhaps it would be more useful to transfer the emphasis on the one hand to health education (with sex education as a component part) and on the other hand to ensuring that the positioning and hours of opening of treatment centres are satisfactory. Nevertheless it has to be acknowledged that the U.K. is dealing more successfully with the epidemic of venereal diseases than are various other countries.

venesection. An old-fashioned term for the cutting of a vein. Removal of blood was once a popular and often irrational form of treatment. One of the large veins at the bend of the elbow was simply exposed and deftly opened by a lancet-stroke, allowing the patient to bleed into a bowl. Blood-letting is perhaps still helpful in such conditions as polycythaemia, or in congestive cardiac failure with marked swelling of the veins, but nowadays it would be carried out by venepuncture, using a wide-bore hollow needle and flexible tubing leading to a receiver. Venepuncture is also in daily use to withdraw blood-samples, and in the reverse direction, to instil replacement blood, transfusion solutions, and drugs.

venom. A general term for the poisonous substances produced by many different creatures, and injected into the body of a victim or adversary, by BITES AND STINGS. Venomous groups include many kinds of insects such as bees, wasps, hornets, and various tropical species, arachnids (spiders and scorpions), reptiles such as snakes and lizards (see SNAKE BITES), spiny fish and jellyfish.

The effects of venom injection may vary from local pain and swelling, as in bee and wasp stings, to rapid prostration and death, which often follows bites by vipers or colubrine snakes (cobras).

ventilation. The process of providing buildings, or individual rooms, with an adequate supply of fresh air.

When people are overcrowded, insufficient ventilation causes 'stuffiness', marked by feelings of oppression and bodily discomfort, with flushing of the cheeks, headache from swelling of the mucous membrane of the nose, nausea, and perhaps fainting and collapse. Such symptoms occur long before oxygen is seriously depleted or carbon dioxide concentration reaches dangerous levels, and are due entirely to the combined physical effects of increased temperature, increased humidity, and lack of air-movement.

Sufficient air-changes must be provided to avoid discomfort. About 28 to 56 cu. m. (1000 to 2000 cu. ft.) of fresh air are required per person per hour, and the appropriate number of air-changes per hour can be worked out from the cubic capacity of the room and the number of occupants. In ordinary dwellings, natural ventilation from windows, doors and chimney vents normally provides all the air-change that is needed, but in factories, offices and public buildings with systems of artificial ventilation, six changes per hour are generally recommended. Steps must be taken to prevent draughts by warming the incoming air and considering the position of inlets.

The katathermometer is used to assess the cooling-power of air in rooms. The dry kata-thermometer measures rate of heat-loss from radiation and convection. The wet kata-thermometer takes accounts of evaporation as well. Comfort for indoor sedentary work calls for a dry kata reading of about 6, representing a

heat-loss from the previously-warmed thermometer of 6 millicalories per sq. cm. per second. If the readings are lower the room is too hot; if higher, it is too cold.

ventriculography. A procedure used in x-ray examination of the brain to visualize the lateral ventricles, which are cavities in the cerebral hemispheres of the brain filled with cerebro-spinal fluid. Brain-tissue and cerebrospinal fluid are of uniform x-ray opacity and an ordinary plate is generally of little help in demonstrating suspected disease. In the technique of ventriculography the fluid is replaced by air or oxygen before x-ray examination, and since air is of different radiographic density it provides a contrast medium to outline the ventricles. Any displacement or alteration in their size and shape helps to determine the site or nature of any disòrder.

The air is normally instilled through a hollow needle passed into the ventricles after a preliminary burr-hole has been made in the skull. An alternative method introduces air after lumbar puncture in the hope that it will rise and enter the ventricles, but this does not always happen.

vermifuge. Any drug used to expel parasitic worms. A similar word, vermicide, implies that the drug actually kills them.

The *British Pharmacopeia* once provided a variety of uncertain remedies of this kind, including male-fern, melon-seeds, quassia, santonin, turpentine and thymol, but a range of really effective synthetic drugs (anthelmintics) is now available. Since worm-infestation (chronic entozoosis) causes much avoidable ill-health, this is an important advance. All these drugs require medical advice and supervision to regulate regimen and adjust dosage to body-weight, since some are mildly toxic.

verruca. A medical term for a WART.

vertebra. The thirty-three vertebrae, united to each other by intervertebral fibro-cartilaginous discs and by ligaments, are the bones which together form the SPINAL COLUMN. Although they conform to a standard pattern, they may be differentiated as the seven cervical, twelve thoracic, five lumbar, five sacral and four coccygeal vertebrae.

Each of the vertebrae has four projections which form the joint with the next vertebra; each also has an arch towards the back which forms the vertebral canal in which lies the spinal cord.

vertigo. A word which means 'turning' or 'spinning' and which is used to describe any sense of unsteadiness or movement experienced by an individual either when he seems to be spinning himself (subjective vertigo), or when the things around him seem to spin (objective vertigo).

Vertigo is always the result of direct or indirect disturbances of the balancing mechanism of the inner ear (labyrinth), of the vestibular nerve connecting the labyrinth to the brain, or of the cerebellum.

The possible causes are thus very numerous. They include diseases of the ear and its central connections; toxaemia from fevers, alcohol or drugs; cardio-vascular abnormalities causing high or low blood-pressure; anaemia; motion sickness; migraine and epilepsy; and organic brain disease, particularly if accompanied by raised intracranial tension.

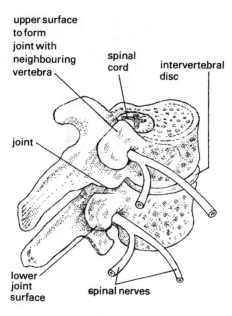

upper surface to form joint with neighbouring vertebra

spinal cord

intervertebral disc

joint

lower joint surface

spinal nerves

Vertebrae

Treatment depends on detailed investigation to determine an exact diagnosis. See also DIZZINESS and MÉNIÈRE'S DISEASE.

vesicles. Small blisters occurring as an eruption on skin or mucous membrane, and conventionally not larger than a pea. If bigger, they are usually called bullae, or just blisters.

The horny layer of the skin is raised by exudation of clear or turbid fluid to form a roughly hemispherical protrusion, sometimes surrounded by a red, inflamed zone.

Vesicles occur in a variety of conditions: (1) specific infections: smallpox; chickenpox; herpes; impetigo; (2) skin diseases: eczema; non-specific pyogenic (pus-forming) infections; (3) parasitism: insect bites; scabies; lice infestation; (4) external irritants, and (5) drugs: iodides; mercury.

Careful study of the type, distribution, and development of vesicles may be of diagnostic help. This is particularly so in differentiating between smallpox and chickenpox. Vesicle contents may also be sampled for microscopic examination and culture to determine any specific microbic or viral cause.

Vincent's angina. A particular form of severe ulcerative inflammation of the mucous membrane of the mouth. In definitive cases two micro-organisms are constantly present: *Bacillus fusiformis* and *Spirillum vincenti*. These appear to act in association, but other factors are involved because the disease tends to be found in people suffering from debilitating general conditions such as continued fevers, blood diseases, metallic poisoning, and vitamin deficiencies. There is always pre-existing dental neglect and inflammation of the gums.

The condition is only mildly infectious with occasional outbreaks in residential institutions.

Numerous cases occurred amongst troops in the First World War and became known as 'trench mouth'.

General symptoms are usually trivial. The gums are red, swollen and ulcerated, and shallow ulcers may form elsewhere in the mouth and pharynx, and on the tonsils, often with an adherent exudate resembling diphtheria. The neck-glands are enlarged and the breath has a characteristic smell.

The occurrence of Vincent's angina should prompt a search for some general disease. Otherwise treatment is by antibiotics combined with suitable antiseptic mouth-washes or local applications. Oxidizing agents such as hydrogen peroxide or potassium chlorate are particularly effective. Thorough dental treatment is also required.

violence. Any tolerable society needs law and order. The mere promulgation of laws is useless unless they are obeyed, and this means either a massive police force and severe punishment, or the inculcation of law-abiding attitudes. There is little evidence that repression curbs violence. Instead, it provokes escalation and necessitates ever more forceful control.

It is painfully obvious throughout the world that there is violence on an increasing scale. Aggressive behaviour is shown by daily reports of vandalism, 'mugging', bomb-attacks, hijacking, kidnapping, bank-raids, carnage on the roads, disrespect for life and property, school indiscipline, and, on a larger stage, by the cruelties inherent in rival political systems, religious feuds, and racial intolerance.

Roots of violence. Psychologists identify at least four basic human needs, unfulfillment of which provokes antisocial behaviour. These are a need for love and security; for new experiences; for praise and recognition; and for responsibility. When basic needs are not met, reaction takes place: fight or flight – attack or withdrawal.

Anger and hate are the usual reactions to rejection and denial of love. With a loving relationship children learn to control their anger; without affection it grows more vicious with increasing strength. A dull, uneventful life induces boredom, frustration, and restlessness. The aimless adolescent seeks new experiences and those forbidden or dangerous particularly attract him. What starts as a 'lark' turns to vandalism and aggression. Violence is predominantly a male activity perhaps because boys and men need challenging and dangerous experiences or because they are more often severely punished and so become more apt to take retaliatory action.

Praise and recognition reward achievement rather that effort. The intellectually slow, culturally disadvantaged, and emotionally deprived are disregarded and seek admiration elsewhere. Acceptance by a gang ministers to self-esteem and it is then a small step to use the safety of a group to 'show-off' and resort to violence.

Denial of responsibility ensures that children fail to develop respect for self, others and property. They become disinclined to wait and work for what they want and to postpone immediate gratification of impulses; and they become contemptuous of the rights of others. Work is often boring and without involvement, and this engenders a craving to discover exciting spare-time outlets for suppressed energies.

Reasons for increasing violence. Criticism and dissatisfaction permeate the present social fabric and affect morals and conduct. The old compact communities, where everyone was known to neighbours and authority, have been disrupted by redevelopment. High-density urban living and population mobility have led to a more impersonal environment. In animal societies, naturalists have shown that over-crowding and noise induce destructive behaviour. Children and adolescents are now physically healthier and stronger and need greater outlets for their energy. Both formal education and the growth of communications have made people more aware of events elsewhere. Unfortunately, the news-media concentrate on violence and sensation, and by Gresham's Law, the bad drives out the good. More general affluence makes relative deprivation increasingly hard to bear. The more glaring the inequalities, the greater the resentment and hostility.

Measures to reduce violence and aggression. If it be true that violence stems from denial of basic emotional needs, corrective measures must be both short-term and long-term. The existing situation demands from society as much concern for the emotional, social and intellectual development of children as it now shows for their physical health. Society must help parents to a knowledge of the essentials of healthy emotional development in their children; provide opportunities for leisure activities; and involve young people in community projects in which they can take pride. To give responsibility to the irresponsible is more difficult but it can be done by encouraging their active participation in the organization and running of social activities and voluntary social projects.

In the long-term a solution lies even more with parent-education, and the slogan 'every child a wanted child', much used in another context, if translated into reality would go far to ensure the basic need for love and security. In relation to the other needs the necessary revolution can be brought about by the determination of all concerned to apply existing social, psychological, and educational knowledge. Interruption of the present vicious circle will help to ensure that the emotionally and intellectually deprived of today do not become tomorrow's parents of yet another deprived generation.

virilism. The development of male characteristics in a woman, with masculine distribution and growth of body and facial hair, deepening of the voice, and cessation of menstruation. Adiposity (excess of fat-containing tissue) is often an additional feature.

As a disease (adrenogenital syndrome), virilism is due to over-secretion of androgenic hormone and this results from changes in the adrenal gland, the endocrine gland which produces this hormone. These changes may be either benign growths (adenoma) or malignant (carcinoma). Surgical treatment is indicated.

Virilism also occurs as a side-effect of corticosteroid drugs, and of testosterone (male hormone) and other anabolic agents with similar properties. This usually calls for adjustment of dosage or change of drug, but androgens based on testosterone are used for some serious conditions such as advanced and inoperable breast-cancer, and masculinization may have to be accepted as a lesser evil.

viruses. Extemely minute infective agents which are only visible by use of the electron microscope. It is helpful to think of their magnitude, by volume, as being roughly one-thousandth that of the bacteria. Pasteur himself suggested that such organisms existed and their reality was demonstrated, shortly after his death in 1895, in connection with tobacco mosaic disease and bovine foot-and-mouth infection.

Most larger infective agents (such as bacteria) can be cultivated in artificial media which do not require cells of living tissue, but no accepted virus has so far been grown in anything simpler than a tissue culture. Inability to multiply independently is thus part of the definition of a virus. This correlation between small size and dependence on living tissues probably means that viruses cannot provide internal enzyme systems for themselves and therefore are forced to rely on those of some convenient host. It is also possible that the virus misdirects in some way the host enzyme systems in its own interests, and that it is this alteration which causes disease in the host.

Research has now identified many specific types and varieties of viruses which are known to be responsible for a wide range of diseases in animals and plants. Conditions of human importance include smallpox, chickenpox, herpes, hepatitis, poliomyelitis, measles, German measles (rubella), mumps, yellow fever, lassa fever and rabies, as well as influenza, the common cold, and other less well-defined affections of the respiratory, gastro-intestinal, nervous and glandular systems.

The influence of viruses in malignant disease is still largely speculative. In 1911 Rous demonstrated that a sarcoma in chickens could be transmitted by cell-free filtrates, and other similar effects have since been produced in mice and other small animals. Human adeno-viruses can also induce tumours in laboratory animals. Whether such experiments are meaningful in relation to human malignant disease remains to be seen, but there is some evidence concerning epidemic lymphoma (a tumour occurring in parts of Africa), which may well have an insect-borne virus concerned in its causation.

In general, drugs and antibiotics have little effect on viral diseases, although there are prospects of future progress. Two products are available commercially: methisazone for smallpox and the complications of smallpox vaccination, and idoxuridine for herpes, especially when the cornea is affected.

Control of important viral diseases depends largely on vaccination. Smallpox vaccination was invented by Edward Jenner as long ago as 1796, but now other vaccines in common use include those against poliomyelitis, measles, rubella, yellow fever, rabies, and influenza. With some viruses, vaccination or an attack produces solid and lasting immunity, but with others, such as influenza and the common cold, results are often brief and uncertain. This is probably due to the existence of several similar viruses only slightly different, and this variation, known as 'antigenic drift' means that a particular vaccine may not be exactly matched to a prevalent infection.

viscera. A collective term for the organs contained within the body-cavities: the chest, abdomen, and pelvis. It is the plural of 'viscus' and can be regarded as equivalent to the ordinary word 'entrails'.

In scientific terminology the prefix 'splanchno-' (from the Greek word for bowels), is used as synonymous with visceral. Thus splanchnology means study of the viscera, and disease of the viscera is generally called splanchnopathology .

visceroptosis. A condition in which the abdominal viscera tend to sag downwards to a lower level than normal.

It is most often seen in women, and is due to loss of tone in the abdominal muscles and to the stretching of suspensory ligaments, and is often caused by the effects of repeated pregnancies. Displacement may be general or limited to individual organs, particularly the stomach, liver, spleen, kidney, or colon. The lower part of the abdomen appears unduly prominent and the patient may suffer dragging pains, indigestion, and constipation, with more indefinite neurasthenic symptoms such as a sense of weight, lassitude, and depression.

In the past there was a vogue for elaborate operations to reposition and resecure the displaced viscera but these had little success. The most satisfactory course is to provide a well-fitted abdominal support and to correct any prominent symptoms – physical or mental – by appropriate medical treatment.

vision. See EYE.

vital statistics. Statistics are numerical data relating to large numbers of specific events, compiled and arrayed to display the significance of such events. Figures of this kind can be related to various aspects of human life in communities, and are therefore used as indices of health and disease, as indicators of fluctuations in health, and as a guide to the relative importance of factors which influence health. As William Farr, the 'father of statistics' said in 1875, 'The exact determination of evils is the first step towards their remedies'.

Statistics related to health and community well-being deal with many topics and vary in usefulness, accuracy, and reliability. A general account of the various types will be found in the article INDICES OF COMMUNITY HEALTH but the term 'vital statistics' is generally understood to comprise those figures which are derived from the statutory registration of births, marriages, and deaths (including foetal deaths). In most countries the bare record of these events is amplified at registration by the collection of other information such as sex, nationality, legitimacy, multiple birth, place of birth, place of residence, marital status, previous marriage, occupation, hospitalization, place of death, age at and cause of death.

As community medicine develops there is obviously scope for the collection of further details, particularly those with social connotations, and some countries do this, but there are difficulties about making registration too elaborate, especially in underdeveloped countries where accurate records of even basic data are hard to achieve.

The mere collection of such figures is meaningless unless they can be related to the population from which they are derived. An accurate census is therefore essential and in many developed countries (e.g., the U.K.) this is normally taken every ten years and the figures for intermediate years are estimated by extrapolation.

Using the census figures and the annual record of events, various useful calculations can be made. The chief of these vital statistics are:

1. Birth rate. The number of live-births per thousand of the population. This is affected by many factors such as the number of young people; age at marriage; social habits; stability of living conditions; contraceptive services; and abortion.

2. Marriage rate. The number of marriages per thousand of the population.

3. Crude death rate. The number of deaths per thousand of the population. Although this rate is of some value in relation to the whole population, it is unhelpful in comparing one locality with another because the relative age-constitutions vary and residents may die and be registered elsewhere. Refinements are needed and these are the corrected or recorded death rate, calculated after allowing for transfers out-and-in to place of usual residence, and the adjusted or standardized death rate, which makes allowance for the age and sex constitution of the local population as compared with the national population.

4. Infant mortality rate. The number of infants dying under 1 year of age per thousand live births. This is a sensitive index of the quality of social conditions and health services.

5. Still-birth rate. The number of still-births per thousand total births (live and still).

6. Perinatal mortality rate. The number of still-births, plus deaths under one week of age, per thousand total births. A useful indication of hazards immediately before and after birth.

7. Neonatal mortality rate. The number of infants dying under one month of age per thousand live births. It is less informative than the perinatal mortality rate.

8. Maternal mortality rate. The number of women dying from causes associated with childbirth per thousand total births. This rate reflects standards of obstetric practice and antenatal care.

Much information can also be derived from manipulation of the death rate figures. Deaths are substantially influenced by occupation and social class. The method of determining, for instance, the occupational mortality involves calculating standard death-rates related to age-groups, for all occupied and retired workers, and then applying these rates to the known numbers and ages of workers in a particular trade as derived from the census. The estimated 'standard deaths' are then compared with the actual occupational deaths and expressed as a standard mortality ratio, the percentage which the actual deaths are of the expected deaths. According to the amount by which this ratio is above or below 100, the health of the particular workers is worse or better than the average. A similar procedure can be applied to any selected category of person identifiable in the census data. The results provide a useful indicator of where measures might be taken to reduce deaths.

vitamin content of foods. Traditionally the amounts of vitamins A and D which are estimated by biological assay are stated in international units and those of the B and C vitamins in milligrams, although the differentiation is no longer necessary: 333 units of vitamin A and 40,000 units of vitamin D each represent a milligram.

Many tables exist purporting to show the exact vitamin content of various foods, and a simplified table giving the protein, fat, carbohydrate and vitamin contents of over fifty common articles of diet is given below. Such tables are useful to persons dealing with large quantities of food but are perhaps of less value for the ordinary householder.

To illustrate let us take the position of a householder who proposes to eat an apple, part of a cabbage and a helping of beef. A table will tell him that 100 g. of apples contain 3 mg. of vitamin C, that 100 g. of spring cabbage contain 60 mg. of that vitamin and that 100 g. of beef contain 35 units of vitamin A. However, before doing arithmetical calculations related to the particular weights of the foods that he is preparing to eat, the householder has various things to remember. Firstly, his concern is with the portion that he intends to eat: there is no point in his weighing the apple before removing the skin and a small bruised portion or weighing the cabbage before removing the outer leaves. Secondly, even when he has weighed only the part that he intends to eat, the table gives him only an average assessment. The amount of vitamin A in his piece of beef will vary appreciably according to how lean or how fat it is, and the vitamin C content of the apple or cabbage will vary with the exact type of the fruit or vegetable, with the climatic conditions under which it was grown, with the degree of ripeness when it was picked, with how long and under what conditions it was stored, and not least – if it is to be cooked – with the method of cooking.

The exact requirement of most vitamins for an adult of average size is known, although more may be required during pregnancy, lactation, strenuous work and illness, and growing children need more than in proportion to body weight. Inadequacy of any vitamin is serious. On the other hand, no quantity of the B and C vitamins has been known to do any harm, harmful excess of A would involve eating very large daily amounts of liver, carrots and spinach, and harmful excess of D would imply a quite inordinate fondness for sardines, herring and salmon. Excess of the fat-soluble vitamins can certainly be produced by over-dosage of vitamin tablets or of cod-liver oil or halibut-liver oil, but with any ordinary diet it is unlikely.

So, to save over-frequent studying of complicated tables, it is perhaps useful to set down the average content of foods rich in the various vitamins, so that, for example, a man who normally eats a helping of liver or a good portion of carrots or spinach can see at a casual glance that he is likely to have enough vitamin A.

Vitamin A. Daily requirement – 2,500 to 5,000 international units. (333 IU equal 1 mg.).

Average number of IU per 100 g.: halibut-liver oil – 1,950,000; cod-liver oil – 105,000; liver – 10,500; carrots – 6,000; spinach – 4,300; butter – 4,000; margarine (reinforced) – 3,000; dried apricots – 1,600; watercress – 1,600; cheese – 1,300; lettuce – 1,280; tomatoes – 980; kidney – 980; eggs – 980; dried prunes – 840; cabbage –

300; sardines – 270; peas and beans – 165; herring – 145; milk – 105.

Vitamin B₁. Daily requirement – 1.5 to 2.3 mg. Average mg. per 100 g.: yeast – 4.3; nuts – 0.9; chicken – 0.7; duck – 0.7; ham – 0.7; boiled rice – 0.7; bacon – 0.6; pork – 0.5; liver – 0.4; wholemeal bread – 0.32; peas – 0.3; egg – 0.14; mutton – 0.14; potatoes – 0.11; spinach – 0.10; beef – 0.07.

Vitamin B₂. Daily requirement – 2.2 to 3.3 mg. Average mg. per 100 g.: yeast – 4.4; liver – 3.0; cheese – 0.5; egg – 0.4; nuts – 0.3; herring – 0.25; bacon – 0.20; beef – 0.20; chicken – 0.20; pork – 0.20; salmon – 0.20; spinach – 0.20; cream – 0.20; wholemeal bread – 0.18.

Nicotinic acid. Daily requirement – 15 to 25 mg.

Average mg. per 100 g.: yeast – 72; liver and kidney – 13; nuts – 9; ham – 6; duck – 6; chicken – 6; pork – 5; mutton – 4; oily fish – 3; beef – 2.5; white fish – 2; wholemeal bread – 2; boiled rice – 1.

Vitamin C. Daily requirement – 70 mg.

Average mg. per 100 g.: blackcurrants – 200; cherries – 200; brussels sprouts – 80; cauliflower – 70; cabbage – 60; strawberry – 60; spinach – 60; orange – 56; lemon – 40; tomato – 24; new potato – 14.

Vitamin D. Daily requirement – 400 to 800 international units. (40,000 IU equal 1 mg.)

Average number of IU per 100 g.: halibut liver oil – 210,000; cod-liver oil – 10,500; salmon – 870; oily fish – 800; tinned salmon – 600; margarine (reinforced) – 350; butter – 60; eggs – 60; cheese – 35; milk – 1.

Shortage of vitamin A is uncommon in adults in developed countries except for people with many dietary pecularities, but can fairly easily occur in children and in particular in babies. Shortage of the B vitamins is fairly frequent among the poorer sections of the community and the elderly, and is also common among heavy consumers of alcohol. Shortage of vitamin C is common in areas in which people eat insufficient fruits and green vegetables, whether from tradition or from the cost of these commodities. Shortage of vitamin D is rare in southern countries (because to a considerable extent it can be manufactured under the skin in the presence of sunlight) but is quite common in northern countries, especially in immigrants from countries of greater sunshine. Exact bodily requirements of vitamin E are not yet known.

In many developed countries multiple vitamin tablets are on sale commercially. A typical one might contain about 2,500 IU of vitamin A (or most of the day's supply), about 0.5 mg. of vitamin B₁ (or about a quarter of the day's supply), possibly a little vitamin B₂ and nicotinic acid (but most tablets lack these either entirely or partially), about 13 mg. of vitamin C (or roughly a quarter of the day's supply) and about 250 IU of vitamin D (or about half of the day's supply). With adequate diet such supplements should theoretically be unnecessary but they can be useful in northern climates during winter months, when in particular little vitamin D is manufactured in the body, vegetables and fruits are scarcer and may have lost some vitamin C by cooking, storage with exposure to light, etc., and intake of the B vitamins may be restricted by cost.

vitamins. In 1906, F.G. Hopkins of Cambridge University reported that young rats fed on pure

PROTEIN, FAT, CARBOHYDRATE AND VITAMIN CONTENT OF EDIBLE PORTIONS OF VARIOUS FOODS

Contents are given per 100g of food. The symbol 'T' represents a trace, and 'IU' means international units. There are many variations. Contents are merely rough averages.

	Protein (g.)	Fat (g.)	Carbohyd. (g.)	Calories	Vit. A (IU)	Vit. B₁ (mg.)	Vit. B₂ (mg.)	Nicotinic Acid (mg.)	Vit. C (mg.)	Vit. D (IU)
Cereals										
White bread	8	1.4	52	240	-	0.07	0.03	0.7	-	-
Wholemeal bread	8	2	47	225	-	0.32	0.18	2.0	-	-
Plain fruit cake	6	16	54	380	T	0.07	0.05	0.8	-	-
Plain biscuits	7	13	75	430	-	T	T	T	-	-
Sweet biscuits	6	31	66	560	-	T	T	T	-	-
Rice (boiled)	2	0.3	30	122	-	0.07	0.07	1.0	-	-
Diary products, etc.										
Butter	0.4	85	1	790	4000	-	-	-	-	60
Margarine	0.2	86	-	790	3000	-	-	-	-	350
Cheese (Cheddar type)	25	35	-	425	1300	0.04	0.5	0.3	-	35
Egg (boiled)	12	12	-	160	980	0.14	0.4	-	-	60
Egg (fried)	14	20	-	240	1150	0.14	0.4	-	-	70
Milk	3.4	3.7	4.8	66	105	0.04	0.14	-	1	1
Cream (single)	2.4	21	3.2	220	700	0.08	0.20	-	T	10
Meat and Poultry										
Bacon (fried)	25	53	-	600	-	0.60	0.20	0.8	-	-
Beef (lean, grilled)	27	12	-	220	35	0.07	0.20	2.5	-	-
Chicken (boiled)	26	10	-	200	-	0.70	0.20	6.0	-	-
Duck (roasted)	23	24	-	320	-	0.70	0.18	6.0	-	-
Ham (lean, boiled)	23	13	-	210	-	0.70	0.20	6.0	-	-
Liver (calf, fried)	29	14	2.5	260	10,500	0.40	3.0	13.0	-	-
Mutton (lean chop)	26	18	-	270	50	0.14	0.18	4.0	-	-
Pork (roasted)	25	23	-	310	-	0.50	0.20	5.0	-	-
Fish										
Cod (steamed)	18	1	-	85	-	0.07	0.14	2.1	-	-
Cod (fried)	21	5	2.5	140	-	0.07	0.12	2.0	-	-
Haddock (steamed)	22	1	-	95	-	0.07	0.14	2.0	-	-
Haddock (fried)	20	8	4	170	-	0.07	0.12	2.0	-	-
Herring (fried)	22	15	2	230	200	-	0.25	3.0	-	800
Salmon (fresh, steamed)	19	13	-	200	150	T	0.20	3.8	-	870
Fruit										
Apple (raw)	0.3	-	11.7	45	14	0.04	-	0.3	3	-
Apple (baked)	0.3	-	10	39	28	-	-	1.4	-	-
Apricot (fresh)	0.6	-	6.7	28	700	T	T	T	11	-
Banana (raw)	1.1	-	19	77	80	0.05	T	T	10	-
Blackberry (raw)	1.3	-	6.5	30	300	T	T	T	21	-
Cherry (raw)	0.6	-	12	48	200	T	T	T	200	-
Dates (dried)	2	-	64	248	98	-	-	-	-	-
Lemon	0.8	-	3.2	15	-	0.04	-	-	40	-
Orange	0.8	-	8.5	35	100	0.07	T	T	56	-
Peach (raw)	0.6	-	9.0	37	700	T	T	T	10	-
Pear (raw)	0.2	-	10	40	10	T	T	T	4	-
Raspberry (raw)	1.0	-	5.6	26	70	T	T	T	30	-
Rhubarb (stewed) without sugar	0.4	-	0.8	5	20	T	-	-	10	-
Strawberry (fresh)	0.6	-	6.2	26	14	T	-	-	60	-
Vegetables										
Beans (Broad, boiled)	4.1	T	7.0	42	-	T	0.10	1.0	27	-
Beans (French, boiled)	0.8	-	1.1	7	200	0.03	0.07	0.7	20	-
Cabbage (Spring, boiled)	1.1	T	0.8	8	290	0.07	0.07	0.3	60	-
Carrot (raw)	0.8	T	5.4	23	6,000	0.07	0.04	0.7	10	-
Carrot (boiled)	0.9	T	4.5	21	5,500	0.05	0.03	0.6	9	-
Leek (boiled)	1.8	T	4.6	25	600	0.05	-	-	20	-
Lettuce (raw)	1.1	T	1.8	11	1,280	0.07	0.07	0.3	14	-
Parsnips (boiled)	1.3	T	13	55	190	0.11	0.07	T	3	-
Peas (fresh, boiled)	5.0	T	8	50	490	0.30		T	3	-
Potatoes (new, boiled)	1.6	T	18	74	-	0.11	0.07	0.1	14	-
Spinach (boiled)	5.1	T	0.9	10	4,000	0.10	0.20	0.4	60	-
Turnip (boiled)	0.9	T	2.8	18	-	T	T	0.1	14	-
Tomato (raw)	0.9	T	2.8	14	980	0.11	T	0.2	24	-

protein, carbohydrate, fat, minerals, and water, in adequate amounts and correct proportions, failed to thrive, but that the addition of only small quantities of milk produced growth. He concluded that foods in their natural state contained substances essential to life although present in only minute quantities. The chemical nature of these substances was then unknown and they were at first called simply 'accessory food factors'. Later they were considered to be nitrogenous compounds, or amines, and they were given the name 'vitamines'. When this assumption was subsequently disproved the terminal 'e' was dropped and the generic term 'vitamin' was adopted. Further research gradually defined several different factors and these were each designated by letters of the alphabet extending at least as far as K, but now with omissions caused by the reclassification of certain elements of the B-complex.

Hopkins' observations merely provided some scientific confirmation for what had been recognized on a practical level for many years: for instance, Captain Cook, in the eighteenth century, had discovered that he could control scurvy in his sailors by giving citrus fruits, and Takaki in 1882 eliminated beri-beri from the Japanese Navy by improving their rice diet. This discovery led the Dutch pathologist Eijkman to experiment with polished and unpolished rice, and he was able to show that the bran contained a factor which prevented and cured the neuritis of beri-beri. This proved to be a starting-point for establishing the nature of DEFICIENCY DISEASES, and ushered in a new era for preventive medicine.

It was however some time before any vitamin was positively identified, although it was soon noted that they fell into two groups as fat-soluble and water-soluble. In the first group vitamin D was identified at the Lister Institute in 1925, and water-soluble vitamin C in 1928 was discovered to be ascorbic acid by Syent-Gyorgy, a Hungarian biochemist and Nobel prizewinner (1937), who is perhaps even better remembered for his profound remark that 'vitamins are what make you ill if you don't take them.'

Since then much has been done to identify, isolate, and synthesize other factors. The present state of knowledge can be broadly summarized as follows:

Vitamin A. Carotene; 'anti-infective' vitamin which is fat-soluble. Sources: fish-liver oils, egg-yolk, liver, dairy products, carrots and green vegetables. Deficiency causes xerophthalmia (corneal degeneration), night-blindness, and susceptibility to infection. Excess may cause severe symptoms, with loss of appetite, periostitis (inflammation of the fibrous membrane covering bones), bone-pains, spontaneous fractures, and enlargement of liver and spleen.

Vitamin B-*complex*. A group of water-soluble vitamins essential to many ENZYME systems concerned in the utilization of carbohydrate, protein, and fat. Although each factor has specific importance there is also overlap and interdependence.

Vitamin B₁. Aneurin or thiamine. Sources: wheat-germ, cereal husks, yeast, egg-yolk, liver, pork, and legumes. Deficiency causes beri-beri or in lesser degrees of deprivation neuritis, mental dullness, cardiac and general weakness.

Vitamin B₂. Riboflavin. Sources: milk, egg-white, liver, offal, beef, tomatoes, and green vegetables. Deficiency causes angular stomatitis (cheilosis, i.e., inflammation of the mucous membrane of the lips and angles of the mouth) and seborrhoea (excess secretion of oil from sebaceous glands) of nose and lips, not infrequently seen in elderly people on a poor diet.

P-P Factor. Pellagra-preventive factor or nicotinic acid (niacin). Sources: yeast, milk, pork, beef and offal. Deficiency causes pellagra.

Vitamin B₆. Pyridoxine or 'anti-dermatitis' factor. Sources: yeast, wheat-germ, milk and vegetables. Deficiency is probably related to pellagra syndrome.

Folic acid (formerly vitamin M). Sources: yeast, spinach, liver. Deficiency causes large celled anaemia as seen in sprue, steatorrhoea, coeliac disease, and pregnancy. In pernicious anaemia it represents the 'extrinsic factor'. It relieves the anaemia but not the associated nerve-degeneration. 'Intrinsic factor' (B₁₂) is also required. Interaction takes place in the liver to produce restoration of satisfactory red-cell formation.

Vitamin B₁₂. Cyanocobalmin: 'intrinsic factor'. Derived from enzyme activity in the stomach. Deficiency causes pernicious anaemia. Interaction with folic acid controls red-cell formation.

Other vitamin B factors are of lesser human importance but their absence causes disease in laboratory animals, or retards bacterial growth. Pantothenic acid (B₃) has effects similar to those of riboflavin and is claimed to be of value in arthritis; biotin neutralizes avidin, a constituent of egg-albumen, which causes dermatitis, emaciation and death in rats fed exclusively on egg-white. Choline, inositol, and para-amino benzoic acid affect bacterial growth.

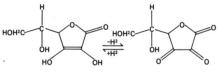

Vitamin C, ascorbic acid

Vitamin C. Ascorbic acid or cevitamic acid. This is water-soluble and not produced or stored in the body; daily needs are increased by fever. Sources: blackcurrants, citrus fruits, other fruits, green vegetables. Deficiency increases capillary permeability and causes scurvy and there is much speculation and untested hypothesis about its role in other conditions. Dr. Linus Pauling, Nobel Laureate, has advocated large doses (1 g. or more per day) for prevention and cure of common colds, and has gained some popular experimental support.

Vitamin D. Calciferol or 'anti-rachitic' vitamin. This is fat-soluble or can be derived from a precursor, ergosterol, by ultra-violet irradiation, and this change can occur in exposed skin. Sources: fish-liver oils, animal fats, egg-yolk, summer milk. Vitamin D controls calcium absorption, and deficiency causes rickets. Pregnant and nursing mothers, and children, require supplies. It is stored by the body and excess can produce hypercalcaemia and kidney damage from calcium deposition.

Vitamin E. Alpha-tocopherol or 'anti-sterility' vitamin, which is fat-soluble. Sources: wheat-germ oil, cereals, egg-yolk, milk and green vegetables. Deficiency effects are not definite in man, but in animals its absence causes testicular degeneration, abortion, muscular and myocardial degeneration, thrombosis, and defects in bones, teeth and pelts. Because of this experimental evidence it is used clinically for treating habitual abortion, menopausal disorders, senile vulvo-vaginitis, male infertility, and peripheral vascular disease. Despite scepticism there is probably much still to learn about vitamin E function in man, and particularly about its role in fat digestion which has implications related to cardio-vascular disease and ageing.

Vitamin K. Phytomenadione, which is water-soluble. Sources: green vegetables mainly, but it can be manufactured in the gut. It is concerned in blood-clotting and deficiency delays clotting and arrest of haemorrhage. Bile-salts are necessary for its absorption, and deficiency states are associated with obstructive jaundice, some types of haemorrhagic disease of the new-born, ulcerative colitis, and feverish wasting diseases, which increase demand and interfere with its manufacture in the gut. Although vitamin K is valuable in selected cases, its use in premature infants needs care to avoid destruction of red blood corpuscles. It is also used as an antidote for anticoagulant drugs and in the treatment of dental haemorrhage.

General. Most people on a normal diet get adequate quantities of vitamins although it may be necessary to supplement the diet at critical periods such as pregnancy, lactation, growth, and acute illness. Exceptions occur chiefly amongst alcoholics, food-faddists, psychotics, mental defectives, impoverished old persons living alone, and sometimes in institutions with bulk-cooking and poor menus. Deficiencies are usually of the B group and if one symptom is recognized it can be assumed that other B factors are minimal too. Those living alone are also prone to scurvy because they do not bother much about fruit and vegetables (see VITAMIN CONTENT OF FOOD).

During illness, deficiencies arise from defective absorption (see DIGESTION) particularly in chronic intestinal disease, after operations on the stomach, and in obstructive jaundice. Indefinite ill-health is often ascribed to vitamin deficiency but not often proven. Even rickets needs care in diagnosis and x-ray confirmation.

Complaints of mental origin may mimic vitamin deficiency, but a feature of deficiency diseases is that they are very rapidly relieved by doses of the appropriate vitamin. If this therapeutic test fails, it can be safely assumed that there is some other cause.

vivisection. Surgical operation on a living animal, usually to advance physiological or pathological knowledge.

In all developed countries vivisection is strictly controlled by law, with limitation of the persons undertaking it and limitation of methods to those that avoid needless suffering. Vivisection is bitterly opposed by many people on emotional rather than rational grounds but is really essential for the advance both of medical and of veterinary science. For instance, Pasteur's experimental vaccination of sheep against anthrax and then inoculation of the sheep with the organism was vivisection but it subsequently saved the lives of multitudes of animals as well as of many people. To give another example, the production of diphtheria antitoxin by giving graded doses of diphtheria toxin to a horse (never large enough to create illness) and then the withdrawal of some blood from the immunized horse (causing no more pain than when a person acts as a blood donor) was vivisection but saved many thousands of lives in the era before diphtheria immunization.

Where vivisection results in the death of an animal the argument is not unlike that between the vegetarian and the eater of flesh. If it is justifiable to slaughter an animal for food, it is perhaps justifiable to kill an animal in order to save both human and animal lives.

vocational adjustment. Any industrial or commercial organization should have three main aims – to achieve maximum production, to limit accidents, and to provide for its employees healthy and happy conditions of work. The interconnection of these three became apparent under the stresses of the First and even the Second World War. For instance, workers and employers under these stresses willingly lengthened working hours and minimized or abolished tea breaks, and then found that, when the lengthening and minimizing had gone beyond a certain point, production fell and accidents and illnesses increased.

In consequence of such happenings, industrial psychology developed rapidly and unobtrusively; and since then it has consolidated its position as an indispensable tool of management for adjusting the worker to the job and the job to the worker.

On the human side, industrial psychology starts off with the selection of the right people for different jobs and then oversees their subsequent progress. At the apprenticeship stage, formal training programmes, based on time-and-motion studies and accurate assessment of work content, have largely replaced casual time-serving methods in which the apprentice was expected to learn largely by watching. Proficiency, trade, and promotion tests help to ensure that capacity and ability are matched to vocational requirements. At management levels also, tests of motivation and personality increasingly influence appointments: in the past we tended to promote a person who had been successful in an entirely different junior job, whereas today we try to assess his competence for the particular new job.

In relation to the machinery and organization of industry, psychology has demonstrated the importance of physical conditions, hours of work, fatigue, monotony, boredom, conditions of employment, and methods of work, and has helped to suggest the vocational adjustments necessary to remedy adverse effects.

Accident prevention has been a particularly fruitful field. A proportion of workers has always been regarded as accident prone, but psychology has elucidated at least some of the factors involved, such as poor co-ordination, slow reaction times, reduced visual acuteness, and the effects of emotional characteristics, where rush, irritation and distraction lead to loss of control and concentration.

vocational guidance. A pupil about to leave school is faced with the problem of deciding upon a career. For a boy, any decision may determine his future until retiral age, while a girl expects to work at least until marriage and perhaps will resume employment later on when family responsibilities decline. If work is to be a source of satisfaction, and not just a necessary evil, the choice of a suitable occupation is of paramount importance. Happiness and success for the individual depends on taking up employment which is congenial and within his capacity, and for the potential employer it is equally essential that abilities and aptitudes should conform to the needs of a particular job.

Inherent in the appointment of guidance and careers teachers in schools, and in the development of arrangements for liaison with youth employment agencies, is a recognition that organized vocational guidance can help to reduce the numbers of occupational misfits. It is also to the general benefit of society that high ability should be fully utilized, and conversely, that resources should not be wasted in attempts to train persons beyond their potential levels of achievement. Personal inclinations cannot, of course, be totally disregarded since ambition and motivation can overcome great difficulties, but it may be just as important to dissuade pupils without the necessary intellectual and physical capacities from embarking on a career which will only bring frustration, as it is to guide those who have no immediate preferences.

Basically, consideration must be given to physical, intellectual, and emotional factors, and these involve advice from the school itself and from the services concerned with school health and child guidance. On the physical side, a child's potentialities may be limited by physique, by the effects of disease or disability, or by sensory defects such as deafness, defective vision, or colour-blindness. Psychological tests assess individual differences of psychological function. Tests of general intelligence measure innate ability in the manipulation of ideas and things. Academic pursuits require intellectual capacity, but practical occupations equally need a high level of aptitude in other directions.

Intelligence tests are supplemented by attainment tests, which measure the skills and knowledge acquired by training and experience, and also by some attempt at personality assessment. A variety of tests now purport to judge emotional adjustment, motivation, and social attitudes. The school-leaver is less likely to have been subjected to these unless some earlier aberrant behaviour has brought him specially to the notice of the Child Guidance Service, but the school authorities are well-placed to make at least some informal assessment of personality. Collation of all this information provides a rational basis for vocational guidance which then seeks to match the aptitudes and abilities of the child to the requirements of a wide range of possible occupations.

In the U.K. there are now formal arrangements by which school-leavers are brought to the notice of the Employment Advisory Service of the Department of Employment. The School Health Service is expected to identify pupils who are 'not unconditionally fit for employment', and to advise the careers officers and their medical support services. Some handicapped children may in fact require the special protection afforded by the Disabled Persons (Employment) Acts 1944 and 1958, and, with the consent of child and parent, this can be organized before a child leaves school.

voice. The larynx or voice box is a part of the respiratory system, situated at the front of the neck. It is a chamber made of cartilage containing the vocal cords, which are two bands of elastic tissue capable of being separated, drawn together, or tensed by muscular action. When the vocal cords vibrate in a current of air expelled from the chest, the result is the sound called voice, or phonation. Modification of this sound by changes in the size and shape of pharynx and mouth, and by positional alterations of tongue, teeth, and lips, is called articulation and produces vowels and consonants, linking to form words, or SPEECH.

Voice has loudness, pitch and timbre. Loudness is dependent on the force with which air is expelled, i.e., it varies with amplitude of vibration. Pitch is related to length and tension of the vocal cords, which is to say that it is determined by frequency of vibration. Length can be altered only slightly. Men normally have longer cords than women and children, and their voices are naturally deeper in the same way as the longer strings of a cello produce deeper notes than the short strings of a violin. Basically length determines range, but within individual range pitch is changed by altering tension, as with a violin string. Timbre depends on the presence and intensity of overtones, which are influenced by the shape and capacity of resonating chambers and these are provided by chest, trachea, pharynx, nose and mouth.

Individual voices are substantially unique since no two persons have identical resonating chambers and articulators. Devices have therefore been made to record 'voice prints' and can be used to identify telephone pests and trap kidnappers telephoning ransom demands. They are also used to study emotional factors influencing speech.

In whispering, a current of air is articulated by the tongue, teeth and lips but the vocal cords are not brought into play.

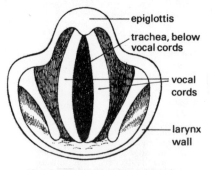

epiglottis

trachea, below vocal cords

vocal cords

larynx wall

Vocal cords viewed from above

volvulus. Intestinal obstruction resulting from a twisting of the bowel. This is usually precipitated by some abnormality of the mesentery, the pleated membrane which supports the bowel; it may be congenitally lax, stretched by over-loaded bowel, or deformed and contracted by disease. Bands or adhesions from previous intra-abdominal disease can also lead to entanglement of the intestinal coils. The pelvic colon, caecum, and small intestine are most commonly involved. Large bowel volvuli tend to occur in older patients with chronic constipation. Those of the small bowel are commoner in children.

The condition is serious because twisting both obstructs the bowel and cuts off its blood-supply, so that gangrene rapidly occurs. Volvulus is an emergency requiring immediate operation.

vomiting. Regurgitation of stomach contents, usually preceded by nausea and salivation. After a deep intake of breath, followed by closure of the glottis (the entrance of the main airway), the stomach is compressed by contraction of the abdominal muscles and descent of the diaphragm so that its contents are squeezed upwards through the oesophagus, pharynx, and mouth. In the projectile vomiting of pyloric stenosis the stomach plays a more active part, contracting forcibly while the pyloric sphincter at the lower opening of the stomach is closed. A similar mechanism produces the regurgitant vomiting of intestinal obstruction.

Vomiting is most usually a reflex act resulting from irritation in the gastro-intestinal tract, but is also produced by the effects of toxaemia on the vomiting centre in the brain, as in poisoning, kidney disease, uraemia, and other metabolic disturbances. Other causes are the psychic effects of anxiety, fear, or disgust, and the over-stimulation of receptors in the inner ear, producing sea-sickness.

Vomiting is also called emesis, and drugs producing it are called emetics. Some, like tartar emetic and salt-solution, act by irritating the stomach. Others, such as apomorphine, act on the brain like toxins.

Cyclical vomiting, or repeated attacks in children occurring without obvious cause, are often ascribed to acidosis. Although ketone bodies may be demonstrable in the urine, acidosis is not a completely satisfactory diagnosis, and possibilities to be considered include migraine, faulty diet particularly related to fat-intake, respiratory infection and psychological causes such as school-phobia and other factors which have given rise to anxiety.

voyeurism. A condition in which a person becomes sexually excited or satisfied by looking at sexual acts or even simply at the genitals of the opposite sex. To a minor extent this is quite a normal phenomenon in part created by the conventional secrecy in which the naked body is held; and it is the main psychological source of the fairly common interest in pornographic pictures. In more extreme varieties it is classed as a PERVERSION and shows itself in the 'Peeping Tom' behaviour, in which the person with this particular sexual deviation attempts to gain satisfaction by looking through bedroom windows or key-holes.

vulva. Those parts of the female REPRODUCTIVE SYSTEM which lie on the body surface.

W

warts. Localized small growths formed on the skin. They vary in size and shape and are in most cases caused by a virus.

The commonest warts or verrucas occur in children and young adults, especially on the hands or less often the face. In many cases they ultimately disappear without treatment. Unless they are very unsightly they are best left untreated.

Plantar warts, on the sole of the foot, quite common in persons frequenting swimming baths, are caused by a fungus and are infectious.

Large, soft, moist warts sometimes occur in the genital area and may cause itching. Treatment, where necessary, varies with the type of wart and its situation.

wasp sting. See BITES AND STINGS.

Wassermann test. The most widely used test for the diagnosis of syphilis, devised by August von Wassermann in 1906. The test ascertains whether blood from the person examined forms antibodies which react with a substance that exists in normal blood. A negative reaction means the patient does not have syphilis, but there are two possible exceptions: (1) a patient who has received considerable antisyphilitic treatment may appear as negative, and (2) during the first two months after infection a patient may still be negative. A positive reaction is normally taken as proof of syphilis, but temporary false positives occur in glandular fever, yaws, leprosy and one or two other conditions.

Most workers nowadays prefer to use the Wassermann and another test simultaneously.

wasting. Shrinkage of muscles and loss of weight occur after prolonged inactivity, as in any disease necessitating bed-rest for a lengthy period. Nowadays, however, a policy of getting patients out of bed much earlier than in the past, together with physiotherapy treatment for persons still confined to bed, make wasting as a consequence of treatment rather un-common.

More common is wasting as a symptom of advanced disease, e.g., as an indication of cancer or tuberculosis. In particular wasting in children may occur as a result of many conditions, from intestinal worms to worry over homework. In general any appreciable loss of weight or in a child failure to gain weight over a sizeable period warrants medical investigation.

water. At one time or another, water – inwardly or outwardly – has been declared a remedy for almost all human ills; and certainly it ranks next to air as the second most urgent of the body's needs. Water accounts for between 50 and 65 per cent of the weight of the body, being nearer the lower figure in the average middle-aged woman (with more fat) and nearer the higher figure in the average young man. Even under conditions when water intake is limited, the daily loss of water seldom falls below 1.7 litres (3 pints): a minimum of 600 ml. (1 pint) in urine without which the body cannot get rid of poisonous waste products; at least 300 ml. (0.5 pint) in evaporation from the lungs; a little in faeces; and anything from 600 ml. (1 pint) upwards in perspiration, with the quantity increasing rapidly if the external temperature is high or if the body is freely exercised. Without water intake we die in three or four days. The minimum intake for continued survival in a temperate climate is about 3 pints (1800 ml.) of which about 1 pint is provided in an average diet (e.g., potatoes are more than half water) and the rest has to be drunk as water, tea, milk, coffee or other liquid. For health an intake of 2 to 2.5 litres (4 to 5 pints) is desirable for the average adult; roughly one-quarter of this is included in food.

Dehydration, or water deficiency exhaustion, occurs in persons deprived of fresh-water intake (e.g., adrift at sea or lost in a desert) or in cases of extreme diarrhoea and vomiting (where the accompanying nausea may prevent drinking). The symptoms include thirst, dryness of mouth and tongue, fatigue and giddiness, and later delirium, coma and death. Minor deficiency through not drinking quite enough is common, and manifests itself in dry skin, pasty appearance and constipation.

Treatment includes rest in a cool room, a high fluid intake if the patient can take it, and intravenous injection of saline solution if the person is unconscious or unable to swallow. Salt depletion often occurs simultaneously with water depletion, and if this is suspected the drink given should contain roughly half a teaspoonful of salt for each tumbler of water.

Since children have smaller reserves of water than have adults, dehydration in children – especially young children – is not uncommon. It should be remembered that any disease involving perspiration or rise of temperature increases the loss of water and that the intake should rise correspondingly.

Insufficiency of water renders it difficult for the kidneys to excrete poisonous products in the urine; and an adequate supply of water helps to prevent constipation and its attendant evils. Whether water is consumed hot or cold and whether it is drunk as water, tea or some other liquid matter little, but it is useful to drink at least a tumblerful each morning and each evening, although elderly people often find that excessive night rising is avoided by taking the evening drink some hours before retiring to bed. It is difficult to take too much water. In general excess is simply excreted, causing no symptoms except increased urination. Water intoxication – with restlessness, muscle twitching and confusion – is an extreme rarity which occurs when the kidneys are defective and cannot cope with the excretory problem.

Oedema (dropsy) is not caused by too much water but by retention of salt, with water retained in the tissues to keep the salt in dilute solution.

While water is necessary and is in general beneficial to health, dangers arise from water that is too hard, too soft, lacking in certain MINERAL SALTS and, worst of all, polluted.

Water which is too hard causes indigestion as well as causing 'furring' of kettles and other domestic utensils. Temporary hardness, created by the water containing a large amount of soluble bicarbonates, can be removed by boiling, but permanent hardness (mainly from chlorides and sulphates) is removable only by fairly elaborate processes. Until recent years it was thought that hard water was completely disadvantageous – necessitating the use of more soap and the frequent replacement of kettles and boilers as well as creating dyspepsia, especially in persons previously accustomed to softer water. Recently, however, it has been shown that soft water is associated with a higher incidence of degenerative heart diseases, and it would appear that one of the minerals in hard water has some protective effect against these conditions.

Soft water can absorb lead from pipes of that metal, and lead gradually accumulates in the body to a level that is poisonous. For many years the use of lead for cold water pipes has been discontinued, but some old lead pipes are still in use. Apart from the land danger soft water is very pleasant for washing and quite pleasant for drinking. It is sometimes alleged to cause constipation, and it is more likely than hard water to be deficient in some of the mineral salts.

The presence or absence of such mineral salts as calcium, magnesium and iron does not really matter: we get our supplies from other sources and the amounts in even the hardest waters are minute. Deficiency of iodine, however, as in parts of Derbyshire and in the Calders area of Scotland, causes simple goitre which can be prevented by adding a small amount of iodine to table salt; and deficiency of fluorine in water is associated with greatly increased incidence of dental caries. See FLUORIDATION.

Where water is polluted it can cause a large number of diseases. Water-borne diseases in man include typhoid, cholera, bacillary dysentery, amoebic dysentery and less commonly bilharziasis, although none of these is conveyed only by water; and in animals anthrax, glanders and hog cholera are all water-borne diseases. A water-borne outbreak is characterized by an explosive outburst, with many cases occurring almost simultaneously. When such an outbreak occurs the public should be warned to boil all water – including water to be used for washing their persons or their dishes – until such time as the source has been identified and the whole water supply adequately sterilized by chlorination.

For external use of water see HYDROTHERAPY.

water, hardness of. The hardness of water depends on its content of calcium and magnesium salts, and the amount of hardness is generally expressed in parts of calcium carbonate per million. In the case of hard water the calcium and magnesium interact with the fatty acids of soap to form an insoluble precipitate, but soft water readily forms a lather with soap.

Temporary hardness, due to calcium and magnesium bicarbonate, can be removed by boiling. Hence the incrustation commonly known as 'furring' in kettles in hard water areas.

Permanent hardness, not removable by boiling, is due to calcium and magnesium sulphates or to magnesium or sodium chlorides. Softening is practicable by special processes, e.g., the Permutit process which uses alumina, silica and sodium, or the Porter-Clark process.

Hard water is a nuisance to housewives, although perhaps less so in the era of detergents than earlier, and it reduces the efficiency and shortens the life of boilers. On the other hand soft water appears to increase the liability to cardio-vascular diseases.

water-borne diseases. The term is normally restricted to diseases caused by infective agents transferred by water. In such cases the water has been polluted or contaminated by faecal matter – as in the use for drinking purposes of water that has already received the sewage or excreta of houses or factories, or water that has been contaminated by floods or heavy rains which carried transport or farm excreta to the drinking water, or water that has been polluted from labour camps or by holiday makers. Water-borne outbreaks in this sense tend to have an abrupt onset, rise very rapidly to a peak of cases, and decline rapidly. Cholera (mainly spread by water), typhoid (sometimes spread by water) and less frequently bacillary dysentery, poliomyelitis, infective hepatitis, Weil's disease (infectious leptospirosis), amoebic dysentery, hookworm infestation and filariasis are examples.

The halogen deficiency diseases (e.g., goitre from lack of iodine in the water and dental caries from deficiency of fluorine) and metallic poisonings (e.g., plumbism from absorption of lead by soft water) are not usually included under the heading of water-borne diseases; and somewhere on the borderline are gastro-intestinal upsets from consumption of bacteriologically satisfactory water containing excessive amounts of vegetable matter.

water brash. A regurgitation of clear acid fluid from the stomach to the mouth, sometimes accompanying HEART-BURN. The cause is excessive secretion of hydrochloric acid by the stomach and temporary loss of control over the sphincter muscle that normally closes the entrance to the stomach. Immediate treatment consists of a short rest and the swallowing of a mild alkali, such as milk of magnesia. If the condition recurs frequently medical inves-tigation may be required.

watering eyes. Tears are normally secreted by the lacrymal duct on the outer side of the eye, pass across the eye with cleansing effect and discharged by a duct on the inner side of the eye to the nose. Watering of the eye may be the result of pressure on the nasal duct (as in some diseases of bone), blockage of the duct (which if left untreated may cause a painful abscess), laxity of the tissues of the lower eyelid (quite common in elderly women) or exposure to wind and cold. Treatment varies with the cause, but in general medical advice is necessary if the condition continues for more than two or three days.

water supply. The water cycle is essentially evaporation, especially from the sea, cloud formation, rainfall, and passage to sea and lakes. Rain at the start of its fall is almost pure water, very soft (and hence useful for washing purposes) and rather insipid (because of the absence of trace elements). As it falls through the atmosphere rain becomes polluted, e.g., in cities it acquires a considerable amount of sulphuric acid and near the sea it gains chlorides. Hence rain water, even if we could collect it from roofs unpolluted by birds and cats, is seldom suitable for drinking. When rain reaches the ground some evaporates, some flows down the incline of the surface and some sinks into the soil, passing downwards until it meets an impermeable layer such as rock.

Water supplies are of three main types – underground water, upland surface water and rivers.

Underground water from a deep well or main spring may have been initially contaminated when falling through the atmosphere or trickling along the ground but has in general been purified by biological processes during its underground journey. It tends to be constant in supply, has very little chance of accidental pollution and is usually hard, having dissolved various minerals during its travels. By contrast water from a shallow well or spring has a danger of drying up in a period of drought and, if polluted at or near the surface (e.g., from a cesspool or farmyard), has had insufficient time for biological processes to act.

Upland surface water flows from moors or mountain slopes to artificial dams and is carried to centres of population by aqueducts. It is generally soft and well aerated. If the gathering ground is reasonably free from people, cattle and dogs, the chance of pollution is slight, and there is usually time for biological processes to effect purification.

River water (e.g., water from the Thames supplying London) is usually hard, because it has had time to absorb trace elements from the ground over which it flows; and where the population is appreciable it is highly polluted, so that purification before use is essential.

Three methods of purification are commonly employed: (1) Storage. This helps greatly – by sedimentation of any impurities, by the sterilizing effects of wind and sun, and by the sheer absence of food on which bacteria can grow. (2) Filtration. Whether sand filters or chemical filters are used, filtration vastly reduces impurities. (3) Sterilization. Although other methods such as the use of ozone have been tried, sterilization by the use of chlorine is increasingly the method of choice.

In Britain and most developed countries the water supplies for sizeable centres of population are absolutely safe, with bacteriological and chemical examination of samples carried out daily or weekly and chlorination increased on the slightest suggestion of any contamination. In remote or undeveloped areas the position is very different, and the fact of water being clear and sparkling is absolutely no indication of whether or not it is contaminated.

For 'camp purification' in such areas there are various commercial preparations available, but perhaps as good as any are potassium permanganate crystals. A few crystals – just enough to turn the water mildly pink – are dropped into the container: if the water turns brown it should be regarded as undrinkable; if, as is usually the case, it remains pink, then in fifteen minutes any contaminating bacteria can be deemed to have been destroyed. If there is reason to suspect vegetables or fruits which are to be eaten without cooking, they in turn can be soaked in water which has been appropriately 'pinked' with the crystals. A minor point to note is that the potassium permanganate crystals introduced should turn the water pink, not red: an overdose will certainly kill any germs but will probably give the traveller a sore throat through action of the disinfectant on his mucous membrane.

wax. A normal secretion of the glands in the skin of the ear canal. In most people the amount of secretion of wax is balanced by extrusion of dried particles, but where secretion is extensive the wax may accumulate and obstruct the passage, causing temporary deafness. Such deafness is particularly liable to occur if water enters the ear during washing and causes the wax to swell.

The instillation of a few drops of hydrogen peroxide into the ears about once a week tends to prevent accumulation of wax. Where it has accumulated to the extent of impairing hearing the wax should be softened by introducing a few drops of sweet oil of almonds (or olive oil), leaving it in place for twenty-four hours with a plug of cotton wool to prevent its exit, and then the ear should be gently syringed to remove the softened wax. Gentleness is essential to prevent damage to the ear drum.

weight. A solitary measurement of weight gives little or no information. If, after allowance has been made for height, bone structure and (in the case of a child) age, the weight of the child or adult is very appreciably above or below the average, the information merely confirms what the doctor or health visitor initiating the weighing already knew; and if the weight, after taking into account the factors already mentioned, is a little above or below the average, there are too many imponderables for the measurement to point to undernutrition or the beginning of a disease associated with loss of weight, or to suggest the start of obesity from hereditary, endocrine, dietetic or other causes. On the other hand, change of weight, as shown by measurements at intervals of two or three months, can provide important information.

The optimum weight for children is a very complex calculation, dependent not only on height but also on age, and is considered in the article on DEVELOPMENT.

Tables of HEIGHT AND WEIGHT of adults are subject to the limitations that average is not 'optimum' and that a person of large frame will clearly have a higher optimum weight than a small-framed person of the same height. While allowance has to be made for the type of frame, insurance companies claim that expectation of life is greatest in persons a few pounds below the average for their height. Being underweight is alleged to increase the chance of death slightly below the age of about 40 years but thereafter to carry no penalty unless it is so marked as to constitute actual malnutrition or to indicate existing disease. Being 10 per cent overweight substantially increases the chance of early death from about 35 years onwards,

and to be 20 per cent overweight increases the mortality risk by about one-third.

For estimation of weight change and even for comparison with tables it is important that there should be little variation in the amount of clothing. In particular the weight of shoes varies considerably, jackets and coats are heavy, and some people contrive to carry a considerable weight in their pockets. Where circumstances necessitate a person being weighed fully dressed an appropriate allowance has to be made for the weight of the clothes.

Pounds converted into kilograms							
lb.	kg.	lb.	kg.	lb.	kg.	lb.	kg.
5	2.3	54	24.5	103	46.6	152	68.8
6	2.7	55	24.9	104	47.1	153	69.3
7	3.2	56	25.4	105	47.5	154	69.7
8	3.6	57	25.8	106	48.0	155	70.2
9	4.1	58	26.3	107	48.4	156	70.7
10	4.5	59	26.8	108	48.9	157	71.1
11	5.0	60	27.2	109	49.3	158	71.6
12	5.4	61	27.7	110	49.8	159	72.0
13	5.9	62	28.1	111	50.2	160	72.5
14	6.3	63	28.6	112	50.7	161	72.9
15	6.8	64	29.0	113	51.1	162	73.4
16	7.2	65	29.5	114	51.6	163	73.8
17	7.7	66	30.0	115	52.1	164	74.3
18	8.2	67	30.4	116	52.5	165	74.7
19	8.6	68	30.8	117	53.0	166	75.2
20	9.0	69	31.3	118	53.4	167	75.6
21	9.5	70	31.7	119	53.9	168	76.1
22	10.0	71	32.2	120	54.3	169	76.5
23	10.4	72	32.6	121	54.8	170	77.0
24	10.9	73	33.1	122	55.2	171	77.5
25	11.3	74	33.6	123	55.7	172	77.9
26	11.8	75	34.0	124	56.1	173	78.4
27	12.2	76	34.5	125	56.6	174	78.8
28	12.7	77	34.9	126	57.0	175	79.3
29	13.1	78	35.4	127	57.5	176	79.7
30	13.6	79	35.8	128	58.0	177	80.2
31	14.1	80	36.3	129	58.4	178	80.6
32	14.5	81	36.7	130	58.9	179	81.1
33	15.0	82	37.1	131	59.3	180	81.5
34	15.4	83	37.6	132	59.8	181	82.0
35	15.9	84	38.1	133	60.2	182	82.4
36	16.3	85	38.5	134	60.7	183	82.9
37	16.8	86	39.0	135	61.1	184	83.4
38	17.2	87	39.5	136	61.6	185	83.8
39	17.8	88	39.9	137	62.0	186	84.3
40	18.1	89	40.3	138	62.5	187	84.7
41	18.6	90	40.8	139	62.9	188	85.2
42	19.0	91	41.3	140	63.4	189	85.6
43	19.5	92	41.7	141	63.8	190	86.1
44	19.9	93	42.2	142	64.3	191	86.5
45	20.4	94	42.6	143	64.8	192	87.0
46	20.7	95	43.0	144	65.2	193	87.4
47	21.3	96	43.5	145	65.7	194	87.9
48	21.8	97	43.9	146	66.1	195	88.3
49	22.2	98	44.4	147	66.6	196	88.8
50	22.7	99	44.9	148	67.0	197	89.2
51	23.1	100	45.3	149	67.5	198	89.7
52	23.6	101	45.7	150	67.9	199	90.2
53	24.0	102	46.2	151	68.4	200	90.7

weight, excessive. See OBESITY.

weight and height. See HEIGHT AND WEIGHT.

weight, loss of. An adult's loss of weight or a child's failure to gain weight as a result of starvation, privation, under-feeding or deliberate dieting (as in the treatment of obesity) is generally easily recognized. Other causes of weight loss include cancer, various diseases of the digestive tract, diabetes mellitus, some diseases of the kidneys, syphilis, tuberculosis, some diseases of the pancreas, a few nervous diseases (e.g., anorexia nervosa) and prolonged errors of diet.

Unless the cause is obvious, medical investigation is desirable; and in general the physician – looking first for common causes – should initially think of the possibility of cancer in the second half of life, of diabetes in persons aged 20 to 50, of tuberculosis in adolescents and young adults, and of gastro-enteritis or defective feeding in infants. Treatment varies with the cause but clearly includes the provision of adequate, appetizing, attractively served meals in circumstances conducive to their enjoyment.

Weil's disease. A serious infectious disease caused by a spirochaete (a corkscrew-like micro-organism) which frequently infects rats and mice and less often cats and dogs. The organism passes from the urine of infected animals to ponds, canals, rivers and swamps; man contracts the disease sometimes by eating food contaminated from such water but more often by the organism passing through the damaged skin of a person bathing or working in infected water. Weil's disease is also called leptospirosis, spirochaetal jaundice and swamp fever.

The incubation period varies from three to twenty-one days but is usually about ten days. The onset of the disease is characterized by high temperatures, rigors, severe headaches, muscle pains and gastro-intestinal disturbances with nausea and vomiting. Jaundice appears about the fifth day. Between 10 and 40 per cent of victims die, the proportion varying largely with the quality of nursing services available, and in the remainder convalescence begins after the second week.

Antibiotics – especially benzylpenicillin and streptomycin – are of some value, but recovery depends in large measure on good nursing and prevention of dehydration.

Weil's disease is in the main preventable. Preventive measures include the use of rubber boots and gloves by workers in water, swamps or mines liable to contamination by the urine of rodents; avoidance of bathing in dubious waters; protection of food from contamination from such water; drainage of swamps; and measures for rodent control.

wet dream. A colloquial term for a discharge of semen and prostatic fluid during sleep, quite common in males at puberty, and scientifically termed a NOCTURNAL EMISSION.

wheal. A small, swollen, burning or itching area of the skin. Weals or wheals (the spelling is variable) may result from sharp blows or from the stings of insects, nettles or jelly fish. See NETTLE RASH.

wheezing. Breathing with difficulty and with a whistling or grating sound. The symptom is found in bronchitis, asthma, some other diseases of the respiratory tract, and congestive heart failure. The cause is either a narrowing of the smaller bronchial tubes (as occurs in asthma) or their partial clogging with mucous (as happens in bronchitis). Treatment is that of the causal condition.

whiplash injury. An injury, not uncommon in car collisions, in which the head and neck are jerked violently backwards. In most cases there is considerable pain and stiffness of the neck. Painkillers will generally relieve the pain but a special supporting collar may be required for several weeks. Occasionally, however, a whiplash injury is so severe as to dislocate a vertebra.

white leg. A term used for two different complications of childbirth.

1. Femoral thrombosis, the formation of a clot in any part of the femoral vein, usually

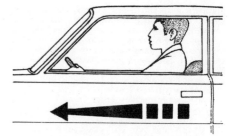

As the car is jerked violently forwards, the head, moving forwards more slowly, is jerked relatively backwards.

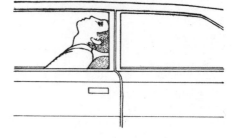

Whiplash injury

appears about nine or ten days after delivery, and is characterized by high temperature, stiffness followed by pain in the leg and some swelling of the affected limb. The vein is tender to the touch and can be felt as a hard line running down the leg. Treatment consists of rest in bed, immobilization of the limb by sandbags on each side, hot boracic fomentations with some lead and opium added, and mild sedatives. The pain usually subsides in a few days and the swelling disappears in two or three weeks.

2. Phlegmasia alba dolens, now rare, is essentially a blockage of the lymphatic vessels at the root of the thigh, with the affected leg becoming greatly swollen, and the skin white and glossy. Treatment is as for femoral thrombosis but the condition may last for several months and in some cases the leg remains permanently swollen.

Both conditions are said to be more common in anaemic women, but the exact causes are still disputed.

whitlow. See HAND.

whooping cough. An acute infection (medically known as pertussis), found mostly in children under the age of 6 years but liable to occur at any age, involving the trachea and bronchi, and characterized by a paroxysmal cough which ends with a crowing, inspiratory 'whoop'. It is caused by *Haemophilus pertussis*, which is transmitted by droplet infection, and the infectivity is greatest during the early catarrhal stage before the typical cough has appeared. The incubation period is seven to ten days.

The initial manifestations, raised temperature and short dry cough, are those of almost any respiratory infection; but in a few days the characteristic paroxysmal cough and whoop appear, and a paroxysm is often followed by vomiting. There is no specific treatment. For the first few days the patient is best kept in bed and given a largely fluid diet; and after he is allowed up he should be isolated from unimmunized children who have not had the disease. Infectivity ends – and the patient may be allowed to associate with susceptible persons – in about three weeks, even though the cough and whoop continue for another fortnight or so.

The disease was formerly very common. For instance, in 1950 there were 157,000 notifications of whooping cough in England and Wales, and of these roughly 1 in every 400 died, most of the deaths being in children under 2 years of age. Antibiotics, increasingly employed in the 1950s and 1960s, do not cure the disease but reduce some of the complications, and so reduce the number of deaths, but not the number of cases.

The big advances in the control of whooping cough were the production of a vaccine (tried out in the Faroe Islands in 1929 but not extensively used until the middle 1950s), the improvement of that vaccine and the persuasion of the public to accept vaccination. By 1971 notifications in England and Wales numbered 15,933, and of these, 23 – or roughly 1 in every 700 – died. In extremely rare cases (e.g., a child suffering from convulsions or with a family history of epilepsy) the vaccine is not advisable because of a very remote chance of brain damage, but to omit vaccination in a child not suffering from such conditions is simply needlessly to run the risk of a serious and occasionally fatal disease.

A vaccine which confers a high degree of immunity is normally combined with the vaccines employed for protection against diphtheria and tetanus. For a normally healthy baby such triple vaccination should be started by the age of 6 months.

Widal test. A blood test for diagnosing typhoid fever, originally devised by Fernan Widal (1862-1929). The test is useful but has two limitations: firstly, that a positive reaction does not usually appear until about the seventh day of the illness, so that a decision to treat a case as typhoid (or to exclude typhoid from the diagnosis) has to be made in advance of the test; and secondly, that a person who is not suffering from typhoid but has had TAB vaccination within recent months may give a slightly positive reaction.

windpipe. The air-passage which extends from the larynx to the point in the upper part of the chest where it divides into the right and left bronchi. The windpipe, which is technically termed the trachea, consists of a fibrous tube kept open by a series of horizontal hoops of cartilage.

womb. The common name for the UTERUS, i.e., the organ in a female mammal in which the offspring are nourished until birth.

women, diseases of. With obvious exceptions, such as diseases of the prostate in men and of the uterus in women, men and women are subject to the same ailments and disabilities, and greater frequency of a condition in one or other sex sometimes provides a clue to causation.

The term 'diseases of women' is, however, normally restricted to illnesses peculiar to women. An alternative term is gynaecological diseases. Examples of such diseases are: cancer, fibroid, displacement or inflammation of the uterus; inflammation, tumour or cyst of the ovaries; salpingitis and other diseases of the uterine tubes; inflammation of the vagina; and disorders of menstruation. While the symptoms vary with the particular disease, common symptoms of gynaecological conditions include – pain below the level of the umbilicus, pain associated with menstruation, pain associated with performance of the sexual act, absence of menstruation, excessive blood loss during menstruation, haemorrhage between menstrual periods, and vaginal discharge. Accurate diagnosis is, of course, a necessary preliminary to treatment.

The branch of medicine specializing in the study of diseases of women is known as gynaecology.

word blindness. A rather vague term for a condition in which, as a result of disease or injury of the speech area of the cerebral cortex or more frequently as a result of disease or injury of the nerve tracts communicating with that area, a person becomes unable to associate meanings with words. According to the nature of the lesion he may on the one hand be able to speak coherently but be unable to appreciate the meaning of written words even though he can spell out the letters composing the words, or he may on the other hand also lose all appreciation of words even as spoken by himself, so that his speech becomes totally unintelligible.

Where word blindness occurs in a previously normal adult the diagnosis is obvious. Where it is suspected in a young child the condition of DYSLEXIA should not be regarded as confirmed until defects of sight, hearing and general intelligence have been eliminated. The treatment of genuine word blindness is not easy but most cases ultimately recover.

World Health Organization. When the charter of the United Nations was adopted at the San Francisco conference of 1945, health would have been overlooked but for the delegations of two countries, Brazil and China. Thanks to their insistence, the World Health Organization (WHO) was created in 1946 – an organization empowered to deal with every aspect of health.

The constitution of the WHO states in its preamble that health is a state of complete physical, mental and social well-being and not merely the absence of disease or infirmity; that the enjoyment of the highest attainable standard of health is one of the fundamental rights of every human being; that promotion and protection of health is of value to all, and that unequal development of these things in some countries is a danger to other countries; that extension to all peoples of the benefits of medical, psychological and related knowledge is essential to the full attainment of health; and that informed opinion and active co-operation on the part of the public are of the utmost importance in the improvement of health. Article 1 of the constitution says, 'the objective of the World Health Organization shall be the attainment by all peoples of the highest possible level of health', and Article 2 lists twenty-two main functions.

The organization, which now has 138 member countries, meets annually to determine policy and approve a budget, but the organization works largely through an Executive Board of twenty-four persons and a Secretariat headed by a Director-General. The work of WHO includes (1) rapid transmission of epidemiological information, standardization of nomenclatures, etc.; (2) provision of help at the request of a government, usually on the basis that the help will include the education and training of staff and that the work will be continued by the country after the WHO aid has ended; and (3) the setting up from time to time of expert advisory committees and panels on many subjects and the publication of reports from these committees and panels. It also provides fellowships which enable doctors, nurses and others to improve their expertise by study in another country.

Probably the most spectacular achievement of WHO has been its attempt – now approaching complete success – to achieve world-wide eradication of smallpox: by 1974 smallpox was believed to be extinct in South America and to remain endemic in only one African and three Asian countries. On malaria eradication it has, in the words of its current Director-General, 'freed well over a thousand million people from the dread of endemic malaria, saved millions of lives and contributed much to economic development.' Simultaneously its publications and technical reports have added to knowledge in many fields, such as (to take examples almost at random) health education, promotion of mental health and reduction of domestic accidents.

Many of its initial tasks inevitably remain uncompleted: malaria, for instance, still kills a million children every year. New health problems also arise periodically: none of us had heard thirty years ago of Lassa fever or of LSD. Yet the World Health Organization moves steadily towards its aim of attaining the highest possible level of health for the people of the world.

worms. A rather ill-defined division of the animal kingdom containing creatures that do not possess appendages. Many species are parasites in the bodies of man and animals, and some of these species cause diseases.

Parasitic ROUND WORMS include the large *Ascaris lumbricoides,* sometimes as long as 40 cm. (16 in.), the whip worm (about 5 cm., or 2 in., long) and the tiny but common thread worm (*Oxyuris vermicularis*) which is a frequent source of anal irritation in children. Parasitic flat worms include the pork and beef TAPEWORMS (*Taenia solium* and *T. saginata*) and the FLUKES responsible for schistosomiasis.

Many worms are transmitted through the eating or drinking of material that contains their eggs, but some diseases, such as FILARIASIS, are passed to man through the bites of blood-sucking insects. Effective treatments for most worm infestations are now available. See VERMIFUGE.

wound. Any breach of the skin with damage to underlying tissues. Wounds are normally classified thus:

1. Clean-cut or incised wounds, caused by a sharp-edged instrument. The edges are definite, and bleeding is generally abundant.

2. Bruised or contused wounds, caused by a blunt instrument. Bleeding is usually scanty or even absent.

3. Punctured wounds or stabs, caused by a pointed instrument. Bleeding may be abundant. If the stab is deep there is danger of involvement of internal organs and also danger of sepsis from the introduction of germs.

4. Torn or lacerated wounds caused by animal bites or contact with moving machinery. The edges are ragged and bleeding is usually scanty.

The classification is not completely satisfactory. For instance, a bullet wound may well be both punctured and lacerated. More important than the type of wound is whether it is clean or potentially septic through introduction of germs.

The main points in the treatment of a wound are: (1) Stop the bleeding if serious: see HAEMORRHAGE. (2) With thoroughly cleaned hands (preferably washed in water containing an antiseptic) cleanse the wound with a mild antiseptic solution or (failing that) water that has been boiled, and apply a sterile dressing, and cover the dressing with a bandage. (3) Keep the part at rest – with a sling or splint if necessary. (4) Treat symptoms of SHOCK. (5) If the wound may have been contaminated by garden or field soil or stable refuse, contact a doctor swiftly so that the patient may receive anti-tetanic serum. See also FIRST AID.

wrinkles. Ridges or folds, especially of the skin of the face, produced through decrease of the natural elasticity of the skin as age advances. The natural process of development of wrinkles is accelerated by prolonged worry, by malnutrition, by excessive use of tea, coffee, alcohol or tobacco, and by lack of fresh air and exercise. There is no reliable cure. Operations to remove wrinkles tend to produce small scars instead of folds, and injection of material under the skin is liable to create deformity. Suitable lotions can often render wrinkles less visible.

wrist. The region between the forearm and the hand. The wrist joint is formed by the lower ends of the radius and ulna and the eight carpal bones. The joint has only fairly moderate sideways movement but very extensive upwards and downwards movement. Both because of the wide range of movement and because a person who falls forward tends to put out his arm and take the strain on his outstretched hand, dislocations and sprains of the wrist are very common. Fracture is also not uncommon (COLLES' FRACTURE). Stiffness of the wrist is sometimes caused by arthritis.

Wrist-drop. In this condition the hand droops at the wrist and there is difficulty in extending the wrist. Probably the commonest type is crutch palsy, where pressure of an inadequately padded crutch in the elbow damages the large nerve of the arm. A similar but more temporary effect is sometimes observed when a person sleeps with the head resting on the upper arm. Other causes include chill and the neuritis created by lead, arsenic or, rarely, alcohol. Forms due to pressure on the nerve or to chill respond to rest, with, if they appear to be lasting too long, the addition of massage or electrical treatment. Where wrist-drop is a result of neuritis induced by poisoning, the source of the poison must, of course, be identified and removed.

writer's cramp. A disease of gradual onset produced by habitual repetitive use of one set of muscles and characterized by pain, weakness and spasm of the muscles concerned. The condition occurs most commonly in manual writers – hence the name – but is also found in typists, seamstresses, musicians and indeed in any occupation demanding precise, finely co-ordinated movements of a set of small muscles, a fact which gives rise to its alternative name of occupational palsy. In a typical case the movements of the pen become more difficult and the writing irregular, the pen is grasped harder and harder and the writing becomes heavier, the hand feels heavy and tired, and ultimately cramp develops almost as soon as writing is started.

Preventive measures include the teaching of unconstricted or less constricted methods of manipulation, the encouragement of the use of either hand, the avoidance of excessive hours at the particular work and the adoption of a policy of gradualness after any appreciable absence. Treatment includes a period of rest, removal of adverse environmental factors, attention to general health and attempts to remove tensions and anxieties. While treatment is completely successful in some cases, in many cases change of occupation is essential, and in a minority occupational palsy occurs also in the new occupation.

wry neck. A condition, technically called torticollis, in which the head is permanently twisted to one side.

1. Wry-neck in infants or young children is often called congenital torticollis but it is seldom truly congenital in the sense of being inherited or resulting from intra-uterine influences. Most commonly it follows injury to one of the sterno-mastoid muscles (which run from base of neck to base of skull) caused during child-birth, especially in breech births. The muscle-fibres are accidentally torn; a swelling filled with blood forms and fibrous tissue grows into it; the relatively inert fibrous tissue restricts muscle growth; and so the muscle becomes shorter than the one on the opposite side of the neck and produces the typical deformity.

2. The condition of ocular torticollis is not usually as marked as the congenital variety and is caused by a weakness or paralysis of one of the muscles controlling the position of the eyes. The head is twisted into the abnormal position in an attempt to keep the eyes parallel and prevent a squint. In this case the sterno-mastoid muscle is not defective and treatment usually involves eye surgery.

3. Spasmodic torticollis, occurring mostly in the middle-aged and more in women than in men, is a condition of doubtful cause. Some cases appear to be of rheumatic origin while others may be due to psychological factors. There is fairly general agreement that no form of surgery is useful and that treatment should start with a period of rest in bed, but there is considerable argument about the value of other forms of treatment – a plain indication that no one form of therapy benefits the majority of patients.

X

xerophthalmia. Dryness and ultimately thickening and opacity of the front of the eye with consequent effect on vision. The condition, rare in highly developed countries, is produced by prolonged deficiency of vitamin A.

x-rays. Electromagnetic radiation consisting of radiated energy of very short wave-length (appreciably shorter than even that of ultra-violet rays) which can penetrate soft tissues and can register on photographic film. Röntgen discovered x-rays in 1895 when experimenting on the passage of electrical currents through tubes containing rarified gases.

Radiological diagnosis. Dense, heavy substances (e.g., bone and various metals) are opaque to x-rays and therefore cast dark shadows, while air and soft tissues are transparent to these rays and so cast no shadows or very light shadows. Because dense substances cast heavy shadows x-rays have obvious value for the detection and exact localization of fractures and of such foreign bodies as bullets and needles. Since the lungs, mainly filled with air, cast very little shadow x-rays can be used to identify abnormalities such as the consolidation of pneumonia or the presence of tuberculosis or cancer in the lung.

Soft tissues which would normally cast little shadow can be rendered temporarily opaque by instillation of a suitable heavy substance: for instance, to confirm the presence or absence of a peptic ulcer the stomach and duodenum can be photographed after the patient has taken a meal containing an adequate amount of barium or bismuth, and the kidney and urinary system can be studied after the injection or swallowing of a compound containing iodine. Conversely, the brain can be studied by injecting air into the ventricles which then show up as white shadows.

In recent decades radiography has become a supremely important diagnostic tool in most branches of medicine and surgery.

Preventive applications. Where an infectious disease is spread largely by mild cases almost without symptoms (e.g., the mild tuberculosis formerly common in the elderly) the development of a system of rapid and inexpensive x-ray photography – mass miniature radiography – provides a useful method of identifying and bringing under treatment persons who may be transmitting the disease. Similarly, where a person's occupation would render him a danger to others if infectious (as in the case of a health visitor, school teacher, midwife or nurse) radiological examination can identify such conditions as early tuberculosis. Again, when tuberculosis has become rare in a country,

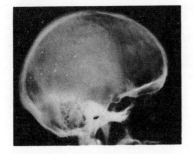

X-ray of normal skull

radiological investigation may be useful in the case of immigrants arriving from a country in which the disease is still widespread.

Therapy with x-rays. While diagnostic examination (even if repeated several times) is harmless, considerable radiological dosage applied for sufficient time can kill cells, so that

x-rays generated at much higher voltage than is used for diagnosis are employed to destroy cancer cells and to suppress over-growth (e.g., in polycythaemia vera and in anchylosing spondylitis). Used either alone or in conjunction with surgery, x-ray treatment has already proved extremely valuable – indeed life-saving – especially for various forms of cancer.

Dangers of x-rays. Sufficiently large doses of radiation destroy all forms of life; and even fairly moderate doses can damage the blood-forming tissues and the sex glands. For patients receiving treatment not only is the dosage carefully regulated but also the rays are directed only to the particular tissues for which they are required. In other words, the patient's blood-forming tissues and sex glands are not at risk. Much care, however, is needed on the part of the operator, who is in constant danger of exposure to radiation. Modern forms of apparatus minimize that risk, but in addition the working hours of radiologists and radiographers are restricted, and they are periodically examined for early indications – such as anaemia – of excessive exposure to x-rays.

Y

yawning. An involuntary reflex action in which the mouth is opened and the breath slowly exhaled. The typical morning yawn is essentially Nature's attempt to stimulate blood circulation and respiration. Yawning during a conversation or while listening to a formal address may imply sleepiness or boredom but more frequently occurs in persons whose blood pressures are low and who normally rely on movement to help the circulation of the blood.

Frequent yawning is usually a sign of insufficient sleep or inadequate exercise.

yaws. An infectious disease – common in South America, the West Indies and parts of Asia and Africa – characterized by lesions in the skin and bones. It is caused by a spirochaete (*Treponema pertenuae*) which closely resembles that of syphilis, but infection is usually transmitted not venereally but by direct contact or on the feet of flies, the contact being generally through abrasions in the skin. The incubation period is three to six weeks.

The primary lesion is a nodule, most often found on the legs or buttocks. Crops of secondary lesions occur, months or even years apart, on any portion of the skin, each batch of nodules tending in the main to subside painlessly but with a nodule occasionally giving rise to an ulcer. Secondary lesions also occur in bones where they cause pain, tenderness and deformity. Sometimes tertiary lesions occur in the form of indolent ulcers and nodules on the skull and breast-bone.

The disease responds quickly to treatment with penicillin and is now becoming rare.

Four spirochaetal diseases are very hard to differentiate: bejel (found mainly in the Middle

East), pinta (found chiefly in the West Indies), yaws, and syphilis. Some experts maintain that all four have evolved from the same organism. However, syphilis is venereally transmitted and the others are not.

yeast. A fungus which ferments sugar and is used in the brewing of beer, the distilling of spirits, the making of wine and the raising of bread. Baker's yeast is prepared by filtering fermenting liquids and compressing the product, and brewer's yeast is a frothy liquid with a bitter taste.

Yeast contains large amounts of the various B vitamins and so tablets of dried yeast are sometimes used in disorders due to deficiency of one or more of these vitamins.

yellow fever. An acute and very serious infectious disease, the dreaded 'yellow jack' of the African trade routes, caused by a virus and transmitted by the bite of a female mosquito (*Aedes egypti*) which breeds in small quantities of water. The incubation period is three to ten days and the disease occurs in two distinct forms. The mild form, found mostly in persons normally resident in areas in which the disease is endemic, is an influenza-like illness characterized by fever, severe headache, nausea and vomiting, with recovery usual in about four days. The severe form has an acute onset with high fever, fast pulse, chills and rigors, severe headache, backache and limb pains, followed by nausea and vomiting, with the vomit sometimes black as a result of the presence of altered blood; there is often an apparent remission about the fourth day with the pulse rate decreasing more than in proportion to the fall of temperature, and then a second phase of high fever, severe vomiting, jaundice, and bleeding from mucous membranes. The fatality rate in the severe form is about 90 per cent, with death usually occurring on the seventh or eighth day. If the patient survives, convalescence begins about the twelfth day.

There is no specific treatment. Sulphonamides and antibiotics are not helpful. Skilled nursing is probably the most important factor in improving the chance of recovery. Small, frequent glucose drinks are useful, and foods of high protein content are said to help if the patient can swallow them; intravenous saline is required if the patient is dehydrated

and vitamin K is sometimes helpful.

Three major measures of prevention are as follows: (1) In areas where the disease is endemic, destruction of mosquitoes and especially of their breeding grounds, e.g., drainage of swamps. (2) Strict anti-mosquito control of all aircraft travelling from an infected area to an area in which the mosquitoes could breed, and vaccination of all travellers on such aircraft. (3) Vaccination of persons travelling to infected areas; such vaccination gives a powerful immunity which lasts for at least six years, but in Britain vaccination is not advocated for children under the age of 9 months.

Z

zinc protamine insulin. A suspension of insulin hydrochloride combined with protamine and zinc. It is slowly liberated and absorbed from the site of injection. A diabetic patient who is unsuitable for modern oral preparations might require three injections of ordinary soluble insulin daily, whereas with a mixture of ordinary soluble insulin and zinc protamine insulin a single daily injection will usually suffice – the soluble insulin beginning to act almost at once and its effect starting to fade after four or five hours, and the protamine zinc insulin beginning to act in about four hours and continuing to do so for at least a further twelve hours, so that the patient has at worst only a few hours each day of excess blood sugar.

zoonosis. A collective term for infections transmitted to human beings from infected animals. Examples are anthrax, plague, rabies, psittacosis, typhus, undulant fever (brucellosis), the bovine type of tuberculosis and many varieties of worm infestation. Measures of prevention vary with the disease but clearly involve the collaboration of medical and veterinary experts. The virtual eradication of the bovine variety of tuberculosis and the progress towards eradication of undulant fever in several developed countries are instances of the success of that collaboration.

zygoma. The arch of bone which forms the prominence of the cheek, to which is attached the masseter muscle of mastication. One of the minor variations in mankind is that the arch is higher in some races than in others.

zymotic diseases. The word 'zymosis' means fermentation and 'zymology' is the science that deals with fermentation. Dr. William Farr (1807-1883) of the English Registrar-General's Department recognized the similarity of fermentation and infection long before that similarity was explained by Pasteur's study of both phenomena. Farr therefore coined the term 'zymotic diseases' for epidemic, endemic and contagious diseases that generally acted in a manner resembling the process of fermentation.

Until the discovery and identification of viruses the term was useful: diseases caused by known organisms (such as tuberculosis, typhoid and malaria) could be described as specific infectious diseases, but a term was needed to cover diseases which behaved in an infectious manner but were thought to be caused either by an unidentified germ or by a mysterious chemical agent. As the viruses responsible for such conditions as smallpox, poliomyelitis and influenza were identified the need for a term embracing organismal and non-organismal infections gradually disappeared, and the term 'zymotic diseases' became archaic. It may, however, be interesting to note that the editor of this book used the term in the title of his MD thesis as late as 1942 because some of the infections that he was studying were not yet proved to be of organismal origin and could not at that time be properly described under any more modern heading.

HEALTH SERVICES OF BRITAIN

The history and problems of services for health and disease are in large measure international. To mention a few examples, the development of hospitals was very similar in various countries of Western Europe, although states that became predominantly non-Catholic were earlier than Catholic countries in separating hospitals from institutions staffed by priests or nuns; the medical derogation of the surgeon as a separate and inferior category occurred in Paris as well as in London; while public health services are often regarded as largely a British creation, they owed much to German thinkers, and some of the early developments in the provision of these services took place in the U.S.A.; Florence Nightingale, founder of professional nursing in Britain, learned the rudiments of nursing skill in Germany; child health clinics arose almost simultaneously in Britain, France and eastern states of the U.S.A.; the idea of health insurance evolved in several different countries at about the same time; and, as vitamins, vaccines and health education decreased deaths of children while better nutrition and better preventive and curative services enabled more and more people to survive into old age, many countries became concerned with the population aspects and the economic factors in health care. Certainly as services developed some countries put more emphasis on the maintenance of health and the prevention of disease (e.g., Sweden) while others concentrated more on treatment of the sick (e.g., Britain); and certainly some opted for a wholly salaried service (e.g., U.S.S.R.), some for a service salaried in respect of nurses and paramedical workers but with doctors and dentists paid fees for items of service provided (e.g., the Netherlands) and some had an elaborate system of medical insurance (e.g., Medicare in the U.S.A.); but on the whole the similarities in the health services and in the health problems of highly developed countries are far greater than the differences.

For topics of clearly multinational significance the reader is referred to articles placed in alphabetical order in this volume. Some topics bearing on health services are COMMUNICATIONS IN THE HEALTH SERVICES, COST OF HEALTH SERVICES, HEALTH EDUCATION, INDICES OF COMMUNITY HEALTH, and POPULATION AND HEALTH. Also certain features in which Britain has perhaps made a unique contribution (e.g., creation of HEALTH VISITORS and of MEDICAL OFFICERS OF HEALTH) are discussed in general articles as well as being mentioned below. The present article attempts to outline British health services under a number of headings, starting with organizational aspects, passing to treatment services at home and in hospital, continuing with services for the maintenance of good health and ending with financial points.

Organization and administration

In the developed countries diagnostic, preventive, and curative services have advanced enormously in recent decades, with a simultaneous increase in complexity. The 'surgeon' and 'physician', the specialists of the last century, have been gradually replaced by a mass of experts, e.g., in the mental field the child psychiatrist, the geriatric psychiatrist, the forensic psychiatrist and the expert in mental subnormality. The nurse has slowly risen to full professional status, and the profession has divided first into hospital general nurses, mental and fever nurses, health visitors, home nurses, midwives, and occupational health nurses, and subsequently has divided to some extent into specialities within each branch, for instance, on the preventive side the health education officer, the geriatric health visitor, the specialist on premature babies, and so on. Other professions have emerged: examples are the clinical psychologist, the radiologist, the medicosocial worker and the physiotherapist. In addition to all this, equipment has become elaborate and expensive: every modern general hospital has its departments of chemical pathology, clinical pathology, bacteriology, cardiology, endocrinology, etc. The promotion of health and the prevention, diagnosis, and treatment of illness have become an enormous industry – which, like other large industries, requires organization and management, but it has to be evaluated not on profits and losses but on its success or failure in improving the health of the population served.

After various insurance schemes had made it possible for an increasing proportion of the population to secure examination and treatment without direct payment, Britain tried in 1948 to co-ordinate its health and disease services in three administrations. Hospitals were grouped into fourteen regions in England and Wales and five regions in Scotland; nineteen Regional Hospital Boards of nominated members were created and the Boards were financed from Central Government funds. Preventive and domiciliary services (such as health visiting, home nursing, domiciliary midwifery, vaccination and immunization, and health services for pre-school and school children) remained with local authorities and were financed from Central Government funds and from the rates levied by the local authorities in more or less equal proportions. General medical, dental, and pharmaceutical services were placed under Executive Councils (consisting of representatives of the local authority, representatives of the professions concerned, and persons nominated by the Secretary of State) financed from central Government funds, but with specific arrangements for general practitioners to be paid a 'capitation fee' for each person on their list, and for dentists to be paid for items of service.

The National Health Service, so established, worked: no political party and no professional association ever suggested its abolition; and early claims of excessive cost were shown to be incorrect by comparison with costs in other developed countries. There were, however, many criticisms, for example, that if a local authority devised a good preventive service (partly at cost to the ratepayers) any saving on prevented disease went to the taxpayers of the whole country; that doctors had too strong a voice on Regional Boards and Executive Councils, and that nurses and other emerging professions were virtually unrepresented on these bodies; and that the private patients of clinical consultants (the majority of whom elected not to work full-time in the NHS) were sometimes admitted to hospital beds to the detriment of other patients awaiting admission.

In 1974 Britain unified the hospital, local authority, and executive council services, placing all three under the control of nominated Boards, each served by an 'Executive Group' consisting of a secretary, a chief medical officer, a chief nursing officer, a chief finance officer, and, for appropriate matters, a chief dental officer and a chief pharmacist. The capitation fee for general medical practitioners and the fee for service for general dental practitioners remained. The alleged aims of the change are greater integration of services, greater stress on prevention of disease, and increased efficiency.

The Health Board and the Executive Group

There are perhaps two points to be noted about the administration pattern. Firstly, there are no Health Boards in districts (and a district may have a population of 100,000 or 200,000 and comprise a half or a quarter of an area), and in areas and regions the persons charged with responsibility for health matters are not elected by the population or responsible to the community but are nominated by the Health Ministers, who must however first obtain recommendations from relevant local authorities, trade unions, professional organizations and voluntary bodies. (Incidentally, boundaries of health districts may not coincide with local government divisions). Secondly, in regions (which do not exist in Scotland), areas and districts, the executive power is placed in the hands of a team of four chief officers – a chief medical officer, a chief nursing officer, a secretary or administrator and a chief finance officer. The exact titles vary in England and Scotland and in areas and districts. The chairman of the medical committee and in some cases the chairman of the nursing committee are also entitled to be present at formal meetings of the Executive Group, and some chief officers – such as the chief dental officers – are entitled to be present when their services are under consideration.

Supporters of the new organization claim that boards of nominated and unpaid members worked admirably for the hospital services in the period 1948-74 and should operate equally well for the integrated services of today, and that the elimination of directly elected members removes the 'parish pump' atmosphere of local authorities, decreases the intrusion of politics and dissociates health services from the common call at times of local authority elections: 'The rates must not increase'. They also maintain that the inclusion of health workers on boards (usually a couple of doctors, a nurse and another person from health occupations) is in accordance with general modern trends.

Opponents of the system suggest that services controlled by elected representatives of the community were more efficient and less expensive, that the Regional Hospital Boards of 1948-74 were extravagant in that they spent quite uncritically whatever funds were allocated by the state, and that, even if a single board could administer the hospitals, it is impossible for a single board of unpaid persons, each of whom has his own daily work as his first priority, to make any detailed scrutiny of the operating and deficiencies of hospital services, domiciliary treatment services and preventive and health educational services serving a population of perhaps a million people – in fact that the Health Boards have such enormous tasks that they can really do little more than rubber stamp the decisions of the Executive Group. Most people seem to accept that the inclusion on the boards of members of various health professions is an improvement on the old Hospital Boards, which were allegedly rather doctor-dominated, but some suggest that the health workers are represented while patients and clients – the consumers – are less adequately represented. Time will doubtless show whether the supporters or the opponents are correct, or whether there is partial truth in each view.

There is in general rather less argument about the theory of executive power resting with a multiprofessional group of chief officers. Nursing is increasingly recognized as a full profession, with nurses outnumbering doctors by about six to one, and with different priorities, problems and professional backgrounds; and only a few backward-looking doctors look nostalgically to the old days when the medical officer of health or the medical superintendent of the hospital was a virtual dictator, while very few people appear to desire the pattern of the British Civil Service, in which the lay administrator holds the responsibility and the professional experts merely serve as advisors to him.

Yet some enquirers ask, why should the chief health education officer and the chief pharmacist not have parity of status with their medical and nursing colleagues? Others wonder whether it is really possible to arrive at concensus decisions, and suspect that, in practice, group administration will mean that the officer with the strongest personality will emerge as the uncrowned king. Again, some thinkers argue that the presence of the chairman of the medical committee at formal meetings of the Executive Group may create difficulties: a consultant or general practitioner who devotes three-quarters of his time to clinical work may well be biassed (e.g., in favour of a possible extension of treatment services rather than a development of preventive or health education services) and is also bound to have less available time for thinking about proposals than have the members of the Executive Group.

To give the consumers a voice there exist Community Health Councils, which can demand information and can make recommendations to Boards, but these councils are alleged to have 'no teeth'; they only have an advisory capacity.

Into the administrative mechanism is built an enormous number of requirements for consultation. While final decision rests with the Board and is often in practice taken by the Executive Group, a decision on most projects or proposed alterations cannot legitimately be taken until the views have been ascertained of any professional committees involved (e.g., the medical and nursing committees), of Community Health Councils, and of various other bodies. Since these committees and councils cannot formulate their views without adequate information, senior officers of the Board spend a great deal of time attending meetings. Additionally, district, area and regional officers have to be in close and frequent communication, and officers of the Department of Health and Social Security (England), the Scottish Home and Health Department (Scotland) and of national planning committees have to be kept in the picture and to give their advice.

Sceptics maintain that the organizational pattern is a bureaucrat's paradise, equipped for endless talk and a minimum of actual decisions, and with the administrative and clerical staff already far outnumbering doctors and threatening to approach the total number of registered nurses. Supporters suggest that an industry employing more than a million people needs a sizeable administrative framework, that the machine functions extremely well, and that it ensures that the best decisions are taken.

General practitioner services

The portion of the Health Service that changed least in 1974 is that of the general practitioners, sometimes called family doctors (though members of a family may have different doctors) or doctors of first approach. The general practitioner (more fully considered in a specific article under that heading) is an unspecialized doctor who requires a wide range of knowledge in order to diagnose and treat a large number of different diseases. He is the lynch-pin of the British treatment services and also takes some interest in disease-prevention and health-promotion. He has access to various laboratory services and is also free to refer a patient to a consultant or to a hospital. Incidentally, such referral is usually to be regarded as a sign of prudence rather than of ignorance: the GP is in effect saying, 'This is a condition serious enough to need the special facilities or the skilled nursing of a hospital', or 'This is an uncommon condition which should be treated by a doctor who has specialized in that type of disease'.

The single-doctor practice of the past is dying out: for one thing, emergency night calls, though far less numerous than some doctors used to allege, occur at irregular intervals, and a doctor who is roused from sleep on two successive nights is clearly tired on the third day – a situation fair neither to himself nor to his patients. The modern trend is increasingly towards group practice by a small number of doctors in partnership, each having his own list of patients but emergency calls at unsocial hours being taken by the particular doctor on duty. Another modern development is the gradual replacement of doctors' consulting rooms (often called 'surgeries' though general practitioners mostly undertake little surgical work except in very remote districts) by health centres which accommodate the GP services and also various preventive and educative services formerly undertaken by Local Health Authorities, e.g., maternal and child health examinations, health education, chiropody and family planning.

Every person is free to choose a personal doctor from those practising in the neighbourhood, although occasionally a GP may refuse to accept a new patient on his list because he already has the maximum number that he is prepared to take or the maximum number that the state will allow him to take. Any dissatisfied patient is free to change his doctor, and similarly a GP is free to remove a patient from his list and to tell him to seek his medical care elsewhere.

The GP is paid by the state for the patients on his list, with extra amounts in certain cases, e.g., higher payment is made for persons of pensionable age (on the ground that they are likely on average to need more of his time) and special payment is made for maternity work. He is therefore legally barred from charging his patient for any service falling within the scope of the National Health Service, but is entitled to make a charge for any service falling outside that scope. For instance, if the patient is unfit for work the GP must supply the required national health insurance certificate without fee, but if the patient asks for a certificate for a private insurance company the doctor is entitled to make a charge.

A person away from home can apply for treatment to any GP in the place where he is temporarily residing, and such treatment is again given without charge, the GP receiving from the state a small payment for such temporary patients.

Private practice remains permissible. In other words, if Mrs White is on Dr Gray's list she cannot enter into an arrangement with Dr Gray for him to treat her in return for fees (because Dr Gray is already being paid from national funds for the medical care of Mrs White), but she can legitimately enter into a financial arrangement with Dr Black (whose list of state-paid patients does not include the name of Mrs White).

There are about 25,000 general practitioners in Britain, so the average practitioner has a list of just over 2,000 patients. Simple arithmetic shows that, if a doctor works for an average of about forty-four hours a week for forty-six weeks a year, he has almost exactly one hour a year available for each person on his list, although of course some people go through many years without ever needing to consult their doctor while others take up several hours in a single month. To conserve professional time the GP normally asks patients to visit the health centre or consulting room unless incapable of doing so, and patients needing home visits are asked to try to notify the practice early in the morning so that the GP can arrange his visits with minimal travelling.

Most surveys have indicated that the majority of people are reasonably satisfied with the GP service. There are, however, some complaints. An unreasonable one which has persisted since 1948 emanates from moderately wealthy people: they allege that when they paid their GP in the old days he visited them at home whereas now he expects them to travel to his premises; but actually the number of general practitioners has increased proportionately more than the population, so that in the 'old days' those who could afford considerable fees manifestly received preferential treatment, to the detriment of other patients who had to be dealt with in even less time than today.

Some people allege that the GP hurries through his consultation with scanty clinical examination, no discussion of the condition and just a hastily scrawled prescription, and that he is prepared to devote much more time to his few private patients. Some argue that with the increasing width of medical knowledge a doctor who professes the entire field of medical science is an anachronism, that the GP has increasingly to refer serious illness to experts and that he is over-trained for simply deciding that patient A should be referred to a heart specialist while patient B only needs a pain-reliever and a few days in bed. Particularly common criticisms relate to communication difficulties and to the absence of guidance by the doctor about measures for the prevention of illness. Lastly, some thinkers query the whole system in which doctor-patient contact begins only after a layman's diagnosis of illness, e.g., a woman consults her doctor because of failing vision and is then found to have cataract as a complication of long-standing undiagnosed diabetes, or a man after many weeks of night sweats and loss of weight decides that he is ill, visits the GP and is discovered to be suffering from advanced tuberculosis of the lung.

All these points have a measure of validity but it is important to note that the majority of people consider that the GP does his job well. Despite criticisms it is likely that the GP will remain the corner-stone of the treatment services.

Another criticism comes from some general practitioners. They maintain that, if people had to pay part of the cost of the service directly, they would no longer waste their doctor's time over trivia. This is undoubtedly true, but any system of direct payment would also deter some patients from seeking early treatment: to avoid a payment which they either could not afford or grudged they would tend to wait to see whether their illness cleared up spontaneously, so that an illness which if diagnosed and treated early might be cured within weeks would not be identified until it was so advanced as to require months of hospital care. Direct payment would in fact negate a basic principle of the National Health Service.

Home nursing services

The nurse who, after some further training, undertakes nursing in the home is still often called the 'district nurse'. The term, however, is becoming confusing because the very senior nursing administrator responsible for the health visiting, home nursing and hospital nursing services of a district (with a population of perhaps 150,000) is called the district nursing officer. 'Community nurse' is sometimes used as an alternative, but that term really includes health visitors as well as home nurses.

The home nursing service – provided without direct charge to recipients – is a valuable part of Britain's health and disease services because, given daily or twice daily visits by skilled nurses, e.g., to give injections or to change dressings, many sick people can be nursed at home by their relatives – to the greater satisfaction of the patients, often to the greater satisfaction of the relatives and with a vast saving to the community on expensive hospital services. Another advantage is that although the home nurse does not have the intensive post-registration education of the health visitor on motivational psychology and the theory and practice of education, she can play quite a useful part in the health education of the families that she is visiting.

In respect of the clinical treatment of individual patients the home nurse works under the direction of the GP, but she is a member of a separate profession with its own priorities and its own senior officers, and she is in no sense under the jurisdiction of the GP.

In some rural areas for geographical reasons (e.g., travelling distances) the tasks of HEALTH VISITOR, domiciliary midwife and home nurse are combined, and because the home nurse was historically the earliest of these appointments the 'triple duty nurse' is often known as the 'district nurse', a curious lowering of status in view of the fact that the home nurse requires less post-registration professional preparation than either the health visitor or the midwife and lower academic entry standards than the health visitor.

The present estimate of the required number of home nurses is about one for every 3,500 to 4,000 population, but increase in the number is probable if greater survival into old age is accompanied by increase in the number of elderly people requiring nursing visits. In 1976 the government, while seeking to prune many services as a matter of economy, specifically exempted home nurses and indicated its aim of increasing the number of home nurses – and also of health visitors – by 6 per cent a year for the next few years. Incidentally, home nursing is the only branch of nursing in which there is not a serious and persisting national shortage, perhaps because the work of a home nurse provides the satisfactions of clinical care without the detailed supervision of hospital nursing, and also provides to a much greater degree than does most hospital nursing the satisfaction of continuity of care for the same patients.

Most surveys have indicated that consumers are well content with the home nursing service. Indeed the bulk of criticisms emanate from home nurses themselves and from some general practitioners: they hanker after the 'triple duty nurse' of the past (still existing in many countries and in rural parts of Britain). Several investigations have shown, however, that (1) to undertake adequate health education and health counselling the health visitor requires advanced preparation and a higher academic entry standard, (2) to enforce that preparation and entry standard on all community nurses would create a serious staff shortage, and (3) the advanced preparation would be largely wasted in respect of the proportion of the time of 'triple duty nurses' devoted to clinical work. So it seems likely that the home nursing service will remain as at present. Indeed the indications are towards a shorter, rather than a longer, post-registration training for home nurses and towards greater use in home nursing of enrolled nurses (with only two years of basic nursing training).

Domiciliary midwifery services

For pregnant women who prefer to be confined at home or who, in a few areas, are unable to secure admission to a maternity hospital, a domiciliary midwifery service is available, again without direct cost to the user. The training of domiciliary and hospital midwives is the same – a three year training in general nursing and a subsequent year's training in midwifery. There is no special preparation for work outside hospital.

With the fall in the birth rate (so that most women who prefer to have their children in hospital can do so) and the increasing popularity of confinement in hospital (where various emergency services are available at need), the domiciliary midwifery service is in some difficulties. If, for example, a population of 10,000 has the annual average of 180 births and if 90 per cent of these births take place in hospital, a single midwife would – if on duty all the time – have only 18 cases a year. But to allow for off-duty we need at least two midwives who, to undertake even 36 cases a year, require a population of 20,000. To stretch each midwife's district further involves - except in compact cities - a vast amount of time spent in travelling; and to seek to involve her for part of her time in hospital midwifery ignores the fact that she may well have opted for domiciliary work to get away from the discipline and routine of hospital. There is no completely satisfactory solution, although some areas are attempting a combination of home nurse and midwife.

Chiropody services

Since many elderly persons suffer from such foot disorders as ingrowing toe nails and corns, and since these defects can render people housebound, creating both shopping problems and problems of loneliness, the chiropody service is important. Whether provided in health centres or clinics for people who can travel, or at home (for those unable to travel) it is – like the other services previously mentioned – supplied without direct charge to the patient. Most chiropodists are salaried employees (like home nurses and health visitors) though some work for sessional fees paid by the Health Board and are free to undertake private work in their own time.

Unfortunately in many parts of Britain there is a serious shortage of qualified chiropodists, so that in these areas people relying on the public service tend to have their feet treated perhaps once in eight weeks when what is really needed to prevent deterioration is about twice that frequency of treatment.

General dental services

Two-thirds of Britain's 18,000 dental officers work as general dentists, the rest working in the school and pre-school dental services (formerly provided by Local Health Authorities), in hospitals and in the armed forces.

As in the case of the GP, a person can choose any general dentist in his neighbourhood and is free to change his dentist, while the dentist is also free to refuse a particular patient. Dental examination is made without charge but dental treatment is not free except to certain groups, e.g., children up to school leaving age, expectant and nursing mothers, and persons receiving supplementary benefit from the Department of Health and Social Security. Apart from such exceptions the patient pays roughly one-half of the cost of treatment and the state makes up the other half.

The majority of general dentists working for the National Health Service also treat patients privately for arranged fees, and essentially the same criticisms – and the same defences against criticisms – arise as in respect of private practice by general practitioners.

While a dentist is quite generously remunerated – receiving on average very much more than a health visitor or health education officer of roughly similar length of training, and nearly as much as a GP – their job is felt by many youngsters to lack interest and glamour; and in many districts there is an appreciable shortage of dentists – an indication that money is not the sole reason why people enter particular lines of work.

A criticism sometimes levelled at general dentists is that some of them show little interest in prevention of dental disease. In the first place this is not wholly true: for example, dentists have spoken and written vigorously in support of rectifying fluoride deficiency in water. And in the second place it has to be remembered that dentists are remunerated for treatment, not for preventive work.

Services of opticians

Tests of eyesight are carried out by ophthalmic medical practitioners (doctors specialized in conditions of the eyes) and by ophthalmic opticians (persons trained in eye testing and in the supplying of glasses). Any person can have his eyes tested free of charge if he first gets a certificate from his GP indicating that he is in need of such testing, but a charge is made for lenses and frames, although some types of spectacles are provided free for children.

Although this portion of the National Health Service is not free, the charges are restricted, part of the cost being met by the State. It is sometimes said that the most obvious benefit of the National Health Service in its first version (1948-74) was the dramatic increase in the number of people wearing suitable glasses.

Pharmaceutical services

A qualified pharmaceutical chemist supplies drugs and appliances prescribed by a doctor and also sells medicines not requiring a medical prescription. When the National Health Service was originally established all prescribed medicines were issued free of charge to the patient but later a prescription charge was introduced and it has been retained. A small sum is payable for each item prescribed and is waived in the case of children under 15 years, expectant and nursing mothers, and old age pensioners, and also in certain long-term illnesses.

When the charge was introduced some people argued that, if a patient needed several items, the fee might bear heavily on persons of low income, and also that, where a patient was likely to need something like thirty to fifty pills for full recovery, a kindly GP might well prescribe the higher number immediately to avoid the patient having to pay for a subsequent possible prescription – so that the cost to the State of unused medicines might well outweigh the money received from prescription charges. However, the public appear to have become accustomed to the charges and there is no present intention to remove them.

Some other community services

Various preventive services, e.g., health visiting and the health education service, are considered later; but brief mention may be made here of some services that are partially preventive and partially curative, e.g., the services of dietitians (for persons substantially overweight or underweight or in need of special diets), of physiotherapists and occupational therapists (for persons in need of special exercises to improve the functioning of muscles or joints), of speech therapists (whose function is obvious) and of orthoptists (for treatment of such defects as squint). All these services are provided without direct charge to the patient.

Allied social services

Under the various Social Services Acts the administration of the home help service, old people's homes, day nurseries and certain institutions for the mentally handicapped passed from Local Health Authorities (later superseded by Health Boards) to the Social Services Committees of local authorities.

The home help service is usually provided on a part-time basis (e.g., two half days per week) for persons who, given some help for heavy household duties, can continue successfully at home, whereas lacking that aid they would require admission to an old people's home or a geriatric or long-stay hospital; and, while the needs and personal wishes of the individual must be considered, it is generally reckoned that if a person requires more than the half-time services of a home help the cost to the community is less if he is cared for in residential accommodation.

The home help service is enormous and still growing. It employs in Britain, mostly as part-time workers, the equivalent of well over thirty thousand full-time workers. Approximately five-sixths of the total time of the service is spent on elderly people (a group that will increase numerically in the next decade), with chronic sickness and maternity covering most of the remaining one-sixth. The service is not free: according to their means recipients are required to pay anything from a negligible charge to the full economic cost.

The home help service is very valuable. As one expert writes, 'By sensible use of the home help service, together with the meals on wheels service (i.e., a service to provide some warm, cooked meals for selected elderly persons), it is often possible to keep an elderly person living on her own for some years longer than would otherwise be possible.'

Since the number of old people – not all of whom need help – is rising steadily, and the number of women of working age is falling, it is increasingly difficult for a local authority to provide all the home helps that it really requires.

Since old people (83 per cent of the consumers) habitually grumble, this important service is by no means free from criticism. Perhaps, however, the most valid criticism arises from persons who ask: should this service, which is clearly neither health work nor social work but something assisting both, have been transferred from Health Departments to Social Work Departments, and should it like the Social Services be subsidized from the local rates or should it, like the Health Service, be subsidized from national taxes? Critics of the transfer point out that the vast majority of recommendations of persons for the service emanate from three types of health worker – health visitors, general practitioners and home nurses – and that increase or decrease in the amount of help needed by a person depends primarily on health changes which again are best appreciated by the health workers. Critics also mention that in most cases either health visitors or home nurses are visiting houses in which home helps work and could smooth out misunderstandings between home help and client, but that the placing of home helps in a separate department necessitates the additional cost of visits by a home helps organizer or a social worker for these purposes. On the other hand, some social workers contend that home helps are an essentially local service and best financed from the local rates. On balance it seems likely that, sooner or later, the home help service will cease to be organized by the Social Work Departments or local authorities and supported by the ratepayers, and will become a part of the National Health Service.

By contrast day nurseries, (e.g., for children whose single parent has to earn a living) and junior and adult centres for the mentally handicapped, are generally recognized as meeting social needs, rather than health needs, and therefore as falling appropriately within the sphere of Social Work Departments.

Old people's homes are intended for elderly persons who are no longer capable of living independently in their own houses but are not in need of the continuous skilled nursing care available in hospital. At their best these homes provide facilities akin to those of a fairly cheap private hotel, but in many homes the accommodation and facilities are poor and the staff inadequate. An old person with only the standard old age pension is left with a small sum per week as pocket money, while a more affluent person is charged a higher amount, going up in appropriate cases to the full economic cost.

The homes are generally recognized as fulfilling a useful and indeed essential function, but criticisms are common. Some people maintain that they are mostly too cheaply equipped and poorly staffed, while others complain that they form a heavy burden on the ratepayers. Some argue that, because an old person may need medical and nursing skills in a geriatric hospital this week, only custodial care in a home for the next fortnight and then another week of hospital attention, the homes and the geriatric hospitals should be under common management. Still others express the view that the system of charges both for old people's homes and for home helps is a disincentive to thrift while persons are in employment: the frugal person who saves for his old age has to pay heavily for these services while the person who spends all his money receives the services for almost nothing.

Some thinkers even believe that the entire separation of health services and social services creates artificial boundaries, that health factors and social factors constantly interact and that the two services should be united.

Hospital services

Despite a great reduction in beds for infectious diseases and tuberculosis in recent decades in consequence of preventive action – 68,000 beds in England, Scotland and Wales in 1936 and barely a quarter of that total now – Britain's hospital beds have increased dramatically over the same period. This increase is explained partly by increased survival into old age (with greater likelihood of illness), partly by increased knowledge (so that some diseases from which people formerly died can now be successfully treated) and partly by the British emphasis on hospital services to the detriment of health education, prevention and community care.

The staffs of hospitals have also increased more than in proportion to the beds, with particular increases in the proportions of doctors of consultant grading and of administrative and clerical staff. At the health services integration of 1974 the hospitals employed some 29,000 doctors of whom 11,500 were graded full consultant: in other words, top-ranking clinical specialists already outnumbered the combined total of health visitors, health education officers and public health medical officers; and there were more doctors working in hospitals than in general practice. Hospitals employed 350,000 qualified or student nurses, of whom almost half were students (raising criticisms about misuse of student nurses as sources of cheap labour) and roughly one-quarter were qualified or student nurses from underdeveloped countries (raising queries about communication difficulties on the one hand and on the other hand fears about the supply of nurses when the developing countries began to provide their own schools of nursing, as they are beginning to do). They employed 274,000 ancillary and domestic workers, 44,000 technicians and 57,000 administrative and clerical staff – and that last total has increased substantially since 1974. In all, the hospitals employed approximately a million persons or about 4 per cent of the working population of Britain.

Hospital treatment is without direct charge to the patient, although a charge is made if the patient requests special facilities (e.g., a private room) and in long-stay cases there is a small charge for board, deducted from the patient's sickness benefit or old age pension. Admission to hospital is usually very speedy in an emergency, e.g., after a road accident, but in non-emergency cases there is often an appreciable gap – of several months or even of a year – between the recommendation for admission and the actual entry of the patient to hospital.

The admitted patient remains a responsible person. He can, for instance, give signed consent for a particular operation or examination, or refuse consent. Operation or examination without the consent of the patient (or, if he is a minor, his parent, or, if he is incapable of giving consent, his available nearest of kin) constitutes an assault, although naturally it is deemed justified in an emergency. Similarly a patient (certified mental patients exempted) has the right to discharge himself at any time, though in fairness he may be required to sign a document stating that he is leaving hospital on his own responsibility and against medical advice.

Refusals and self-discharges are rarities however. A patient goes to hospital to secure treatment, not to refuse it.

In hospital the ward administration is in the charge of a nursing officer (formerly known as the ward sister, but the term is inappropriate for a person who may be of either sex). He or she is assisted by staff nurses (fully qualified), enrolled nurses (with shorter training), student nurses (taking their three year training), pupil nurses (taking a shorter two year course), nursing auxiliaries and ward orderlies. Treatment is in the charge of a clinical consultant (a doctor recognized as a full specialist in the particular branch). He may be assisted by a senior registrar (i.e., a highly qualified and experienced doctor who hopes shortly to be appointed as a consultant), a registrar (usually with a postgraduate qualification) and a house physician or house surgeon (both being recently qualified young doctors starting their medical career).

Radiology departments, biochemical and bacteriological laboratories, occupational therapy departments and so forth are available as support services; and links with the community are provided – both while the patient is in hospital and after his discharge – in some areas by liaison health visitors and in other areas by medico-social workers (the almoners and psychiatric social workers of the past).

If the total staff of a hospital appears large it has to be remembered that sick patients require services for twenty-four hours a day and for seven days a week. To illustrate the point let us think of the nursing staff needed for a twelve-bedded ward in an acute hospital. In that ward the number of patients will vary from ten to twelve, because even if there is a substantial waiting list for the particular disease it is not practicable to have all the beds occupied every day: Mrs Smith was expected to be discharged on Thursday but made such rapid recovery that she can go home on Tuesday, and Miss Jones was expected to linger till about the weekend but dies on the same Tuesday, but the next two patients on the waiting list have to be notified and perhaps arrangements made for ambulances to call for them on Thursday. If that ward with ten to twelve patients needs two nurses at all times – and there are many tasks that require two nurses – then for a complete week it would at first appear to need roughly eight and a half nurses if each works for forty hours. But nurses like other people need annual leave and have illnesses, so we actually require for that ward a permanent full-time staff of ten nurses, assuming that in the year each averages seven weeks absence between annual leave and illness. In other words, for that acute ward we require roughly the same number of whole-time nurses as the average number of patients in the ward. Similar arguments apply in respect of doctors, laboratory technicians, porters, domestics and so on. Indeed for some conditions the numbers mentioned would be utterly inadequate. For instance, a heart transplant operation requires for at least a fortnight something like the whole-time services of five doctors and seventeen nurses.

Britain's general hospitals and many of its special hospitals (e.g., children's hospitals and orthopaedic hospitals) have a very high reputation and are generally reckoned among the best in the world. Yet the hospital services in this country receive far more criticism than do either the services for home treatment or the preventive services. Apart from the question of private beds, considered later, some of the main criticisms are here summarized. (1) It is alleged that long-stay geriatric hospitals and mental hospitals – together constituting more than one-half of all

hospital beds – are commonly housed in the oldest and poorest buildings, are given the minimum of equipment, have inadequate nursing staffs, and often have low standards of medical and nursing care. (2) It is said that the routine of acute general hospitals was organized to suit the convenience of the consultants at a time when they were 'honoraries' giving their services free and at times unsuitable for their private patients, and that the traditional organization lingers on, e.g., with patients being roused at very early hours so that washing, breakfast and bed-making can be completed before the hour at which consultants wish to start their visits. (3) It is stated that for at least a quarter of his 168 hour week a seriously ill patient is nursed by overseas people with whom he may have difficulty in communicating because of their accents or because of their limited knowledge of English. (4) It is also stated that about half the nursing is done by unqualified student nurses who naturally lack full nursing skills. All these criticisms have a measure of validity, and the last two simply indicate the severe and still increasing shortage of nurses and emphasize the fact that (unlike some other countries) Britain has failed to make nursing as financially attractive to prospective students as are other professions.

A fifth criticism has been increasingly raised in recent years – namely whether the best use of limited funds is to spend about 60 per cent of them on hospitals (to cure or alleviate serious illness), over 30 per cent on treatment services outside hospital and supportive social services (both mainly for persons already ill or incapacitated), about 5 per cent on ambulance services, and only a little over 2 per cent on all the services designed to improve and maintain health and to prevent or reduce the frequency of disease. Yet people who are ill demand and require treatment, and perhaps any fall in hospital expenditure can come only after successful expansion of preventive services.

See also MENTAL HOSPITALS in the alphabetical text.

The private patient controversy

While about half Britain's consultant doctors work full-time for the state and are therefore debarred from accepting private patients, the remainder have part-time contracts (e.g., for seven sessions a week) with the remainder of their time free for private work. Since any patient, public or private, may need skilled medical treatment at any hour of any day, the allocation of time is of course theoretical: the consultant cannot say that he will devote Monday afternoons and Thursday mornings to private patients and the rest of his time to public patients.

Private patients pay the consultant for his services and, if treated as private patients in a public hospital, pay the hospital roughly the economic cost of their care.

The controversy about private patients has become one of the main items of health politics. Some of the arguments on both sides may be briefly outlined.

Opponents say: – (1) It is improper for the

same doctor to treat both public and private patients: since he cannot do better than his best, he is under a constant temptation to give rather less than his best to public patients in order to induce persons who can afford fees to opt for private treatment; and in other professions we would not be happy with, for instance, a school teacher who taught some pupils for salary and others for private fees. (2) Where beds or staff are scarce public patients often have to wait for months for admission but private patients usually seem able to secure prompt admission and treatment. (3) Private patients make more demands than do public patients (e.g., consultants request more laboratory investigations for them and the patients make more requests for nursing attention) but nurses, technicians, paramedical workers, domestics and even junior doctors receive no extra remuneration for the additional work, the consultant being the only gainer. (4) Private patients are the very people most likely to point out errors or defects, so their treatment as public patients in public wards would enable them to point out features that seemed unsatisfactory or could be improved. (5) The consultant who notionally spends one-quarter of his time on private patients often actually gives them half of his total time: there is a natural temptation to devote more time to a patient who is paying a large sum of money than to a patient treated at public expense.

Supporters say: – (1) The private patient pays primarily for privacy and for treatment at the time that is suitable for him; it is quite incorrect to suggest that the consultant gives better treatment to persons who pay him fees. (2) Where the private patient secures priority of admission – as has been proved in some cases – this is a defect of the system which should be rectified, not an indictment of private practice as a whole. (3) The private patient saves the country money, both by enabling the consultant to work less than full-time for the National Health Service and by making a contribution towards the running of the hospital. (4) The allegation that nurses and paramedicals receive no additional payment is based simply on jealousy; they are paid salaries for full-time work and should be unconcerned about what the consultant makes in time not paid by the state. (5) To transfer private patients to nursing homes or specially built private hospitals would entail additional cost (e.g., duplication of x-ray departments) and would waste the time of the consultant in frequently travelling between public and private hospitals. (6) While nurses and paramedicals may deem the remuneration of a full-time consultant high, it is really so low that if all private work were banned quite a number of consultants would emigrate to countries that give better rewards.

With the British genius for compromise it seems likely that some reduction will be made in the number of private beds, that a joint public and private waiting list will be evolved to secure equality of treatment in respect of admission to hospitals, and that a method may be devised of paying a small honorarium to nurses and paramedical workers caring for private patients.

Perhaps, however, factors other than the views of consultants and the opposing views of various other health workers will play a part in deciding what happens. On the one hand, if the present scarcity of nurses becomes even greater (e.g., through developing countries establishing their own colleges of nursing) the sheer lack of facilities in public wards may create in affluent persons an increasing demand for private treatment and a willingness to pay fees not only to the doctor but also to nurses and other workers. On the other hand, if differentials in remuneration decline in Britain – as happened to some extent with the £6 a week limitation on increase in earnings in 1975 and the £4 a week limitation in 1976 – there may be a sharp drop in the number of persons prepared to pay for private treatment.

Maternal and child health services

Pregnancy is a normal physiological process but in the later decades of the nineteenth century in Britain about one live-born infant in every seven died before reaching the age of 12 months (as well as an uncounted number of pregnancies ending in still-births) and nearly one pregnancy in every ten ended in the mother's death. The situation was not very much better than when Euripedes – 2,300 years earlier – made the heroine of his tragedy, Medea, say, 'I would rather stand in the battle line thrice than once bear a child'. Inevitably in the later nineteenth century and the first half of the twentieth century services for the improvement of maternal and child health developed with a strong preventive slant and, although maternity hospitals passed to hospital boards in 1948, these services remained largely in the hands of local authorities until the 1974 integration.

Antenatal care, which prevents many of the complications of pregnancy and childbirth, involves initial medical examination to check that the expectant mother has no undetected illness, various specific tests (e.g., of blood for anaemia and for rhesus factor estimation), health education on diet and on general management of pregnancy, subsequent monthly medical examinations, attention to teeth and any other potential problems, reasonably frequent counselling visits by health visitor or midwife or both, and provision both of health education sessions and of sessions for psychoprophylaxis or relaxation exercises.

Confinement in hospital is usually advised for all first births, for women with any abnormality, for mothers with three or more children, for women over 35 years of age and for women whose home circumstances are unsuitable for home confinement. Fully 90 per cent of expectant mothers in Britain now have their babies in hospital. The remainder are delivered at home, usually by domiciliary midwives who can call in the appropriate general practitioner at need.

Post-natal examination, about a month after the birth, is deemed important for the prevention of various conditions, such as subsequent chronic backache.

Over the last quarter of a century a deliberate attempt has been made to interest general practitioners in antenatal care, obstetrics and post-natal care; those with appropriate experience in matters pertaining to childbirth are paid a special fee for undertaking these functions.

Child health care is largely a matter of (1) educative home visits by health visitors (discussed later), and (2) periodical examinations at health centres, child health clinics or the consulting rooms of the GP. In the first four weeks after birth (in which two-thirds of the remaining infant deaths now occur) special attention is devoted to haemolytic disease of the new-born (rhesus incompatibility), neonatal cold injury (for the very young baby is particularly susceptible to serious drops in the temperature of a room), screening tests (e.g., for phenylketonuria and for congenital dislocation of the hip), and care of premature babies (usually in special units). Subsequently, although periodical examinations are desirable to measure physical and mental development, the health visitor – both in the home and in clinics, health centres or consulting rooms – is the parents' main advisor on health maintenance, offering guidance on such matters as infant feeding, weaning, immunizations, accident prevention and the provision of a domestic atmosphere that will promote the emotional and social – as well as the physical – development of the child. In most cases parents are also encouraged to attend parentcraft sessions where groups can discuss with health visitors and other health professionals problems of child management, the prevention of various diseases, the introduction of suitable toys, the need for playmates when the child is old enough, the value and limitations of nurseries and play-groups and the preparation of the four-year-old for the change from home to school.

These services between them have played the major part in reducing maternal deaths as a result of child-bearing from more than one mother in every eleven to less than one in five thousand and in reducing infant deaths during the first twelve months from one in seven to one in seventy – incomparably the biggest health advance in any century.

While guidance on nutrition, personal hygiene and immunization remains important, it is increasingly being realized that the first half dozen years of life are the most important period for emotional and mental development, as well as for physical growth, and it is likely that the biggest contribution of health visitor home visits and of child health clinics in the next twenty years will lie in the fostering of personalities strong enough to withstand the normal stresses of life.

See also in the alphabetical text INFANT WELFARE and MATERNAL AND CHILD WELFARE.

Family planning services

Family postponement is important for couples who desire to save a little money before one ceases work to look after a baby, and also for unmarried persons who are not prepared to avoid sexual intercourse. Family spacing is important to prevent mothers becoming exhausted and children being neglected by

reason of numbers and nearness in age. Family limitation is important to avoid the increased risks associated with pregnancy over the age of 36 (e.g., more maternal illness and a higher proportion of babies suffering from mongolism) and the difficulties of parents reaching retirement age before the youngest child is independent. Family avoidance is vital for carriers of serious hereditary disease. As for national aspects, Britain is already overcrowded and the population is still increasing by about two million people every ten years, and since population far outstrips our food production Britain already has to import foods to the value of over £3,000 millions a year, or roughly one pound a week for every man, woman and child in the country.

Yet until 1967 family planning services were provided only by a relatively small number of voluntary clinics (mostly under the auspices of the Family Planning Association) and by a tiny handful of forward-looking local authorities. An Act of 1967 empowered local authorities to provide contraceptive advice and treatment on both medical and social grounds; and family planning is now a recognized part of the health services of Britain.

However, many areas are subject to criticism because they have done little more than make services available. Clearly the provision of services alone, without considerable simultaneous health education as to their desirability, would lead to their being used by the intelligent and educated but largely ignored by the unintelligent and illiterate.

Health visiting services

Just as the general practitioner is the cornerstone of treatment services, so the health visitor (whose visits are likewise without any direct cost to the clients) is the corner-stone of disease-preventing and health-promoting services.

A qualified nurse with higher academic qualifications than are needed for general nursing and with post-qualification specialized full-time training in psychology, sociology and health teaching, she - and since 1973 in some cases he - is essentially the general purpose family health counsellor and medico-social adviser. About 10 per cent of health visitors are specialized, e.g., undertaking liaison with hospitals to ensure that the latter have full information about the patient's home conditions and that the patient's prescribed routine continues after he leaves hospital, or acting as specialist advisers to colleagues on such subjects as health education of groups, problems of one-parent families, care of premature babies, or the physical and emotional problems of the elderly. The remaining 90 per cent are family health visitors, charged with responsibility for maintaining and improving the health of the people. To reduce duplicate visiting and possible contradictory advice, health visitors and general practitioners increasingly work together, not with one subordinate to the other but as experts in different lines, with different priorities, but between them tackling the health problems and disease problems of the same collection of people.

The health visitor's work for the physical health and in recent years also the emotional health of babies, toddlers and in some cases school children is universally recognized as a vital component of the health services; she has the incalculable built-in advantage that, whereas other medical, nursing and social workers normally establish contact only after the patient or client seeks help, the health visitor by tradition visits at discretion. So she can often identify and cope with emerging problems before they have become known to the client. She can in fact prove the truth of the old adages that a stitch in time saves nine and that prevention is better and cheaper than cure. As far back as 1917 an official report of what was later called the Ministry of Health described the health visitor as 'the most important element in any scheme for maternity and child welfare'.

Her work in maintaining the health of elderly persons has gained wide recognition in the last dozen years, but some people mistakenly think her concerned only with the two ends of life. Actually she is available (subject to limitations of time) to the entire community. A detailed study published in 1973 showed that 71 per cent of health visitor visits were to families with young children, 18 per cent to households containing old people and no young children, and 11 per cent to households containing neither children nor old people. Incidentally the same study showed that 60 per cent of health visitor visits were initiated by the health visitor, 16 per cent were made at the request of clients, 9 per cent at the request of general practitioners, and the remainder following suggestions from various sources. Another investigation of the same year revealed that health visitors undertook more education of groups than did all other health and disease workers combined.

The required number of health visitors is estimated by the health authorities at one per 3,000 population, although some investigators have claimed that for adequate discharge of their important duties a figure of one per 2,250 population would be more realistic. Yet, perhaps because local authorities were more interested in treatment and social support than in prevention and health education, very few areas at the 1974 integration of health services had much more than one per 4,000 population and some had only about one per 5,000. Recognizing the importance of the health visiting service, the Government in 1976, when financial stringency was compelling it to reduce many services, committed itself to seeking to achieve at least a 6 per cent annual increase for some years in the number of health visitors; and to that end polytechnics and other institutions of higher education were encouraged to provide more courses for suitable nurses aspiring to become health visitors.

The linking of health visitors and general practitioners in recent years has been criticized on three grounds: (1) that general practice (where a dozen doctors may visit patients in one short street) is inefficiently organized and that a health visitor dealing with the persons in a practice spends considerably more time travelling than when she had an equal number of clients in a compact district; (2) that the health visitor with a compact district knew the district including the interactions of neighbours (e.g., if a child developed a preventable disease she could use that illness as a lever to step up appropriate preventive measures in nearby families, and if the household on the immediate left of noisy new neighbours showed strain she could watch the mental health of the household on the immediate right of the newcomers) – advantages that disappear when she deals with a practice population; and (3) that, since the doctor's primary interest is in cure, alleviation or support, he may unintentionally push his health visitor colleague in these directions, to the detriment of health education, health counselling and the early recognition and rectification of problems. There is a measure of truth in these criticisms, but there is a big advantage in the reduction of duplicate visiting – in either doctor or health visitor being able to say to the other, 'I visited Mrs. A yesterday and I think she is all right for a week or so, but I also visited Mr. B and suggest that he needs a visit from you.'

In the 1960s the introduction of men into health visiting was as controversial as had been the introduction of women doctors earlier. Protagonists claimed that suitably trained men could do most health visiting duties and had a special role both in the health education of male adolescents and in the health maintenance of old men. Antagonists said that health visiting was a female profession and that husbands would resent their wives being visited by men. Aberdeen pioneered men in 1962 designating them 'Male Health Visiting Officers' since they could not at that time legally be called health visitors. Belfast, Liverpool and Bolton followed, and after much argument men were formally admitted to the health visiting profession in 1972.

Since 1962 the regulation of health visitor preparation and the approval of health visitor courses have been entrusted to a U.K. body, established by statute, the Council for the Education and Training of Health Visitors. This is interesting and perhaps significant, since in all other branches of nursing and midwifery there are separate controlling bodies for England and Wales, Scotland and Northern Ireland.

See also HEALTH VISITOR in the alphabetical text.

School health services.

Children of school age (5 to 16) constitute one-fifth of the population and on numerical grounds alone it is clearly a matter of national concern that steps should be taken to foster their physical and mental health, both to enable them to derive full advantage from their educational opportunities and to ensure that they later realize their full potential in adult life. As an organized group, accessible and under control for eleven years at an important stage of their development, they are an obvious target for systematic attempts to improve health.

As now organized the school health service – a part of the National Health Service (not of the education service, though clearly health workers and teachers must collaborate closely) – provides a highly developed preventive service designed to ensure that the well-being of children is supervised throughout their school career, and that any necessary action is taken to safeguard or enhance their health, to secure early treatment of remediable defects and to minimize the physical and educational handicaps imposed by disability.

The school health service has medical and nursing aspects. The medical aspects include full routine examination of all children after school entry and again shortly before they attain school leaving age, medical examination of any child where the parent, the teacher or the school nurse deems it desirable because of suspected physical or mental illness, identification of children with defects or disabilities (e.g., of vision, of hearing, of posture, or of nutrition), arrangements for the correction of defects or if necessary modification of the educational regime in such a way as to minimize the foreseeable effects of any irremediable handicap, and advice on matters of school hygiene. The school nurse in addition to taking part in these tasks seeks to screen every pupil (preferably twice a year) for evidence of mental or physical disease as well as for uncleanliness or infestation, sees that immunizations are up to date, investigates outbreaks of infection, studies children with frequent absences, maintains an unobtrusive watch on the health of all children, and – if she is a health visitor – may play an important part in health education (either teaching classes herself or acting as an expert 'resource person' behind the teacher) and may visit the homes of selected children to advise and help the parents.

Other workers in the school health service include dental officers and dental hygienists (the latter being qualified to carry out simple routine procedures such as scaling and small fillings), orthoptists (specialists in training eye-muscles, e.g., to rectify a squint) and audiometricians (specialists in the testing of hearing).

The medical part of the service has been criticized on the ground that defects are sometimes missed. The allegation is factually correct. However expert the medical officer – and over the years he acquires an unrivalled knowledge of children who are not seriously ill – a single ten-minute examination is insufficient to guarantee the identification of every defect in any system of the body; but the overwhelming majority of defects requiring treatment or special educational measures are found, and it is highly unlikely that any other type of doctor could identify a larger proportion of defects in the available time. A paediatrician, for instance, would start with a wide knowledge of seriously ill children but virtually no experience of the beginnings of departure from health; and a general practitioner (with few children of any particular age-group in his practice) would normally have seen children only when illness was sufficiently advanced for the parents to recognize it. In any case it seems likely that the 1974 integration of health services will in

the fullness of time lead to a combination of the former local authority clinical medical officer (concerned with pre-school and school children who are not ill and in most cases not in the process of becoming ill) and the former hospital paediatrician (concerned with children sent to him because they are sufficiently ill to be referred to the hospital).

The nursing part of the service has been criticized on the grounds that (1) if the school nurse is a qualified health visitor she 'wastes' part of her time on tasks that any qualified nurse without further specialized training could do, e.g., identification of deviations from normality, scrutiny of immunization states, cleanliness inspections and advice on personal hygiene and school hygiene; and (2) if she is not a health visitor she is unequipped to undertake health education and to offer unobtrusive and tactful advice to senior pupils and to parents. The simple answer to the criticism is that in the large schools that are developing as part of the modern educational pattern there is ample room for both a school health visitor and a school nurse, and already national salary scales make provision for these separate professions.

A more serious but possibly temporary difficulty has arisen in connection with health education in schools. Until 1975 there was a shortage both of health visitors and of teachers, and many individual schools arrived at a division of health education acceptable to both parties, often on the lines that the younger pupils needed the teacher's expertise in the teaching of children and the older pupils required the health visitor's greater knowledge of health and disease. With a sudden surplus of unemployed young teachers in 1976 and 1977 teachers began, not unreasonably, to say – 'All teaching in schools should be done by qualified teachers; a graduate (e.g., in biology or history) spends a year learning how to teach children; he may during that year get some education in health and disease, and if so he is the person in the school competent to teach health.' In reply, equally not unreasonably, doctors and health visitors began to say – 'Just as the prospective history teacher spends years learning his subject, we spend years learning about health and disease; a person who tries to teach emotional health, genetics and inter-personal relations after a few days or weeks of rudimentary instruction is likely to do more harm than good'. Probably the finding of a long-term solution can be left to the good sense of the professions concerned.

Environmental health services.

The sanitary inspector or public health inspector – renamed the environmental health officer in 1974 – has a four-year training in sanitary law, housing requirements, food inspection and elementary bacteriology, and has important responsibilities in respect of maintaining a healthy environment. Until 1974 he worked under the general direction of the medical officer of health; and in outbreaks of infectious disease – especially food-borne infections – there was very close collaboration between public health doctors, health visitors and sanitary inspectors.

One of the major changes of the 1974 integration was to remove medical officers and health visitors from the jurisdiction of local authorities, linking them with other doctors and nurses under the authority of health boards, but to leave environmental health officers as employees of local authorities, with the chief officer in any district designated as director of environmental health.

This separation implies that environmental health officers will have to be prepared to undertake health education and persuasion on environmental hygiene (as opposed to mere enforcement of laws and regulations) and will have to acquire the skills for these difficult tasks. It also implies that they will have to tackle in food-borne outbreaks the far from easy task of obtaining food histories from patients and contacts, who – apart from sometimes having poor memories about what they ate days or even weeks previously – are sometimes reluctant to divulge the shops from which they made purchases or the persons with whom they shared meals.

The change had the complete and enthusiastic approval of the environmental health officers but it is perhaps too early to say whether the complete separation of environmental health from personal health is in the long-term interest of the community. Indeed, already the separation has been followed by an attempt at a new linkage: arrangements have been made whereby each local authority has available to it the advice on environmental hygiene of a community medicine specialist; but the doctor is paid by the health board and his duties towards the local authority are purely advisory, not executive.

The community medicine specialist

The MEDICAL OFFICER OF HEALTH, who vanished in the U.K. in 1974 (except curiously in the Isle of Man) but still exists in many English-speaking countries, is more fully discussed in the alphabetical part of this book, but a brief description here is essential to facilitate understanding of his partial successor, the community medicine specialist.

To cope with infections and to deal with problems of polluted water supplies, impure food and bad housing, Liverpool and London appointed medical officers of health in 1847 and 1848 respectively. Other cities followed, e.g., Aberdeen and Edinburgh in 1862, and before the end of the century every county and large town was required to appoint a doctor with a post-graduate qualification in public health as its full time medical officer of health.

He became the administrative head of the local authority's public health department, at first concerned mainly with environmental and epidemiology services but in due course extending to include maternity and child health services and the school health service. He also had responsibility for the local authority's infectious and tuberculosis hospitals, and for maternity hospitals. By 1930 he headed a very large department in which

persons engaged in personal health services (e.g., health visitors and domiciliary midwives) numerically far outstripped persons employed on environmental health (e.g., sanitary inspectors), while the staffs of local authority hospitals vastly outnumbered the total community staff.

In the 1930s local authorities began to provide general hospitals, and in due course had responsibility for more than two-thirds of the country's hospital beds. So the public health department, headed by the medical officer of health (the MOH), had charge of virtually all the health and disease workers except for general medical and dental practitioners (independent contractors), district nurses (employed by voluntary agencies until 1948 or sometimes later) and the staffs of voluntary hospitals. But several trends of opinion began to appear: (1) Many thinkers advocated amalgamation of local authority and voluntary hospitals. (2) Linkage seemed desirable between on the one hand consultants in voluntary hospitals (giving services free and making their living through private patients) and general practitioners (paid by private patients and by national health insurance remuneration) and on the other hand doctors employed full time in local authority hospitals and in the pre-school and school services; but consultants and general practitioners were very reluctant to be placed under the control of the medical officer of health and many doctors employed by local authorities felt that the latter paid inadequate salaries. (3) Both health visitors and sanitary inspectors were increasing in numbers and in professional stature and were beginning to resent being directed by another profession, and to some extent the same was true of hospitals nurses. (4) With very large hospital responsibilities some medical officers of health became largely hospital administrators, with little time for interest in preventive and health-promoting services.

The foundation of the National Health Service in 1948 reflected the first two trends. All hospitals – local authority and voluntary – were transferred to regional hospital boards. So the MOH had no responsibility for either hospital beds or general medical, dental or pharmaceutical services. However, with health visitors' functions extending to include the elderly, with district nursing becoming a local authority function, with the creation of the home help service and the day nursery service and with the gradual development of health education, after-care services, health screening and health centres, the responsibilities of the MOH remained very wide, and in some towns and counties he had additional duties as director of social welfare although these extra duties were removed in the early 1970s.

With the 1974 reorganization by which all health services except environmental health passed to the Health Boards, the post of MOH ceased to exist. Essentially, with the recognition of nursing as a full profession the large portion of his work concerned with co-ordination and direction of health visiting and home nursing services passed to the chief nursing officer of the area or district, the sanitary portion passed to the director of environmental hygiene of the district local authority, and the strictly medical portion passed to the chief administrative medical officer of the area or district and the various community medicine specialists, while his general planning functions passed to the Executive Group (consisting of a doctor, a nurse, an administrator and a finance officer).

The area or district medical officer or chief medical officer (MO) – terminology varies – who heads the community medicine team is sometimes regarded as a combination of the MOH of 1973 and the senior administrative medical officer of a hospital board in 1973, or as a reincarnation of the MOH of 1947. However, by far the largest numbers of professional staff both in the community and in the hospitals are now under control and direction of the area or district nursing officer; and while the MOH had ultimate responsibility for all his services, the area or district MO is a member of a team of equals.

Varying according to the size of the area or district there are in the community medicine team a number of community doctors of consultant status and remuneration, designated community medicine specialists (CMS). One, for example, may be CMS for pre-school and school health services, another CMS for epidemiology and for liaison with the environmental health department of the district local authority, a third CMS for medico-social problems and for liaison with the social work department of the regional local authority, and a fourth CMS for records and research. Each CMS is assisted by 'clinical medical officers' who in the future are likely to be replaced by trainee consultants (corresponding with the registrars and senior registrars of clinical medicine and surgery) but are at present mainly former public health medical officers who failed to obtain consultant posts at the time of integration. To give one illustrative example, the CMS for pre-school and school health services has obvious similarities to the 1973 principal or senior MO responsible for local authority child health services but with the difference that he is not responsible for health visiting and nursing services.

It is probably too early to attempt any evaluation of the new service, but a few factual points can be made. (1) The 1974 integration was followed by considerable economy cuts in 1975 and 1976 and by massive national unemployment, so that – apart from the temporary difficulty of many people having to adapt to new jobs and to work out new lines of communication – sizeable improvements in health statistics or in provision of health services should not at first be expected and in general cannot be found. (2) Whether in consequence of these economy cuts or otherwise some areas of (possibly temporary) deterioration can be found, e.g., in 1975 decreased uptake of family planning facilities in England and in 1976 – despite government commitment to increase numbers – a substantial fall in the number of student health visitors in Scotland. (3) The prospective CMS has longer professional preparation than had the prospective public health MO and after appointment has higher status and salary. (4) Many of the current criticisms emanate from public health medical officers who expected but did not receive

promotion to consultant grading, and these criticisms commonly relate to the new inability to co-ordinate services by instructing or directing health visitors and environmental health officers; but, irrespective of organizational changes, these professions had reached maturity and could not have continued to be organized and supervised by members of a different profession; and indeed before the 1974 changes some medical officers of health had ensured that their chief nursing officers and chief public health inspectors were virtually independent. (5) The 1974 integration has at least removed the last remnants of the old tension between curative and preventive doctors, which had its origin in the fact that in the past curative doctors depended for their livelihood on the illnesses of patients while preventive workers were seeking to reduce the amount of illness in the community.

Health education services

During the twentieth century the U.K. appears to be passing gradually but fairly steadily from regarding health education as a frill to deeming it the most important and possibly the most difficult branch of all health services and all education services.

The subject of HEALTH EDUCATION in general – systematic attempts to alter attitudes and behaviour in directions conducive to health or to the avoidance of disease – is more fully discussed in the alphabetical text, but can be considered under four heads – education of individuals, education of groups, education by mass media, and organizational aspects.

In health education of individuals Britain led the world by creating and periodically enlarging a profession of health visitors whose primary aim is alteration of attitudes and behaviour. Increasingly health education of individuals is also being attempted by some general practitioners and some nurses (though both of these have other priorities and lack the health visitor's special training in the subject) and by some hospital nurses and doctors (though patients are seldom in the frame of mind for successful health education and not often in hospital long enough for systematized counselling). For the most part the improvements in the health of mothers, pre-school children and school children in the last seventy years are due to health education of individuals, e.g., on antenatal care, preparation for childbirth, feeding and weaning of babies, family planning, child nutrition, children's developmental needs, immunization, physical and mental hygiene, and so on. Difficulties arise, however, from persisting shortages of staff: even with a considerable increase in health visitors in recent years and the further increase both in health visitors and in home nurses sought by the Health Ministries, there will never be enough health educators to do the entire job of health improvement by one-to-one discussion.

Health education of groups presupposes either that people are prepared to come together for discussion and information (as in classes for prospective parents, discussion groups for parents of young children, courses on health subjects of topical interest, and pre-retirement classes) or that there is a captive audience (e.g., school pupils and students in universities, polytechnics and colleges of education). This form of health education has developed enormously in the last twenty years, with the largest parts played by health visitors – who do more group teaching than all other health professions combined – and school teachers. Difficulties include – (1) the neglect until very recently of middle-aged persons and of persons verging on old age; (2) the false idea – still prevalent in some quarters – that all that is needed to educate on an aspect of physical or mental health is ability to speak and technical knowledge of the subject, whereas really knowledge of motivational psychology and of the attitudes and cultural and social pressures of the group taught is vital for successful health education; (3) the practice of health education by some persons with a faulty approach (e.g., in some schools strongly anti-smoking teachers have found that their vigorous attempts to discourage smoking have resulted in a sharp increase in cigarette consumption; (4) the tendency – still quite prevalent – to transform health education into a depressing series of negatives (e.g., don't overeat, don't overdrink, don't smoke, don't have illicit sexual relations), and (5) perhaps the recent separation of environmental health from the rest of the health and disease services.

The role of books, leaflets, posters, radio and television programmes, newspaper articles, etc., is perhaps not yet fully understood. At the least these constitute important reinforcements to individual and group teaching and can also produce useful once-only actions (e.g., in emergency situations). Whether mass media alone can create long-term changes of attitude and behaviour is still arguable.

Until very recently health education in most parts of the U.K. was rather unsystematized. Thus a health visitor might be teaching a group of parents about the need for reasonable permissiveness and the importance of children learning to make their own decisions, and stressing perhaps the importance of pocket money and of its being spent at the child's discretion; a school teacher might simultaneously be trying to persuade the children of these parents not to smoke, and a dental officer might be pointing out that sweet-eating harms teeth and causes obesity, while a medical officer might be trying to discourage the purchase of fireworks. Clearly, while health visitors, teachers, doctors and dentists remain professional officers with their own priorities, some organization and co-ordination was needed. Furthermore, since health education is highly complex and difficult, its practitioners required refresher courses from time to time – to raise their morale and to give them any new information about promotion of health, causes of specific diseases, motivational psychology and teaching techniques.

Nationally this co-ordination and education of the educators is undertaken in England and Wales by the Central Council for Health Education and in Scotland by two bodies, the Scottish Health Education Unit (responsible

for mass media work and for large-scale campaigns) and the Scottish Council for Health Education (responsible for refresher courses and training). In towns and counties and in the regions that succeeded them there was very little co-ordination of health education and very little provision of courses for health and education staffs, with a handful of outstanding exceptions (such as Aberdeen and Croydon), until the Health Ministries in 1974 advised the newly created Health Boards to appoint health education officers to a number of approximately one for every 50,000 population (a proportion based on the previous establishments of Aberdeen and Croydon) and incited various universities and health visitor schools to provide courses of training for prospective health education officers. The latter might be health visitors, teachers, doctors, dentists or other members of health or education professions but should – before acceptance for training – have had some experience in health education and have suitable qualities of personality. Both training and subsequent appointments were curtailed as a result of the financial situation of 1975 and 1976, but this curtailment is manifestly temporary since on a long-term basis health education clearly reduces diseases and saves money.

The actual health education of prospective parents, parents of pre-school and young school children, school pupils, adolescents, adults and persons approaching pensionable age will obviously continue to be undertaken by health visitors, school teachers, other health board staff, environmental health officers (in respect of hygiene) and perhaps social workers, but clearly the appointment of health education officers as co-ordinators, stimulators and providers of resources should do much to advance health education and so to reduce the prevalence both of disease and of the impaired physical or mental health which – without constituting clinical disease – interferes with the enjoyment of life and with the efficient performance of work. Perhaps, indeed, with all respect to the remarkable advances in clinical medicine and surgery, the appointment of health education officers ranks next to the creation of health visitors in the important steps towards the improvement of physical and mental health.

National health insurance

In the early years of this century there was growing dissatisfaction with the medical services generally available to the community in Britain. Many people could not afford to pay for medical attention and contract practice had developed through friendly societies or clubs to which insured members paid weekly contributions in order to secure attendance and treatment during illness. In 1909 the Report of the Royal Commission on the Poor Law pointed out the inadequacies of medical care and recommended an extension of contract practice, but a Minority of the Commission influenced by Beatrice and Sidney Webb favoured a salaried medical service run by local authorities. However, in

1911 David Lloyd George, Chancellor of the Exchequer in the Liberal Government of that day, sponsored the enactment of a National Health Insurance Act described in its preamble as 'an Act to provide for insurance against loss of health, and for the prevention and cure of sickness and for purposes incidental thereto'.

. The original Act, which came into force on 15th January, 1913, and later amendments to it were subsequently consolidated by the National Health Insurance Act of 1924.

The scope of this legislation was limited since it only covered persons employed in manual labour under a contract of service and other persons employed at remuneration originally not in excess of £250, although this figure gradually reached £420 by 1948. The cost of the scheme was met by weekly contributions paid partly by the insured person and partly by the employer with a contribution from the Exchequer. Originally these contributions were 4d, 3d, and 2d respectively which gave rise to the popular political catch-phrase of the time – '9d for 4d'.

The benefits provided were medical attendance and treatment (including the cost of medicines), sickness benefit, disablement benefit and maternity benefit. The scheme was administered by the Central Government Departments in England and Wales and in Scotland, with the help of the Approved Societies, which were self-governing associations of insured persons. The funds for medical attendance and treatment were disbursed by Local Insurance Committees and for all other benefits by the Approved Societies. The scheme did not provide any form of hospital or specialist treatment nor did it cater for dependents but the Approved Societies besides their official function of paying out the cash benefits continued to provide and extend cover for dependants as part of their ordinary business. The incorporation of the Approved Societies in the scheme introduced inequalities since they were commercial concerns adjusting premiums to risks and some were in a much better position to provide supplementary benefits – for dental, ophthalmic, hospital or convalescent treatment – than others.

Although these arrangements were reasonably satisfactory at their inception they were obviously insufficiently comprehensive and on a number of occasions proposals were made to extend arrangements so as to cover dependants and to provide hospital and specialist facilities. The inadequacies became more apparent as time went on and increasingly from 1939 inflation caused a rise in the costs of medical treatment and added to the difficulties of already impoverished voluntary hospitals. In preparation for post-war reconstruction Sir William Beveridge in 1942 was invited to prepare a report on a plan for a comprehensive reconstruction of all forms of social insurance.

In the plan which he proposed he made three assumptions: (1) that children's allowances must be paid, (2) that there must be comprehensive health and rehabilitation services, (3) that there should be maintenance of adequate employment.

The first and third assumptions are irrelevant here, but the second was accepted by the Government and the result was the National Health Service Act 1946 (1947 in Scotland) which provided from the appointed day in 1948 a complete general medical, general dental, pharmaceutical and hospital service for the whole community and expanded the preventive, social, and environmental services provided by the local authorities. This was really the end of 'Health Insurance' in the strict sense in this country because Beveridge said that restoration of a sick person to health was a duty of the State and that the National Health Service should be organized not by the Ministry concerned with social insurance but by Departments responsible for the health of the people, and that the Service should be available where needed without contribution conditions. It thus became, and in principle still is, something not specifically earned by an insurance contribution but a necessary service for every citizen provided free by the State out of the general revenue from taxation.

The fact that the single insurance contribution now covers all kinds of social insurance and has been called upon to some extent to provide for part of the cost of the National Health Service does not invalidate this basic philosophy of health provision.

Costs and staffing

In 1974 Britain's health service cost approximately 5.7 per cent of the national gross product, as compared with a cost of 5.9 per cent in France, 7.4 per cent in the U.S.A. and 8.3 per cent in West Germany. Approximately three-fifths of the costs were on hospitals which at the 1974 integration employed 790,000 staff: 350,000 qualified or student nurses, 274,000 ancillary and domestic workers, 57,000 administrative and clerical staff, 44,000 technicians and 29,000 doctors of whom 11,500 were graded as full consultants. Another quarter of the total costs were on what were then called Executive Council Services, with pharmaceutical services the largest item, general medical practitioners (25,000 in all) the second largest and general dental practitioners (12,000 in all) the next largest. One-ninth of the total costs were on social work departments (in which home helps and staffs of children's nurseries and old people's homes counted for some 90,000 persons). Of the remaining one-twentieth of the total cost roughly half went on ambulance services and home nursing, leaving exactly 2.7 per cent available for health promotion and disease prevention services, such as antenatal and child health clinics, immunization, family planning, health visitors, dietitians, health education officers, and so on.

From different quarters the services have been criticized as (1) too expensive, and certainly in a country of just over fifty million people (including children and old age pensioners) one million seems a large proportion to employ on sickness and health; (2) too cheap, and certainly we spend less in proportion than various other countries: there is a grave and persisting shortage of nurses and our hospitals are carrying on largely by misuse of the labour of student nurses and in particular of student nurses from developing countries, so that a quarter of the nursing of patients is undertaken not merely by students who are unqualified but often by students from foreign countries and with communication difficulties; and (3) having wrong priorities, e.g., fewer health visitors and health education officers combined than the total number of full clinical consultants. For a fuller discussion of these points see COSTS OF HEALTH SERVICES in the alphabetical text.

Outlook

To make a forecast in years of inflation, economy cuts and massive unemployment is difficult, but a few points can be made with confidence. (1) With the establishment of chairs of nursing in several universities and with some young nurses holding an honours degree plus a postgraduate diploma (e.g., in health visiting) and in some cases a higher degree (e.g., M.Sc. or Ph.D.) there is no possibility of reversion to medical domination of health and disease services: the multiprofessional management team is certain to persist. (2) Since prevention is normally cheaper than cure, the financial difficulties of the U.K. should increase – not diminish – the emphasis on health education and disease prevention, and the numbers of health education officers and health visitors should continue to rise. (3) Even if the salaries of nurses and paramedical workers are raised to the level of professions of similar length and intensity of training, staff shortages will continue and will therefore result in increasing emphasis on domiciliary as against institutional services, but this trend may be lessened by further advances in medical knowledge. (4) Sooner or later there will either be an amalgamation of health and social services or a transfer to health services of some services (e.g., home helps) at present administered by social work departments. (5) Despite many criticisms the general outlook for the health and disease services is favourable: Britain's services are among the best in the world and are likely so to continue.

ILLUSTRATION ACKNOWLEDGEMENTS

British Optical Association: 440
Department of Graphic Design, Glasgow School of Art: 261
Department of Medical Illustration, Westminster Medical School: 25b, 195b, 414b, 458
Department of Medical Photography and Illustration, Southern General Hospital, Glasgow: 2, 7b, 32a, 32b, 43, 49a, 49b, 59, 68, 96, 99, 118, 195a, 195c, 237, 267, 276, 286, 303, 319, 351, 353, 393, 413, 484, 487
Mary Evans Picture Library: 9, 317
Fox Photos Ltd.: 290
Greater Glasgow Health Board: 149a, 149b
Health and Safety Executive: 344
Historical Picture Service: 155
Mr. Alec Hope: 88b
Keystone Press Agency: 255
Mr. Ken MacLean: 88a
Mr. Tom Macnair, Deanstone Drive Further Education Day Centre, Glasgow: 404
Mansell Collection: 248, 253, 258, 399
The National Portrait Gallery, London: 27, 117
National Society for Mentally Handicapped Children: 323
Natural History Photographic Agency: 272
Oxfam: 287
Popperfoto: 30b, 141, 205, 228, 280b, 310
Radio Times Hulton Picture Library: 39a, 207a, 278, 337, 358
The Society of Chiropodists, London/Camera Talks Ltd.: 202
Spinal Paralysis Service, Edenhall Hospital, Musselburgh: 35b
John Topham Picture Library: 347

The letters a, b, c following some of the page numbers indicate the order on pages with more than one illustration; the illustrations are ordered from the top of the left hand column to the bottom of the right hand column.